SURGICAL RADIOLOGY

A COMPLEMENT IN RADIOLOGY AND IMAGING TO THE SABISTON
DAVIS-CHRISTOPHER TEXTBOOK OF SURGERY

Volume II

Edited by

J. GEORGE TEPLICK, M.D., F.A.C.R.

Professor and Director, Division of General
Diagnosis, Department of Diagnostic Radiology,
Hahnemann Medical College and Hospital, Philadelphia

MARVIN E. HASKIN, M.D., F.A.C.R., F.A.C.P.

Professor and Chairman, Department of Diagnostic Radiology,
Hahnemann Medical College and Hospital, Philadelphia

1981

W. B. SAUNDERS COMPANY • Philadelphia • London • Toronto

W. B. Saunders Company: West Washington Square
Philadelphia, PA 19105

1 St. Anne's Road
Eastbourne, East Sussex BN21 3UN, England

1 Goldthorne Avenue
Toronto, Ontario M8Z 5T9, Canada

Library of Congress Cataloging in Publication Data

Main entry under title:

Surgical radiology.

1. Surgery.   2. Diagnosis, Radioscopic.   3. Imaging
systems in medicine.   I. Teplick, J. George.   II. Haskin,
Marvin E.   III. Textbook of surgery. [DNLM: 1. Surgery
2. Radiography. W0100 S9626]

RD31.S925   617'.07572   78–20730

ISBN 0–7216–8782–3 (v. II)

SURGICAL RADIOLOGY   ISBN   0-7216-8782-3

Last digit is the print number: 9   8   7   6   5   4   3   2   1

To
SELMA AND PAM

for their love, patience, and encouragement

CONTRIBUTORS

VOLUME II

KURT AMPLATZ, M.D.

Professor of Radiology, University of Minnesota Hospitals. Staff, University of Minnesota Hospitals, Variety Club Heart Hospital, Minneapolis, Minnesota.

Carotid Occlusive Disease, Subclavian Steal Syndrome, Takayasu's Arteritis, Buerger's Disease, Raynaud's Syndrome, Circulatory Problems of the Upper Extremity

PETER R. BREAM, M.D.

Associate Professor of Radiology, University of Alabama School of Medicine, Birmingham, Alabama. Radiologist, St. Vincent's Medical Center, Jacksonville, Florida.

Congenital Heart Disease, Acquired Valvular Heart Disease, Postoperative Findings Common to Acquired and Congenital Heart Disease

KLAUS M. BRON, M.D., F.A.C.R.

Professor of Radiology, University of Pittsburgh School of Medicine. Chief, Vascular Radiology, Presbyterian-University Hospital, Pittsburgh, Pennsylvania.

Leriche Syndrome, Femoral Bypass, Arterial Injuries, Acute Arterial Occlusion, Arteriovenous Fistula, Technique of Abdominal-Femoral Arteriography

WILFRIDO R. CASTAÑEDA-ZUÑIGA, M.D.

Assistant Professor of Radiology, University of Minnesota Medical School. Attending Radiologist, University of Minnesota Hospitals. Consultant Radiologist, Veterans Administration Hospital, St. Paul, Minnesota.

Buerger's Disease, Raynaud's Syndrome, Circulatory Problems of the Upper Extremity

RONALD A. CASTELLINO, M.D.

Associate Professor of Radiology, Stanford University School of Medicine, Stanford, California.

Cardiac Homotransplants

PAUL R. CIPRIANO, M.D.

Assistant Professor of Radiology, Stanford University School of Medicine, Stanford, California. Attending Radiologist, Stanford University Hospital and Veterans Administration Hospital, Palo Alto, California.

Cardiac Neoplasms

ROBERT A. CLARK, M.D.

Assistant Professor of Radiology, University of Cincinnati Medical Center. Staff, Cincinnati General Hospital, Cincinnati, Ohio.

The Surgical Treatment of Pulmonary Tuberculosis; Radiologic Aspects

DAVID P. COLLEY, M.D.

Assistant Professor of Radiology, University of Cincinnati Medical Center. Staff, Cincinnati General Hospital, Cincinnati, Ohio.

The Surgical Treatment of Pulmonary Tuberculosis; Radiologic Aspects

IRVING EHRLICH, B.S., M.D.

Radiologist, St. Joseph Hospital, Reading, Pennsylvania.

Cardiac Pacemakers

LARRY P. ELLIOTT, M.D.

Professor of Radiology; Director, Division of Cardiac Radiology, University of Alabama School of Medicine, Birmingham, Alabama.

Congenital Heart Disease, Acquired Valvular Heart Disease, Postoperative Findings Common to Acquired and Congenital Heart Disease

KENT ELLIS, M.D.

Professor of Radiology, College of Physicians and Surgeons, Columbia University. Attending Radiologist, Presbyterian Hospital in the City of New York, New York, N.Y.

The Pericardium

DAVID S. FEIGIN, M.D., L.C.D.R., M.C., U.S.N.R.

Assistant Professor of Radiology, University of California, San Diego, School of Medicine. Formerly Chief, Division of Diagnostic Radiologic Pathology, Armed Forces Institute of Pathology; Assistant Professor of Radiology, Uniformed Services University of the Health Sciences, Washington, D.C. Chief, Chest Radiology, Veterans Administration Medical Center, San Diego; Radiologist, Hospital of the University of California, San Diego, California.

Disorders of the Chest Wall

GUSTAVE FORMANEK, M.D., C.Sc.

Associate Professor of Radiology, University of Minnesota Hospitals. Staff, University of Minnesota Hospitals, Variety Club Heart Hospital, Minneapolis, Minnesota.

Carotid Occlusive Disease, Subclavian Steal Syndrome, Takayasu's Arteritis

GORDON GAMSU, M.D.

Associate Professor of Radiology; Attending Radiologist, University of California Medical Center, San Francisco, California.

Tracheostomy, Tracheobronchial Tumors and Tumorlike Conditions, Carcinoma of the Lung

LAWRENCE R. GOODMAN, M.D.

Associate Professor; Head of Chest Radiology, Hahnemann Medical College and Hospital, Philadelphia, Pennsylvania.

Tracheostomy, Thoracic Trauma

RONALD GRAHAM GRAINGER, M.D., F.R.C.P., F.R.C.R., F.A.C.R. (Hon.), F.R.A.C.R. (Hon.)

Honorary Clinical Lecturer, University of Sheffield. Consultant Radiologist, The Royal Hallamshire Hospital, Sheffield, England.

The Mediastinum

DIANA F. GUTHANER, M.D., M.B., M.R.C.P. (U.K.), F.R.C.R., F.A.C.C.

Assistant Professor of Radiology, Stanford University Medical Center, Stanford, California. Cardiovascular Radiologist, Stanford University Hospital; Veterans Administration Hospital, Palo Alto, California.

Cardiac Catheterization, The Coronary Circulation, Bypass Graft Angiography, Ventricular Aneurysms

BAO-SHAN JING, M.D.

Clinical Professor of Radiology, University of Texas Medical School at Houston. Professor and Radiologist, Department of Diagnostic Radiology, The University of Texas System Cancer Center, M. D. Anderson Hospital and Tumor Institute, Houston, Texas.

Disorders of the Lymphatic System

STEPHEN L. KAUFMAN, M.D.

Assistant Professor of Radiology, Johns Hopkins University School of Medicine. Attending Radiologist, Johns Hopkins Hospital, Baltimore, Maryland.

Visceral Ischemic Syndromes

DONALD LATHAM KING, M.D.

Professor of Radiology, College of Physicians and Surgeons, Columbia University. Attending Radiologist, Presbyterian Hospital in the City of New York. New York, N.Y.

The Pericardium

WILLIAM C. KLINGENSMITH, III, M.D.

Associate Professor, University of Colorado Health Sciences Center. Director, Division of Nuclear Medicine, University Hospital, University of Colorado Health Sciences Center, Denver, Colorado.

Liver Homotransplantation

MORRIS N. KOTLER, M.D., F.R.C.P.

Professor of Medicine; Director, Non-Invasive Laboratory, Hahnemann Medical College and Hospital, Philadelphia, Pennsylvania.

Clinical Echocardiography

ERICH K. LANG, M.D., M.S.

Professor of Radiology, LSU Medical Center and Tulane School of Medicine. Chairman, Department of Radiology, LSU Medical Center. Director, Department of Radiology, Charity Hospital of New Orleans. New Orleans, Louisiana.

Thoracic Outlet Syndrome, Aneurysms of the Chest and Neck, Surgical Renovascular Hypertension

MICHAEL S. LEVINE, M.D.

Attending Radiologist, Leesburg General Hospital, Leesburg, Florida.

Aneurysms of the Abdominal Aorta, Visceral Branches, and Arteries of the Lower Extremities

ALAN R. LIST, M.D.

Assistant Professor, Department of Radiology, LSU Medical Center. Radiologist, Charity Hospital of New Orleans. New Orleans, Louisiana.

Surgical Renovascular Hypertension

JOHN E. MADEWELL, M.D.

Chairman and Registrar, Department of Radiologic Pathology, Armed Forces Institute of Pathology. Professor of Radiology, Uniformed Services University of the Health Sciences, Washington, D.C.

Disorders of the Chest Wall

RANDOLPH P. MARTIN, M.D.

Associate Professor of Medicine (Cardiology). Director, Noninvasive Laboratory, University of Virginia School of Medicine, Charlottesville, Virginia.

Cardiac Neoplasms

WALLACE T. MILLER, M.D.

Professor of Radiology, University of Pennsylvania School of Medicine. Chief, Chest Section, Department of Radiology, Hospital of the University of Pennsylvania, Philadelphia, Pennsylvania.

Abscess and Fungal Infections, The Pleura and its Disorders, Bronchiectasis

GARY S. MINTZ, M.D.

Assistant Professor of Medicine, Cardiovascular Institute, Hahnemann Medical College and Hospital. Attending Physician, Hahnemann Hospital, Philadelphia, Pennsylvania.

Clinical Echocardiography

ROBERT A. NOVELLINE, M.D.

Assistant Professor of Radiology, Harvard Medical School. Associate Radiologist, Massachusetts General Hospital, Boston, Massachusetts.

Disorders of Veins

IVO OBREZ, M.D., Sc.D.

Professor of Radiology, University of Ljubljana School of Medicine. Chief, Cardiovascular Section, Institute of Roentgenology, Ljubljana, Yugoslavia.

The Coronary Circulation

WAYNE PARRY

Instructor in Medicine; Chief Technician, Non-Invasive Laboratory, Hahnemann Medical College and Hospital, Philadelphia, Pennsylvania.

Clinical Echocardiography

CHARLES PUTMAN, M.D.

Chairman and Professor, Department of Radiology, Duke University Medical Center, Durham, North Carolina.

Thoracic Trauma

CARL E. RAVIN, M.D.

Associate Professor of Radiology, Duke University School of Medicine. Director, Diagnostic Radiology, Duke University Medical Center, Durham, North Carolina.

Assisted Circulation

SHELDON A. ROEN, M.D.

Assistant Professor of Radiology; Chief, Section of Radiological Special Procedures, University of Miami School of Medicine, Miami, Florida.

Aneurysms of the Abdominal Aorta, Visceral Branches, and Arteries of the Lower Extremities

BARRY A. SACKS, M.D.

Instructor in Radiology, Harvard Medical School. Chief, Vascular Radiology, Beth Israel Hospital, Boston, Massachusetts.

Fat Embolism Syndrome, Pulmonary Embolism

JORGEN U. SCHLEGEL, M.D., Ph.D.

Professor and Chairman, Department of Urology, Tulane University School of Medicine. Chief of Staff, Tulane Medical Center. Chief of Service, Department of Urology, Tulane Medical Center, Charity Hospital, and Veterans Administration Hospital, New Orleans, Louisiana.

Surgical Renovascular Hypertension

BERNARD L. SEGAL, M.D.

Professor of Medicine, Hahnemann Medical College and Hospital. Medical Director, Likoff Cardiovascular Institute, Hahnemann Medical College and Hospital, Philadelphia, Pennsylvania.

Clinical Echocardiography

STANLEY S. SIEGELMAN, M.D.

Professor of Radiology; Director, Diagnostic Radiology, Johns Hopkins University School of Medicine, Baltimore, Maryland.

Visceral Ischemic Syndromes

JAMES F. SILVERMAN, M.D.

Associate Professor of Clinical Radiology, Stanford University School of Medicine, Stanford, California.

Cardiac Homotransplants

MORRIS SIMON, M.D.

Professor of Radiology, Harvard Medical School. Director of Clinical Radiology, Beth Israel Hospital, Boston, Massachusetts.

Fat Embolism Syndrome, Pulmonary Embolism

ARTHUR S. SOUZA, JR., M.D.

Instituto Radiodiagnostico, São Paulo, Brazil.

Postoperative Findings Common to Acquired and Congenital Heart Disease

JOHN O. TAUBMAN, M.B., Ch.B., M.R.C.P.E., D.M.R.D., F.R.C.P.

Associate Professor; Director, Division of Diagnostic Radiology, University Hospital, University of Colorado Health Sciences Center, Denver, Colorado.

Liver Homotransplantation

INA L. TONKIN, M.D.

Associate Professor of Radiology, University of Tennessee College of Medicine. Attending Cardiovascular Radiologist, University of Tennessee Medical Center and LeBonheur Children's Medical Center, Memphis, Tennessee.

Congenital Heart Disease, Acquired Valvular Heart Disease Postoperative Findings Common to Acquired and Congenital Heart Disease

WILLIAM J. TUDDENHAM, M.D.

Professor of Radiology, University of Pennsylvania School of Medicine. Director, Department of Radiology, Pennsylvania Hospital, Philadelphia, Pennsylvania.

Iatrogenic Lesions of the Lungs

MANUEL VIAMONTE, JR., M.D.

Professor of Radiology, University of Miami School of Medicine, Miami, Florida. Chairman and Director, Department of Radiology, Mount Sinai Medical Center, Miami Beach, Florida.

Aneurysms of the Abdominal Aorta, Visceral Branches, and Arteries of the Lower Extremities

SIDNEY WALLACE, M.D.

Clinical Professor in Diagnostic Radiology, The University of Texas Medical School at Houston. Professor in Program in Radiology Technology Education, School of Allied Health Sciences. Professor of Radiology; Head, Clinical Section, Department of Diagnostic Radiology, The University of Texas System Cancer Center, M. D. Anderson Hospital and Tumor Institute, Houston, Texas.

Disorders of the Lymphatic System

W. RICHARD WEBB, M.D.

Assistant Professor of Radiology, University of California, San Francisco, School of Medicine. Attending Radiologist, University of California Medical Center, San Francisco, California.

Tracheobronchial Tumors and Tumorlike Conditions, Carcinoma of the Lung

LEWIS WEXLER, M.D., F.A.C.C.

Professor of Radiology, Stanford University Medical School. Chief of Cardiovascular Radiology, Stanford University Hospital, Stanford, California.

Cardiac Catheterization, The Coronary Circulation, Bypass Graft Angiography, Ventricular Aneurysm, Cardiac Neoplasms

AUDREY R. WILSON, M.D.

Director, Division of Angiography, Assistant Professor of Radiology, Hahnemann Medical College and Hospital, Philadelphia, Pennsylvania.

Renal Allografts

JEROME F. WIOT, M.D.

Professor and Chairman of Radiology, University of Cincinnati Medical Center; Staff, Cincinnati General Hospital, Cincinnati, Ohio.

The Surgical Treatment of Pulmonary Tuberculosis; Radiologic Aspects

FOREWORD

This new three-volume work on surgical radiology fills a much needed role and is a very welcome addition to this field. Drs. Teplick and Haskin are to be highly commended for their comprehensive approach to all aspects of radiologic diagnosis in surgical patients. These authors have been unusually thorough in their coverage of the entire field of surgery and have included each of the surgical specialties in this impressive undertaking.

In 1967 Teplick and Haskin met a pressing need with the introduction of a two-volume work designed as a radiologic companion to the Beeson-McDermott *Textbook of Medicine*. This innovative concept added much to the famous text with which it was to be jointly used. Carefully and exhaustively illustrated, these two volumes were extremely well received; a second edition was published in 1971, and a third edition appeared in 1976. The success of these editions is a matter of record, and it is easy to predict that the new surgical companion text will also be widely used and be rapidly recognized as a timely addition to the surgical armamentarium.

Since the discovery of x-rays by Roentgen in 1895, massive strides have been made in the field of radiology. A number of subspecialties have developed and now constitute an established part of this discipline. In the first volume of this series on surgical radiology, special emphasis has been placed upon the newer aspects of radioisotope techniques in surgical diagnosis, the role of ultrasound in surgical patients, and the expanding indications for the use of computerized tomography. Each of these sections is presented in a clear and concise manner with excellent illustrations. This extensive work by Teplick and Haskin emphasizes the expanding role of the radiologist not only in *diagnostic* but also in therapeutic procedures. The passage of a variety of catheters, needles, and tubes with the use of image intensification permits a multidimensional approach to the *treatment* of a number of specific disorders. Techniques that have proved highly effective in radiologic management include removal of gallstones; biopsy of pulmonary, mediastinal, and other masses; dilatation of stenotic lesions of the arterial system; control of massive hemorrhage by selective arteriography and perfusion of vasoconstrictors; direct embolization of bleeding sites; selective chemotherapeutic and embolic infusion of neoplasms; and a variety of additional procedures. Each of these serves as an example of the ever-increasing importance of the radiologic sciences to diagnosis and treatment in modern medicine.

There is little doubt that this three-volume series will be very favorably received by all members of the surgical and allied professions, and much praise is due the editors and contributors for this comprehensive and highly useful text.

DAVID C. SABISTON, JR.

PREFACE

These three volumes are designed to provide a single source of radiologic information related to surgical conditions. In addition to preoperative radiographic diagnosis, emphasis is placed on radiographic appearances following surgery and on radiographic findings associated with surgical complications.

In the main, this is planned to be a radiologic compendium for hospital practice, embracing knowledge unique to the hospital environment, including the emergency room, recovery room, and intensive care units. The emphasis, therefore, is quite different from that of the usual radiologic textbook. A recurring theme is comparative pre- and postoperative radiographic appearances, with appropriate attention to complications following surgery.

The explosive development of both newer techniques and the modalities of ultrasound, computed tomography, Chiba needle aspiration biopsy, and nuclear medicine has made closer cooperation between the clinician and the radiologist imperative for integrating the necessary imaging studies of surgical patients and those who are candidates for surgery. These modalities are discussed in detail and illustrated profusely throughout these volumes. In addition, special detailed sections on newer and updated imaging modalities precede the chapters on specific disorders in Volume I.

The general organization follows that of the Davis-Christopher *Textbook of Surgery,* edited by D. C. Sabiston, Jr., M.D. The numerous contributors to *Surgical Radiology* have been selected for their demonstrated interest and experience in subjects appropriate to the scope of these volumes.

Volume I comprises general abdominal conditions, including the acute abdomen and disorders of the gastrointestinal and biliary tracts, liver, pancreas, and spleen. Chapter 1 discusses radiographic considerations of the acute care unit. Contributions by 27 individual authors or collaborating groups and about 1800 illustrations are contained in Volume I.

Contained in Volume II are the disorders of the lungs, pleura, chest wall, mediastinum, heart, and entire vascular system. This volume concludes with a section discussing renal, hepatic, and cardiac transplantation.

Volume III includes endocrine, pediatric, head and neck, neurosurgical, musculoskeletal, breast, and genitourinary disorders. The increasingly important role of interventional radiology is discussed in a separate chapter.

Each volume contains a separate index, and a combined index of the three volumes appears in Volume III.

Surgical Radiology should prove a most useful addition to the armamentarium of the hospital radiologist, the clinician, and the surgeon as well as the entire resident staff.

We gratefully acknowledge the assistance and guidance of John Hanley, President of the W. B. Saunders Company. We would especially like to thank Mildred Strehle for her patience, graciousness, and many kindnesses. We are also grateful for Constance Burton's fine editorial assistance.

J. GEORGE TEPLICK, M.D.
MARVIN E. HASKIN, M.D.

CONTENTS

VOLUME II

Volume II

19

THE LUNGS, PLEURA, AND CHEST WALL

Part I
Tracheostomy

LAWRENCE R. GOODMAN, M.D.
GORDON GAMSU, M.D.

The advent of positive-pressure ventilation via an artificial airway has markedly increased the number of patients undergoing both endotracheal intubation (see Chapter 1) and tracheostomy. Tracheostomy is most often indicated when prolonged ventilatory support is needed in patients with respiratory failure. Tracheostomies are also performed to bypass upper airway obstruction and to improve tracheal toilet in patients who have difficulty in mobilizing their secretions.

IMMEDIATE COMPLICATIONS

A well-penetrated radiograph should be obtained immediately following surgery to evaluate tube position and postoperative complications. The tube should measure approximately two thirds the width of the trachea and lie along the long axis of the trachea.[8] The tip should be approximately one half to two thirds the distance from the stoma to the carina. When a cuff is present, it is visualized as an oval lucency within the tracheal air column. If the cuff acutely distends the trachea, the pressure within the balloon is too high (Fig. 19–1). In prolonged intubations of patients receiving positive-pressure breathing, gradual dilatation of the trachea may be unavoidable.

The chest radiograph obtained immediately following tracheostomy should also be observed for evidence of postoperative complications. Mediastinal widening may be the first indication of mediastinal hemorrhage. Caution should be used in interpreting mediastinal widening on portable anteroposterior chest radiographs because changes

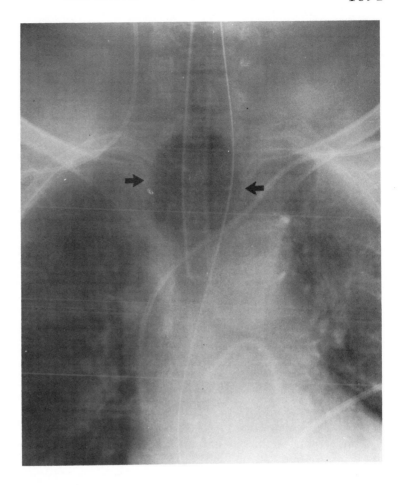

Figure 19–1. Acute tracheal dilatation. The balloon of an endotracheal tube cuff is markedly distending the trachea (arrows). Malfunction of the release valve had not been appreciated.

in patient positioning or target-film distance may magnify the mediastinum. Pneumothorax is usually secondary to violation of the pleural space during tracheostomy rather than tracheal perforation. A small amount of gas in the neck is not uncommon following tracheostomy. Large amounts of subcutaneous or mediastinal gas require further consideration, however. Air may dissect into the fascial planes of the neck and mediastinum from the tracheostomy stoma. Laceration of the tracheal wall may allow dissection of air into the mediastinum. When high-peak inspiratory pressures are being used, pulmonary barotrauma may result in a pneumomediastinum. The development of a pneumomediastinum in a patient on assisted ventilation must always be considered a significant radiographic finding.[17] Pneumomediastinum is diagnosed radiographically by the observation of separation of the parietal mediastinal pleura from the mediastinum and the visualization of mediastinal structures not normally discernible within the cardiomediastinal silhouette (Fig. 19–2).

Areas of pulmonary consolidation appearing soon after a tracheostomy or intubation may be caused by aspirated blood or aspiration pneumonia or may be secondary to retained secretions causing airway obstruction and atelectasis.

LATE COMPLICATIONS

Late complications of tracheostomy and endotracheal intubation are due to injury to the glottis and trachea during intubation and include stenosis, malacia, hemorrhage,

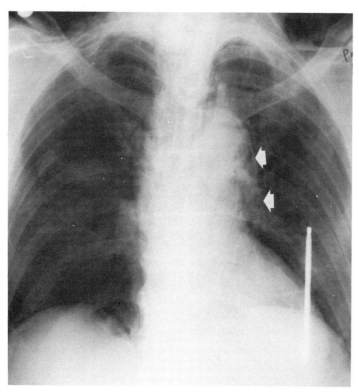

Figure 19–2. Post-tracheostomy air leak. Subcutaneous emphysema was noted clinically after a difficult tracheostomy. The initial tracheostomy tube insertion was paratracheal. The radiograph demonstrates marked bilateral subcutaneous emphysema in the neck and a pneumomediastinum (arrows). The patient's temperature was normal. A pneumothorax was evident several hours later.

and fistula. Although improved cuff design and clinical management have reduced tracheal injuries, the ability to maintain critically ill patients for prolonged periods has increased the incidence of tracheal injury.[2, 16] Five to fifteen per cent of tracheostomized patients acquire clinically significant tracheal obstruction after the tube has been removed.

Trachael wall injury is caused by pressure either from the cuff or from the tracheal tube itself.[3] The common factor in cuff trauma is the lateral wall pressure on the trachea, which often exceeds capillary perfusion pressure and results in necrosis of the tracheal wall. Histologic inflammatory changes have been noted at 24 to 48 hours. Mucosal ulceration can occur within seven days.[9, 16] Continued ulceration and inflammation may result in exposure of the tracheal cartilaginous rings in one to three weeks. Fragmentation and total loss of cartilage can occur in two to three weeks. Tracheal wall damage may result in exuberant granulation tissue or granuloma formation. Alternatively, fibrous tissue can result in stricture of the trachea. If damage to the cartilage rings occurs, a focal area of tracheomalacia may result.[10] Rarely, deep injury of the tracheal wall causes perforation into an adjacent structure.

Tracheostomy tubes angulated anteriorly and to the right may erode through the tracheal wall into the adjacent innominate artery, causing fatal hemorrhage. Tubes angulated posteriorly may erode through the posterior tracheal membrane into the esophagus or mediastinum. If food particles are recovered from tracheal secretions or unexplained pneumonia develops in patients on long-term intubation, the possibility of tracheoesophageal fistula should be considered. Investigation should be undertaken with a barium swallow, with the cuff deflated. Careful fluoroscopic monitoring is necessary to demonstrate the fistula and to ensure that aspiration is not occurring via the larynx. Alternatively, a tube can be placed in the esophagus and the contrast agent instilled directly opposite the site of the suspected fistula. Water-soluble contrast agents are extremely irritating to the lungs and should not be employed in the investigation of a tracheoesophageal fistula.

The most frequent long-term complication of tracheostomy or prolonged endotracheal intubation is tracheal stenosis.[1, 5, 9, 10] The condition is frequently overlooked because the symptoms are mistakenly attributed to the progression of the patient's concomitant lung disease. Thus, a potentially correctable lesion may be missed. Symptoms may suggest upper airway obstruction or may be nonspecific. In any patient who has been intubated or has had a tracheostomy and who exhibits wheezing, "asthma," stridor, exertional dyspnea, difficulty in clearing secretions, a persistent cough, or hemoptysis, the diagnosis of tracheal stenosis should be considered. Although symptomatic obstruction may occur years after intubation, symptoms most frequently surface within the first few months after extubation. Advances in tracheal surgery have greatly increased the need for accurate radiographic evaluation of the site, the severity, and, especially, the length of the tracheal lesion.

Fixed or Rigid Tracheal Stenosis

After tracheostomy, fixed obstruction from scarring may occur anywhere between the vocal cords and the carina. The majority of lesions are at the level of the tracheal stoma, the tracheostomy cuff, or the tube tip.[1, 9–11] At the stoma, obstruction may be due to scarring of the anterior wall or the anterior and lateral walls or to the formation of a "granulation ball" on the anterior wall (Fig. 19–3). Stenosis at the site of the balloon cuff

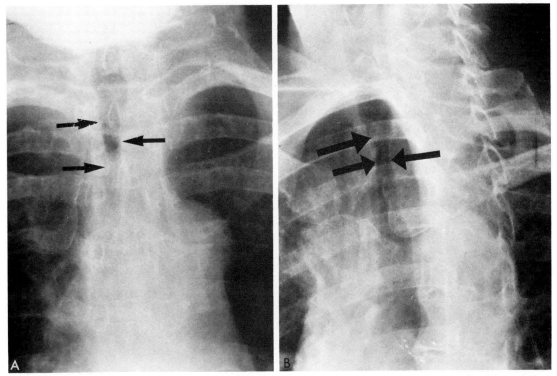

Figure 19–3. Tracheal stenosis. Posteroanterior *(A)* and oblique *(B)* radiographs reveal mild to moderate narrowing at the level of the stoma (arrows).

often produces a short segment of circumferential narrowing. The tracheal lumen may be eccentric or central. The lesion is often intrathoracic and may not be visible on plain radiographs of the neck (Fig. 19–4 and 19–5). Stenosis produced by the tip of the endotracheal or tracheostomy tube most often involves the anterior tracheal wall.

Obstruction of the subglottic area is rare following a properly performed tracheostomy. However, subglottic stenosis often follows a high tracheostomy through the cricoid cartilage (Fig. 19–6). Prolonged endotracheal intubation is more frequently associated with glottic and subglottic lesions (Figs. 19–7 and 19–8).[10, 16]

Tracheomalacia

Iatrogenic tracheomalacia associated with previous intubation or surgery on the trachea is defined as a focal area of abnormal tracheal wall compliance. The cartilage and other supporting structures of the trachea must be damaged to produce this lesion. The most common site of acquired tracheomalacia is immediately caudad to the internal orifice of a tracheostomy stoma (Figs. 19–9 and 19–10). Tracheomalacia is also found adjacent to areas of scarring and fixed stenosis. Diagnosis may be extremely difficult, especially in determining the length of the segment of tracheomalacia.[6, 7, 18]

Text continued on page 1100

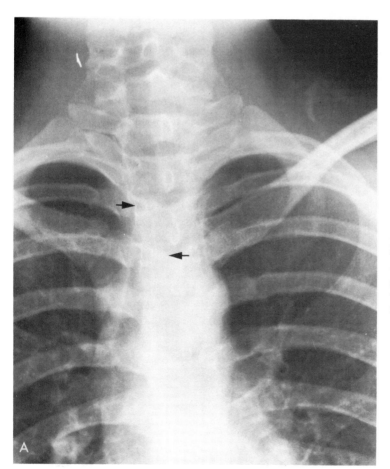

Figure 19–4. Tracheostenosis following tracheostomy. *A,* Posteroanterior chest radiograph demonstrates that the tracheal air column is absent for about 2 cm at the level of the clavicles (arrows). There is also a slight narrowing of the trachea at the level of the stoma (C_7 to T_1). Surgical clips in the neck serve as a reference marker.

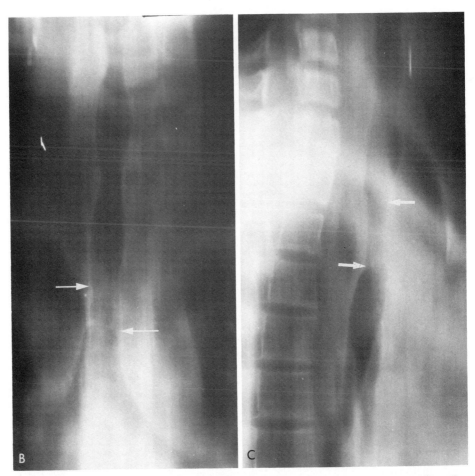

Figure 19–4 *Continued.* *B* and *C*, Anteroposterior and lateral tomograms confirm the approximately-50-per cent stenosis of the midtrachea (arrows) and the slight narrowing at the stomal site. The vocal cords are normal. (*From* Goodman, L. R.: Pulmonary support and monitoring apparatus. *In* Goodman, L. R., and Putman, C. E. (eds.): Intensive Care Radiology: Imaging in the Critically Ill. St. Louis, C. V. Mosby Company, 1978.)

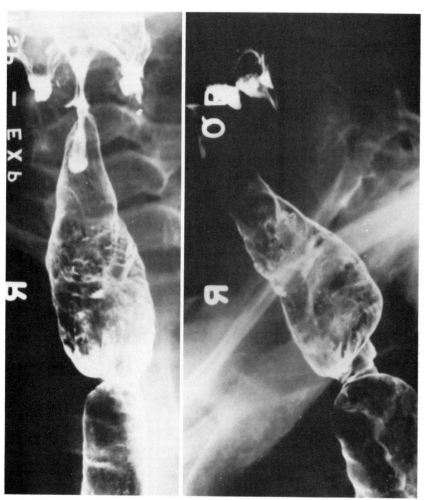

Figure 19–5. Tracheal stenosis at cuff. A tantalum tracheogram demonstrates circumferential narrowing of the trachea at the thoracic inlet, which is present in two projections.

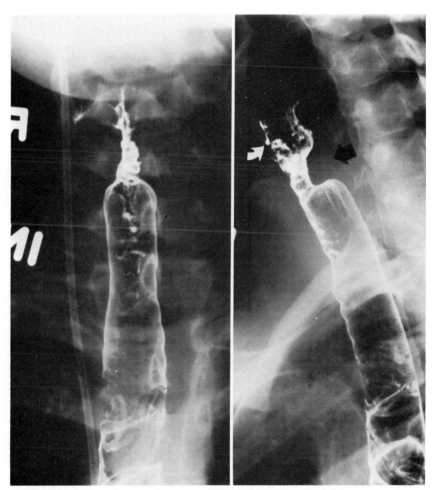

Figure 19–6.   Subglottic stenosis following a tracheostomy through the cricothyroid membrane. Severe tracheal stenosis involving the undersurface of the vocal cords is present in frontal and lateral projections of a tantalum tracheogram. The anterior commissure is visible (curved arrow).

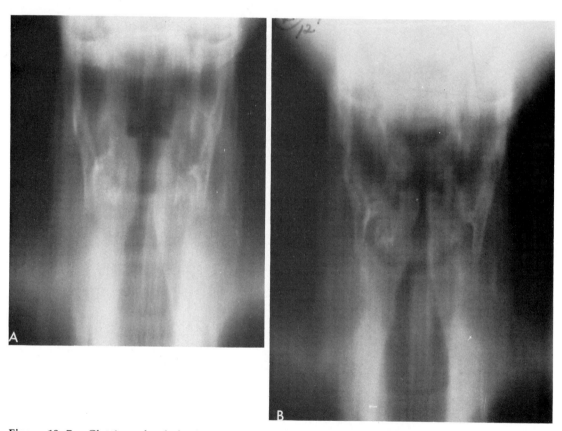

Figure 19–7. Glottic and subglottic stenosis. Dyspnea occurred approximately 15 years after endotracheal intubation. *A,* Deep inspiration. There is limited abduction of the vocal cords and asymmetric narrowing of subglottic arch. *B,* Phonation ("E") — relatively normal adduction of vocal cords. The subglottic stenosis is unchanged.

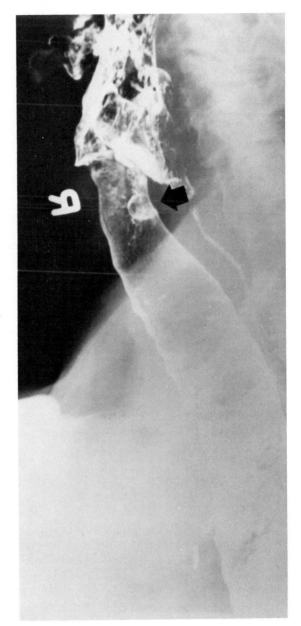

Figure 19–8. Subglottic granuloma following prolonged postoperative assisted ventilation. A lateral projection of a tantalum tracheogram shows a subglottic granuloma (arrow).

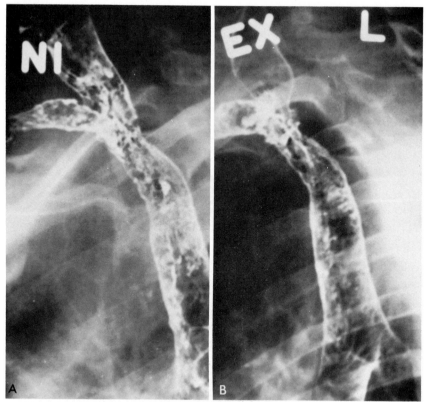

Figure 19–9. Tracheomalacia. Inspiration and expiration views in the oblique projection of a tantalum tracheogram of a patient with a tracheostomy. Airway obstruction developed whenever the tracheostomy was removed. *A,* The inspiratory radiograph reveals a reasonably normal-caliber trachea. *B,* The expiratory radiograph demonstrates marked tracheomalacia immediately caudad to the tracheostomy stoma.

EVALUATION OF PATIENTS WITH SUSPECTED TRACHEAL OBSTRUCTION

Evaluation requires a combined structural and functional determination of the site, severity, and length of the tracheal stenosis, as well as of the tracheal dynamics of the involved segment. Both physiologic and radiologic studies are necessary.[7]

Pulmonary function studies with maximal forced inspiratory and expiratory flow-volume loops should always be obtained.[12, 14] Significant stenosis almost always shows an abnormality in the flow-volume loop. The characteristic abnormalities are a plateau in the midportion of the vital capacity on either the inspiratory or the expiratory curve or on both. One exception to this rule is found in patients with severe peripheral airways disease. In this circumstance, flow rates are insufficient to detect the tracheal lesion.

In patients with rigid lesions, plain radiographs of the trachea usually detect the site of stenosis. The intrinsic contrast of air within the trachea can provide considerable information. Anteroposterior and lateral views of the neck, and anteroposterior, lateral, and oblique views of the chest are useful in delineating the severity of the stenosis (see Fig. 19–3).[8, 11, 13] Tomography or xerotomography of the entire trachea in both the anteroposterior and the lateral views further defines the lesion. A lead marker at the level

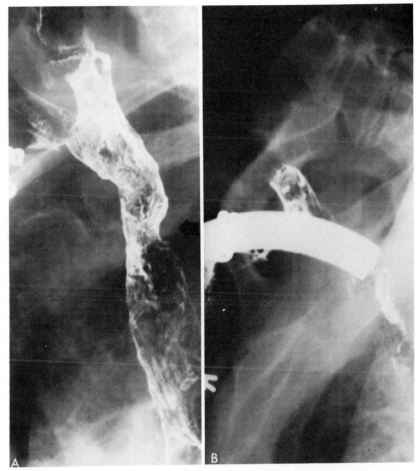

Figure 19–10.   Tracheomalacia. A lateral view of a tantalum tracheogram of a patient with a tracheostomy. *A,* With the tracheostomy tube removed, indrawing of the posterior tracheomembrane, producing stenosis, is apparent. *B,* When the tracheostomy tube is replaced, the impingement of the tip of the tracheostomy tube on the posterior membrane is apparent.

of the stoma facilitates localization (see Figs. 19–4 and 19–7). In difficult cases, positive-contrast tracheography offers optimal visualization. Metallic tantalum is the contrast agent of choice but is not generally available (see Figs. 19–5, 19–6, and 19–8). Propyliodone (Dionosil) is the contrast agent, most frequently used but it may cause mucosal edema and further compromise the lumen. As a general rule, narrowing of at least 50 per cent of the cross-sectional area of the trachea must be present before symptomatic airway obstruction occurs.

Tracheomalacia should be suspected whenever the patient's symptoms are out of proportion to the plain radiographic findings, or when the flow-volume loop indicates a more severe stenosis than that demonstrated by the plain radiographs. To demonstrate tracheomalacia, the trachea must be studied during full inspiration, full expiration, and the Valsalva and Müller maneuvers. Cine or video tape recording of the fluoroscopy assists greatly in evaluation. In studying these dynamic changes, positive-contrast tracheography may provide information not obtainable by other methods (see Figs. 19–9 and 19–10).[7, 18]

RADIOGRAPHY FOLLOWING THERAPY

Recent advances in the surgical techniques of tracheal resection and end-to-end anastomosis have markedly improved the outlook for patients with iatrogenic tracheal stenosis and tracheomalacia. In the immediate postoperative period, complications of radiographic interest include mediastinal infection or hemorrhage and disruption of the anastomosis. Radiographs following successful resection reveal shortening of the trachea commensurate with the length of trachea resected (Fig. 19–11).[9] Excessive granulation tissue at the suture lines and restenosis are uncommon but do occur (Fig. 19–12). Repeated dilatation of the trachea is now performed less frequently but is still undertaken for short-segment stenosis in those patients for whom surgery is not feasible. Perforation of the trachea, with the development of a tracheal sinus into the mediastinum, is an uncommon complication.

Soft silicon stents in the shape of a T may be used to facilitate cervical tracheal reconstruction or to attempt to retard further narrowing of a stenotic segment (Fig. 19–13).[15]

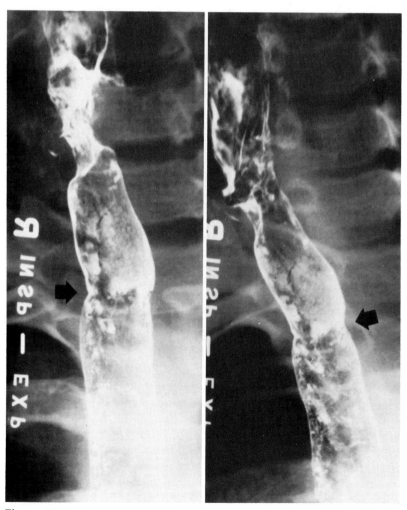

Figure 19–11. Postresection tracheogram. Frontal and lateral radiographs of the trachea taken from a tantalum tracheogram of a patient after the resection of 4 cm of the trachea. The trachea is of relatively normal caliber, with a minor indentation at the anastomosis site (arrows).

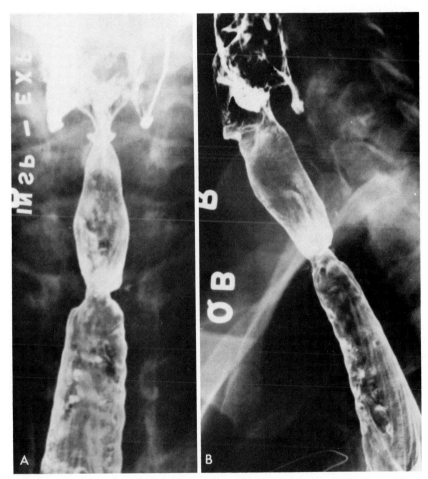

Figure 19–12. Postresection stenosis. A tantalum tracheogram of a patient with increasing dyspnea following tracheal resection. Frontal *(A)* and oblique *(B)* views from a tracheogram reveal restenosis at the site of previous resection. The large wire suture is from an earlier median sternotomy.

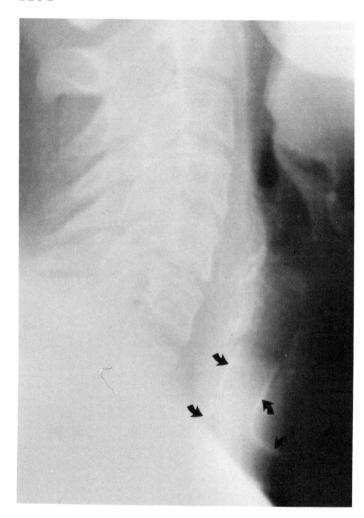

Figure 19–13. Tracheal stent. A T-shaped silicon stent (arrows) dilates a stenotic area in the cervical trachea.

References

1. Andrews, M.J., and Pearson, F.G.: An analysis of 59 cases of tracheal stenosis following tracheostomy with cuffed tube and assisted ventilation, with special reference to diagnosis and treatment. Br. J. Surg. *60*:208–212, 1973.
2. Ching, N.P.H., Ayres, S. M., Spina, R.C., et al.: Endotracheal damage during continuous ventilatory support. Ann. Surg. *179*:123–127, 1974.
3. Cooper, J.D., and Grillo, H.C.: Experimental production and prevention of injury due to cuffed tracheal tubes. Surg. Gynecol. Obstet. *129*:1235–1241, 1969.
4. Dane, T.E.B., and King, E.G.: A prospective study of complications after tracheostomy for assisted ventilation. Chest *67*:398–404, 1975.
5. Fishman, N.H., Dedo, H.H., Hamilton, W.K., et al.: Postintubation tracheal stenosis. Ann. Thorac. Surg. *8*:47–56, 1969.
6. Gamsu, G., and Nadel, J.A.: New technique for roentgenographic study of airways and lungs using powdered tantalum. Cancer *30*:1353–1357, 1972.

7. Gamsu, G.: The trachea in health and disease in diagnostic radiology. *In* Margulis, A.R., and Gooding, C.A. (eds.): San Francisco, University of California, 1976, pp. 537–552.
8. Goodman, L.R., and Putman, C.E.: Intensive Care Radiology: Imaging of the Critically Ill. St. Louis, The C.V. Mosby Company, 1978.
9. Grillo, H.C.: Reconstruction of the trachea. Experience in 100 cases. Thorax *28*:667–679, 1973.
10. Harley, H.R.S.: Laryngotracheal obstruction complicating tracheostomy or endotracheal intubation with assisted respiration. Thorax *26*:493–533, 1971.
11. James, A.E., Jr., Macmillan, A.S., Jr., Eaton, S.B., et al.: Roentgenology of tracheal stenosis resulting from cuffed tracheostomy tubes. Am. J. Roentgenol. *109*:455–466, 1970.
12. Kryger, M., Bode, F., Antic, R., et al.: Diagnosis of obstruction of the upper and central airways. Am. J. Med. *61*:85–93, 1976.
13. Macmillan, A.S., Jr., James, A.E., Jr., Stitik, F.P., et al.: Radiological evaluation of post-tracheostomy lesions. Thorax *26*:696–703, 1971.
14. Miller, R.D., and Hyatt, R.E.: Evaluation of obstructing lesions of the trachea and larynx by flow-volume loops. Am. Rev. Respir. Dis. *108*:475–481, 1973.
15. Montgomery, W.W.: T tube tracheal stent. Arch. Otolaryngol. *82*:320–321, 1965.
16. Mulder, D.S., and Rubush, J.L.: Complications of tracheostomy: relationship to long term ventilatory assistance. J. Trauma *9*:389–402, 1969.
17. Rohlfing, B.M., Webb, W.R., and Schlobohm, R.M.: Ventilator-related extra-alveolar air in adults. Radiology *121*:25–31, 1976.
18. Stitik, F.P., Bartelt, D., James, A.E., Jr., et al.: Tantalum tracheography in upper airway obstruction: 100 experiences in adults. Am. J. Roentgenol. *130*:35–42, 1978.

Part II

Thoracic Trauma

CHARLES E. PUTMAN, M.D.
LAWRENCE R. GOODMAN, M.D.

INTRODUCTION

The radiologist evaluating the severely traumatized patient must make numerous critical diagnostic decisions with a minimum of radiographic studies. In no other area of medicine is such important diagnostic information obtained from such a limited imaging format. Until the patient's condition is stabilized, the radiologist must rely primarily on the anteroposterior chest radiograph to evaluate the nature and extent of thoracic trauma.

This chapter discusses the evaluation of skeletal, pulmonary, and cardiac injury following blunt or penetrating chest trauma, with emphasis on the anteroposterior radiograph. If possible, the patient should be erect or semi-erect, with the back flat against the cassette and the shoulders rolled forward. Care should be taken to avoid rotation because many critical decisions are based on the perceived shift of the mediastinum, trachea, and heart. A minimal distance of 40 inches should be established and maintained through subsequent examinations to allow meaningful radiographs for comparison. With both stationary and portable equipment, high kilovoltage and short exposures minimize motion and are preferred.

The anteroposterior erect radiograph is usually adequate to delineate most fractures, pneumothorax and pneumomediastinum, pleural effusions, lung contusions, and atelectasis. In addition, clues to severe visceral injury to the tracheobronchial tree, the esophagus, and the cardiovascular system may appear on the initial radiographs. Only after careful scrutiny of technically adequate anteroposterior radiographs and initial stabilization of the patient are further radiographic studies warranted.

FRACTURES OF THE RIBS, STERNUM, AND CLAVICLE

The traumatic fracture of a rib or of several contiguous ribs, although painful, is seldom of great clinical significance by itself. In addition to the frontal radiograph, oblique radiographs of the injured ribs are required. A lead shot over the contused or painful area facilitates evaluation. Pneumothorax, no matter how small, is especially important in traumatized patients requiring ventilatory support, since a small air leak may rapidly be converted into a tension pneumothorax. On occasion, air is seen in the soft tissues of the chest, associated with a closed fracture of the ribs, without a demonstrable pneumothorax. One must assume a pleural laceration has occurred and be alert for the occurrence of delayed pneumothorax.

Flail chest, the paradoxical motion of a segment of the chest wall, may follow severe deceleration or crush injuries. The inappropriate motion of the chest wall with respiration is usually diagnosed clinically, although severe soft tissue hematoma may obscure the diagnosis. The free segment of the chest wall may be the result of multiple unilateral fractures, multiple bilateral fractures, or a combination of rib, sternal, and costochondral fractures (Fig. 19–14). The flail segment indicates both a potentially dangerous impairment of lung function and the severe nature of the chest trauma. Atelectasis, contusion, laceration, and pneumothorax are frequent. Evidence of trauma to the cardiovascular system, the tracheobronchial tree, and the esophagus must be sought.

Although fractures of the upper and lower three ribs are not usual, associated

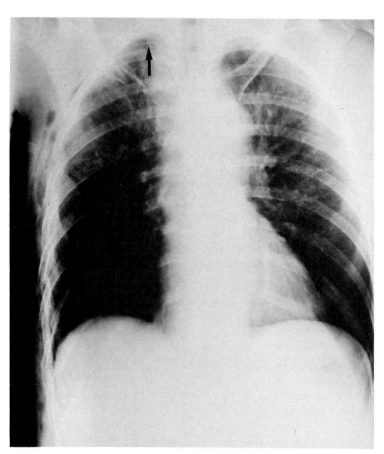

Figure 19–14. Flail chest. An anteroposterior chest radiograph of a patient with a crushing injury to the right chest. There are extensive subcutaneous emphysema, fractures of the first through the tenth axillary ribs on the right, and a small apical pneumothorax (arrow). Even on this suboptimal radiograph one can see the oligemia in the right lung and the relative plethora in the left lung. Shortly after this film was taken the patient acquired the extensive opacification of the right hemithorax that is consistent with bleeding. The initial radiograph of a flail chest may show minimal changes, but subsequent complications, such as parenchymal bleeding, hemothorax, and tension pneumothorax, are not unusual.

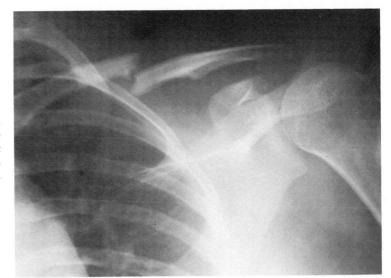

Figure 19–15. Clavicular fracture. A midshaft displaced clavicular fracture in a young football player. This was considered to be a benign fracture until the patient returned 24 hours later with signs and symptoms of a left branchial plexus injury.

visceral injuries are common and potentially lethal. Fractures of the upper three ribs are frequently associated with injury to the major vascular structures, trachea, major bronchi, and nerves.[9] An unpublished survey by one of the authors (C.E.P.) indicates that subclavian artery or vein laceration, brachial plexus injury, or aortic rupture is associated with first or second rib fractures in one third of cases. Similarly, one third of patients with tracheobronchial injuries have upper rib fractures. Patients with fractures of the first and second rib have a hospital mortality rate of 15 per cent and 27 per cent respectively, an indication of the severity of associated intra- and extrathoracic injuries.[40]

The presence of fractures of the lower three ribs suggests the possibility of injury to the liver or spleen. These injuries are particularly hazardous because of the dangers of delayed hemorrhage. In addition to lower rib fractures, the upper abdomen must be scrutinized for evidence of splenomegaly, upper abdominal hematomas, or blood in the flanks. The absence of rib fractures does not rule out significant upper abdominal injury.

Clavicular and scapular fractures are usually considered to be benign injuries. Their presence in a patient who has sustained blunt chest trauma should alert the radiologist to potentially more serious injury, including brachial plexus and vessel wall injury (Fig. 19–15).

Fractures of the sternum often go unrecognized and usually are associated with other thoracic cage injuries. Pneumomediastinum and pneumothorax may be related to sternal fractures. If the sternal fracture is comminuted, pericardial or cardiac injury is a distinct possibility (Fig. 19–16). Costal cartilage fractures often accompany sternal fractures, are difficult to diagnose radiographically, and are usually more painful and debilitating than a fractured sternum.[18]

The majority of sternoclavicular dislocations involve anterior dislocation of the clavicle and pose little serious threat to the patient. The uncommon retrosternal dislocation may cause symptomatic impingement on the trachea, esophagus, great vessels, and superior mediastinal nerves. Radiographic evaluation of this area is difficult. With the patient prone, angulation of the tube 35 degrees toward the head demonstrates the sternoclavicular articulation with little interference from the spine.[20] Fluoroscopy, oblique radiography, and tomography are often required (Fig. 19–17). Lee

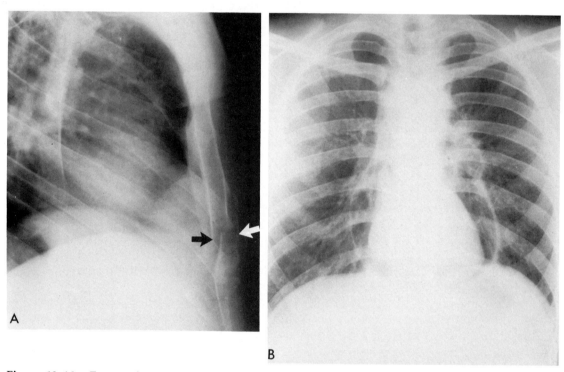

Figure 19–16. Fractured sternum — pneumopericardium. *A,* This sternal fracture (arrows) followed a steering wheel injury. Note the retrosternal hematoma. *B,* A posteroanterior radiograph demonstrates a large pneumopericardium in the same patient. Later, associated pneumomediastinum developed, but the patient remained asymptomatic. The angiocardiogram was normal, and the pneumopericardium resolved over the next several days.

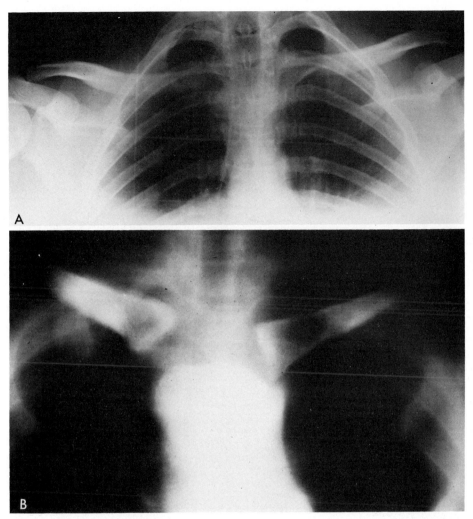

Figure 19–17. Subluxation of the clavicle. *A,* A posteroanterior view of the upper chest in a young male patient who sustained blunt thoracic trauma. There appears to be asymmetry of the sternoclavicular joints, but even with fluoroscopy a definitive diagnosis of subluxation could not be made. *B,* An anteroposterior tomogram of the same patient reveals definite subluxation of the right sternoclavicular joint. This can be a painful and demobilizing injury.

and Gwinn recently described a new view for diagnosing clavicular dislocation (Fig. 19–18).[22]

PNEUMOTHORAX

Although a large pneumothorax or tension pneumothorax can be diagnosed from a supine or semi-erect radiograph, a potentially important air leak may be missed without a horizontal beam radiograph (Fig. 19–19). On the supine films, a small pneumothorax may present as a lucency medial or inferior to the lung or in the costophrenic angle. If upright radiographs cannot be obtained, a lateral decubitus radiograph with the side in question elevated can delineate air in the pleural space (Fig. 19–20). Regardless of the type of examination, care must be taken to exclude artifacts

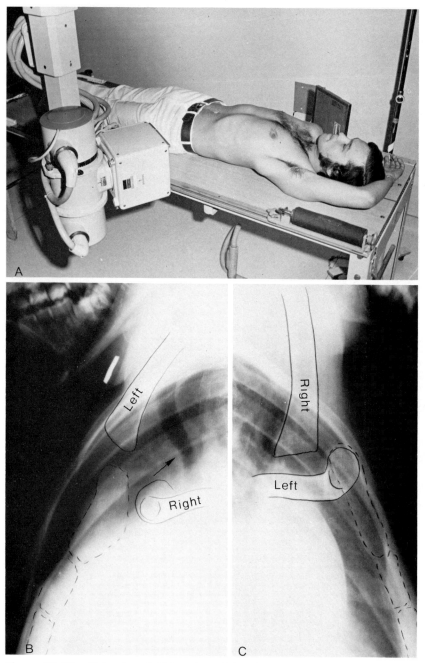

Figure 19–18. Retrosternal dislocation of the clavicle. *A,* The position of the x-ray tube, patient, and grid cassette for a clavicular view is shown. The central beam is parallel to the table top, centered on the sternoclavicular joint, and directed along the axis of the clavicle. A grid cassette is placed against the far shoulder perpendicular to the x-ray beam. *B,* With the film against the right shoulder, the medial end of the right clavicle lies posterior to the manubrium and indents the trachea (arrow). The normal left clavicle is in direct alignment with the manubrium. *C,* When the cassette is against the left shoulder, the head of the left clavicle projects through the manubrium, whereas the axis of the right is behind the sternum. (*From* Lee, F. A., and Gwinn, J. L.: Retrosternal dislocation of the clavicle. Radiology *110:*631–634, 1974.)

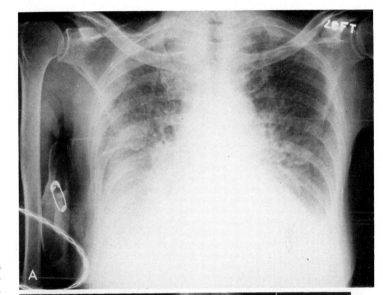

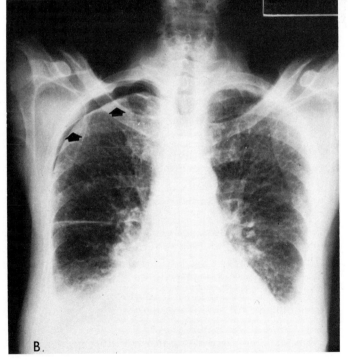

Figure 19–19. Pulmonary edema and pneumothorax. *A,* An anteroposterior chest radiograph of a patient with overt congestive heart failure secondary to the injudicious use of fluids following abdominal injury. *B,* A posteroanterior chest radiograph taken immediately after the anteroposterior radiograph reveals an unexpected right pneumothorax (arrows). The presence of bilateral pleural effusions is also confirmed. Films taken with the patient in various positions may be necessary to define small collections of pleural air or fluid.

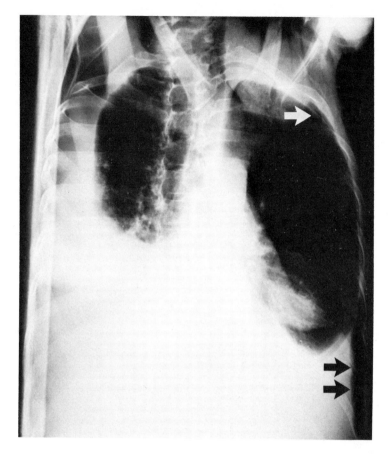

Figure 19–20. Hemothorax and hemopneumothorax. A right lateral decubitus film in a patient with multiple injuries. A large right effusion is present. The arrows point to a left pneumothorax not seen on the standard anteroposterior radiograph. An associated left effusion is also noted.

resulting from skin folds, bandages, bed sheets, tubes, and so forth that may mimic a pneumothorax.

The physiologic significance of a pneumothorax does not necessarily correspond to the amount of air in the pleural space. It is also difficult on an anteroposterior film alone to estimate the size of the pneumothorax. A classification of minimal, moderate, or severe should suffice, since the surgeon's estimate of the patient's cardiopulmonary status and extrathoracic injuries determines the mode of treatment. The exception is the tension pneumothorax with a collapsed lung, mediastinal shift, and depressed diaphragm (Fig. 19–21), which requires immediate treatment.

In the majority of cases, a pneumothorax associated with blunt or penetrating trauma is simply due to a laceration of the visceral pleura with the escape of air into the pleural space. However, a pneumothorax that is large or persistent or associated with mediastinal or subcutaneous emphysema or large effusions suggests injury to the organs of the mediastinum as well.

Traumatized patients requiring intubation and positive-pressure breathing are likely to acquire barotrauma, including pneumomediastinum and pneumothorax.[8] Frequent radiographic assessment is required if early signs of barotrauma are to be detected (see Chapter 1).

The radiographic assessment of chest tube placement can usually be made on the anteroposterior radiograph. The tube for the drainage of air is ideally in the apex and the tube for the drainage of fluid at the base posteriorly. In the adhesion-free chest, these tubes usually function adequately even when they are not ideally positioned. In cases in which the tubes are not functioning well, decubitus, cross-table lateral, and oblique films better define the relationship of the tube to the area to be drained. All tubes should have a radiopaque marker for radiographic localization.

PNEUMOMEDIASTINUM

In a recent review of 200 consecutive cases of significant blunt thoracic trauma, 40 per cent of the patients had subcutaneous emphysema or pneumomediastinum on their initial chest radiograph. In this subgroup, two thirds had an associated pneumothorax, and ten had a variety of major injuries to their larynx, esophagus, or tracheobronchial tree. In ten other patients, isolated pneumomediastinum was present without apparent cause; it is assumed that the trauma led to rupture of distal airways or alveoli, and air dissected along the bronchovascular sheaths into the mediastinum (Fig. 19–22). A pneumomediastinum should not be assumed to be a benign finding, especially a severely traumatized patient, because air within the mediastinum may rupture into the pleural space and cause a pneumothorax or tension pneumothorax. Tension pneumomediastinum is rare in adults but may be lethal if not recognized early.

Any increase in mediastinal or subcutaneous air requires explanation. Endoscopy, tomography, and contrast studies may be necessary to exclude the diagnosis of injury to the larynx, bronchus, or esophagus (see Figs. 19–29 and 19–32). Mediastinal air may dissect caudally and result in pneumoretroperitoneum and pneumoperitoneum. The converse, that is, air from below the diaphragm entering the thorax, is very rare.

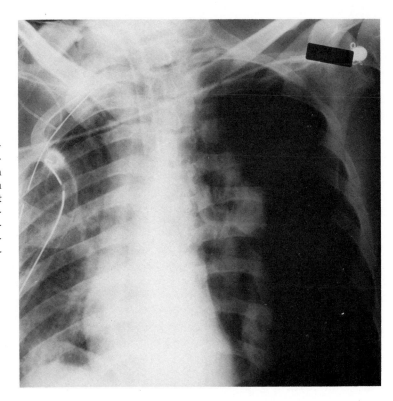

Figure 19–21. Tension pneumothorax. An anteroposterior radiograph demonstrates a tension pneumothorax on the left, with almost total collapse of the left lung, depression of the left hemidiaphragm, and shift of the mediastinum to the right. The right-sided chest tubes and endotracheal tube are in good position.

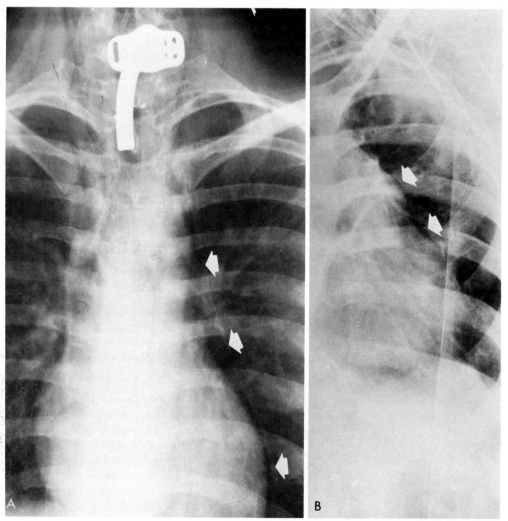

Figure 19–22. Pneumomediastinum. *A*, A large lucency is seen adjacent to the left heart border, delineated by the visceral and parietal pleura (arrows). Subcutaneous air is seen in the neck. *B*, A small lucent area is seen adjacent to the left border of the heart, delineated by the visceral and parietal pleura (arrows). No air was seen in the neck. This was an unexpected finding in a patient receiving positive pressure therapy. (*From* Goodman, L. R.: Cardiopulmonary disorders. *In* Goodman, L. R., and Putman, C. E. (eds.): Intensive Care Radiology. St. Louis, The C. V. Mosby Company, 1978.)

PLEURAL EFFUSIONS

Many cases of spontaneous pneumothorax are associated with a small hydrothorax, and almost all cases of traumatic pneumothorax are associated with a hemothorax of variable size. An isolated hemothorax is most often the result of a laceration of the pulmonary parenchyma or a bleeding intercostal artery. Rupture of a major pulmonary vessel is usually fatal before the patient receives medical attention. Pulmonary parenchymal bleeding is usually self-limited because of low pressure in the pulmonary circuit. Persistent rapid bleeding into the thorax is most often secondary to a lacerated intercostal or internal mammary artery or injury to the aorta and great vessels.

Radiographic findings may vary with the amount and viscosity of the pleural fluid. On the anteroposterior supine radiograph, a uniform increase in density may be the only clue to a unilateral effusion. Blunting of the costophrenic angle, thickening of the lateral pleural stripe, or fluid in the minor fissure may also be present. On the supine or semi-erect radiograph, fluid may accumulate in the medial pleural space and appear as a triangular paraspinous mass.[37] This is especially frequent on the left side. In doubtful cases, a second projection must be obtained. A lateral decubitus radiograph with the side in question dependent is ideal (see Fig. 19–20); an anteroposterior upright (see Fig. 19–19) or the opposite decubitus film is usually adequate to demonstrate a shift of fluid, however.

Ultrasonograms can be helpful in diagnosing fluid when the patient cannot be moved and when one cannot distinguish between pleural thickening, peripheral lung disease, and pleural fluid loculation (Fig. 19–23). Ultrasonography is also helpful as a guide to thoracentesis or chest tube placement when pleural adhesions exist.

PULMONARY CONTUSION AND LACERATION

A pulmonary contusion presents as a nonsegmental fluffy infiltrate within hours of the injury.[38] It is most often on the side of the trauma, although contralateral injury may occur. Rib fractures are absent in the majority of patients. The infiltrates may progress for the first 12 to 24 hours, followed by definite clearing over the next 2 to 3 days and complete resolution within 1 to 2 weeks (Fig. 19–24). The failure of the infiltrate to follow this characteristic x-ray sequence suggests an endobronchial lesion, an infection, recurrent bleeding, or a pulmonary hematoma (Fig. 19–25).[10, 31]

Pulmonary lacerations from blunt or penetrating trauma may have varied presentations. Hematomas are caused by parenchymal lacerations which may be single or multiple.[39] Radiographic signs of the laceration or hematoma are usually masked initially by the associated contusion. As the contusion infiltrate resolves, the hematoma appears as a spheric or elliptic radiodensity, with or without an air-fluid level. As the lesion decreases in size, the blood clot may shrink and a crescent of air may appear around the clot.[31, 41] The hematoma usually disappears in three to five weeks. On occasion, the hematoma organizes, and a nodular density indistinguishable from other coin lesions persists on the radiograph (Fig. 19–26).

Following a laceration, the edges of the lung may retract without marked bleeding and present on the radiograph as an enlarging air-containing, thin-walled cyst (Fig. 19–27). The lucency tends to shrink over a period of several weeks, either disappearing completely or leaving a linear scar in the lung.[14] In missile injuries, especially high-velocity injuries, a lucent hole, representing the lacerated tissue, may be seen within the lung contusion. Lacerations that follow penetrating trauma resolve more slowly and are more prone to infection because the tracts contain necrotic tissue and foreign matter and are often contaminated. On occasion, the "hole" in the lung persists as a radiographic sequela long after clinical resolution of the patient's problems.[21, 36]

TRACHEOBRONCHIAL INJURY

Laceration or disruption of the trachea or proximal bronchi is a potentially serious injury that is frequently overlooked following a severe deceleration or crush injury. In many patients, extrathoracic or other serious intrathoracic injuries divert attention from the airways. In another 10 per cent, there are no physical and radiographic signs of intrathoracic injury on initial presentation. Finally, in some patients with incomplete

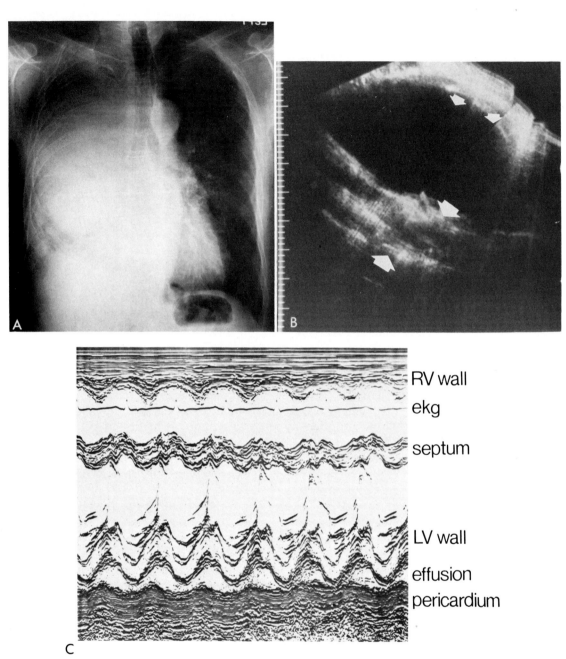

Figure 19–23. Hemothorax and hemopericardium. *A,* A posteroanterior radiograph of a patient hit in the right chest by a large crane. Almost complete opacification of the right hemithorax is noted. Decubitus films were of little benefit in distinguishing pleural from parenchymal disease. Although the right heart border is not seen, there does not appear to be significant enlargement of the cardiac silhouette. *B,* Ultrasound scan of the fourth intercostal space on the right with the patient in the left lateral decubitus position. A large pleural effusion is identified by the small arrows. Deeper echoes (large arrows) are related to the collapsed lung. *C,* Echocardiogram of the same patient confirms the presence of an associated small pericardial effusion. Pericardial collections may be difficult to define in the presence of large pleura effusions, particularly on the left.

Figure 19–24. Pulmonary contusion. A posteroanterior chest radiograph taken immediately after blunt chest trauma reveals peripheral patchy infiltration in the left lung and a fractured left clavicle. There was no history of gastric aspiration, and the radiographic appearance was almost normal within 24 hours. A presumptive diagnosis of lung contusion was made.

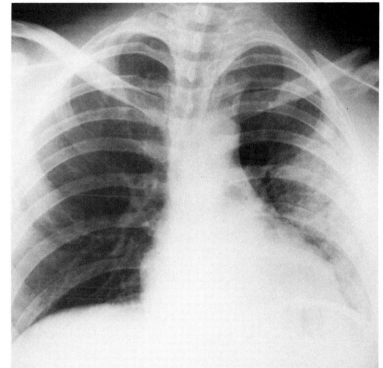

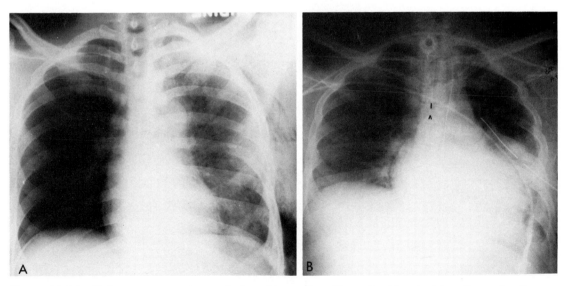

Figure 19–25. Pulmonary contusion and pleural laceration. The patient jumped four floors, landing on his left side. *A,* Diffuse unilateral pulmonary edema pattern, presumably representing contusion. Fractures of ribs 5 to 9 are present, with severe subcutaneous emphysema and no pneumothorax. *B,* Pulmonary edema pattern cleared within 24 hours, revealing retrocardiac consolidation resulting from hemorrhage. A prophylatic chest tube was placed on the left. The tracheostomy tube is too close to the carina.

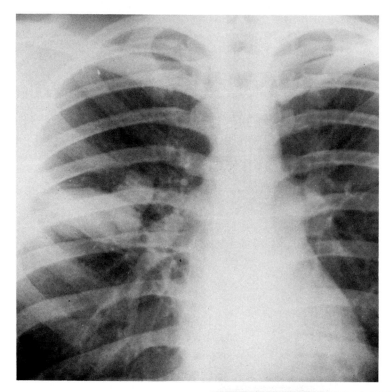

Figure 19–26. Pulmonary hematoma. A posteroanterior radiograph taken three weeks after right-sided blunt chest trauma. The homogenous rounded density near the minor fissure replaces the more confluent air-space process that appeared on the initial radiograph. This hematoma slowly resolved during the next six months.

Figure 19–27. Pulmonary contusion and laceration. An anteroposterior chest radiograph of a young patient who was thrown from a moving car and landed on the left chest. A parenchymal density with a large central lucency is noted in the left lower lobe. There are no penetrating injuries and no rib fractures. The lucency represents a laceration of lung parenchyma from nonpenetrating trauma.

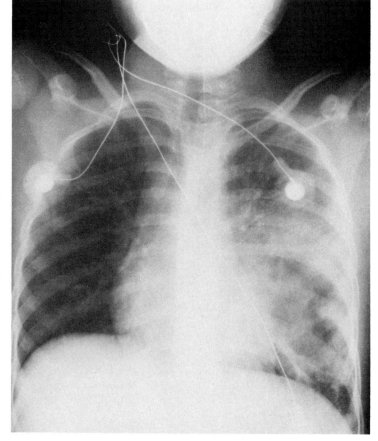

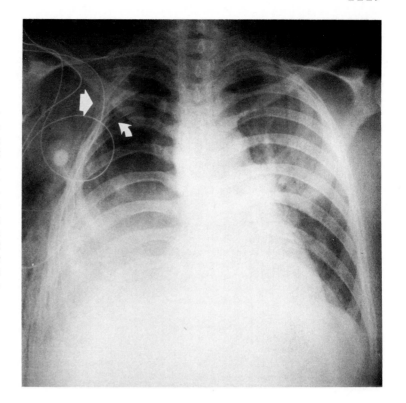

Figure 19–28. Fractured bronchus. An anteroposterior radiograph of a young female injured in a motorcycle accident. The first four ribs on the right are fractured, and there is a homogenous density involving most of the right hemithorax. Subcutaneous emphysema (arrow) and pneumothorax (curved arrow) are also present on the right, with an area of apparent lung contusion in the left upper lobe. Bronchoscopic examination showed the right main stem bronchus to be completely avulsed.

tears, initial symptoms resolve spontaneously and resurface months or years later with evidence of bronchial stenosis.[5, 7]

Most injuries occur within 2 to 5 cm of the carina. In those patients with complete disruption of the bronchus or a large tear, a characteristic pattern emerges. The initial radiograph demonstrates fractures of the upper ribs and air in the mediastinum, pleura, and subcutaneous tissues (Fig. 19–28). A sharp cut-off of the bronchial air column may be visible. The air leak may continue despite tube drainage, and the lung becomes progressively atelectatic. With complete disruption, the lung is no longer tethered to the hilum by the rigid bronchus. On the supine radiograph the lung may collapse away from the hilum, and on the erect film it may fall to the diaphragm (Fig. 19–29).

In cases of less severe tracheobronchial injury, the air leak may be absent or seal itself, and areas of atelectasis may resolve. As the bronchus heals and scars, the patient may present with distal infection or collapse long after the injury.

Because surgical repair with the preservation of lung tissue may be possible only in the first week or two after the injury, prompt diagnosis is critical. Any chest trauma patient with upper rib fractures, unexplained air leaks, or atelectasis should be evaluated early. Tomography, bronchoscopy, and bronchography are the procedures of choice.

DIAPHRAGMATIC INJURY

Other serious skeletal, cardiopulmonary, and upper abdominal injuries often accompany diaphragmatic rupture, frequently obscuring the diagnosis. Diaphragmatic laceration without herniation of abdominal contents usually escapes radiographic diagnosis, although slight abnormalities in diaphragmatic contour may be present on the radiograph.[6, 17, 24]

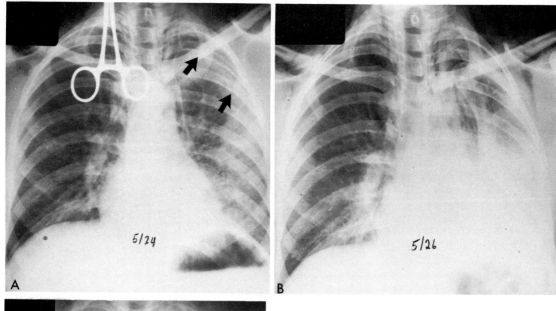

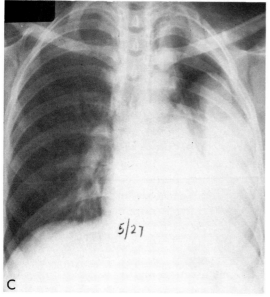

Figure 19–29. Fractured bronchus. *A,* An anteroposterior radiograph taken soon after an auto accident on May 24. Left-sided subcutaneous emphysema, pneumomediastinum, and small left pneumothorax with patchy infiltrate in the left lower lobe are evident. The left third and fourth posterior ribs are fractured (arrows). A surgical clamp is lying over the right upper chest. *B,* An anteroposterior radiograph taken 36 hours after the accident shows increasing subcutaneous emphysema and pneumothorax. There is further opacification of the left hemithorax, with deviation of the lung laterally. *C,* An anteroposterior radiograph (erect) taken 72 hours after the accident with increasing pneumothorax and total opacification of left lung. The lung appears to fall toward the diaphragm. At surgery, the complete transection of the left main stem bronchus was noted.

When there has been rupture and herniation into the chest (95 per cent on the left), a gas-filled viscus or soft-tissue mass is frequently seen above the diaphragm (Fig. 19–30). A nasogastric tube may also be seen entering the chest (Fig. 19–31). Nonspecific signs of traumatic herniation include obscuration and apparent elevation of the diaphragm, pleural effusion, atelectasis, and contralateral shift of the mediastinum.[19] Orally administered contrast agents followed through to the colon help to visualize the relationship of the gastrointestinal tract to the diaphragm. Fluoroscopy of the diaphragm may be misleading because of adjacent thoracoabdominal disease. In an acute situation, several hundred cubic centimeters of air injected into the peritoneal cavity rise into the hemothorax if the diaphragm is lacerated. A combined liver-spleen-lung scan provides information on the liver and spleen and their relationship to the lung base.

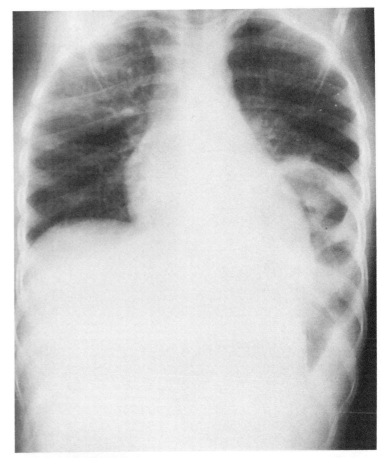

Figure 19–30. Traumatic hernia of the diaphragm. An anteroposterior chest radiograph of a young patient thrown from a horse. The patient complained of the sensation of fullness in the left chest and abdominal pain. There is an apparent elevation of the left hemidiaphragm with a collection of bowel or stomach gas in the left chest. At surgery, the partial disruption of the diaphragm was found.

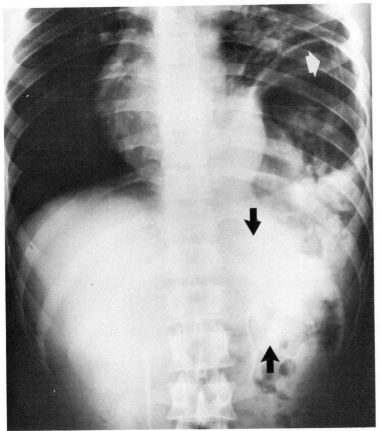

Figure 19–31. Traumatic diaphragmatic hernia. An anteroposterior chest and abdominal radiograph of a patient with multiple injuries after being hit by a truck. There is obliteration of the normal diaphragmatic surface, the stomach being elevated into the chest. The nasogastric tube (white arrow) is in an abnormal position, and there is slight superior displacement of the contrast-filled left kidney (black arrows). Patchy left lung infiltrates and the contralateral shift of the mediastinum are noted. All of these findings are characteristic of diaphragmatic rupture. At surgery, the stomach, omentum, and splenic flexure were found to be herniated through an 8-inch tear. The spleen was also lacerated.

1121

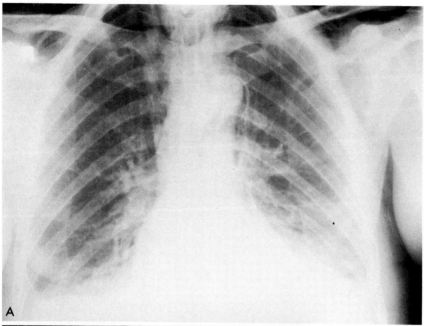

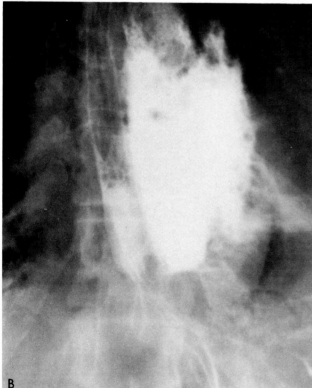

Figure 19–32. Esophageal tear. *A,* An anteroposterior radiograph of a 45-year-old painter who fell from a roof. Subcutaneous emphysema, pneumomediastinum, and bibasilar infiltrates are present on the initial film. *B,* A spot radiograph taken after a water-soluble contrast esophagogram reveals the extravasation of dye into the mediastinum and pleural space. At surgery, a 6-cm tear was noted in the esophageal wall. The patient acquired mediastinitis, empyema and sepsis and died two weeks after initial surgery.

Early recognition allows surgical repair, with the return of pulmonary function to normal, and prevents the possibility of delayed complication. A patient with an undiagnosed diaphragmatic laceration may present months or years later with an obstructed or strangulated hernia or with an asymptomatic lower thoracic mass visible on the radiograph.

ESOPHAGEAL TRAUMA

It is extremely unusual to sustain isolated esophageal injury from blunt trauma; usually this entity is associated with fatal injuries, such as aortic rupture or lethal cardiac contusion.[42] Radiographic findings of esophageal rupture consist of subcutaneous emphysema, mediastinal widening, pneumomediastinum, left lower lobe atelectasis, and a left-sided hemothorax. Orally administered water-soluble contrast medium usually shows extravasation into the mediastinum or pleural space or both (Fig. 19–32). Esophagography demonstrates 50 per cent of cervical perforations and 75 per cent of thoracic esophageal perforations.[23] If the initial study does not define a laceration and there is persistent clinical or indirect radiographic evidence of esophageal rupture, a repeat contrast examination is indicated. Delayed rupture usually occurs in areas of hematoma or contusion related to the initial blunt trauma. The irritation of a nasogastric tube or the inadvertent intubation of the esophagus during an attempt at endotracheal intubation adds further stress to the previously damaged esophagus.

A post-traumatic pneumatocele in the inferior pulmonary ligament can simulate a ruptured esophagus. The inferior pulmonary ligament consists of two sheets of pleura separated by alveolar tissue. It extends downward in a sheetlike fashion from the inferior margin of the pulmonary hilus to the level of the diaphragm.[29] Presumably, alveoli adjacent to the ligament rupture into the ligament, causing air to be localized in a characteristic triangular configuration (Fig. 19–33). Esophagography with water-

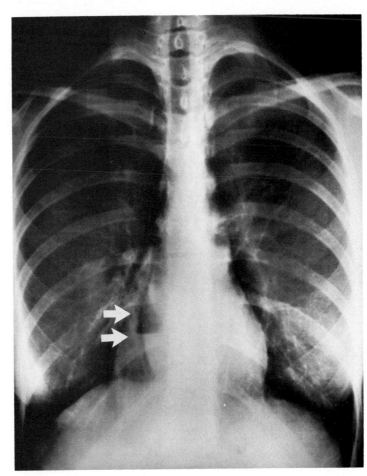

Figure 19–33. Air in the inferior pulmonary ligament. A posteroanterior radiograph of a young patient taken soon after an auto accident. A triangular collection of air is seen along the right heart border (arrows). No subcutaneous air was noted, and the decubitus film revealed no other air deposits in the right pleural space. An esophagogram was normal. This air, presumably located within the inferior pulmonary ligament, slowly disappeared over the next few days, with no complications. It is more usual to see the post-traumatic pneumatocele involving the left inferior pulmonary ligament.

soluble contrast is necessary to differentiate this entity from esophageal rupture. Post-traumatic pneumatoceles require no further treatment and usually resolve over a period of several weeks.[30]

AORTIC TRAUMA

Following blunt chest trauma or a penetrating injury, widening of the mediastinal contour may have numerous origins, including aortic or great vessel rupture, disruption of small mediastinal arteries and veins, and esophageal and tracheobronchial injuries. Although the majority of patients with aortic laceration die before reaching the hospital, the diagnosis of aortic injury must be rapidly excluded before other causes of mediastinal widening are sought. Care must be used in interpreting mediastinal widening on the anteroposterior supine radiograph. Ayella et al. have suggested that tilting the patient slightly beyond the vertical position results in a radiograph that more closely approximates a posteroanterior film.[2, 3]

In addition to mediastinal widening, other signs of aortic rupture include a mediastinal mass, a pleural effusion (usually left), and deviation of the trachea or esophagus to the right.[15, 16, 26] An extrapleural cap, resulting from blood dissecting between the left apical parietal pleura and the rib cage, may be an early sign of a vascular leak (Fig. 19–34).[33] When the tear involves the intima and media, the radiograph may be normal in a small percentage of patients (Fig. 19–35).[32]

Unstable patients who are clearly bleeding into the chest are usually operated on without further work-up. In other patients suspected of having aortic rupture, aortography is required for confirmation and for evaluation of the extent of rupture, the site or sites of injury, and the status of the brachiocephalic vessels (Fig. 19–36). Speed is of the essence, because secondary rupture and exsanguination occur within 24 hours in one third of cases. The approach and technique should be determined by the experience of the angiographer and the condition of the patient. In order to definitely exclude the diagnosis of a ruptured aorta, the films should be obtained in at least two projections and scrutinized carefully before the study is terminated. The angiographic signs include (1) minimal irregularity in the contour of the aortic isthmus; (2) linear translucencies indicative of an intimal flap; (3) the complete transection of the aorta with extravasation of contrast into the mediastinum or pleural space; and (4) the presence of a false aneurysm, with contrast material remaining within this cavity after the remainder of the aorta has cleared. The majority of patients with aortic injuries who survive long enough to have angiography have lacerations at the aortic isthmus.

TRAUMA TO THE HEART

Blunt injuries to the anterior chest, severe crush injuries, or penetrating trauma may result in cardiac tamponade, laceration, or contusion. Although serious injury to the heart may occur without other signs of thoracic injury, multiple anterior rib fractures, sternal fractures, pneumopericardium, or congestive heart failure should alert the radiologist to a possible traumatic cardiac lesion.[35]

The rapid accumulation of blood in the pericardial space often causes cardiac tamponade and severe hemodynamic impairment without altering the radiographic appearance of the cardiac silhouette. If time permits, ultrasonic examination is a sensitive, noninvasive method for the documentation of small but significant collec-

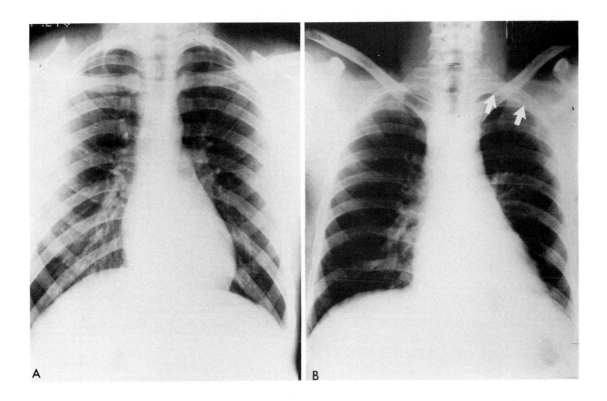

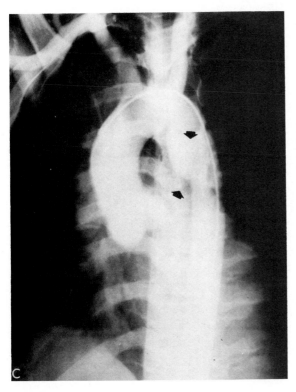

Figure 19–34. Aortic laceration. *A*, A posteroanterior chest radiograph taken four years prior to an automobile accident is normal. *B*, A posteroanterior chest radiograph taken two hours after the accident reveals minimal widening of the superior mediastinum and the presence of the left apical cap (arrows), which was not present on the previous examination. *C*, A retrograde aortogram confirms the presence of an aortic rupture; the arrows delineate the linear intimal flap. The diagnosis of rupture was confirmed at surgery.

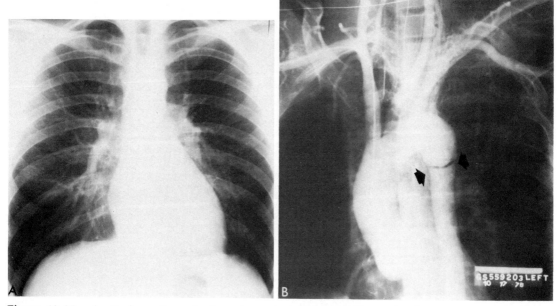

Figure 19–35. Aortic laceration. *A,* A posteroanterior chest radiograph of a patient following an automobile accident. This radiograph is considered normal. *B,* An aortogram was performed because of unequal pulses in the upper extremities and vague chest pain. The arrows point to the intimal flap at the isthmus of the aorta.

tions of pericardial fluid. In addition, echocardiography can evaluate cardiac function, valvular status, and chamber size (see Fig. 19–23).[34]

Cardiac contusions frequently follow blunt trauma, presenting most often as an acute arrhythmia or with the electrocardiographic changes of an acute myocardial infarction. Ventricular aneurysms of the contused segment are an unusual sequela. Any unusual contour of the heart border in the months or years following cardiac contusion suggests the presence of an aneurysm (Fig. 19–37). Diagnosis requires fluoroscopy and, in most cases, hemodynamic and angiographic evaluation.[11, 25]

Penetrating cardiac injuries, such as bullet or knife wounds, are usually fatal. On occasion, fluoroscopic localization is necessary to determine the site of a foreign body within the heart. Cardiac catheterization and angiocardiography are usually necessary to diagnose intracardiac damage and plan a surgical approach. If an intracardiac or intravascular foreign body is documented, a radiograph should be obtained in the operating room after the patient is anesthetized and positioned in order to be certain that the object has not moved farther along the vascular tree. One of the authors (L.R.G.) has seen three cases of fruitless explorations because the bullet in the cardiovascular system had migrated in the interval between the last preoperative radiographic examination and the operation. The bullets were eventually found in a brachial artery, a femoral artery, and a pulmonary artery (Fig. 19–38).

POST-TRAUMATIC PULMONARY INSUFFICIENCY

The parenchymal changes most commonly seen in the traumatized patient are due to atelectasis (collapse of a segment, lobe, or entire lung), contusion, hemorrhage, aspiration, or iatrogenic pulmonary edema.

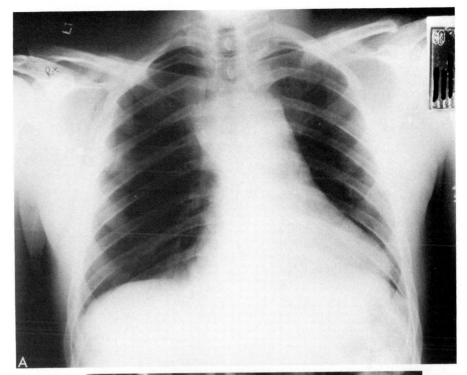

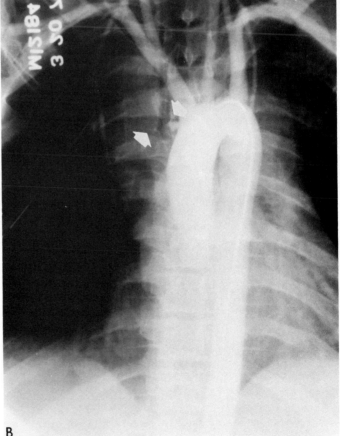

Figure 19–36. Innominate artery laceration. *A*, An anteroposterior chest radiograph of a 33-year-old male injured in a bobsled accident. There is widening of the superior mediastinum and prominence of the cardiac shadow. *B*, An aortogram performed shortly after the anteroposterior chest radiograph reveals extravasation of contrast media near the innominate artery at its origin (arrows). At surgery, the diagnosis of laceration of this vessel was confirmed.

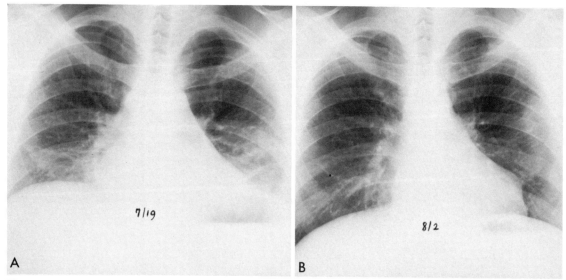

Figure 19–37. Post-traumatic ventricular aneurysm. *A,* A posteroanterior radiograph of a young male involved in an auto accident. The initial radiograph reveals patchy basilar densities (contusion) and a small left pleural effusion. *B,* A posteroanterior radiograph taken two weeks later reveals an unusual configuration of the left heart border. Angiocardiogram and surgery confirmed the presence of a post-traumatic left ventricular aneurysm.

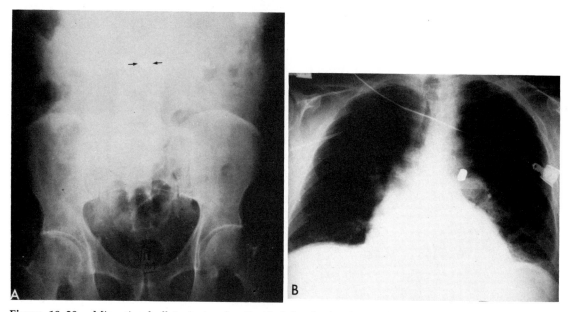

Figure 19–38. Migrating bullet. *A,* A suboptimal abdominal radiograph reveals a bullet over the spine (arrows). At surgery, lacerations of the liver, small bowel, superior mesenteric vein, and inferior vena cava were repaired. The bullet was not found at surgery. *B,* A postoperative radiograph shows the bullet in the left pulmonary artery. The spent bullet presumably came to rest in the inferior vena cava and embolized to the lung. (Courtesy of A. Slovin, M.D., Long Island, New York.)

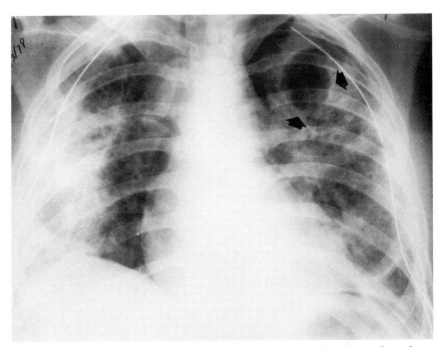

Figure 19–39. Fat emboli. An anteroposterior chest radiograph taken three days after major skeletal injury reveals bilateral pneumothoraces, left upper lobe laceration (arrows), and parenchymal consolidation. These changes were presumed to be due to pulmonary hemorrhage, but progressive pulmonary insufficiency ensued. An open lung biopsy showed multiple fat emboli, with areas of alveolar and interstitial edema.

The development of a symmetric air space process in the first few hours after chest trauma commonly follows the injudicious use of plasma expanders or may follow transfusion reaction. The development of a similar process 24 hours after injury should alert the radiologist to the possibility of fat embolism or adult respiratory distress syndrome (ARDS). Both of these entities are discussed in detail in other chapters and are only briefly discussed in this section.

The clinical triad of petechiae, neurologic dysfunction, and pulmonary insufficiency in a patient with severe skeletal trauma suggests the presence of fat embolism. More often than not, such patients have a persistently normal chest radiograph or nonspecific patchy infiltrates occurring unilaterally or bilaterally (Fig. 19–39). A few patients have a patchy air space consolidation that progresses to a pulmonary edema pattern indistinguishable from cardiac failure except that the pulmonary vessels and heart are normal in size. If the patient survives and associated cardiopulmonary problems are minimized, the radiographs often return to their baseline state within seven to ten days.[28]

The adult respiratory distress syndrome, or post-traumatic pulmonary insufficiency, has a wide variety of possible causes and occurs after a variety clinical insults.[1, 4, 12, 27] The radiographic features of the chest are nonspecific but usually follow a predictable pattern in most patients.[13, 28] One to three days after injury, interstitial edema may develop in the presence of a normal cardiac silhouette and pulmonary vasculature. Hemodynamic measurements are usually necessary to exclude acute left heart failure. A diffuse alveolar filling process develops, which progressively becomes more confluent over the next several days (Fig. 19–40). Once the basic radiographic pattern is established, sequential radiographs usually show minimal changes for a

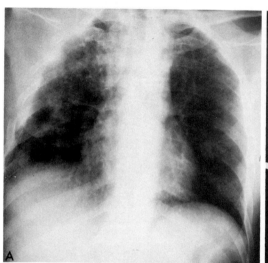

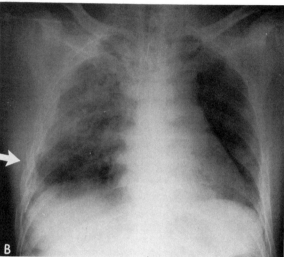

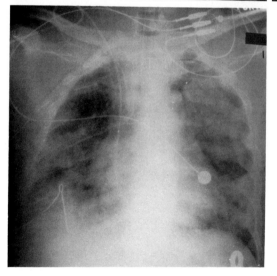

Figure 19–40. Flail chest, pulmonary contusion, and adult respiratory distress syndrome following a three-story fall. *A,* Multiple fractures of the third through the seventh ribs as well as a costochondral fractures caused a flail chest. Note the patchy contusion on the right. *B,* The following day, contusion increased and hematoma is visible. Subcutaneous air is seen laterally (arrow). *C,* A pneumothorax developed on the right, necessitating the use of a chest tube. The patient became increasingly difficult to ventilate, and by the fourth day bilateral consolidation was present, consistent with ARDS or fat embolization from his pelvic fractures. The Swan-Ganz catheter, in the left pulmonary artery, recorded normal wedge pressures.

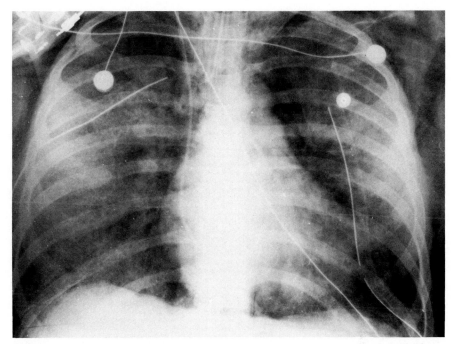

Figure 19–41.   Adult respiratory distress syndrome. An anteroposterior chest radiograph, taken 48 days after an automobile accident, of a patient with severe pulmonary insufficiency. Note the diffuse air-space process, the normal heart, and the lack of pleural effusions. Chest tubes are in place because of a pneumothorax stemming from the high ventilatory pressures required for ventilation. The Swan-Ganz pressures are normal, and the endotracheal tube is in a good position. The clinical course and radiographic findings are characteristic of the adult respiratory distress syndrome.

week or more (Fig. 19–41) unless there are complications such as superimposed pneumonia, cardiac or renal failure, barotrauma, or oxygen toxicity. If the patient survives this acute phase, the radiograph may return to its normal baseline state over the next three to six weeks, or focal linear densities representing interstitial scarring or fibrosis may persist. Careful attention to radiographic technique and comparison radiographs allow the radiologist to identify subtle improvements or complications that occur during this protracted interval. The diagnosis of ARDS is one of exclusion; specific, correctable causes must be sought and therapy instituted. Because many specific diseases in the post-traumatic period mimic or contribute to this syndrome, an ongoing dialogue between the radiologist and clinician is definitely required (see Chapter 1).

References

1. Arens, J. F.: Shock lung. South. Med. J. *65*:206–208, 1972.
2. Attar, S., Ayella, R. J., and McLaughlin, J. S.: The widened mediastinum in trauma. Ann. Thorac. Surg. *13*:435–499, 1972.
3. Ayella, R., Hankins, J., Turney, S., et al.: Ruptured thoracic aorta due to blunt trauma. J. Trauma *17*:199–205, 1977.
4. Bergofsky, E. H.: Pulmonary insufficiency after non-thoracic trauma: shock lung. Am. J. Med. Sci. *265*:93–101, 1972.
5. Burke, J. F.: Early diagnosis of traumatic rupture of the bronchus. J.A.M.A. *181*:682–686, 1962.

6. Carter, B. N., Ginseffi, J., and Felson, B.: Traumatic diaphragmatic hernia. Am. J. Roentgenol. Radium Ther. Nucl. Med. 65:56–72, 1951.
7. Chesterman, J. T., and Satsangi, P. N.: Rupture of the trachea and bronchi by closed injury. Thorax 21:21–27, 1966.
8. Cohn, R.: Non-penetrating wounds of the lungs and bronchi. Surg. Clin. North Am. 52:585–595, 1972.
9. Conn, J. H., Handy, J. D., and Fain, W. R.: Thoracic trauma: analysis of 1022 cases. J. Trauma 3:22–40, 1963.
10. Crawford, W. O., Jr.: Pulmonary injury in thoracic and non-thoracic trauma. Radiol. Clin. North Am. 11:527–541, 1973.
11. DeMuth, W. E., and Zinsser, H. F.: Myocardial contusion. Arch. Intern. Med. 115:434–442, 1965.
12. Dyck, D. R., and Zylak, C. J.: Acute respiratory distress in adults. Radiology 106:497–501, 1973.
13. Eaton, R. J., Senior, R. M., and Pierce, J. A.: Aspects of respiratory care pertinent to the radiologist. Radiol. Clin. North Am. 11:93–107, 1973.
14. Fagan, C. J., and Swischuck, L.: Traumatic lung and paramediastinal pneumatoceles. Radiology 120:11–18, 1976.
15. Flaherty, T. T., Wegner, G. P., and Crummy, A. B.: Non-penetrating injuries to the thoracic aorta. Radiology 92:541–546, 1969.
16. Glickman, M.: Special radiologic procedures. In Goodman, L. R., and Putman, C. E. (eds.): Intensive Care Radiology: Imaging of the Critically Ill. St. Louis, The C. V. Mosby Company, 1978.
17. Grage, T., McClean, L., and Campbell, G.: Traumatic rupture of the diaphragm. Surgery 46:669–681, 1959.
18. Grimes, O. F.: Non-penetrating injuries to the chest wall and esophagus. Surg. Clin. North Am. 52:597–609, 1972.
19. Hill, L. D.: Injuries of the diaphragm following blunt trauma. Surg. Clin. North Am. 52:611–624, 1972.
20. Kattan, K. R.: Modified view for use in roentgen examination of the sternoclavicular joints. Radiology 108:8, 1973.
21. LaRose, J. H.: Cavitation of missile tracks in the lung. Radiology 90:995–998, 1968.
22. Lee, F. A., and Gwinn, J. L.: Retrosternal dislocation of the clavicle. Radiology 110:631–634, 1974.
23. Love, L., and Berkow, A. E.: Trauma to the esophagus. Gastrointest. Radiol. 2:305–321, 1978.
24. Minagi, H., Brody, W. R., and Laing, F. C.: The variable roentgen appearance of traumatic diaphragmatic hernia. J. Can. Assoc. Radiol. 26:124–128, 1977.
25. Maynard, A. de L., Brooks, H. A., and Fronix, C. J.: Penetrating wounds of the heart. Arch. Surg. 90:680–686, 1965.
26. Pate, J. W., Butterick, O. D., and Richardson, R. L.: Traumatic rupture of the thoracic aorta. J.A.M.A. 203:1022–1024, 1968.
27. Petty, T. L., and Ashbaugh, D. G.: The adult respiratory distress syndrome. Chest 60:233–239, 1971.
28. Putman, C. E.: Adult respiratory distress syndrome. In Goodman, L. R., and Putman, C. E. (eds.): Intensive Care Radiology: Imaging of the Critically Ill. St. Louis, The C. V. Mosby Company, 1978.
29. Rabinowitz, J. G., and Wolf, B. S.: Roentgen significance of the pulmonary ligament. Radiology 87:1013–1020, 1966.
30. Ravin, C., Smith, W., Lester, P., et al.: Post-traumatic pneumatocele in the inferior pulmonary ligament. Radiology 121:39–41, 1976.
31. Reynolds, J., and Davis, J. T.: Injuries of the chest wall, pleura, lungs, bronchi and esophagus. Radiol. Clin. North Am. 4:383–401, 1966.
32. Sandor, F.: Incidence and significance of traumatic mediastinal hematoma. Thorax 22:43–63, 1967.
33. Simeone, J. F., Minagi, H., and Putman, C. E.: Traumatic disruption of the thoracic aorta: significance of the left apical cap. Radiology 117:265–268, 1975.
34. Soulen, R. L., Lapayowker, M. S., and Jimenez, J. L.: Echocardiography in diagnosis of pericardial effusion. Radiology 86:1047–1051, 1966.
35. Soulen, R. L., and Freeman, E.: Radiologic evaluation of traumatic heart disease. Radiol. Clin. North Am. 9:285–297, 1971.
36. Spees, E. K., Strevey, T. E., Geiger, J. P., et al.: Persistent traumatic lung cavity resulting from medium and high velocity missiles. Ann. Thorac. Surg. 4:133–142, 1967.
37. Trackler, R. T., and Brunkler, R. A.: Widening of the left paravertebral pleural line on supine chest roentgenograms in free pleural effusions. Am. J. Roentgenol. Radium Ther. Nucl. Med. 96:1027–1034, 1966.
38. Williams, J. R., and Bonte, F. J.: Pulmonary damage in non-penetrating chest injury. Radiol. Clin. North Am. 1:439–448, 1963.
39. Williams, J. R., and Bonte, F. J.: The roentgenological aspect of non-penetrating chest injuries. Springfield, Illinois, Charles C Thomas, Publisher, 1961.
40. Wilson, J. M., Thomas, A. W., Goodman, P. C., et al.: Severe chest trauma: morbidity implication of 1st or 2nd rib fracture in 120 patients. Arch. Surg. 113:846–849, 1978.
41. Wiot, J. F.: The radiologic manifestations of blunt chest trauma. J.A.M.A. 231:500–503, 1975.
42. Worman, L. W., Hurley, J. D., and Pembuton, A. H.: Rupture of the esophagus from external blunt trauma. Arch. Surg. 85:333–338, 1962.

Part III
Lung Abscess and Fungal Infections

WALLACE T. MILLER, M.D.

LUNG ABSCESS

Lung abscess is a local area of suppuration and cavitation of the lung secondary to infection by a necrotizing organism. It may be divided into three groups: (1) abscess secondary to pneumonia with no predisposing factors, (2) abscess associated with aspiration, and (3) abscess associated with malignancy or immunosuppression or both.

This condition occasionally occurs as a complication of pneumonia in an otherwise healthy person. The organisms responsible are *Staphylococcus, Pseudomonas, Proteus, Klebsiella,* and *Escherichia coli.*[34] The incidence of this type of abscess has decreased considerably since the advent of antibiotics.[32]

Lung abscess has often been associated with aspiration. Presumably, the patient aspirates debris from the mouth and pharynx into the bronchus, with the subsequent development of pneumonia and lung abscess. This is probably the mechanism for the frequent development of lung abscess in alcoholics.[2, 26, 32, 34] In many alcoholics, aspiration is well documented through a history of stupor, coma, or delirium tremens. In others, however, it is difficult to document aspiration, and it is possible that other factors contribute to the high incidence of lung abscess in alcoholics. Partial immunosuppression is one such factor.

Other causes of aspiration are epilepsy, anesthesia, esophageal obstruction, cerebral vascular accident, encephalopathy, and minor surgery — particularly dental extraction or tonsillectomy.[26, 34] The aspirated organisms are those commonly present in the normal mouth and upper respiratory area — alpha-hemolytic streptococci, *Neisseria,* coagulase-negative staphylococcis, and various gram-negative bacilli and chloroform organisms.[2, 26]

A third major group of patients who acquire lung abscess are those with underlying malignancy or those who are immunosuppressed, either naturally or secondary to drug therapy for malignancy. Patients receiving radiation therapy and steroid therapy are particularly susceptible to the development of lung abscess.[26] The elderly and the alcoholic patient fall into this group owing to depression of their immune defense mechanisms.

Whereas most lung abscesses are related to one of these three groups, some are occasionally secondary to an infected bleb or bulla, an infected sequestration, or a poorly draining segment of lung. Solitary or multiple lung abscesses may also occur from hematogenous embolization of septic material.

Clinical Presentation

The usual symptoms are cough, sputum production, chills and fever, chest pain, and hemoptysis.[34] Hemoptysis can be a fairly common finding, with an incidence as high as 52 per cent in some series.[32] Clubbing of the fingers may occur in as much as 20 per cent of the cases.[32]

The development of hemoptysis and purulent sputum in a patient who is undergoing therapy for pneumonia frequently heralds the presence of a lung abscess.[35]

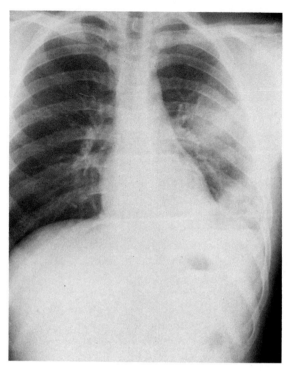

Figure 19–42. Lung abscess secondary to aspiration. The patient is a 20-year-old male with pulmonary consolidation that occurred after the extraction of wisdom teeth. Two large areas of consolidation are present in the left lung, and small areas of central cavitation can be seen. This is early in the course of lung abscess formation. Subsequently, the cavities become larger and thin walled.

In infants, symptoms often include high fever, tachypnea, cyanosis, and septic shock.

Radiographic Characteristics

Radiographically, lung abscess is almost invariably preceded by pneumonia. This is manifested by an area of dense consolidation in one or more pulmonary segments or lobes. Over a period of days to weeks the pulmonary consolidation becomes more localized and dense, and a localized collection of air develops in the midst of a densely consolidated segment (Fig. 19–42). Erect or decubitus films taken at this time may demonstrate an air-fluid level, which is the pathognomonic feature (Fig. 19–43). Initially, lung abscess tends to be thick walled and to have irregular margins. As the abscess matures, the walls become thin and the outline of the cavity smooth.

Abscesses may be single or multiple. Rapid appearance of multiple, well-demarcated, and relatively thin-walled cavities strongly suggests septic emboli (Fig. 19–44).[9] Although most patients initially have pneumonia and acquire a lung abscess later, occasionally a patient has an established lung abscess as the initial clinical presentation. These patients tend to be alcoholic or immunosuppressed.[23]

Because of the high incidence of aspiration as the cause of lung abscess, one might expect most lung abscesses to be in the lower lobe. Interestingly, this is not true, the upper lobes being commonly involved.[32, 34] There is a greater likelihood of occurrence in the right lung than in the left and in posterior lung segments than in anterior lung segments,[32, 34] but lung abscess can occur in any portion of the lung, and the location is of little value in differential diagnosis.

Lung abscess must be distinguished from cavitary malignancy (generally primary

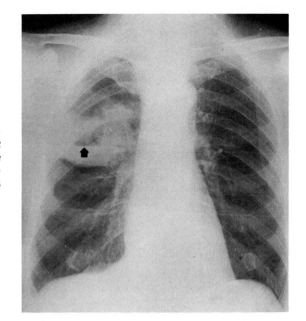

Figure 19–43. Lung abscess in an immunosuppressed patient. This 37-year-old male with chronic myelogenous leukemia acquired an infiltrate in the right upper lobe, which subsequently became cavitary. A well-developed air-fluid level (arrow) is present in the thick-walled cavity.

but occasionally secondary), from tuberculosis, and from fungal infections, all of which may have an identical radiographic appearance. This differentiation must be made by clinical means. In the very young patient, a pneumatocele may simulate lung abscess, but pneumatoceles tend to be very thin walled and to change size rapidly, features not typical of lung abscess.

In cases of severe lung abscess, thrombosis of the lobar pulmonary artery may occur, with subsequent infarction of the entire lobe. This severe type of lung abscess has been called gangrene of the lung. It is characterized by a large, thin-walled cavity that follows the outline of a lobe (Fig. 19–45). It generally requires surgical therapy, although occasionally it can respond to prolonged antibiotic therapy.[22]

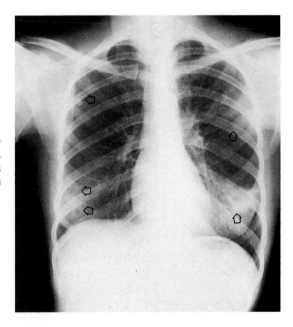

Figure 19–44. Septic emboli. Scattered nodules are seen throughout both lung fields (arrows), cavitation visible in several. These nodules appeared rapidly in this patient with a diverticular abscess. This is a typical course for septic emboli.

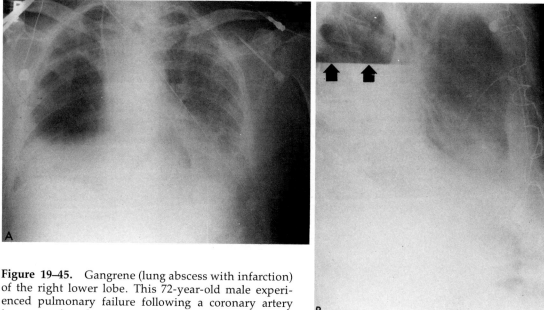

Figure 19–45. Gangrene (lung abscess with infarction) of the right lower lobe. This 72-year-old male experienced pulmonary failure following a coronary artery bypass graft and subsequently acquired an infiltrate in the right lower lobe. This rapidly developed a rather thin-walled cavity with an extensive air-fluid level. The outlines of the cavity are seen on the posteroanterior film *(A)*, and the air-fluid level is well demonstrated on the lateral film *(B)* (arrows). The cavity completely fills the space that is ordinarily occupied by the right lower lobe. This is a typical picture of lobar gangrene.

Therapy

The treatment of lung abscess is prolonged antimicrobial therapy with the appropriate antibiotic.[4, 8, 16] It is important to obtain organisms for culture. Bronchoscopy may be useful in this regard and also in establishing drainage of the abscessed cavity if drainage is poor.[8] In past years surgery was a primary therapy for the treatment of lung abscess,[3] but it is now generally reserved for the treatment of the complications of lung abscess — empyema or a chronic abscess that is not responsive to drug therapy.[35]

Prognosis

Incidence of lung abscess has declined since the advent of antibiotic therapy. The mortality rate of the uncomplicated lung abscess has also declined, from approximately 25 per cent 10 to 15 years ago to 5 per cent or less with prolonged antimicrobial therapy.[35] In those patients whose abscesses complicate some underlying malignant disease, however, or result from natural or drug-induced immunosuppression, the mortality rate is 75 to 90 per cent.[8, 20, 26]

ACTINOMYCOSIS AND NOCARDIOSIS

Actinomyces and *Nocardia* have been considered to be fungi by many microbiologists in the past. It now seems certain that *Actinomyces* and *Nocardia* are bacteria that share two properties with fungi: the formation of hyphae and the use of spores for dissemination. This distinction from fungi is important because therapy is quite different than that for mycotic infections.[33]

Actinomycosis is caused by the organism *Actinomyces israelii,* a rod-shaped bacterium found commonly in dental caries and at gingival margins in patients with poor oral hygiene. It is anaerobic and microaerophilic and therefore requires special culture techniques.[33] The characteristic clinical finding of actinomycosis is the presence of "sulfur granules" in draining material from abscesses and sinuses. These sulfur granules are dense clusters of microorganisms.[25] Although the mere presence of sulfur granules is highly suggestive of the diagnosis, culture is required for confirmation.[17] The most frequent manifestation of actinomycosis is osteomyelitis of the mandible. Pulmonary actinomycosis is relatively uncommon.

Radiographically, pulmonary actinomycosis is most commonly manifested as an area of pneumonia in one lung, generally in the periphery. Adequate therapy is curative. With inadequate treatment, because of minimal symptoms or lack of recognition of the causative organism, lung abscess, empyema, chest wall invasion, and osteomyelitis of the ribs are frequent sequelae (Fig. 19–46). Occasionally, the only radiographic manifestation may be a chest wall mass without associated pulmonary disease.[17] Therapy for actinomycosis is long-term penicillin. Surgery may be necessary to treat empyema and chest wall abscess.[28]

Nocardiosis is generally caused by *Nocardia asteroides.* Unlike *Actinomyces, Nocardia* is found to inhabit the soil and is worldwide in distribution.[5] In tropical climates, species of this organism are a common cause of mycetoma of the foot (madura foot).

Nocardiosis may be primary in man and as such may have a radiographic appearance similar to that of pneumonia, lung abscess, tuberculosis, or empyema.[5] Most commonly, it has a nonspecific appearance and resembles any other pneumonia.[5] Secondary nocardiosis is now much more common than primary disease. *Nocardia* occurs as a secondary invader in patients with underlying malignancy or in those

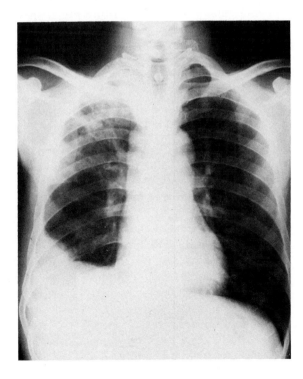

Figure 19–46. Actinomycosis. The chest radiograph of a 42-year-old male with a low-grade fever and cough. There is patchy consolidation in the right upper and lower lobes, with fluid in the right pleural space. This was subsequently found to be pulmonary actinomycosis with empyema.

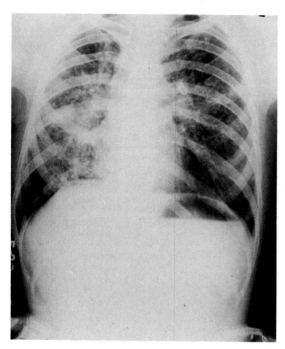

Figure 19–47. Nocardiosis (opportunistic invader). This 47-year-old female with leukemia acquired fever and cough. At autopsy, diffuse patchy changes in both lung fields were found to be secondary to *Nocardia*. The radiographic findings are nonspecific and could be associated with any of a large number of opportunistic invaders.

receiving immunosuppressive therapy.[12] As with other opportunistic invaders, recognition depends primarily upon culture of the organism, since radiographically *Nocardia* is indistinguishable from any other type of bacterial or even fungal pneumonia (Fig. 19–47). The presence of nodular pulmonary infiltrates might represent *Nocardia*, but it also suggests a fungus as the opportunistic invader. Needle aspiration biopsy is sometimes useful in obtaining organisms.[5] Nocardiosis requires long-term treatment with sulfonamides, generally Sulfadiazine.[33]

FUNGAL INFECTIONS

Fungal diseases of the lung are being recognized with increasing frequency. They may be divided into four main groups.

1.   Insignificant subclinical infection. This involves primarily coccidioidomycosis and histoplasmosis, which cause mild, self-limited diseases that heal spontaneously with no apparent sequelae.

2.   Severe primary invasive fungal infection. Most commonly, *Blastomyces* and *Cryptococcus*, occasionally, Histoplasma and *Coccidioides*, and rarely, *Aspergillus* can primarily involve the lung and result in a severe and often life-threatening illness. The incidence of these diseases is low.

3.   Secondary invasive fungal infection. In patients with natural or drug-induced immunosuppression secondary to neoplasm, debilitating illness, or drug therapy, opportunistic infection with a variety of fungi can occur. *Aspergillus, Monilia, Mucor*, and even *Coccidioides* and *Histoplasma* have been implicated as secondary invaders in the immunosuppressed patient.[5]

4.   *Hypersensitivity pneumonitis secondary to infection with fungi and actinomycetes.* Various fungi and actinomycetes that are not invasive may occasionally cause signifi-

cant pulmonary disease by acting as antigens. Three types of lung disease are apparent: asthma; diffuse alveolar-interstitial lesions (extrinsic allergic alveolitis); and bronchial obstruction secondary to a hypersensitivity reaction to *Aspergillus* (allergic bronchopulmonary aspergillosis).[30]

Epidemiology

Most of the fungi causing human disease are inhabitants of the soil; disease is usually exogenous and is caused by direct inhalation of the organism.[6]

Candidiasis, on the other hand, is considered endogenous, since *Candida* is among the normal flora of the gastrointestinal tract to the human and is not found in the soil.[6] Actinomycosis is also usually an endogenous infection, whereas nocardiosis is of exogenous origin.[12]

Histoplasmosis

Histoplasmosis is the most common of the fungal diseases in North America; it occurs in the central and eastern portions of North America, particularly in the Ohio, Mississippi, and St. Lawrence River Valleys. In endemic areas, *positive skin tests for Histoplasma* may be found in 80 per cent of the population.[14]

PRIMARY HISTOPLASMOSIS. This condition is generally asymptomatic or manifested by transient flulike symptoms. The chest radiograph may show one or more poorly defined areas of pulmonary consolidation, often associated with hilar adenopathy; pleural effusion is rare.[21] The primary disease may occasionally be more severe, occurring in the form of acute lobar pneumonia, diffuse bronchopneumonia, or miliary densities similar to miliary tuberculosis. This is termed disseminated histoplasmosis (Fig. 19–48) and may occasionally progress to acute disseminated disease and death, most commonly in the very young and very old.[15]

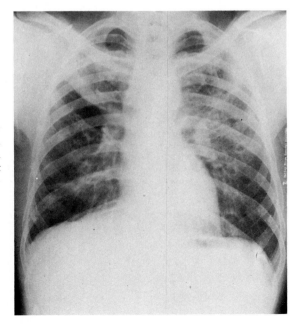

Figure 19–48. Disseminated histoplasmosis. The patient is a 52-year-old male with cough, fever, and weight loss. Patchy consolidation is present in both lung fields. This appearance was found to represent pulmonary histoplasmosis; the disease was eradicated with amphotericin B.

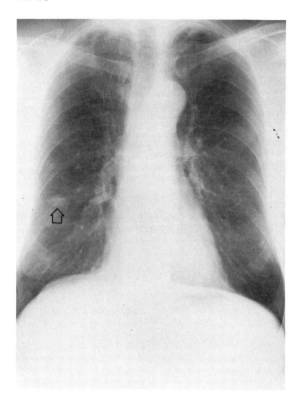

Figure 19–49. Histoplasmosis as a solitary nodule. A well-demarcated nodule was seen in the right lower lobe (arrow) in this 42-year-old male. At surgery, a histoplasmoma was discovered.

SOLITARY PULMONARY NODULE. A relatively common form of pulmonary histoplasmosis, the nodule is usually sharply circumscribed and 1 to 3 cm in diameter (Fig. 19–49). The lesions are, of course, quite difficult to differentiate from other solitary nodules in the lung and, particularly in older patients, may require surgery for diagnosis. Calcification, often central, often occurs in the chronic lesion.

MULTIPLE PULMONARY NODULES. Occasionally, histoplasmosis may present as multiple pulmonary nodules (Fig. 19–50), usually in people who have been heavily exposed to organisms contaminated by bird excreta.[15, 29] These nodules tend to regress spontaneously, a fact that may be a clue to the character of the illness. The nodules are generally mistaken for metastatic tumor. Healing is often characterized by small diffuse calcifications.

CHRONIC HISTOPLASMOSIS. This may occasionally occur as a localized area of consolidation, usually in the upper lobe. Cavitation commonly occurs. It may closely simulate tuberculosis radiographically.[15, 19] A solitary nodule is a frequent manifestation of the chronic disease (see Fig. 19–49). Hilar and mediastinal adenopathy may also occur, and sclerosing mediastinitis with obstruction of the superior vena cava may develop in chronic histoplasmosis (Fig. 19–51).[19, 31]

OPPORTUNISTIC INVASION. Histoplasmosis can occasionally occur as an opportunistic invader.[13] In this instance, it generally has the nonspecific appearance of a rapidly progressive pneumonia.

TREATMENT. No therapy is required for most cases of self-limited histoplasmosis. For the treatment of cases of disseminated histoplasmosis or of the chronic pneumonic or cavitary form, amphotericin B has proved efficacious.[24] Surgery may be useful in treating chronic cavitary disease.[27]

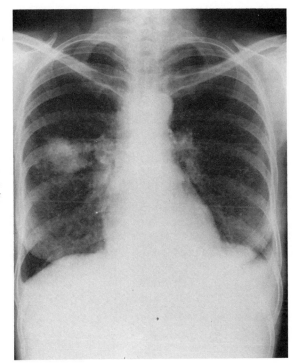

Figure 19–50. Histoplasmosis as multiple nodules. One large nodule is present in the right midlung field, and multiple smaller nodules are disseminated throughout both lung fields. The diagnosis of histoplasmosis was confirmed on lung biopsy.

Coccidioidomycosis

Coccidioidomycosis is prevalent in the southwestern United States. It is caused by the soil fungus *Coccidioidomyces immitis*. The rate of infection is high in endemic areas, the incidence of positive skin tests being greater than 50 per cent.[1]

Most patients with coccidioidomycosis are completely asymptomatic or have a mild flulike syndrome.[10] The radiographic findings are similar to those of histoplasmosis; patients may have multiple patchy or single areas of pneumonic infiltration

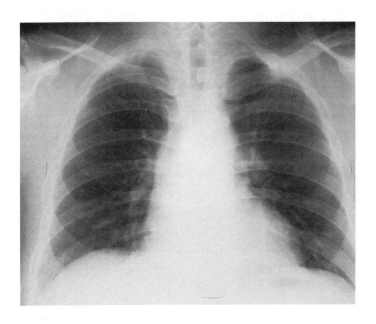

Figure 19–51. Sclerosing mediastinitis secondary to histoplasmosis. This 27-year-old male presented with superior vena caval obstruction. This chest radiograph shows slight widening of the mediastinum. Venography showed obstruction of the superior vena cava. Surgery revealed mediastinal fibrosis, with granulomas compatible with histoplasmosis. Sclerosing mediastinitis is an uncommon complication of histoplasmosis.

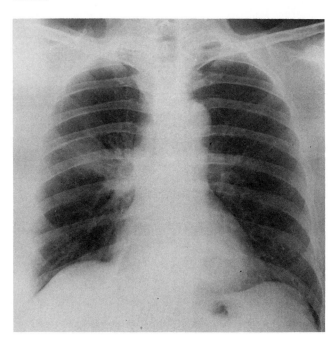

Figure 19–52. Coccidioidomycosis. A patchy alveolar infiltrate is present in the superior segment of the right lower lobe, with associated right hilar adenopathy. This appearance represents coccidioidomycosis.

(Fig. 19–52), lymphadenopathy (Fig. 19–53), and occasionally, pleural effusions (Fig. 19–54). The primary pneumonitis generally clears up spontaneously; in approximately 5 per cent there may be a residual chronic lesion.[10] This chronic lesion can be either cavitary or solid and, when cavitary, is characteristically, but not always, thin walled. Two thirds of these lesions occur in the lower lobes.[10] Rarely, a miliary pattern is seen.

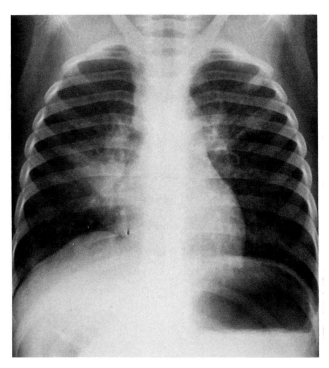

Figure 19–53. Coccidioidomycosis with mediastinal adenopathy. The patient is a seven-year-old boy with several pulmonary nodules and rather extensive right hilar and mediastinal adenopathy secondary to coccidioidomycosis. Histoplasmosis can have a similar appearance. Primary tuberculosis must also be considered in the differential diagnosis.

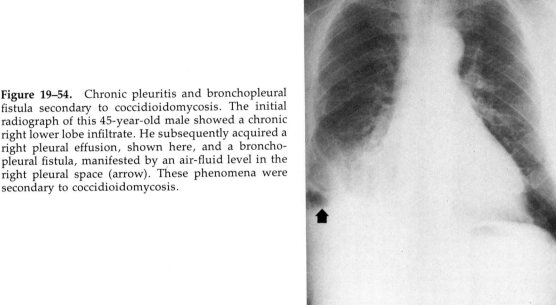

Figure 19–54. Chronic pleuritis and bronchopleural fistula secondary to coccidioidomycosis. The initial radiograph of this 45-year-old male showed a chronic right lower lobe infiltrate. He subsequently acquired a right pleural effusion, shown here, and a broncho-pleural fistula, manifested by an air-fluid level in the right pleural space (arrow). These phenomena were secondary to coccidioidomycosis.

Most patients do not require drug therapy, but for acutely ill patients and for those with chronic disease, amphotericin B may be curative.[1] As in all cases of solitary nodules, surgery may be required for the diagnosis of the solitary nodular form. Surgery may also be useful in treating chronic cavitary lesions that are not responsive to drug therapy.

Blastomycosis

North American blastomycosis is caused by *Blastomyces dermatitidis*. Like histoplasmosis and coccidioidomycosis, it is endemic in North America, principally the Mississippi and Ohio River valleys and the South Central and Middle Atlantic states.[7]

Unlike histoplasmosis and coccidioidomycosis, blastomycosis is usually an invasive, progressive disease. The patient's symptoms are variable, often insidious but occasionally acute. The radiographic picture is nonspecific and may demonstrate a mass (Fig. 19–55), an infiltrate, a cavity, multicentric lesions, and even disseminated disease.[7] Diagnosis is made by culture of the organism. Once the diagnosis is established, therapy is mandatory. Two therapeutic agents are available — 2-hydroxystilbamidine and amphotericin B) Disseminated disease with bone and skin involvement is common, and the five-year mortality rate is approximately 20 per cent.[36]

South American blastomycosis is caused by *Blastomyces brasiliensis* and although endemic in Brazil has been reported in a number of other Central and South American countries. All North Americans with proven South American blastomycosis have acquired the disease in South America.[11] South American blastomycosis involves organs other than the lungs extensively, including the skin, the lymphatics, the mucous membranes, and the gastrointestinal tract.[11] In the lungs it may cause localized or diffuse infiltrates. Bilateral infiltrates are much more common than unilateral ones and

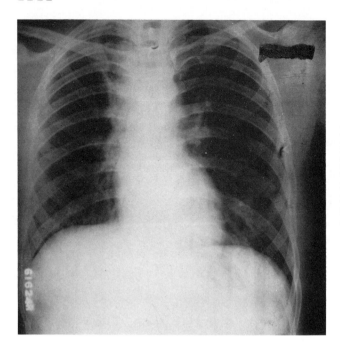

Figure 19–55. Blastomycosis. The patient is a 47-year-old male with chronic cough and fever. A mass is apparent in the right upper lobe along the mediastinum, with a dense infiltrate in the right lung adjacent to the mediastinum. The diagnosis of blastomycosis was confirmed by sputum smear and culture.

are frequently cavitary. Occasionally, multiple nodules may be seen. Emphysema and fibrosis almost always follow the pulmonary lesions.[11] Sulfa drugs or amphotericin B are used for treatment.[11]

Aspergillosis

Aspergillosis is generally caused by *Aspergillus fumigatus* and has at least four different clinical presentations: (1) secondary noninvasive aspergillosis, (2) allergic aspergillosis, (3) secondary invasive aspergillosis, and (4) primary invasive aspergillosis.[37]

1. *Secondary noninvasive aspergillosis (mycetoma).* In this form, the organism tends to invade a pre-existing pulmonary cavity and form a rounded mass of hyphae (fungus ball). This mass usually lies free in the cavity, and can change location as the patient changes position. (Fig. 19–56). This type of lesion is generally asymptomatic but may result in massive hemoptysis, in which case surgical therapy is indicated.[18] Drug therapy is contraindicated. This form of aspergillosis is commonly seen in association with sarcoidosis[18] and may be seen secondary to pre-existing tuberculosis, lung cyst, or bronchiectasis.

2. *Allergic aspergillosis.* In this type, there is a hypersensitivity reaction of the bronchial tree to the usually innocuous *Aspergillus*.[30] As a consequence, the patient acquires mucous plugs containing hyphae of aspergilli. Clinical characteristics of this group of patients are asthma and blood eosinophilia of mild to moderate degree.[37] Diagnosis is made by special staining of the bronchial plugs, which may be obtained through the sputum, or by bronchoscopy. Radiographically, these patients characteristically have plugging of their bronchi and a pattern that resembles clusters of grapes or a finger in a glove (Fig. 19–57). They may have consolidation or cavitation (Fig. 19–58). Treatment is long-term steroid therapy. Therapy with amphotericin B is contraindicated.

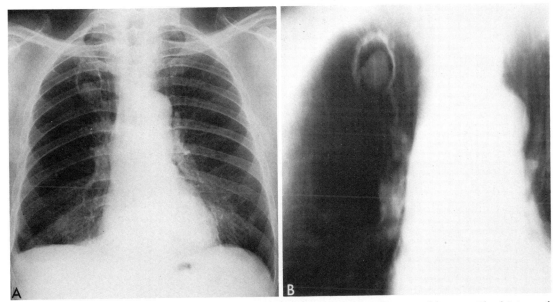

Figure 19–56.   Secondary noninvasive aspergillosis (mycetoma). This 58-year-old man with a history of tuberculosis acquired a nodule in the right upper lobe cavity. *A,* On the erect film, the nodule lies in the lower portion of the cavity. *B,* On the tomogram, made in the supine position, the nodule is seen to lie in the middle of the cavity, a position that indicates the nodule's mobility. This is characteristic of the fungus ball seen in secondary noninvasive aspergillosis.

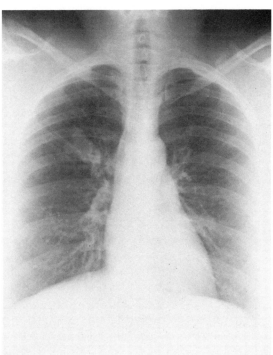

Figure 19–57.   Allergic aspergillosis. The patient is a 37-year-old female with chronic asthma and blood eosinophilia of 9 per cent. The nodular, "finger-in-glove" appearance of the matted mycelia is shown, as well as a mucous plug in the right upper lobe.

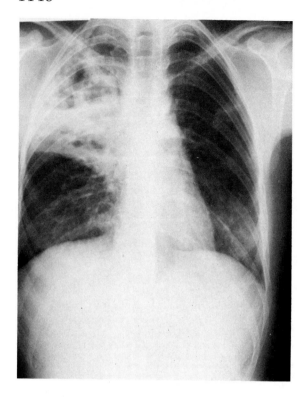

Figure 19–58. Allergic aspergillosis. Chronic consolidation is present in the right upper lobe of a 17-year-old asthmatic patient. Multiple air-fluid levels, indicative of abscess formation are seen. This is a less characteristic appearance of allergic aspergillosis.

3. *Secondary invasive aspergillosis.* In this instance, *Aspergillus* is a secondary invader of the immunosuppressed patient.[5] Radiographically, this type of aspergillosis resembles a non-specific pneumonia or tuberculosis. Diagnosis is made by sputum smear and culture, and amphotericin B is used for treatment.

4. *Primary invasive aspergillosis.* This is the rare instance in which the ubiquitous and usually harmless *Aspergillus* becomes invasive, presumably secondary to inoculation with large numbers of fungi. This most commonly occurs in the agrarian population. Diagnosis is made by smear and culture of the organism, and treatment is with amphotericin B.[37] Radiographic findings are nonspecific, demonstrating a pneumonic consolidation indistinguishable from other types of pneumonia or tuberculosis.

Opportunistic Fungal Disease

Patients with chronic disease states and malignancy as well as those receiving immunosuppressive, antibiotic, or corticosteroid therapy may be infected by any one of a number of fungi. The common invaders in these cases are *Aspergillus, Monilia, Mucor,* and *Cryptococcus,* but occasionally other fungi have been reported.[5, 23] Radiographs of the patient with an opportunistic fungal infection generally demonstrate a pneumonic infiltrate (Fig. 19–59). This may be cavitary (Fig. 19–60) and is sometimes nodular (Fig. 19–61). A nodular appearance is the one radiographic characteristic that can suggest that an opportunistic invader is a fungus. In most instances the character of the organism cannot be suspected on the basis of the radiographic findings. Sputum smear and culture are necessary to make the diagnosis. When the diagnosis is established, appropriate antifungal drugs are necessary for treatment. The mortality

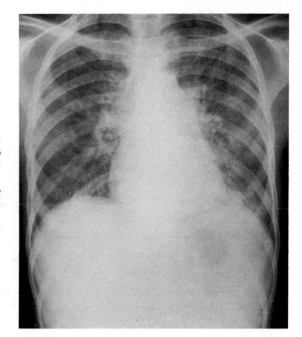

Figure 19–59. Opportunistic infection (cryptococcosis). Patchy consolidation is seen in both lungs but particularly in the left lower lobe of this 35-year-old female with acute myelogenous leukemia. *Cryptococcus* was cultured from the sputum, and the patient improved with amphotericin B.

rate in these patients is high, owing to the combination of the underlying problem and a serious invasive fungal infection.[5]

Extrinsic Allergic Alveolitis

Hypersensitivity reactions in the lung can result from various types of mold spores and *Actinomyces*. A partial list of these diseases includes farmer's lung, bagassosis, and

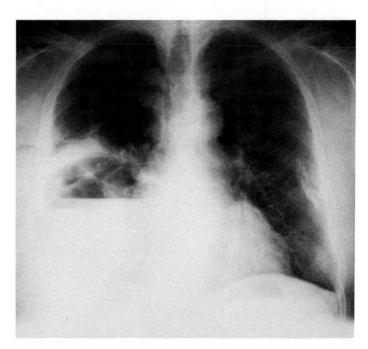

Figure 19–60. Opportunistic infection (aspergillosis). This 34-year-old man with Hodgkin's disease acquired an infiltrate and subsequently a cavity in the right lower lobe. This proved to be aspergillosis.

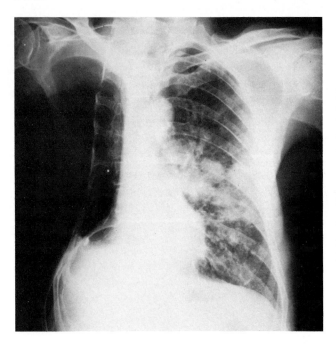

Figure 19–61. Opportunistic infection (moniliasis). This 62-year-old man underwent an extensive thoracoplasty on the right side for tuberculosis and was chronically ill and debilitated. He acquired nodular infiltrates in the left lung, which proved to be moniliasis. Nodular infiltrates of this type strongly are suggestive of fungus or *Nocardia*. The infectious process must be differentiated from metastatic tumor, the clinical clue being the sudden onset of symptoms and the rapid development and progression of the pulmonary infiltrates.

mushroom worker's disease — all due to various forms of thermophilic *Actinomyces*; maple bark disease due to craniosporum corticale; mold worker's lung due to *Aspergillus clavatus*; and sequoiosis due to various fungi.[30] Clinically, these patients may have respiratory symptoms several hours after intense exposure or may slowly acquire respiratory symptoms over a prolonged period due to recurrent occupational exposure.

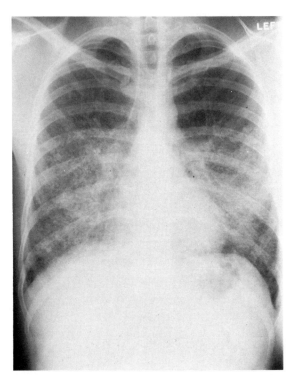

Figure 19–62. Allergic alveolitis (mushroom worker's disease). Diffuse nodulation is present throughout the interstitium of both lungs. This picture is characteristic of allergic alveolitis, which in this instance is an allergic reaction to thermophilic *Actinomyces*, associated with mushroom picking.

Pathologically, there is edema in the alveoli and interstitial infiltrates of plasma cells and lymphocytes in the interstitium.[30] Radiographically, these patients may display fine, nodular, interstitial infiltrates (generally seen in the chronic form) (Fig. 19–62) or diffuse, hazy, alveolar infiltrates resembling pulmonary edema (generally seen in the acute form). Intermittent exposure may produce a confusing picture of episodic infiltrates and clearing. Treatment is the removal of the patient from exposure to the offending antigen. Steroids are occasionally beneficial.[30]

References

1. Albert, B. L., and Sellers, T. F., Jr.: Coccidioidomycosis from fomites: report of a case and review of the literature. Arch. Intern. Med. 112:253–261, 1963.
2. Barnett, T. B., and Herring, C. L.: Lung abscess. Initial and late results of medical therapy. Arch. Intern. Med. 127:217–227, 1971.
3. Bartlett, J. G., Gorbach, S. L., Tally, F. P., et al.: Bacteriology and treatment of primary lung abscess. Am. Rev. Respir. Dis. 109:510–518, 1974.
4. Bartlett, J. G., and Gorbach, S. L.: Treatment of aspiration pneumonia and primary lung abscess. Penicillin G vs. clindamycin. J.A.M.A. 234:935–937, 1975.
5. Bragg, D. G., and Janis, B.: Radiographic presentation of pulmonary opportunistic inflammatory disease. Radiol. Clin. North Am. 11:357–369, 1973.
6. Buechner, H. A., Seabury, J. H., Campbell, C. C., et al.: The current status of serologic, immunologic and skin tests in the diagnosis of pulmonary mycoses. Report of the committee on fungus diseases and subcommittee on criteria for clinical diagnosis. American College of Chest Physicians. Chest 63:259, 1973.
7. Busey, J. F.: North American blastomycosis. In Buechner, H. A. (ed.): Management of Fungus Disease of the Lungs. Springfield, Illinois, Charles C Thomas, Publisher, 1971, p. 24.
8. Chidi, C. C., and Mendelsohn, H. J.: Lung abscess. A study of the results of treatment based on 90 consecutive cases. J. Thorac. Cardiovas. Surg. 68:168–172, 1974.
9. Curry, J., and Wier, J. A.: Histoplasmosis: a review of one hundred consecutively hospitalized patients. Am. Rev. Tuberc. Pulm. Dis. 77:749–763, 1958.
10. Einstein, H. E.: Coccidioidomycosis. In Buechner, H. A. (ed.): Management of Fungus Disease of the Lungs. Springfield, Illinois, Charles C Thomas, Publisher, 1971, p. 86.
11. Fountain, F. F., and Sutliff, W. D.: Paracoccidioidomycosis in the U.S. Am. Rev. Respir. Dis. 993:89–93, 1969.
12. Frazier, A. R., Rosenow, E. C., III, and Robert, G. D.: Nocardiosis. A review of 25 cases occurring during 24 months. Mayo Clin. Proc. 50:657–663, 1975.
13. Furcolow, M. L.: Tests of immunity in histoplasmosis. N. Engl. J. Med. 268:357–361, 1963.
14. Furcolow, M. L.: Environmental aspects of histoplasmosis. Arch. Environ. Health 10:4–10, 1965.
15. Furcolow, M. L., and Buechner, H. A.: Histoplasmosis. In Buechner, H. A. (ed.): Management of Fungus Disease of the Lungs. Springfield, Illinois, Charles C Thomas, Publishers, 1971, p. 145.
16. Gopalakrishna, K. V., and Lerner, P. I.: Primary lung abscess. Analysis of 66 cases. Cleveland Clin. Q. 42:3–13, 1975.
17. Harvey, J. C., Cantrell, J. R., and Fisher, A. M.: Actinomycosis: its recognition and treatment. Ann. Intern. Med. 46:868–885, 1957.
18. Israel, H. L., and Ostrow, A.: Sarcoidosis and aspergilloma. Am. J. Med. 47:243–250, 1969.
19. Loewen, D. F., Procknow, J. J., and Loosli, C. G.: Chronic active pulmonary histoplasmosis with cavitation. A clinical and laboratory study of thirteen cases. Am. J. Med. 28:252–280, 1960.
20. Mark, P. H., and Turner, J. A. P.: Lung abscess in children. Thorax 23:216–220, 1968.
21. Murray, J. F., and Howard, D.: Laboratory acquired histoplasmosis. Am. Rev. Respir. Dis. 93:47, 1966.
22. O'Reilly, G. V., Dee, M., and Otteni, G. V.: Gangrene of the lung. Successful medical management of three patients. Radiology 126:575, 1978.
23. Pappas, G., Schröter, G., Brettschneider, L., et al.: Pulmonary surgery in immunosuppressed patients. J. Thorac. Cardiovasc. Surg. 59:882–887, 1970.
24. Parker, J. D., Sarosi, G. A., Doto, I. L., et al.: Treatment of chronic pulmonary histoplasmosis. A National Communicable Disease Center Cooperative Mycoses Study. N. Engl. J. Med. 283:225–229, 1970.
25. Payne, W. S., Cardoza, F., and Weed, L. A.: Chronic draining sinuses of the chest wall. Surg. Clin. North Am. 53:927–936, 1973.
26. Perlman, L. V., Lerner, E., and D'Esopo, N.: Clinical classification and analysis of 97 cases of lung abscess. Am. Rev. Respir. Dis. 99:390–398, 1969.
27. Polk, J. W.: Treatment of pulmonary histoplasmosis. Dis. Chest 56:149–151, 1969.

28. Prather, J. R., Eastridge, C. E., Hughes, F. A., Jr., et al.: Actinomycosis of the thorax: diagnosis and treatment. Ann. Thorac. Surg. 9:307–312, 1970.
29. Procknow, J. J.: Pulmonary histoplasmosis in a farm family — fifteen years later. Amer. Rev. Respir. Dis. 95:171–188, 1967.
30. Salvagio, J. E., and Buechner, H. A.: Pulmonary hypersensitivity diseases associated with actinomycetes and fungi. In Buechner, H. A. (ed.): Management of Fungus Disease of the Lungs. Springfield, Illinois, Charles C Thomas, Publisher, 1971, p. 3.
31. Schowengerdt, C. G., Suyemoto, R., and Main, F. B.: Granulomatous and fibrous mediastinitis — a review and analysis of 180 cases. J. Thorac. Cardiovasc. Surg. 57:365–379, 1969.
32. Schweppe, H. I., Knowles, J. H., and Kane, L.: Lung abscess: an analysis of Mass. General Hospital cases from 1943 through 1956. N. Engl. J. Med. 265:1039–1043, 1961.
33. Seabury, J. H.: Actinomycosis and nocardiosis. In Buechner, H. A. (ed.): Management of Fungus Disease of the Lungs. Springfield, Illinois, Charles C Thomas, Publisher, 1971.
34. Shafron, R. D., and Tate, C. F., Jr.: Lung abscess — a five year evaluation. Dis. Chest 53:12–18, 1968.
35. Takaro, T.: Lung abscess and fungal infections. In Sabiston, D. C., Jr. (ed.): Davis-Christopher Textbook of Surgery. Philadelphia, W. B. Saunders Company, 1977, p. 2074.
36. Witorsch, P., and Utz, J. P.: North American blastomycosis: a study of 40 patients. Medicine 47:169–200, 1968.
37. Zimmerman, R. A., and Miller, W. T.: Pulmonary aspergillosis. Am. J. Roentgenol. 109:505–517, 1970.

Part IV

The Pleura and its Disorders

WALLACE T. MILLER, M.D.

The pleura is a serous membrane that invests the lung and lines the thoracic cavity. Histologically, the pleural surface consists of a uniform layer of flattened mesothelial cells without a basement membrane, resting upon a layer of loose connective tissue. The visceral pleura is thin and elastic and is intimately connected to the lung by fibrous prolongations of the deeper layer of connective tissue. The parietal pleura is thicker and is easily separated from the chest wall by the underlying layer of loose areolar tissue. The subpleural areolar tissue contains lymphatic channels, veins, arteries, and a rich network of capillaries. The visceral pleura extends between the lobes of the lung, lining the major and minor intralobar fissures. The pleura may also extend into anomalous fissures, when these exist.[38]

Normally, only a potential space exists between the parietal and the visceral pleura. This becomes a true space when the pleural layers are separated by air or fluid.

Because of the inherent elasticity of the lungs, which tend to recoil inward toward the hila, negative intrapleural pressures ordinarily exist. During inspiration, pressures of −6 to −12 cm of water are present; during expiration, pressures of −4 to −8 cm of water exist. Extremes of +40 cm of water may be seen during a Valsalva maneuver or −40 cm of water during a Müller maneuver. The pleural pressure is slightly more negative at the apices than at the bases.[28]

PNEUMOTHORAX

The presence of air in the pleural cavity is pneumothorax. In most instances, air arrives in the pleural cavity secondary to some iatrogenic maneuver — thoracentesis, thoracostomy, and so forth. It can also result from penetrating or nonpenetrating

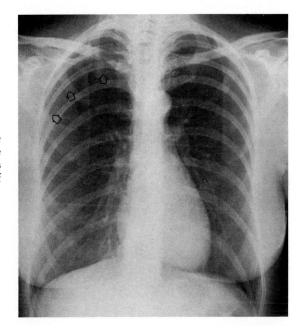

Figure 19–63. Spontaneous pneumothorax. The visceral pleura can be seen sharply outlining the partially collapsed right lung (arrows). Spontaneous pneumothorax is characteristically a disease of young males and is idiopathic.

trauma. Pneumothorax is a common accompaniment of rib fracture, in which case it is secondary to laceration of the visceral pleura by sharp fragments of the fractured rib. It may also occur after blunt trauma in the absence of rib fracture, presumably secondary to shearing of the lung parenchyma or a small bronchus.

Spontaneous pneumothorax occurs in the absence of trauma and is generally the result of the rupture of a subpleural cyst, bleb, or bulla. This occurs most commonly in men in the third and fourth decades[19] and recurs in approximately 30 per cent of cases.[2]

Whereas most patients with spontaneous pneumothorax are young and have no coexisting lung disease, spontaneous pneumothorax can complicate a variety of pulmonary disorders; most commonly tuberculosis,[31] asthma,[37] eosinophilic granuloma of the lung,[20] and carcinoma of the lung.[10] It has also been reported to occur with sarcoidosis;[1] pulmonary metastases, particularly osteosarcoma;[13] and various types of chronic interstitial pulmonary fibrosis.[4] Chronic pneumothorax indicates a *bronchopleural fistula* and may be caused by a variety of the diseases mentioned previously (see Fig. 19–67).

Symptomatically, most patients with spontaneous pneumothorax present with chest pain, dyspnea, or both.[23]

Radiographically, pneumothorax is characterized by the presence of the sharp line of visceral pleura outlining the partially collapsed lung (Fig. 19–63). This is generally apparent on the routine chest radiograph, but if it is not seen and pneumothorax is suspected, a radiograph made with the chest in full expiration may demonstrate the pneumothorax. The volume of the thoracic cage is reduced in expiration, making the air in the pleural space greater relative to the amount of air in the contracted lung. This causes the lung to retract farther from the lateral chest wall.

Pneumothorax is often associated with fluid in the pleural space and appears as a fluid level. This makes the pneumothorax more readily recognizable (see Fig. 19–67B).

In a patient with prior pleural scarring, the lung may not collapse uniformly, creating a loculated pneumothorax. This may be difficult to differentiate from a pulmonary bleb or bulla (Fig. 19–64). This distinction is important, since a bleb obvi-

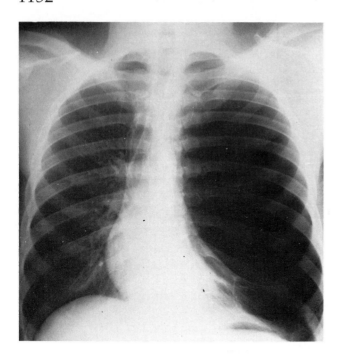

Figure 19–64. A bulla simulating pneumothorax. A large bulla is seen in the left upper lobe, displacing the remainder of the lung. This differs from a pneumothorax in that the sharp edge of the collapsed lung cannot be seen.

ously should not be treated with a chest tube. Loculated pneumothorax is generally recognizable by adhesions that extend from the visceral lung surface to the parietal pleura.

Tension pneumothorax (Fig. 19–65) causes enlargement of the ipsilateral hemithorax and displacement of the mediastinum toward the contralateral side. The involved lung is usually totally collapsed. Tension pneumothorax is a life-threatening

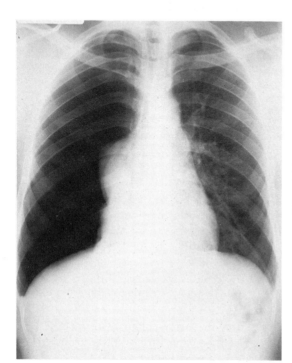

Figure 19–65. Tension pneumothorax. Air fills the right pleural space and the mediastinum is shifted toward the left. The right hemithorax is large, and the lung is totally collapsed.

situation and may require emergency needle aspiration prior to the institution of more permanent therapeutic measures.

The treatment of a spontaneous pneumothorax depends upon a number of factors. A small (5 to 20 per cent) asymptomatic pneumothorax may require observation only.[38] Occasionally, larger pneumothoraces may be treated by needle aspiration. More commonly, they require closed drainage with a tube thoracostomy.[29]

PLEURAL EFFUSION

Pleural effusion is the presence of fluid within the pleural space. This fluid may be a transudate, exudate, pus, blood, chyle, or any combination of these. The identification of the character of the fluid, generally by thoracentesis, is of utmost importance in establishing the cause of the pleural effusion.

In a normal person, there is a constant transudation and absorption of fluid within the pleural cavity. Six hundred to 1000 cc of fluid may be formed and absorbed in a single day.[36] The formation of pleural fluid and its reabsorption are related to the hydrostatic pressure in the systemic capillaries that supply the parietal pleura, the negative intrapleural pressure, the colloid osmotic pressure of the pleural fluid, the permeability of the subpleural capillaries and lymphatics, and the diaphragmatic and intercostal muscle activity.[5, 36] Abnormal amounts of fluid may accumulate when there is an increase in hydrostatic pressure (congestive heart failure), a decrease in colloid osmotic pressure (low protein states), or an increase in capillary permeability (pleural tumor or inflammation).

While it is useful to think of pleural effusion in terms of altered physiologic states, it is also helpful to consider the various pathologic entities that may cause these physiologic alterations. A partial list of these pathologic conditions is given in Table 19–1.

Of the various causes of pleural effusion, the most common is congestive heart failure. This is generally manifested radiographically by the associated presence of increased pulmonary vascular markings and cephalization of the pulmonary blood flow; that is, the upper lobe vessels are greater in size than the lower lobe vessels, a

TABLE 19–1. PATHOLOGIC ENTITIES LEADING TO PLEURAL EFFUSIONS

1. Congestive heart failure
2. Infection
   A. Viral
   B. Bacterial (including tuberculosis)
   C. Fungal
3. Neoplasm
   A. Primary
      (1) Benign mesothelioma
      (2) Malignant mesothelioma
   B. Secondary
      (1) Bronchogenic carcinoma
      (2) Carcinoma of the breast
      (3) Lymphoma
      (4) Other primary neoplasms
4. Pulmonary infarct
5. Collagen vascular disease
   A. Lupus erythematosus
   B. Rheumatoid arthritis
   C. Periarteritis nodosa
6. Subdiaphragmatic processes
   A. Subdiaphragmatic abscess
   B. Acute pancreatitis
   C. Peritoneal dialysis
   D. Ascites
7. Low protein states
   A. Chronic liver disease
   B. Chronic renal disease
   C. Intestinal malabsorption
   D. Starvation
8. Miscellaneous
   A. Sarcoidosis
   B. Drug reactions
   C. Myxedema

reversal of the normal physiologic state (see Fig. 19–71). Cardiomegaly is also generally present. Effusions secondary to congestive heart failure are frequently bilateral and when unilateral are almost invariably right-sided.[24] This fluid is a transudate with a low protein level and low level of specific gravity (less than 1.016).

Most infectious processes that involve the pleura are characterized by pleural fluid with a high white cell count and high protein content and, consequently, a high specific gravity (greater than 1.016). In cases of tuberculous pleural effusion, the white cells in the fluid are usually predominantly lymphocytes, whereas in acute bacterial emphyema, they are predominantly polymorphonuclear leukocytes. In viral infections, the cells are usually lymphocytes. Because of the high protein content of infectious effusions, they are frequently loculated (Figs. 19–66 and 19–67).

In most instances, the organism can be cultured from the pleural fluid. In cases of tuberculosis, a pleural biopsy frequently reveals granulomas.[34] Consequently, pleural biopsy is indicated in unexplained pleural effusions.

Neoplasm is the most common cause of massive pleural effusion (Fig. 19–68).[25, 33] The diagnosis of a malignant pleural effusion can sometimes be suggested radiographically by the presence of pleural nodules (see Fig. 19–73). The diagnosis is generally determined by the character of the pleural fluid. Pleural biopsy or thoracentesis generally yields malignant cells.[25] Malignant pleural effusions are frequently serosanguineous and usually exudative in character, with a high protein content, high specific gravity, and moderately high white cell count.

Pulmonary infarction is another frequent cause of pleural effusion. Often associated radiographically with consolidation within the lung field, it may be difficult to differentiate from pneumonia. The pleural effusion is exudative, with a high protein content and a high specific gravity. It is often bloody, with a fairly high cell count, generally of red blood cells.

The collagen vascular diseases, particularly rheumatoid arthritis and lupus, may be manifested by pleural effusion. In cases of lupus, the effusions are frequently

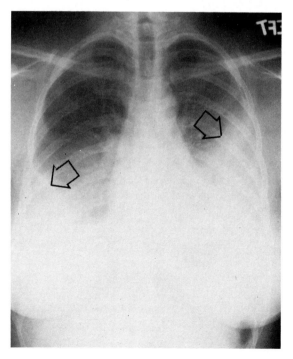

Figure 19–66. Bilateral empyema. Loculated collections of fluid are noted in both hemithoraces (arrows). The shape of this fluid collection, its border convex toward the hilum, suggests that it is loculated. On decubitus films, a small amount of free fluid was demonstrated, but most of the fluid was loculated. The organism in this instance was *Hemophilus influenzae*; in most instances the offending organism is *Staphylococcus* or a gram-negative bacterium.

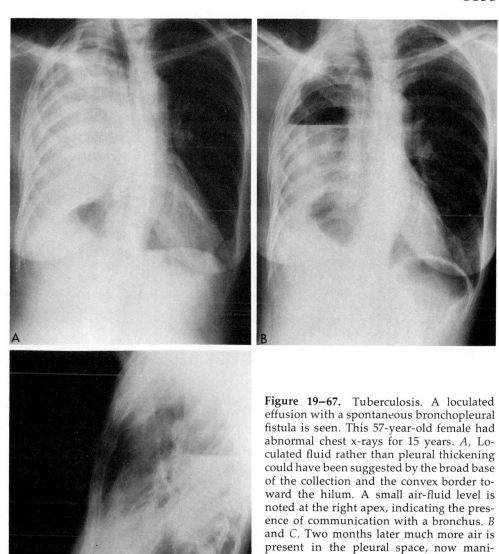

Figure 19–67. Tuberculosis. A loculated effusion with a spontaneous bronchopleural fistula is seen. This 57-year-old female had abnormal chest x-rays for 15 years. *A,* Loculated fluid rather than pleural thickening could have been suggested by the broad base of the collection and the convex border toward the hilum. A small air-fluid level is noted at the right apex, indicating the presence of communication with a bronchus. *B* and *C,* Two months later much more air is present in the pleural space, now manifested by a large air-fluid level and a decreased amount of loculated fluid. At this time, both the sputum and the pleural fluid were positive for *Mycobacterium tuberculosis* infection. This had apparently remained quiescent for 15 years as a loculated pleural effusion.

bilateral and may be associated with pericardial effusion (Fig. 19–69).[39] There is seldom associated lung disease; when it is present, it is nonspecific in character. In the case of rheumatoid disease, pleural effusions are more commonly seen in men, in spite of the predominance of rheumatoid arthritis in females.[9] The effusions are usually unilateral (Fig. 19–70), high in protein and specific gravity, and low in glucose. They may occasionally be associated with the pulmonary manifestations of rheumatoid disease, such as interstitial fibrosis or pulmonary nodules, but more often these are absent.[9]

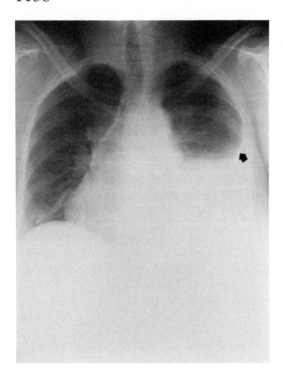

Figure 19–68. Malignant pleural effusion. A large pleural effusion is present in the left hemithorax, with a characteristic meniscus (arrow). Most malignant effusions are due to metastatic carcinoma. In this instance, the effusion was secondary to myeloma.

Radiographically, pleural effusions are recognizable by blunting of the costophrenic sulci (see Figs. 19–68 to 19–70). The fluid usually exhibits a meniscus shape laterally on the posteroanterior film and posteriorly on the lateral film. Thus it has a border that is downwardly concave. Commonly, a pleural effusion as great as 300 cc may not be

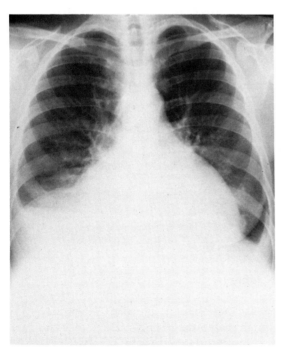

Figure 19–69. Pleural and pericardial effusions secondary to lupus erythematosus. This 27-year-old female has small bilateral pleural effusions with a characteristic meniscus. The cardiac silhouette is enlarged. Echocardiography revealed a moderate pericardial effusion to be the cause of the cardiac enlargement. Both pericardial and pleural effusions are commonly seen in lupus.

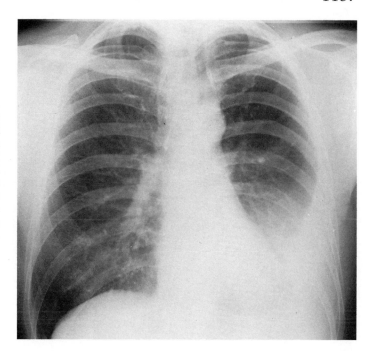

Figure 19–70. Rheumatoid effusion. The patient is a 27-year-old male with a loculated effusion along the left lateral chest wall. The patient had known rheumatoid arthritis. The loculation of the effusion is suggested by its lateral position in the chest and its convex border toward the hilum. Loculation is characteristically seen when the effusion has a high protein content. No pulmonary manifestations of rheumatoid disease are present.

apparent on the posteroanterior film,[8] but effusions of 100 cc are generally apparent on the lateral film, and decubitus films may demonstrate as little as 25 cc of free pleural fluid.[16]

Large pleural effusions may occasionally accumulate beneath the lung so that the lung retains its normal shape, particularly on the posteroanterior film (Fig. 19–71). Such effusions as great as 1000 cc may not blunt the lateral costophrenic sulcus, but will generally produce blunting of the posterior costophrenic sulcus on the lateral film (Fig. 19–72). On the left side, it may cause an increased distance between the stomach bubble and the lower border of the lung.[32] A decubitus film will readily confirm the presence of an infrapulmonary effusion.

Loculated pleural effusion may sometimes be difficult to differentiate from consolidation within the lung. Characteristically, loculated effusions have a broad base at the pleural margin and a smooth, convex surface directed toward the hilum (see Figs. 19–66 and 19–67A). In some instances, it may be impossible to differentiate a loculated pleural effusion from an intrapulmonary problem, such as a bronchogenic carcinoma. Loculation tends to occur in pleural effusions with a high protein content.

Hemothorax is the collection of blood in the pleural cavity. Radiographically, this is indistinguishable from an ordinary pleural effusion. It is generally associated with some form of trauma, surgical or otherwise, but can sometimes be seen in cases of neoplasm or pulmonary infarction.

Surgical management of hemothorax depends upon the amount of blood accumulated and the presence of continued bleeding. If the hemothorax is small, nothing need be done. In cases of larger amounts of blood accumulation, tube thoracostomy may be indicated; and in cases of active bleeding, open thoracostomy is generally required.[38]

The accumulation of chyle in the pleural cavity, chylothorax, is generally the result of traumatic disruption of the thoracic duct. It may be due to blunt chest injury, penetrating wounds, or surgery. Twenty per cent of cases of chylothorax are iatrogenic, and 80 per cent stem from gunshot wounds, automobile accidents, stab wounds, and blunt trauma.[38] Tumors, most commonly lymphomas and metastatic carcinoma, are also

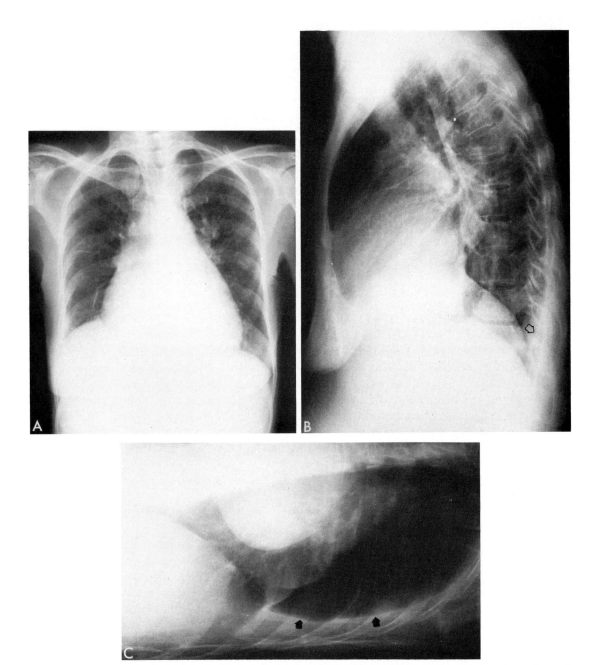

Figure 19–71. Infrapulmonary effusion secondary to congestive heart failure. *A,* The heart is enlarged, and there is cephalization of the pulmonary vasculature. These findings suggest chronic congestive heart failure. *B,* There is no blunting of the right costophrenic sulcus on the lateral film. Only a small meniscus is seen posteriorly (arrow). *C,* A decubitus film shows a moderate amount of free pleural fluid (arrows) in the right pleural space. Fluid may collect beneath the lung (infrapulmonary effusion) and be difficult to detect without the aid of a decubitus film.

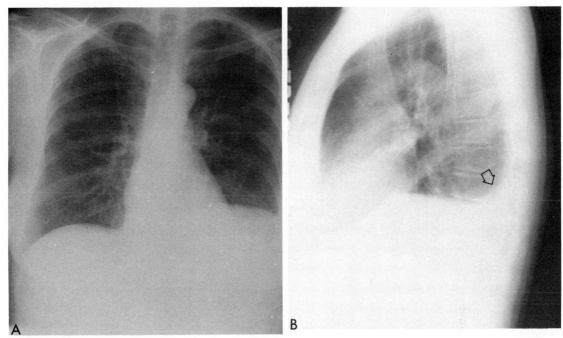

Figure 19–72. Infrapulmonary effusion secondary to *Candida* infection. This 35-year-old female was immunosuppressed secondary to drug therapy for chronic myelogenous leukemia. She first acquired a small left lower lobe infiltrate and then a chronic left pleural effusion. *A,* On the posteroanterior film, the left costophrenic sulcus is not definitely blunted. *B,* On the lateral film, there is definite blunting of the posterior costophrenic sulcus (arrow). A left decubitus film revealed a moderate pleural effusion on the left.

an occasional cause of chylothorax.[3] Chylous effusion, like hemothorax, is indistinguishable radiographically from other causes of pleural effusions. The diagnosis is indicated by the presence of large amounts of fat in the pleural fluid.

Empyema is the collection of pus in the pleural space. Because of the high protein content of the fluid and the inflammatory response of the pleura, loculation is frequent (Fig. 19–66). Another clue to the existence of pus in the pleural space is the presence of pneumonia or lung abscess in the lung, since this is the usual factor leading to the development of empyema.[22]

Occasionally, empyema may be due to a penetrating chest wound, a benign pleural effusion infected by iatrogenic needle aspiration or surgery, the intrapleural extension of a subphrenic abscess, or the rupture of a mediastinal structure, such as the esophagus.

At present, the most common organism responsible for empyema is *Staphylococcus aureus;* it is closely followed by the gram-negative organisms — *Pseudomonas, Klebsiella, Escherichia coli,* and *Aerobacter aerogenes.*[40] Empyema is frequently associated with other debilitating conditions. Vianna found that more than half of his patients with empyema had alcoholism, some form of chronic lung disease, or another pre-existing debilitating condition, such as tuberculosis, diabetes, or malignancy. Empyema may be an infectious complication of long-term steroid therapy.[40] At one time, empyema was most frequently seen as a complication of pneumonia in otherwise healthy patients, but with the advent of antibiotics, empyema in the nondebilitated patient has decreased dramatically.

The identification of the organism is generally accomplished by Gram's stain and culture of the pleural aspirate. Empyema must be treated rapidly with the appropriate antibiotics. Frequent pleural fluid cultures should be obtained to determine the clinical efficacy of the antibiotic regimen.[38]

In addition to the institution of antibiotic therapy, the pleural space should be drained. Occasionally, this can be accomplished by repeated thoracentesis, but closed chest tube drainage usually must be employed. Open pleural drainage is frequently necessary. This requires the resection of a short segment of rib and the insertion of a large-bore tube into the cavity, which is left open to atmospheric pressure.[38]

In some instances, decortication of the lung, followed by closed chest tube drainage, may be necessary to evacuate the empyema adequately and expand the remaining lung. This is not advocated as the primary treatment for empyema but is used in complicated cases in which closed or open tube drainage has not been successful.[26]

The mortality rate of patients with empyema is high because of the severity of the condition and its frequent association with underlying debilitating diseases. Vianna found a mortality rate of 18 per cent in a group of 41 patients.[40]

PLEURAL THICKENING

Pleural thickening can be localized or diffuse. It frequently occurs at the apices and is presumably related to aging, although it can be secondary to prior inflammatory disease, such as tuberculosis. The presence of a large unilateral apical pleural cap should suggest the possibility of superior sulcus (Pancoast) tumor, although frequently it is secondary to benign disease.

Blunting of the costophrenic sulci by pleural thickening is a frequent result of a prior pleural effusion and may be difficult to differentiate from a pleural effusion without a decubitus film. Prior pulmonary infarction is another cause of localized pleural thickening. Blunting of a lateral costophrenic sulcus without blunting of the costophrenic sulcus posteriorly is almost always due to pleural thickening rather than to fluid.

Multiple nodular areas of pleural thickening along the lateral chest wall are strongly suggestive of asbestosis, particularly when they are bilateral.[18] This is frequently associated with pleural calcification and almost never with pleural effusion. Nodular pleural changes resulting from asbestosis must be differentiated from those caused by metastatic tumor and pleural mesothelioma, but in the latter diseases, the involvement is usually unilateral.

Generalized pleural thickening can be unilateral or bilateral. When bilateral, it almost always is indicative of asbestosis, although it is occasionally seen in cases of metastatic tumor. When unilateral, extensive pleural thickening is indicative of a prior hemothorax or pyothorax and is commonly a manifestation of prior tuberculosis. Extensive unilateral pleural thickening may also be associated with pleural calcification. Chronic pleural thickening with a border that is convex toward the hilum suggests the presence of a loculated pleural effusion, even when present for many years (see Fig. 19–67). Active tubercle bacilli can frequently be found in such chronic loculated collections.

PLEURAL TUMORS

Various types of metastatic tumor may involve the pleura. Metastatic tumor may cause diffuse pleural nodulation (Fig. 19–73), pleural effusion, or both. The tumors that

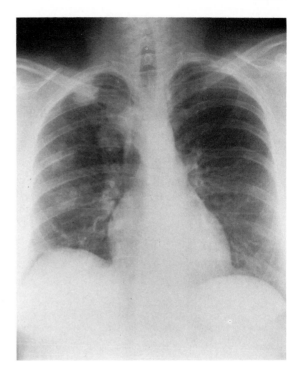

Figure 19–73. Pleural nodulation secondary to metastatic tumor. Multiple nodules are seen in the left hemithorax. They have a broad base, and only one side of the nodule is seen to be sharply outlined, characteristics of pleural nodules. All are located in one hemithorax, a feature strongly suggestive of pleural, rather than pulmonary, disease. These pleural nodules were metastases from a nonresectable breast carcinoma.

most commonly cause pleural metastases are carcinomas of the lung and of the breast.[25] A large number of other primary tumors may involve the pleura, including carcinomas of the ovary, stomach, rectum, bladder, and pancreas, and various types of sarcomas.[25] Lymphoma also frequently involves the pleura,[14] and leukemia may occasionally cause a pleural effusion.

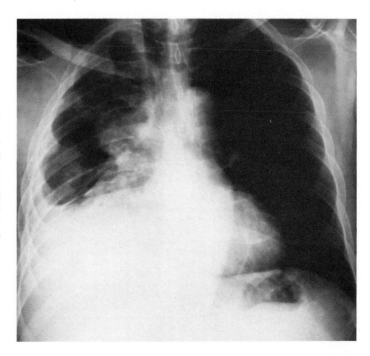

Figure 19–74. Pleural nodules and pleural effusion secondary to malignant mesothelioma. A pleural effusion is present on the right, and nodules are seen along the right lateral chest wall. These were secondary to diffuse mesothelioma. This 48-year-old male had prior exposure to asbestos and had some pleural calcification in the diaphragmatic pleura on the left, which is not obvious on the reproduction.

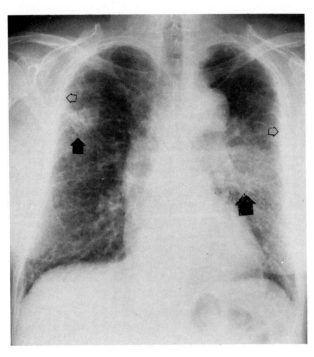

Figure 19–75. Bilateral primary lung carcinoma in a patient with asbestosis. This 72-year-old man had a history of asbestos exposure. Diffuse interstitial lung disease is present, and there is a large nodule in the left lung field (closed arrow) and a small nodule in the right lung field (closed arrow). Minor diffuse pleural thickening is noted along both lateral chest walls (open arrows). The interstitial lung disease and the pleural thickening are secondary to asbestosis. Primary carcinoma of the lung has a high association with asbestosis and smoking. Simultaneous bilateral primary carcinomas are unusual.

Various treatments for metastatic pleural effusions have been used. Hormonal therapy, radiation therapy, and the obliteration of the pleural space by the instillation of various sclerosing agents have all been tried, with varying degrees of success.[17, 21, 27]

Primary tumors of the pleura (pleural mesothelioma) can be divided into two types —local and diffuse. Local mesothelioma is almost always benign and histologically is

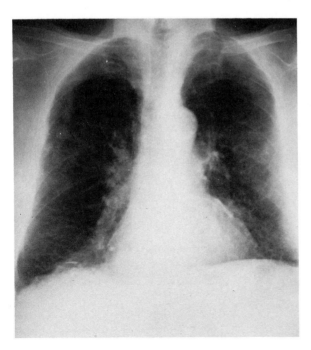

Figure 19–76. Asbestosis. Diffuse interstitial lung disease is evident, and small nodules are present along both lateral chest walls. There are small areas of calcification in the pericardium and in the diaphragmatic pleura on the right side. These changes are secondary to asbestosis. The nodular changes in the pleura (arrows) could suggest the diagnosis of mesothelioma, but uncomplicated asbestosis commonly causes nodular pleural disease. Mesothelioma is frequently accompanied by pleural effusion.

usually a fibrous mesothelioma.[6] These patients are generally asymptomatic but may complain of arthralgia, clubbing of the fingers, or fever.[11] Localized mesothelioma is generally amenable to surgical resection.

Diffuse mesothelioma, on the other hand, is usually fatal. Radiographically, it is characterized by pleural nodulation, pleural effusion, or both (Fig. 19–74). It is generally, but not always, unilateral.[7] There is a clear association between diffuse mesothelioma and asbestosis.[12, 30] There is also a clear association between asbestosis and lung carcinoma (Figs. 19–75 and 19–76).

References

1. Aho, A., Heinivaara, O., and Mähönen, H.: Boeck's sarcoid as a cause of spontaneous pneumothorax. Ann. Med. Intern. Fenn. 47:163–167, 1958.
2. Avery, M.E., Riley, M.C., and Weiss, A.: The course of bronchiectasis in childhood. Bull. Johns Hopkins Hosp. 109:20–34, 1961.
3. Bessone, L.N., Ferguson, T.B., and Burford, T.H.: Chylothorax, collective review. Ann. Thorac. Surg. 12:527–550, 1971.
4. Beyer, A., Richter, K., and Eribo, O.: Zwei Verlaufsbeobachtungen eines Hamman-Rich-Syndromes mit rezidivierendem Spontanpneumothorax (Two observations of the Hamman-Rich syndrome with recurrent spontaneous pneumothorax). Fortschr. Rontgenstr. 94:568–579, 1961.
5. Black, L.F.: The pleural space and pleural fluid. Subject review. Mayo Clin. Proc. 47:493–506, 1972.
6. Blount, H.C., Jr.: Localized mesothelioma of the pleura. A review with six new cases. Radiology 67:822, 1956.
7. Borow, M., Conston, A., Livornese, L., et al.: Mesothelioma following exposure to asbestos: a review of 72 cases. Chest 64:641–646, 1973.
8. Bowen, A.: Quantitative roentgen diagnosis of pleural effusions. Radiology 17:520, 1931.
9. Carr, D.T., and Mayne, J.G.: Pleurisy with effusion in rheumatoid arthritis, with reference to the low concentration of glucose in pleural fluid. Am. Rev. Respir. Dis. 85:345–350, 1962.
10. Citron, K.M.: Spontaneous pneumothorax complicating bronchial carcinoma. Tubercle 40:384–386, 1959.
11. Clagett, O.T., McDonald, J.R., and Schmidt, H.W.: Localized fibrous mesothelioma of pleura. J. Thorac. Surg. 24:213–230, 1952.
12. Demy, N.G., and Adler, H.: Asbestosis and malignancy. Am. J. Roentgenol. 100:597–602, 1967.
13. D'Ettorre, A., and Babini, L.: Pneumothorax from pulmonary metastases. Ann. Radiol. Diagn. 38:595–601, 1965.
14. Fisher, A.M.H., Kendall, B., and Van Leuven, B.D.: Hodgkin's disease. A radiological survey. Clin. Radiol. 13:115–127, 1962.
15. Hartweg, H.: Das Rontgenbild des Thorax bei den chronischen Leukosen (The roentgenogram of the thorax in chronic leukoses). Fortschr. Rontgenstr. 92:477–490, 1960.
16. Hessen, I.: Roentgen examination of pleural fluid: a study of the localization of free effusions, the potentialities of diagnosing minimal quantities of fluid and its existence under physiological conditions. Acta Radiol. (Suppl.) 86:1–80, 1951.
17. Hickman, J.A., and Jones, M.C.: Treatment of neoplastic pleural effusions with local instillations of quinacrine (mepacrine) hydrochloride. Thorax 25:226–229, 1970.
18. Hourihane, D.O., Lessof, L., and Richardson, P.C.: Hyaline and calcified pleural plaques as an index of exposure to asbestos. A study of radiological and pathological features of 100 cases with a consideration of epidemiology. Br. Med. J. 1:1069–1074, 1966.
19. Hyde, L.: Benign spontaneous pneumothorax. Ann. Intern. Med. 56:746–751, 1962.
20. Kittredge, R.D., Geller, A., and Finby, N.: The reticuloendothelioses in the lung. Am. J. Roentgenol. 100:588–592, 1967.
21. Leininger, B.J., Barker, W.L., and Langston, H.T.: A simplified method for management of malignant pleural effusion. J. Thorac. Cardiovasc. Surg. 58:758–763, 1969.
22. LeRoux, B.T.: Empyema thoracis. Br. J. Surg. 52:89–99, 1965.
23. Lindskog, G.E., and Halasz, N.A.: Spontaneous pneumothorax. A consideration of pathogenesis and management with review of seventy-two hospitalized cases. Arch. Surg. 75:693–698, 1957.
24. Logue, R.B., Rogers, J.V., Jr., and Gay, B.B., Jr.: Subtle roentgenographic signs of left heart failure. Am. Heart J. 65:464–473, 1963.
25. Maher, G.G., and Berger, H.W.: Massive pleural effusion: malignant and nonmalignant causes in 46 patients. Am. Rev. Respir. Dis. 105:458–460, 1972.
26. Mayo, P., and McElvein, R.B.: Early thoracotomy for pyogenic empyema. Ann. Thorac. Surg. 2:649–657, 1966.
27. Meyer, P.C.: Metastatic carcinoma of the pleura. Thorax 21:437–443, 1966.

28. Milic-Emili, J., Henderson, J.A.M., Dolovich, M.B., et al.: Regional distribution of inspired gas in the lung. J. Appl. Physiol. 21:749–759, 1966.
29. Mills, M., and Baisch, B.F.: Spontaneous pneumothorax — a series of 400 cases. Ann. Thorac. Surg. 1:286–297, 1965.
30. Newhouse, M.L., and Wagner, J.C.: Validation of death certificates in asbestos workers. Br. J. Industr. Med. 26:302–307, 1969.
31. Oshiro, M., Nagano, K., and Izumi, T.: Clinical statistics of 75 cases of spontaneous pneumothorax with special reference to the cause of the disease. Jpn. J. Tuberc. 10:25, 1962.
32. Petersen, J.A.: Recognition of infrapulmonary pleural effusion. Radiology 74:34–41, 1960.
33. Rabin, C.B., and Blackman, N.S.: Bilateral pleural effusion. Its significance in association with a heart of normal size. J. Mount Sinai Hosp. 24:45, 1957.
34. Schub, H.M., Spivey, C.G., Jr., and Baird, G.D.: Pleural involvement in histoplasmosis. Am. Rev. Respir. Dis. 94:225–232, 1966.
35. Smith, A.R.: Pleural calcification resulting from exposure to certain dusts. Am. J. Roentgenol. 67:375–382, 1952.
36. Stewart, P.B.: The rate of formation and lymphatic removal of fluid in pleural effusions. J. Clin. Invest. 42:258–262, 1963.
37. Sugita, K., and Koya E.: Bronchial asthma and spontaneous pneumothorax. Jpn. J. Dis. Chest 6:1188, 1962.
38. Takaro, T.: The pleura and empyema. In Sabiston, D.C. (ed.) Davis-Christopher Textbook of Surgery. Philadelphia, W.B. Saunders Company, 1977, p. 2087.
39. Taylor, T.L., and Ostrum, H.: The roentgen evaluation of systemic lupus erythematosus. Am. J. Roentgenol. 82:95–107, 1959.
40. Utley, J.R., Parker, J.C., Hahn, R.S., et al.: Recurrent benign fibrous mesothelioma of the pleura. J. Thorac. Cardiovasc. Surg. 65:830–834, 1973.
41. Williams, J.R., and Bonte, F.J.: The Roentgenological Aspect of Nonpenetrating Chest Injuries. Springfield, Illinois, Charles C Thomas, Publisher, 1961.

Part V

Bronchiectasis

WALLACE T. MILLER, M. D.

"Bronchiectasis" literally means *dilated bronchi*. In actuality, the term implies a more specific finding — irreversible, localized dilatation of the bronchi secondary to the destruction of the muscular and elastic tissue of the bronchial walls. Once a common disorder, bronchiectasis is now a relatively infrequent medical problem. This decrease in the incidence of bronchiectasis has been traced to the introduction of broad spectrum antibiotics in the early 1950's.[8, 10]

The effort to manage bronchiectasis played an important role in the development of thoracic surgery. The development of pulmonary resection was stimulated by this effort, and the first successful pneumonectomy was performed by Rudolph Nissen in 1931 on a 12-year-old girl with bronchiectasis.[20]

ETIOLOGY AND PATHOPHYSIOLOGY

The most important factor in the development of bronchiectasis is the presence of infection.[29] In all likelihood, obstruction is generally a secondary factor.[6] The obstruction may be caused by a foreign body, tenacious plugs of mucopurulent material, tumor, or extrabronchial compression.[3] Etiologically, there are three types of bronchiectasis: postinfectious bronchiectasis, congenital bronchiectasis, and bronchiectasis associated with immune-related diseases.

Postinfectious Bronchiectasis

Although all bronchiectasis is certainly postinfectious, patients with this type of bronchiectasis have had a recognized episode of infection that resulted in the development of bronchiectasis. Foremost among the postinfectious group is childhood bronchiectasis. The vast majority of cases can be traced to an episode of infection in early childhood. In one series 50 per cent of the patients indicated that their symptoms began before the age of three.[5] Other authors have reported that 65 to 70 per cent of bronchiectasis occurs before the age of 20.[21, 23] The etiologic factor in these children is generally bacterial pneumonia, but asthma, whooping cough, measles, and other contagious diseases may also be responsible.[8] The bronchiectasis that generally accompanies the Swyer-James (idiopathic hyperlucent lung)[28] or MacLeod (congenital hypoplasia of the pulmonary artery)[18] syndrome is thought to be secondary to an acute infection that occured in infancy or childhood.[9]

Although most bronchiectasis is associated with childhood pneumonia, adult pneumonia may also be a factor in the development of bronchiectasis. This is particularly likely when the pneumonia is necrotizing. It is a common cause of the development of bronchiectasis in the right middle lobe (right middle lobe syndrome) and lingula.[24]

Tuberculosis may also lead to bronchiectasis. Interestingly, tuberculous bronchiectasis generally does not require surgical management.[8] This may be due to the fact that it is usually in the upper lobes, allowing good postural drainage in the upright position.

The presence of a foreign body is an occasional etiologic factor in the development of obstructive pneumonia and subsequent bronchiectasis. This is much more frequent in children but can occur in adults, particularly in elderly people.

Congenital Bronchiectasis

Congenital bronchiectasis is a rare entity, and some authors doubt its existence. However, certain congenital diseases that cause defects in the supporting structures of the bronchi, abnormal secretions, or abnormal ciliary action definitely predispose to the development of bronchiectasis.[13] Included in this group are cystic fibrosis of the pancreas and Kartagener's syndrome (situs inversus, sinusitis, and bronchiectasis). Although in both of these conditions the bronchiectasis is acquired, it develops because of the congenital inability of patients with these diseases to handle bronchial secretions adequately.[7]

A common problem following lobectomy or segmentectomy for localized bronchiectasis is the development of bronchiectasis in segments that were previously found normal by bronchography.[12] This generally occurs in the absence of a documented infectious episode. Thus it seems that many people who acquire bronchiectasis have a congenital defect in the bronchial wall, which makes them more susceptible to this disease process.

Bronchiectasis in Immune-Related Diseases

Immune-related diseases are another cause of bronchiectasis. They can be divided into two major groups: immune deficiency syndromes and hypersensitivity states. The immune deficiency syndromes are marked by a deficiency of gamma globulin; they include both congenital and acquired agammaglobulinemia and dysgammaglobulinemia.[27] The most common hypersensitivity state is allergic aspergillosis, a complication of asthma.[30] This is characterized by severe elevations of IgA and by the presence of central, rather than peripheral, bronchiectasis. The entities that have in the past been called mucoid impaction of the bronchus[26] and plastic bronchitis[14] probably fall into this category.

PATHOLOGY

In a classic paper written in 1950, Reid described the pathologic characteristics of bronchiectasis and defined three classifications of the condition on the basis of the severity of bronchial dilatation and bronchiolar obliteration.[22] There is a close correlation between the pathologic description and the radiographic (bronchogram) findings.

Group 1 — Cylindric Bronchiectasis

In this classification, the bronchi are regular in outline, with a slight increase in their diameter distally; their lumina end squarely and abruptly. The smaller bronchi are frequently filled with purulent material and do not fill well with bronchographic contrast material (Fig. 19–77).

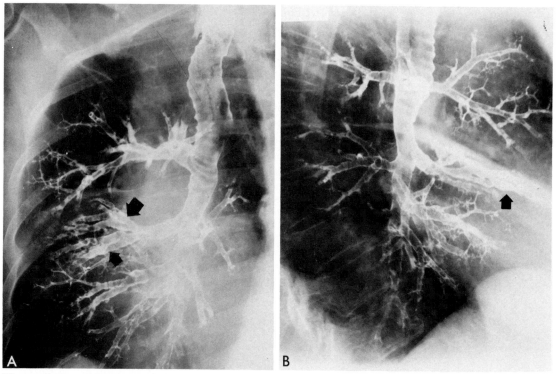

Figure 19–77. Cylindric bronchiectasis. Oblique (*A*) and lateral (*B*) films made following a bronchogram demonstrate cylindric bronchiectasis in the right middle lobe (arrows). The bronchi are widened, do not taper normally, and end abruptly. These changes are most obvious on the lateral film. There is also loss of volume of the right middle lobe and some consolidation of the right middle lobe secondary to chronic disease. Minimal bronchiectatic changes are noted in some of the right lower lobe bronchi.

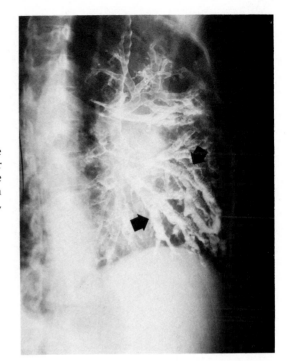

Figure 19–78. Varicose bronchiectasis. Extensive varicose bronchiectasis involves the lingula and lower lobe bronchi (arrows). There is dilatation of the bronchi, with irregular constriction of the lumina in multiple areas. The bronchi do not taper normally, and the smaller peripheral bronchi are not filled.

Group 2 — Varicose Bronchiectasis

The dilatation of the bronchi is greater in this group than in group I, and the outlines of the bronchi are irregular owing to local constrictions. There is obliteration of the lumina of the smaller peripheral bronchi by fibrous tissue (Fig. 19–78).

Group 3 — Saccular or Cystic Bronchiectasis

There is marked dilatation of the bronchi in this group, with extensive dilatation of the bronchial walls resulting in multiple cystlike enlargements of the bronchial tree. There is extensive obliteration of the peripheral bronchi by fibrosis (Fig. 19–79).

The elastic tissue of the bronchi involved by bronchiectasis and the muscular coats of the bronchial wall undergo destruction and are replaced by fibrous tissue. The degree of wall destruction and replacement by fibrous tissue becomes progressively greater as the condition progresses from cylindric to saccular.

Chronic inflammatory changes in the lung associated with bronchiectasis lead to the extreme enlargement of the bronchial arteries and to numerous anastomoses of these vessels with the pulmonary arteries in the diseased lung segments.[16] These pathologic findings explain the hemoptysis that is often a troublesome clinical symptom in patients with bronchiectasis.

CLINICAL FINDINGS

The characteristic clinical findings of bronchiectasis are cough and the production of purulent sputum. Hemoptysis occurs in approximately 50 per cent of older patients[9]

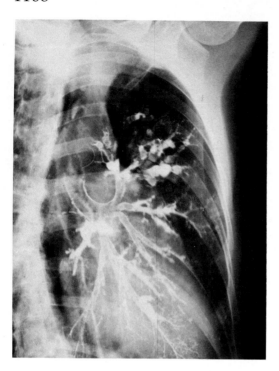

Figure 19–79. Saccular or cystic bronchiectasis. Cystic bronchiectasis involves the left upper lobe bronchi (arrows) in this patient with cystic fibrosis of the pancreas. The left upper lobe bronchi demonstrate cystic dilatation, with incomplete filling of the peripheral bronchi. Minimal changes are also noted in the lingula and in the superior and lateral basal segments of the left lower lobe.

and may occasionally be massive. Patients with advanced cases may acquire cor pulmonale[3] and, rarely, brain abscess or amyloidosis. Digital clubbing has been reported in up to 25 per cent of patients with bronchiectasis.[15]

Pulmonary function tests vary considerably. There is a high association of chronic bronchitis, and consequently it is often difficult to determine whether the altered pulmonary function is due to bronchiectasis or chronic bronchitis. Usually, mild disease causes little or no functional impairment. Patients with more advanced disease exhibit pulmonary function similar to obstructive disease, which is characterized by a decrease in the timed vital capacity, a reduction of diffusing capacity, an impairment in mixing, and an increase in the functional residual volume.[4]

As might be expected, radionuclide ventilation studies reveal uneven ventilation and air trapping, and radionuclide perfusion studies show diminution of perfusion in the involved segments.[1]

RADIOGRAPHIC FINDINGS

Although some authors have reported a high incidence of positive findings on the chest radiograph,[11] in most instances the plain film findings are either nonexistent or nonspecific. The exception is the chest radiograph of the patient with cystic bronchiectasis. This condition is almost invariably manifested radiographically by evidence of volume loss and a honeycomb pattern in the area of the involved lung segment (Fig. 19–80). Cylindric or varicose bronchiectasis may be exhibit volume loss of a lung segment and chronic stranding or patchy consolidation of that segment. These findings are nonspecific. Occasionally, the outlines of the dilated bronchi may be visible within a consolidated and partially atelectatic segment.

The diagnosis of bronchiectasis usually requires bronchography. Although fiberoptic bronchoscopy has largely replaced bronchography, bronchiectasis is still a solid indication for bronchography. It is important to avoid bronchography during or immediately after an episode of acute pneumonia, since postinflammatory changes secondary to pneumonia may simulate bronchiectasis on a bronchogram obtained at this time. This phenomenon has been called "reversible bronchiectasis" or "pseudo-bronchiectasis." These changes revert to normal in one to three months.[2, 19]

The bronchogram may be performed by introducing a catheter through the nose and glottis and into the tracheobronchial tree, or percutaneously through the cricothyroid membrane and into the tracheobronchial tree. The usual contrast medium is oily propyliodone (Dionosil). Careful demonstration of the bronchi of both lungs is necessary, particularly if surgical therapy of bronchiectasis is contemplated. All abnormal bronchi must be identified before a decision is made to proceed with surgical removal of the involved segments.

The pathologic changes of tubular, varicose, and saccular bronchiectasis described by Reid can all be demonstrated bronchographically (see Figs. 19–77 to 19–79). It is important to fill the small peripheral bronchi during bronchography, since the clubbed appearance of cylindric bronchiectasis may be simulated by incompletely filled bronchi.

TREATMENT

Diffuse bronchiectasis is best treated medically with postural drainage and antibiotics for exacerbations.[8] Expectorants and the cessation of smoking may also be useful.

Localized bronchiectasis may be treated surgically. The following are the indications for surgery outlined by Lindskog and Hubbell: (1) symptoms of a degree sufficient to cause discomfort, inconvenience, or complications; (2) the existence of localized

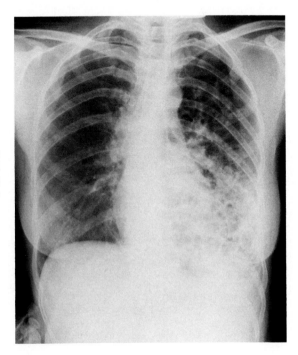

Figure 19–80. Cystic bronchiectasis. Multiple cystlike areas are seen in the left lower lung field and left midlung field (honeycomb lung). These cystic changes represent the cystic dilatation of the bronchi. The right lung is normal.

bronchiectatic changes conclusively demonstrated by bronchography; (3) an adequate cardiorespiratory reserve; and (4) the absence of concurrent disease of a magnitude to contraindicate major surgery.[17] The results are best when surgery is performed for the correction of localized unilateral disease, but the surgical treatment of bilateral disease has good results in some cases. Occasionally, operation on the most severely involved side of patients with bilateral disease results in the cessation of symptoms, so that the contralateral disease does not require resection.[25]

Sealy et al. reported that 80 per cent of patients with localized bronchiectasis were relieved of all symptoms following surgery and 36 per cent of those with multisegmental disease were symptom-free after surgery.[25] However, in a long-term follow-up, Field observed little difference between the condition of the patients who had been treated medically and that of the patients whose bronchiectasis had been treated surgically.[8] This suggests that the long-term results of surgical therapy for bronchiectasis may not be as favorable as other authors have reported. Certainly, patients with extensive disease are best treated medically. Those patients who are symptomatic owing to localized disease may do well with surgical therapy.

References

1. Bass, H., Henderson, J. A. M., Heckscher, T., et al.: Regional structures and function in bronchiectasis. A correlative study using bronchography and ^{133}Xe. Am. Rev. Respir. Dis. 97:598–609, 1968.
2. Blades, B., and Dugan, D. J.: Pseudobronchiectasis. J. Thorac. Surg. 13:40–48, 1944.
3. Campbell, G. S.: Bronchiectasis. In Sabiston, D. C., Jr. (ed.): Davis-Christopher Textbook of Surgery. Ed. 11. Philadelphia, W. B. Saunders Company, 1977, p. 2098.
4. Cherniack, N. S., and Carton, R. W.: Factors associated with respiratory insufficiency in bronchiectasis. Am. J. Med. 41:562–571, 1966.
5. Clark, N. S.: Bronchiectasis in childhood. Br. Med. J. 1:80–88, 1963.
6. Croxatto, O. C., and Lanari, A.: Pathogenesis of bronchiectasis. Experimental study and anatomic findings. J. Thorac. Surg. 27:514–528, 1954.
7. Culiner, M. M.: Intralobar bronchial cystic disease, "the sequestration complex" and cystic bronchiectasis. Dis. Chest 53:462, 1968.
8. Field, C. E.: Bronchiectasis. Third report on a follow-up study of medical and surgical cases from childhood. Arch. Dis. Child. 44:551, 1979.
9. Fraser, R., and Paré, J. A. P.: Diagnosis of the Diseases of the Chest. Philadelphia, W. B. Saunders Company, 1970, p. 1044.
10. Glauser, E. M., Cook, C. D., and Harris, G. B. C.: Bronchiectasis: a review of 187 cases in children with follow-up pulmonary function studies in 58. Acta Paediatr. Scand. (Suppl.) 165, 1, 1966.
11. Gudbjerg, C. E.: Bronchiectasis. Radiological diagnosis and prognosis after operative treatment. Acta Radiol. (Suppl.) 143:1–146, 1957.
12. Helm, W. H., and Thompson, V. C.: The long term results of resection for bronchiectasis. Quart. J. Med. 27:353, 1958.
13. Hentel, W. L., Longfield, A. N., and Gordon, J.: A re-evaluation of bronchiectasis using fume fixation. 1. The bronchoalveolar structure: a preliminary study. Dis. Chest 41:41–45, 1962.
14. Johnson, R. S., and Sita-Lumsden, E. G.: Plastic bronchitis. Thorax 15:325–332, 1960.
15. Laurenzi, G. A.: A critical reappraisal of bronchiectasis. Med. Times 98:89, 1970.
16. Liebow, A. A., Hales, M. R., and Lindskog, G. E.: Enlargement of the bronchial arteries and their anastomoses with the pulmonary arteries in bronchiectasis. Am. J. Pathol. 25:211–231, 1949.
17. Lindskog, G. E.., and Hubbell, D. S.: An analysis of 215 cases of bronchiectasis. Surg. Gynecol. Obstet. 100:643–650, 1955.
18. MacLeod, W. M.: Abnormal transradiancy of one lung. Thorax 9:147–153, 1954.
19. Nelson, S. W., and Christoforidis, A.: Reversible bronchiectasis. Radiology 71:375–382, 1958.
20. Nissen, R., and Wilson, R. H. L.: Pages in the History of Chest Surgery. Springfield, Illinois, Charles C Thomas, Publisher, 1960, p. 35.
21. Perry, K. M. A., and King, D. S.: Bronchiectasis: a study of prognosis based on a follow-up of 400 patients. Am. Rev. Tuberculosis 41:531–548, 1940.
22. Reid, L. M.: Reduction in bronchial subdivision in bronchiectasis. Thorax 5:233–247, 1950.
23. Riggins, H. M.: Bronchiectasis; morbidity and mortality of medically treated patients. Am. J. Surg. 54:50–67, 1941.

24. Sanderson, J. M., Kennedy, M. C. S., Johnson, M. F., et al.: Bronchiectasis: results of surgical and conservative management, a review of 393 cases. Thorax 29:407–416, 1974.
25. Sealy, W. C., Bradham, R. R., and Young, W. G., Jr.; The surgical treatment of multisegmental and localized bronchiectasis. Surg. Gynecol. Obstet. 123:80–90, 1966.
26. Shaw, R. R.: Mucoid impaction of bronchi. Thorac. Surg. 22:149–163, 1951.
27. Suhs, R. H., Dowling, H. F., and Jackson, G. G.: Hypogammaglobulinemia with chronic bronchitis or bronchiectasis. Treatment of five patients with long term antibiotic therapy. Arch. Intern. Med. 116:29–38, 1965.
28. Swyer, P. R., and James, G. C. W.: A case of unilateral pulmonary emphysema. Thorax 8:133–136, 1953.
29. Tannenberg, J., Pinner, M., and Hills, B.: Atelectasis and bronchiectasis. An experimental study concerning their relationship. J. Thorac. Surg. 11:571, 1962.
30. Zimmerman, R. A., and Miller, W. T.: Pulmonary aspergillosis. Am. J. Roentgenol. 109:505–517, 1970.

Part VI

The Surgical Treatment of Pulmonary Tuberculosis; Radiologic Aspects

ROBERT A. CLARK, M.D.
DAVID P. COLLEY, M.D.
JEROME F. WIOT, M.D.

Pulmonary tuberculosis is a disease treated primarily by chemotherapy, since modern antituberculosis drugs are effective. Surgical therapy is usually reserved for cases of medical treatment failure or the complications of chronic disease. The various radiographic appearances of tuberculosis remain important to the surgeon in order to define those cases requiring surgery and to recognize postoperative complications.

HISTORICAL ASPECTS: COLLAPSE THERAPY

Before the advent of effective chemotherapy, the active treatment of pulmonary tuberculosis was directed toward putting the affected lung at rest or collapsing it mechanically. Collapse therapy was primarily directed toward the compression or obliteration of cavities.

Attempts to put the lung at rest consisted of producing paralysis of the diaphragm by crushing the phrenic nerve (Fig. 19–81), or decreasing diaphragmatic motion by the repeated production of pneumoperitoneum (Fig. 19–82). The latter method required the periodic intraperitoneal injection of air and was never considered truly effective.

Collapse therapy included induced pneumothorax, extrapleural compression by inert substances (plombage), and surgical thoracoplasty. Pneumothorax therapy frequently failed because pleural-parenchymal adhesions often prevented adequate collapse. Plombage consisted of filling the extrapleural space — between the ribs and the pleura — with a sufficient volume of inert material to collapse the adjacent lung. When plastic (lucite) spheres were used, characteristic multiple perfectly round, cavity-like lucencies were seen on the radiograph (Fig. 19–83). These spheres were often not entirely watertight, and small amounts of fluid sometimes collected in each sphere (Fig. 19–84), simulating infection and tissue breakdown in the view of the uninitiated.

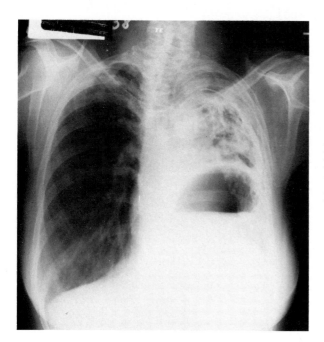

Figure 19–81. Phrenic crush. The left diaphragm is paralyzed and elevated following a surgical crushing of the left phrenic nerve. This greatly limits excursion of the diseased left upper lobe and helps promote healing.

Figure 19–82. Marked elevation of both hemidiaphragms (arrows) following instillation of intraperitoneal air as collapse therapy.

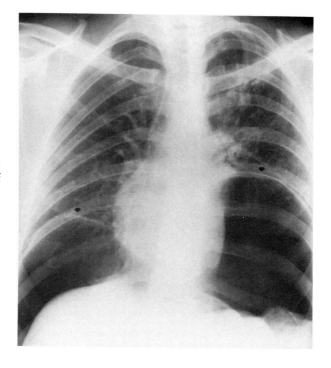

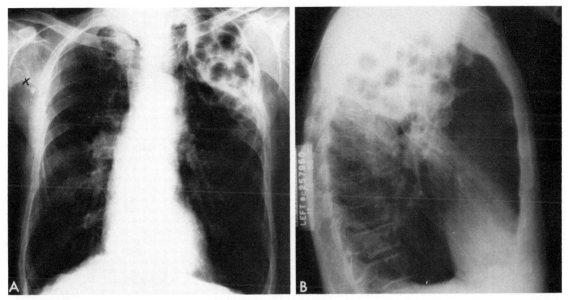

Figure 19–83. *A* and *B,* Extrapleural plombage. The round lucencies in the left upper thorax are lucite balls inserted extrapleurally.

Plombage with paraffin (oleothorax) produced a water-density extrapleural mass, although late calcification could occur (Fig. 19–85*A*). Rarely, a bronchoextrapleural fistula was a late complication of oleothorax (Fig. 19–85*B*). This was due to either the reactivation of the tuberculosis or the direct erosion of a bronchus by the paraffin.

The most popular procedure was surgical thoracoplasty. This consisted of the removal of multiple ribs and the collapse of the chest wall and the affected lung, producing a characteristic deformity (Fig. 19–86). The evaluation of disease activity in the collapsed upper lobe required tomography.

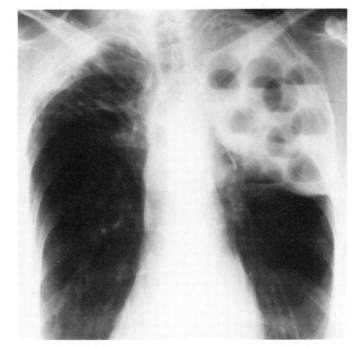

Figure 19–84. The varying fluid levels and "ping-pong ball" appearance of plastic sphere plombage are characteristic.

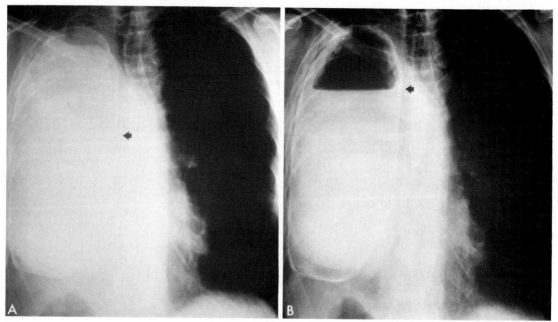

Figure 19–85. *A*, Calcified rim of extrapleural paraffin plombage (arrow). *B*, The large air-fluid level indicates a complicating broncho-extrapleural fistula (arrow), which developed several years later.

Because many patients who have undergone these procedures are still encountered, the recognition of the radiographic appearances is important.

RADIOGRAPHIC TECHNIQUES

The posteroanterior and lateral radiographs are the basic projections necessary to evaluate the chest. Special techniques, such as lordotic views, fluoroscopy, and

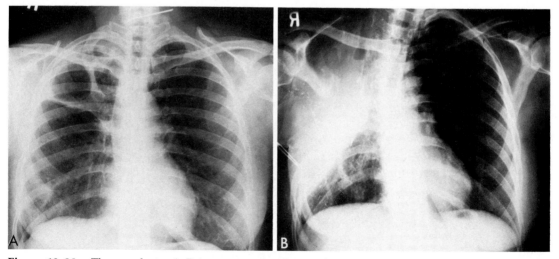

Figure 19–86. Thoracoplasty. *A*, Prior to surgery, a large tuberculous cavity is seen in the right upper lobe. *B*, After thoracoplasty, there is a characteristic deformity of the chest wall with compression of the right upper lobe.

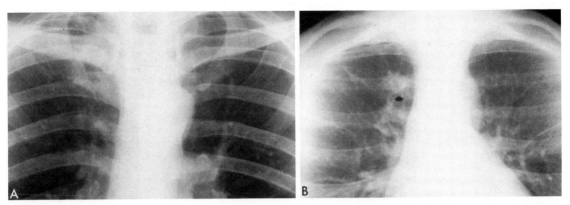

Figure 19–87. *A,* A subtle increase in density posterior to the head of the right clavicle may be overlooked or ignored on the standard frontal projection. *B,* The lordotic view displaces the clavicle superiorly, clearly revealing the underlying right apical density (arrow).

tomography, are helpful to more effectively visualize lesions suspected on the standard chest radiographs.

Since pulmonary tuberculosis so often involves the lung apices, lesions may be obscured by overlying ribs or clavicle in the standard views. The lordotic projection of the chest, which is produced by angling the x-ray beam cephalad in the anteroposterior direction, may more clearly demonstrate these apical lesions (Fig. 19–87).

Fluoroscopy also can be used to rotate lesions away from overlying bones for better visualization. In addition, mediastinal lymph node enlargement can be determined if barium esophagography is performed at the time of fluoroscopy.

Tomography is an excellent technique for the evaluation of tuberculous lesions. This technique may be used to evaluate cavity detail in the presence of surrounding fibrosis and contraction (Fig. 19–88). Likewise, calcifications or air bronchograms

Figure 19–88. An intracavitary fungal ball (aspergilloma) is outlined tomographically in the left upper lobe (arrow).

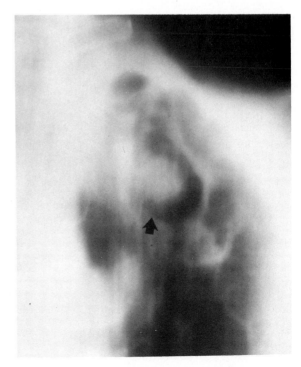

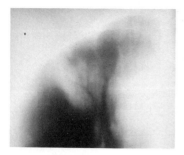

Figure 19–89. Well-defined air bronchogram is seen in an otherwise solid right upper lobe density on this tomographic image. This finding virtually excludes neoplasm. This lesion proved to be active tuberculosis. Enlarged mediastinal nodes are also present.

within mass lesions are demonstrated best by tomography (Fig. 19–89). Diagnostically this is important, since the presence of either calcium or an air bronchogram within a mass virtually excludes the possibility of malignancy.

Although it has been utilized successfully in the past to image bronchial abnormalities, bronchography is rarely performed in cases of tuberculosis today. Tomography and, occasionally, bronchoscopy are usually sufficient to visualize bronchial stenosis, obstruction, or bronchiectasis.

Preoperative Diagnosis

Primary tuberculosis is characterized by a small pulmonary infiltrate, which may involve any area of the lung. This pneumonic process drains via the lymphatics, which appear as linear densities, into enlarged hilar lymph nodes. The pulmonary infiltrate and the enlarged nodes compose the "primary complex" (Fig. 19–90). Healing may result in the complete clearing of the pulmonary lesions or may leave a nodule (tubercle), which may calcify. Occasionally the lymph node enlargement may persist (Fig. 19–91).

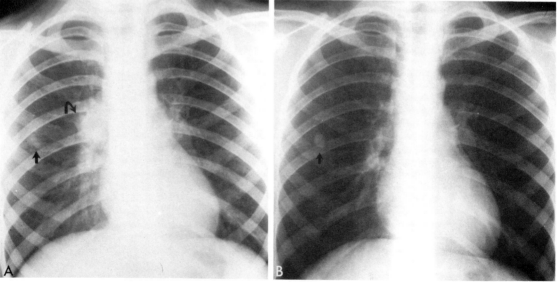

Figure 19–90. *A,* Regional lymphadenitis in the right hilum (curved arrow) with an associated peripheral infiltrate (straight arrow) constitute the "primary (Ghon) complex" in this patient. *B,* Four years later, the lymph node enlargement has disappeared and the peripheral infiltrate (arrow) has become smaller, now containing tiny flecks of calcification.

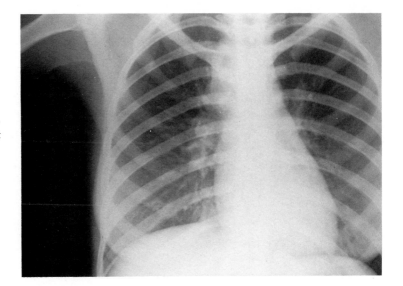

Figure 19–91. Persistent para-tracheal lymph node enlargement from tuberculosis.

Reinfection tuberculosis is characterized by upper lobe involvement, often with caseation, necrosis, and fibrosis. Lobar consolidation occurs, and multiple lobe involvement is frequent (Fig. 19–92). The process is typically progressive and often leads to cavitation. The cavities are round or irregular and usually have thick walls (Fig. 19–93*A*). Fluid levels are infrequent. Thin-walled cavities are more often seen with the atypical mycobacteria and may be confused with emphysematous blebs (Fig. 19–93*B*).

Adequately treated reinfection tuberculosis usually heals, leaving residual nodules and fibrous strands (Fig. 19–94). Fibrous contraction collapse of a lobe or segment may also occur. The organisms can remain dormant, however, particularly with inadequate therapy, and recavitation may occur.

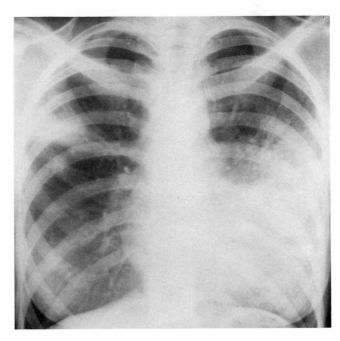

Figure 19–92. Minimal right upper lobe involvement, but extensive left lower lobe and lingular consolidation, are characteristic of multilobular tuberculosis.

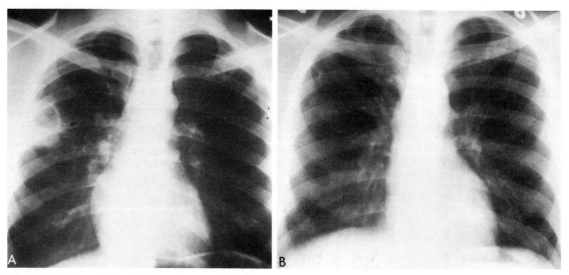

Figure 19–93. *A,* Air-fluid level seen in thick-walled (arrow) tuberculous cavity. *B,* Contrast the pencil-sharp, thin-walled right apical pleural cavity with the cavity demonstrated in *A.* This was secondary to *Mycobacterium kansasii.*

Miliary tuberculosis is an acute tuberculous reinfection characterized by numerous nodules, 3 to 5 mm in size, spread throughout the lungs (Fig. 19–95). The lesions are exudative and may clear rapidly with drug treatment.

Indications for Resection

None of the types of tuberculosis discussed previously require surgical therapy. Certain radiographic appearances of reinfection tuberculosis are indications for surgery in the proper clinical setting, however.

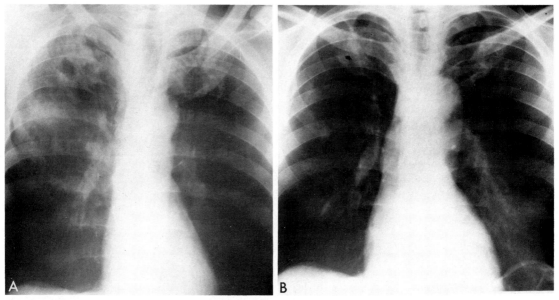

Figure 19–94. *A,* Bilateral apical acute tuberculosis was treated adequately. *B,* Three years later, fibrous scarring and apical nodules (arrow) remain.

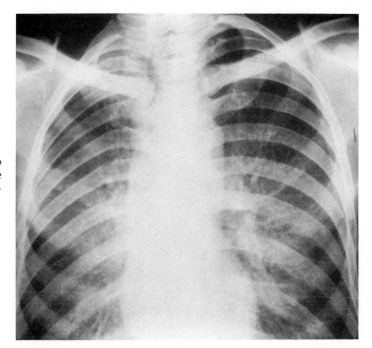

Figure 19–95. Bilateral diffuse, 3- to 5-mm nodules are seen throughout the lung parenchyma in this case of miliary tuberculosis.

Persistent cavitary disease with positive sputum smears despite adequate chemotherapy is a recognized indication for surgery (Fig. 19–96). The presence of cavities can be best demonstrated using tomography. The two most likely causes of persistent cavitary disease are atypical mycobacteria and drug-resistant organisms.

Recurrent hemoptysis requiring resection may result from several sources. Caseating tuberculous pneumonia may erode blood vessels directly. An eroded blood vessel

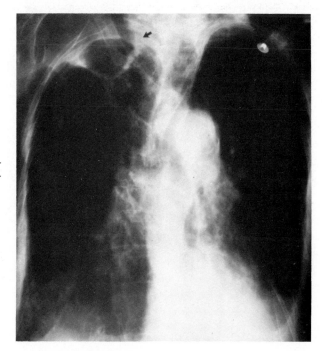

Figure 19–96. This apical cavity (arrow) persisted with positive sputum smears despite adequate triple-drug chemotherapy.

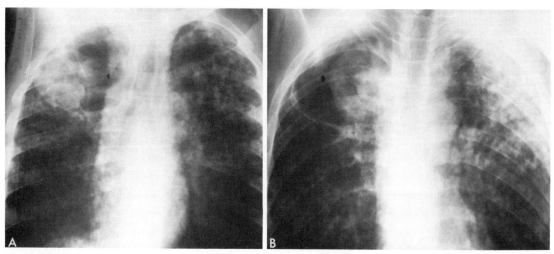

Figure 19–97. *A* and *B*, Right and left lateral decubitus views clearly demonstrate the mobility of the large irregular mass (arrows) in an old tuberculous cavity. At operation this was found to be clotted blood.

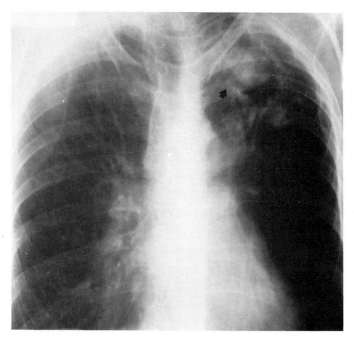

Figure 19–98. Intracavitary *Aspergillus* fungal ball (arrow) associated with hemoptysis.

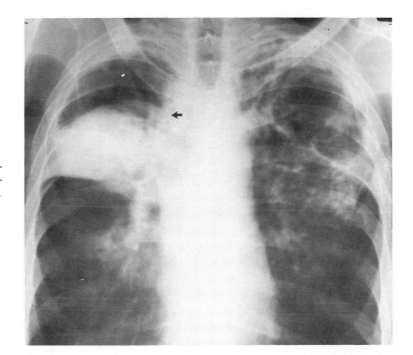

Figure 19–99. A surgically verified fungal ball floating in an intracavitary hemorrhage (arrow).

may hemorrhage into a pre-existing cavity (Fig. 19–97) the clot forming a mobile mass lesion within the cavity. The acute appearance of such a mass should suggest the diagnosis. The differential diagnosis includes an intracavitary fungal ball, which may also be associated with hemoptysis (Fig. 19–98). A fungal ball and hemorrhage may coexist, resulting in an intracavitary mass and fluid level (Fig. 19–99). Broncholithiasis also may be associated with hemoptysis and is most accurately identified by tomography.

Lobar or segmental collapse requiring resection may result from fibrotic contraction or bronchial obstruction. Broncholithiasis and endobronchial tuberculosis are obstructing lesions that are best demonstrated by tomography (Fig. 19–100).

Spontaneous bronchopleural fistula, pneumothorax, pleural effusion, and empyema are other complications that can be identified radiographically and that may require surgical therapy (Fig. 19–101).

Pulmonary mass lesions without central calcifications must be resected to exclude malignancy (Fig. 19–102). The enlargement or growth of a mass lesion is not always indicative of neoplasm. A granuloma with central calcification can enlarge (Fig. 19–103).

Postoperative Complications

The appearance of the chest following resection for tuberculosis is similar to that following any other lung resection. Certain complications are more specific following resection for tuberculosis, however, and their radiographic recognition is important.

A recurrent infiltrate or cavitation following surgery is usually the result of the bronchogenic spread of organisms (Fig. 19–104). The typical pathologic appearances of reinfection tuberculosis may ensue.

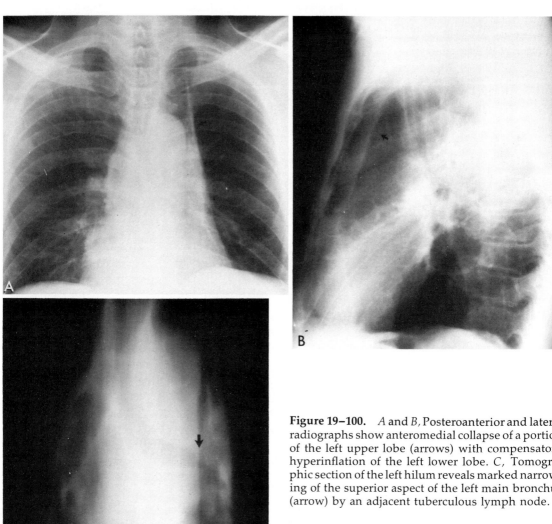

Figure 19–100. *A* and *B,* Posteroanterior and lateral radiographs show anteromedial collapse of a portion of the left upper lobe (arrows) with compensatory hyperinflation of the left lower lobe. *C,* Tomographic section of the left hilum reveals marked narrowing of the superior aspect of the left main bronchus (arrow) by an adjacent tuberculous lymph node.

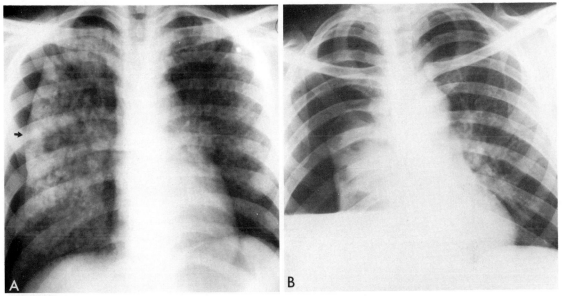

Figure 19–101. *A,* Typical widespread pattern of multiple small (3- to 5-mm) miliary nodules with associated spontaneous pneumothorax (arrow). *B,* Large pneumothorax with collapsed right lung and tuberculous empyema seen as a fluid level.

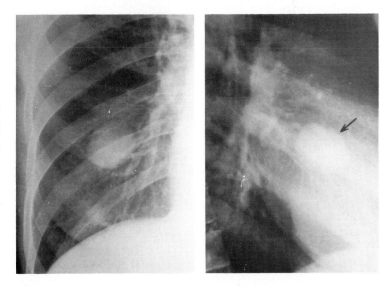

Figure 19–102. A noncalcified right middle lobe nodule (arrow) removed surgically proved to be a healed tuberculous nodule. This type of nodule cannot be distinguished from neoplasm radiographically.

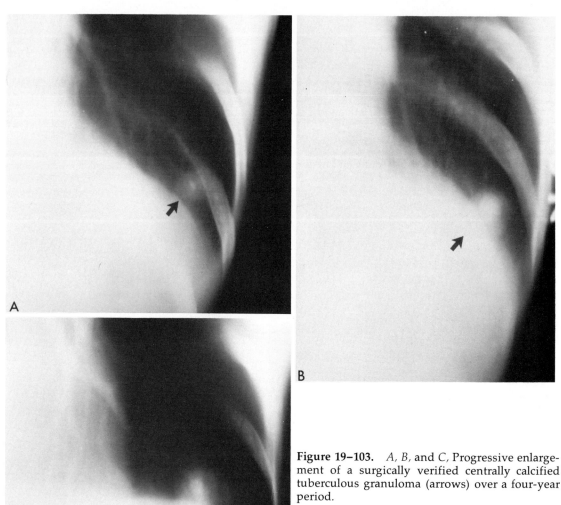

Figure 19–103. *A, B,* and *C,* Progressive enlargement of a surgically verified centrally calcified tuberculous granuloma (arrows) over a four-year period.

Empyema occurs with or without bronchopleural fistula. A persistent hemithorax air space and persistent subcutaneous emphysema respectively signal bronchopleural or bronchopleural-cutaneous fistulas (Fig. 19–105). Bronchopleural fistulas may be demonstrated directly by bronchography, with contrast material communicating with the pleural space (Fig. 19–106). Alternatively, contrast material instilled through a thoracostomy tube into the pleural space may communicate with bronchi (Fig. 19–107). The direct demonstration of the fistula aids in the planning of the surgical approach.

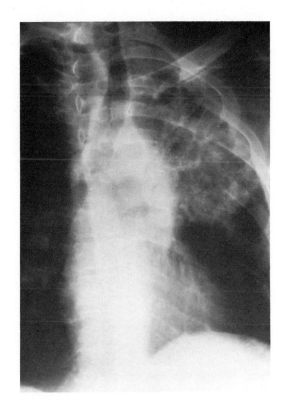

Figure 19–104. Extensive left upper lobe destruction due to tuberculous cavitation in a patient who had previously undergone a partial left upper lobe resection (note surgical sutures).

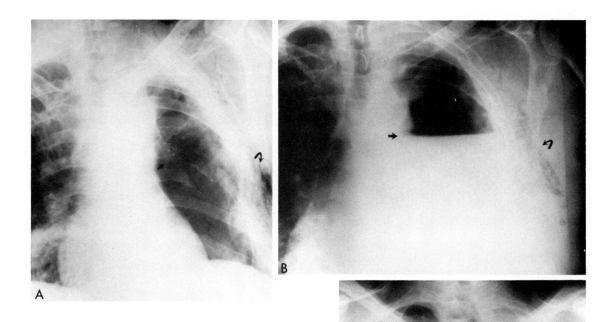

Figure 19–105. *A,* Subcutaneous air (curved arrow) outlines a portion of the pectoralis muscle in this post-surgical patient with a bronchopleural-cutaneous fistula (straight arrow). *B,* Twenty-four hours later hydrothorax develops (straight arrow) with persistent subcutaneous emphysema (curved arrow). *C,* Two weeks later a persistent, loculated hydropneumothorax (arrows) persists owing to a bronchopleural fistula.

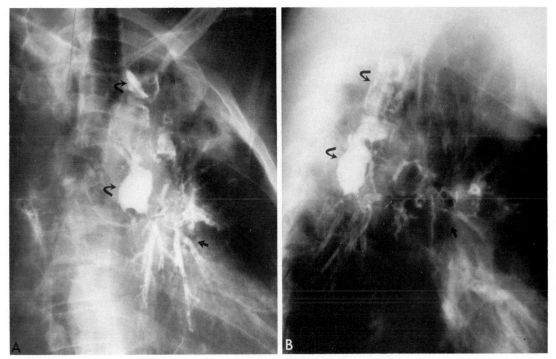

Figure 19–106. *A* and *B*, Bronchography demonstrates leakage of contrast material into the pleural space (curved arrows) as well as normal bronchi (straight arrow).

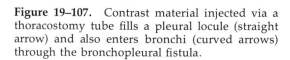

Figure 19–107. Contrast material injected via a thoracostomy tube fills a pleural locule (straight arrow) and also enters bronchi (curved arrows) through the bronchopleural fistula.

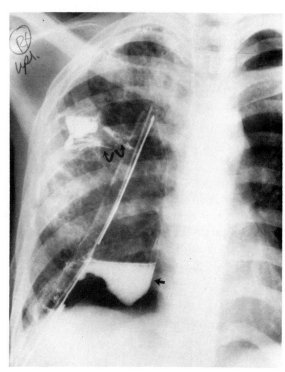

References

1. DeLarue, N. C., and Gale, G.: Surgical salvage in pulmonary tuberculosis. Ann. Thorac. Surg. *18*:38–51, 1974.
2. McLaughlin, J. S., and Hankins, J. R.: Current aspects of surgery for pulmonary tuberculosis. Ann. Thorac. Surg. *17*:513–525, 1974.
3. Seibert, C. E., and Tabrisky, J.: Lucite extraperiosteal plombage. Roentgenologic review of late complications. Am. J. Roentgenol. *100*:593–596, 1967.
4. Steele, J. D.: The surgical treatment of pulmonary tuberculosis. Ann. Thorac. Surg. *6*:484–502, 1968.
5. Wiot, J. F., and Spitz, H. B.: Pulmonary tuberculosis. *In* Potchen, E. J. et al. (eds.): Principles of Diagnostic Radiology. New York, McGraw-Hill, Inc., 1971.

Part VII
Tracheobronchial Tumors and Tumorlike Conditions

W. RICHARD WEBB, M.D.
GORDON GAMSU, M.D.

A large variety of tumors, both benign and malignant, arise within the tracheobronchial tree. Although certain lesions have a characteristic radiographic appearance, which often leads to a correct diagnosis, tumors differing histologically can present with identical radiographic features if they involve similar portions of the respiratory tract.

In this section, the radiographic diagnosis of tumors occurring in the trachea, large central bronchi, and peripheral bronchi and bronchioles is discussed, with emphasis on the features that various tumors share regardless of their cell type. For each of these three locations, there is a discussion of the radiographic methods useful in detecting neoplastic lesions, the frequency of the major radiographic findings, and some general radiographic signs of value in distinguishing certain tumors. In general, the symptoms, the methods used for diagnosis, and the treatment depend more on the tumor's location than on its histologic makeup.[96]

THE NORMAL TRACHEA

Anatomically, the trachea is relatively short, measuring 10 or 11 cm in length.[65] It extends inferiorly from the cricoid cartilage at the level of the sixth cervical vertebra to the carina at the upper margin of the fifth thoracic vertebral body.[65] Often the inferior surfaces of the opposed vocal cords are visible on frontal radiographs taken during breath holding; the trachea begins approximately 1 cm below these subglottic "shoulders," which provide an excellent radiographic landmark (Fig. 19–108).

Radiographically, the tracheal walls are parallel, except for smooth indentions on the left at the level of the aortic arch and on the right at the tracheobronchial angle caused by the azygous vein. The tracheal diameter ranges from 11 to 30 mm in adults, averaging 17.5 mm on posteroanterior radiographs and 19.5 mm on lateral radiographs.[52] The trachea is supported by 16 to 20 cartilaginous "rings," which are incomplete posteriorly and most accurately described as C-shaped.[65] These rings give a

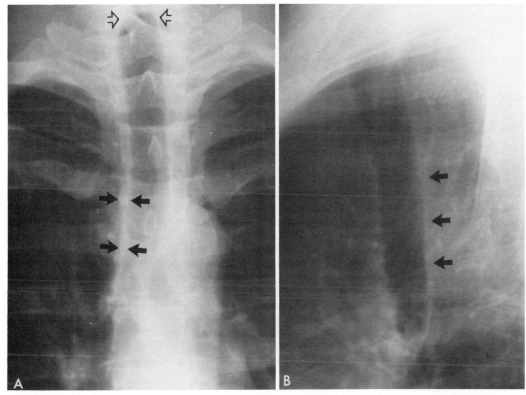

Figure 19–108.   Normal trachea. *A,* On the posteroanterior radiograph, the trachea begins 1 cm below the well-defined subglottic "shoulders" (open arrows), and the right paratracheal stripe, representing a combination of tracheal wall, mediastinal contents, and pleura, is clearly seen (closed arrows) below the thoracic inlet. *B,* Serration of the tracheal wall, due to impressions made by the tracheal rings, is present anteriorly on the lateral radiograph. A normal posterior paratracheal stripe is also seen (arrows). Both paratracheal stripes usually measure less than 3 mm in width.

serrated contour to the tracheal air column, most apparent anteriorly on the lateral radiograph (see Fig. 19–108).

The tracheal wall itself is visualized radiographically as a discrete structure, or "stripe," of soft tissue density in two areas; in both, air within the adjacent lung provides the necessary radiographic contrast. The right paratracheal stripe is most helpful in diagnosing tracheal lesions. It is seen on frontal radiographs above the azygous vein and below the clavicle and is made up of the tracheal wall, mediastinal contents, and pleura (see Fig. 19–108).[130] In a large majority of normal patients, the right paratracheal stripe measures 3 mm or less.

The posterior paratracheal stripe or band is seen above the carina on the lateral film (see Fig. 19–108).[8, 136] In addition to the tracheal wall, the pleura and the esophagus make up this density; it normally measures 3 to 3.5 mm in width.[8, 136]

Although thickening of either stripe may reflect an abnormality of lung, pleura, or mediastinal structures (Fig. 19–109), the possibility of a tracheal lesion must be considered in the differential diagnosis.

TRACHEAL TUMORS

Primary neoplasms of the trachea are rare and occur much less frequently than tumors of laryngeal or bronchial origin.[88] In adults, malignant lesions of the trachea are

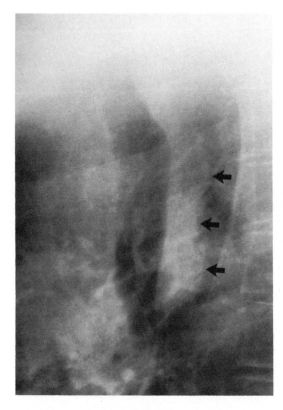

Figure 19–109. Thickened posterior paratracheal stripe. A mass is visible on this lateral radiograph narrowing the upper trachea from behind, and the posterior paratracheal stripe (arrows) measures more than 1 cm in width. Both the mass lesion and the thickened paratracheal stripe are the result of the invasion of the tracheal wall by an esophageal carcinoma.

slightly more common than benign tumors or tumorlike conditions. In a series of 503 tracheal tumors diagnosed in adults, 273 (54 per cent) were malignant and 230 (46 per cent) were benign.[56] In children, more than 90 per cent of tracheal tumors are benign.[56]

Malignant Tumors

Carcinomas account for 80 to 90 per cent of tracheal malignancies.[56, 79] Most frequent are squamous cell carcinoma, derived from tracheal epithelium, and adenoid cystic carcinoma (cylindroma) arising from mucous glands in the tracheal wall. In a

TABLE 19–2. THE RELATIVE FREQUENCY OF MALIGNANT TRACHEAL TUMORS*

Tumor	Number	Percentage
Epithelial origin		
Squamous cell carcinoma	24	45.2
Small cell undifferentiated carcinoma	2	3.8
Adenocarcinoma	1	1.9
Mucous gland origin		
Adenoid-cystic carcinoma	19	35.8
Mucoepidermoid carcinoma	1	1.9
Mesenchymal origin		
Leiomyosarcoma	3	5.7
Lymphoma	2	3.8
Plasmacytoma	1	1.9
Total	53	100.0

*Modified from Houston, H. E., Payne, W. S., Harrison, E. G., Jr., and Olsen, A. M.: Primary cancers of the trachea. Arch. Surg. 99:132–139, 1969.

study by Houston, 24 (51 per cent) of 47 tracheal carcinomas were squamous cell lesions, and 19 (40 per cent) were adenoid cystic carcinomas (Table 19–2).[79] Other series show squamous cell carcinoma to be more common, accounting for 67 to 73 per cent of malignant tracheal tumors.[69, 82, 88] Sarcomas arising in the mesenchymal elements of the tracheal wall, lymphoma, and plasmacytoma make up 11 to 18 per cent of tracheal malignancies.[56, 79]

Benign Tracheal Tumors

A large variety of benign conditions involve the trachea, but in a majority of cases, benign tracheal lesions are not truly neoplastic but inflammatory (polyps, scleroma), infiltrative (amyloidosis), or perhaps degenerative (tracheobronchopathia osteochondroplastica).[51, 56] In adults, osteochondromas (tracheobronchopathia osteochondroplastica) predominate, accounting for 30 per cent of benign lesions, followed by papillomas (18 per cent), and fibromas (13 per cent).[56] In children, papillomas account for nearly 60 per cent of benign tumors; fibromas and angiomas make up 23 per cent and 15 per cent respectively.[56] Other tracheal tumors include chondroma, hamartoma, leiomyoma, granular cell myoblastoma, and lipoma, none of which is common.[51, 56, 88, 103]

Clinical Diagnosis

The symptoms of tracheal tumor are nonspecific and can mimic a variety of diseases. Most symptoms are related to airway obstruction.[56, 88] Cough occurs in 33 to 85 per cent of patients, hemoptysis in 27 to 66 per cent, and dyspnea in 20 to 73 per cent.[69, 79, 88] Weight loss and dysphagia suggest malignancy.[69, 88]

The delay in diagnosis following the onset of symptoms averages ten months[88] and, not surprisingly, tends to be longer in patients with slow-growing or benign tumors. Furthermore, intratracheal masses can grow to a large size before symptoms become evident, and 50 to 75 per cent of the tracheal lumen must be occluded before wheezing and dyspnea are noted.[51] Tumors located in the proximal trachea can cause laryngeal dysfunction and hoarseness; hoarseness occurs in 13 to 27 per cent of patients with tracheal neoplasm.[69, 79] Lower tracheal tumors may prolapse into the right or left main bronchi, causing pulmonary collapse or obstructive pneumonitis.[56]

Pulmonary function tests are of value in defining airway obstruction in patients with tracheal neoplasm. In particular, the performance of flow-volume loops can be extremely helpful.[53] Contrary to forced vital-capacity maneuvers, in which air flow is measured in relation to time, flow-volume curves measure the rate of flow relative to the lung volume level at which flow is occurring. In the absence of emphysema and chronic bronchitis, flow-volume loops are sensitive to obstruction of large airways and are accurate in determining the severity and location of tracheal lesions.[53]

Radiographic Diagnosis

ROUTINE CHEST RADIOGRAPHS. These are of limited value in the detection of tracheal tumors.[51, 82, 88] The penetration of the mediastinum on standard posteroanterior radiographs is often insufficient to allow adequate visualization of the tracheal lumen, and on the lateral view only the lower trachea is well seen. In a study by Karlan et al. of 11 patients with tracheal tumors (Table 19–2), routine posteroanterior and lateral radiographs were interpreted as being prospectively abnormal in only four cases.[88] In none of these four was an endotracheal mass lesion detected on the frontal radiograph,

TABLE 19–3. RADIOGRAPHIC DIAGNOSIS OF TRACHEAL TUMORS IN 11 PATIENTS*

Examination	Number	Abnormal	Number with Normal Routine Examination
Routine	11	4	—
High KVP technique	7	6	4
Oblique	2	2	1
Thoracic inlet	3	2	1
Lateral cervical soft tissues	1	1	1
Tomography	8	8	7

*Modified from Karlan, M. S., Livingston, P. A., and Baker, D. C., Jr.: Diagnosis of tracheal tumors. Ann. Otol. Rhinol. Laryngol. *82:*790–799, 1973.

and in three cases a mediastinal mass was the sole radiographic abnormality. Endotracheal mass lesions visible on routine radiographs may be overlooked, however, if the entire tracheal shadow is not carefully examined.[82] In 5 of Karlan's 11 patients, an endotracheal mass was seen when films were viewed retrospectively.

HIGH-KILOVOLTAGE (KVP) RADIOGRAPHS. In the posteroanterior projection, these allow better penetration of the dense mediastinum than is possible on standard radiographs.[88] Many institutions now use the high-kilovoltage technique exclusively for chest radiographs. In Karlan's study, six of seven high-kilovoltage examinations had abnormal findings.[88] Even with high-kilovoltage technique, however, overlying structures may obscure tracheal detail.

OBLIQUE VIEWS. Oblique views of the chest project the trachea away from obscuring mediastinal structures, particularly the spine, and are often helpful in visualizing endotracheal lesions (see Table 19–3).

CONED-DOWN VIEWS. Coned-down views of the thoracic inlet and cervical soft tissues assist in the diagnosis of proximal tracheal tumors (see Table 19–3).

TOMOGRAPHY. In the posteroanterior or lateral projection, this is perhaps the most valuable standard radiographic study for the diagnosis of tracheal masses.[51, 82, 88, 107] Tomography is accurate and easy to perform and results in no morbidity. In a series reported by Houston et al. only 13 (24 per cent) of 53 tracheal tumors were visible on routine chest examination.[79] Tomography was performed in 18 cases, however, and was of diagnostic assistance in 16; in 13 of the 16 cases of abnormal tomograms, the routine radiographs had been considered normal. Similar figures were reported by Karlan (see Table 19–3).[88]

PLAIN XEROGRAPHY OR XEROTOMOGRAPHY. These techniques assist further in the diagnosis of tracheal tumors; the greater latitude, contrast, and edge enhancement permitted by xeroradiography allow excellent visualization of small tracheal masses, which is not possible with conventional means.[72]

POSITIVE-CONTRAST TRACHEOGRAPHY. Positive-contrast tracheography using iodinated oil, barium suspension, or tantalum powder gives the best definition of endotracheal masses and their site or origin (see Figs. 19–115, 19–133, 19–140, and 19–142).[51] Furthermore, the dynamic relationship of the mass and the airway can be appreciated using this technique, an understanding that aids in the explanation of symptoms of tracheal obstruction and in the differentiation of neoplasms from benign strictures. Tracheography is not without hazards, however, and deaths have been reported.[82] Tomography followed by bronchoscopy and biopsy is more often the procedure of choice for patients with a suspected tracheal tumor.[82, 88]

Localized Lesions of the Trachea

Localized tracheal tumors appear radiographically as mass lesions of soft tissue density obscuring a portion of the tracheal air column. Tumors most often arise in the posterior or lateral wall, and oblique views may be necessary to visualize lesions in profile. Masses are most often sessile and eccentric, producing an asymmetric narrowing of the tracheal lumen (Fig. 19–110). However, they may be polypoid and entirely intraluminal.[51, 79, 82] Annular, or "napkin ring," lesions of the trachea commonly result from congenital or acquired stricture but are seen in approximately 10 per cent of patients with tracheal carcinoma;[79] benign tumors do not produce annular narrowing. Benign tracheal tumors are rarely extrinsic to the tracheal lumen. In general, masses with an irregular or lobular contour and sessile masses with ill-defined margins are malignant lesions (see Fig. 19–110).[82] Malignant tumors may extend into the mediastinum (Fig. 19–111). Direct extension of tumor into the mediastinum occurred in 9 of 30 squamous cell carcinomas reported by Hajdu et al.[69] and a mediastinal mass was radiographically visible in 8 of 20 patients with tracheal neoplasm studied by Karlan.[88]

The lower third of the trachea is the most common location of tracheal tumors;[56] 35 to 44 per cent occur in this location.[69, 79, 88] Squamous cell carcinoma is particularly common in the distal trachea, and more than half of squamous lesions occur within

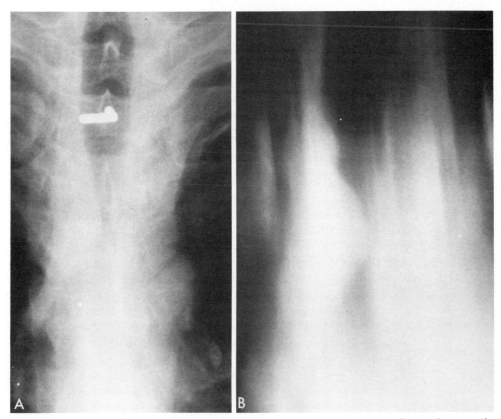

Figure 19–110. Localized tracheal narrowing. *A,* On a posteroanterior radiograph, a sessile and eccentric mass is seen arising from the right tracheal wall, thickening the right paratracheal stripe. *B,* An anteroposterior tomogram demonstrates lobulation of the tumor mass and suggests malignancy. Biopsy revealed an adenoid cystic carcinoma (cylindroma).

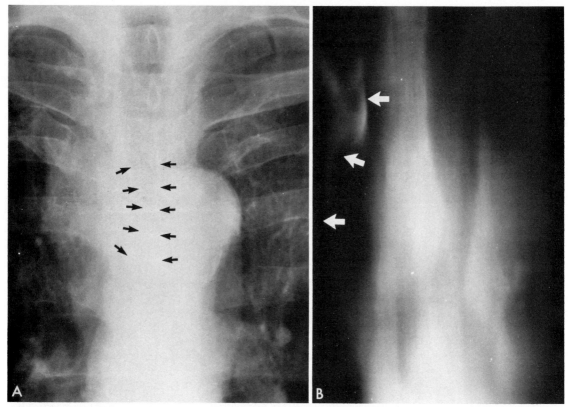

Figure 19–111. Distal tracheal lesion with a large mediastinal mass. *A,* A posteroanterior radiograph shows a large right mediastinal mass associated with narrowing of the distal trachea (arrows). *B,* An anteroposterior tomogram, following the injection of radiographic contrast material in the right antecubital vein, defines the lateral displacement and partial obstruction of the superior vena cava (arrows) by the mass lesion. Localized and eccentric narrowing of the airway, just above the carina, suggests a lesion arising from the tracheal wall. A biopsy showed squamous cell carcinoma, a common tumor in this location.

several centimeters of the carina (see Fig. 19–111). If squamous cell lesions are excluded, however, the proximal trachea is the most common site of tracheal neoplasm.[69]

It may be difficult on radiologic grounds to distinguish between a primary tracheal neoplasm and a neoplasm arising in adjacent cervical or mediastinal structures and involving the trachea by direct extension. Carcinomas of the thyroid gland, the esophagus, and the lung are most commonly responsible for secondary invasion of the tracheal wall (Fig. 19–112).[65] In patients with esophageal carcinoma, symptoms of esophageal obstruction usually predominate, but carcinomas of the lung and the thyroid can present initially with symptoms suggestive of primary tracheal tumor.[66] Tracheal invasion usually results in an asymmetric, irregular tracheal narrowing; an associated mediastinal mass is frequently seen. Polypoid intraluminal masses are rare, but they do occur.[66]

Tracheal compression due to a mediastinal mass that does not invade the tracheal wall is a common occurrence. In such cases, the masses produce a smooth, concentric impression upon the tracheal lumen; irregularity and lobulation indicates invasion of the trachea itself. Displacement of the trachea away from the mass lesion is common.

A fixed inflammatory stricture can radiographically simulate an annular neoplasm of the tracheal wall, making differentiation difficult.[65] Strictures, however, often demonstrate a smooth, tapered narrowing and lack the abrupt shoulders and nodularity

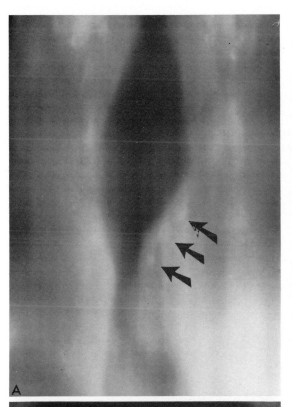

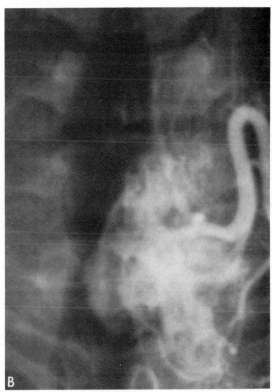

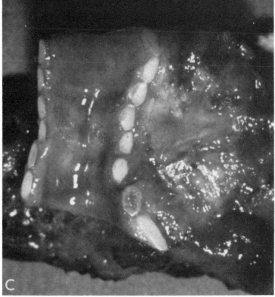

Figure 19–112. Tracheal invasion by thyroid carcinoma. Anteroposterior tomogram of the cervical trachea (*A*) and a thyrocervical arteriogram (*B*) show a 2-cm lobulated mass in the left thyroid lobe, invading the tracheal wall and causing the inward displacement of three calcified tracheal rings (arrows). Hemoptysis was the only complaint of this 27-year-old man, and a mass was not palpable clinically. *C,* Following circumferential resection of six tracheal rings, the surgical specimen shows tumor invasion of the tracheal wall. The histologic diagnosis was mixed follicular and papillary thyroid carcinoma.

of neoplastic lesions. A variable stricture can be easily distinguished from a neoplastic or infiltrative lesion with positive-contrast tracheography. The diameter of a variable stricture varies during inspiration and expiration and during Valsalva's and Müller maneuvers, whereas neoplastic lesions or fixed strictures remain unchanged.[53]

Multiple or Diffuse Tracheal Lesions

Multiple, discrete masses arising within the trachea are uncommon, but occur frequently in patients with squamous papillomatosis. In one survey, 25 of 26 patients with this disease had multiple lesions.[25] In addition, 3 of 30 patients with squamous cell carcinoma studied by Hajdu had a multicentric tumor with two coincidental primary neoplasms.[69] In both series, however, the multiple lesions were small and difficult or impossible to recognize radiographically. In most cases, endoscopy was necessary for diagnosis.[25, 69]

Diseases producing generalized thickening of the tracheal wall and narrowing of the tracheal lumen are more easily diagnosed on chest radiographs. Although examples of infiltrating carcinoma with wall thickening have been reported,[69, 79] generalized

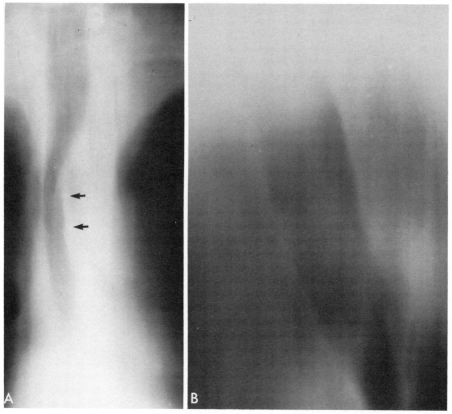

Figure 19–113. Saber-sheath trachea. Anteroposterior (*A*) and lateral (*B*) tomograms of a 71-year-old man with chronic obstructive pulmonary disease reveal marked coronal narrowing of the intrathoracic trachea with a normal or increased sagittal diameter. A long tracheal segment is involved. Although some nodularity is present, and suggesting tumor, the adjacent tracheal wall appears of normal width (arrows) when contrasted with the mediastinal fat. A smooth narrowing is more common.

thickening of the tracheal wall usually indicates a benign process, most commonly tracheobronchopathia osteochondroplastica, amyloidosis, or scleroma.[25, 51]

Thickening of the tracheal wall is best diagnosed by the examination of the paratracheal stripes; the observation of the right paratracheal stripe is most helpful in this regard. A right paratracheal stripe measuring more than 4 mm in width is abnormal[30] and, although a nonspecific finding, if associated with narrowing of the tracheal air column, strongly suggests tracheal infiltration. In addition, lesions thickening the tracheal wall often give an irregular or lumpy contour to the air column (Fig. 19–113), which is not seen with extratracheal conditions, such as pleural fluid, that result in uniform thickening of the paratracheal stripe.

Two benign, non-neoplastic conditions produce generalized tracheal narrowing: "saber-sheath trachea" and polychondritis. Their differentiation from infiltrative conditions, however, is usually possible on clinical and radiographic grounds.

SABER-SHEATH TRACHEA.   This is a relatively common condition often associated with chronic obstructive pulmonary disease and characterized by the narrowing of the intrathoracic trachea in the coronal plane.[62] In the sagittal plane, the tracheal lumen is normal or increased in diameter, and the trachea assumes a flattened contour resembling a sword's scabbard (see Fig. 19–113).[62] In itself, this condition is not symptomatic. It may reflect a degeneration of the tracheal wall. In patients with a saber-sheath trachea, the right paratracheal stripe is normal or slightly thickened. In some patients, the narrowing produces a nodular appearance, which may simulate tumor (see Fig. 19–113).

POLYCHONDRITIS.   This is a rare systemic disease affecting cartilage throughout the body, most notably in the nose, the ears, and the joints.[85] The cartilage of the tracheobronchial tree is also involved; it is slowly replaced by fibrous tissue. Marked narrowing of the trachea can occur, leading to respiratory failure and death. Radiographs reveal generalized, smooth narrowing of the trachea and major bronchi (Fig. 19–114).[85]

Surgery

Tracheal tumors not involving the tracheal wall can be removed endoscopically.[65] Squamous papillomas and inflammatory polyps are often treated in this manner.[25]

Localized tumors arising from or invading the tracheal wall should be removed by tracheal resection.[64, 65] Until recently, it was believed that only 2 cm of trachea could be removed without causing undue stress on the anastomotic site.[40, 64, 65] Thus, lesions larger than 2 cm were removed by lateral or fenestral resections and the resulting defects closed by a variety of materials serving as patch grafts.[56] Dermal grafts supported with wires, fascia lata, pericardium, costal periosteum, or autologous bronchial wall have been used along with a variety of plastic sheets or meshes. These techniques have met with some success, but in many cases early leakage with fatal mediastinitis or scarring with eventual tracheal obstruction has resulted.[65] Similarly, circumferential tracheal resection with the substitution of a solid prosthesis or tracheal homograft often results in serious or fatal complications.

Circumferential tracheal resection with an end-to-end anastomosis is currently considered to be the treatment of choice for tracheal tumors.[64, 65] A combination of cervical flexion and upward mobilization of the carina and lung hila permits more than half of the trachea to be resected and the ends approximated without undue tension on the anastomosis. Laryngeal release, in which the larynx is dissected from its superior attachments, has also been advocated.[40] Complex procedures have been devised to

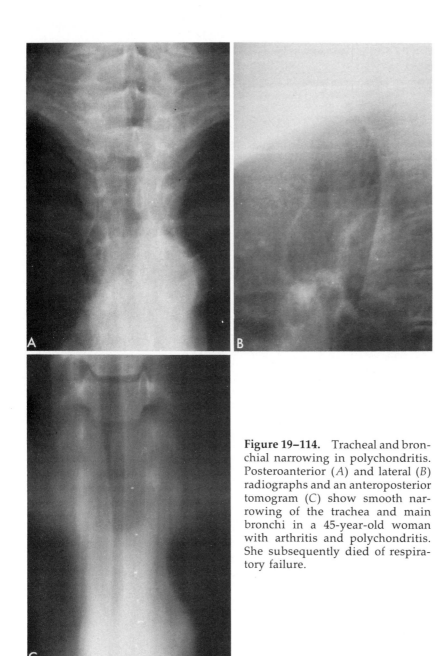

Figure 19–114. Tracheal and bronchial narrowing in polychondritis. Posteroanterior (A) and lateral (B) radiographs and an anteroposterior tomogram (C) show smooth narrowing of the trachea and main bronchi in a 45-year-old woman with arthritis and polychondritis. She subsequently died of respiratory failure.

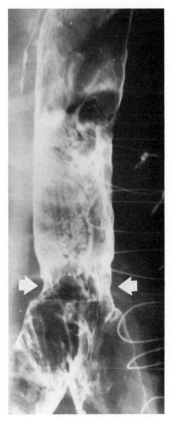

Figure 19–115. Normal postoperative trachea. A tantalum tracheogram, obtained following the circumferential resection of a 5-cm segment of the distal trachea for a granular cell myoblastoma, shows slight tracheal narrowing (arrows) at the site of the anastomosis. This narrowing was invisible on the plain radiograph.

allow the resection of lesions not limited to the trachea. Laryngotrachectomy can be performed for tumors involving both the larynx and the upper trachea; this procedure is often combined with a mediastinal tracheostomy.[64, 65] Lesions involving the carina can be resected, with the reimplantation of the mainstem bronchi into the remaining tracheal stump.

Following the circumferential resection of a short tracheal segment, it may be difficult on routine or tomographic examinations to detect the site of anastomosis unless stricture or polyps have resulted (Fig. 19–115). If a long segment of trachea has been resected, there may be a visible elevation of the hilar structures and carina, with narrowing of the carinal angle (Fig. 19–116). The larynx may descend to the thoracic inlet, particularly if laryngeal release has been performed.

The results of circumferential tracheal resection for malignancy have been good. Of 29 patients with primary tracheal tumors studied by Grillo, ten had disease too extensive for resection, and eight underwent various types of complex resection.[64] Of 11 patients who underwent resection and reanastomosis performed for curative purposes, nine are living and have no recurrent disease. These nine patients have been monitored for two to twelve years after surgery.

The potential complications of circumferential tracheal resection include suture line separations with mediastinitis; tracheal stenosis; suture line granulations requiring endoscopic removal; and rarely, tracheoinnominate artery fistula or tracheoesophageal fistula.[64, 65] Mediastinitis is characterized radiographically by mediastinal widening, pneumomediastinum, and occasionally, air-fluid levels. In patients with this complication, positive-contrast tracheography, preferably using iodinated oil, may

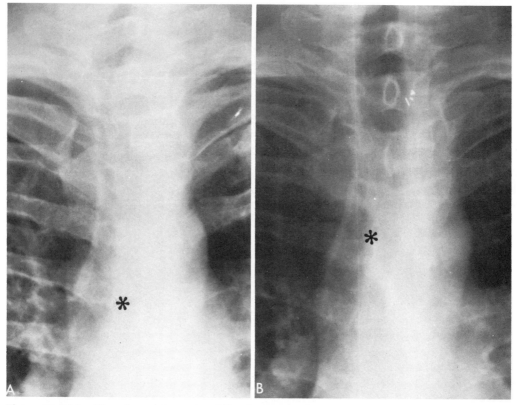

Figure 19–116. Elevation of the carina following tracheal resection. A, A preoperative postero-anterior radiograph of a man with thyroid carcinoma invading the proximal trachea (see Fig. 19–112). The carina (asterisk) is in a normal position, well below the aortic arch. B, After the circumferential resection of a 4-cm tracheal segment, a posteroanterior radiograph shows carinal elevation (asterisk) relative to the aorta. Furthermore, the carinal angle has decreased, and both main bronchi appear more vertical than they did on the preoperative films.

demonstrate the site of the anastomotic dehiscence and the extent of the infection in the mediastinal space. Most patients with tracheoesophageal fistula show radiographic evidence of recurrent aspiration in the lower lobes, with pneumonia or abscess formation; tracheography or, more often, esophagography is used to confirm this diagnosis. The diagnosis of tracheal stenosis is discussed elsewhere in these volumes.

BRONCHIAL TUMORS

Tumors involving the large central bronchi (the left and right main bronchi, the lobar bronchi, and the segmental bronchi) are far more common than tracheal tumors. In general, the differential diagnosis is similar to that already described for tracheal masses. In this location, however, bronchogenic carcinoma accounts for more than 90 per cent of neoplastic lesions; bronchial adenomas, particularly adenoid cystic carcino-mas, are relatively uncommon.[2, 122] The most frequent benign tumors occurring within the central bronchi are lipoma, fibroma, and hamartoma.[25, 103] In one series, however, only 11 of these benign neoplasms were encountered during 11,626 bronchoscopies performed in a ten-year period;[45] in this same period, more than 2000 bronchogenic carcinomas are likely to occur. Granular cell myoblastoma, leiomyoma, chondroma, neurogenic tumors, papilloma, tracheobronchopathia osteochondroplastica, amyloidosis, and bronchogenic cyst also can occur within or adjacent to the central bronchi.[25, 45, 103, 114]

Clinical Diagnosis

The nonspecific symptoms of an endobronchial tumor include cough and hemoptysis[45, 103] and are most common in patients with bronchogenic carcinoma and bronchial adenoma. Obstructing bronchial tumors can result in dyspnea, local wheezing, and symptoms of pneumonia, including chest pain, fever, and expectoration of purulent sputum.[28, 45, 103]

The cytologic examination of sputum samples or of material obtained by bronchial brushing uncovers approximately 70 per cent of centrally located bronchogenic carcinomas but is of little value in the diagnosis of patients with benign lesions.[28, 55] Fibroscopic bronchoscopy with transbronchial biopsy allows accurate diagnosis of a variety of endobronchial lesions, both benign and malignant, and is extremely useful in the evaluation of patients with suspected bronchial neoplasm.[131]

Radiographic Diagnosis

PLAIN CHEST RADIOGRAPHS. These demonstrate abnormal findings in approximately two thirds of patients with bronchial neoplasms. In half of these, a mass lesion is visible; in the remainder, the radiographic findings suggest bronchial obstruction.[22, 25, 114]

Tumors arising from the bronchial wall may be primarily extrinsic to the bronchial lumen. In such cases, they are visible as nodular mass lesions in the hilar region or central portions of the lung. More commonly, however, bronchial tumors project into the bronchial lumen, and bronchial obstruction often results.[25, 103]

PARTIAL BRONCHIAL OBSTRUCTION. This prevents mucous transport and the cleansing of the distal bronchial tree. Partial bronchial obstruction thus contributes to the development of pneumonia (obstructive pneumonitis) and, in some cases, bronchiectasis (Fig. 19–117) or abscess formation (Fig. 19–118).[25, 45, 103] Radiographs reveal homogeneous or patchy consolidation limited to a lobe or a segment, reflecting the distribution of the obstructed bronchus.[28, 161] Obstructive pneumonia can clear up following appropriate antibiotic treatment, but it often recurs. Occasionally, mucus accumulates distal to an obstructing lesion and results in radiographically visible mucous plugs. These appear as fingerlike, branching, or ropy densities following the distribution of the bronchial tree. Bronchograms of patients with recurrent pneumonia may reveal severe bronchiectasis.[45] If bronchiectasis is present, lesions otherwise resectable through the bronchoscope are usually removed with the affected lung.[45]

COMPLETE BRONCHIAL OBSTRUCTION. This condition often results in the collapse of the distal lung, and in most cases a lobe or segment is airless 24 hours after the obstruction of its bronchus.[74, 91, 141] A collapsed and consolidated lung distal to an obstruction is known as drowned lung (Fig. 19–119); consolidation results primarily from edema fluid.[91, 141] Air bronchograms, radiographic signs of alveolar consolidation, are characteristically absent in such patients. Air within the bronchial lumen, which is necessary for the visualization of an air bronchogram, is resorbed and replaced by fluid following complete bronchial obstruction. Felson, however, reports that 9 (10 per cent) of 85 patients with bronchial obstruction by tumor had radiographically visible air

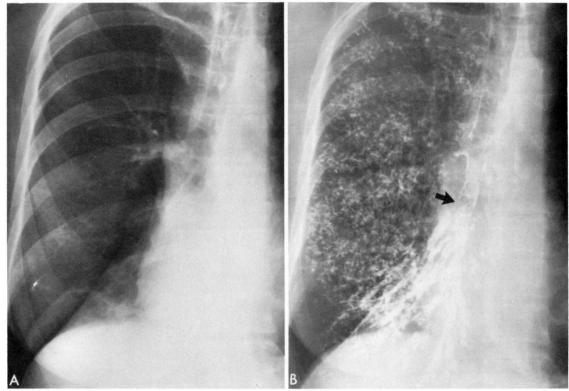

Figure 19–117. Endobronchial mass producing bronchiectasis. *A,* A posteroanterior view of the right lung shows right lower lobe atelectasis. *B,* A right lower lobe bronchogram reveals a small, spherical endobronchial mass (arrow) with partial bronchial obstruction and distal bronchiectasis. The endobronchial mass was a carcinoid bronchial adenoma.

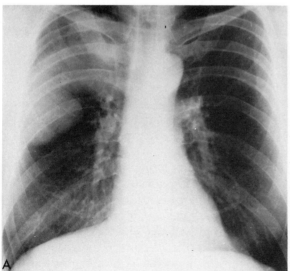

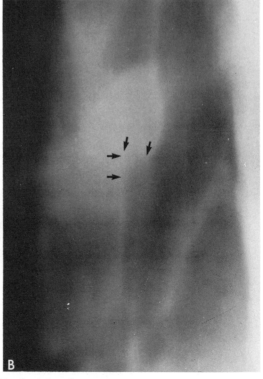

Figure 19–118. Lung abscess resulting from bronchial obstruction. *A,* A posteroanterior radiograph of a 47-year-old man shows a large mass in the right upper lobe, proven pathologically to be a lung abscess. *B,* A V-shaped occlusion of the right upper lobe bronchus (arrows) is visible on an oblique tomogram of the right hilum. At surgery, a squamous cell carcinoma was found originating in the right upper lobe bronchus. Bronchiectasis was also found distal to the obstruction.

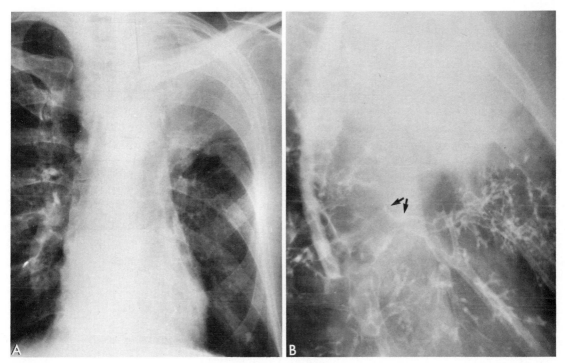

Figure 19–119. Drowned lung. *A,* Left upper lobe collapse and consolidation, primarily due to fluid, are seen on a posteroanterior radiograph of a 75-year-old woman. *B,* A bronchogram shows occlusion of the left upper lobe bronchus (arrows) by an endobronchial mass, producing a convex meniscus pointing toward the hilum. This appearance usually indicates a bronchial adenoma or benign tumor. Resection revealed a carcinoid bronchial adenoma.

bronchograms.[50] Presumably, these patients had intermittent, rather than complete, bronchial obstruction.

In a minority of patients, the obstruction of a bronchus results in distal air trapping leading to hyperexpansion of the lung, a condition known as obstructive emphysema. This is caused by one of two mechanisms. First, a partially obstructive endobronchial lesion can result in a check-valve effect. A check-valve obstruction allows air to enter the lung distal to an obstructing lesion as the bronchus dilates during inspiration but prevents air from leaving the lung on expiration, during which the bronchus contracts around the endobronchial mass.[7] Depending on the site of the obstruction, air trapping due to a check-valve obstruction can occur within a segment, a lobe, or an entire lung.

The second mechanism that causes obstructive emphysema is collateral ventilation, or ventilation by other-than-normal bronchial pathways.[102] Segments of lung distal to a total bronchial obstruction can be ventilated from normally aerated adjacent lung segments via the intra-alveolar pores of Kohn or the direct bronchoalveolar communications commonly referred to as the canals of Lambert.[102] Because these collateral pathways are small, resistance to rapid airflow is great, and the collaterally ventilated lung segment or lobe traps air during normal respiration. Collateral ventilation can occur at the segmental or lobar level but cannot occur from one lung to the other. Consequently, when air trapping occurs within an entire lung a partial or check-valve obstruction of the main bronchus must be present.

At full inspiration, the lung volume is near normal in patients with obstructive emphysema, and the radiographic diagnosis of this phenomenon is most easily made

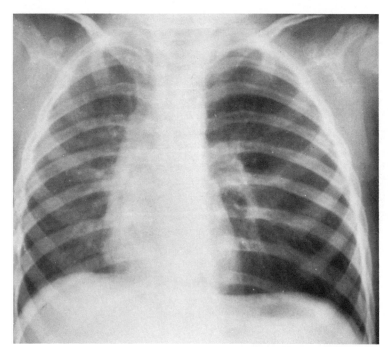

Figure 19–120. Air trapping produced by a check-valve bronchial obstruction. A posteroanterior radiograph taken during expiration in a two-year-old child shows air trapping within the left lung due to the impaction of a peanut impacted in the left main bronchus. Hyperlucency, mediastinal shift to the right, and poor diaphragmatic motion are evident.

through dynamic studies.[7, 102] Films taken at full inspiration and during or after a forced expiration often enable a correct diagnosis (Fig. 19–120). Timed filming during a forced vital-capacity maneuver (FEV_1) provides additional information, and fluoroscopy with rapid expiration or "sniffing" may be extremely helpful in subtle cases. Air trapping within a lobe or lung prevents a normal decrease in lung volume during expiration and limits the excursion of the ipsilateral hemidiaphragm. In the comparison of one side with the other, a difference in diaphragmatic excursion exceeding 1.5 cm is uncommon in normal patients.[162] A shift of the mediastinal structures away from the side where air trapping is present also occurs with expiration, and mediastinal "rocking" from side to side may be seen at fluoroscopy during rapid breathing.[7] Hyperlucency of a lobe or a segment trapping air is common following expiration, and a shift in the position of major or minor fissures is sometimes seen. Lateral decubitus films may also be employed to diagnose air trapping and are particularly useful in the diagnosis of children because they require minimal cooperation from patients. In the decubitus position, the dependent lung should show a significantly decreased volume compared with that of the opposite side. If a decrease in volume is not apparent, air trapping is probably present (Fig. 19–121).

TOMOGRAPHY. This technique assists greatly in the visualization of endobronchial lesions and should be performed on patients with radiographic evidence of bronchial obstruction, even if a mass is not evident on routine radiographs (see Fig. 19–118).[94] A number of tomographic projections have been utilized to define specific portions of the tracheobronchial tree.[23, 94] However, tomographic evaluation of central bronchial structures is generally limited to a combination of three standard projections: anteroposterior, 55 degree posterior oblique, and lateral. Anteroposterior tomograms allow the best definition of lesions involving the right and left main bronchi. Oblique tomograms provide excellent visualization of lobar and segmental bronchi, particularly the upper lobe bronchi and their anterior and apical divisions, the right middle lobe

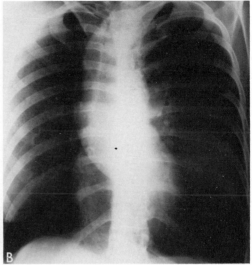

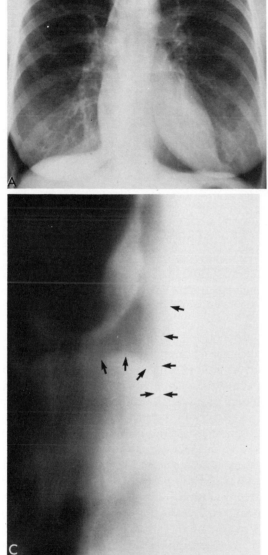

Figure 19–121. Air trapping produced by a bronchial adenoma. *A,* A posteroanterior radiograph shows an ill-defined hilar mass in a 52-year-old woman with hemoptysis and right-sided wheezing. *B,* On a right lateral decubitus film, there is little decrease in volume of the right lung owing to air trapping. *C,* A right hilar tomogram shows a 3-cm oval mass expanding and obstructing the lumina (arrows) of the right main bronchus and bronchus intermedius. The histologic diagnosis was mucoepidermoid bronchial adenoma.

bronchus, and the lingular bronchus (Fig. 19–122). Lateral tomography gives the best definition of the lower lobe bronchi.

XEROTOMOGRAPHY. This method further improves the visualization of endobronchial masses (see Fig. 19–122). In a study by Ting et al. of 14 patients with central bronchogenic carcinoma, only 50 per cent were diagnosed using conventional tomography, whereas 86 per cent were correctly diagnosed following xerotomograms.[141]

BRONCHOGRAPHY. This technique has been used extensively in the diagnosis of lesions occurring in the central bronchi, particularly bronchogenic carcinoma. Its

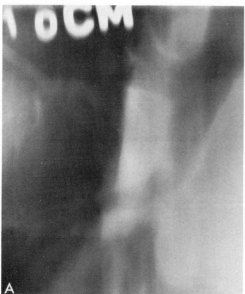

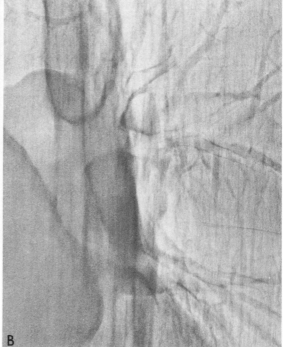

Figure 19–122. Normal oblique tomograms. A standard tomogram (*A*) and a xerotomogram (*B*) of the right hilum provide excellent detail of the right upper and middle lobe bronchi. The resolution of the xerogram exceeds that of the plain film tomogram and allows visualization of small bronchi not visible on conventional films. (The xerotomogram appears reversed because of the method used in its processing.)

accuracy in detecting and diagnosing bronchogenic carcinoma ranges from 89 to 94 per cent and in cases of central lesions approaches 100 per cent.[55, 122, 161] This procedure may result in morbidity, however, and in recent years, bronchography has been largely replaced by fiberoptic bronchoscopy with forceps or brush biopsy of bronchoscopically or radiographically visible lesions.

In addition to their value in detecting and localizing endobronchial masses not visible on plain radiographs, tomography and bronchography may define characteristics of the tumor and its effect on the airway lumen, thereby helping to differentiate benign from malignant lesions.[149] A number of radiographic signs seem to suggest malignancy.[55, 122] These include bronchial amputation, with the abrupt termination of the bronchial lumen in a convexity pointing away from the hilum; sharp cutoff of a bronchus (Fig. 19–123), asymmetric narrowing of the bronchial lumen; and rattail narrowing of the bronchial lumen, with the termination of the bronchus in a V-shaped collection of contrast material (see Figs. 19–118 and 19–123).[122] A smooth, rounded filling defect or bronchial amputation with a convexity pointing toward the hilum most often indicates a bronchial adenoma[122, 141] but also can be seen with any benign endobronchial neoplasm (see Fig. 19–119).

Inflammatory lesions, particularly granulomatous strictures, can closely mimic the bronchographic appearance of bronchogenic carcinoma. Furthermore, bronchial obstruction may result from cases of chronic or unresolved pneumonia, but obstruction from this cause is often distinguishable from carcinomatous obstruction.[18] Multiple nonobstructing endobronchial lesions usually suggest bronchial papillomatosis, amyloidosis, tracheobronchopathia, or multiple metastases.

RADIONUCLIDE SCANNING. Radionuclide scanning with aerosols, perfusion agents, and tumor-detecting agents has met with some success in the diagnosis of

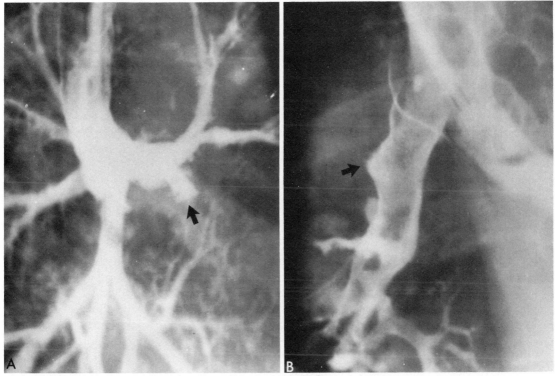

Figure 19–123. Bronchographic abnormalities in cases of bronchogenic carcinoma. The bronchograms of two patients with bronchogenic carcinoma show abrupt amputation (arrow) of the lingular bronchus (A) and an obstruction of the right upper lobe bronchus (B) with a V-shaped appearance (arrow). These findings are distinct from those seen with bronchial adenoma.

endobronchial neoplasm, particularly bronchogenic carcinoma. The use of radionuclides is discussed in detail elsewhere.

Surgery

Polypoid or pedunculated tumors may sometimes be resected through the bronchoscope, leaving the patient symptom-free.[25] Chronic infection distal to an obstructing lesion, however, often requires the removal of a segment or a lobe for a complete cure.[2, 96]

Normal radiographic findings following partial or complete pneumonectomy and the radiographic appearance of postsurgical complications are discussed elsewhere.

PERIPHERAL TUMORS: SOLITARY NODULES

Neoplastic lesions arising from subsegmental bronchi and bronchioles are often asymptomatic and are detected radiographically as solitary, peripheral nodules.[96] Although they can result in the obstruction of small bronchi, the amount of lung affected is small, and the radiographic signs of atelectasis, obstructive pneumonitis, or air trapping are insignificant.[13] Bronchogenic carcinomas account for nearly 80 per cent of resected solitary lung tumors, and bronchial adenomas make up more than 6 per cent.[13, 114] Of 2958 resected nodules studied by Bateson including 1616 granulomas, 169 (13 per cent) were hamartomas, and 105 (8 per cent) were cysts. Other benign tumors are much less common.

Radiographic Diagnosis

Plain radiographs, tomograms, xerograms, and sometimes, computerized tomography and bronchography are used in the radiographic evaluation of solitary pulmonary nodules.[10, 86, 97, 104] Attempts at radiographic diagnosis are directed primarily at the differentiation of benign from malignant lesions. Although a number of radiographic signs have been reported that make the diagnosis of benignancy or malignancy more likely in individual cases, only a few signs have a sufficient degree of specificity to affect treatment.[13]

The radiographic visualization of a calcification within a solitary pulmonary nodule indicates, with rare exceptions, benign disease.[112] More specifically, the presence of a dense central or laminated calcification virtually excludes the diagnosis of malignancy (see Fig. 19–127).[13, 112] A bronchogenic carcinoma (scar carcinoma) arising adjacent to a calcified granuloma sometimes incorporates the calcific density, producing a malignant mass with a dense calcification. In such cases, however, the calcification is usually eccentric rather than central (Fig. 19–124). Bronchogenic carcinomas themselves occasionally calcify, but this calcification is often stippled and invisible radiographically.[112] Of 72 patients with a malignant solitary pulmonary nodule studied by O'Keefe et al., ten had a calcification visible on radiographs of the resected specimen, but only one of these calcifications was visible on standard chest radiographs.[112] In the same series,

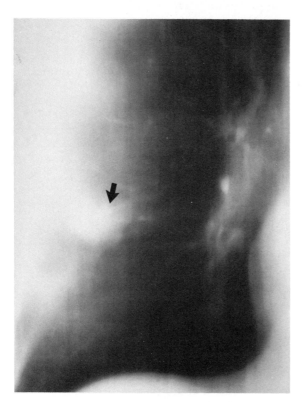

Figure 19–124. Eccentric calcification in a case of bronchogenic carcinoma. An anteroposterior tomogram shows an ill-defined right lower lobe mass with a dense but eccentric calcification (arrow). Excision disclosed a squamous cell carcinoma incorporating a calcified granuloma.

67 of 135 benign lesions, consisting mostly of granulomas and hamartomas, contained calcifications, 46 of which were visible radiographically. Metastatic malignant tumors, particularly osteogenic sarcoma, chondrosarcoma, and thyroid carcinoma, can show stippled or homogeneous calcification.

Fluoroscopy at low kilovoltage and tomography greatly assist in the visualization of calcifications within a mass lesion.[104, 112] Furthermore, xerotomography may show calcium not seen on standard tomograms.[97] Computerized tomography has also been used for this purpose, but its relatively poor resolution, its tendency toward statistical variation in transmitted radiation, and its partial volume averaging make it difficult to diagnose small calcifications with certainty.[86]

The rate at which a solitary nodule grows in size or doubles in volume (doubling time) has been used to determine the likelihood of its being malignant.[109, 110] In general, if a nodule doubles in volume in less than one month or more than 18 months, it is benign.[109, 110] Overlapping of growth rates of benign and malignant lesions, however, particularly among rapidly growing nodules, makes the use of doubling time as an absolute indicator of malignancy hazardous (see Fig. 19–127). It is generally accepted, however, that if a nodule does not grow over a period of two years, it is benign and resection is not necessary. Only rare exceptions to this rule have been reported.[109]

In summary, a pulmonary nodule may be considered benign if it demonstrates a dense central or laminated calcification on plain radiographs or tomograms or if it is unchanged in size over a period of two years. Although neither of these findings is an absolute indicator of benign disease, thoracotomy, which bears a small, but definite, risk of death may be deferred. In each case, the risk of not operating on a potentially malignant lesion must be weighed against the risk of operative mortality. The radiographic diagnosis of solitary pulmonary nodules is discussed in more detail elsewhere (pp. 1248–1250).

Solitary pulmonary nodules in patients younger than 35 are rarely malignant,[152] and some authors consider surgery unwarranted in patients less than 30 years of age.[110] In such cases, needle aspiration biopsy, with the excision of the nodule (if the biopsy indicates a malignancy) or frequent follow-up radiographs (if the biopsy specimen proves benign), is an alternative to immediate thoracotomy.[110]

In older patients, pulmonary nodules often require surgical excision for diagnosis, and wedge resections or segmentectomies are usually done in patients whose lesions are benign.[96] In cases of malignant nodules, more radical surgery, often lobectomy or pneumonectomy, is required, depending on the location and the extent of the tumor.[28] The radiographic appearance following resectional surgery and of common postsurgical complications are reviewed elsewhere (pp. 1259–1262).

Bronchial Adenoma and Benign Tumors of Trachea and Bronchi

Bronchial adenoma, benign tumors of the tracheobronchial tree, and tumorlike congenital malformations of the respiratory tract constitute a dissimilar group of lesions. Although the clinical and radiographic manifestations of different lesions can be identical to some extent, their distribution within the tracheobronchial tree, their tendency to cause bronchial obstruction, and their overall appearance vary. Furthermore, the surgical approach to individual lesions can differ.

BRONCHIAL ADENOMA

Bronchial adenomas are uncommon and constitute less than 5 per cent of tumors affecting the tracheobronchial tree.[27] In fact, three recent surveys report the incidence of bronchial adenoma relative to other respiratory tract tumors to be only 0.6 per cent and 1.2 per cent.[24, 44, 99] They arise from the epithelium of mucous glands within the bronchial wall and based on their cell of origin are divided into two distinct groups: carcinoid tumors and so-called salivary gland–type lesions.[22, 44] Carcinoid tumors arise from neuroectodermal (Kulchitsky) cells and account for 85 to 90 per cent of adenomas occurring within the bronchial tree.[22, 24, 44, 57] They rarely occur in the trachea.[27] Salivary gland–type tumors, so named because of their histologic similarity to tumors arising within the salivary glands, are subdivided into adenoid cystic carcinomas or cylindromas, and mucoepidermoid carcinomas.[44, 99] Adenoid cystic carcinoma makes up only 6 to 12 per cent of bronchial adenomas but accounts for 95 per cent of adenomas arising from the tracheal wall (see Fig. 19–110).[27, 44, 57, 61]

Although originally considered to be benign tumors, bronchial adenomas are most appropriately thought of as adenocarcinomas of low-grade malignancy.[24, 44] They are slow growing and locally invasive. Carcinoid tumors metastasize to regional lymph nodes in 15 per cent of the cases, and 5 per cent have distant metastases.[24, 61] Adenoid cystic carcinomas are more malignant, and metastases are three times as common as with carcinoid tumors.[24, 44] Mucoepidermoid carcinomas exhibit the most benign course, and although they can be locally invasive, they rarely metastasize.[24, 92]

Bronchial adenomas occur most commonly in patients 40 to 60 years of age; the mean age ranges from 48 to 51 years.[22, 24, 44, 57, 99] The occurrence of bronchial adenomas in patients younger than 20 years is not uncommon, however, and half of the patients are less than 50 at the time of diagnosis.[22, 57]

More than 80 per cent of the bronchial adenomas occur centrally, in the main, lobar, or segmental bronchi;[24, 44, 61] only 1 per cent are intratracheal. They are highly vascular, and hemoptysis is a common presenting complaint.[22, 24, 44] Their location in the bronchial wall beneath the lining epithelium is responsible for the frequency of bronchial obstruction observed in patients with this lesion.[44, 57, 92] Nearly half of the bronchial adenomas are associated with radiographic signs of obstruction, primarily atelectasis or consolidation (Table 19–4), typically limited to a lobe or a segment (see Fig. 19–117).[22, 24, 44, 57] Atelectasis and consolidation are often intermittent, and recurrent episodes of infection result in bronchiectasis or lung abscess. Bronchiectasis is present pathologically in more than one third of the patients but is less often visible radiographically.[22] Obstructive emphysema (see Fig. 19–121) was seen in 3 of 72

TABLE 19–4. RADIOGRAPHIC FEATURES OF BRONCHIAL ADENOMA

Radiographic Features	Bower[22]	Donahue et al.[44]	Giustra and Stassa[57]	Lawson et al.[92]
Hilar mass	6 (21%)	12 (35%)	26 (31%)	—
Atelectasis or consolidation	15 (54%)	15 (43%)	39 (46%)	53 (74%)
Peripheral mass	8 (29%)	6 (17%)	24 (29%)	13 (18%)
Bronchiectasis	3 (11%)	1 (3%)	—	25 (35%)
Abscess	2 (7%)	—	—	—
Normal	1 (3%)	1 (3%)	6 (7%)	3 (4%)
Tracheal mass	1 (3%)	0	1 (1%)	0
Total patients	28	35	84	72

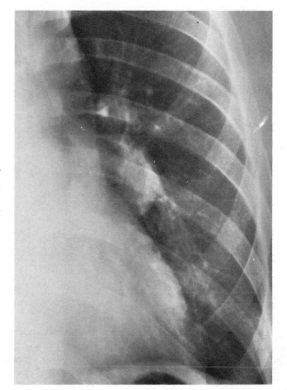

Figure 19–125. Bronchial adenoma producing a hilar mass. A posteroanterior radiograph of the left lung shows a lobulated hilar mass representing a mucoepidermoid bronchial adenoma. This is larger than most bronchial adenomas that present as mass lesions.

patients studied by Lawson et al.[22, 92] Central bronchial adenomas, with or without findings of obstruction, may be visible as discrete mass lesions in, or near, the hila (Fig. 19–125).[44] These masses, which are usually less than 4 cm in diameter, can be difficult to recognize without tomography.[57, 61, 92]

Peripheral mass lesions, which are not associated with the findings of obstruction, occur in approximately 20 per cent of the cases.[22] They are often well defined, round or oval, and slightly lobulated in contour.[13, 57] Rarely, calcification and ossification occur.[57, 92]

Bronchography is often used in the diagnosis of bronchial adenomas because of their central location.[57] In most cases, they have a large endobronchial component and appear bronchographically as intraluminal masses obstructing the bronchus in which they arise, producing a convex meniscus pointing toward the hilum (see Fig. 19–119).[57, 147] Also, lesions that are largely endobronchial can expand the bronchus as they grow, resulting typically in a flaring of the bronchial lumen at the point of its obstruction (see Fig. 19–121).[92] In one survey, five of seven patients with bronchial adenoma demonstrated this finding.[147]

The local extension of bronchial adenomas beyond the bronchial wall occurs commonly, and endoscopic removal of visible tumor is usually not curative.[44] Endoscopic removal is often followed by local recurrence or metastasis.[44] Surgical excision of the tumor, its bronchus, and the distal lung is the treatment of choice for bronchial adenoma. Because this tumor occurs centrally in the large majority of cases, either pneumonectomy or lobectomy is usually required.[22, 24, 44] A small percentage of bronchial adenomas are resectable by segmentectomy. Local radiation can be of some value, particularly in patients with adenoid cystic carcinoma, but bronchial adenomas are relatively radioresistant.[44] Chemotherapy is rarely employed.[44]

For patients treated surgically, the prognosis is good.[22, 24] In two recent surveys, the ten-year survival rate of patients treated primarily by surgery averaged 66 per cent.[44, 99] The complications of pneumonectomy and lobectomy are discussed elsewhere (pp. 1259–1262). Following resection, distant metastasis is more common than local recurrence at the primary site. Bone metastases, either lytic or blastic, are readily recognized radiographically.[57, 99]

CONGENITAL AND DEVELOPMENTAL LESIONS

Developmental lesions of the respiratory tract are divided pathologically into hamartomas, teratomas, bronchopulmonary anomalies, and vascular malformations. Only those lesions entering into the differential diagnosis of pulmonary mass lesions are discussed in detail in this chapter. With the exception of cystic adenomatoid malformation, each is most commonly diagnosed in adults.

Hamartoma

CHONDROMATOUS HAMARTOMAS. These are benign tumors containing various connective tissue elements that are found normally in the lung and bronchi, but these elements are present in a disorganized state.[12, 96] As their name implies, these tumors always contain cartilage. Also found in varying amounts are fibrous tissue, fat, smooth muscle, myxomatous tissue, and epithelial tissue.[116] Hamartomas most likely originate

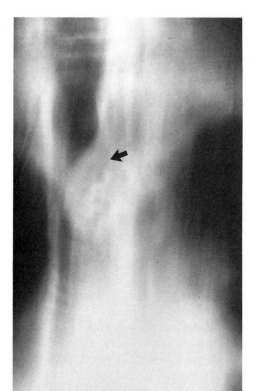

Figure 19–126. Endotracheal hamartoma. An anteroposterior tomogram of the trachea shows a 2.5-cm mass arising from the left tracheal wall and extending into both the tracheal lumen and the mediastinum. Conglomerate, or "popcorn," calcification is evident. An area of lucency within the mass (arrow) may represent fat.

within embryonic rests in the bronchial wall,[96] but Bateson has recently hypothesized that they derive from undifferentiated mesenchymal tissues and represent true neoplasms rather than congenital malformations.[15, 137] They account for more than 75 per cent of benign lung tumors.[5]

Despite their bronchial origin, only 5 to 15 per cent of chondromatous hamartomas present as endobronchial masses with evidence of partial or complete bronchial obstruction (Fig. 19–126).[12, 103, 137] In most cases, chondromatous hamartomas appear radiographically as solitary pulmonary nodules, and they account for 6 to 8 per cent of

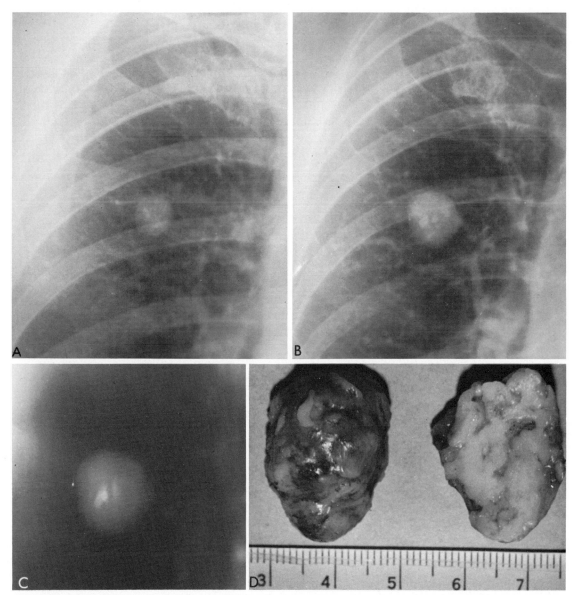

Figure 19–127. Pulmonary hamartoma. *A,* A posteroanterior view of the right upper lobe of a 52-year-old woman demonstrates a well-defined oval nodule measuring 14 mm in diameter. A small, eccentric calcification is visible. *B,* Three years later, the nodule has almost doubled in diameter and appears lobulated. *C,* A tomogram shows two areas of dense calcification. *D,* The resected lesion was a typical hamartoma containing a large amount of cartilage. Such relatively rapid growth is not uncommon.

resected lung nodules.[13, 135] Peripheral hamartomas are usually 1 to 4 cm in diameter, well-defined, sharply circumscribed, and often lobulated (Fig. 19–127).[12, 21] Radiographically visible calcification of cartilage is reported to occur in as many as 32 to 34 per cent of all chondromatous hamartomas,[12, 112] and the frequency of calcification increases with the tumor's size.[12] Several authors have concluded that radiographically visible calcification is uncommon,[68, 116] but this most likely reflects the relatively small size of the lesions in their series. Calcification is seen in only 9 per cent of nodules less than 3 cm in diameter but is present in 75 per cent of those 5 cm or larger.[12] Calcification can be stippled or conglomerate; conglomerate, or "popcorn," calcification is characteristic of hamartomas and is rarely seen with other lesions.[12, 13, 96, 112] Accumulations of fat can produce lucent or pseudocavitary areas within the tumor mass, usually visible only on tomograms (see Fig. 19–126).[12, 21] Rarely, cystic, air-filled hamartomas have been reported.[39]

Hamartomas are most commonly diagnosed in patients older than 50 years of age and are twice as common in men as in women.[12, 96] They are rare in children, and less than 10 per cent occur in patients younger than 40.[12, 96] In most cases, hamartomas grow slowly, increasing in diameter 0.5 to 5 mm per year (see Fig. 19–127).[87, 135] Rapid growth can occur, however, thereby causing hamartomas to be confused with bronchogenic carcinoma.[128] Endobronchial lesions can be resected bronchoscopically, unless infection has caused destruction of the distal lung; peripheral tumors when noncalcified require excision for diagnosis.[103, 135]

Congenital Cystic Adenomatoid Malformation

This condition is most appropriately considered a hamartoma.[78] It is nonneoplastic, however, and distinct from the chondromatous lesions already discussed. Pathologically, a cystic adenomatoid malformation is a mass of disorganized pulmonary tissue containing numerous cysts lined by bronchial epithelium; the alveoli are poorly developed, and cartilage is absent.[70, 78] Usually cysts occupy a single lobe.[70, 78] The developmental defect resulting in cystic adenomatoid malformation is unknown, but the morphologic characteristics of this lesion indicate that it forms after lobar architecture is established at five weeks of embryonic age but before cartilage appears at six weeks.[70] A cystic adenomatoid malformation is present from birth and is most commonly diagnosed in neonates.[70]

Cysts within the malformation commonly communicate with the bronchial tree and therefore contain air that is visible on chest radiographs.[95] In a majority of cases, multiple air-filled cysts are scattered throughout a mass of soft tissue density.[70, 78] In one study, this finding was noted in 11 (73 per cent) of 15 patients.[95] Less frequently, a single air-filled cyst predominates, simulating congenital lobar emphysema.[95] Regardless of its presentation, a malformation communicating with the bronchial tree and containing air expands the lobe or lung in which it occurs, and there is often a mediastinal shift away from the affected side. Presumably, air trapping within cysts results from the absence of bronchial cartilage and the collapse of bronchial walls during expiration.[70] A noncommunicating malformation contains fluid and does not undergo progressive enlargement. It appears radiographically as a large mass lesion.[95]

The compression of normal lung results in symptoms of respiratory distress, often in the first few hours of life. The mortality rate is high unless prompt resection of the malformation is performed.[70] Following excision, the normal lung expands and the mediastinum returns to a normal position. Surviving infants undergo normal growth and development, without late sequelae.[33, 70]

Teratoma

A majority of intrathoracic teratomas are found in the mediastinum.[14] Intrapulmonary teratomas are rare; only 16 cases have been reported in detail.[151] Teratoma is distinguishable from hamartoma in that it contains various tissue elements not normally found within the lung, most commonly skin and hair.[3, 54] It has been diagnosed in patients ranging from 16 to 68 years of age, and although it is said to occur more commonly in women, it does not demonstrate a strong sex predominance.[151] Expectoration of hair (trichoptysis) is pathognomonic of teratoma.[54]

Pulmonary teratomas most often appear as lobulated mass lesions larger than 5 cm in diameter usually in the lung periphery.[29, 151] Radiographically, the masses contain lucent areas of fat and dense conglomerate calcifications.[29] Of 14 cases in which the tumor's location was specified, nine occurred in the left upper lobe.[3, 151] This location, in close proximity to the thymus, suggests that thymic anlage migrating with the lung bud during embryogenesis is responsible for the occurrence of these lesions.[29, 54] In only three cases were the tumors closely associated with a bronchus.[14, 54, 151] Collier et al. reported a cystic, squamous cell–lined teratoma that contained air because of a free bronchial communication. In another case, a small endobronchial teratoma resulted in distal bronchiectasis.[14] Six of sixteen reported pulmonary teratomas were malignant,[3, 54, 151] but the possibility of metastasis from an extrathoracic tumor must be excluded before a lesion can be considered as primary within the lung.[3] Barrett, cited by Gautam, has reported a surviving patient who was free of tumor 17 years after the excision of a malignant pulmonary teratoma.

Bronchopulmonary Anomalies

BRONCHOPULMONARY SEQUESTRATION. This is a congenital pulmonary malformation caused by the sequestration from normal lung, and subsequent abnormal development, of a portion of the embryonic lung. It consists of disorganized pulmonary parenchyma without normal bronchial or pulmonary arterial connections and contains ectatic and cystic bronchial structures.[127, 146] Although its exact origins remain undetermined, it is generally conceded that sequestration results from the abnormal budding of the foregut during the period when the lung, bronchi, and pulmonary vessels are forming.[127, 146] Occasionally, the sequestra communicate with the upper gastrointestinal tract, another foregut derivative.[127, 146] Sequestrations usually receive their blood supply from systemic arteries, and arteriography is necessary prior to surgical excision in order to visualize the major arterial branches.[146] Fatal intraoperative hemorrhage can result if systemic arteries are accidentally cut during resection.[127, 146] Bronchography is also of value in diagnosis and usually demonstrates the displacement and draping of normal bronchi around a mass lesion (Fig. 19–128).[127, 146] Two main forms of sequestration, intralobar and extralobar, have been described.[146] Although these forms have pathologic similarities, clinically and radiographically they differ significantly in several clinical and radiographic characteristics (Table 19–5).

INTRALOBAR SEQUESTRATION. This form is the most common. In this malformation, the sequestered portion of the lung lies within the visceral pleura of a normal lobe.[153] It is most frequent on the left, and two thirds occur adjacent to the diaphragm in the posterobasal segment of the left lower lobe.[127, 146] In nearly 75 per cent of cases, arterial supply is from the descending thoracic aorta, and with rare exceptions, pulmonary veins provide venous drainage.[127, 153] Uncomplicated intralobar sequestration most often appears radiographically as a homogeneous, well-defined, round or triangular mass lesion (see Fig. 19–128).[146] Rarely, uncomplicated sequestra contain air,

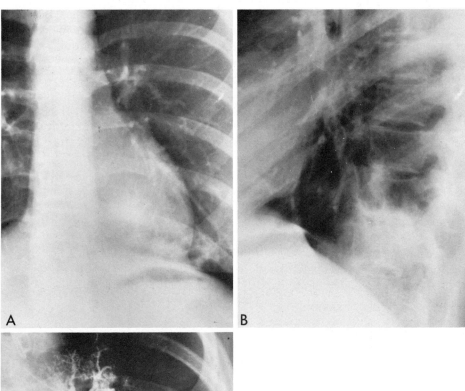

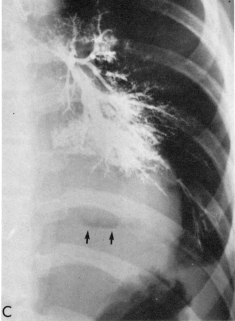

Figure 19–128. Intralobar pulmonary sequestration. Posteroanterior (*A*) and lateral (*B*) radiographs of a young woman with recurrent left lower lobe pneumonia show an ill-defined area of consolidation medially in the region of the posterobasal segment. *C,* A bronchogram demonstrates the displacement of normal bronchial structures around the area of the density, which is now seen to contain an air-fluid level (arrows). Subtracted films from an arteriogram demonstrate an anomalous artery arising from the thoracic aorta, supplying the left lung base

Legend continued on the opposite page

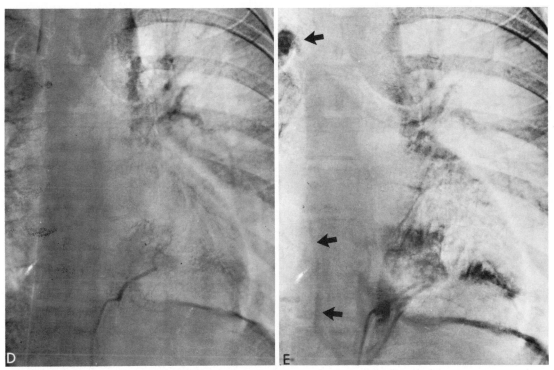

Figure 19–128 *Continued.* (D), with venous drainage (arrows) via the azygous system (E). Azygous drainage is rare with intralobar sequestration and is much more common with extralobar lesions. An intralobar sequestration, however, was found at surgery.

presumably owing to collateral ventilation or small communications with the bronchial tree.[36, 127] Air-filled sequestra may be difficult to visualize radiographically, because of their intimate association with normally aerated lung. Infection is common and the possibility of sequestration must be considered in patients with recurrent pneumonia in one portion of the lung. Following infection, a major communication with the bronchial tree often occurs, and single or multiple air- and fluid-filled cysts become visible, with a variable amount of surrounding pulmonary parenchymal consolidation. A single large cyst resembling a lung abscess can predominate. These cysts may fill at bronchography.[36]

EXTRALOBAR SEQUESTRATION. This form consists of ectopic pulmonary tissue enclosed within its own pleural envelope.[127, 146] In 90 per cent of cases, it is associated

TABLE 19–5. FEATURES DISTINGUISHING INTRALOBAR AND
EXTRALOBAR SEQUESTRATIONS*

	Intralobar	Extralobar
Pleural covering	Within the visceral pleura	Isolated pleural envelope
Usual origin of arterial supply	Thoracic aorta	Abdominal aorta
Usual venous drainage	Pulmonary veins	Systemic (azygous) veins
Bronchial communication	Occasional	Rare
Location	Left lower lobe (60%)	Left base (90%)
Associated diaphragmatic hernia	Rare	Common
Infection	Common	Rare
Age at diagnosis	Adulthood	Infancy or childhood

*Modified from Sade, R. M., Clouse, M., and Ellis, F. H., Jr.: The spectrum of pulmonary sequestration. Ann. Thorac. Surg. *18*:644–658, 1974.

with the left hemidiaphragm, but it may lie within the abdomen; eventration of the left hemidiaphragm can coexist.[127] In contrast to intralobar sequestration, the extralobar form rarely becomes infected. In infants, however, the displacement and compression of normal lung can result in respiratory distress. Extralobar sequestration appears radiographically as a soft tissue mass. Its arterial supply is most commonly from the abdominal aorta, and it drains into systemic veins, usually the azygous system.[127]

BRONCHOGENIC CYST. This results from the abnormal budding of the bronchial tree from the ventral foregut during embryonic development.[124] The cysts are lined with bronchial epithelium and contain serous fluid or mucoid material when uninfected.[120, 124] Uncomplicated cysts occasionally communicate with the esophagus or bronchial lumen,[17] and some cysts have a systemic arterial supply similar to that of sequestration.[120] In fact, Culiner regards bronchogenic cyst to be closely related to sequestration, as one manifestation of the so-called sequestration complex.[36] Bronchogenic cysts most often appear radiographically as well-defined round, oval, or slightly lobulated nodules of soft tissue density.[73, 120, 124] They account for 3.5 per cent of resected solitary pulmonary nodules.[13] Cysts are most common in the lower lobes and central portions of both lungs and range from 1 to 10 cm in diameter (Fig. 19–129).[73, 124] Occasionally, a bronchogenic cyst results in bronchial obstruction.

In a majority of patients, bronchogenic cysts become infected and communicate with the bronchial tree; infected cysts contain air and frequently demonstrate air-fluid levels radiographically.[124] Of 32 pulmonary bronchogenic cysts studied by Rogers and Osmer, 12 (38 per cent) were air filled when first seen, and nine subsequently developed an air-fluid level.[124] Seven (22 per cent) presented with air-fluid levels, and thirteen (40 per cent) had homogenous mass lesions. Typically, air-filled bronchogenic cysts are thin walled (1 or 2 mm) and sharply defined.[120, 124] Infected cysts can lose their sharp definition, however, because of the inflammatory consolidation of surrounding lung (Fig. 19–130). Symptoms are usually limited to patients with developing infection and bronchial communication.[73, 124].

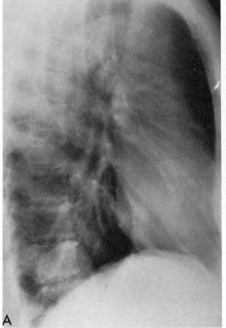

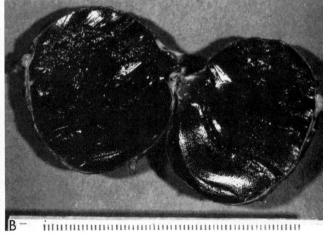

Figure 19–129. Uninfected bronchogenic cyst. *A,* A lateral radiograph of an asymptomatic 45-year-old woman shows a well-defined, lobulated mass lesion in the posterior left lower lobe. *B,* A pathologic specimen reveals an uninfected bronchogenic cyst containing dark, mucoid material.

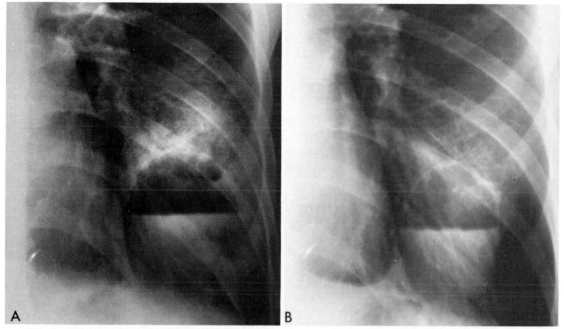

Figure 19–130. Infected bronchogenic cyst. *A,* A posteroanterior radiograph of a 30-year-old man with cough and fever demonstrates an ill-defined bronchogenic cyst containing an air-fluid level in the left lower lobe. Consolidation surrounds the cyst, obscuring its margins. *B,* Four months later, following antibiotic therapy, the cyst is thin-walled and sharply defined. The air-fluid level persists because bronchial communication is present.

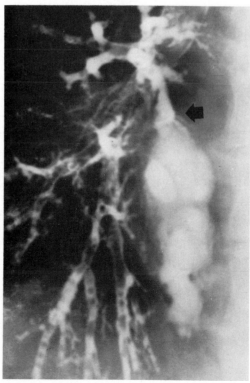

Figure 19–131. Bronchographic filling of a bronchogenic cyst. A right lower lobe bronchogram shows filling of a multiloculated bronchogenic cyst from a branch of the superior segment bronchus (arrow).

Bronchography, although of limited value in the differential diagnosis of broncho-genic cyst, helps in detecting and localizing possible associated bronchiectasis. Six of eighteen patients with bronchogenic cysts studied bronchographically showed filling of cysts by contrast material (Fig. 19–131); each contained air on plain radiographs.[124] Bronchography showed the displacement of normal bronchi by the cyst in ten patients and demonstrated bronchiectasis in two.[124] In patients with a bronchogenic cyst, bronchiectasis can result from bronchial compression or from an associated develop-mental defect of the bronchial walls referred to as congenital cystic bronchiectasis.[36]

Vascular Malformations

CONGENITAL ARTERIOVENOUS FISTULA.   This is an abnormal communication of the pulmonary artery and vein within the lung.[77] It is postulated that this malformation results from the deficient formation or abnormal dilatation of pulmonary capillaries owing to a developmental defect in the capillary wall.[58] From 35 to 67 per cent of cases are associated with Osler-Weber-Rendu disease (hereditary hemorrhagic telangiecta-sis), in which arteriovenous malformations are found throughout the skin, mucous membranes, and viscera.[42, 58, 98, 106]

Pulmonary arteriovenous fistula is twice as common in women as in men and is most often diagnosed in patients of middle age;[77] in a study by Dines et al. the mean age at diagnosis was 41 years.[42] Symptoms or physical findings generally reflect the right-to-left shunting of unoxygenated blood through the arteriovenous communica-tion. The most common symptoms are dyspnea, palpitation, hemoptysis, and chest pain; positive physical findings include an audible bruit, clubbing, and cyano-sis.[42, 58, 106] In general, fistulas less than 2 cm in diameter on chest radiographs are asymptomatic.[42] Furthermore, according to Dines et al., single fistulas are less common-ly symptomatic (37 per cent) or associated with positive physical findings (68 per cent) than multiple fistulas (59 per cent symptomatic and 86 per cent with positive physical findings).[42] Cerebrovascular accidents associated with cyanosis and polycythemia, and embolization through the fistula from systemic veins are serious complications. Rupture can occur with hemothorax.[58, 98, 108]

Pulmonary arteriovenous malformations can occur in several forms. A simple arteriovenous fistula supplied by one feeding artery and drained by one pulmonary vein is most common.[42] Radiographically, this simple fistula appears as a peripheral, well-defined round, oval, or serpentine density, often with large vessels extending to the hilum (Fig. 19–132).[42, 106] In some cases, fluoroscopy demonstrates pulsation of the fistula or a change in its size with respiratory maneuvers. Tomography can accurately define the vascular nature of this lesion, but pulmonary arteriography is necessary for a final diagnosis.[106] Furthermore, both lungs must be examined at arteriography; fistulas are multiple in 35 per cent of the patients and bilateral in 8 per cent.[42] Pathologically, a simple fistula is a dilated, thin-walled sac, usually in a subpleural location.[98] More than two thirds are located in the lower lobes.[42, 58, 98] Fistulas can enlarge over a period of months or years; a radiographically visible increase in size was noted in 11 (17 per cent) of Dines' 63 patients.[42] A rapid increase in size can occur.[77] Complex arteriovenous fistulas with multiple arterial and venous communications have been reported. These can be large and are often symptomatic.

Pulmonary telangiectasia is an uncommon form of arteriovenous malformation characterized by innumerable minute fistulas scattered diffusely throughout both lungs.[75] Symptoms are common and progressive and cyanosis is present in all patients. Diagnosis is usually made in childhood.[37, 75] In a review of sixteen patients, the chest radiographs were normal in three.[37] In 13 patients with abnormal radiographs, the findings were generally limited to an abnormal pattern or distribution of pulmonary vessels. Nodular densities were unusual. A coarse, spidery appearance of the peripheral vessels, vascular tortuosity, and hypervascularity have all been reported.[37] Pulmonary arteriograms may seem normal if magnification views are not obtained.[129] Abnormal arteriographic findings include beaded or tortuous vessels, bulging small arteries and veins in the lung periphery, small aneurysmal sacs, and multiple ill-defined areas of

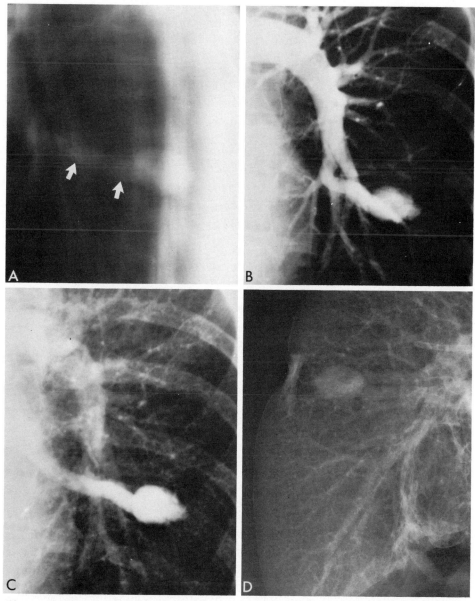

Figure 19–132. Arteriovenous fistula. *A*, A lateral tomogram of the left lower lobe in an asymptomatic young man with a left lower lobe nodule shows a well-defined oval 2-cm nodule, with a large vascular structure (arrows), extending toward the left atrium. Pulmonary arteriography demonstrates a simple arteriovenous fistula with a single supplying artery (*B*) and vein (*C*). *D*, A radiograph of the inflated left lower lobe taken after resection clearly shows the fistula with a parallel artery and vein extending from the hilum.

vascular blush associated with the early filling of veins.[37, 129] Treatment is difficult, and the prognosis is poor.[75]

Surgery is the treatment of choice for pulmonary arteriovenous fistula, and some authors regard the presence of a lesion as an indication for its excision.[98, 106] Others recommend a more conservative approach, with surgery limited to patients with (1) symptoms and one or more enlarging fistulas, (2) symptoms and large shunts, or (3) a history of Osler-Weber-Rendu disease. Each of these conditions is associated with an increased incidence of death in patients treated by nonsurgical means.[42, 58] At operation, an attempt is made to limit the amount of lung tissue removed; in some cases, multiple fistulas, unrecognized at the time of surgery, enlarge and become clinically significant after the resection of the dominant lesion.[106] The local dissection of fistulas, with the ligation and division of their branches, is particularly advantageous when multiple lesions must be removed.[19] Of 36 patients treated surgically and followed for an average of eight years, 31 were considered well, with no progression of symptoms or recurrence of lesions; four experienced worsening of dyspnea and cyanosis owing to the enlargement of their fistulas; and one died of a cerebrovascular accident of undetermined cause.[42] In the same series, 27 patients were treated without surgery. Seven of these experienced enlargement of their fistulas, and four died from causes attributable to their vascular lesions.[42]

MISCELLANEOUS TUMORS

Polyps

SQUAMOUS PAPILLOMA.   Papilloma represents an abnormal proliferation of stratified squamous, or sometimes, ciliated columnar epithelium forming a polypoid mass within the airway lumen.[25, 48, 96] These lesions are supported by a core of fibrovascular tissue connecting them to the tracheal or bronchial wall.[25] They are benign and thought to be of viral origin; malignant change rarely occurs.[48, 63]

Papilloma is the most common laryngeal tumor of childhood, and laryngeal papillomas occasionally occur in adults.[96, 125] Laryngeal lesions are often multiple and spread locally.[103, 125] In children, papillomas are successfully treated by surgical excision or regress at puberty.[48, 63, 125] In 2 per cent of the patients, however, lesions spread distally to involve the tracheobronchial tree, a condition referred to as tracheobronchial papillomatosis.[96, 139] The trachea is most often involved,[125] and of 26 patients surveyed by Caldarola et al. the trachea alone was affected in 21, the trachea and bronchi in 3, and bronchi alone in 2.[25] Tracheal and bronchial papillomas rarely occur without previous laryngeal disease.[139]

The involvement of the trachea often produces symptoms, hoarseness due to laryngeal disease being the most common. Hemoptysis also occurs.[25, 96, 125] In most cases, the lesions are multiple and small, ranging from 3 to 6 mm in diameter, but they can be large, resulting in tracheal obstruction.[25] Plain radiographs are rarely of value. Tomograms or contrast tracheography are necessary for diagnosis.[25, 96]

The extension of papillomas to the bronchi, bronchioles, and lung parenchyma is rare,[125] only ten cases being reported in a recent review.[140] The interval between the diagnoses of laryngeal lesions and bronchial spread ranges from 1 to 36 years. Although laryngeal lesions are most common in children younger than five, the average age of patients with tumors involving the bronchial tree is 15.[125, 140] Bronchial obstruction results in wheezing, atelectasis, and recurrent pneumonia. Papillomas may be visualized as nodular mass lesions within the lung, and they often cavitate, with progressive

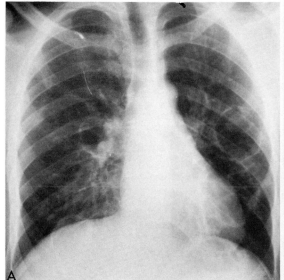

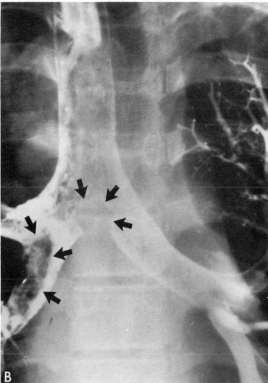

Figure 19–133.   Tracheobronchial papillomatosis. *A,* A posteroanterior radiograph of a 16-year-old girl with bronchopulmonary spread of laryngeal papillomatosis. This radiograph shows numerous large cysts due to cavitation and expansion of papillomas. *B,* A bronchogram demonstrates a large papilloma at the carina and in the right main bronchus and bronchus intermedius (arrows). Such an appearance is characteristic of this progressive disease.

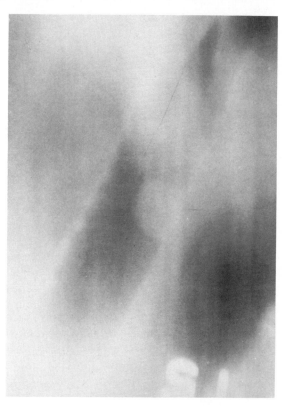

Figure 19–134.   Tracheal polyp. A lateral tomogram in a 66-year-old man shows a well-defined 1.5-cm polyp arising from the posterior tracheal wall. This lesion is sessile and larger than most papillomas.

expansion of thick- or thin-walled cysts (Fig. 19–133).[125, 140] Bronchography can show endobronchial masses, and the filling of cysts has been reported.[125, 140]

Bronchoscopic excision of tracheal or bronchial papillomas is the treatment of choice, but the lesions recur following resection in more than 90 per cent of patients.[25, 103] In Caldarola's series, as many as 52 procedures were required for the removal of papillomas.[25] Tracheostomy may be required for associated laryngeal lesions that produce airway obstruction.[96, 125, 139] Cystic pulmonary lesions are not usually associated with symptoms and, unless they are infected, no treatment is necessary.[140]

INFLAMMATORY POLYPS. Inflammatory polyps of the tracheobronchial tree are characterized histologically by a loose connective tissue core covered by normal bronchial epithelium.[87] They lack the squamous overgrowth typical of papillomas, and, in general, occur in older persons.[25, 126, 133] These lesions may be polypoid or sessile and are larger than squamous papillomas (Fig. 19–134).[25] In most patients, polyps range from 0.5 to 2 cm in diameter;[25] in one reported case an endobronchial polyp measured 8 cm in length.[154] Occasionally, polyps are multiple.[87] The findings of bronchial obstruction are common. Following excision, polyps do not recur.

Granular Cell Myoblastoma

Granular cell myoblastoma is a rare tumor; approximately 50 cases involving the tracheobronchial tree and lung have been reported.[132, 148] Despite its name, this tumor does not derive from muscle cells; a neural origin is most likely.[26, 89] Cases have occurred in patients ranging from 8 to 59 years of age, the majority in patients from 30 to 49.[158]

These tumors arise in relation to the bronchial wall, and most are present as masses within major bronchi.[26, 96] The symptoms and radiographic findings of bronchial obstruction are common.[26, 96] Tracheal involvement can occur (Fig. 19–135), often with extension into mainstem bronchi.[158] Multiple endotracheal or endobronchial masses are present in approximately 10 to 15 per cent of the patients.[132, 148] Granular cell myoblastoma is rarely present as a solitary pulmonary nodule, and the lesions range from several millimeters to more than 6 cm in diameter.[26, 132]

In approximately 30 per cent of the cases, tumors extend locally, permeating the bronchial wall and peribronchial tissues, and infiltration of the pulmonary parenchyma has been reported.[103, 148] Because of this, endobronchial resection is often incomplete and tumors may recur.[148] The complete excision of the lesion, segmental resection, lobectomy, or pneumonectomy is often performed, depending on the site of the tumor.[89, 132] Distant metastases do not occur.[96]

Lipoma

Tracheobronchial lipoma originates in the collections of fat found in the walls of cartilage-containing airways.[35, 80, 96] It has been diagnosed in patients ranging from 29 to 64 years of age, and nearly 90 per cent of the cases occur in men.[35, 80, 115] By 1968, 32 cases had been recorded.[35] Lipomas are most common in the main or lobar bronchi and typically lie within the bronchial lumen.[96, 111, 115] Endobronchial lesions are usually oval, measuring several centimeters in length. The symptoms and radiographic findings of bronchial obstruction are common, and obstructive pneumonitis and bronchiectasis are often found (Fig. 19–136).[96, 111] Occasionally, a lipoma extends in a dumbbell fashion to lie primarily outside of the bronchus.[35, 45] These tumors may be

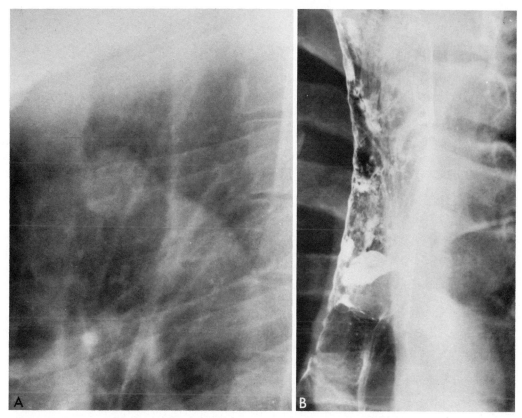

Figure 19–135. Granular cell myoblastoma. *A,* A 2-cm polypoid intratracheal mass is visible on the lateral radiograph of a 29-year-old man with dyspnea and wheezing. *B,* A tantalum tracheogram, in the right posterior oblique position, clearly shows the mass, which is capped by a collection of contrast. Endotracheal or endobronchial involvement is characteristic of this tumor.

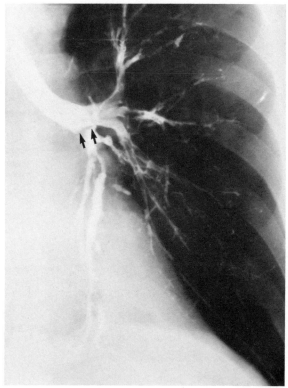

Figure 19–136. Endobronchial lipoma. An endobronchial mass, proven to be a lipoma, is visible (arrows) obstructing the left lower lobe bronchus, resulting in distal bronchiectasis. In patients with this tumor, bronchiectasis usually requires lobectomy.

large. The fatty nature of lipomas is rarely appreciated on chest radiographs, and a correct diagnosis prior to surgery is rarely made.[103]

A number of cases have been treated by bronchoscopic excision of the endobronchial tumor. In no case has there been a recurrence. The common finding of destructive disease in the distal lung tissue may necessitate lobectomy or pneumonectomy, however.[80, 103, 111]

Lipomas may occur in an extrapleural location, but these tumors are distinct clinically from the endobronchial lesions.[96, 103] Liposarcoma of the lung is rare.[96]

Leiomyoma

Leiomyoma of the lung and tracheobronchial tree is a rare tumor; a review of the literature in 1969 revealed only 24 cases.[159] It is thought to arise from smooth muscle found in the walls of bronchi or perhaps blood vessels.[1, 103] It has been reported in patients ranging from 4 to 63 years of age[158] and is most common in women.[1, 96, 144] Of the 24 cases reviewed by Weitzner, 10 were endobronchial and 14 occurred within the pulmonary parenchyma.[159] Among patients with endobronchial lesions, symptoms are common and often due to obstructive pneumonia; bronchiectasis may result.[144] In such patients, radiographic findings are limited to signs of airway obstruction.[144] Pulmonary parenchymal leiomyomas are usually asymptomatic.[96, 103] They appear radiographically as well-defined, peripheral mass lesions and range from 2 to 13 cm in diameter.[159] Calcification is rare, and cavitation does not occur. Because lesions often involve the lung parenchyma, segmental resection or lobectomy is often required.[96, 144]

Leiomyosarcoma is more common than leiomyoma; more than 50 cases have been reported.[67] The average age of patients is the same as that of patients with leiomyoma,

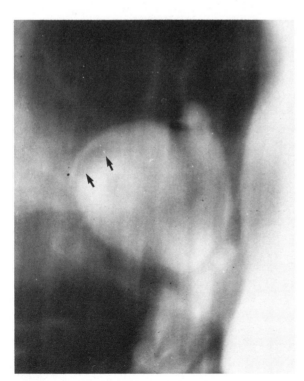

Figure 19–137. Pulmonary leiomyosarcoma. A well-defined mass with an area of cavitation (arrows) is visible in a 24-year-old man. Except for the cavitation, this appearance is similar to that of leiomyoma.

but leiomyosarcoma is twice as common in men as in women. Patients are without exception symptomatic.[1, 67, 119] A nodular pulmonary mass, generally larger than a leiomyoma, is seen in a majority of cases.[67, 119] Cavitation may occur (Fig. 19–137).[67] Endobronchial obstruction with atelectasis occurred in 5 of 16 patients reviewed by Agnos and Starkey.[1] Hilar lymph node metastasis does not occur. The treatment is surgical excision; the survival rate after resection is better than that in cases of bronchogenic carcinoma.[67, 119]

So-called multiple pulmonary leiomyomas associated with smooth muscle tumors of the uterus most likely represent pulmonary metastases from a low-grade uterine leiomyosarcoma.[9, 96]

Fibroma and Fibrosarcoma

Fibroma can involve the lung or tracheobronchial tree but is rare.[31, 45, 90] Patients range in age from 24 to 84 years of age.[96] Pulmonary parenchymal lesions are most common in the right lower lobe and are usually asymptomatic.[31, 90] Tracheal or bronchial lesions produce symptoms and signs of obstruction.[31] Malignant transformation to fibrosarcoma can occur, and segmental excision or lobectomy is recommended.[96] Endobronchial resection may be followed by recurrence.[31]

Fibrosarcomas, regardless of their location, are usually symptomatic.[45, 67, 156] Of 13 cases reported by Guccion and Rosen, 3 were endobronchial and 10 were found within the lung parenchyma.[67] Endobronchial lesions are most common in children and young adults, whereas pulmonary masses are found in patients of middle age.[67, 156] Pulmonary lesions are usually round and well defined, measuring 3.5 to 9 cm in diameter, but they may exceed 20 cm.[67, 156] They are slow growing, and the prognosis following excision may be good.[67] A survival of 24 years has been reported.[67]

Chondroma And Chondrosarcoma

True chondromas, containing only cartilage, are exceedingly rare, and their relationship to the more common chondromatous hamartomas is uncertain.[114, 155] They occur most commonly as endobronchial lesions, and they can calcify.[15, 114] Chondrosarcoma is also rare: 17 cases were recorded in a recent review. This tumor occurs much more commonly as a pulmonary mass lesion than as a mass within the tracheal or bronchial lumen.[39, 121] In general, pulmonary lesions have a poor prognosis, 10 in one review of 12 patients with pulmonary chondrosarcomas dying within one year of diagnosis.[39] Tracheal and bronchial lesions may be associated with longer survival, but only two cases have been reported.[39]

Neural Tumors

Neurogenic tumors of the lung and tracheobronchial tree, either benign or malignant, are rare.[2, 34, 43] Among benign tumors are neurilemmoma, neurofibroma, and neuroma;[103] they are most often present as well-defined solitary nodules within the lung parenchyma, but endobronchial lesions have been reported.[2, 43, 114] These tumors, particularly when multiple, may be associated with neurofibromatosis.[96, 103] They are thought to arise from sympathetic nerve fibers that accompany arterioles or bronchioles.

Vascular Tumors

Vascular lung tumors are classified, according to their cell of origin, as sclerosing hemangioma, hemangiopericytoma, and hemangioendothelioma.[157] Although they all contain vascular channels, these tumors are solid. Unlike arteriovenous fistulas, vascular lung tumors rarely exhibit pulsation at fluoroscopy or opacification during angiography.

SCLEROSING HEMANGIOMA.   Sclerosing hemangioma is a rare benign tumor; only 19 well-documented cases were recorded in a revent review.[157] It is characterized by the proliferation and sclerosis of small vessels, and areas of hemorrhage are common. Because of histologic similarities, this tumor is often grouped with postinflammatory lesions; at present, its origin remains uncertain.[103] More than 75 per cent of the cases occur in women, most often between 30 and 60 years of age, and hemoptysis results in 40 per cent. Radiographically, the lesion appears as a homogeneous nodule ranging from 1.9 to 9 cm in diameter, nearly half occurring in the right lower lobe (Fig. 19–138). Bronchial involvement is unusual, and bronchial obstruction is not characteristic of this tumor. Excision is necessary for diagnosis; recurrence has not been reported.[157]

HEMANGIOPERICYTOMA.   This tumor contains a profuse proliferation of capillaries, surrounded by neoplastic accumulations of pericytes.[101] Twenty-eight cases of hemangiopericytoma originating in lung tissue were reviewed by Meade et al.[101] Nearly two thirds occur in women, and patients range in age from 18 to 73 years. The tumors tend to be peripheral, varying in size from 2 to 15 cm. Calcification does not occur. In several cases reported by Feldman and Seaman, pulsation was visible at fluoroscopy or surgery, and in one patient a slight tumor blush was visible at angiography.[49] These have not been consistent findings, however, and the vascular channels within the tumor may

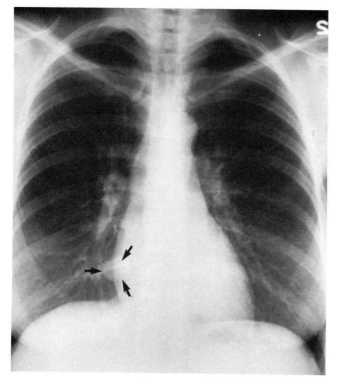

Figure 19–138.   Sclerosing hemangioma. An asymptomatic 40-year-old woman shows a well-defined right lower lobe nodule on a posteroanterior radiograph. This nodule was found to represent a sclerosing hemangioma at surgery. Hemoptysis is a common presenting complaint in patients with this tumor. (*From* Webb, W. R., and Gamsu, G.: Sclerosing hemangioma of the lung. Br. J. Radiol. *50*:213–215, 1977. Reproduced by permission.)

be bloodless.[101] Hemangiopericytoma can be benign or malignant, and excision is the treatment of choice.[49, 101] The mortality rate from recurrence averages 40 per cent.[101]

HEMANGIOENDOTHELIOMA. Hemangioendothelioma, or angiosarcoma, occurs rarely within the lung. It usually appears as a pulmonary mass lesion[150] and may result from the malignant transformation of benign angioma. Metastases are common.

Chemodectoma

Chemodectoma is a nonchromaffin paraganglioma, but it may be confused histologically with bronchial adenoma or hemangioma.[59, 105] It occurs as a peripheral solitary nodule, and symptoms are uncommon.[59, 105] Pulmonary chemodectoma is rare, mediastinal tumors being more frequent.[96] Microscopic pulmonary lesions resembling chemodectoma have been reported but are invisible radiographically and have no clinical significance.[59]

TUMORLIKE CONDITIONS AND PSEUDOTUMORS

Postinflammatory Pseudotumor

Postinflammatory pseudotumors of the lung are not uncommon and accounted for 7 of 130 benign tumors reviewed by Arrigoni et al.[5] They are considered to represent the reparative phase of an inflammatory process, although a history of previous inflammatory disease is sometimes lacking.[96, 103, 113] Depending on their dominant histologic features, these tumors have been referred to as xanthomas, xanthofibromas, histiocytomas, xanthogranulomas, plasma cell granulomas, and pseudolymphomas.[5, 32, 14] Nearly one third occur in children.[113] Some cases begin as acute pneumonia, but more than 50 per cent are asymptomatic.[113] Postinflammatory pseudotumors most often appear as single or multiple well-defined pulmonary nodules, and they may be large.[32] Rarely do endobronchial lesions occur.[4, 32] Although pseudotumors may be confused histologically with malignant lesions, they do not metastasize and rarely recur following excision.[96, 113]

Plasma Cell Granuloma

In an excellent survey, Bahadori and Liebow reviewed the characteristics of 40 patients with plasma cell granuloma.[11] Most affected patients are less than 30 years of age at the time of diagnosis; the tumor is particularly common among children. Twenty-four patients were asymptomatic and without a history of prior disease. In 23 patients, plasma cell granulomas appeared radiographically as solitary, circumscribed, round or oval nodules; in ten, the nodules were well defined (Fig. 19–139). The masses ranged up to 12 cm in diameter, and calcification or cavitation was seen in several. Thirteen additional patients had ill-defined densities or densities suggesting atelectasis. In many cases, the masses surrounded bronchi, producing bronchial compression, or extended endobronchially. Distal bronchiectasis was occasionally present. Serial radiographs often demonstrated an increase in the size of the lesions over a period of months or years. In the large majority of patients, plasma cell granuloma behaves as a benign tumor. Lesions may recur, however, if incompletely resected and can invade the mediastinum, thereby compressing normal structures.[11]

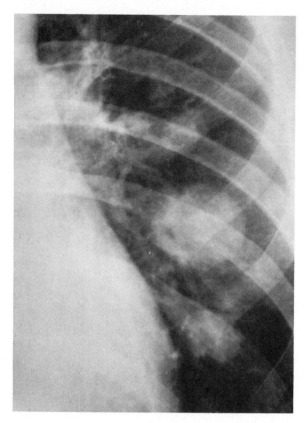

Figure 19–139. Multiple plasma cell granulomas. Posteroanterior view of the left lung in a 35-year-old asymptomatic man demonstrates multiple well-defined pulmonary nodules. Biopsy revealed numerous plasma cells. Plasma cell granulomas are solitary lesions in a large majority of cases.

Pseudolymphoma

This is a distinct form of postinflammatory pseudotumor.[32] It consists of a mixed cellular infiltration by many mature lymphocytes and is characterized by true lymphoid germinal centers.[81] In general, patients with pseudolymphoma are older than those with other forms of pseudotumor, ranging in age from 38 to 80.[81] Radiographically, pseudolymphoma produces ill-defined areas of segmental or nodular consolidation that extend peripherally.[32, 81] Air bronchograms are almost always present, distinguishing this lesion from other pseudotumors.[32, 81] Hilar and mediastinal adenopathy and pleural effusion do not occur.[81] Treatment should be conservative; patients are usually asymptomatic and the lesion is self limited.

Amyloidosis

The deposition of amyloid material within the respiratory tract can result in three forms of disease: (1) tracheobronchial amyloidosis, (2) pulmonary parenchymal masses, and (3) the diffuse infiltration of the pulmonary interstitium.[30, 76, 160] The involvement of the lung or tracheobronchial tree is common in patients with primary amyloidosis but is rarely seen in patients with disease secondary to chronic inflammation or malignancy.[76] In many patients, amyloidosis is limited to the respiratory system.[6] Patients are generally older than 50 at the time of diagnosis, and the condition occurs most frequently in men.[30, 76]

TRACHEOBRONCHIAL AMYLOIDOSIS.   This can occur as a solitary endotracheal or endobronchial mass, or it can produce generalized infiltration of the tracheobronchial tree.[6, 25, 138] The solitary endotracheal masses usually involve the larynx and subglottic region and produce airway obstruction.[76, 138] Diffuse involvement is less common, but more than 20 cases have been reported.[6, 76] Symptoms include cough, hemoptysis, obstruction of airways, and recurrent pneumonia.[6, 76] Radiographs of patients with a solitary mass are nonspecific (Fig. 19–140).[138] With the diffuse form of tracheobronchial amyloidosis, radiographs show generalized, irregular narrowing of the trachea and main bronchi, with thickening of the right paratracheal stripe, owing to the infiltration of the tracheal wall.[30, 60, 76] Tomography and bronchography are often helpful in demonstrating the extent of disease and in further evaluating its appearance; multiple eccentric or concentric strictures are associated with multiple nodular masses and bronchial obstructions.[30, 60, 76] Tracheobronchial amyloidosis most often involves the trachea and contiguous main bronchi, but isolated bronchial lesions have been reported. The treatment is bronchoscopic removal of the obstructing amyloid deposits.[6, 76] Repeated bronchoscopies are often necessary.[60] The redeposition of amyloid occurs at an unpredictable rate, and recurrences are frequent.[60] Bleeding is a complication of endoscopic removal and can be fatal.[60]

NODULAR AMYLOIDOSIS.   This condition is characterized by single or, more often, multiple pulmonary masses.[76, 145] The nodules usually range from 2 to 6 cm in diameter and are well-defined and round or oval.[76, 145] They are often located peripherally and can demonstrate calcification or cavitation.[6] Stippled calcification is said to occur in half of the cases but can be difficult to recognize without tomography.[76, 145] The nodules grow slowly in most cases but may enlarge rapidly and can recur following excision.[76] Hilar adenopathy is sometimes seen.[76, 160]

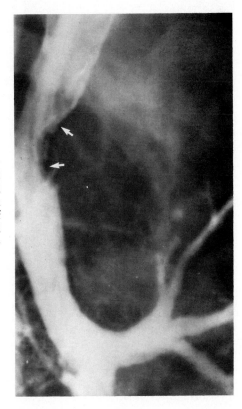

Figure 19–140.   Tracheobronchial amyloidosis. A left bronchogram, in a 16-year-old boy with a cough, wheezing, and shortness of breath, shows slight narrowing of the distal trachea with a sessile mass partially obstructing the left main bronchus (arrows). Bronchoscopic biopsy was diagnostic of amyloidosis. Repeated bronchoscopic excisions of amyloid tissue were necessary to alleviate the symptoms of obstruction.

INTERSTITIAL AMYLOIDOSIS. This is usually associated with disseminated disease.[76] Radiographs show interstitial thickening and honeycombing.[76]

Tracheobronchiopathia Osteochondroplastica

This condition is characterized by numerous cartilaginous and bony nodules within the submucosal tissues of the trachea and main bronchi.[16, 25] Is is relatively common, accounting for nearly 30 per cent of the benign tracheal tumors in adults,[56] and 17 per cent of the benign lesions involving the trachea and bronchi;[25] by 1974, 245 cases had been reported.[100] The origin of tracheobronchiopathia osteochondroplastica is unknown. The condition may result from metaplasia of elastic tissues in the tracheal wall or from a degenerative process, or it may be an end stage of tracheobronchial amyloidosis.[16, 76, 100] It is most common in men, and patients are usually more than 50. Symptoms are often lacking, but cough, hoarseness, mild dyspnea, and hemoptysis occur in some patients.[16]

Radiographs demonstrate narrowing of the trachea, with thickening of its wall and the projection of numerous irregular nodules into the tracheal lumen;[100] the posterior tracheal wall is usually spared (Fig. 19–141).[25, 100] In most patients, similar abnormalities affect the major bronchi. The calcification and ossification of submucosal nodules are

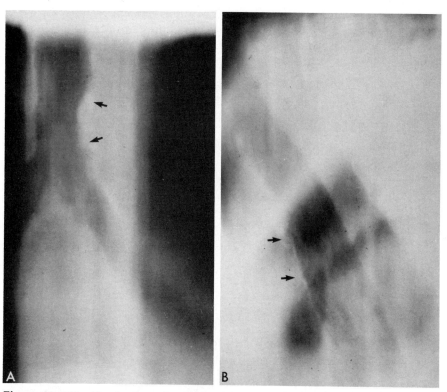

Figure 19–141. Tracheobronchopathia osteochondroplastica. Anteroposterior (A) and lateral (B) tomograms of a 64-year-old man show irregular narrowing of the lumen and main bronchi. Calcified nodules are present within the tracheal wall (arrows), but the posterior (membranous) portion of the trachea is, characteristically, spared. These nodules consist of cartilage and bone, perhaps reflecting a degenerative or metaplastic process.

characteristic features.[100] Except for the calcification, the radiographic appearance closely simulates tracheobronchial amyloidosis. This condition has also been confused with saber-sheath trachea.[134]

No specific treatment has evolved for tracheobronchiopathia; in general, therapy is nonsurgical and directed at the symptoms of airway obstruction or infection.[100, 134] The progression of symptoms is not common.

Scleroma

Scleroma is a chronic inflammatory disease of the upper respiratory tract. It is common in people of the Near East, Eastern Europe, Russia, and South America.[51, 71, 93] Thought to be bacterial in origin, it results in granulomatous lesions involving the nose, pharynx, larynx, and trachea.[51] Radiographically, tracheal involvement can take two forms.[71] Generalized diffuse mucosal thickening, with narrowing of the tracheal air column, is the more common, occurring in 12 of 14 patients studied by Handausa and Elwi (Fig. 19–142).[71] The other form, localized tumor masses, is occasionally seen.[51, 71]

Ectopic Tissue

INTRAPULMONARY LYMPH NODES. These are normally found near the hila, extending to the third- and fourth-order bronchi.[47, 117] Occasionally, peripheral, subpleural aggregations of lymphoid tissue become large, with a well-defined capsule. These are radiographically visible as small, circumscribed, peripheral pulmonary nodules.[20, 47] Subpleural lymph nodes made up 4 of 887 asymptomatic resected solitary pulmonary nodules reported by Steele;[142] nearly 20 cases have been reported. Visible lymph nodes are most common in the lower lobes (Fig. 19–143).[20, 96] They may grow in response to chronic inflammation.[47]

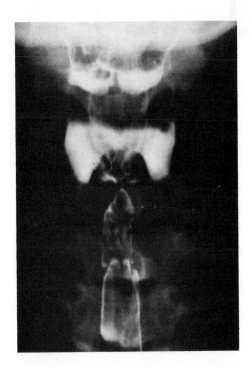

Figure 19–142. Tracheal scleroma. Laryngotracheogram in a young man with respiratory distress shows narrowing of the proximal trachea due to scleroma. The larynx is normal, but it is often involved in this disease.

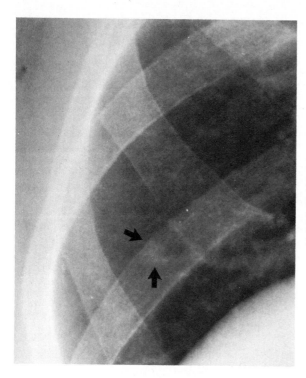

Figure 19–143. Intrapulmonary lymph node. A small well-defined nodule (arrows) is visible in the right lower lobe on this posteroanterior radiograph. This nodule, representing an intrapulmonary lymph node, was unchanged in size during a period of several years but was removed along with a right lower lobe adenocarcinoma. Intrapulmonary lymph nodes are most often found in the lower lobes.

ENDOMETRIOSIS. This condition of the lung and bronchi is rare, the literature of 1968 reporting only five cases in which endometrial tissue within the lung was associated with the symptoms and radiographic findings of lung disease.[83] The origin of endometrial tissue in the lung parenchyma is unknown but may be embolic; in women dying during, or shortly after, pregnancy, microscopic deposits of endometrium are sometimes seen within the lung. Pulmonary endometriosis presents as a pulmonary mass lesion, up to 4 cm in diameter, or as an endobronchial lesion accompanied by signs of bronchial obstruction.[83, 123] The masses are often subpleural. It has been suggested that some peripheral deposits of endometrium within the lung may derive from the more common pleural lesions that result from the direct spread of endometrial tissue from the abdomen.[83] Pulmonary masses may be cystic and thin walled. In one patient, a pulmonary density was visible only during episodes of menstruation associated with hemoptysis.[123]

SPLENOSIS. This condition results from the autotransplantation of splenic tissue from the abdomen to the pleural space following trauma to the spleen and left diaphragm.[38, 41] Nodules of splenic tissue grow in the pleural space, producing single or multiple nodules that are indistinguishable radiographically from lung masses. Splenosis occurs only on the left and is diagnosed 10 to 32 years following the splenic injury.[38] Splenosis is generally asymptomatic; rarely is the diagnosis made before surgery. In one reported case, however, in a man with an apparent left lung mass, a preoperative diagnosis of splenosis was made, using a radioisotope liver-spleen scan.[41]

References

1. Agnos, J. W., and Starkey, G. W. B.: Primary leiomyosarcoma and leiomyoma of the lung. Review of the literature and report of two cases of leiomyosarcoma. N. Engl. J. Med. *258*:12–17, 1958.

2. Aletras, A., Bjork, V. O., and Fors, B.: Benign broncho-pulmonary neoplasms. Dis. Chest 44:498–504, 1963.
3. Ali, M. Y., and Wong, P. K.: Intrapulmonary teratoma. Thorax 19:228–235, 1964.
4. Armstrong, P., Elston, C., and Sanderson, M.: Endobronchial histiocytoma. Br. J. Radiol. 48:221–222, 1975.
5. Arrigoni, M. G., Woolner, L. B., Bernatz, P. E., et al.: Benign tumors of the lung. A ten year surgical experience. J. Thorac. Cardiovasc. Surg. 60:589–599, 1970.
6. Attwood, H. D., Price, C. G., and Riddell, R. J.: Primary diffuse tracheobronchial amyloidosis. Thorax 27:620–624, 1972.
7. Aytac, A., Yurdakul, Y., Ikizler, C., et al.: Inhalation of foreign bodies in children. Report of 500 cases. J. Thorac. Cardiovasc. Surg. 74:145–151, 1977.
8. Bachman, A. L., and Teixidor, H. S.: The posterior tracheal band: a reflector of local superior mediastinal abnormality. Br. J. Radiol. 48:352–359, 1975.
9. Bachman, D., and Wolff, M.: Pulmonary metastases from benign-appearing smooth muscle tumors of the uterus. Am. J. Roentgenol. 127:441–446, 1976.
10. Bachynski, J. E.: Selective bronchography of solitary mass lesions in the lung. J. Can. Assoc. Radiol. 22:65–70, 1971.
11. Bahadori, M., and Liebow, A. A.: Plasma cell-granulomas of the lung. Cancer 31:191–208, 1973.
12. Bateson, E. M., and Abbott, E. K.: Mixed tumors of the lung, or hamarto-chondromas. A review of the radiological appearances of cases published in the literature and a report of fifteen new cases. Clin. Radiol. 11:232–247, 1960.
13. Bateson, E. M.: An analysis of 155 solitary lung lesions illustrating the differential diagnosis of mixed tumors of the lung. Clin. Radiol. 16:51–65, 1965.
14. Bateson, E. M., Hayes, J. A., and Woo-Ming, M.: Endobronchial teratoma associated with bronchiectasis and bronchiolectasis. Thorax 23:69–76, 1968.
15. Bateson, E. M.: Histogenesis of intrapulmonary and endobronchial hamartomas and chondromas (cartilage-containing tumors): a hypothesis. J. Pathol. 101:77–82, 1970.
16. Bergeron, D., Cormier, Y., and Desmeules, M.: Tracheobronchopathia osteochondroplastica. Am. Rev. Respir. Dis. 114:803–806, 1976.
17. Bergstrom, J. F., Yost, R. V., Ford, K. T., et al.: Unusual roentgen manifestations of bronchogenic cysts. Radiology 107:49–54, 1973.
18. Berkmen, Y. M.: Bronchial obstruction in unresolved pneumonia and its differentiation from broncho-genic carcinoma. Radiology 105:309–313, 1972.
19. Bjork, V. O.: Local extirpation of multiple bilateral pulmonary arteriovenous aneurysms. J. Thorac. Cardiovasc. Surg. 53:293–296, 1967.
20. Blakely, R. W., Blumenthal, B. J., and Herbert, L. F.: Benign intrapulmonary lymph node presenting as coin lesion. South. Med. J. 67:1216–1218, 1974.
21. Bleyer, J. M., and Marks, J. H.: Tuberculomas and hamartomas of the lung: comparative study of 66 proved cases. Am. J. Roentgenol. Radium Ther. Nucl. Med. 77:1013–1022, 1957.
22. Bower, G.: Bronchial adenoma. A review of twenty-eight cases. Am. Rev. Respir. Dis. 92:558–563, 1965.
23. Brown, L. R., and DeRemee, R. A.: 55° oblique hilar tomography. Mayo Clin. Proc. 51:89–95, 1976.
24. Burcharth, F., and Axelsson, C.: Bronchial adenomas. Thorax 27:442–449, 1972.
25. Caldarola, V. T., Harrison, E. G., Clagett, O. T., et al.: Benign tumors and tumor-like conditions of the trachea and bronchi. Ann. Otol. Rhinol. Laryngol. 73:1042–1061, 1964.
26. Campbell, D. C., Jr., Smith, E. P., Jr., Hood, R. H., Jr., et al.: Benign granular-cell myoblastoma of the bronchus. Review of the literature and report of a case. Dis. Chest 46:729–733, 1964.
27. Cleveland, R. H., Nice, C. M., Jr., and Ziskind, J.: Primary adenoid cystic carcinoma (cylindroma) of the trachea. Radiology 122:597–600, 1977.
28. Cohen, S., and Hossain, M. S.: Primary carcinoma of the lung. A review of 417 histologically proved cases. Dis. Chest 49:67–74, 1966.
29. Collier, F. C., Dowling, E. A., Plott, D., et al.: Teratoma of the lung. Arch. Pathol. 68:138–142, 1959.
30. Cook, A. J., Weinstein, M., and Powell, R. D.: Diffuse amyloidosis of the tracheobronchial tree. Bronchographic manifestations. Radiology 107:303–304, 1973.
31. Corona, F. E., and Okeson, G. C.: Endobronchial fibroma. An unusual case of segmental atelectasis. Am. Rev. Respir. Dis. 110:350–353, 1974.
32. Cox, I. L., Chang, C. H. J., and Mantz, F.: Pseudotumor of the lung. A case report and review stressing radiographic criteria. Chest 67:723–725, 1975.
33. Crawford, T. J., and Cahill, J. L.: The surgical treatment of pulmonary cystic disorders in infancy and childhood. J. Pediatr. Surg. 6:251–255, 1971.
34. Crofts, N. F., and Forbes, G. B.: Malignant neurilemmoma of the lung metastasizing to the heart. Thorax 19:334–337, 1964.
35. Crutcher, R. R., Waltuch, T. L., and Ghosh, A. K.: Bronchial lipoma. Report of a case and literature review. J. Thorac. Cardiovasc. Surg. 55:422–425, 1968.
36. Culiner, M. M.: Intralobar bronchial cystic disease, the "sequestration complex" and cystic bronchiecta-sis. Dis. Chest 53:462–469, 1968.
37. Currarino, G., Willis, K. W., Johnson, A. F., et al.: Pulmonary telangiectasia. Am. J. Roentgenol. 127:775–779, 1976.

38. Dalton, M. L., Jr., Strange, W. H., and Downs, E. A.: Intrathoracic splenosis. Case report and review of the literature. Am. Rev. Respir. Dis. *103*:827–830, 1971.

39. Daniels, A. C., Conner, G. H., and Francis, H. S.: Primary chondrosarcoma of the tracheobronchial tree. Report of a unique case and brief review. Arch. Pathol. *84*:615–624, 1967.

40. Dedo, H. H., and Fishman, N. H.: Laryngeal release and sleeve resection for tracheal stenosis. Ann. Otol. Rhinol. Laryngol. *78*:285–296, 1969.

41. Dillon, M. L., Jr., Koster, J. K., Coy, J., et al.: Intrathoracic splenosis. South. Med. J. *70*:112–114, 1977.

42. Dines, D. E., Arms, R. A., Bernatz, P. E., et al.: Pulmonary arteriovenous fistulas. Mayo Clin. Proc. *49*:460–465, 1974.

43. Diveley, W., and Daniel, R. A., Jr.: Primary solitary neurogenic tumors of the lung. J. Thorac. Surg. *21*:194–201, 1951.

44. Donahue, J. K., Weichert, R. F., and Ochsner, J. L.: Bronchial adenoma. Ann. Surg. *167*:873–884, 1968.

45. Donoghue, F. E., Andersen, H. A., and McDonald, J. R.: Unusual bronchial tumors. Ann. Otol. Rhinol. Laryngol. *65*:820–828, 1956.

46. Doppman, J., and Wilson, G.: Cystic pulmonary hamartoma. Br. J. Radiol. *38*:629–631, 1965.

47. Ehrenstein, F. I.: Pulmonary lymph node presenting as an enlarging coin lesion. Am. Rev. Respir. Dis. *101*:595–599, 1970.

48. Elliott, G. B., Belkin, A., and Donald, W. A. J.: Cystic bronchial papillomatosis. Clin. Radiol. *13*:62–67, 1962.

49. Feldman, F., and Seaman, W. B.: Primary thoracic hemangiopericytoma. Radiology *82*:998–1008, 1964.

50. Felson, B.: Chest Roentgenology. Philadelphia, W. B. Saunders Company, 1973, p. 61.

51. Fleming, R. J., Medina, J., and Seaman, W. B.: Roentgenographic aspects of tracheal tumors. Radiology *79*:628–636, 1962.

52. Fraser, R. G., and Paré, J. A. P.: Diagnosis of Diseases of the Chest. Ed. 2. Philadelphia, W. B. Saunders Company, 1977, p. 56.

53. Gamsu, G., Borson, B., Webb, W. R., et al.: Structure: function correlation in tracheal stenosis. Am. Rev. Respir. Dis. (Suppl.), *115*:328, 1977.

54. Gautam, H. P.: Intrapulmonary malignant teratoma. Am. Rev. Respir. Dis. *100*:863–865, 1969.

55. Genoe, G. A.: Diagnosis of bronchogenic carcinoma by means of bronchial brushing combined with bronchography. Am. J. Roentgenol. Ther. Nucl. Med. *120*:139–144, 1974.

56. Gilbert, J. G., Mazzarella, L. A., and Feit, L. J.: Primary tracheal tumors in the infant and adult. Arch. Otolaryngol. *58*:1–9, 1953.

57. Giustra, P. E., and Stassa, G.: The multiple presentations of bronchial adenomas. Radiology *93*:1013–1019, 1969.

58. Gomes, M. R., Bernatz, P. E., and Dines, D. E.: Pulmonary arteriovenous fistulas. Ann. Thorac. Surg. *7*:582–591, 1969.

59. Goodman, M. L., and Laforet, E. G.: Solitary primary chemodectomas of the lung. Chest *61*:48–50, 1972.

60. Gottlieb, L. S., and Gold, W. M.: Primary tracheobronchial amyloidosis. Am. Rev. Respir. Dis. *105*:425–429, 1972.

61. Greene, R., McLoud, T. C., and Stark, P.: Other malignant tumors of the lung. Semin. Roentgenol. *12*:225–237, 1977.

62. Greene, R.: "Saber-sheath" trachea: relation to chronic obstructive pulmonary disease. Am. J. Roentgenol. *130*:441–445, 1978.

63. Greenfield, H., and Herman, P. G.: Papillomatosis of the trachea and bronchi. Am. J. Roentgenol. Radium Ther. Nucl. Med. *89*:45–50, 1963.

64. Grillo, H. C.: Reconstruction of the trachea. Experience in 100 consecutive cases. Thorax *28*:667–679, 1973.

65. Grillo, H. C.: Congenital lesions, neoplasms, and injuries of the trachea. *In* Sabiston, D. C., Jr., and Spencer, F. C.: Gibbon's Surgery of the Chest. Philadelphia, W. B. Saunders Company, 1976, p. 256.

66. Grimes, O. F., and Bell, H. G.: The significance of hemoptysis in carcinoma of the thyroid gland. Surgery *24*:401–408, 1948.

67. Guccion, J. G., and Rosen, S. H.: Bronchopulmonary leiomyosarcoma and fibrosarcoma. A study of 32 cases and review of the literature. Cancer *30*:836–847, 1972.

68. Gudbjerg, C. E.: Pulmonary hamartoma. Am. J. Roentgenol. Radium Ther. Nucl. Med. *86*:842–849, 1961.

69. Hajdu, S. I., Huvos, A. G., Goodner, J. T., et al.: Carcinoma of the trachea. Clinicopathologic study of 41 cases. Cancer *25*:1448–1456, 1970.

70. Halloran, L. G., Silverberg, S. G., and Salzberg, A. M.: Congenital cystic adenomatoid malformation of the lung. A surgical emergency. Arch. Surg. *104*:715–719, 1972.

71. Handousa, P., and Elwi, A. M.: Some clinicopathological observations on scleroma. J. Laryngol. Otol. *72*:32–47, 1958.

72. Harle, T. S., Hevezi, J. M., Rogers, L. F., et al.: Xerotomography of the tracheobronchial tree. Am. J. Roentgenol. Radium Ther. Nucl. Med. *124*:353–357, 1975.

73. Healy, R. J.: Bronchogenic cysts. Radiology *57*:200–203, 1951.

74. Henry, W. J., and Miscall, L.: Rapidly reversible atelectasis due to change in position. J. Thorac. Cardiovasc. Surg. 41:686–688, 1961.
75. Higgins, C. B., and Wexler, L.: Clinical and angiographic features of pulmonary arteriovenous fistulas in children. Radiology 119:171–175, 1976.
76. Himmelfarb, E., Wells, S., and Rabinowitz, J. G.: The radiological spectrum of cardiopulmonary amyloidosis. Chest 72:327–332, 1977.
77. Hoffman, R., and Rabens, R.: Evolving pulmonary nodules: multiple pulmonary arteriovenous fistulas. Am. J. Roentgenol. Radium Ther. Nucl. Med. 120:861–864, 1974.
78. Holder, T. M., and Christy, M. G.: Cystic adenomatoid malformation of the lung. J. Thorac. Cardiovasc. Surg. 47:590–597, 1964.
79. Houston, H. E., Payne, W. S., Harrison, E. G., Jr., et al.: Primary cancers of the trachea. Arch. Surg. 99:132–139, 1969.
80. Hutcheson, J. B., Ashe, W. M., and Paulson, D. L.: Lipomas of the bronchus. A presentation of two cases and an analysis of the literature. J. Thorac. Surg. 35:638–642, 1958.
81. Hutchinson, W. B., Friedenberg, M. J., and Saltzstein, S.: Primary pulmonary pseudolymphoma. Radiology 82:48–56, 1964.
82. Janower, M. L., Grillo, H. C., MacMillan, A. S., Jr., et al.: The radiological appearance of carcinoma of the trachea. Radiology 96:39–43, 1970.
83. Jelihovsky, T., and Grant, A. K.: Endometriosis of the lung. A case report and brief review of the literature. Thorax 23:434–437, 1968.
84. Jensen, K. G., and Schiodt, T.: Growth conditions of hamartoma of the lung. Thorax 13:233–237, 1958.
85. Johnson, T. H., Mital, N., Rodnan, G. P., et al.: Relapsing polychondritis. Radiology 106:313–315, 1973.
86. Jost, R. G., Sagel, S. S., Stanley, R. J., et al.: Computed tomography of the thorax. Radiology 126:125–136, 1978.
87. Kahn, B., and Amer, N. S.: Multiple bronchial polyps. Chest 57:279–283, 1970.
88. Karlan, M. S., Livingston, P. A., and Baker, D. C., Jr.: Diagnosis of tracheal tumors. Ann. Otol. Rhinol. Laryngol. 82:790–799, 1973.
89. Korompai, F. L., Awe, R. J., Beall, A. C., et al.: Granular cell myoblastoma of the bronchus: a new case, 12 year follow-up report, and review of the literature. Chest 66:578–580, 1974.
90. Kovarik, J. L., and Ashe, S. M. P.: Intrapulmonary fibroma. Am. Rev. Respir. Dis. 88:539–542, 1963.
91. Lansing, A. M.: Radiological changes in pulmonary atelectasis. Arch. Surg. 90:52–56, 1965.
92. Lawson, R. M., Ramanathan, L., Hurley, G., et al.: Bronchial adenoma: review of an 18 year experience at the Brompton Hospital. Thorax 31:245–253, 1976.
93. Lund, W. S.: A fatal case of scleroma. J. Laryngol. Otol. 74:791–796, 1960.
94. McLeod, R. A., Brown, L. R., Miller, W. E., et al.: Evaluation of the pulmonary hila by tomography. Radiol. Clin. North Am. 14:51–84, 1976.
95. Madewell, J. E., Stocker, J. T., and Korsower, J. M.: Cystic adenomatoid malformation of the lung. Morphologic analysis. Am. J. Roentgenol. Radium Ther. Nucl. Med. 124:436–448, 1975.
96. Madewell, J. E., and Feigin, D. S.: Benign tumors of the lung. Semin. Roentgenol. 12:175–186, 1977.
97. Maklad, N. F., and Ravikrishmam, K. P.: Xerotomography of peripheral lung lesions. Chest 69:516–518, 1976.
98. Mansour, K. A., Hatcher, C. R., Logan, W. D., et al.: Pulmonary arteriovenous fistula. Am. Surg. 37:203–208, 1971.
99. Marks, C., and Marks, M.: Bronchial adenoma. A clinicopathologic study. Chest 71:376–380, 1977.
100. Martin, C. J.: Tracheobronchopathia osteochondroplastica. Arch. Otolaryngol. 100:290–293, 1974.
101. Meade, J. B., Whitwell, F., Bickford, B. J., et al.: Primary hemangiopericytoma of lung. Thorax 29:1–15, 1974.
102. Menkes, H. A., and Traystman, R. J.: Collateral ventilation. Am. Rev. Respir. Dis. 116:287–309, 1977.
103. Miller, D. R.: Benign tumors of lung and tracheobronchial tree. Ann. Thorac. Surg. 8:542–560, 1969.
104. Miller, W. E., Crowe, J. K., and Muhm, J. R.: The evaluation of pulmonary parenchymal abnormalities by tomography. Radiol. Clin. North Am. 14:85–93, 1976.
105. Mostecky, H., Lichtenberg, J., and Kalus, M.: A non-chromaffin paraganglioma of the lung. Thorax 21:205–208, 1966.
106. Moyer, J. H., Glantz, G., and Brest, A. N.: Pulmonary arteriovenous fistulas. Physiologic and clinical considerations. Am. J. Med. 32:417–435, 1962.
107. Muhm, J. R., and Crowe, J. K.: The evaluation of tracheal abnormalities by tomography. Radiol. Clin. North Am. 14:95–104, 1976.
108. Muri, J. W.: Arteriovenous aneurysm of the lung. Am. J. Surg. 89:265–271, 1955.
109. Nathan, M. H., Collins, V. P., and Adams, R. A.: Differentiation of benign and malignant pulmonary nodules by growth rate. Radiology 79:221–232, 1962.
110. Nathan, M. H.: Management of solitary pulmonary nodules. An organized approach based on growth rate and statistics. J.A.M.A. 227:1141–1144, 1974.
111. Ochsner, S., LeJeune, F. E., and Ochsner, A.: Lipoma of the bronchus. Report of a case. J. Thorac. Surg. 33:371–378, 1957.
112. O'Keefe, M. E., Good, C. A., and McDonald, J. R.: Calcification in solitary nodules of the lung. Am. J. Roentgenol. Radium Ther. Nucl. Med. 77:1023–1033, 1957.
113. Pearl, M.: Post-inflammatory pseudotumor of the lung in children. Radiology 105:391–395, 1972.

114. Peleg, H., and Pauzner, Y.: Benign tumors of the lung. Dis. Chest 47:179–186, 1965.
115. Plachta, A., and Hershey, H.: Lipoma of the lung. Review of the literature and report of a case. Am. Rev. Respir. Dis. 86:912–916, 1962.
116. Poirier, T. J., and Van Ordstrand, H. S.: Pulmonary chondromatous hamartomas. Chest 59:50–55, 1971.
117. Pripstein, S., Culiner, M. M., and Brodey, P. A.: Roentgenographic demonstration of peripheral intrapulmonic lymphadenopathy. Radiology 121:280, 1976.
118. Proctor, D. F.: The upper airways. II. The larynx and trachea. Am. Rev. Respir. Dis. 115:315–342, 1977.
119. Ramanathan, T.: Primary leiomyosarcoma of the lung. Thorax 29:482–489, 1974.
120. Reed, J. C., and Sobonya, R. E.: Morphologic analysis of foregut cysts in the thorax. Am. J. Roentgenol. Radium Ther. Nucl. Med. 120:851–860, 1974.
121. Rees, G. M.: Primary chondrosarcoma of lung. Thorax 25:366–371, 1970.
122. Rinker, C. T., Garrotto, L. J., Lee, K. R., et al.: Bronchography. Diagnostic signs and accuracy in pulmonary carcinoma. Am. J. Roentgenol. Radium Ther. Nucl. Med. 104:802–807, 1968.
123. Rodman, M. H., and Jones, C. W.: Catamenial hemoptysis due to bronchial endometriosis. N. Engl. J. Med. 266:805–808, 1962.
124. Rogers, L. F., and Osmer, J. C.: Bronchogenic cyst. A review of 46 cases. Am. J. Roentgenol. Radium Ther. Nucl. Med. 91:273–283, 1964.
125. Rosenbaum, H. D., Alavi, S. M., and Bryant, L. R.: Pulmonary parenchymal spread of juvenile laryngeal papillomatosis. Radiology 90:654–660, 1968.
126. Rowlands, D. T., Jr.: Fibroepithelial polyps of the bronchus: a case report and review of the literature. Dis. Chest 37:199–202, 1960.
127. Sade, R. M., Clouse, M., and Ellis, F. H., Jr.: The spectrum of pulmonary sequestration. Ann. Thorac. Surg. 18:644–658, 1974.
128. Sagel, S. S., and Ablow, R. C.: Hamartoma: on occasion, a rapidly growing tumor of the lung. Radiology 91:971–972, 1968.
129. Sagel, S. S., and Greenspan, R. H.: Minute pulmonary arteriovenous fistulas demonstrated by magnification pulmonary arteriography. Case report. Radiology 97:529–530, 1970.
130. Savoca, C. J., Austin, J. H. M., and Goldberg, H. I.: The right paratracheal stripe. Radiology 122:295–301, 1977.
131. Schoenbaum, S. W., Pinsker, K. L., Rakoff, S. J., et al.: Fiberoptic bronchoscopy. Complete evaluation of the tracheobronchial tree in the radiology department. Radiology 109:571–575, 1973.
132. Schulster, P. L., Khan, F. A., and Azueta, V.: Asymptomatic pulmonary granular cell tumor presenting as a coin lesion. Chest 68:256–258, 1975.
133. Sears, H. F., Michaelis, L. L., Minor, G. R., et al.: Endobronchial polyp. A case presentation. J. Thorac. Cardiovasc. Surg. 70:371–375, 1975.
134. Secrest, P. G., Kendig, T. A., and Beland, A. J.: Tracheobronchopathia osteochondroplastica. Am. J. Med. 36:815–818, 1964.
135. Shah, J. P., Choudhry, K. U., Huvos, A. G., et al.: Hamartomas of the lung. Surg. Gynecol. Obstet. 136:406–408, 1973.
136. Shields, J. B., and Holtz, S.: The retrotracheal space. Radiology 120:19–23, 1976.
137. Sibala, J. L.: Endobronchial hamartomas. Chest 62:631–634, 1972.
138. Simon, J. L.: Primary amyloid tumor of the trachea. A case report. Radiology 103:555–556, 1972.
139. Singer, D. B., Greenberg, S. D., and Harrison, G. M.: Papillomatosis of the lung. Am. Rev. Respir. Dis. 94:777–781, 1966.
140. Smith, L., and Gooding, C. A.: Pulmonary involvement in laryngeal papillomatosis. Pediatr. Radiol. 2:161–166, 1974.
141. Spain, D. M.: Acute non-aeration of lung: Pulmonary edema versus atelectasis. Dis. Chest 25:550–558, 1954.
142. Steele, J. D.: The Solitary Pulmonary Nodule. Springfield, Illinois, Charles C Thomas, Publisher, 1964, p. 6.
143. Strutynsky, N., Balthazar, E. J., and Klein, R. M.: Inflammatory pseudotumors of the lung. Br. J. Radiol. 47:94–96, 1974.
144. Taylor, T. L., and Miller, D. R.: Leiomyoma of the bronchus. J. Thorac. Cardiovasc. Surg. 57:284–288, 1969.
145. Teixidor, H. S., and Bachman, A. L.: Multiple amyloid tumors of the lung. A case report. Am. J. Roentgenol. Radium Ther. Nucl. Med. 111:525–529, 1971.
146. Telander, R. L., Lennox, C., and Sieber, W.: Sequestration of the lung in children. Mayo Clin. Proc. 51:578–584, 1976.
147. Templeton, A. W., Moffat, R., and Nelson, D.: Bronchography and bronchial adenomas. Chest 59:59–61, 1971.
148. Teplick, J. G., Teplick, S. K., and Haskin, M. E.: Granular cell myoblastoma of the lung. Am. J. Roentgenol. Radium Ther. Nucl. Med. 125:890–894, 1975.
149. Ting, Y. M., Doust, B. D., and Chuang, V. P.: Xerotomographic diagnosis of central bronchogenic carcinoma. Chest 67:172–175, 1975.
150. Tralka, G. A., and Katz, S.: Hemangioendothelioma of the lung. Am. Rev. Respir. Dis. 87:107–115, 1963.

151. Trivedi, S. A., Mehta, K. N., and Nanavaty, J. M.: Teratoma of the lung: report of a case. Br. J. Dis. Chest 60:156–159, 1966.
152. Trunk, G., Gracey, D. R., and Byrd, R. B.: The management and evaluation of the solitary pulmonary nodule. Chest 66:236–239, 1974.
153. Turk, L. N., III, and Lindskog, G. E.: The importance of angiographic diagnosis in intralobar pulmonary sequestration. J. Thorac. Cardiovasc. Surg. 41:299–305, 1961.
154. Vontz, F. K., and Vitsky, B. H.: Giant bronchial polyp treated by emergency thoracotomy. Chest 66:102–104, 1974.
155. Walsh, T. J., and Healy, T. M.: Chondroma of the bronchus. Thorax 24:327–329, 1969.
156. Webb, W. R., and Hare, W. V.: Primary fibrosarcoma of the bronchus. Am. Rev. Respir. Dis. 84:881–889, 1961.
157. Webb, W. R., and Gamsu, G.: Sclerosing hemangioma of the lung. Br. J. Radiol. 50:213–215, 1977.
158. Weitzner, S., and Oser, J. F.: Granular cell myoblastoma of bronchus. Am. Rev. Respir. Dis. 97:923–930, 1968.
159. Weitzner, S.: Leiomyoma of the lung. Report of a case. Am. Rev. Respir. Dis. 100:63–66, 1969.
160. Wilson, S. R., Sanders, D. E., and Delarue, N. C.: Intrathoracic manifestations of amyloid disease. Radiology 120:283–289, 1976.
161. Wilt, K. E., Andrews, N. C., Meckstroth, C. V., et al.: The role of bronchography in the diagnosis of bronchogenic carcinoma. Dis. Chest 35:517–523, 1959.
162. Young, D. A., and Simon, G.: Certain movements measured on inspiration-expiration chest radiographs correlated with pulmonary function studies. Clin. Radiol. 23:37–41, 1972.

Part VIII

Carcinoma of the Lung

GORDON GAMSU, M.D.
W. RICHARD WEBB, M.D.

Since the turn of the century the incidence of bronchogenic carcinoma has increased alarmingly. Formerly rarely encountered, this neoplasm has established itself in the Western Hemisphere as the most common fatal malignancy in males.[13] The prevalence varies widely among countries and racial groups. It is estimated that the incidence of bronchogenic carcinoma in the United States in 1980 will be more than 80,000 cases, and the United Kingdom and Finland will have even higher death rates than America.[36, 40, 74]

Strong evidence indicts the inhalation of carcinogenic substances as a major cause of the increasing incidence of bronchogenic carcinoma. Numerous studies indicate a correlation between smoking and lung cancer.[29, 37] The risk increases directly in proportion to the number of cigarettes smoked. Well-differentiated squamous cell carcinoma, oat cell carcinoma, and to a lesser extent, adenocarcinoma, all demonstrate an increased incidence with increased cigarette consumption.[87] The inhalation of a variety of substances found in industry and mining has been incriminated in the development of bronchogenic carcinoma. Primary among these substances is asbestos, which is found extensively in industry and construction.[25, 71] An estimated 4.5 million Americans have been significantly exposed to asbestos fibers. The risk that bronchogenic carcinoma will occur in these people is probably six to ten times that of the general population and perhaps 60 to 90 times higher when combined with heavy cigarette smoking. Arsenic, radioactive materials, anthracite and silica, bichromates, and chloromethyl methyl ether have been implicated as industrial, mining, or environmental carcinogens.[8, 23, 28] There is always a prolonged interval between the initiation of exposure to the carcinogenic agent and the development of lung cancer. Underlying these environmental factors are racial predisposition and possibly immunologic responses to the various stimuli.

CLINICAL PRESENTATION

Bronchogenic carcinoma has its peak incidence in people between the ages of 55 and 60 years; the disease is rare in those younger than 35 years. In about 10 per cent of patients, the lesion is detected initially on a chest radiograph of an asymptomatic individual.[20] At centers where screening of asymptomatic people is performed, about half of the lung cancers are detected by sputum cytology and half by chest radiographs.[34]

A cough, usually productive, is the presenting symptom in 75 per cent of cases.[35, 45] The majority of patients are heavy smokers, and most have a history of chronic cough. Any change in the pattern of cough or sputum production should be considered significant.

Hemoptysis is present in about 50 per cent,[35, 45] most frequently in the form of bloody streaking of the sputum.

Less commonly the condition presents as an unresolved pneumonia, dysphagia from nodal metastases to the periesophageal area, or localized wheezing from an endobronchial lesion.

The extension of a peripheral neoplasm to the pleural surface may cause pleuritic chest pain and a pleural friction rub. Pleural effusions are not uncommon with bronchogenic carcinoma. A serous pleural effusion is most often the result of obstruction of hilar nodes and, less commonly, of involvement of the pleura. A bloody effusion usually indicates the extension of the tumor into the pleural space.

Spread to the mediastinum can be by direct extension or by the involvement of lymph nodes. The structures within the mediastinum most likely to be involved are the superior vena cava, recurrent laryngeal nerves, pericardium, and heart.[70, 76] Superior sulcus tumors tend to invade directly into the extrapleural structures at the thoracic inlet. Pain and shoulder weakness are the most frequent symptoms. Horner's syndrome and arm swelling are variably present.[77]

The distant dissemination of bronchogenic carcinoma occurs via the bloodstream or the lymphatic system. A small proportion of patients initially present with distant metastases. Lung cancer tends to metastasize to the liver, adrenals, bone, kidneys, and brain. Osteolytic bone lesions in distal extremities originate most commonly from a primary lung carcinoma.

NONMETASTATIC EXTRATHORACIC MANIFESTATIONS

Nonmetastatic extrathoracic syndromes are not uncommon in cases of bronchogenic carcinoma. These may be endocrine or metabolic, neuromuscular, skeletal and connective tissue, or vascular and hematologic (Table 19–6). They may antecede pulmonary findings by months or even years.

Endocrine and Metabolic Syndromes

Bronchogenic carcinomas often secrete abnormal hormones and enzymes because they contain cells originating in the primitive neural crest. These cells retain the

TABLE 19–6. EXTRATHORACIC MANIFESTATIONS OF BRONCHOGENIC CARCINOMA

Endocrine and Metabolic
  Cushing's syndrome
  Hypercalcemia
  Excessive antidiuretic hormone
  Carcinoid syndrome
  Estrogen excretion

Neuromuscular
  Peripheral neuropathy
  Cortical cerebellar degeneration
  Carcinomatous myopathy
  Subacute spinocerebellar degeneration
  Mental aberration

Skeletal and Connective Tissue
  Clubbing
  Pulmonary hypertrophic osteoarthropathy
  Acanthosis nigricans
  Dermatomyositis

Vascular and Hematologic
  Migratory thrombophlebitis
  Nonbacterial verrucal endocarditis
  Anemia
  Fibrinolytic purpura

potential for the production of polypeptide hormones. Carcinomas containing these cells can secrete sufficient hormone to produce clinical endocrine syndromes.[9, 58] In many, the hormone is immunologically different from the primary hormone. The frequency of endocrine syndromes is reported to be 12.1 per cent in all cases of bronchogenic carcinoma and 21.1 per cent in cases of oat cell carcinoma. In many instances metastases, especially to the liver have occurred before the onset of the endocrine syndrome.

Neuromuscular Syndromes

Bronchogenic carcinoma is the major cause of carcinomatous neuropathies.[11] Although the pathogenesis has not been established, antibody production against neural and muscular tissues has been postulated. The incidence varies from 4 to 16 per cent.[38, 52] Symptoms from the neuropathy may antecede the discovery of the carcinoma by as much as three years.[52] In the majority of cases, however, advanced disease is present. In one third of patients the onset of the syndrome occurs at a time when the chest radiograph is normal; in another third no extrathoracic metastases can be found. In a large series, Morton et al. found that oat cell carcinoma was the cell type in 56 per cent of the patients with one of these syndromes.[52] In 22 per cent, squamous carcinoma was the cause, in 16 per cent, large cell undifferentiated carcinoma, and in 5 per cent, adenocarcinoma. Alveolar cell carcinoma is much less commonly associated with these syndromes. The spectrum of neuromuscular dysfunction includes lesions simulating myasthenia gravis, polymyositis, neuropathies, cerebellar disease, and psychoses.

Skeletal and Connective Tissue Syndromes

Pulmonary osteoarthropathy is found in about 3 per cent of patients with bronchogenic carcinoma, being most commonly associated with squamous cell carcinoma and occasionally with adenocarcinoma.[63] Pain, clubbing of the fingers and toes, local tenderness, edema, and warmth of the distal extremities are present. Radiographs demonstrate periosteal new bone along the distal extremities of the involved bones (Fig. 19–144).[24] Relief of symptoms commonly follows the resection of the primary neoplasm. Osteoarthropathy may antecede the discovery of the lung neoplasm by up to two years.

Acanthosis nigricans and scleroderma are rare accompaniments of bronchogenic carcinoma.

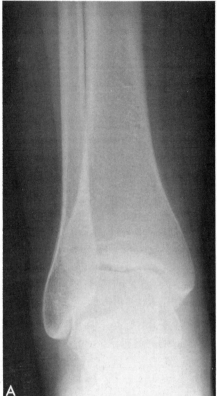
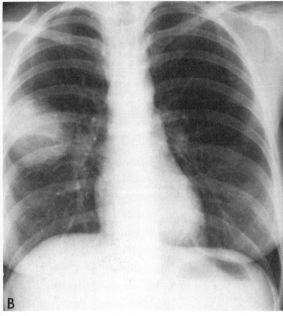

Figure 19–144. Hypertrophic osteoarthropathy. *A,* A view of the right ankle of a 31-year-old woman demonstrates periosteal new bone formation along the fibula from hypertrophic osteoarthropathy. *B,* A chest radiograph shows a large squamous cell carcinoma in the right midlung field.

Vascular and Hematologic Syndromes

Vascular and hematologic abnormalities are uncommon associations of bronchogenic carcinoma. Migratory thrombophlebitis involving unusual areas and resistant to therapy suggests the presence of a neoplasm. Bronchogenic carcinoma is the most common cause of this syndrome in men.[46] Thromboembolic phenomena may be associated with elevated platelet counts and may also occur in the absence of thrombocytosis.

Anemia, purpura, and intravascular coagulopathies have been described, but their origin is obscure and they are rare.

HISTOLOGIC CELL TYPES

Four primary histologic types of bronchogenic carcinoma are recognized.[20, 21, 41] Squamous cell (epidermoid) carcinoma, with an incidence ranging from 35 to 75 per cent, is the most frequent. Adenocarcinoma is the second most common, composing from 4 to 25 per cent of the cases. The remaining of 30 to 40 per cent are anaplastic tumors, with a ratio of two small cell carcinomas to one large cell undifferentiated carcinoma. Bronchioloalveolar cell carcinoma is usually categorized histologically as adenocarcinoma. The clinical and radiologic presentation of bronchioloalveolar cell carcinoma warrants a separate discussion, however. This cell type makes up only 1 to 2 per cent of carcinomas in most series.

Squamous Cell Carcinoma

Squamous cell carcinoma can occur both centrally and peripherally. The central lesions arise predominantly in segmental bronchi; they are less common in lobar bronchi, mainstem bronchi, and the trachea. Because of the site of origin, atelectasis is the most common presentation of squamous cell carcinoma, followed by a large parenchymal mass (greater than 4 cm), a small mass (less than 4 cm), and a hilar mass. Cavitation occurs in about 10 per cent. A pleural effusion is present in about 3 per cent, usually accompanied by other radiographic findings.

Adenocarcinoma

Second in frequency, adenocarcinoma invariably arises in the periphery of the lung. The usual presentation is a lung mass, which is less than 4 cm in diameter in two thirds of the cases and larger in one third. Hilar prominence, segmental collapse, and cavitation are all less frequent than with squamous cell carcinoma. A pleural effusion may occur, but is uncommon.

Small Cell Undifferentiated Carcinoma.

This tumor probably arises from the Kutchitsky cell, which is of neural origin and is found throughout the bronchial tree.[7] The tumor is composed of small undifferentiated cells. Although oat cell carcinoma is only one of the forms of small cell undifferentiated carcinoma, these terms are often used interchangeably. Small cell undifferentiated carcinoma usually arises centrally, and a hilar mass or hilar prominence is present in more than 50 per cent of cases. The other 50 per cent show either a parenchymal mass (usually less than 4 cm in diameter) or an area of collapse or pneumonitis. The prognosis in small cell undifferentiated carcinoma is so poor that many physicians consider resection contraindicated for any centrally located lesion.[82] Peripheral small cell undifferentiated carcinomas may have a somewhat better prognosis. This tumor type is the dominant cause of nonmetastatic neoplastic syndromes.

Large Cell Undifferentiated Carcinoma

Large cell undifferentiated carcinoma is the least common of the four main cell types of bronchogenic carcinoma, with an incidence of 10 to 15 per cent in most studies. The tumor is composed of large cells without differentiation. It tends to arise from the bronchi within the pulmonary parenchyma and therefore most commonly presents as either an area of pneumonitis, an area of collapse, or a mass larger than 4 cm in diameter. Large cell undifferentited carcinoma is the most likely diagnosis when a bronchogenic carcinoma presents radiographically as a large peripheral mass.

Alveolar Cell Carcinoma

Alveolar cell carcinoma, or bronchioloalveolar cell carcinoma, is an unusual tumor arising from bronchiolar epithelium. There is evidence to suggest that this neoplasm often arises in association with an area of scarring in the lung or diffuse pulmonary fibrosis. The pathologic distinction between alveolar cell carcinoma and adenocarcinoma has not been fully resolved. Alveolar cell carcinoma has two distinctive clinical and radiographic patterns.[49]

LOCALIZED ALVEOLAR CELL CARCINOMA. The localized form of alveolar cell carcinoma constitutes 60 to 90 per cent of cases. The lesion presents as a circumscribed mass between 1 and 10 cm in diameter. In a small minority of cases, the localized form may demonstrate extremely slow growth and may be visible radiographically for many years before the correct diagnosis is considered. Alveolar cell carcinoma may permeate the lung parenchyma, sparing the peripheral bronchi passing through the lesion. Air may be visible within these bronchi, producing air bronchograms and providing an important clue to the correct diagnosis (Fig. 19–145). In about half of the cases of localized alveolar cell carcinoma, a linear band of tissue or a tail may be seen extending from the lesion to the adjacent pleural surface. Although this finding may also be seen in granulomatous processes, it should arouse suspicion of an alveolar cell carcinoma. Less commonly, alveolar cell carcinoma fills a number of segments or lobes of a lung and has the radiographic appearance of a pneumonia. The prognosis for localized alveolar cell carcinoma is relatively good.

DIFFUSE ALVEOLAR CELL CARCINOMA. The diffuse form of alveolar cell carcinoma is unusual and may be secondary to a localized form. Alveolar cell carcinoma probably spreads to one or both lungs by a combination of lymphatic and transbronchial dissemination in a fashion similar to that of pulmonary tuberculosis. The diffuse pattern varies from one portion of the lung to another. The dominant radiographic feature is often ill-defined small nodules. As the lesions coalesce, more discrete areas of pulmonary consolidation become visible (Fig. 19–146). Lymphatic permeation may produce the appearance of lymphangitic carcinomatosis. Pleural effusions, cavitation, and hilar and mediastinal lymphadenopathy are all rare. The diffuse form of alveolar cell carcinoma has an extremely poor prognosis, with virtually no patients surviving more than three years.[49]

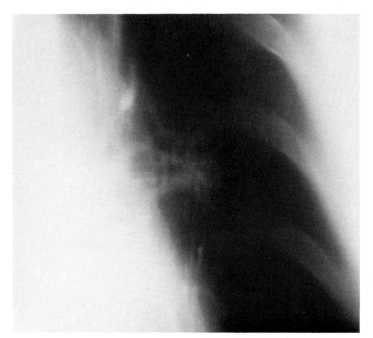

Figure 19–145. Alveolar cell carcinoma. A coned-down view of the left midlung field from a tomogram shows an ill-defined mass containing air bronchograms. Histologically, the lesion was found to be a focal alveolar cell carcinoma.

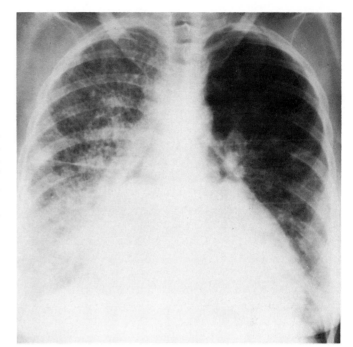

Figure 19–146. A 36-year-old woman with diffuse alveolar cell carcinoma. A consolidative and nodular process is present in the right lung and, to a lesser extent, in the left lung. An air-fluid level in the pericardium follows a pericardiocentesis for cardiac tamponade from a malignant effusion.

RADIOGRAPHIC FEATURES

The radiographic features of bronchogenic carcinoma are determined by the size of the lesion, its site of origin, and its growth and dissemination. About 60 per cent of bronchogenic carcinomas present with a single radiographic feature. Forty per cent demonstrate a combination of findings that represent spread of the tumor.[14] The time of detection also influences the radiographic pattern of presentation. Radiographs of asymptomatic subjects tend not to show a multiplicity of findings. Sputum cytologic screening may uncover lesions that are not visible on plain chest radiographs.[61]

At the time of detection, most bronchogenic carcinomas are no longer amenable to surgical cure. Of 1000 cases described by Mountain, 54 per cent had hilar involvement, and an additional 35 per cent had mediastinal involvement.[53] One must always be alert to the possibility of central spread when interpreting the radiographs of patients suspected of having bronchogenic carcinoma.

Atelectasis

The sequelae of obstruction of a bronchus are the most common radiographic features of bronchogenic carcinoma.[14, 42, 66] The majority of central bronchogenic carcinomas arise from an endobronchial location.[19] Most commonly, the area of collapse is segmental, but a lobe or a whole lung may be involved (Figs. 19–147 and 19–148). Rarely, a right mainstem bronchus lesion results in the collapse of the right upper and middle lobes, while the right lower lobe remains inflated. The degree of volume loss of the subtended lung parenchyma is variable. The lung may be completely airless and reduced to its minimal volume. Alternatively, the obstructed lung may become filled with desquamated material, mucus, and fluid, and lose little of its volume. In both

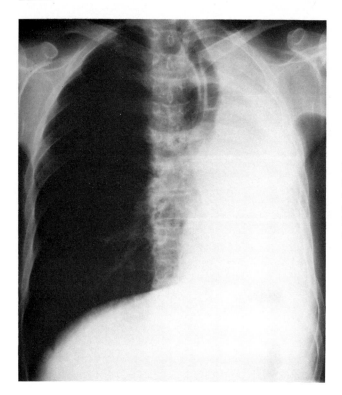

Figure 19–147. Atelectasis. A frontal radiograph of a 53-year-old male demonstrates complete collapse of the left lung. An abrupt cut-off of the proximal left mainstem bronchus is evident and was due to a poorly differentiated squamous cell carcinoma.

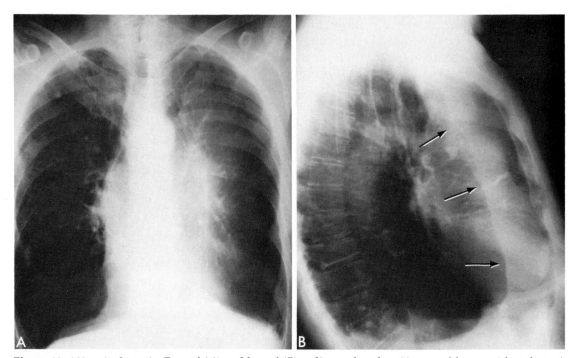

Figure 19–148. Atelectasis. Frontal (*A*) and lateral (*B*) radiographs of an 80-year-old man with atelectasis of the left upper lobe. *A*, On the frontal projection an ill-defined density overlies the upper left hemithorax. Evidence of previous granulomatous disease is present. *B*, On the lateral radiograph the anteriorly displaced major fissure is visible (arrows).

instances the absence of air bronchograms is suggestive of obstruction of the proximal bronchus.

Occasionally the completely obstructed segment of lung remains aerated, presumably by collateral ventilation. The bronchi distal to the segment may then become filled with mucus, producing plugs. The radiographic appearance is of ropy densities following the course of the bronchial tree. The obstructing neoplasm proximal to the mucous plugs may be overlooked unless further investigation is undertaken.

Obstructive Pneumonitis

Bronchial obstruction predisposes to infection in the subtended segment. Obstructive pneumonitis or abscess formation can result. Again, the obstructing proximal neoplasm may not be evident, and therapy for the infection often produces clinical and radiologic improvement. Pneumonia in elderly patients should always be watched until complete radiologic clearing has occurred (Figs. 19–149 to 19–151). Further investigation should be undertaken if resolution remains incomplete.

Hyperinflation

Although it arises from the bronchus, bronchogenic carcinoma rarely produces hyperinflation or air trapping in the distal lung parenchyma. Hyperlucency of the lung resulting from diminished blood within the vessels and parenchyma of the lung can be observed on radiographs obtained at full inspiration. The volume of the hyperlucent segment or lobe is usually mildly reduced. Radiographs obtained in expiration infrequently show air trapping.

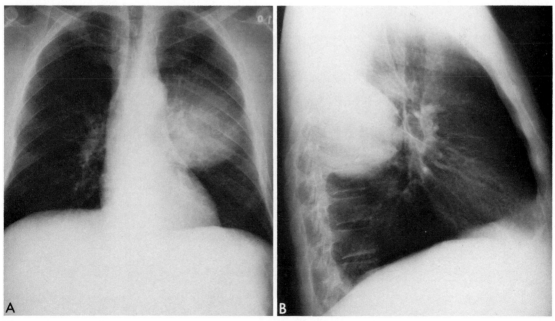

Figure 19–149.   Obstructive pneumonitis. Frontal (*A*) and lateral (*B*) radiographs of a patient with obstructive pneumonitis of the superior segment of the left lower lobe. Obstruction was from a small bronchogenic carcinoma situated at the orifice of the superior segmental bronchus. *B,* On the lateral projection, upward bowing of the left major fissure is evident.

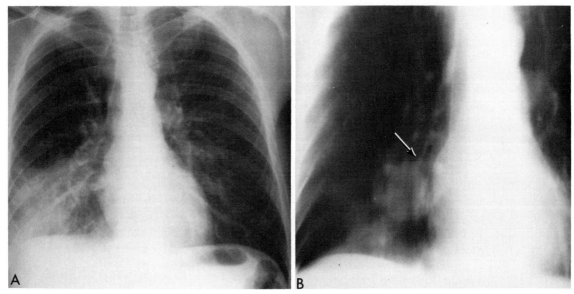

Figure 19–150. Pneumonia from carcinoma. *A,* A frontal radiograph of a middle-aged man demonstrates a right lower lobe pneumonia. *B,* A tomogram following incomplete clearing of the pneumonia demonstrates a large squamous cell carcinoma partially obstructing the right lower lobe segmental bronchi (arrow).

Solitary Pulmonary Nodules

Although a large body of statistical and clinical information is now available on the single pulmonary nodule, controversy still persists about the management of patients with a nodule. The reason for disagreement is that although there is a better prognosis

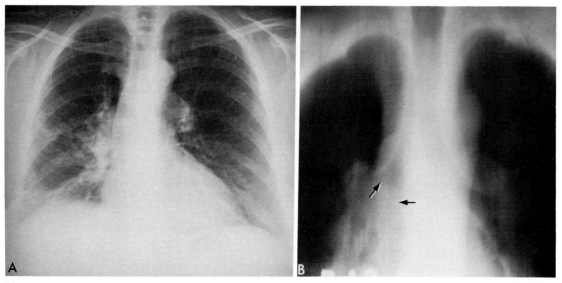

Figure 19–151. Pneumonia due to carcinoma. *A,* A frontal radiograph of a 49-year-old woman demonstrates patchy consolidation in the right lower and middle lobes. The right hilus is prominent. *B,* A frontal tomogram demonstrates a large mass arising from the bronchus intermedius and partially obstructing the right lower and upper lobes (arrows).

for bronchogenic carcinoma presenting in this manner, there is also a reluctance to subject asymptomatic patients to an unnecessary thoracotomy.

The radiographic criteria for classifying a lesion as a single pulmonary nodule have not been entirely agreed upon. The determination of which patients belong in this category therefore varies. The size of a single pulmonary nodule is usually considered to be from 1 to 6 cm in diameter. The minimal size is usually accepted as being twice the diameter of the nearest blood vessel. The maximal size is often not detailed. The shape of the single pulmonary nodule is usually considered to be round or oval. The major criterion for considering a lesion a nodule is its margin or edge. This is variously described as circumscribed or sharp. Surrounding atelectasis or pneumonitis usually excludes the lesion from this category. Single pulmonary nodules may contain calcification and may be cavitary. Tomography is a valuable technique for evaluating most single pulmonary nodules. The differential possibilities of a single pulmonary nodule are numerous (Table 19–7).

The management of the single pulmonary nodule is based on a variety of factors, and arguments can be marshaled for and against radiographic monitoring of the lesions, various biopsy procedures, or immediate thoracotomy.[47, 64, 80, 83] In the most general terms, nodules can be considered benign if they are unchanged in appearance over a two-year period, contain dense or central calcification, or occur in patients younger than 35 years of age.

Employing a combination of radiologic, clinical, and laboratory information, Garland, in one study, and Edwards et al., in another, were able to distinguish benign from malignant pulmonary nodules in more than 90 per cent of patients.[26, 32] The degree of certainty required for the management of the single pulmonary nodule does not allow even this uncertainty. (Fig. 19–152). Demonstrable biologic stability or negative cytologic samples from the lesion remain the criteria for observing the nodule with serial radiographs. Needle aspiration is the method of choice in the evaluation of most nodules that are not densely or centrally calcified or that occur in patients older than 35 or in patients without prior radiographs for comparison.

TABLE 19–7. THE SOLITARY PULMONARY NODULE

Origin	Calcification	Cavitation
Bronchogenic cyst*	Rare	Common
Sequestration*	No	Common
Arteriovenous fistula	Phleboliths	No
Bronchial atresia	No	No
Tuberculoma*	Common	Rare
Histoplasmoma*	Common, central	Rare
Coccidioidomycoma*	Unusual	Common
Hydatid	Rare	Common
Bronchial adenoma*	Rare	Rare
Hamartoma*	Common	No
Other benign tumors	Rare	No
Bronchogenic carcinoma*	Rare, peripheral	Not uncommon
Metastasis*	Rare	Uncommon
Alveolar cell carcinoma	No	Rare
Plasmacytoma	No	No
Hematoma*	No	Common
Rheumatoid nodule	No	Common
Amyloidosis	Rare	Rare
Wegener's granuloma	Rare	Uncommon

*These are more common lesions.

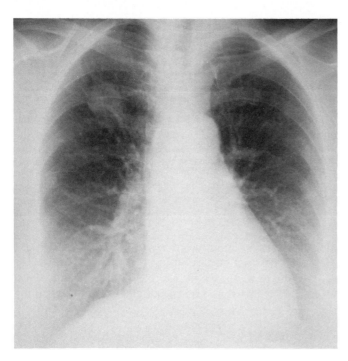

Figure 19–152. Carcinoma — single nodule. A frontal radiograph of a 69-year-old woman demonstrates a 2-cm, ill-defined, right upper lobe nodule. The nodule had not been present on a film taken two years previously. Right upper lobe lobectomy revealed that the mass was an adenocarcinoma.

Serial radiographs enable the determination of the rate of growth of pulmonary nodules. Nathan et al. have demonstrated that most malignant lung lesions have an exponential growth pattern.[57] Growth can be expressed in terms of "doubling time," defined as the time the tumor takes to double its volume. Most malignant nodules have doubling time between 37 and 465 days.[57] Although extensively described, in our experience, doubling time has not been of practical value in selecting patients for observation.

A synchronous or metachronous malignancy (pulmonary or extrapulmonary) does influence the management of the single pulmonary nodule. The lung nodule is a second primary lung neoplasm in a significant proportion of patients when the other malignancy is a squamous cell carcinoma or adenocarcinoma.[15, 16] An assumption of a solitary metastasis to the lung should not be entertained in most circumstances. The pulmonary nodule must be evaluated for a possible alternative cause. Sometimes whole-lung tomography or a CT scan will demonstrate a multiplicity of nodules, when only a solitary nodule was seen on regular films. Multiple nodules are more likely to be metastases.

Central Mass

From 12 to 35 per cent of bronchogenic carcinomas present initially as enlargement of one hilus.[14, 42] Hilar enlargement may result from a tumor arising in one of the bronchi within the hilus, or a peripheral bronchogenic carcinoma may have hilar nodal enlargement as its presenting radiographic feature. Occasionally a neoplasm within the hilus may not cause a radiographic change in the contour of the hilar structures on the posteroanterior or lateral radiographs but may give an increased density to the hilus. This radiographic characteristic is often difficult to detect and is based on a subjective comparison of the densities of the two hila. A 55 degree hilar tomogram may resolve the uncertainty.

Mediastinal Enlargement

Mediastinal widening as the only radiographic presentation of bronchogenic carcinoma is unusual (Fig. 19–153). Bronchogenic carcinoma, usually small cell undifferentiated carcinoma, arises within the mediastinum in less than one per cent of cases.[42, 53] Anterior, paratracheal, subcarinal, or middle mediastinal nodes may be involved. In the absence of an associated pulmonary lesion, bronchogenic carcinoma is not often considered a likely possibility. Lymphoma; sarcoidosis; metastasis from the thyroid, kidney, or breast; or melanoma are more likely causes of this radiographic presentation. Superior vena caval obstruction, diaphragmatic paralysis, or vocal cord paralysis may be the presenting clinical symptom.

Superior Sulcus Tumors

A group of pulmonary neoplasms arising in the subpleural apex of the lung was first described by Pancoast.[60] Their name is derived from the sulcus, or groove, formed by the subclavian artery at the lung apex. Squamous cell carcinoma is the commonest of these neoplasms, but they may be derived from any of the four histologic types. Superior sulcus tumors tend to cross the pleura and invade the adjoining tissue, including the ribs, spine, and nerves. Shoulder or arm pain is the most common clinical symptom. Horner's syndrome or muscle atrophy may be present owing to the involvement of the superior sympathetic nerves or brachial plexus.

Superior sulcus tumors present radiographically with a variable-sized mass at the apex of one lung. A minor degree of asymmetry of the normal apical soft tissues may be the only abnormal finding. Detailed bone radiographs, including magnification views, are useful in detecting minor degrees of bone destruction. In our experience, computed

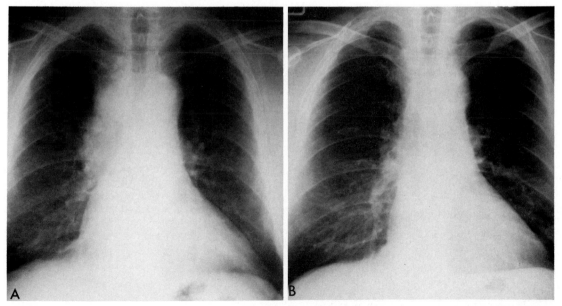

Figure 19–153. *A,* Radiation therapy. A small cell undifferentiated carcinoma in a 56-year-old man presenting as a mediastinal mass. A large mass is present in the right paratracheal region. The right hilus is also enlarged. *B,* One year following radiation therapy to the mediastinum, striking regression of the mass has occurred.

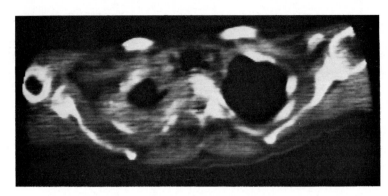

Figure 19–154. Pancoast tumor. A CT scan through the apex of the lungs of a middle-aged woman with right shoulder pain. Asymmetry of the soft tissues is visible, with destruction of the vertebral body and the rib. The lucency in the center of the lesion was a cavity within the squamous cell carcinoma, producing a Pancoast syndrome.

tomography scans are of considerable value in evaluating the paraspinous component of the soft tissue mass and may demonstrate bone destruction of the ribs and spinous elements not apparent on conventional radiographs (Fig. 19–154).

Cavitation

The incidence of cavitation in patients with bronchogenic carcinoma is between 5 and 16 per cent.[14, 42] Approximately 80 per cent of cavitary bronchogenic carcinomas are squamous cell, 10 per cent are large cell undifferentiated, and the remainder are adenocarcinomas or alveolar cell carcinomas (Fig. 19–155).[17] Cavitation in cases of small cell undifferentiated carcinoma is exceedingly rare, even when the tumor reaches large proportions.

The usual cause of cavitation is necrosis and excavation of the tumor, which produce a thick-walled cavity with an irregular inner surface. Very occasionally a

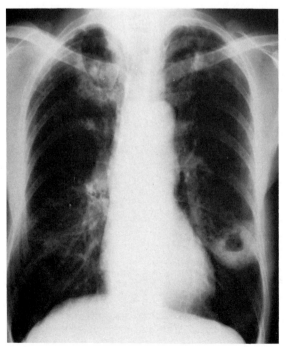

Figure 19–155. Cavitating carcinoma. A frontal radiograph of a 62-year-old man demonstrates a thick-walled cavitating mass in the left lower lung field. Bilateral fibronodular disease is present in both upper lobes, with upward retraction of the left hilum and upward displacement of the minor fissure. A left lower lobe lobectomy revealed a squamous cell carcinoma.

thin-walled cystic bronchogenic carcinoma is found. Two causative mechanisms are possible, and both probably occur. Extreme necrosis and excavation of the tumor may result in a thin-walled cyst. Alternatively, the neoplasm may arise in the wall of a bronchogenic cyst or other lung cyst. Cavitation is not a function of the size of the tumor; lesions 1 cm in diameter may cavitate, whereas a carcinoma as large as 10 cm in diameter may not.

Occasionally a lung abscess distal to an obstructing neoplasm establishes a communication with the bronchial tree. Excavation of the abscess can then produce a cavity distal to the neoplasm. This phenomenon is particularly likely to occur after radiation therapy. Rarely, the area of dense radiation fibrosis that exists following radiation therapy cavitates, although no carcinoma is present. In this circumstance, differentiation from recurrent tumor becomes extremely difficult, and the radiographs may be misleading.

Large Peripheral Mass

The incidence of the presentation of bronchogenic carcinoma as a parenchymal mass larger than 4 cm in diameter is about 18 per cent with squamous cell carcinomas, 25 per cent with adenocarcinomas, 40 per cent with large cell undifferentiated carcinomas, 8 per cent with small cell undifferentiated carcinomas, and 30 per cent with alveolar cell carcinomas.[42, 49, 82] The mass is usually irregular in outline but may at times be strikingly well defined in contour. Many carcinomas that present as a large mass have radiographically evident strands of tissue extending toward the hilus, representing the infiltration of the interstitium of the lung by malignant cells. Cavitation may occur in these large masses. Air bronchograms are not visible except occasionally with alveolar cell carcinomas.

Normal Chest Radiograph

Sputum cytologic screening of subjects at high risk for the development of bronchogenic carcinoma has shown that some patients have malignant cells in their sputum although their chest radiographs are normal.[34, 61] Painstaking fibrobronchoscopy performed while the patient is under general anesthesia can reveal the occult neoplasm in the majority of cases.[50] In the few patients in whom this technique is unsuccessful, tomography may reveal a neoplasm not visible on the plain radiographs. Prior to the advent of fibrobronchoscopy, bronchography was advocated for the localization of the occult neoplasms,[43] but this procedure is no longer recommended. In a few patients insufflated tantalum powder has demonstrated delayed mucociliary clearance at the site of the neoplasm and from the bronchi distal to it.[31]

METASTASES

Mediastinal Metastases

Lymphatic spread is usually to the hila, mediastinum, or supraclavicular lymph nodes. Bronchogenic carcinoma is the cause of the superior vena cava syndrome in 75 per cent of cases. Esophageal obstruction may result from extrinsic compression. The early radiographic manifestations of mediastinal spread are subtle changes in the

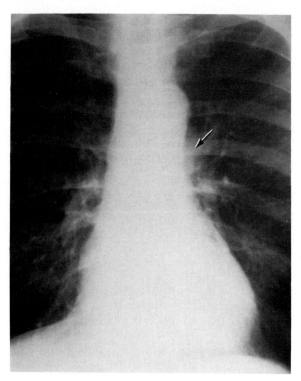

Figure 19–156. Mediastinal metastatic adenopathy. A frontal radiograph of a 51-year-old man with hoarseness and left vocal cord paralysis demonstrates a lateral convexity of the aortopulmonary window (arrow). This radiographic finding indicates involvement of mediastinal lymph nodes between the pulmonary artery and the aorta. The cause of the enlarged nodes proved to be an undifferentiated small cell carcinoma. A parenchymal lung lesion could not be demonstrated.

mediastinal contours (Fig. 19–156). Special attention must be given to the aortopulmonary window and the right paratracheal stripe.[68] Frontal, lateral, and oblique tomography may all assist in detecting mediastinal involvement. Recently, computed tomography has been advocated for the detection of mediastinal spread.[21] This technique appears to be extremely sensitive and accurate. It is not unlikely in the near future that CT studies of the mediastinum will be used routinely to determine whether definitive surgery is feasible.

Pulmonary Metastases

Bronchogenic carcinoma spreads via the lymphatic system and the blood stream. The more common appearance of metastatic dissemination to the lungs is that of lymphangitic carcinomatosis (Fig. 19–157). Less commonly, multiple pulmonary nodules signifying hematogenous dissemination occur. An alternative route of spread is seen in cases of diffuse alveolar cell carcinoma, which may apparently metastasize via the bronchial tree.

Pleural Metastases

A pleural effusion is present at the time of diagnosis in 2 to 5 per cent of patients with bronchogenic carcinoma.[14, 42] Most patients with a pleural effusion have a nonresectable lesion. Serous effusion is most frequent and usually indicates hilar lymph node involvement with lymphatic blockage. Oat cell carcinoma most frequently produces a serous pleural effusion. Malignant cells in the pleural fluid indicate extension of tumor into the pleural space. A hemorrhagic pleural effusion with or without

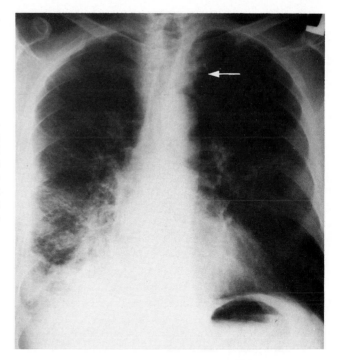

Figure 19–157. Lymphangitic carcinomatosis. A frontal radiograph of a patient with a left upper lobe cavitating squamous cell carcinoma (arrow). The widening of the right paratracheal stripe indicates mediastinal adenopathy. The diffuse density in both lungs, predominantly in the right lower lobe, represents lymphangitic carcinomatosis.

malignant cells invariably indicates direct invasion of the pleura and nonresectability.[12] A spontaneous pneumothorax is rare with bronchogenic carcinoma and is usually the result of the direct invasion of the visceral pleura. Occasionally, airway obstruction from a proximal lesion causes the rupture of a subpleural bleb, producing a pneumothorax.

Chest Wall Metastases

The direct extension of bronchogenic carcinoma to the chest wall or spine rarely occurs at the time of initial presentation, except in the case of superior sulcus tumors. By the time patients with pulmonary tumors come to autopsy, about 10 per cent have chest wall involvement by direct extension or hematogenous dissemination.

Extrathoracic Metastases

Small cell undifferentiated carcinoma grows rapidly and has a tendency to metastasize early. Squamous cell carcinoma may grow rapidly but tends to metastasize late. Adenocarcinoma, on the other hand, may grow slowly but metastasize early.

The skeletal system becomes involved by metastatic tumor in about 30 per cent of patients with bronchogenic carcinomas.[56] Squamous cell carcinoma and large cell undifferentiated carcinoma tend to cause osteolytic lesions; small cell undifferentiated carcinoma and adenocarcinoma may produce osteolytic or osteoblastic metastases. The bones most commonly involved are the vertebrae, pelvic bones, and proximal long bones. Metastases to the distal extremities are unusual, but bronchogenic carcinoma is the most common neoplasm to metastasize to these sites.

The soft tissue organs most likely to be affected by metastases from bronchogenic carcinoma are the lumph nodes, liver, adrenals, kidneys, and brain. Almost any organ of the body may eventually be involved, and metastases are found in 95 per cent of patients at autopsy.

STAGING OF BRONCHOGENIC CARCINOMA

The staging of bronchogenic carcinoma at the time of its detection is useful for determining the prognosis, planning therapy, exchanging information, and assessing the results of therapy.

The prognosis in cases of bronchogenic carcinoma is strongly influenced by the cell type, the state of the disease at the time of detection, and the presence or absence of symptoms.

In general terms, there are three stages of bronchogenic carcinoma; (1) a peripheral lesion without regional or distant dissemination, (2) spread to regional lymph nodes, and (3) distant metastases. In an excellent article by Mountain et al., the survival of patients with bronchogenic carcinoma is related to staging based on a "TNM" classification. "T" relates to the primary neoplasm and has five subgroups. "N" relates to regional lymph node involvement and has three subgroups. "M" relates to distant metastases and has two subgroups.[54] The five-year survival rate of all patients with bronchogenic carcinoma is about 15 per cent; 40 to 50 per cent of patients with asymptomatic peripheral pulmonary nodules survive five years, whereas virtually none with centrally arising lesions or with mediastinal or distant metastases survive that length of time. Most patients with nonresectable lesions or distant metastases die within six months, and few live longer than one year.

At present, approximately 50 per cent of patients with bronchogenic carcinoma undergo a thoracotomy, with some anticipation of cure. Only a little more than half of these have a resection with a prospect of long-term survival. Only about half of the later group survives more than five years. This dismal picture attests to our inability to diagnose the disease early and to select those patients with a reasonably high chance of surgical cure.[51] Rapidly increasing experience with CT scans of the mediastinum, and also of the lung, pleura and chest wall should greatly improve proper patient selection.

Radiologic Techniques in Diagnosis and Staging

The plain chest radiograph remains the most practical radiologic method for the detection and localization of pulmonary neoplasms. Chest radiographs should be obtained at relatively high (120 to 150) kilovoltage with a system capable of short (5 to 15 msec) exposures. Modifications to the routine posteroanterior and lateral projections have been used with varying success. Oblique radiographs are promoted by those experienced with this technique and may detect lesions not visible on the two routine projections. Expiratory and forced expiratory radiographs have not proved worthwhile, although an occasional endobronchial lesion shows air trapping on expiration. High kilovoltage (350 kvp) has been adopted in a few centers, and although promising, the technique still requires refinement.

Tomography used to be employed in almost all cases of suspected bronchogenic carcinoma. Whole-lung tomography helps to define the lesions, confirm or exclude the possibility of calcification within the lesion, detect other lung lesions, and evaluate the hila and mediastinum. Fifty-five degree oblique and lateral tomograms of the hila (Fig. 19–158) are the most useful methods available for detecting hilar adenopathy.[13, 72]

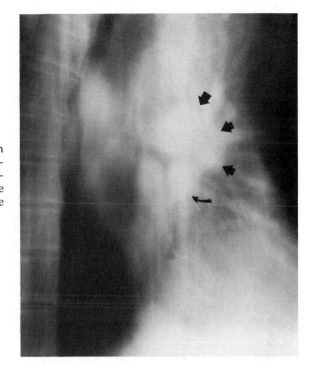

Figure 19–158. Metastatic hilar adenopathy. An oblique tomogram through the left hilus demonstrates enlarged nodes surrounding the left pulmonary artery (straight arrows). An enlarged node is situated between the upper and lower lobe bronchi (curved arrow).

Xerotomography is capable of defining the bronchial tree farther into the lung periphery than regular film tomography. In our experience, xerotomography has not added appreciably to the information provided by plain film tomography. Chest fluroscopy is rarely useful except in the evaluation of suspected diaphragmatic paralysis.

Bronchography is of limited value in the evaluation of suspected bronchogenic carcinoma. Occasionally, a slowly resolving pneumonia may have the appearance of a mass on plain chest radiographs. The bronchographic demonstration of normal bronchi within the lesion reduces the likelihood that a neoplasm is present and allows continued radiographic observation of the lesion (Fig. 19–159). Bronchographic features suggestive of a carcinoma are a "rattailed" bronchus within the lesion, the abrupt termination of a bronchus at the edge of a mass, and an annular constricting lesion. Fibrobronchoscopy has all but replaced bronchography in the differentiation of malignant from inflammatory lesions. Bronchoscopy enables the performance of a biopsy under direct vision or brush biopsy with fluoroscopic assistance. Localization by a radiologist at the time of a brush biopsy is most helpful. Lesions beyond the reach of the fibroscope or bronchial brushes are most easily handled by transthoracic needle aspiration.

A number of angiographic procedures have been proposed for the evaluation of bronchogenic carcinoma but have not gained widespread acceptance. They have been used in the differentiation of malignant from benign masses and in attempts to stage bronchogenic carcinoma. Bronchial and pulmonary angiography are capable of suggesting the malignancy of a lesion. Most primary carcinomas of the lung obtain their blood supply from the bronchial circulation and have diminished pulmonary artery branches around the lesion. Occluded or stenotic pulmonary arteries in the vicinity of a lesion are suggestive of a neoplasm.

Pulmonary angiography, azygography, and superior vena cava angiography have been used to assess the mediastinum for the staging of bronchogenic carcinoma.[27, 48]

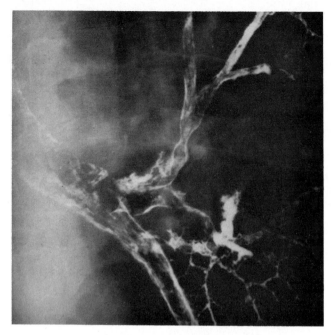

Figure 19–159. Bronchogram of carcinoma. A view of the left hilus from a tantalum bronchogram of a middle-aged patient with hemoptysis and positive sputum cytologic findings demonstrates a narrowing of the apical posterior segmental bronchus. The plain radiographs of the chest and chest tomograms were normal. The lesion proved to be a small annular squamous cell carcinoma.

Opacification of these vascular structures may give indirect evidence of enlarged nodes that are too small to change the contour of the mediastinum on plain radiographs or tomograms. The displacement, obstruction, or intraluminal invasion by the tumor of mediastinal vascular structures is usually evidence of nonresectability. With all these vascular studies, as with bronchography, the evidence is indirect, and significant false positive and false negative results occur. Mediastinoscopy accompanied by mediastinal node biopsy has to a large extent replaced angiography.

Ventilation and perfusion lung scans have been advocated for the assessment of the resectability of lung neoplasms, but they are of little value. In the patient with diminished respiratory reserve, perfusion scans can provide information on differential lung function and assist in the planning of pulmonary resection.[10, 59]

Gallium-67 citrate, when injected intravenously, labels a high proportion of bronchogenic carcinomas. Unfortunately, the label is not specific for neoplasm; inflammatory lesions also take up the isotope. Recent studies have recommended gallium scanning for the selection of patients with a radiographically normal mediastinum for mediastinoscopy.[4] The authors of these reports conclude that if the primary lesion and the mediastinum concentrate gallium, mediastinoscopy should be undertaken.[4] If the primary tumor concentrates gallium but the mediastinum does not, the patient should undergo thoracotomy without mediastinoscopy. This approach requires further validation but may diminish the number of unnecessary mediastinoscopies. Alternative approaches to the selection of patients for mediastinoscopy have been proposed based on the cell type and the location of the lesion.[2, 85]

Computed tomography has been advocated for the routine assessment of all patients suspected of having bronchogenic carcinoma.[21, 72] The sensitivity of computed tomography in the detection of pulmonary nodules is greater than that of plain film tomography.[55] There is no good rationale for performing computed tomography on all single pulmonary nodules, however.[69] The evaluation of the hila is easier and better with routine tomography, in most circumstances. CT can detect normal lymph nodes in the mediastinum and enlarged nodes not seen with other radiologic techniques. When the plain chest radiographs are normal, we consider CT should be used routinely to select patients for mediastinoscopy. If enlarged nodes are present in the pretracheal space, mediastinoscopy should be undertaken. Patients with a normal CT scan of the mediastinum should go directly to thoracotomy. Superior sulcus tumors are elegantly displayed by computed tomography, as are peripheral masses that have invaded the chest wall. CT brain scans may help exclude the possibility of cerebral metastases before surgery is performed.

RADIOLOGIC BIOPSY TECHNIQUES

Aspiration biopsy has become firmly established as a method of investigating peripheral masses suspected of being neoplastic.[75, 79, 88] The minimum size of a lesion capable of being biopsied varies with the skill of the operator. In our experience, biopsy specimens can be taken from lesions as small as 1 cm. Confirmation that the tip of the needle is within the lesion requires two projections. Biplane fluoroscopy is the most convenient method, but single-plane fluoroscopy and cross-table radiographs are acceptable.

Needle biopsy of the lung is a safe procedure. Pneumothorax occurs in about 20 per cent of patients but requires intercostal tube evacuation in only a small percentage. The dissemination of malignant cells due to an aspiration biopsy probably does not occur. The results of needle aspiration are 85 to 90 per cent positive for malignant cells. The accuracy in identifying the cell type is high in cases of squamous cell carcinoma and adenocarcinoma but low in instances of undifferentiated tumor.

The bronchial brushing of lung masses, employing a control-tipped catheter or preshaped catheter, yields results equal to or better than those of bronchial brushing through a fibrobronchoscope. The mobility of the control-tipped catheter is greater than that of a fibroscope. The direct visualization of the central airways has advantages, however, and in most institutions, fibrobronchoscopy and brushing have replaced brushing with catheters.[65]

POSTOPERATIVE APPEARANCE

The normal appearance of the chest radiograph following segmentectomy, lobectomy, or pneumonectomy depends on the amount of pulmonary tissue resected.

With segmentectomy or lobectomy, the volume of the hemithorax is reduced. The remaining lobe or lobes usually expand to fill the space occupied by the resected portion of the lung. The ipsilateral hemidiaphragm is often elevated, and the mediastinum is variably shifted toward the side of resection. The increase in volume of the remaining pulmonary tissue (compensatory hyperexpansion) results in the reorientation of pulmonary arteries and major bronchi, often visible radiographically when the amount of lung removed is significant. Following upper-lobe lobectomy, the lower-lobe bronchus and artery rotate outward and upward as the lower lobe expands superiorly. The arteries and bronchi appear more widely spaced than normal. Following lower-lobe lobectomy, the upper-lobe pulmonary arteries rotate outward and downward. Shift of the diaphragm and mediastinum is relatively limited by fixed structures, and the reorientation of vessels often provides the most important clue to the recognition of lobectomy when a clinical history is lacking. The ipsilateral hilus is usually distorted and smaller than its counterpart. A small pneumothorax may be visible for days following the removal of the chest tube.[73]

Pneumonectomy results in a large, air-filled space, bounded by parietal pleura. The "empty" hemithorax contains gas and a variable amount of fluid producing a single large air-fluid level (Fig. 19–160A). In the absence of complications, air is slowly absorbed and the pleural space progressively fills with fluid.[5, 18] Eventually the space is obliterated by connective tissue (Fig. 19–160B). Postoperative radiographs show filling of the pleural space with fluid within 16 to 24 weeks, but this may vary from 3 weeks to nine months and is usually associated with a gradual decrease in the volume of the hemithorax. The decreasing volume is reflected by a mediastinal shift toward the evacuated hemithorax (Fig. 19–160C). Diaphragmatic elevation occurs but is difficult to recognize because of the fluid.

Any displacement of the heart and mediastinum to the contralateral side apparent more than two weeks following pneumonectomy indicates excessive fluid accumulation and should raise the suspicion of empyema or delayed bleeding. A drop in the level of the pleural fluid from one examination to the next suggests the presence of a bronchopleural fistula or empyema, particularly when associated with mediastinal shift

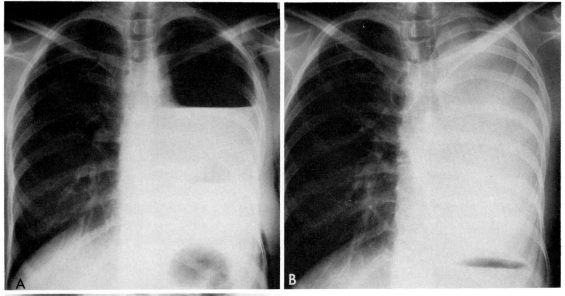

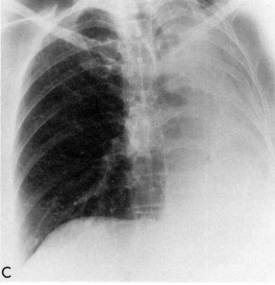

Figure 19–160. Pneumonectomy—postoperative changes. *A,* A frontal radiograph taken shortly after a left pneumonectomy was performed. An air-fluid level, with mild displacement of the mediastinum to the side of the pneumonectomy, is normal. *B,* Four months later, the lung has filled with fluid, and replacement with areolar tissue has occurred. The mediastinum has shifted further toward the side of the pneumonectomy. *C,* A frontal radiograph taken four years following a pneumonectomy for a left bronchogenic carcinoma in different patient. Marked volume loss of the left hemithorax has occurred. The right lung herniates over the midline to the left side. The heart is completely obscured within the opaque left hemithorax. A decrease in the intercostal spaces on the left is also a normal finding.

toward the opposite side. The decrease in fluid is apparently due to its expectoration via the tracheobronchial tree. A transient drop in the level of pleural fluid during the first few weeks after surgery was seen in 17 per cent of patients studied by Christiansen et al. and probably reflects the absorption of fluid from the pleural space.[18] A bronchopleural fistula did not develop in these patients, and they continued to show progressive volume loss on the side of the pneumonectomy.

Bronchopleural fistula and empyema are relatively common complications of resectional surgery in patients with pulmonary neoplasms.[3, 5, 18, 86] These complications can result from inadequate surgical closure of the bronchus or visceral pleura, devitalization and breakdown of the bronchial stump, or intraoperative contamination of the pleural space by exogenous or endogenous bacteria in bronchial secretions or infected lymph nodes. Although they are often associated, a bronchopleural fistula can occur without concurrent or subsequent infection of the pleural space. An uncomplicated bronchopleural fistula most commonly occurs following partial pneumonectomy. Silver et al. found that 23 per cent of 75 patients who had had a lobectomy or segmentectomy had a persistent postoperative pneumothorax, suggesting the presence of bronchopleural fistula.[73] Only two of the patients subsequently acquired an empyema. Bronchopleural fistulas are less frequent following pneumonectomy, occurring in 4.6 to 10 per cent of patients; empyema occurs in 2.2 to 6.9 per cent of patients following pneumonectomy for bronchogenic carcinoma.[5, 18, 45]

Following lobectomy, a majority of persistent pleural spaces resulting from bronchopleural fistula close without treatment, a process averaging 80 days but ranging from 17 days to more than 9 months.[18, 39] The length of time required for closure depends on the size of the fistula, its rate of healing, the volume of the space, and the compliance of the adjacent lung. A noninfected pleural space should slowly decrease in size on serial radiographs. If the remaining lung is of poor compliance owing to fibrosis, the space may be obliterated by fluid with little decrease in the volume of the hemithorax. A persistent increase in the gas within the hemithorax or a sudden pneumothorax in a patient whose lung has re-expanded indicates a recurrence of the bronchopleural fistula.

Empyema is a dread complication of thoracic surgery and usually necessitates vigorous therapy with drainage of the pleural space. The mortality rate of patients with postoperative empyema ranges from 16 to 28 per cent.[39, 45] Bronchopleural fistula and empyema most often occur one to two weeks after surgery but may have a delayed onset, occurring months later. Chest pain, dyspnea, and cough productive of frothy or blood-tinged sputum are the most common symptoms of bronchopleural fistula. Spiking fever is usually present when an empyema develops. An increase in the volume of a fluid-filled hemithorax following pneumonectomy or an increasing pleural effusion following a lesser resection suggests empyema (Fig. 19–161). Thoracentesis is usually necessary for diagnosis. Increasing pleural thickening following pulmonary resection may be the result of aspergillosis infection of the pleural space; differentiation from recurrent neoplasm is extremely difficult. In our experience, CT has proved accurate in delineating localized empyemas following pulmonary resection. The encapsulated fluid can be distinguished from the pleural peel and free pleural fluid. CT can assist in localizing the fluid for thoracentesis.

Fistulograms, with the injection of contrast material into the pleural cavity, may be useful in localizing the site of a bronchopleural fistula. Water-soluble contrast materials are extremely irritating to the airway and should be avoided. Bronchographic contrast material may be injected into the pleural space under strict aseptic conditions. Fluoroscopic control, with the rotation of the patient into all positions, is necessary to determine the site of a peripheral air leak. When the bronchopleural fistula is due to a bronchial stump dehiscence, bronchography is the method of choice for localization.

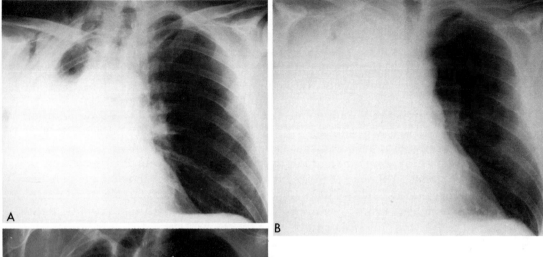

Figure 19–161. Postpneumonectomy empyema. *A,* A portable radiograph five days following a right-sided pneumonectomy for bronchogenic carcinoma. The heart and mediastinum have shifted to the right. *B,* Two weeks later the heart and mediastinum have returned to the midline, indicating volume expansion of the right hemithorax. This finding is distinctly abnormal. A small amount of gas is still present in the right hemithorax. Aspiration of the right hemithorax demonstrated an empyema. *C,* One month after drainage of the right empyema with an Eloesser flap, the heart and mediastinum have again shifted to the side of the pneumonectomy.

Again, bronchographic contrast materials should be used. Bronchoscopy or thoracentesis with the injection of methylene blue dye confirms the presence of bronchopleural fistula but is not capable of localizing the site of the air leak.

Recently, automatic mechanical stapling devices have been used for the closure of the bronchus, pulmonary arteries, veins, and lung parenchyma in patients undergoing pulmonary resection. A number of small metal staples are inserted simultaneously in rows several centimeters long, taking the place of standard surgical sutures. Staples are associated with fewer postoperative complications than standard sutures. In a study by Hood et al., only 2 per cent of 289 patients underoing lobectomy or a lesser resection experienced a prolonged air leak, indicating a bronchopleural fistula.[39] Two of sixty patients acquired a bronchopleural fistula following pneumonectomy, but in each case, carcinoma had recurred in the bronchial stump. On postoperative radiographs, the metal staples have a characteristic appearance.

RADIATION PNEUMONOPATHY

Radiation pneumonitis, more recently termed radiation pneumonopathy or radiation pleuropneumonitis, has been known for some time. The first reports appeared in the 1920's shortly after the advent of kilovoltage equipment capable of penetrating and delivering significant doses to the internal structures of the thoracic cavity. A historical review, with clinical and pathologic descriptions, is given by Rubin and Casarett.[67]

Patients with bronchogenic carcinoma treated with radiation therapy by necessity have the lung tissue immediately surrounding the tumor irradiated. Most will develop pneumonopathy, and in many it is moderately symptomatic. Fatal radiation pneumonitis is rare in the treatment of bronchogenic carcinoma.

Histopathologic Changes in the Lung

The morphologic changes in lung tissue following irradiation occur on a continuum but can be divided in the first six months into three phases.[33] An exudative phase is seen during the first 30 days; a pneumonic phase lasts from the second to the third month; and a reparative phase occurs between the third and sixth to ninth month. In the exudative phase, endothelial and epithelial damage appears with interstitial edema, alveolar proteinosis, and hyaline membranes. In about 40 per cent of cases, capillary congestion and platelet aggregation may be present. In the pneumonic phase, alveolar type 2 pneumocytes proliferate and, together with alveolar macrophages, fill the air spaces. Capillary damage is extensive, and collagen deposition begins. In the reparative phase, multiple cells proliferate, with profound reconstruction of the lung architecture. Mast cells, among others, predominate, and collagen production leads to fibrosis. At six to nine months and beyond, fibrosis of the alveolar walls develops, with marked reduction in the number, size, and volume of the alveoli. The number of patent capillaries and small vessels is markedly reduced. With higher doses of irradiation, complete fibrotic replacement of the lung may occur.

Alterations in Pulmonary Function

Usually at the time of the onset of clinical symptoms — one to two months after irradiation — changes in pulmonary function occur. During the exudative phase, decreased ventilation and perfusion to the irradiated area as well as ventilation-perfusion mismatch are found. The decrease in pulmonary blood flow reaches a maximum by 100 to 150 days.[62] Many studies have demonstrated changes in pulmonary mechanics when large volumes of lung are irradiated. Total lung capacity, vital capacity, and forced expiratory volumes are reduced. Diffusing capacity and lung compliance may also be diminished. The fall in pulmonary compliance usually occurs with the radiographic appearance of the pneumonic phase and persists into the chronic fibrotic phase. Radioisotopic studies of regional blood flow appear to be the most sensitive indicators of functional damage and may show abnormalities before radiographic changes appear.

Clinical Features

The clinical syndrome related to radiation pneumonopathy varies with the volume of lung irradiated and the dose delivered. In general, doses of less than 2000 rads applied to small volumes of lung do not produce symptoms. With larger lung volumes or higher doses the initial findings may be clinical or radiographic. Symptoms usually occur six weeks to three months following irradiation, the initial symptom usually being a cough, which may be mild or severe.[67] Dyspnea, low-grade fever, and tachypnea may be prominent features. Following whole lung irradiation, severe dyspnea, cyanosis, marked tachypnea, and fever may occur, progressing to death. Patients having irradiation of less than 50 per cent of the volume of their lungs show a gradual decrease in symptoms as the process evolves from the exudative to the fibrotic phase. Corticosteroid treatment may dramatically reduce the symptoms. With the exception of tachypnea and occasional cyanosis and pleural friction rub, the physical findings are usually normal.

Radiographic Findings

The radiographic findings of radiation pleuropneumonitis generally coincide with the onset of symptoms, which occurs 6 to 12 weeks following the completion of treatment[30, 62] The first manifestation is an ill-defined, hazy increase in density in the irradiated field that obscures the pulmonary vasculature. This may progress to pulmonary consolidation with air bronchograms or to a nodular or acinar pattern. The radiographic changes have a relatively sharp edge and are limited to the field of irradiation (Fig. 19–162A).

Patients receiving a dose just sufficient to cause pneumonitis may show complete radiographic resolution. In the majority of patients, however, the pneumonic changes progress to chronic and usually irreversible fibrosis. The appearance changes from consolidation to dense linear streaks radiating from the area of involvement. Marked cicatricial volume loss occurs, and retraction toward the area of scarring results. In the lower lobes the diaphragm is elevated. Hilar retraction and elevation occur with upper lobe irradiation. The mediastinum may shift toward the irradiated side. The permanent changes of fibrosis take 6 to 24 months to evolve (Fig. 19–162B and C). Radiation changes after two years are unusual; should changes occur at this time an alternative process should be considered.

Pleural or pericardial effusions are uncommon. Cavitation is usually from necrosis of the tumor but rarely occurs without residual cancer being evident in the wall of the cavity. Spontaneous pneumothorax is an unusual complication of radiation pneumonopathy. Other complications are usually associated with tumor destruction and include bronchial obstruction, rib fractures, and tracheoesophageal fistula. Respiratory insufficiency due to radiation fibrosis of large volumes of lung is uncommon. Chronic pericarditis and pleurisy with chronic effusions do occur but are also uncommon.

The possibility of radiation changes outside the field of irradiation has been extensively discussed. These changes can almost always be attributed to an alternative process, such as infection.

Modifying Factors in Radiation Pneumonitis

The three interdependent primary factors in the development of clinical radiation pneumonopathy are the volume of lung irradiated, the radiation time, and the dose.[81] Irradiation of one third to one half of a lung usually produces symptomatic disease. Whole-lung irradiation can lead to severe symptoms and even death. The dose required for the treatment of bronchogenic carcinoma invariably produces regional changes in perfusion and regional radiographic changes but may cause no symptoms. Although the total dose is important, the number of fractions into which the dose is divided is even more important. The greater the number of fractions, the lower is the damage from irradiation. A number of chemotherapeutic drugs, given before, during, or after

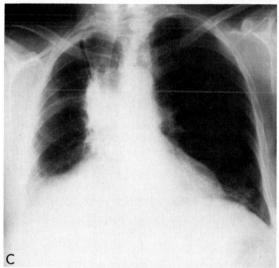

Figure 19–162. Radiation changes. *A,* A frontal radiograph of a middle-aged woman nine weeks following right mediastinal radiation therapy. A dosage of 4960 rads was given over a period of 39 days in a 9- by 8-cm field. Moderately dense consolidation to the right of the mediastinum within the radiation field is part of the pneumonic phase of radiation pneumonopathy. *B,* Ten months later, there is a marked increase in density of the area, with volume loss and retraction, which is evidence of radiation fibrosis. *C,* One year later, further retraction and volume loss in the area of radiation fibrosis has occurred.

irradiation, potentiate or add to the effect of irradiation. Among these are actinomycin-D, bleomycin, cyclophosphamide, vincristine, and Adriamycin.

RECURRENCE OF BRONCHOGENIC CARCINOMA

The metastatic potential of lung cancer is high. Between 35 and 70 per cent of patients who die within one month after pulmonary resection have either metastatic spread or persistence of tumor in the thorax at autopsy.[78, 84] Within one year after resection, the incidence rises to 85 per cent. Postmortem studies provide the main evidence of the distribution of recurrence but do not indicate the site of the initial reappearance of the tumor. Recurrence within the hemithorax of the previous resection occurs in 50 to 88 per cent of patients.[1, 78] Mediastinal nodal involvement is slightly less common, being present in 77 to 86 per cent of cases. Spread to the contralateral lung, brain, and distant lymph nodes is next in frequency, occurring in 25 to 40 per cent of

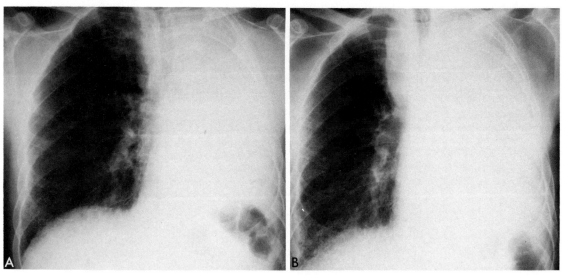

Figure 19–163. Postoperative tumor recurrence. *A,* A frontal radiograph of a 60-year-old man four months following a left pneumonectomy for a squamous cell carcinoma. The mediastinum is displaced toward the side of pneumonectomy. The cardiac silhouette is not visible. Pulmonary fibrosis is present at the right base. *B,* Three months later the mediastinum has shifted to the midline. A right paratracheal mass is present, with narrowing of the intrathoracic trachea. The tumor has recurred within the left hemithorax and mediastinum.

patients. Metastases also frequently occur to the adrenals, liver, kidneys, pericardium, and bone.

When patients present with a recurrent tumor in the hemithorax in which lobectomy was performed, the radiographic appearance is most commonly that of enlarged hilar or mediastinal lymph nodes. Lymphangitic carcinomatosis in the residual ipsilateral lung may be the initial radiographic appearance. Ipsilateral pleural effusion is not an uncommon initial finding. Spread to the opposite lung may be in the form of multiple pulmonary nodules or of linear and small nodular densities representing lymphangitic carcinomatosis. Recurrence in the ipsilateral hemithorax after pneumonectomy is difficult to detect radiologically. A shift of the mediastinum to the opposite side may indicate a tumor mass in the evacuated hemithorax (Fig. 19–163). A recent report describes a case of a tumor mass within the ipsilateral hemithorax detected by computed tomography.[21] The tumor was denser than the normal fibroadipose tissue present after pneumonectomy. Mediastinal tumor becomes evident only when contralateral nodes enlarge and alter the contour of the mediastinum. Symptoms will usually draw attention to metastases to distant organs, including the brain, bone and liver.

References

1. Abadir, R., and Muggia, F. M.: Irradiated lung cancer. An autopsy analysis of spread pattern. Radiology *114*:427–430, 1975.
2. Acosta, J. L., and Manfredi, F.: Selective mediastinoscopy. Chest *71*:150–154, 1977.
3. Adler, R. N., and Plaut, M. E.: Post-pneumonectomy empyema. Surgery *71*:210–214, 1972.
4. Alazraki, N. P., Ramsdell, J. W., Taylor, A., et al.: Reliability of Gallium scan chest radiography compared to mediastinoscopy for evaluating mediastinal spread in lung cancer. Am. Rev. Respir. Dis. *117*:415–420, 1978.

5. Andersen, J. C., Egedorf, J., and Stougard, J.: The pleural space succeeding pneumonectomy. A roentgenological and clinical study of 167 cases of bronchogenic carcinoma. Scand. J. Thorac. Cardiovasc. Surg. 2:70–73, 1968.

6. Barker, W. L., Langstron, H. T., and Naffah, P.: Postresectional thoracic spaces. Ann. Thorac. Surg. 2:299–310, 1966.

7. Baylin, S. B., Abeloff, M. D., Wieman, K. C., et al.: Elevated histaminase (diamine oxidase) activity in small-cell carcinoma of the lung. N. Engl. J. Med. 293:1286–1290, 1975.

8. Blot, W. J., and Fraumeni, J. F., Jr.: Arsenical air pollution and lung cancer. Lancet 2:142–144, 1975.

9. Bower, B. F., and Gordon, G. S.: Hormonal effects of nonendocrine tumors. Annu. Rev. Med. 16:83–118, 1965.

10. Boysen, P. G., Block, A. J., Olsen, G. N., et al.: Prospective evaluation for pneumonectomy using the 99mtechnetium quantitative perfusion lung scan. Chest 72:422–425, 1977.

11. Brain, W. R.: The neurological complications of neoplasms. Lancet 1:179–184, 1963.

12. Brinkman, G. L.: The significance of pleural effusion complicating otherwise operable bronchogenic carcinoma. Dis. Chest 36:152–154, 1959.

13. Brown, L. R., and DeRemer, R. A.: 55° oblique hilar tomography. Mayo Clin. Proc. 51:89–95, 1976.

14. Byrd, R. B., Carr, D. T., Miller, W. E., et al.: Radiographic abnormalities in carcinoma of the lung as related to histological cell type. Thorax 24:573–575, 1969.

15. Cahan, W. G.: Multiple primary cancers, one of which is lung. Surg. Clin. North Am. 49:323–335, 1969.

16. Cahan, W. G., Castro, E. B., and Hajdu, S. I.: The significance of a solitary lung shadow in patients with colon carcinoma. Cancer 33:414–421, 1974.

17. Chaudhuri, M. R.: Primary pulmonary cavitating carcinoma. Thorax 28:354–366, 1973.

18. Christiansen, K. H., Morgan, S. W., Karich, A. F., et al.: Pleural space following pneumonectomy. Ann. Thorac. Surg. 1:298–304, 1965.

19. Cohen, S., and Hossain, M. S.: Primary carcinoma of the lung. A review of 417 histologically proved cases. Dis. Chest 49:67–74, 1966.

20. Collins, N. P.: Bronchogenic carcinoma. Importance of the cell type. Arch. Surg. 77:925–932, 1958.

21. Crowe, J. K., Brown, L. R., and Muhm, J. R.: Computed tomography of the mediastinum. Radiology 128:75–87, 1978.

22. De Villiers, A. J., and Windish, J. P.: Lung cancer in a fluorspar mining community. I: Radiation, dust, and mortality experience. Br. J. Ind. Med. 21:94–109, 1964.

23. Diner, W. C.: Hypertrophic osteoarthropathy. J.A.M.A. 181:555–557, 1962.

24. Dutra, F. R., and Carney, J. D.: Asbestosis and pulmonary carcinoma. Arch. Environ. Health 10:416–423, 1965.

25. Early diagnosis of lung cancer. Br. Med. J. 2:710–711, 1968.

26. Edwards, W. M., Cox, R. S., Jr., and Garland, L. H.: The solitary nodule (coin lesion) of the lung. Am. J. Roentgenol. 88:1020–1042, 1962.

27. Engelman, R. M., Schafer, P. W., and Higgins, G. A., Jr.: Pulmonary angiography in lung cancer suspects. J. Thorac. Cardiovasc. Surg. 57:356–364, 1969.

28. Figueroa, W. G., Raszkowski, R., and Weiss, W.: Lung cancer in chloromethyl methyl ether workers. N. Engl. J. Med 288:1096–1097, 1973.

29. Fletcher, C. M., and Horn, D.: Smoking and health. W.H.O. Chron. 24:345–370, 1970.

30. Fried, J. R., and Goldberg, H.: Post-irradiation changes in lungs and thorax: a clinical, roentgenological and pathological study, with emphasis on late and terminal stages. Am. J. Roentgenol. 43:877–895, 1940.

31. Gamsu, G., and Nadel, J. A.: New technique for roentgenographic study of airways and lungs using powdered tantalum. Cancer 30:1353–1357, 1972.

32. Garland, L. H.: The differential diagnosis of solitary pulmonary nodules. Chicago Med. Soc. Bull. 60:805–812, 1958.

33. Gross, N. J.: Pulmonary effects of radiation therapy. Ann. Intern. Med. 86:81–92, 1977.

34. Grzybowski, S., and Coy, P.: Early diagnosis of carcinoma of the lung. Cancer 25:113–120, 1970.

35. Gupta, A. K., Pryce, D. M., and Blenkinsopp, W. K.: Pre-operative length of history and tumour size in central and peripheral bronchial carcinomata. Thorax 20:398–404, 1965.

36. Hammond, E. C.: Lung cancer death rates in England and Wales compared with those in the U.S.A. Br. Med. J. 2:649–654, 1958.

37. Hammond, E. C., and Wynder, E. L.: Cigarette smoking and lung cancer in Canada. Can. Med. Assoc. J. 82:372–377, 1960.

38. Hinds, J. R., and Hitchcock, G. C.: Adenocarcinoma of the lung. Thorax 24:10–17, 1969.

39. Hood, R. M., Kirksey, T. D., Calhoon, J. H., et al.: The use of automatic stapling devices in pulmonary resection. Ann. Thorac. Surg. 16:85–96, 1973.

40. Korpela, A., and Magnus, K.: The incidence of lung cancer in Finland and Norway. Br. J. Cancer 15:393–408, 1961.

41. Kreyberg, L., Liebow, A. A., Euhlinger, E., et al.: Histological typing of lung tumors. Geneva, World Health Organization, 1967.

42. Lehar, T. J., Carr, D. T., Miller, W. E., et al.: Roentgenographic appearance of bronchogenic adenocarcinoma. Am. Rev. Respir. Dis. 96:245–248, 1967.

43. Lerner, M. A., Rosbash, H., Frank, H. A., et al.: Radiologic localization and management of cytologically discovered bronchial carcinoma. N. Engl. J. Med. 264:480–485, 1961.

44. Le Roux, B. T.: Empyema thoracis. Br. J. Surg. 52:89–99, 1965.
45. Le Roux, B. T.: Bronchial carcinoma. Thorax 23:136–143, 1968.
46. Lieberman, J. S., Borrero, J., Urdaneta, E., et al.: Thrombophlebitis and cancer. J.A.M.A. 177:542–545, 1961.
47. Lillington, G. A.: The solitary pulmonary nodule — 1974. Am. Rev. Respir. Dis. 110:699–707, 1974.
48. Low, L. R., Keyting, W. S., and Daywitt, A. L.: Azygography in management of carcinoma of the lung. Radiology 81:96–100, 1963.
49. Marco, M., and Galy, P.: Bronchioloalveolar carcinoma. Clinicopathologic relationships, natural history, and prognosis in 29 cases. Am. Rev. Respir. Dis. 107:621–629, 1973.
50. Marsh, B. R., Frost, J. K., Erozan, Y. S., et al.: Occult bronchogenic carcinoma. Endoscopic localization and television documentation. Cancer 30:1348–1352, 1972.
51. Mittman, C., and Bruderman, I.: Lung cancer: to operate or not? Am. Rev. Respir. Dis. 116:477–496, 1977.
52. Morton, D. L., Itabashi, H. H., and Grimes, O. F.: Nonmetastatic neurological complications of bronchogenic carcinoma: the carcinomatous neuromyopathies. J. Thorac. Cardiovasc. Surg. 51:14–29, 1966.
53. Mountain, C. F.: Surgical prospects and priorities for clinical research. Cancer Chemother. Rep. 4:19–24, 1973.
54. Mountain, C. F., Carr, D. T., and Anderson, W. A. D.: A system for the clinical staging of lung cancer. Am. J. Roentgenol. 120:130–138, 1974.
55. Muhm, J. R., Brown, L. R., and Crowe, J. K.: Detection of pulmonary nodules by computed tomography. Am. J. Roentgenol. 128:267–270, 1977.
56. Napoli, L. D., Hansen, H. H., Muggia, F. M., et al.: The incidence of osseous involvement in lung cancer, with special reference to the development of osteoblastic changes. Radiology 108:17–21, 1973.
57. Nathan, M. H., Collins, V. P., and Adams, R. A.: Differentiation of benign and malignant pulmonary nodules by growth rate. Radiology 79:221–231, 1962.
58. Nathanson, L., and Hall, T. C.: A spectrum of tumors that produce paraneoplastic syndromes. Lung tumors: how they produce their syndromes. Ann. N. Y. Acad. Sci. 230:367–377, 1974.
59. Olsen, G. N., Block, A. J., and Tobias, J. A.: Prediction of postpneumonectomy pulmonary function using quantitative macroaggregate lung scanning. Chest 66:13–16, 1974.
60. Pancoast, H. K.: Superior pulmonary sulcus tumor: tumor characterized by pain, Horner's syndrome, destruction of bone and atrophy of hand muscles. J.A.M.A. 99:1391–1396, 1932.
61. Pearson, F. G., Thompson, D. W., and Delarue, N. C.: Experience with the cytologic detection, localization, and treatment of radiographically undemonstrable bronchial carcinoma. J. Thorac. Cardiovasc. Surg. 54:371–382, 1967.
62. Prato, F. S., Kurdyak, R., Sailbil, E. A., et al.: Physiological and radiographic assessment during the development of pulmonary radiation fibrosis. Radiology 122:389–397, 1977.
63. Rassam, J. W., and Anderson, G.: Incidence of paramalignant disorders in bronchogenic carcinoma. Thorax 30:86–90, 1975.
64. Ray, J. F., III, Magnin, G. E., Smullen, W. A., et al.: The coin lesions story: update 1976. Chest 70:332–336, 1976.
65. Richardson, R. H., Zavala, D. C., Mukerjee, P. K., et al.: The use of fiberoptic bronchoscopy and brush biopsy in diagnosis of suspected pulmonary malignancy. Am. Rev. Respir. Dis. 109:63–66, 1974.
66. Rigler, L. G.: The earliest roentgenographic signs of carcinoma of the lung. J.A.M.A. 195:655–657, 1966.
67. Rubin, P., and Casarett, G. W.: Clinical Radiation Pathology. Philadelphia, W. B. Saunders Company, 1968, pp. 423–470.
68. Savoca, C. J., Austin, J. H. M., and Goldberg, H. I.: The right paratracheal stripe. Radiology 122:295–301, 1977.
69. Savoca, C. J., and Gamsu, G.: Review of Muhm, J. R., Brown, L. R., and Crowe, J. K.: Detection of pulmonary nodules by computed tomography. Am. J. Roentgenol. 128:267–270, 1977. In Invest. Radiol. 12:474–475, 1977.
70. Selby, H. M., Luomanen, R., and Sherman, R. S.: The x-ray appearance of oat-cell cancer of the lung. Radiology 81:817–822, 1963.
71. Selikoff, I. J., Bader, R. A., Bader, M. E., et al.: Asbestosis and neoplasia. Am. J. Med. 42:487–496, 1967.
72. Shevland, J. E., Chiu, L. C., Schapiro, R. L., et al.: The role of conventional tomography and computed tomography in assessing the resectability of primary lung cancer: a preliminary report. J. Comput. Assist. Tomogr. 2:1–19, 1978.
73. Silver, A. W., Espinas, E. E., and Byron, F. X.: The fate of the postresection space. Ann. Thorac. Surg. 2:311–326, 1966.
74. Silverberg, E., and Holleb, A. I.: Cancer statistics, 1974–worldwide epidemiology. CA 24:2–21, 1974.
75. Sinner, N.: Transthoracic needle biopsy of small peripheral malignant lung lesions. Invest. Radiol. 8:305–314, 1973.
76. Sobel, M., Rodman, T., and Pastor, B. H.: The incidence and clinical significance of cardiac involvement in bronchogenic carcinoma. Am. J. Med. Sci. 240:739–748, 1960.
77. Spengler, D. M., Kirsh, M. M., and Kaufer, H.: Orthopaedic aspects and early diagnosis of superior sulcus tumor of lung (Pancoast). J. Bone Joint Surg. 55A:1645–1650, 1973.

78. Spjut, H. J., and Mateo, L. E.: Recurrent and metastatic carcinoma in surgically treated carcinoma of lung. An autopsy survey. Cancer 18:1462–1466, 1965.
79. Stevens, G. M., Weigen, J. F., and Lillington, G. A.: Needle aspiration biopsy of localized pulmonary lesions with amplified fluoroscopic guidance. Am. J. Roentgenol. 103:561–571, 1968.
80. Trunk, G., Gracey, D. R., and Byrd, R. B.: The management and evaluation of the solitary pulmonary nodule. Chest 66:236–239, 1974.
81. Wara, W. M., Phillips, T. L., Margolis, L. W., et al.: Radiation pneumonitis: a new approach to the derivation of time-dose factors. Cancer 32:547–552, 1973.
82. Weiss, R. B.: Small-cell carcinoma of the lung: therapeutic management. Ann. Intern. Med. 88:522–531, 1978.
83. Weiss, W., and Boucout, K. R.: The prognosis of lung cancer originating as a round lesion. Am. Rev. Respir. Dis. 116:827–836, 1977.
84. Weiss, W., and Gillick, J. S.: The metastatic spread of bronchogenic carcinoma in relation to the interval between resection and death. Chest 71:725–729, 1977.
85. Whitcomb, M. E., Barham, E., Goldman, A. L., et al.: Indications for mediastinoscopy in bronchogenic carcinoma. Am. Rev. Respir. Dis. 113:189–195, 1976.
86. Williams, N. S., and Lewis, C. T.: Bronchopleural fistula: a review of 86 cases. Br. J. Surg. 63:520–522, 1976.
87. Wynder, E. L., Mabuchi, K., and Beattie, E. J., Jr.: The epidemiology of lung cancer. Recent trends. J.A.M.A. 213:2221–2228, 1970.
88. Zelch, J. V., Lalli, A. F., McCormack, L. J., et al.: Aspiration biopsy in diagnosis of pulmonary nodule. Chest 3:149–152, 1973.

Part IX

Thoracic Outlet Syndrome

ERICH K. LANG, M.D.

The symptoms associated with a variety of conditions such as cervical rib syndrome, first thoracic rib syndrome, scalenus anticus syndrome, hyperabduction syndrome, costoclavicular syndrome, and pectoralis minor syndrome are attributable to compression of the brachial plexus, the subclavian-axillary artery, the vein in the thoracic outlet region, or all three.[1, 2, 6, 14, 16, 20]

Since both vascular and neural structures are subject to compression, symptoms may be neurologic, vascular, or both.[14] Symptoms attributable to neural compression, however, are encountered more often.[4] These consist of pain, paresthesia, and numbness usually involving the fingers and hands and most commonly following an ulnar nerve distribution.[15, 19] Advanced neurologic conditions may cause sensory deficits, motor weakness, and muscle atrophy.[18]

Symptoms caused by arterial compression may mimic those of nerve compression and include numbness, fatigue, paresthesia, ischemic pain, motor weakness, and in extreme cases, distal gangrene.[8, 15] Diminution or absence of the brachial and radial pulse and a bruit heard over the subclavian artery are objective findings indicating arterial compression. Symptoms and objective findings tend to be accentuated in certain positions and by exercise.[1]

Symptoms of venous compression include pain, cyanosis, swelling, and distal edema.

Although such prominent clinical manifestations imply compression of neurovascular structures in the thoracic outlet area, they do not permit localization of the precise site of compression.[7, 8, 15] Surgical procedures deployed to correct conditions of anatomic tightness and compression must be directed toward a specific anatomic site, however.[4, 5, 16, 19] Therefore, the precise nature and location of the offending lesion and, particularly, coexistence of multiple lesions must be identified preoperatively.[4, 5, 8]

A meticulous history is most important to exclude patients with a systemic condition such as a collagen-vascular or metabolic disorder, osteoarthritis, or tumor of the spinal cord which can mimic the symptom complex of the neurovascular compression syndrome.[4, 7, 19, 20, 21]

Compression of neural or vascular structures may occur in the neck, at the level of the first rib, in the scalenus anticus tunnel, in the costoclavicular space, and even as far laterally as at the point of crossing of the pectoralis minor tendon traversing to the coracoid process.[14] To delineate the mechanism and site of obstruction, three specific diagnostic maneuvers have been advocated.

1. *The Adson maneuver* is designed to identify compression of the subclavian artery and brachial plexus by the scalene muscles against the first rib.[1] The radial pulse is monitored while the patient extends the neck, turns the chin toward the side under investigation, and sustains a maximal inspiration.[1] Reduction or disappearance of the radial pulse constitutes a positive test.[9] If the radial pulse is reduced without turning of the chin toward the side under investigation, the presence of a cervical rib should be suspected.[1, 2, 4, 13, 19]

2. *The costoclavicular compression maneuver* is designed to assess diminution of the costoclavicular space and resultant compression of the subclavian artery by the subclavius muscle, the clavicle itself, or the first rib.[14] The radial pulse is monitored while the patient assumes an exaggerated military position, the shoulders drawn backward and downward.[2, 5, 6, 8, 16] Reduction or disappearance of the radial pulse constitutes a positive test.

3. *The hyperabduction maneuver* is felt to be specific for assessing arterial compression by the pectoralis minor tendon.[2, 16, 19] Reduction or disappearance of the radial pulse during passive movement of arm into a hyperabduction position represents a positive finding.

Adjunct examinations, such as chest roentgenograms, may be used to substantiate the clinical diagnosis. The mere coexistence of objective findings, such as a cervical rib, and subjective symptoms compatible with thoracic outlet syndrome does not constitute definitive evidence for this diagnosis, however.[8] Most rudimentary or cervical ribs found on routine chest roentgenograms are asymptomatic, whereas symptoms mimicking those of thoracic outlet syndrome may be attributable to coexistent osteoarthritis, a cervical disc, or other conditions.[7, 15, 18, 21]

Available clinical examinations and laboratory studies (plethysmography, chest roentgenograms, and so forth) cannot sufficiently establish the nature and site/or presence of multiple obstructing lesions. Moreover, this diagnosis cannot be established by exploration under general anesthesia because many of these conditions become manifest only if the tonus of the involved muscles is normal and not relaxed. Therefore, antegrade arteriography is needed to examine the patient in a variety of positions utilizing normal and increased muscle tonus in order to affirm the diagnosis.[3, 8, 11, 13, 17]

ANATOMY

The subclavian artery exits from the thorax behind the sternoclavicular joints, passing over the first rib between the scalenus medius and scalenus anticus muscles. More laterally, the subclavian artery passes under the subclavius muscle and clavicle and enters the axilla and is now known as the axillary artery. The axillary artery passes

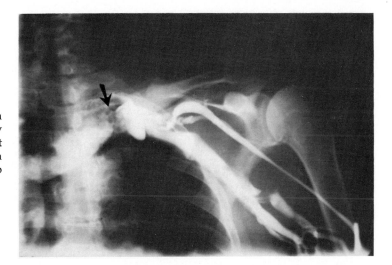

Figure 19–164. Note compression of the subclavian vein (arrow) by the scalenus anticus muscle against the clavicle. At this point, the vein crosses over the first rib anterior to the scalenus anticus muscle.

posterior to the tendon of the pectoralis minor muscle and then becomes the brachial artery.[13, 14]

The axillary vein passes behind the costocoracoid ligament and pectoralis minor tendon accompanying the artery; upon reaching the edge of the first rib, however, the subclavian vein passes over the first rib anterior to the scalenus anticus muscle (Fig. 19–164).

The anterior rami of the cervical spinal nerves, C_5, C_6, C_7, C_8, and T_1, exit through the intervertebral foramina and form trunks that pass through the scalene triangle accompanying the subclavian artery.[14, 18, 19] Two trunks composing the heads of the median nerve form a scissorlike encirclement of the axillary artery as it passes beneath the pectoralis minor tendon. The rami from C_8 and T_1 form the lowest trunk, which runs posterior to the subclavian artery and causes the groove on the first rib, which is often erroneously attributed to the artery.

The arteries, veins, and brachial plexus are subject to compression at the following sites: (1) the interscalene triangle (artery and nerves); (2) the space between the scalenus anticus muscle and the clavicle (vein); (3) the space between the first rib and the clavicle, or costoclavicular space (artery, vein, and nerves); (4) the space defined by the costocoracoid fascia (artery, vein, and nerves); and (5) the space beneath the pectoralis minor tendon (artery, vein, and nerves).

In addition, compression may be attributable to cervical ribs; a fibrous band from the cervical rib attaching to the undersurface of the first rib can compromise this space and cause compression of the subclavian artery against the first rib.[4-6, 20] A long transverse process of C_7 may function like a cervical rib. Acquired lesions of the clavicle or the first rib, such as an abundant callus, may likewise cause compression.[9] Abnormally short first thoracic ribs may attach to the sternum by ligaments, which in turn may cause compression of the lower components of the brachial plexus.

Compression in the thoracic outlet area may also be caused by tumors, particularly Pancoast tumors.[18]

ARTERIOGRAPHIC DIAGNOSIS

Selective subclavian arteriography via a transfemoral approach is advocated, since it permits examination in various stress positions and since an antegrade injection of

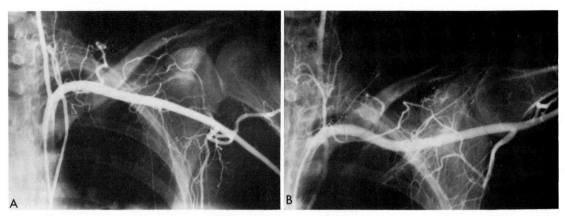

Figure 19–165. *A,* Arteriograms recorded in a neutral position demonstrate normal caliber of the subclavian and axillary arteries throughout their passage through the thoracic outlet. *B,* Arteriograms recorded in Lang's (modified hyperabduction) position demonstrate a normal caliber of subclavian and axillary arteries without evidence of compression (typical normal appearance under stress positions).

contrast medium simulates conditions of normal blood flow.[3, 11, 13, 17] Because of resultant turbulence and spasm of the artery (proximity to the puncture site), retrograde transaxillary injections may mask or falsify lesions. Moreover, it is difficult to have the patient assume various test positions and maintain a sterile field at the site of the axillary artery puncture.

A baseline study is performed with the patient in a neutral position; that is, the patient is placed in a relaxed supine position on the examining table and the injection is administered using a contrast medium bolus of about 15 ml (Fig. 19–165*A*). This series is designed to assess intrinsic arterial lesions, thrombosis of the artery, and poststenotic or aneurysmal dilation of the artery heralding a hemodynamically significant obstruction (Fig. 19–166).[11, 13]

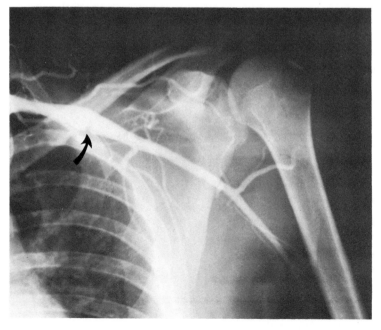

Figure 19–166. A fusiform dilatation of a segment of the subclavian artery traversing the costoclavicular space is noted. The defect along the inferior circumference of the artery suggesting a valvelike structure or intimal fold (arrow) was caused by marked localized intimal hyperplasia. Surgical excision and vasoplasty corrected this hemodynamically significant lesion. (From Lang, E. K.: *In* Abrams, H. L. (Ed.): Angiography. Ed. 2. Boston, Little, Brown & Company, 1971.)

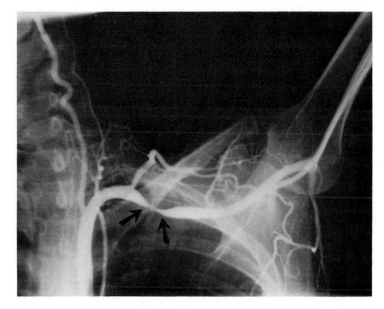

Figure 19–167. Compression of the subclavian artery passing through the interscalene triangle is documented on this arteriogram recorded in hyperabduction position (Allen's maneuver). The ridge-like effacement of the undersurface of the artery is due to compression of the vessel against the anterior first rib (arrows).

The second injection series is recorded while the patient executes the Adson maneuver. The patient is seated upright in front of a film changer. He extends the neck, turns the chin toward the side to be examined, and sustains deep inspiration during the injection of 10 ml of contrast medium and roentgenographic recording. Serialographic documentation at a rate of two roentgenograms per second for two seconds usually suffices.

This series is primarily intended to demonstrate compression in the interscalene triangle due to inherent tightness or to fibrous bands that may originate from a cervical rib and insert onto the undersurface of the first rib.

A third injection of contrast medium is recorded with the patient in a position simulating the hyperabduction maneuver (Allen's maneuver). The patient is placed supine on the examining table, and the humerus of the side to be examined is abducted

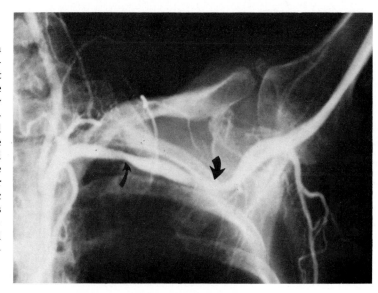

Figure 19–168. An arteriogram recorded in hyperabduction position demonstrates a torsion effect and resultant narrowing of the lumen of the subclavian artery while passing through the interscalene triangle (small arrow) and effacement and compression of the axillary artery in the costocoracoid space while passing beneath the tendon of the pectoralis minor (large arrow). The hemodynamic significance of both lesions is attested by segments of post-stenotic dilatation with increased density of contrast medium indicating stasis.

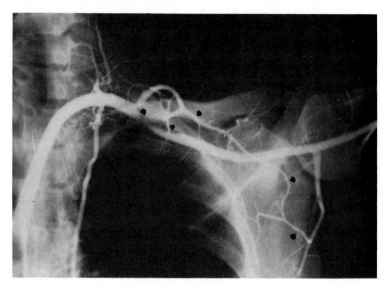

Figure 19–169. An arteriogram recorded in Lang's (modified hyperabduction) position demonstrates almost complete cutoff of the subclavian artery passing through the scalene triangle. The degree of compression is greater than in Adson's and Allen's maneuvers. The almost complete obstruction to antegrade flow results in activation of a collateral bypass network via the suprascapular, circumflex scapular, and subscapular into the posterior circumflex humeral artery (arrows). The impression upon the superior circumference of the subclavian artery is attributable to pressure by the subclavius muscle (arrows).

90 degrees, with the forearm pointing upward. The head is then turned to the contralateral side, and deep inspiration is maintained during the injection of contrast medium and roentgenographic recording.[11, 13]

This arteriographic series is used for assessment of the subclavian artery passing through the interscalene triangle and costoclavicular space and of the axillary artery crossing beneath the pectoralis minor tendon (Figs. 19–167 and 19–168).

Lang's maneuver may be substituted for the series obtained in a hyperabduction maneuver. For this examination, the patient is placed supine on the examining table, and the humerus of the side to be examined is abducted 90 degrees while the patient lifts a 5-pound weight 2 inches above the table top. The head is turned sharply to the contralateral side, and recording of the injection of contrast medium is once again carried out while deep inspiration is maintained. Examination in this position tends to accentuate the angiographic findings observed in Allen's maneuver and can be used for the assessment of potential compression sites in the interscalene triangle, the costoclavicular space, and the costocoracoid space at the point where the axillary artery crosses beneath the pectoralis minor tendon (Fig. 19–169).[11, 13]

In some instances, if a lesion is not demonstrated with the patient in the routine positions described, arteriograms should also be performed with the patient in a position in which he experiences maximal symptoms, provided this is technically feasible.[13]

ARTERIOGRAPHIC FINDINGS AND INTERPRETATION

Although arteriograms show gradients of compression effect, these findings do not necessarily parallel the severity of symptoms and do not allow prognostication. Mere torsion of the subclavian artery at its point of emersion from the scalene tunnel as seen on stress-position arteriograms does not necessarily indicate a pathologic condition.[13] A characteristic ridgelike compression effect on the inferior circumference of the subclavian artery indicates tightness in the interscalene triangle and compression of the vessel against the anterior first rib (see Fig. 19–167).[11, 13]

An impression upon the superior circumference of the subclavian artery coupled with the characteristic ridgelike compression of its inferior circumference indicates

Figure 19–170. Arteriograms in Allen's and Lang's maneuvers demonstrate a complete cutoff of the subclavian artery at its point of emergence from the scalene triangle. Antegrade flow to the afflicted extremity is maintained via a collateral network over the suprascapular and subscapular arteries into the posterior circumflex humeral artery. Note reconstitution of flow in the distal segment of the axillary artery (arrow). (From Lang, E. K.: *In* Abrams, H. L. (Ed.): Angiography. Ed. 2. Boston, Little, Brown & Company, 1971.)

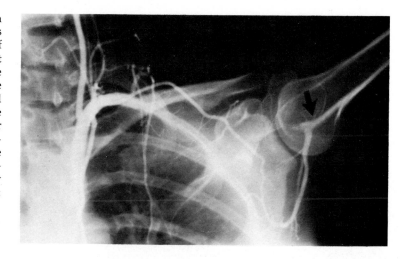

diminution of the costoclavicular space, with pressure exerted against the subclavian artery from above by the subclavius muscle and resultant compression of the vessel against the anterior first rib (see Fig. 19–169). Abnormalities of the clavicle, such as abundant callus formation or malunion, may accentuate such findings.[9, 11, 13, 16] Arteriographic demonstration of an antegrade collateral bypass network (via the suprascapular, circumflex scapular, and subscapular arteries into the posterior circumflex humeral artery) strongly suggests the hemodynamic significance of the documented lesion and the resultant substantial reduction of flow across the compromised segment (Fig. 19–170). Moreover, a hemodynamically significant lesion should be demonstrable in at least two stress positions (Adson's, Allen's, and Lang's maneuvers). Not infrequently, a complete compression and cessation of antegrade flow may be observed when the patient is in one of the stress positions (see Fig. 19–170).

Figure 19–171. Compression of the axillary artery at its point of crossing beneath the pectoralis minor tendon (in Lang's maneuver) indicates tightness of the costocoracoid space (arrow). In this patient, the compromise in the costocoracoid space is attributable to a hematoma restricted behind the costocoracoid fascia.

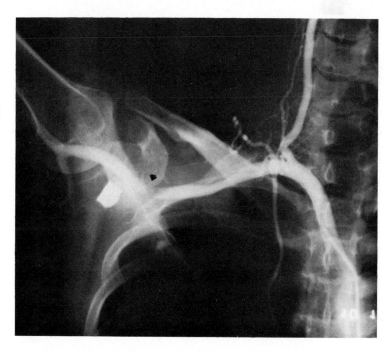

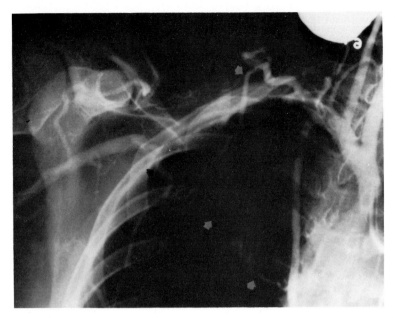

Figure 19–172. Complete occlusion of the right subclavian artery from its point of emergence from the scalene triangle to the point of crossing beneath the pectoralis minor tendon encouraged development of an excellent antegrade collateral network via the internal mammary and intercostal branches of the transverse cervical artery. Note excellent reconstitution of flow in the axillary artery. (Courtesy of E. K. Lang and Angiography, Second Ed. Edited by Herbert L. Abrams. Boston, Little, Brown & Company, 1971.)

Compression of the axillary artery at the point where it crosses beneath the pectoralis minor tendon is often demonstrable only in Allen's or Lang's position and indicates tightness in the costocoracoid space (see Fig. 19–168, Fig. 19–171).

Even in patients with severe clinical symptoms, loss of pulse, and complete compression of the subclavian artery on arteriograms, gangrene is quite uncommon.

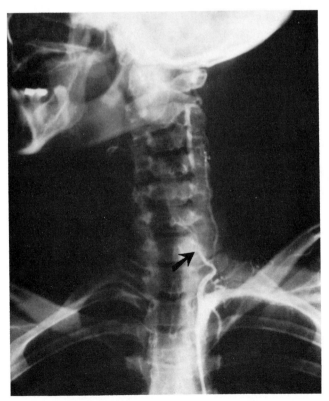

Figure 19–173. Note the sharp cutoff of the left vertebral artery at its point of entry into the intervertebral foramen of the sixth cervical vertebra (arrow). The artery is compressed at its point of passage between the tendons of the longus colli and anterior scalene muscles. Reconstitution of flow in the distal vertebral artery via collaterals from the ascending cervical artery is noted. (Courtesy E. K. Lang and Angiography, Second Ed. Edited by Herbert L. Abrams. Boston, Little, Brown & Company, 1971.)

This is attributable to effective antegrade collateral flow via the suprascapular, circumflex scapular, and subscapular arteries into the posterior circumflex humeral artery as well as via the descending ramus of the transverse cervical artery to the posterior circumflex humeral artery. These antegrade collateral pathways can retain, in the radial artery, a flow rate of 8 to 15 per cent of normal, despite complete obstruction of a segment of the subclavian artery (see Fig. 19–170). This antegrade collateral pathway is readily demonstrated on arteriograms; the magnitude of collateral flow can be assessed objectively on radioisotope flow studies.[11-13] The total flow to the distal extremity is expressed on radionuclide flow studies by the integral area under the curve.[12] The delay in the arterial appearance of the radionuclide and the multipeaked deflection reflect the dissipation of the radionuclide bolus forced to pass through the collateral system.

Both temporary and permanent occlusion of the subclavian or axillary artery in the scalene triangle, the costoclavicular space, or the axilla result in the immediate activation of this antegrade collateral pathway (see Fig. 19–170, Fig. 19–172).[9]

The vertebral artery is subject to compression at its point of entry into the neural foramen of the sixth cervical vertebra while passing between the tendons of the longus colli and anterior scalene muscle. Its compression is provoked by the turning of the patient's head to the contralateral side.[10] A typical basilar insufficiency syndrome results if the flow from the contralateral vertebral artery is inadequate. This may occur with a congenitally small or diseased vessel or if the contralateral vertebral artery does not connect to the basilar artery (Fig. 19–173).

Preoperative assessment of thoracic outlet syndromes by arteriography has greatly improved diagnostic accuracy, particularly in the identification of multiple coexistent lesions. Surgical treatment results have likewise improved.

References

1. Adson, A. W., and Coffey, J. R.: Cervical rib: a method of anterior approach for relief of symptoms by division of the scalenus anticus. Ann. Surg. 85:839, 1927.
2. Bateman, J. E.: Neurovascular syndromes related to the clavicle. Clin. Orthop. 58:75–82, 1968.
3. Benzian, S. R., and Mainzer, F.: Erect arteriography: its use in thoracic outlet syndrome. Radiology 111:275–277, 1974.
4. Dale, W. A.: Thoracic outlet syndrome in vascular surgery. Baltimore, University Park Press, 1975.
5. DeBruin, T. R.: Costoclavicular space enlargement: eight methods for relief of neurovascular compression. Int. Surg. 46:340–360, 1966.
6. Falconer, M. A., and Weddell, G.: Costoclavicular compression of the subclavian artery and vein: relation to the scalenus anticus syndrome. Lancet 2:538–543, 1943.
7. Fox, A. J., Lin, J. P., Pinto, R. S., et al.: Myelographic cervical nerve root deformities. Radiology 116:355–361, 1975.
8. Gilroy,J., and Meyer, J. S.: Compression of the subclavian artery as a cause of ischaemic brachial neuropathy. Brain 86:733–746, 1963.
9. Haimovici, H.,and Caplan, L. H.: Arterial thrombosis complicating the thoracic outlet syndrome: arteriographic considerations. Radiology 87:462–464, 1966.
10. Husni, E. A., Bell, H. S., and Storer, J.: Mechanical occlusion of the vertebral artery: a new clinical concept. J.A.M.A. 196:475–478, 1966.
11. Lang, E. K.: Arteriographic diagnosis of the thoracic outlet syndrome. Radiology 84:296–303, 1965.
12. Lang, E. K.: Quantitative assessment of flow in antegrade and retrograde collateral channels serving the brachiocephalic area. Radiology 87:457–461, 1966.
13. Lang, E. K.: Arteriography of thoracic outlet syndrome. In Abrams, H. L. (ed.): Angiography. Ed. 2. Boston, Little, Brown & Company, 1971.
14. Nichols, H. M.: Anatomic structures of the thoracic outlet. Clin. Orthop. 51:17–25, 1967.
15. Overton, L. M.: The causes of pain in the upper extremities: a differential diagnosis study. Clin. Orthop. 51:27, 1967.
16. Riddell, D. H.: Thoracic outlet syndrome: thoracic and vascular aspects. Clin. Orthop. 51:53–64, 1967.
17. Rosenberg, J. C.: Arteriographic demonstration of compression syndromes of the thoracic outlet. South. Med. J. 59:400–403, 1966.

18. Schlesinger, E. B.: The thoracic outlet syndrome from a neurosurgical point of view. Clin. Orthop. *51*:49–52, 1967.
19. Silver, D.: Thoracic outlet syndrome. *In* Sabiston, D. C., Jr. (ed.): Davis-Christopher Textbook of Surgery. Ed. 11. Philadelphia, W. B. Saunders Company, 1977.
20. Taveras, J. M., and Wood, E. H.: Diagnostic Neuroradiology. Baltimore, The Williams & Wilkins Company, 1964.
21. Tomsick, T. A., Ahlstrand, R. A., and Kisel, T. M.: Thoracic outlet syndrome associated with rib fusion and cervical thoracic scoliosis. J. Can. Assoc. Radiol. *25*:211–213, 1974.

Part X
Disorders of the Chest Wall

DAVID S. FEIGIN, M.D., L.C.D.R., M.C., U.S.N.R.
JOHN E. MADEWELL, M.D.

INTRODUCTION

An unusual variety of imaging techniques are available for the evaluation of disorders of the chest wall and of the postoperative chest wall.[25] Plain film roentgenograms are most useful in showing obvious soft tissue swelling and gross involvement of bone (Fig. 19–174). In any patient with known disease of the lungs, pleura, or mediastinum, films should always be obtained to the area in the chest wall where pain or swelling is present. Overpenetration often allows visualization of bone abnormalities (Figs. 19–175 and 19–176). Tomography is often useful when bone involvement is

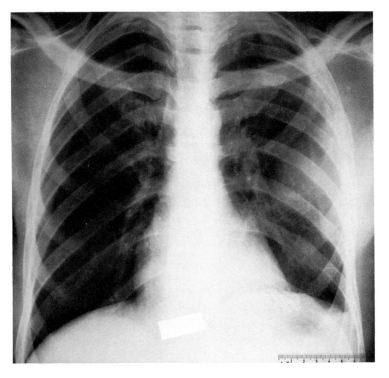

Figure 19–174. Malignant reticuloendothelial neoplasm in the left chest wall. This 38-year-old man presented with a superficial mass in the left lateral chest wall. The frontal roentgenogram shows an ill-defined extrapleural mass in the left hemithorax, with erosion of the anterior third left rib. The soft tissues on the left side of the chest are more dense than those on the right, and the soft tissue planes appear displaced laterally. A small left pleural effusion is also present. (AFIP Neg. No. 76-2770.)

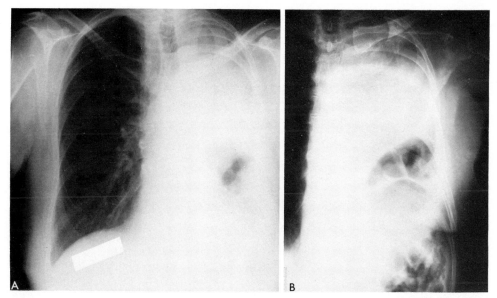

Figure 19–175. Normal postoperative appearance and malignant thymoma of the chest wall. This 74-year-old woman had had a left pneumonectomy 15 years earlier for a lesion that was originally thought to be a benign fibrous tissue tumor. Her illness at the time these roentgenograms were taken was heralded by a superficial mass over the anterior portion of the left chest. *A,* The frontal roentgenogram shows no definite abnormality other than the effects of the pneumonectomy. *B,* An overpenetrated view of the left chest shows the previous resection and partial regeneration of the left sixth posterior rib. This is a normal postoperative appearance following a thoracotomy. The new superficial mass did not involve the deeper tissues of the chest wall. (AFIP Neg. No. 77-8597.)

subtle or difficult to detect because of massive soft tissue or intrathoracic involvement (Fig. 19–177). Tomography may thus be helpful in cases of localized pain in which specific plain films show no abnormalities.

Xerography demonstrates soft tissues, especially fascial planes, much more readily than plain film roentgenography or tomography (Fig. 19–178). Thus, it may be used in evaluating the extent of soft tissue masses and the progress of postsurgical healing. Computed tomography may also show the extent of chest wall lesions and the presence of bone involvement.[68, 70] Specific diagnoses may be possible if the lesion has a characteristic density or appearance, as does a lipoma (Fig. 19–179).[39]

Arteriography is usually not helpful in the differential diagnosis of chest wall masses involving soft tissues or bone or both. Nevertheless, arteriography (Fig. 19–180) may aid in the determination of the extent of involvement of a lesion, and, thereby, in the selection of the most appropriate therapy.[41] Angiography also shows the extent of major vessel involvement and the degree of vascularity within the lesion.

Nuclear medicine procedures may help to determine the extent of a lesion, the degree of bone involvement, and the presence of additional lesions in areas where symptoms are absent.[135] Bone scans with phosphate agents, especially when used sequentially, can show the presence and extent of bone involvement better than other imaging techniques (Fig. 19–181). Nevertheless, it may be impossible to differentiate bone and soft tissue involvement using technetium-labeled phosphate agents. Gallium-67 may demonstrate the presence and extent of inflammatory processes as well as of many neoplastic processes involving both bones and soft tissues of the chest wall (see Fig. 19–207). Unfortunately, the use of gallium-67 in the postoperative chest is limited

Text continued on page 1284

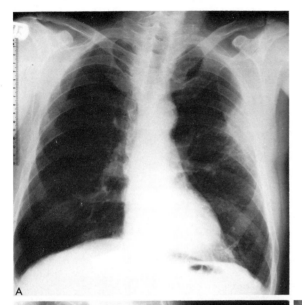

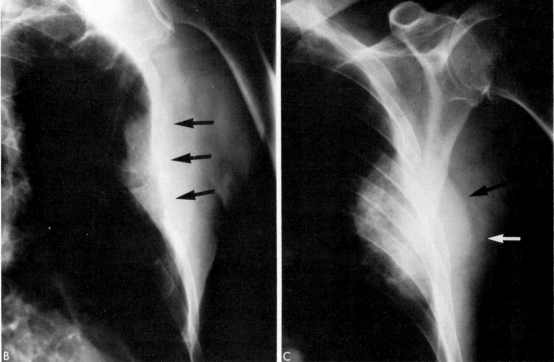

Figure 19–176. Bronchogenic, pleomorphic carcinoma of the chest wall and pleura. This 71-year-old man noted increasing pain along the left chest for six months. *A,* The frontal roentgenogram of the chest shows an ill-defined mass in the lateral portion of the left midlung field; it appears pleural based, although there is no evidence of pleural thickening. *B,* The oblique view shows marked thickening of the soft tissues of the chest wall and partial destruction of the adjacent ribs (arrow). *C,* An overpenetrated frontal view shows more clearly the partial destruction of the third and fourth lateral left ribs, as well as the marked soft tissue thickening (arrows) in the chest wall. (AFIP Neg. No. 77-3639.)

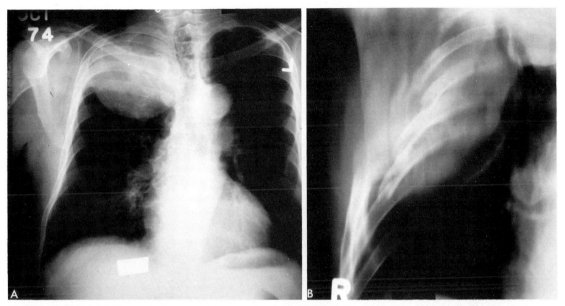

Figure 19–177. Malignant pleomorphic neoplasm in the right upper chest. This 58-year-old man was noted to have a right upper lung field mass on a routine roentgenogram. *A*, An initial frontal roentgenogram shows a well-circumscribed right upper lobe mass with no evidence of bone or chest wall involvement. *B*, A frontal tomogram taken 15 months later shows destruction of several right upper lateral ribs and marked displacement of soft tissue planes in the anterolateral chest wall. (AFIP Neg. No. 76-7585.)

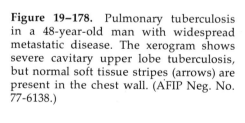
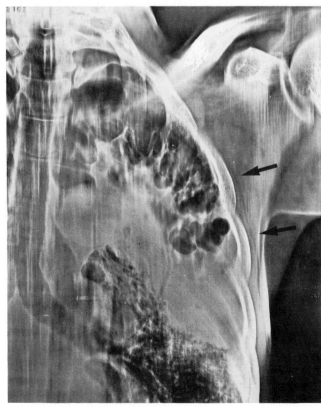

Figure 19–178. Pulmonary tuberculosis in a 48-year-old man with widespread metastatic disease. The xerogram shows severe cavitary upper lobe tuberculosis, but normal soft tissue stripes (arrows) are present in the chest wall. (AFIP Neg. No. 77-6138.)

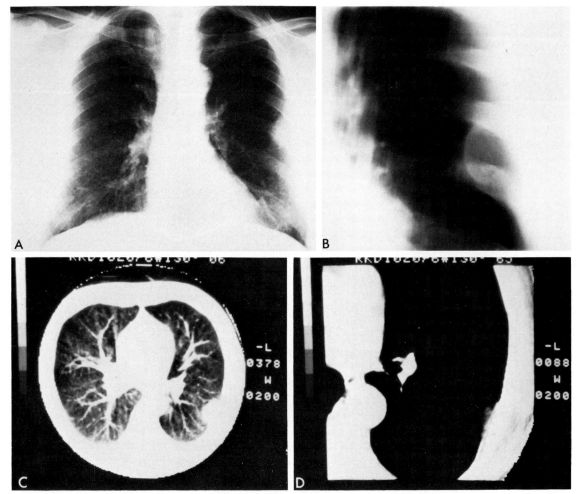

Figure 19–179. Lipoma of the left chest wall. This 67-year-old man was discovered to have a left chest mass on a routine roentgenogram. *A,* The frontal roentgenogram shows a pleural-based mass in the lateral portion of the left midlung field. *B,* An oblique tomogram shows the smooth margin and the low density of the lesion, with a lack of rib involvement. *C,* A computed tomogram shows no involvement of the adjacent lung and no generalized pleural thickening associated with the lesion. *D,* The computed tomogram of the chest wall (higher CT number) shows lack of involvement of bone and soft tissues. (AFIP Neg. No. 77-9030.) (*From* Faer, M. J., Burnham, R. E., and Beck, C. L.: Transmural thoracic lipoma: demonstration by computed tomography. Am. J. Roentgenol. *130*:161–163, 1978. Reproduced by permission.)

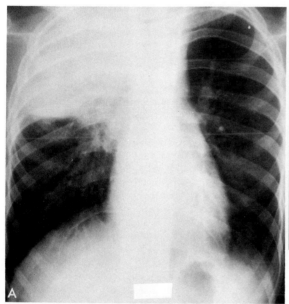

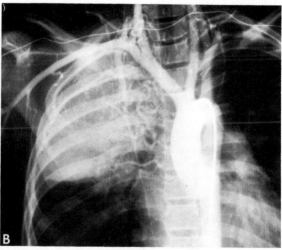

Figure 19-180. Actinomycosis in the right upper chest of a 13-year-old girl. *A,* The frontal roentgenogram shows massive infiltration of the right upper lobe, with no evidence of chest wall or bone involvement. *B,* The frontal view of the aortogram shows abnormal vasculature in the posterior chest wall, with hypertrophied vessels. These findings indicate that the inflammatory process involved the chest wall, a finding that was confirmed at surgery. (AFIP Neg. No. 75-11126.)

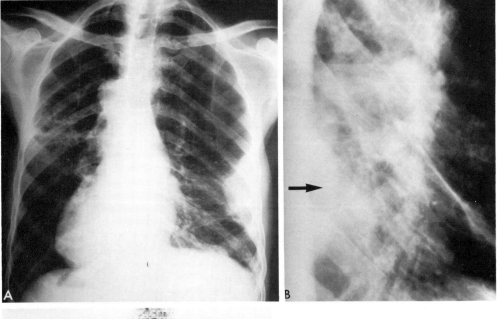

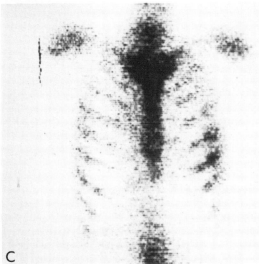

Figure 19–181. Malignant neoplasm, probably mesothelioma, in a 48-year-old man with situs inversus who presented with left-sided chest pain. *A,* The frontal roentgenogram shows an irregular extrapleural mass along the left chest wall, with thickening of the soft tissue stripe lateral to the rib cage. *B,* An oblique close-up view shows pleural thickening and localized rib destruction (arrow). *C,* A technetium polyphosphate bone scan demonstrates increased uptake in two left lateral ribs, indicating the involvement of at least one rib that showed no roentgenographic abnormality. (AFIP Neg. No. 77-6138.)

by its increased local uptake in all areas of recent surgery, whether these areas are diseased or not.

It is important, however, to recognize that although all these modalities may provide significant morphologic information about a chest wall disorder, the differential diagnosis of chest wall lesions is exceedingly difficult and biopsy is almost invariably necessary to diagnose a chest wall mass or determine the specific cause of symptoms referable to the chest wall.[42]

CONGENITAL MALFORMATIONS OF RIBS AND STERNUM

Sternal deformities may cause grotesque changes in the external appearance of the chest wall. They can be associated with physiologic and psychologic problems, necessitating surgical correction.[51, 89, 102, 104] Sternal deformities are of three principal types: depression deformities (pectus excavatum), protrusion deformities (pectus carinatum), and sternal clefts.

Depression Deformities (Pectus Excavatum)

This is a deformity of the anterior chest characterized by a sharp posterior concavity of the sternum, with a deep indentation at the distal aspect just adjacent to the xyphoid. The attached anterior cartilage margins also dip posteriorly. There are two major types: One has a deep deformity or pocket involving predominantly the central and distal parts of the sternum; the manubrium is in a normal position. The second type is characterized by a broad, flatter deformity that may run from nipple to nipple and involve the manubrium. In this type the anteroposterior chest diameter may narrow, and the intrathoracic space is often significantly compromised. The impairment of cardiac function that may be associated with pectus excavatum is one of the physiologic indications for surgery.

Clinically, this deformity produces a concavity with a peripheral slope (Fig. 19–182). The rest of the chest wall development is normal, and therefore, surgical correction of the anomaly is relatively uncomplicated. Radiographically, pectus excavatum is best demonstrated on the lateral film as a deep anterior central depression on concavity in the middle and distal sternum (Fig. 19–182). The anteroposterior diameter of the chest may be narrow, and as a result the frontal view of the chest may show a shift, usually to the left, or enlargement of the cardiac silhouette.

Pectus excavatum can be associated with congenital heart disease, homocystinuria, Marfan's syndrome,[91] the systolic click–late systolic murmur syndrome,[136] congenital bowing of the tibia,[8] and idiopathic mitral valve prolapse.[115] Pectus excavatum is associated with the last condition in 60 per cent of the cases.[115]

An unusual variant of pectus excavatum is chondromanubrial prominence with chondrogladiolar depression. There is a marked manubrial protrusion with sternal depression in this anomaly (Fig. 19–183). The surgical approach differs slightly from that for the typical pectus excavatum in that both the protrusion and the depression must be corrected.[110]

Pectus excavatum is usually found in patients with an asthenic habitus[80] and may be familial.[114, 144] Occasionally, pectus excavatum is asymmetric because of sternal axis deviation. This deviation is usually characterized by the turning of the anterior surface of the sternum toward the smaller hemithorax, which is usually on the right.[110] This deformity may also be associated with hypoplasia or absent ribs on the smaller hemithorax side.

Protrusion Deformities (Pectus Carinatum)

Pectus carinatum is a congenital anomaly of the sternum that occurs less frequently than pectus excavatum. The gross configuration may be severely deforming and an indication for operative correction. Physiologic studies of patients with protrusion deformities have been few, and physiologic compromise has been less well documented than with pectus excavatum. The sternum is usually broad; occasionally a double xyphoid is found.[105] The sternum is elongated and joined to the xyphoid at an abnormally sharp angle, which causes the sternal protrusion. The xyphoid may be parallel to the displaced sternum or angulated posteriorly.

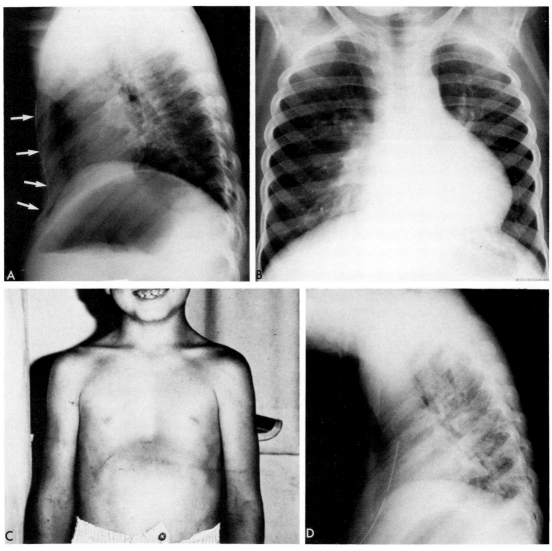

Figure 19–182. Pectus excavatum. The patient is a young boy with a chest deformity characterized by an anterior concavity in the chest wall. *A,* The lateral chest view with barium on the cutaneous surface of the chest wall demonstrates the concavity to be a depressed sternum (arrows). The ribs in the mid-clavicular line are anterior to the sternum but angle posteriorly to join the midline depressed sternum. *B,* The frontal roentgenogram of the chest shows displacement of the mediastinum and heart to the left. *C,* A clinical photograph of the patient's chest shows the shallow anterior concavity extending from nipple to nipple. *D,* The postoperative lateral chest view with a tube in the anterior chest shows the repositioned sternum and the lucent retrosternal space resulting from surgical relocation of the depressed sternum. (Courtesy of J. Alex Haller, M. D., Baltimore, Maryland.)

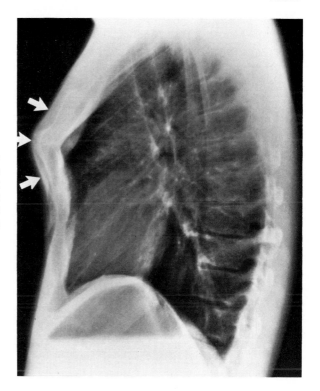

Figure 19–183. Chondromanubrial prominence with chondrogladiolar depression. The lateral chest view shows the marked anterior protrusion of the manubristernae (arrows) and a more typical excavatum deformity involving the lower part of the sternum. (Courtesy of J. Alex Haller, M. D., Baltimore, Maryland.)

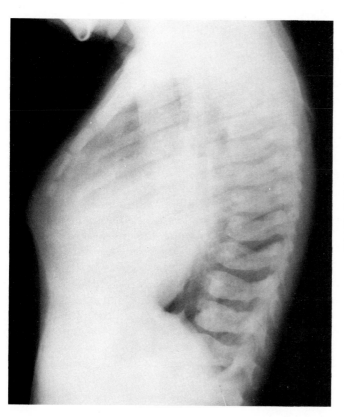

Figure 19–184. Pectus carinatum. This young child presented with protrusion of the anterior chest wall. The lateral roentgenogram demonstrates the anterior displacement of the sternum. This is usually most marked in the inferior sternum.

Clinically, the defect is characterized by protrusion of the sternum and symmetrical prominence of the costal cartilages. Occasionally, this congenital anomaly is familial or associated with congenital heart disease. Radiologically, the lateral film shows a prominent anteriorly displaced sternum, most marked at its inferior end (Fig. 19–184).

Cleft Sternum

There are three types of sternal clefts: localized superior, localized inferior, and complete. The last is the rarest of the three types as well as the most severe. The superior cleft involves the manubrium and gladiolus, usually extending to the level of the third or fourth interspace. A superior cleft has a characteristic V- or U-shaped clinical appearance, the edge of the cleft and the central depression of the skin being easily visible. In cases of this type, the heart is usually normal.

The inferior sternal cleft is frequently associated with the pentalogy of defects called Cantrell's syndrome.[19, 88] There is wide separation in the distal portion of the sternum, usually associated with a soft tissue raphe running from the defect to the umbilicus or omphalocele.[3, 60] Also present are a ventral crescent defect in the diaphragm and a deficiency of the diaphragmatic pericardium in which the pericardial cavity communicates with the peritoneal cavity. In addition, there is usually an intrinsic cardiac defect, most frequently a ventricular septal defect, which may be independent or a part of a more complex deformity, such as tetralogy of Fallot.

The complete sternal cleft is a rare anomaly usually associated with defects in the ventral abdominal wall, diaphragm, and pericardium but not with intracardiac defects.[113]

Roentgenograms are rarely obtained of patients with cleft sternum, since it is usually obvious clinically. The medial bony edge of the sternal cleft can be seen on plain films, but it is best shown on tomograms.[72] The superior and complete clefts also have laterally displaced clavicles.

Rib Deformities

Most anomalies of the ribs are incidental and of no clinical significance. These rib anomalies may, however, be confused with intrathoracic and chest wall disease. Unlike rib anomalies, sternal anomalies are often disfiguring and may require surgical correction for a variety of cosmetic, psychologic, and physiologic reasons.

Rib deformities are frequent findings in people who are otherwise normal, occurring in 2.8 per cent of the population.[133] These anomalies probably result from irregular segmentation during the first half of the division of the mesoderm into somites as the rib grows out from the vertebra.[133] The most common rib anomaly is bifurcation (Fig. 19–185). Others include cervical rib, rudimentary first rib, flaring, fusion, and bridging (Fig. 19–186). These anomalies most frequently affect the upper ribs and are rare in the lower ribs. Of this group, the cervical rib is most likely to produce symptoms of compression of the nerves or vessels, but it is more often an incidental finding on a chest roentgenogram. Hypoplasia or even aplasia of the first rib can occur and is associated with hypertrophy of the second rib and a more slanted clavicle.[21] Other uncommon rib anomalies include pseudoarthrosis and synchondrosis of the first rib.[16, 44]

Rib and other skeletal anomalies may also indicate the presence of underlying

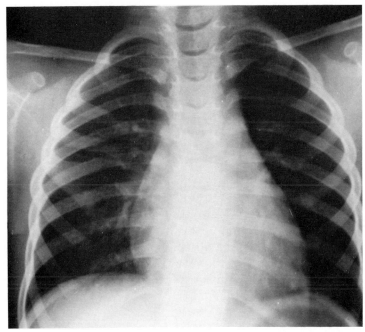

Figure 19–185. Rib deformity: bifurcation of the right fourth rib. A two-year-old girl with a palpable mass in the right anterior chest wall. The frontal roentgenogram demonstrates flaring and widening of the anterior portion of the right fourth rib. The widening extends from the anterior margin laterally for approximately 3 cm. There is also superior displacement and inferior erosion of the anterior margin of the right third rib. This is due to the misshapen, widened right fourth bifid rib. (AFIP Neg. Nos. 77-5964-3.)

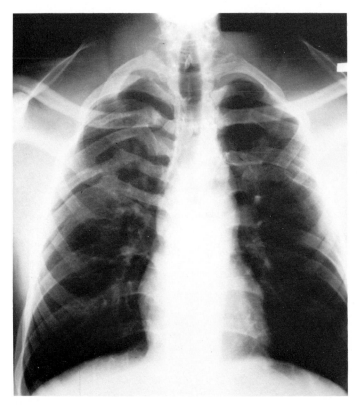

Figure 19–186. Multiple rib anomalies. This young man had no symptoms stemming from these lesions. The frontal roentgenogram shows bilateral numerous rib anomalies with fusion, bridging, bifurcation, and hypoplasia.

developmental or hereditary disease. Best known of this group is the basal cell nevus syndrome. Rib anomalies are present in 75 per cent of patients with this condition.[46] The most common rib anomaly seen is an upper thoracic bifid rib, but rib splaying on the anterior ends; short, broad, vestigial synchondrosis; partial agenesis to the posterior; and cervical ribs may be associated. This syndrome has also been associated with other chest wall bony abnormalities, such as deformed clavicles and scapulae[46] and mild pectus excavatum.[71] These patients most commonly present to dental surgeons with maxillary and mandibular swelling due to keratocysts;[101] the chest abnormalities are usually incidental.

Rib anomalies may be an indication of other less common syndromes, such as Klippel-Feil syndrome, Down's syndrome, Poland syndactyly, Brachmann–de Lange syndrome, neurofibromatosis, and Melnick-Needle syndrome. The last two of these are usually associated with thin, narrow ribs (ribbonlike).[64, 77, 82] In neurofibromatosis especially, the thin ribs are usually associated with scoliosis and are most prominent near the apex of the scoliosis on the side of the convexity. The thinning involves the proximal shaft of the ribs and may occur as scoliosis progresses.[77] It is not due to direct pressure from neurofibromas.[64] Rib anomalies never suggest a specific underlying syndrome, but if clinical information warrants it, an evaluation may be performed.

ACQUIRED DEFORMITIES

Scoliosis and kyphoscoliosis are chest wall deformities with a wide variety of causes. Infections, especially tuberculosis (Fig. 19–187) are now far less common causes than previously, making idiopathic scoliosis the most common form. Scoliosis is generally divided into nonstructural and structural types. The nonstructural, or

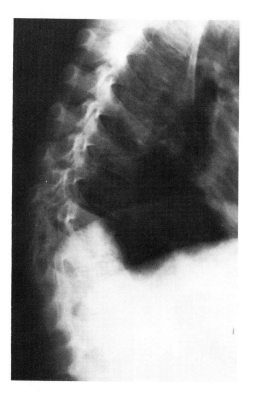

Figure 19–187. Tuberculosis of the thoracic spine (T_{11} and T_{12}) in a 44-year-old woman who had back pain in the thoracic area for several years. This lateral roentgenogram of the lower thoracic spine shows complete destruction of the T_{11}-to-T_{12} disc space, with bony fusion between T_{11} and T_{12} and kyphoscoliosis. (AFIP Neg. Nos. 70-11939-1.)

postural, form is usually caused by temporary postural influences and is the easiest form to correct. Structural scoliosis involves a definite morphologic abnormality that leads to changes in the shape of vertebrae. The two forms may be distinguished roentgenographically by obtaining views of the spine with the patient bent to each side. Nonstructural scoliosis exhibits symmetic motion, whereas structural scoliosis results in asymmetric motion.

Structural scoliosis is usually acquired, although congenital cases, caused by hemivertebrae, other vertebral anomalies, and arthrogryposis, also occur.[121] Causes of acquired structural scoliosis include asymmetric paralysis, such as occurs in poliomyelitis and cerebral palsy; neurofibromatosis; mesenchymal disorders such as Marfan's disease and rheumatoid arthritis;[111] trauma; surgical procedures, including thoracoplasty; and radiation therapy.

A strong association has been established between scoliosis and congenital heart disease.[67, 106, 145] The specific cause of scoliosis in this case remains unknown and does not appear to be related to such variables as the location of the heart, the size of the aortic arch, the presence of cyanosis, or the patient's surgical history. Recently, coarctation of the aorta has also been found to be associated with an increased incidence of scoliosis.[98] Nonetheless, most cases of scoliosis in children and adolescents are idiopathic.[30, 103]

The assessment of scoliosis involves the taking of roentgenograms of the entire spine with the patient standing or bending maximally. The measurement of curvature is often accomplished by Cobb's technique, in which perpendiculars are drawn to the inferior surface of the bottom vertebrae and the superior surfaces of the top vertebrae that are involved in the curve. The angle formed by the intersection of these perpendiculars measures the degree of angulation of the curve.[30] Roentgenograms also aid in the determination of the prognosis, because scoliosis is usually progressive only until both iliac apophyses are fused.

The stage of scoliosis at the time of its recognition determines its treatment. Nonstructural scoliosis and mild structural scoliosis can be treated by bed rest and exercise. Slightly more severe structural scoliosis is treated by traction, plaster casting, or the use of the Milwaukee (Blount's) brace. For severe structural scoliosis, surgery is often necessary. Spinal fusion is usually accomplished by the splitting and chipping of spinous processes and laminae and the subsequent imposition of small grafts posterior to the denuded laminae (Hibbs' technique). Spinal fusion is often aided by the imposition of Harrington's rods (Figs. 19–188, and 19–189), which are used to stabilize the reduced curvature. Another surgical technique that is sometimes used is the resection of proximal portions of the ribs on the concave side of the curvature.

The progress of all patients with scoliosis is measured by periodic roentgenograms of the spine using the previously described method. Dramatic results are not uncommon (see Figs. 19–188 and 19–189).

An important consequence of the treatment of scoliosis is the compression of the duodenum by the superior mesenteric artery, a phenomenon known as the cast syndrome.[9, 49] The syndrome has most often been seen in patients treated with body casts, but also it is observed in patients treated with the Milwaukee brace, Harrington's rod, or traction. The patients complain of abdominal distention and severe vomiting. Plain films of the abdomen demonstrate gastric dilatation and distention of the first two portions of the duodenum (Fig. 19–190). Contrast studies of the upper gastrointestinal tract may be difficult to obtain with the patient in a body cast, but when performed they demonstrate normal mucosal patterns in the stomach and duodenum and a sharp cutoff of the third portion of the duodenum by extrinsic linear compression. Paralytic ileus may also be demonstrable in the patients with recent surgery.

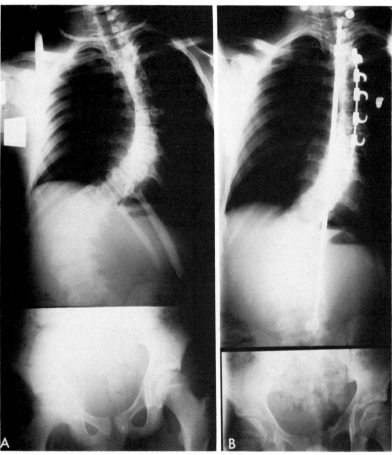

Figure 19–188. Idiopathic structural scoliosis. *A,* Preoperative frontal roentgenogram of the entire spine shows severe scoliosis of the thoracic and lumbar regions. *B,* Marked improvement with reduction of curves is evident following surgical placement of Harrington rods and spinal fusion. (AFIP Neg. No. 9-2175.)

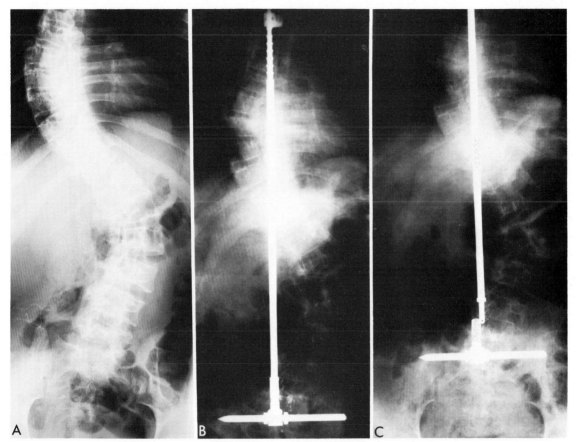

Figure 19–189.   Idiopathic structural scoliosis. *A,* A preoperative view of the thoracolumbar spine shows the thoracic curve to the right and lumbar curve to the left. *B,* A similar view taken after spinal surgery and the placement of a Harrington rod. *C,* A similar view taken several months later shows the rod to have slipped out of its inferior connection. The device was subsequently removed. (AFIP Neg. No. 9-2176.)

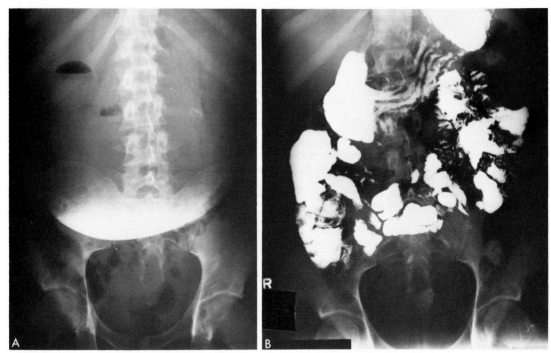

Figure 19–190. Body cast syndrome. The patient is a 20-year-old man with pain attributed to a herniated intervertebral disc. He complained of severe abdominal pain and vomited repeatedly prior to admission. *A,* A supine abdominal film obtained after barium ingestion shows massive distention of the stomach. *B,* An upper gastrointestinal series obtained after decompression shows sharp cutoff of the duodenal barium column to the right of spine. (*From* Berk, R. N., and Coulson, D. B.: The body cast syndrome. Radiology *94*:303–306, 1970. Reproduced by permission.)

The occurrence of the cast syndrome may be related to hyperextension of the spine and laxity of the abdominal muscles resulting in the displacement of the intestine into the pelvis, with traction on the mesentery and vessels.[73] Immobility, rapid weight loss, and other factors may also contribute. Nonsurgical therapy, including nasogastric suction; intravenous fluids; frequent position changes, especially of the prone patient; and occasionally, cast removal, is usually sufficient for the alleviation of symptoms. Rarely, however, duodenojejunostomy may be necessary to relieve severe obstruction and prevent airway obstruction or gastric perforation with peritonitis.

Fractures of ribs or vertebrae may be the cause of significant deformity of the chest wall. Usually, however, such deformity gradually diminishes as growth of ribs continues.

TUMORS OF RIBS AND STERNUM

Although metastatic disease of the bony chest wall is common, primary neoplasms are unusual.[5, 43, 57, 58, 97, 140] The usual symptoms of a lesion are pain and pathologic fracture, but the lesion may be asymptomatic. The incidental finding of a neoplastic mass is more common in the ribs than in other bones because such masses are often discovered on routine chest radiographs. Sternal neoplasms are usually symptomatic masses rather than incidental findings.[11]

Because of the frequency of metastatic tumors involving the chest wall, additional lesions should always be sought when a bone lesion is discovered in the ribs or sternum. If no source of primary tumor is found, surgical removal is generally recommended.[17] An *en bloc* resection rather than a biopsy is generally performed because many chest wall tumors, especially chondrosarcomas, may present with a variety of histologic patterns and there is a high risk of sampling error, causing inaccurate diagnosis.

Although approximately half of rib neoplasms are benign,[57] the rapid growth of any chest wall tumor must always suggest the possibility of malignancy. This also applies to lesions previously found to be benign because of the possibility that such a lesion might have undergone malignant change.

Benign Tumors

FIBROUS DYSPLASIA. This is the most common bone tumor or tumorlike condition of the ribs.[127] It is often classified as a benign bone tumor, but it probably

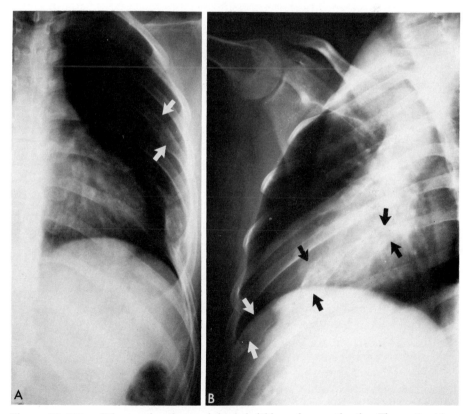

Figure 19–191. Fibrous dysplasia of the left fifth and seventh ribs. The patient is a 24-year-old woman with mild left chest pain and lumps noted on the left anterior chest in the area of the fifth and seventh ribs. *A,* A frontal roentgenogram of the chest shows two lytic lesions, one short lesion (arrows), involving the posterolateral aspect of the left fifth rib, and the other involving a long segment of the left seventh rib from the midposterior rib to the costochondral junction. *B,* The oblique view demonstrates the enlongate lesion in the left seventh rib (arrows). Both lesions have expanded the bone with a thin cortical rim, encasing the major portion of the lesions. (AFIP Neg. Nos. 73-967-7 and 73-967-2.)

originates as a developmental abnormality of the bone-forming mesenchyme, together with filling of the medullary cavity by fibrous tissue and the formation of poor trabeculae.[2]

Fibrous dysplasia is most common in the second and third decades of life.[57] The lesions are usually found in asymptomatic patients.[54] Both monostotic and polyostotic lesions occur, although the solitary lesion is much more common. When fibrous dysplasia is polyostotic, it may be associated with skin pigmentation and endocrine disturbances — Albright's syndrome. Lesions of fibrous dysplasia may demonstrate progressive growth[150] and rarely undergo malignant transformation.[65, 147]

Roentgenographically, fibrous dysplasia most commonly presents as a long lesion in a long bone, but lesions may also be found in the ribs,[69, 116] where they usually involve a significant portion of the rib (Fig. 19–191). The appearance is that of a focal lytic lesion, possibly with a region of local expansion. The cortex is usually intact but may be quite thin over a localized area of expansion. Occasionally, focal expansion may become marked and present with a "soap bubble" appearance. Whether mild or marked, the expansion is usually symmetric and fusiform. The lytic lesions may gradually increase in density to a ground-glass appearance, or occasionally, late in the development of the lesion, they may progress to homogeneous sclerosis.

CARTILAGE TUMORS. Cartilaginous benign tumors (chondromas) represent approximately 2.7 per cent of the benign tumors of the ribs[57] and are also found in the sternum. Chondromas of the chest wall are either enchondromas or osteochondromas. When the lesion arises in the marrow space, leading to the expansion of the bone, the term "enchondroma" is used. If, however, the tumor arises eccentrically and grows as a projection from the bone, the term "osteochondroma" is applied. Both of these forms are common tumors of the ribs and are less common in the sternum. Both types may progress to giant masses while remaining benign.[96] These large cartilaginous masses may cause pressure erosion of the adjacent ribs.

A rib enchondroma most commonly occurs in the anterior aspect adjacent to the costochondral junction.[57, 97] The lesion presents as a small lytic area with or without pain. It is circular or oval in shape and usually displays a sclerotic margin. Focal expansion of the rib may occur (Fig. 19–192). The cartilage matrix may mature and calcify, creating a stippled pattern of calcific density that is specific for the enchondroma (Fig. 19–193). If no calcification is present within the lesion, the appearance is nonspecific and surgical resection is generally necessary for diagnosis.

Enchondromas are the most common primary tumors of the sternum. They may arise in any region of the sternum, but they are most common in the manubrium.[93] The tumor may present as an asymptomatic or painful mass. The mass is generally hard, nodular, and fixed to the bony chest wall. A large sternal enchondroma, which is usually accompanied by a prominent firm soft tissue mass, may have fluctuant areas when palpated.

Osteochondromas of ribs, like enchondromas, are most commonly located in the anterior aspect of the rib (Fig. 19–194).[57] They occur most frequently in adults but are occasionally found in infants.[62, 118] Although they are usually solitary lesions, they may be multiple, as in multiple familial osteochondromatosis. An important feature of osteochondromas of the ribs and sternum, which also applies to all osteochondromas of the central skeleton, is the strong tendency for such lesions to evolve into chondrosarcomas.[109] The growth of an osteochondroma after adjacent epiphyseal plates are closed should always suggest the possibility that malignant change has occurred.

EOSINOPHILIC GRANULOMA. Eosinophilic granuloma is a localized form of histiocytosis X.[74] It may represent an inflammatory histiocytic lesion rather than true

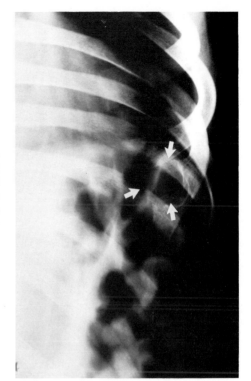

Figure 19–192. Enchondroma of the left sixth rib. The patient is a 10-year-old asymptomatic boy with a lesion noted on chest film obtained for trauma. This coned-down frontal roentgenogram of left lower chest shows a circular, lytic, expanding lesion in the anterior left sixth rib (arrows). There is a sclerotic shell and no calcification. This location is common in cartilage tumors. (AFIP Neg. No. 74-14791-2.)

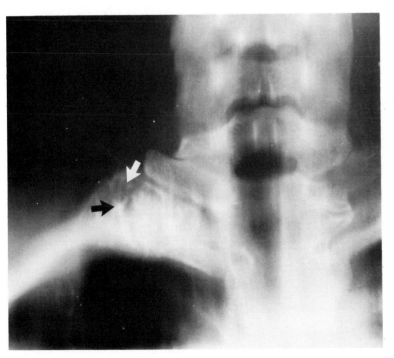

Figure 19–193. Enchondroma of the right first rib. This 26-year-old man presented with a dull ache in the right upper chest. The frontal view of the chest (not shown) demonstrated a swelling of the posterior aspect of the right first rib. Tomograms show the intramedullary lytic lesion in the posterior aspect of the rib, with the stippled areas of calcification typical of cartilage tumors (arrows). (AFIP Neg. No. 77-300-1.)

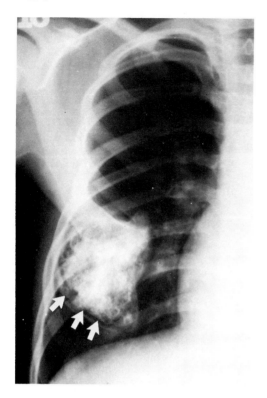

Figure 19–194. Osteochondroma of the right fifth rib. The patient is an 8-year-old boy with a slow-growing anterior chest wall mass present since birth. He has other, similar, lesions in the femur and pubis as well as a family history of osteochondromatosis. This frontal roentgenogram of the chest shows a large lesion involving the anterior aspect of the right fifth rib, with stipple calcifications. The mass has grown beyond the rib and caused secondary pressure erosion of the superior aspect of the right sixth rib (arrows). This finding signifies slow growth. (AFIP Neg. No. 72-13034-4.)

neoplasm. When located in the ribs, however, these lesions mimic the appearance of true bony neoplasms on roentgenograms, and surgical resection is generally necessary to confirm the diagnosis. Eosinophilic granuloma classically occurs in patients younger than ten, but the lesion is not uncommon in adults. Solitary lesions are most common, but multiple lesions throughout the skeleton may be present.[94] Patients usually present with symptoms of local pain and tenderness for a few weeks or months.[81]

The roentgenographic appearance is that of a growing, destructive lesion of the rib, which is generally discovered as an irregular small lytic lesion. The lesion originates in the medullary cavity and is usually central, causing erosion of the endosteal surfaces of the cortex and, occasionally, cortical expansion (Fig. 19–195). Periosteal reaction, which

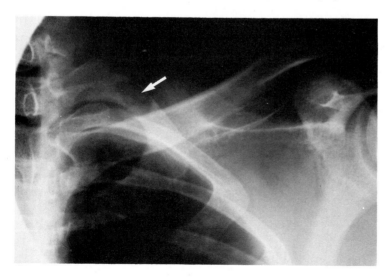

Figure 19–195. Eosinophilic granuloma of the left first rib in a 33-year-old man who had had upper left chest pain for several weeks. A coned-down view of the left upper chest wall reveals an oval lytic lesion in the posterior left first rib. There is a density in the lytic lesion representing a sequestrum (arrow) and a pathologic fracture. No soft tissue mass is present. The margins of the lytic process are sharp and well defined, with no sclerosis. (AFIP Neg. No. 69-2917.)

is common in eosinophilic granuloma of long bones, is infrequent with the rib lesion. Periosteal reaction does frequently occur, however, when the lesion undergoes pathologic fracture, which is not an uncommon occurrence.[81] Varying amounts of peripheral sclerosis may be present around the lytic focus of the lesion.[29]

GIANT CELL TUMOR AND ANEURYSMAL BONE CYST. Giant cell tumors are uncommon rib lesions that usually present as painful masses involving the posterior aspect of the rib. The bone lesion may be associated with a large soft tissue mass, which may project externally on the chest wall or be visualized as an extrapleural mass on a roentgenogram of the chest.

The roentgenographic appearance is that of a localized lytic lesion, which is commonly fusiform in shape, often causing cortical expansion. The prominent soft tissue mass is usually obvious on the roentegenograms (Fig. 19–196). Although giant cell tumors in the long bones usually appear as eccentric metaphyseal lesions, eccentricity is not usually observed in the rib lesions. The lytic lesion usually appears to be expanding symmetrically. Some areas of the cortical shell around the expansile lesion of a giant cell tumor of the rib may be completely destroyed, while other areas remain with a septate or trabeculated appearance. Pathologic fractures are not uncommon.

The distinction between giant cell tumors and aneurysmal bone cysts is controversial;[13, 31, 66, 76] it is not clear whether these represent the same or separate entities. The histologic differentiation between these lesions may be difficult. Radiographically, the appearances of giant cell tumor of ribs and aneurysmal bone cysts are similar.

HEMANGIOMA. Hemangiomas may occur in ribs as expansile, elongated, lytic lesions. Roentgenographically, they usually have a reticulated appearance, owing to reinforced thick trabeculae (Fig. 19–197), which is similar to the classic appearance seen in hemangiomas of the vertebral bodies. Occasionally, the rib lesions may expand

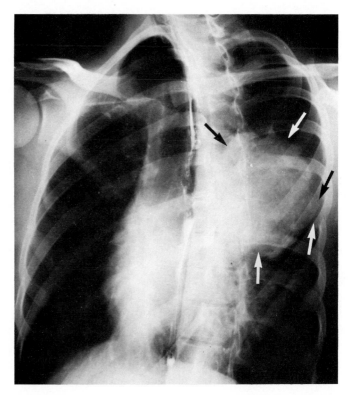

Figure 19–196. Giant cell tumor in the left seventh rib in a 22-year-old woman who had had pain in the left chest. An oblique view of the chest shows destruction of the posterior left seventh rib with a large soft tissue mass (arrows). About the soft tissue mass, especially in its inferior aspect, there is a thin sclerotic shell. This is the most common location and radiographic pattern seen in cases of giant cell tumors of the ribs. There are no adjacent rib erosions. Incidentally, note the barium within the esophagus. (AFIP Neg. No. 67-10782.)

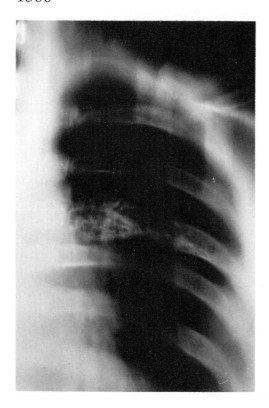

Figure 19–197. Hemangioma of the left fifth rib. This 21-year-old woman presented with a full sensation in the left upper chest. A tomogram of the left upper chest demonstrates a lytic, expanded lesion of the posterior left fifth rib involving a 7-cm segment. There is a reticulated or coarse trabecular appearance, which is typical of hemangiomas. (AFIP Neg. No. 76-595-1.)

focally to a marked degree, causing a "soap bubble" appearance. Although hemangiomas may occur in any portion of the rib, the posterior aspect is the most common location.[18, 57]

OTHER BENIGN TUMORS. Bone cysts also cause lytic lesions in the ribs, with fusiform expansion and a sharply defined cortical margin. Pathologic fractures occur frequently because of the thinned cortical shell. Unless pathologic fracture has occurred, the lesion is generally asymptomatic.

Nonossifying fibromas (fibroxanthomas) may also occur as lytic rib lesions. As in long bones, nonossifying fibromas in ribs appear oval and eccentric. They usually display a well-developed sharp margin with a sclerotic rim.

Osteomas, in contrast to the lytic lesions of the ribs, present with dense bony sclerosis.[126]

Other rare lesions that may occur in the ribs and the sternum include interosseous ganglion,[15] neurilemmoma,[28, 40] osteoid osteoma,[57] and osteoblastoma. None of these lesions is associated with specific roentgenographic findings.

Malignant Tumors

In contrast to benign tumors, malignant bony tumors of the chest wall usually cause the destruction of bone, resulting in ill-defined borders and large soft tissue masses. They may, however, mimic the appearance of benign tumors on roentgenograms, when they present as localized lesions with sclerotic rims. Most malignancies with this deceptive roentgenographic pattern have arisen from pre-existing benign

Figure 19–198. Metastatic carcinoma from the breast in a 59-year-old woman several years after surgery for breast carcinoma. She presented with chest wall discomfort, pain, and some areas of local rib tenderness. The frontal roentgenogram demonstrates multiple lytic areas of metastatic disease in the ribs, scapulae, and clavicles. The lytic areas are well circumscribed, with several pathologic fractures in the left lower rib cage. Also noted is slight subpleural thickening, due to bleeding, and linear densities in the lower lung fields, due to pulmonary lymphangiectatic spread of the tumor. (AFIP Neg. No. 214640-2B.)

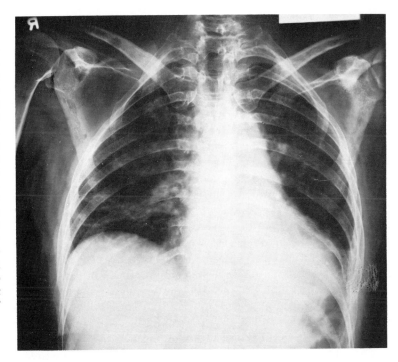

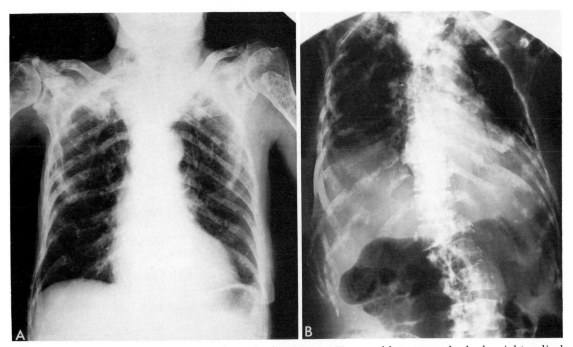

Figure 19–199. Metastatic carcinoma from the breast in a 67-year-old woman who had a right radical mastectomy for carcinoma of the breast. She presented three years postoperatively with pain in both hips, which rapidly progressed to diffuse bone pain. *A,* The frontal roentgenogram demonstrates the area of the prior mastectomy and diffuse osteolytic as well as osteoblastic metastasis throughout the ribs, clavicle, scapula, and upper humeri. There are usually no soft tissue masses associated with these bony metastatic deposits, as demonstrated in this case. *B,* View of the chest and abdomen taken nine months after *A,* which demonstrates the progression of both lytic and blastic metastasis throughout the skeleton. (AFIP Neg. Nos. 77351-2 and 77351-3.)

tumors. The most common example of this transformation is the evolution of benign cartilage tumors, such as enchondromas, into chondrosarcomas.

METASTASES. Metastatic disease is the most common malignancy involving the bones of the chest wall, especially the ribs. These metastases most commonly originate from carcinomas. The high incidence of osseous metastatic disease in the chest wall is the result of its predilection for red marrow areas. Such areas are found in both ribs and sternum throughout most of life.

The roentgenographic appearance of chest wall metastatic bone disease is typically that of multiple lytic lesions (Fig. 19–198), but of course a solitary metastatic lesion can also occur. Blastic metastases are less common than lytic lesions and are most frequently seen in prostatic adenocarcinoma. Both lytic and blastic lesions may appear in patients with primary malignancies of the breast (Fig. 19–199) or the prostate gland or with lymphoma. Whether lytic or blastic, metastatic lesions are usually poorly circumscribed and are commonly associated with pathologic fractures.

PLASMACYTOMA AND MYELOMA. Myeloma involves bone by infiltration and destruction. When solitary, the lesion is called a plasmacytoma, but the lesions are usually multiple. The plasmacytoma is a solitary destructive lesion of bone with expansion and an adjacent soft tissue mass. The bony expansion may be marked, with thick ridging around the periphery causing a "soap bubble' appearance (Fig. 19–200). Plasmacytomas frequently become multiple myeloma, the multiple lesions appearing a few months to several years following the discovery of the plasmacytoma.

The lesions of multiple myeloma can vary widely in size and shape within a single patient. The lytic lesions may occasionally be surrounded by sclerotic margins. Diffuse osteoporosis of the bony skeleton may accompany multiple myeloma and lead to vertebral compression fractures.[6, 52] The ribs and the sternum are common sites of involvement by multiple myeloma, and pathologic fractures are especially frequent in the ribs. A soft tissue mass is frequent in multiple myeloma but uncommon in rib

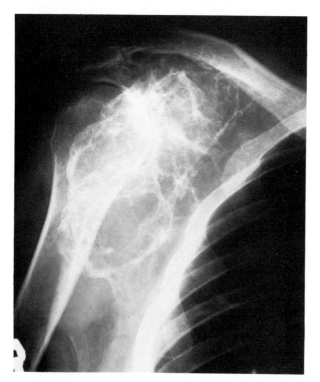

Figure 19–200. Plasmacytoma of the scapula in a 58-year-old man with progressive right shoulder pain, a decrease in range of motion of several months' duration, and a mass in the right shoulder. An anteroposterior view of the right shoulder demonstrates a large, expansile, lytic lesion of the scapula. There is an intact sclerotic shell with multiple loculated areas within the lesion. This is a frequent radiographic pattern in cases of plasmacytoma. (AFIP Neg. No. 74-9036-2.)

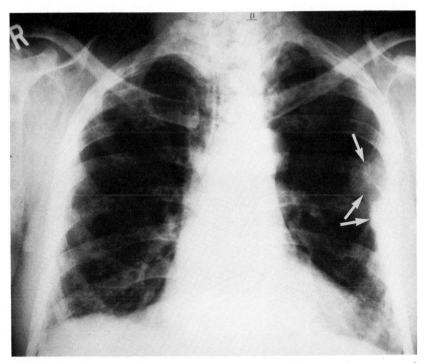

Figure 19–201. Multiple myeloma in a 44-year-old man who presented with pneumonia, anemia, and chest pain. The frontal roentgenogram of the chest shows multiple lytic lesions throughout the ribs, scapula, and clavicle, with patchy osteosclerosis throughout the marrow space. In the left lateral chest, multiple lytic lesions show the adjacent pleural-based soft tissue masses frequently seen in cases of multiple myeloma (arrows). (AFIP Neg. No. 70-9112-3.)

metastases, an important distinction.[147] These soft tissue masses may become large and present as extrapleural masses on chest roentgenograms (Fig. 19–201).

CHONDROSARCOMA. The most common primary bone malignancy of the chest wall is chondrosarcoma. It most commonly occurs in an adult, as a large destructive lesion, especially on a rib, with a prominent soft tissue mass. A chondrosarcoma may, however, also originate from a pre-existing benign cartilage tumor. The possibility of such malignant transformation often necessitates the surgical resection of a lesion that has been present for many years. Resection should be undertaken whenever pain or a change in appearance occurs in a benign cartilaginous lesion of the chest wall. Roentgenographically, chest wall chondrosarcomas may be completely radiolucent, but they commonly contain stippled areas of calcification that suggest their cartilaginous origin (Fig. 19–202).

EWING'S SARCOMA. Ewing's sarcomas of the chest wall usually occur in patients younger than 20. In fact, 80 per cent of cases occur in children younger than 13, and the condition is rare in people older than 40. The lesion is usually painful and associated with a large soft tissue mass on the external chest wall or an extrapleural mass visualized on the chest roentgenogram.[12, 146] When it occurs in a rib, Ewing's sarcoma is usually characterized by diffuse bone destruction and a prominent soft tissue mass (Fig. 19–203). A distinctive feature of Ewing's sarcoma is the "onionskin" periosteal reaction, which is unusual in other rib tumors. However, the roentgenographic appearance of Ewing's sarcoma as well as its clinical setting is often similar to that of osteomyelitis.

Text continued on page 1307

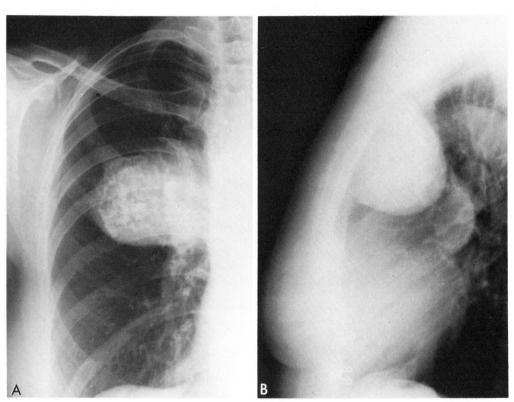

Figure 19–202. Chondrosarcoma of the right second rib. This 74-year-old woman had a mass in the right anterior chest wall for three years. It had grown more rapidly in the last 12 months. *A*, The frontal roentgenogram of the chest shows a large mass arising from the anterior aspect of the right second rib, with stippled and curvilinear calcification, suggesting a cartilage tumor. There is no bony shell or cortical rim about the large mass. *B*, The lateral chest roentgenogram shows the origin of this mass growing internally with a broad-based extrapleural configuration. The surface of the mass is smooth, with no infiltration of the adjacent lung. (AFIP Neg. Nos. 67-2745-1 and 67-2745-2.)

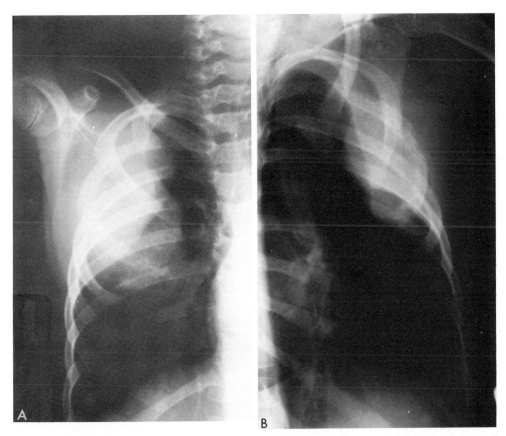

Figure 19–203. Ewing's sarcoma of the right third rib in a 6-year-old girl. She presented with pain, swelling, and a mass in the right upper chest. *A,* Frontal roentgenogram demonstrates a large soft tissue mass extending into the adjacent lung, with a sharp margin superiorly and an ill-defined margin inferiorly. Also evident is a "moth-eaten" pattern of bone destruction involving a long segment of the right third rib. *B,* Oblique view of the chest with bony technique shows the moth-eaten bony destruction and periosteal reaction (arrows). The extrapleural component of the tumor extends up into the apex. (AFIP Neg. Nos. 67-7878-1 and 67-7878-2.)

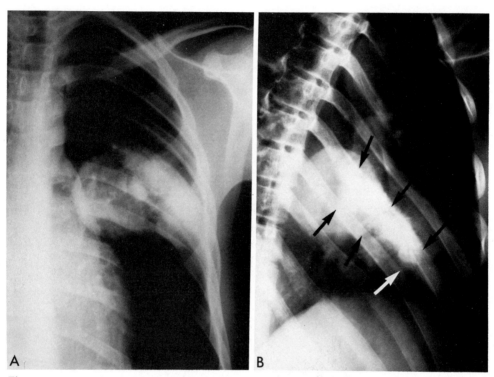

Figure 19–204.   Osteosarcoma of the left sixth rib. This 15-year-old male presented with a painful mass of the left posterior chest wall. *A,* Frontal roentgenogram of the chest demonstrates a large pleural-based mass growing from the posterolateral left sixth rib. *B,* Oblique view of the left chest best shows the extensive involvement of the intramedullary space and the adjacent soft tissue mass with homogenous sclerosis typical of osteosarcoma (arrows). The peripheral margin of the soft tissue sclerosis is spiculated, causing a pseudo-sunburst appearance. This is due to the partial mineralization of the more central mature malignant osteoid from the osteosarcoma. (AFIP Neg. Nos. 74-10591-1 and 74-10591-2.)

OSTEOSARCOMA. Osteosarcomas represent 2.9 per cent of primary rib tumors.[57] They occur in young people and are associated with pain and a palpable mass. The soft tissue mass of osteosarcoma is not usually as prominent, either clinically or roentgenographically, as in chondrosarcoma or Ewing's sarcoma.

The roentgenographic appearance of osteosarcoma in the chest wall may be lytic, blastic, or mixed. When lytic, its appearance is similar to that of other malignant lesions. When blastic or mixed, however, a homogeneous increase in density may be present both in the bone and in the surrounding soft tissue mass (Fig. 19–204). The homogeneous osseous density in osteosarcomas is thus easily distinguishable from the stippled density found in cartilaginous tumors.

OTHER MALIGNANT TUMORS. Other, less frequent, malignant neoplasms of the bony chest wall include fibrosarcomas, various sarcomas, and lymphomas, including Hodgkin's disease. Such lesions display a nonspecific appearance of bone destruction. The appearance of these rib lesions is similar to those in extrathoracic bones.

TUMORS OF SOFT TISSUES

Lipoma and Liposarcoma

Lipomas are common tumors of soft tissue but are unusual in the chest wall.[132] They may originate deep within the soft tissues of the chest wall, however, especially just outside the parietal pleura.[137] In this location they may appear as smooth extrapleural masses on roentgenograms or as masses limited to the chest wall that cannot be demonstrated by conventional radiographic techniques. They often manifest slow growth.

Lipomas are histologically and chemically identical to normal fatty tissue. Unlike normal fat, lipomas are not available to the body economy and may actually increase in size during starvation.[132] Some lipomas contain bone marrow elements and are called myelolipomas.

Lipomas of the chest have been divided into three groups by Heuer: (1) hourglass-shaped tumors with both intrathoracic and extrathoracic components connected by a thin isthmus of tissue between the ribs; (2) anterior mediastinal masses that may extend into the neck; and (3) wholly intrathoracic masses, including those of the mediastinum.[55, 56] When chest wall lipomas are roentgenographically visible, they fall into Heuer's first category (see Fig. 19–179; Fig. 19–205). These are characterized roentgenographically by smooth walls and an extrapleural appearance. Since they are partly surrounded by air-containing lung, their less-than-water density is not usually roentgenographically appreciated. The portion of the lipoma within the chest wall is usually of insufficient size to manifest a density less than that of surrounding soft tissues, although the displacement of normal structures may be visualized. The intrathoracic portion may change in shape with respiration[47] or change in position.[137] Pressure erosion of the adjacent ribs may also occur.[112] Computed tomography may be helpful in evaluation (see Fig. 19–179).[58] However, despite all these characteristics, most extrapleural lipomas are indistinguishable from other soft tissue masses of the chest wall.[120]

One form of lipoma that is more common in the chest wall is the spindle cell lipoma.[37] More than half of these occur in the soft tissues of the shoulder or back, and most of the remaining cases occur in the posterior neck soft tissues. In contrast to most lipomas, which are more common in females than in males, spindle cell lipomas occur almost exclusively in men older than age 45. The histologic differention of spindle cell lipoma from liposarcoma may be difficult.

An interesting variant of the benign lipoma is the hibernoma. These are tumors of brown fat that resemble the brown fat of the human embryo and that of the interscapular gland of hibernating animals. Human embryos contain brown fat in the neck and axillae as well as in the interscapular regions, the mediastinum, and elsewhere.[84] When visulaized roentgenographically, hibernomas resemble benign lipomas with an intrathoracic component.[92] No malignant counterpart has been described for this entity. Like lipomas, hibernomas may grow slowly.

Liposarcomas may occur in patients of any age but are far more common in adults

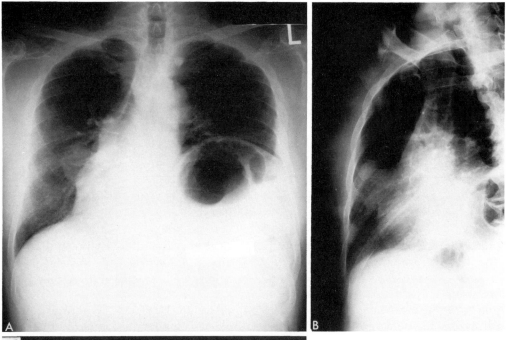

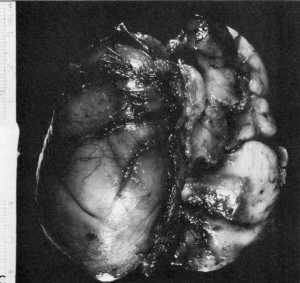

Figure 19–205. Lipoma of the chest wall. This 70-year-old man had no symptoms related to this lesion. *A,* The frontal roentgenogram shows a smooth mass in the right midlung field that appears less dense than adjacent soft tissue structures. The elevation of the left hemidiaphragm is not related to this lesion. *B,* The oblique view shows the mass to be continuous with the chest wall as well as with the pericardium. *C,* A specimen photograph shows the fatty mass after dissection from the chest wall, with its smooth border (toward the left) abutting the parietal pleura. (AFIP Neg. Nos. 77-10376 and 77-10366.)

than in children.[34] There is general agreement that liposarcomas arise *de novo* rather than from benign lipomas. Liposarcomas of the chest wall are far less common than benign lipomas. Most liposarcomas occur in the gluteal regions, thighs, lower extremities, and retroperitoneum. They have been reported in the anterior chest wall and axilla[33] and may give rise to either distant or local metastases. The most common sites of metastases include the lungs and pleura and the liver.[132] Roentgenographically, liposarcomas resemble other malignant tumors of the chest wall and may be exceedingly destructive to normal chest wall structures. Decreased density from fat content is only rarely evident.

Fibrous Tumors

The benign form of fibrous tissue tumors in soft tissues has been termed fibromatosis by Stout and Lattes to distinguish this group of benign fibroblastic proliferative lesions from the self-limited scar.[132] Although many forms of fibromatosis are common lesions, the involvement of the chest wall is unusual.[27]

Fibromatosis may be divided into two categories: those occurring in children, probably congenitally and those occurring in adults, considered acquired. Many of the lesions in both categories occur in the dermal or subcutaneous tissues of the chest wall and thus present as superficial masses, which are rarely evaluated roentgenographically. The deep fibromatoses are most commonly found in the paraspinal regions, where they present as ill-defined densities on roentgenograms[27] or are roentgenologically inapparent. They have not been reported to cause secondary defects in bone, nor do they cause intrathoracic masses. Their sizes range from 1 to 12 cm.

The fibromatoses often interlace with surrounding soft tissue and are as ill defined grossly as they are roentgenographically. Approximately 85 per cent of resections demonstrate disease in the margins of the resected tissue.[27] Nevertheless, only one third of fibromatoses recur locally, which suggests that complete resection is not always necessary.

Fibrosarcoma is the malignant counterpart of benign fibromatosis. This is usually found in the superficial soft tissues, but it can occur in the deep soft tissues, especially those of the leg.[138] A variable number (probably about 10 per cent) of fibrosarcomas occur in the chest wall.[132] Their origin is obscure. Lieberg has reported one case that began as a hemophilic cyst.[75] The degree of malignancy seems to correlate with the size of the lesion. Small fibrosarcomas usually do not lead to metastatic disease except after repeated episodes of surgery. Lesions that are very large at the time of initial detection are associated with a poor prognosis. The complete surgical removal of a fibrosarcoma is necessary, since recurrence is common when the tumor has not been completely resected.[138] The most common site of metastatic disease is the lung, in which the metastases generally appear as multiple, well-demarcated, parenchymal masses of uniform size. Of all fibrosarcomas, approximately 75 per cent recur, and 10 per cent metastasize to the lungs or other organs.[129] Full-lung tomograms should be obtained before the performance of definitive surgery.[99] Approximately one quarter of all patients with fibrosarcoma die of this disease; the disease is more malignant in adults than in children.[131, 132]

Roentgenographically, fibrosarcomas are sharply demarcated masses that often become large (Fig. 19–206). Calcifications may be present; invasion and erosion of bone are common findings. When fibrosarcomas are very large it may be impossible to determine whether they originate from the chest wall or from a lung, the mediastinum, or the pleura. Fibrosarcomas cannot be differentiated roentgenographically from other

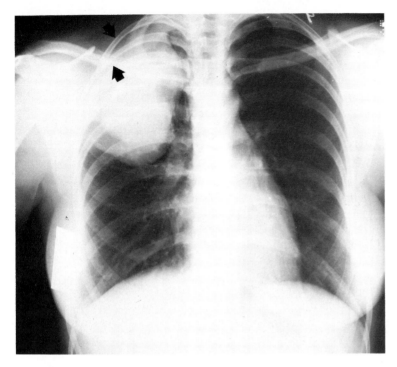

Figure 19–206. Round cell tumor of the right upper chest in a 23-year-old woman with a seven-month history of increasing right shoulder pain. The frontal roentgenogram shows an extrapleural right upper chest mass, with mild thinning of the posterolateral portions of the right second and third ribs (arrows). The smooth remodeling of the ribs is consistent with a soft tissue, rather than bony, origin for this tumor. (AFIP Neg. No. 72-17759.)

sarcomas of the chest wall; however, angiography may distinguish the most malignant portions of the tumor by their increased vascularity.[148]

Malignant fibrous histiocytomas and similar lesions also occur in the chest wall. These tumors resemble both reticulum cell sarcomas and other benign and malignant fibrous lesions. They are more common in adults than in children and occur most frequently in the posterior chest wall. Malignant fibrous histiocytomas were first described by O'Brien and Stout in 1964.[90] These tumors are highly malignant, metastases occurring in about one third of the cases.[124] Their roentgenographic appearance is very similar to that of fibrosarcomas and other malignant fibrous tumors (Fig. 19–207).

Many variant forms of malignant fibrous histiocytomas have been recently described. The myxoid variant appears to behave in a more benign fashion than the typical form.[143] Other variants include the malignant histiocytoma and epithelioid sarcoma,[124] both of which are more aggressively malignant than the typical malignant fibrous histiocytoma. There are no descriptions of roentgenographic differences among these lesions. Complete surgical resection is emphasized in the treatment of all.

Extra-abdominal desmoid (musculoaponeurotic fibromatosis) is an aggressive benign fibrous tumor. This term was originally used to describe fibromatoses of the abdominal wall of women who had recently been pregnant.[132] The tumors resemble hyperplastic scars and usually interdigitate with surrounding muscle in a manner similar to that of other fibromatoses. Many authors consider extra-abdominal desmoids to be well-differentiated fibrosarcomas, which they resemble roentgenographically as well as histologically.

More than 10 per cent of extra-abdominal desmoids are found in the chest wall.[4, 35] They generally occur in young women, and about half recur locally following resection. Recurrence seems to be more likely in very young patients. Sixty-three per cent of the patients whose cases were studied by Enzinger experienced trauma before the

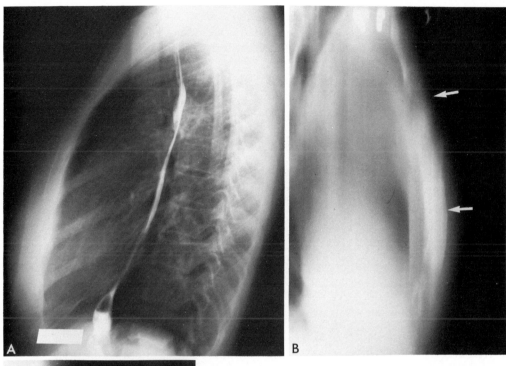

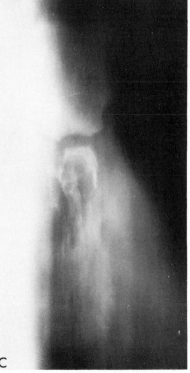

Figure 19–207. Malignant fibrous histiocytoma of the anterior chest wall in a 27-year-old woman with increasing anterior chest pain. *A,* The lateral chest roentgenogram shows mild widening of the soft tissues anterior to the sternum. The lower portion of the bony sternum is not well visualized, but no definite bone erosion is seen. *B,* A lateral tomogram of the sternum shows irregular cortical thickening in the lower portion of the sternum (lower arrow) and poor visualization of the lower manubrium and upper sternal body (upper arrow). *C,* An oblique tomogram of the sternum reveals multiple lytic lesions and cortical destruction in the upper portion of the body of the sternum. (AFIP Neg. No. 73-11079.)

appearance of the lesion but this history was not well documented in many of these cases.[35] The progression and prognosis are variable, ranging from aggressive entrapment of nerves and arteries to spontaneous regression.

Extra-abdominal desmoids generally appear roentgenographically as large, ill-defined tumors in the soft tissues of the shoulder. They may also occur elsewhere in the chest wall. In Enzinger's series, only two were visible as intrathoracic masses (Fig. 19–208).

An unusual fibrous tumor is the elastofibroma.[132] This tumor is always found anterior to the lower portion of the scapula in relation to the latissimus dorsi and rhomboideus muscles, in elderly people. Cases of bilateral involvement have been reported.

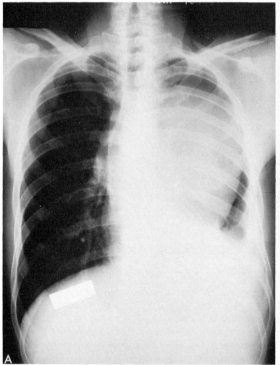
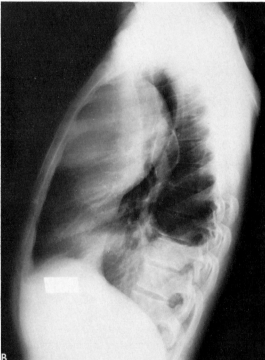
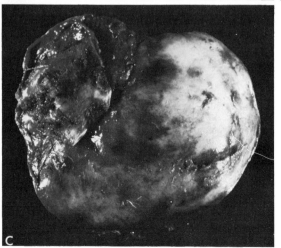

Figure 19–208. Desmoid fibroma of the left chest. This 34-year-old man presented with a three-week history of dull pain in the left posterior chest. A, The frontal roentgenogram shows a large left chest mass with left pleural effusion. B, The lateral roentgenogram shows the smooth border of the mass's posterior surface and the displacement of adjacent left lung structures. C, A specimen photograph shows the smooth border of the intrathoracic portion of this mass on its right side. (AFIP Neg. Nos. 77-9028 and 77-10365.)

Vascular Tumors

Benign hemangiomas are usually divided into capillary and cavernous types,[132] both of which are more common in distal extremities than in the chest wall. Capillary hemangiomas are composed of capillaries alone, whereas cavernous hemangiomas contain widely dilated vessels. Most hemangiomas of the soft tissues are cavernous.[53] The infrequent hemangiomas in the chest wall may contain calcified phleboliths (Fig.

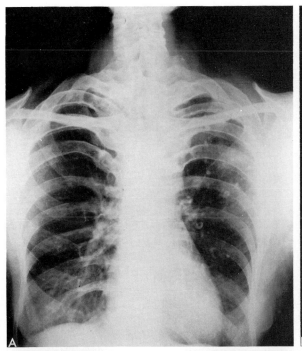
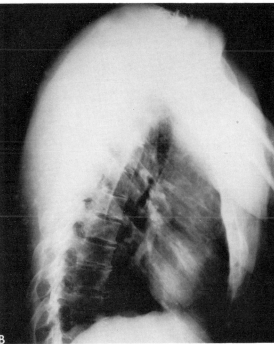
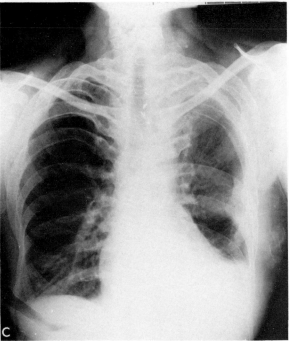

Figure 19–209. Hemangioma of the chest wall. This 52-year-old woman had noted a mass over the left posterior chest wall for more than 30 years and was admitted because of increasing weakness in her legs. The mass was found to be compressing the spinal cord and was removed during three surgical procedures. *A,* The frontal view shows phleboliths overlying the left lung field, simulating granulomatous disease of the lung. *B,* The lateral view shows the phleboliths to lie in a mass of the posterior chest wall. *C,* The postoperative frontal view shows pleural effusion, pleural thickening, surgical clips, and sutures as well as postoperative rib changes. (AFIP Neg. No. 52-5175.) (*From* Hodges, P.: Archives Surg., *64:*777–782, 1952. Reproduced by permission.)

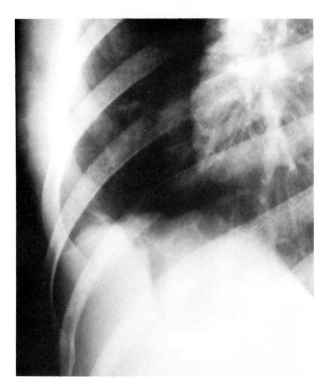

Figure 19–210. Vascular tumor, possible hemangioendothelioma, of the right tenth rib. This 13-year-old boy was radiographed because of local tenderness. The oblique roentgenogram shows the frontolateral portion of the right tenth rib to have a long region of erosion on its inferior surface, with a smooth residual border but with loss of normal trabeculation and increased irregular ossification within the rib. A soft tissue mass projects into the thoracic cavity from this region. At surgery, the neoplasm was found to have originated from the intercostal artery, growing along the vessel, with consequent bony erosion and growth disturbance. (AFIP Neg. No. 73-1004.)

19–209) or may cause hypertrophy of adjacent soft tissues or bone.[92] Bone erosion rather than hypertrophy may also be noted (Fig. 19–210). Hemangiomas may recur locally but do not metastasize.

Hemangiopericytomas can be found anywhere in the soft tissues in both adults and children.[132] These tumors originate from the pericytes, which are unique cells found spiraling around the outside of capillaries and postcapillary venules.[79] Hemangiopericytomas may be benign or malignant, and it may be impossible to determine malignancy from the histologic appearance of the lesion. Location does not appear to be important in the forecasting of the outcome of the condition, however. Most hemangiopericytomas occur in the thigh and the groin.

In the chest wall, hemangiopericytomas are found in the deep soft tissues, especially in the back. Chest wall masses may present as intrathoracic masses through the displacement of the pleura or the invasion of the pleura and lung.[79] Primary cases in lung tissue have also been reported.[48] Speckled calcification may be found within the mass, and the erosion of bone, typical of soft tissue chest wall masses, also occurs. One recent report suggests that the angiographic pattern of radially arranged branching arteries seen in these masses may be distinctive.[149]

Malignant hemangiopericytomas metastasize most commonly to a lung. Between 35 and 50 per cent metastasize,[38, 132] and about 20 to 25 per cent of the patients die of their disease.

Other rare, vascular tumors in the chest wall include angiosarcomas, Kaposi's sarcoma,[132] lymphangiomas, and other tumors originating in the lymphatic system.

Neural Tumors

Most neural tumors in the chest occur in the mediastinum, especially the posterior mediastinum.[107] Neural tumors of all types, however, may originate from intercostal nerves or other nerves within the chest wall. They are more common in the posterior chest wall. Malignant neural tumors are exceedingly difficult to differentiate from benign tumors by roentgenographic techniques.

Neural tumors fall into two categories: those of sympathetic origin and those of nerve sheath origin.[1] Those involving the chest wall are usually of nerve sheath origin and may be classified as neurilemmomas (schwannomas) or neurofibromas. Neurilemmomas are more common[107] and grow as lateral masses on the parent nerves, compressing them. In contrast, the growth of neurofibromas diffusely expands their parent nerves, and axons may often be identified within the tumor masses.

Neurilemmomas and neurofibromas are virtually identical roentgenographically, appearing as firm, well-circumscribed, spherical masses. They often cause pressure erosion of the adjacent ribs or other bones and may also spread the adjacent ribs.[107] Bone destruction is more common in the malignant neural tumors (Fig. 19–211), and ragged destruction of bone is strongly suggestive of malignancy.

The only neural tumors of sympathetic origin commonly found in the chest wall are neuroblastomas and ganglioneuroblastomas, the most malignant tumors of the sympathetic series. These are most often seen in children (Fig. 19–212) and may be very large (Fig. 19–213), involving the pleura, the lung, and the mediastinum extensively.

Malignant neural tumors of nerve sheath origin are called malignant schwannomas. Approximately 15 per cent of malignant schwannomas occur in the trunk, approximately one third of these occurring on the anterior chest wall.[24] These masses may be superficial or deep and are roentgenographically indistinguishable from their benign counterparts. Metastases occur most often to the lungs and spread via the hematogenous route. There is a five-year survival rate of approximately 50 per cent. Although many malignant schwannomas, like their benign counterparts, occur as

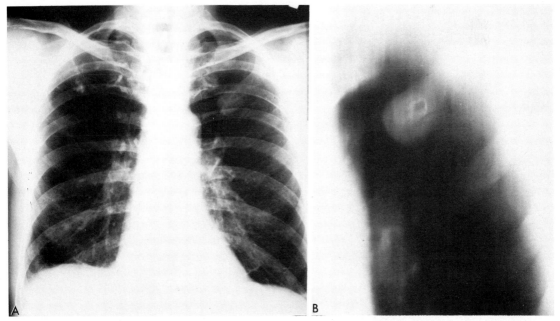

Figure 19–211. Neurilemmoma of the left upper chest wall in a 61-year-old man without known symptoms. *A,* The frontal roentgenogram shows a round mass surrounded by air in the left upper lung field adjacent to the second anterior rib. *B,* The frontal tomogram shows proximity of the mass to the rib, with no evidence of rib destruction or erosion. At surgery, the mass was found to be just inside the rib, indenting the parietal pleura (AFIP Neg. No. 78-346.)

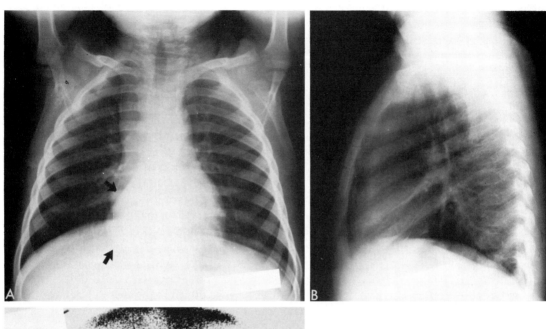

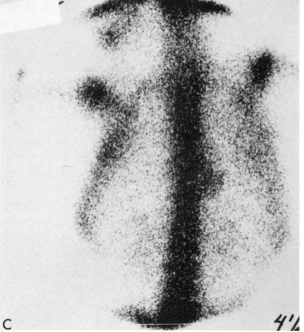

Figure 19–212. Ganglioneuroblastoma of the posterior mediastinum and chest wall in a 19-month-old boy who was radiographed incidentally. *A,* The frontal roentgenogram of the chest shows widening of the mediastinum toward the right. An extrapleural mass (arrow) overlies the right side of the heart and extends below the dome of the diaphragm, strongly suggesting a posterior location. *B,* The lateral view does not clearly show the mass. No bone involvement is manifested. *C,* The posterior view of a gallium-67 radionuclide scan shows increased uptake in the region of the mass seen on the frontal roentgenogram.

Legend continued on the opposite page

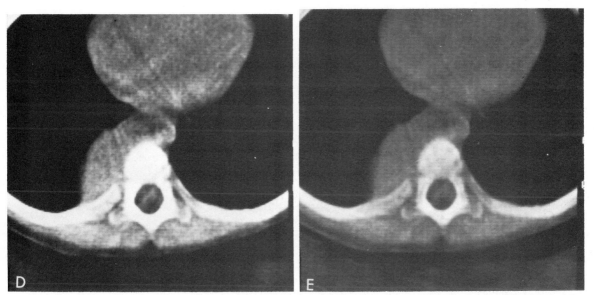

Figure 19–212 Continued. D, A computed tomogram clearly shows the extent of the mass. E, A computed tomogram at a higher window setting shows marked demineralization of the vertebral body and right rib, with widening of the costovertebral joint. The superficial soft tissues do not appear involved. In this case, the chest wall involvement was visualized only by computed tomography. (AFIP Neg. No. 77-10375.)

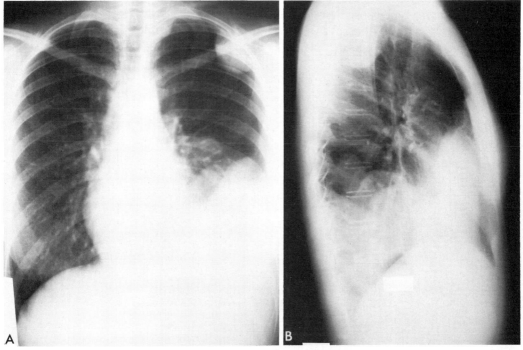

Figure 19–213. Neuroblastoma of the mediastinum and chest wall. This 21-year-old woman complained of progressive left chest pain over a period of three months. A, The frontal roentgenogram shows a multilobulated mass involving the lower portions of the left thoracic cavity, chest wall, and mediastinum. A separate extrapleural lesion is apparent in the left upper thorax. B, The lateral view demonstrates an extensive lobular mass obscuring the left hemidiaphragm and most of the heart shadow. At surgery, this malignant tumor was found to involve the pericardium, diaphragm, lung, and chest wall, with metastases to several organs, including the pleura. (AFIP Neg. No. 72-12636.)

asymptomatic masses, the involvement of the brachial plexus or pleura may cause pain. Horner's syndrome can result from benign or malignant nerve sheath tumors.[1]

Malignant schwannomas are common in von Recklinghausen's disease (neurofibromatosis).[24] Approximately one quarter of the patients with malignant schwannomas have the stigmata of neurofibromatosis.[45] A schwannoma is more likely to be malignant when the patient has von Recklinghausen's disease.[107] In addition to bone erosion and destruction, which especially involve ribs, scoliosis may be found in these patients. This is characteristically a kyphoscoliosis, involving the lower thoracic region with a marked kyphotic predominance. The scoliosis may be secondary to growth disturbances or to the presence of abnormal vertebrae.[61] Meningomyoceles also occur in patients with von Recklinghausen's disease with greater than normal frequency.

Patients with von Recklinghausen's disease have an increased incidence of soft tissue sarcomas in addition to nerve sheath tumors. These sarcomas include rhabdomyosarcomas, liposarcomas, and unclassified sarcomas.[23]

Muscle Tumors

The most common tumor of muscular origin found in the deeper tissues of the chest wall is rhabdomyosarcoma. The four categories of rhabdomyosarcoma are the embryonal, the botryoid, the pleomorphic, and the alveolar.[63] This classification is based primarily upon histologic distinctions, although clinically some of these groups differ markedly.

Embryonal and botryoid rhabdomyosarcomas occur most commonly in children. The embryonal type is usually found in the head, the neck, and the urogenital tract, but it may also occur in other areas, including the chest wall.[132] Embryonal rhabdomyosarcomas may occur at any time in childhood, the average age at onset being nine years.[125]

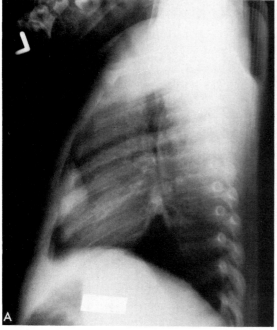
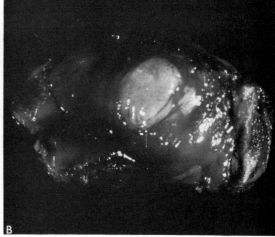

Figure 19–214. Embryonal rhabdomyosarcoma. The patient is a 14-month-old boy with a superficial mass on the right side of anterior chest wall. *A*, Lateral chest view. The mass is visualized just behind the lower portion of the sternum, exhibiting extrapleural signs. The soft tissue stripe of the sternum is not disturbed because the mass proved to be to the right of the sternum. The mass was not clearly visualized on frontal or oblique views of the chest. *B*, Specimen photograph. A well-demarcated tumor is seen through the parietal pleura of the anterior chest wall. (AFIP Neg. Nos. 76-563 and 75-15366.) (Courtesy of The Johns Hopkins Hospital, Baltimore, Maryland.)

Although the period of survival is usually only a few months,[126] a few long-term survivors have been reported.[63] The embryonal tumors are well-circumscribed masses that may be visualized in the thoracic space (Fig. 19–214). The appearance of calcification within these tumors is unusual, but bone erosion is often visualized.

The botryoid form is usually polypoid or grapelike and is found in children with an average age of seven years.[125] This highly fatal tumor is rare in the chest wall.

The pleomorphic and alveolar forms of rhabdomyosarcoma are generally found in adults. The latter is most common in adolescents and young adults (average age, 23 years), and the pleomorphic type is more frequent in adults of middle age. Like the childhood forms, the adult forms are usually fatal, although some pleomorphic rhabdomyosarcomas may grow very slowly. These adult tumors appear as well-circumscribed soft tissue masses with no distinguishing features. Calcification is uncommon, but bone erosion is frequent.

With the exception of the alveolar type, rhabdomyosarcomas occur much more often in males. Unlike other sarcomas, rhabdomyosarcomas commonly involve lymph nodes,[124] and sometimes lymphadenopathy is the earliest finding. Lung and pleural metastases are also common; the pancreas and bone are involved less often. Because of the frequency of local invasion and distant metastases, radical surgery combined with aggressive radiotherapy and chemotherapy is generally advocated.[125]

Other tumors of muscular origin are leiomyoma, leiomyosarcoma, and rhabdomyoma.[99, 127]

INFECTIONS OF THE CHEST WALL

Pyogenic Abscess and Osteomyelitis

Pyogenic infection of the chest wall, with or without the involvement of bone, is similar to such disease elsewhere in the body. Acute abscess formation occurs, with obvious pain and swelling; the abscess may be secondary to local trauma or hematogenous in origin.[144] Pyogenic infections of the lung or the pleura may spread rapidly, soon involving the soft tissues and bones of the chest wall.[142]

Osteomyelitis of the ribs generally begins with a soft tissue mass, loss of the deep fascial planes, and subsequent periosteal elevation.[137] Infection is usually present for seven to ten days before bone destruction is visualized on plain roentgenograms.[144] Tomography may show erosive changes (Fig. 19–215) before they can be visualized on plain roentgenograms. The typical findings of the later stages include involucra, and spread to the adjacent ribs and other bones is common (Fig. 19–216). Sclerosis adjacent to lytic regions is also a usual finding in the advanced stages. Mild infections or those inadequately treated may lead to chronic osteomyelitis (Brodie's abscess formation) (Fig. 19–217).

Osteomyelitis involves the sternum much less often than the ribs.[129] Previous trauma, poor nutrition, or antecedent infection are predisposing factors. Postoperative sternal osteomyelitis has frequently been seen after median sternotomies[129, 130, 133, 135, 136, 139, 145] and following bone marrow aspiration.[132] Hematogenous osteomyelitis involving the sternum is unusual; its highest incidence is in heroin addicts.[7, 69, 83] A wide variety of organisms, especially gram-negative bacteria, may be the cause of this type of hematogenous osteomyelitis. Unusual causative organisms, such as fungi, have been found, especially in patients with wounds or recent surgery.[108, 123] A soft tissue mass, the loss of deep fascial planes, and the displacement of the anterior pleural stripe are common findings in sternal osteomyelitis (Fig. 19–218).

Text continued on page 1323

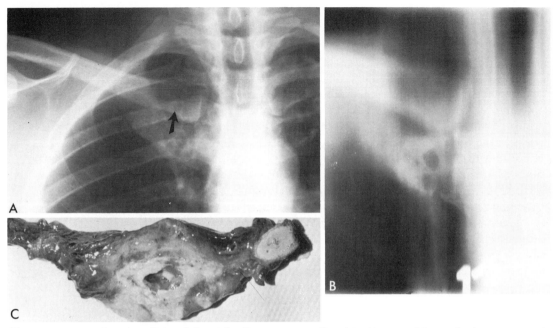

Figure 19–215. Osteomyelitis of the right first anterior rib. This 33-year-old man had a one-month history of a tender mass over the right sternoclavicular region. *A*, The frontal chest roentgenogram shows subtle cortical thinning in the anterior right first rib, with cystic lesions (arrow) near the costochondral junction anteriorly. *B*, A frontal tomogram shows the cystic lysis of the anterior first rib, with minimal erosion of the adjacent sternum. The clavicle appears normal. No periosteal reaction is seen. *C*, A specimen photograph shows the resected rib with a large cyst in its center and dense fibrous connective tissue surrounding the thin cortex of bone. (AFIP Neg. Nos. 72-7215 and 72-5617.)

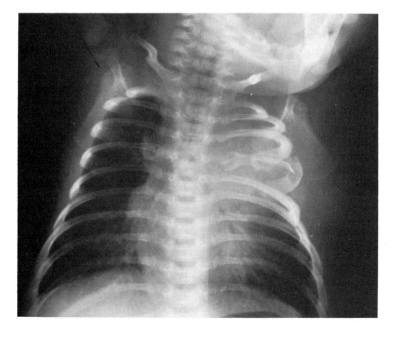

Figure 19–216. Osteomyelitis of the left upper ribs in a two-month-old boy with a two-day history of fever, cough, and shortness of breath. The frontal roentgenogram shows an alveolar infiltrate in the left upper lung field compatible with pneumonia. There is a marked soft tissue thickening, spreading the upper five left ribs. The destruction of the lateral and posterior regions of the left fourth rib, with marked periosteal reaction and cortical thickening, is also evident. These ribs were resected. This osteomyelitis was thought to have originated from the direct spread of the pulmonary infection. (AFIP Neg. No. 59-2454.)

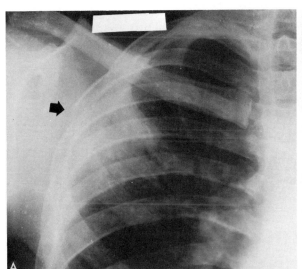

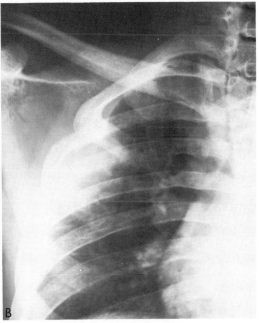

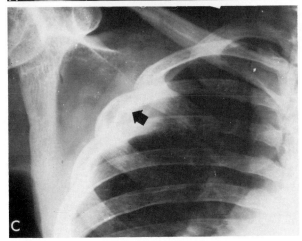

Figure 19–217. Chronic osteomyelitis of the right third rib. This 20-year-old male had sickle cell disease and right upper chest pain for several weeks. *A,* The initial roentgenogram shows mild lysis and an indistinct lateral cortex (arrow) of the right third rib. *B,* One week later, there is increased irregularity of the cortex, with loss of the trabecular pattern in the same region. *C,* Nine weeks later, the lateral cortex appears far sharper, but both outer and inner cortices are thickened and the trabecular pattern remains indistinct. Periosteal reaction remains on the medial surface (arrow). (AFIP Neg. No. 54-13095.)

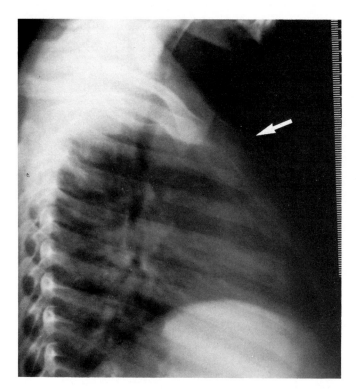

Figure 19–218. Osteomyelitis of the manubrium of the sternum. This three-year-old boy had a one-week history of a painless presternal mass. The lateral roentgenogram shows soft tissue swelling superficial to the upper sternum (arrow). The manubrium is expanded, with thinning of the cortex and diffuse lysis. This lesion is typical of hematogenous osteomyelitis. (AFIP Neg. No. 67-4023.)

Figure 19–219. Osteomyelitis of the right clavicle in a five-year-old girl with a four-day history of swelling over the right clavicle. The frontal roentgenogram shows a marked periosteal reaction and cortical thinning, with a large region of irregular lysis in the central portion of the right clavicle. Soft tissue swelling, with loss of the normal fascial planes adjacent to the right clavicle, is also evident. (AFIP Neg. No. 71-5041.)

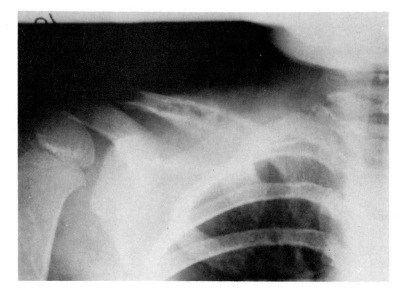

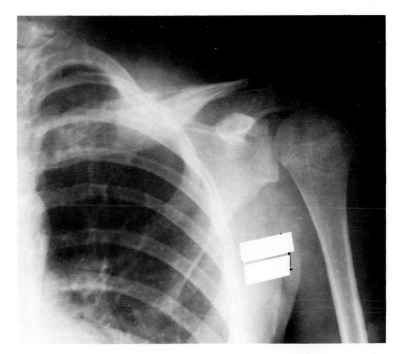

Figure 19–220. Osteomyelitis of the left clavicle in an 11-year-old girl with marked local swelling. The frontal roentgenogram shows lamellated periosteal reaction, with marked expansion of the proximal portion of the left clavicle. The cortex is markedly thinned, especially superiorly. There is soft tissue swelling and loss of fascial planes. (AFIP Neg. No. 62-4745.)

Clavicular osteomyelitis is also relatively uncommon. The medial end of the clavicle is most commonly involved in hematogenous infection.[100] The entire clavicle or the midshaft may also be involved.[125] Hematogenous osteomyelitis of the clavicle is usually associated with the involvement of other bones.[86] The findings are similar to those of osteomyelitis in other bones (Figs. 19–219 and 19–220). Osteomyelitis of the scapula has been reported rarely,[22] mostly as a consequence of hematogenous osteomyelitis in children. Erb palsy with arm weakness may be a consequence of this involvement.

Chest Wall Tuberculosis

Tuberculosis is the most frequent inflammatory process of the ribs and is second only to metastatic disease as a cause of rib destruction.[134] Rib involvement nevertheless accounts for only 5 per cent of all cases of bone tuberculosis.[26, 122]

Clinically, rib tuberculosis is usually not associated with active pulmonary disease. The rib lesion may be asymptomatic, or it may produce local pain and swelling.[134] Rib involvement is often associated with tuberculosis of other bones, especially the spine. Tuberculosis of the dorsal spine can spread, involving the adjacent posterior ribs, but usually rib involvement occurs via the hematogenous route. Sinus formation or chest wall abscess or both occur in about 25 per cent of the cases.[122]

The radiologic picture may vary. The involvement of the "shaft," the most common form of rib tuberculosis, usually produces a demarcated area of destruction (Figs. 19–221 and 19–222). Cortical expansion and a cystic appearance can develop. One or more ribs may be involved. Pathologic fracture is rare.

Sometimes, a multicystic appearance, with sclerotic margins and without bone expansion, is seen. Direct extension from a cold abscess of vertebral tuberculosis may

Text continued on page 1327

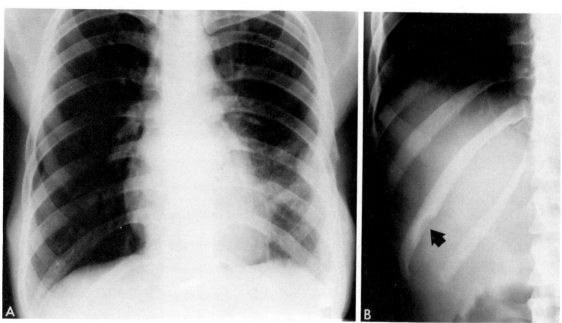

Figure 19–221. Bilateral tuberculosis of the ribs in a 26-year-old woman with a history of malaise for four months. *A,* The frontal roentgenogram of the chest shows an extrapleural mass in the lateral portion of the left midlung field, with lysis of the adjacent portion of the left sixth lateral rib and superficial soft tissue swelling. *B,* An overpenetrated view of the lower chest and upper abdomen shows a lytic lesion in the right eleventh posterolateral rib appearing as a smooth region of erosion and surrounding ill-defined sclerosis (arrow). The patient had no known history of pulmonary tuberculosis. (AFIP Neg. No. 68-10302.)

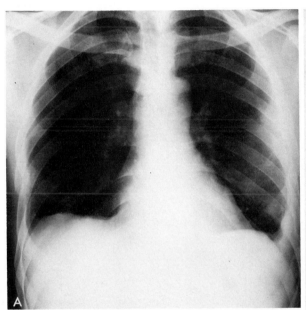

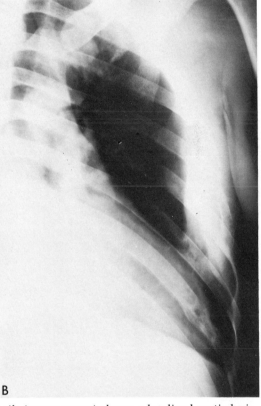

Figure 19–222. Tuberculosis of the chest wall and ribs. This 31-year-old man presented with pain in the left chest wall. *A,* The frontal chest roentgenogram shows diffuse pleural thickening with nodularity, which is greater on the left than on the right but involves both costophrenic angles as well as the left lateral chest wall. *B,* An oblique view shows the inflammatory involvement of two ribs. One rib (upper arrow) shows a localized cystic lysis, with cortical thinning and some periosteal reaction. The other rib (lower arrow) shows another localized cystic lesion, with some expansion and marked cortical thinning. Although the upper rib lesion was contiguous with the tuberculous empyema, the lower rib lesion was remote from the pleural involvement. (AFIP Neg. No. 68-7554.)

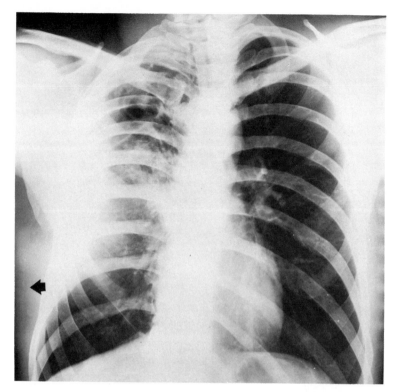

Figure 19–223. Tuberculosis of the right upper lobe and chest wall. The frontal roentgenogram shows right upper lobe empyema and pulmonary parenchymal involvement, with blunting of the right costophrenic angle. The chest wall involvement is manifested by the marked lateral deviation of the fascial planes inferior to the right scapula (arrow) in comparison with those on the left. No bone involvement was found. (AFIP Neg. No. 54-26877.)

Figure 19–224. Actinomycosis. The patient is a 42-year-old male with history of persistent pneumonia with purulent sputum production of three months' duration. The frontal roentgenogram shows infiltrate in right middle and right lower lobes. The inferior border of the right posterior ninth rib is eroded (arrow). (AFIP Neg. No. 63-6934.)

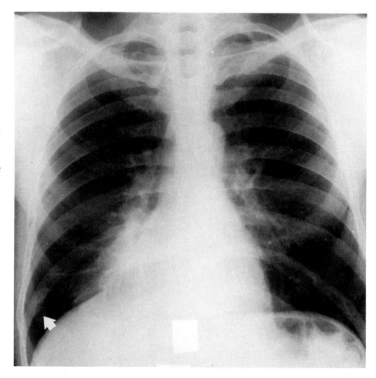

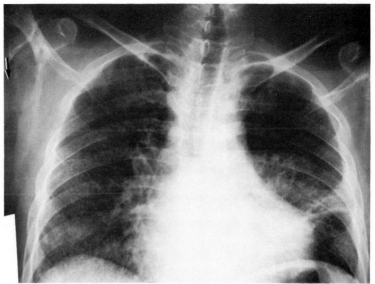

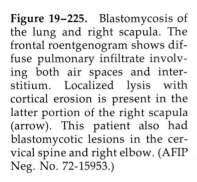

Figure 19–225. Blastomycosis of the lung and right scapula. The frontal roentgenogram shows diffuse pulmonary infiltrate involving both air spaces and interstitium. Localized lysis with cortical erosion is present in the latter portion of the right scapula (arrow). This patient also had blastomycotic lesions in the cervical spine and right elbow. (AFIP Neg. No. 72-15953.)

involve one or more adjacent ribs. Costochondral tuberculosis usually presents as a sharply demarcated area of rib destruction associated with a local soft tissue mass.

Chest wall tuberculosis may occur without rib involvement (Fig. 19–223). This often results from the direct extension of pleural disease, with or without active pulmonary tuberculosis.

Actinomycosis and Other Organisms

Actinomycosis of the chest wall usually occurs by direct extension of active disease from the lung and pleura (see Fig. 19–180; Fig. 19–224).[95] The disease may remain indolent for long periods. Fistulous tracts to the chest wall are frequently encountered. Actinomycosis is differentiated from tuberculosis by active pulmonary pleural disease and often by the degree of its spinal involvement. Vertebral actinomycosis usually spares the intervertebral disc, whereas spinal tuberculosis markedly narrows the disc space.

Many unusual organisms infrequently involve the chest wall. Coccidioidomycosis, blastomycosis (Fig. 19–225), brucellosis, cryptococcosis, sporotricosis, candidiasis,[123] and *Yersinia* pseudotuberculosis[117] have been reported. Most of these infections resemble tuberculosis and actinomycosis in their indolence and are generally distinguishable only by appropriate microbiologic investigation.

References

1. Ackerman, L. V., and Taylor, F. H.: Neurogenous tumors within the thorax. Cancer 4:669–691, 1951.
2. Aegerter, E., and Kirkpatrick, J. A.: Orthopedic Diseases. Philadelphia, W. B. Saunders Company, 1963.
3. Aytac, A., and Saylam, A.: Successful surgical repair of congenital total cleft sternum with partial ectopia cordis. Thorax 31:466–469, 1976.

4. Baffi, R. R., Didolkar, M. S., and Bakamjian, V.: Reconstruction of sternal and abdominal wall defects in a case of desmoid tumor. J. Thorac. Cardiovasc. Surg. 74:105–108, 1977.
5. Barrett, N. R.: Primary tumours of rib. Br. J. Surg. 178:113–132, 1955.
6. Batts, M.: Multiple myeloma, review of forty cases. Arch. Surg. 39:807–823, 1939.
7. Bayer, A. S., Chow, A. W., Louie, J. S., et al.: Sternoarticular pyoarthrosis due to gram-negative bacilli. Arch. Intern. Med. 137:1036–1040, 1977.
8. Beals, R. K., and Fraser, W.: Familial congenital bowing of the tibia with pseudoarthrosis and pectus excavatum. J. Bone Joint Surg. 58A:545–548, 1976.
9. Berk, R. N., and Coulson, D. B.: The body cast syndrome. Radiology 94:303–306, 1970.
10. Beiser, G. D., Epstein, S. E., Stampfer, M., et al.: Impairment of cardiac function in patients with pectus excavatum, with improvement after operative correction. N. Engl. J. Med. 287:267–272, 1972.
11. Beltrami, V., and Gidaro, G.: Resection and reconstruction of the sternum: case report. Thorax 31:350–353, 1976.
12. Bergstrand, H.: Four cases of Ewing sarcoma in ribs. Am. J. Cancer 27:26–36, 1936.
13. Biesecker, J. L., Marcove, R. C., Huvos, A. G., et al.: Aneurysmal bone cysts; a clinicopathologic study of 66 cases. Cancer 26:615–625, 1970.
14. Biesecker, G. L., Aaron, B. L., and Mullen, J. T.: Primary sternal osteomyelitis. Chest 63:236–238, 1973.
15. Binet, E. F., and Markarian, B.: Correlation conferences in radiology and pathology: asymptomatic clavicular lesion. N. Y. State J. Med. 75:1710–1712, 1975.
16. Bowie, E. R., and Jacobson, H. G.: Anomalous development of the first rib simulating isolated fracture. Am. J. Roentgenol. 53:161–165, 1945.
17. Brindley, G. V., Jr.: Primary malignant tumors of the chest wall (excluding primary cutaneous neoplasms). Ann. Surg. 153:684–696, 1961.
18. Bucy, P. C., and Capp, C. S.: Primary hemangioma of bone with special reference to roentgenologic diagnosis. Am. J. Roentgenol. 23:1–33, 1930.
19. Cantrell, J. R., Haller, J. A., and Ravitch, M. M.: A syndrome of congenital defects involving the abdominal wall, sternum, diaphragm and heart. Surg. Gynecol. Obstet. 107:602–614, 1958.
20. Cerat, G. A., McHenry, M. C., and Loop, F. D.: Median sternotomy wound infection and anterior mediastinitis caused by bacteroides fragilis. Chest 69:231–232, 1976.
21. Cohn, B. N. E.: Congenital absence of ribs. Am. J. Roentgenol. 52:494–499, 1944.
22. Cunningham, D. G.: Hematogenous osteomyelitis of the scapula presenting as Erb's palsy. Ill. Med. J. 147:439–440, 1975.
23. D'Agostino, A. N., Soule, E. H., and Miller, R. H.: Sarcomas of the peripheral nerves and somatic soft tissues associated with multiple neurofibromatosis (von Recklinghausen's disease). Cancer 16:1015–1027, 1963.
24. Das Gupta, T. K., and Brasfield, R. D.: Solitary malignant schwannoma. Ann. Surg. 171:419–428, 1970.
25. Das Gupta, T. K., and Ghosh, B. C.: Principles of diagnosis and management of soft tissue sarcomas. Surg. Annu. 7:115–136, 1975.
26. Davidson, P. T., and Horowitz, I.: Skeletal tuberculosis. Ann. Med. 48:77–84, 1970.
27. Dehner, L. P., and Askin, F. B.: Tumors of fibrous tissue origin in childhood. Cancer 38:888–900, 1976
28. Divertie, M. D., and Dahlin, D. C.: Neurilemmoma of rib. Dis. Chest 44:635–637, 1963.
29. Dundon, C. C., Williams, H. A., and Laipply, T. C.: Eosinophilic granuloma of bone. Radiology 47:433–444, 1946.
30. Duthie, R. B., and Ferguson, A. B., Jr.: Mercer's Orthopedic Surgery. Ed. 7. Baltimore, The Williams & Wilkins Company, 1973, pp. 451–476.
31. Edling, N. P. G.: Is the aneurysmal bone cyst a true pathologic entity? Cancer 18:1127–1130, 1965.
32. Emanuel, B., and Young, N.: Recurrent osteomyelitis of the sternum. Ill. Med. J. 152:110–112, 1977.
33. Enterline, H. T., Culberson, J. D., Rochlin, E. B., et al.: Liposarcoma. Cancer 13:932–950, 1960.
34. Enzinger, F. M., and Winslow, D. J.: Liposarcoma. Virchows Arch. Anat. 335:367–388, 1962.
35. Enzinger, F. M., and Shiraki, M.: Musculo-aponeurotic fibromatosis of the shoulder girdle (extra-abdominal desmoid). Cancer 20:1131–1140, 1967.
36. Enzinger, F. M., and Shiraki, M.: Alveolar rhabdomyosarcoma. Cancer 24:18–31, 1969.
37. Enzinger, F. M., and Harvey, D. A.: Spindle cell lipoma. Cancer 36:1852–1859, 1975.
38. Enzinger, F. M., and Smith, B. H.: Hemangiopericytoma. Hum. Pathol. 7:61–82, 1976.
39. Faer, M. J., Burnam, R. E., and Beck, C. L.: Transmural thoracic lipoma: demonstration by computed tomography. Am. J. Roentgenol. 130:161–163, 1978.
40. Fawcett, K. J., and Dahlin, D. C.: Neurilemmoma of bone. Am. J. Clin. Pathol. 47:759–766, 1967
41. Finck, E. J., and Moore, T. M.: Angiography for mass lesions of bone, joint, and soft tissue. Orthop. Clin. North Am. 8:999–1010, 1977.
42. Forrester, D. M., and Becker, T. S.: The radiology of bone and soft tissue sarcomas. Orthop. Clin. North Am. 8:973–998, 1977.
43. Gayler, B. W., and Donner, M. W.: Radiographic changes of the ribs. Am. J. Med. Sci. 253:586–619, 1967.
44. Gershon-Cohen, J., and Delbridge, R. E.: Pseudoarthrosis, synchondrosis and other anomalies of the first ribs. Am. J. Roentgenol. 53:49–54, 1945.

45. Ghosh, B. C., Huvos, A. G., and Fortner, J. G.: Malignant schwannoma. Cancer 31:184–190, 1973.
46. Gorlin, R. J., Vickers, R. A., Kelln, E., et al., The multiple basal-cell nevi syndrome. Cancer 18:89–103, 1965.
47. Gramiak, R., and Koerner, H. J.: A roentgen diagnostic observation in subpleural lipoma. Am. J. Roentgenol. 98:465–467, 1966.
48. Greene, R., McCloud, T. C., and Stark, P.: Other malignant tumors of the lung. Semin. Roentgenol. 12:225–238, 1977.
49. Griffiths, G. L., and Whitehouse, G. H.: Radiological features of vascular compression of the duodenum occurring as a complication of the treatment of scoliosis (the cast syndrome). Clin. Radiol. 29:77–83, 1978.
50. Grmoljez, P. F., Barner, H. H., Wilman, V. L., et al.: Major complications of median sternotomy. Am. J. Surg. 130:679–681, 1975.
51. Haller, A. J., Jr., Katlic, M., Shermeta, D. W., et al.: Operative correction of pectus excavatum: an evolving perspective. Ann. Surg. 184:554–557, 1976.
52. Heiser, S., and Schwartzman, J. J.: Variation in the roentgen appearance of the skeletal system in myeloma. Radiology 58:178–191, 1952.
53. Heitzman, E. R., Jr., and Hones, J. B.: Roentgen characteristics of cavernous hemangioma of striated muscle. Radiology 74:420–427, 1960.
54. Henry, A.: Monostotic fibrous dysplasia. J. Bone Joint Surg. 51:300–306, 1969.
55. Heuer, G. J.: The thoracic lipomas. Ann. Surg. 98:801–819, 1933.
56. Heuer, G. J., and Andrus, W. D.: The surgery of mediastinal tumors. Am. J. Surg. 50:146–224, 1940.
57. Hochberg, L. A.: Primary tumors of the rib, review of the literature and presentation of eleven cases not reported previously. Arch. Surg. 67:566–594, 1953.
58. Hochberg, L. A., and Crastnopol, P.: Tumors of the ribs. Dis. Chest 28:406–414, 1955.
59. Hoeboek, A.: Polyostotic fibrous dysplasia of bone. Acta Radiol. 36:145–154, 1951.
60. Hoffman, E.: Surgical correction of bifid sternum using marlex mesh. Arch. Surg. 90:76–80, 1965.
61. Holt, J. F., and Wright, E. M.: The radiologic features of neurofibromasosis. Radiology 51:647–653, 1948.
62. Hopkins, S. M., and Freitas, E. L.: Bilateral osteochondroma of the ribs in an infant: an unusual cause of cyanosis. J. Thorac. Cardiovasc. Surg. 49:247–249, 1965.
63. Horn, R. C., Jr., and Enterline, H. T.: Rhabdomyosarcoma: a clinicopathological study and classification of 39 cases. Cancer 11:181–199, 1958.
64. Hunt, J. C., and Pugh, D. G.: Skeletal lesions in neurofibromatosis. Radiology 76:1–19, 1961.
65. Huvos, A. G., Higinbottham, N. L., and Miller, T. R.: Bone sarcomas arising in fibrous dysplasia. J. Bone Joint Surg. 54A:1047–1056, 1972.
66. Jaffe, H. L.: Tumors of bone, general discussion. In Tumors of Bone and Soft Tissue, A Collection of Papers Presented at the Eighth Annual Clinical Conference on Cancer, 1963, at the University of Texas M. D. Anderson Hospital and Tumor Institute, Houston, Texas. Chicago, Year Book Medical Publishers, Inc., 1963, p. 47.
67. Jordan, C. E., White, R. I., Jr., Fischer, K. C., et al.: The scoliosis of congenital heart disease. Am. Heart J. 84:463–469, 1972.
68. Jost, R. G., Sagel, S. S., Stanley, R. J., et al: Computed tomography of the thorax. Radiology 126:125–136, 1978.
69. Kelly, P. J.: Osteomyelitis in the adult. Orthop. Clin. North Am. 6:983–989, 1975.
70. Kollins, S. A.: Computed tomography of the pulmonary parenchyma and chest wall. Radiol. Clin. North Am. 15:297–308, 1977.
71. Koutnik, A. W., Kolodny, S. C., Hooker, S. P., et al.: Multiple nevoid basal cell epithelioma, cyst of the jaw and bifid rib syndrome: Report of a case. J. Oral Surg. 33:686–689, 1975.
72. Larsen, L. L., and Ibach, H. F.: Complete congenital fissure of the sternum. Am. J. Roentgenol. 87:1062–1063, 1962.
73. Leigh, T. F.: Acute gastric dilatation. J.A.M.A. 172:1376–1381, 1960.
74. Lichtenstein, J.: Histiocytosis X, integration of eosinophilic granuloma of bone, "Letterer-Siwe disease" and "Schuller-Christian disease" as related manifestations of a single nosologic entity. Arch. Pathol. 56:84–102, 1953.
75. Lieberg, O. U., Penner, J. A., and Bailey, R. W.: Fibrosarcoma presenting as a pseudotumor of hemophilia. J. Bone Joint Surg. 57:422–444, 1975.
76. Locher, G. W., and Kaiser, G.: Giant-cell tumors and aneurysmal bone cysts of ribs in childhood. J. Pediatr. Surg. 10:103–108, 1975.
77. Loop, J. W., Akeson, W. H., and Clawson, D. K.: Acquired thoracic abnormalities in neurofibromatosis. Am. J. Roentgenol. 93:416–424, 1965.
78. McCormick, T. L., Kuhns, L. R., and Perry B. L.: Radiographic changes in children following cardiac surgery performed by splitting the sternum. Radiology 118:141–143, 1976.
79. McMaster, M. J., Soule, E. H., and Ivins, J. C.: Hemangiopericytoma. Cancer 36:2232–2244, 1975.
80. Master, A. M., and Stone, J.: The heart in funnel shaped and flat chests. Am. J. Med. Sci. 217:392–400, 1949.
81. Maurer, E., and DeStefano, G. A.: Eosinophilic granuloma of rib. J. Thorac. Surg. 17:350–356, 1948.
82. Melnick, J. C., and Needles, C. F.: An undiagnosed bone dysplasia. A family study of 4 generations and 3 generations. Am. J. Roentgenol. 97:38–48, 1966.

83. Mir-Sepasi, M. H., Gazzaigga, A. B., and Bartlett, R. H.: Surgical treatment of primary sternal osteomyelitis. Ann. Thorac. Surg. *19*:698–703, 1975.
84. Morgan, A. D., Jepson, E. M., and Billimoria, J. D.: Intrathoracic hibernoma. Thorax *21*:186–192, 1975.
85. Morrey, B. F., Bianco, A. J., Jr., and Rhodes, K. H.: Septic arthritis in children. Orthop. Clin. North. Am. *6*:923–934, 1975.
86. Morrey, B. F., and Bianco, A. J.: Hematogenous osteomyelitis of the clavicle in children. Clin. Orthop. *125*:24–28, 1977.
87. Mosavy, S. H., and Dabagh, H.: Primary sternal osteomyelitis: a case report. Am. Surg. *42*:923–924, 1976.
88. Murphy, D. A., Aberdeen, E., Dobbs, R. H., et al.: The surgical treatment of a syndrome consisting of thoraco-abdominal wall, diaphragmatic, pericardial, and ventricular septal defects, and a left ventricular diverticulum. Ann. Thorac. Surg. *6*:528–534, 1969.
89. Naef, A. P.: The surgical treatment of pectus excavatus: An experience with 90 operations. Ann. Thorac. Surg. *21*:63–66, 1976.
90. O'Brien, J. E., and Stout, A. P.: Malignant fibrous xanthomas. Cancer *17*:1445–1458, 1964.
91. Ochsner, A., and DeBakey, M.: Chone-chondrosternum — report of a case. A review of the literature. J. Thorac. Surg. *8*:469–511, 1939.
92. Omell, G. H., Anderson, L. S., and Bramson, R. T.: Chest wall tumors. Radiol. Clin. North Am. *11*:197–214, 1973.
93. O'Neal, L. W., and Ackerman, L. V.: Cartilaginous tumors of ribs and sternum. J. Thorac. Surg. *21*:71–107, 1951.
94. O'Neill, J. F., Skromak, S. J., and Casey, P. R.: Eosinophilic granuloma of ribs, review of literature and report of two cases with four and six and one-half year follow-up, respectively. J. Thorac. Surg. *29*:528–540, 1955.
95. Oosthuizen, S. F., and Fainsinger, M. H.: Pulmonary actinomycosis. Br. J. Radiol. *22*:152–155, 1949.
96. Pandey, S.: Giant chondromas arising from the ribs. J. Bone Joint Surg. *57B*:519–522, 1975.
97. Pascuzzi, C. A., Daklin, D. C., and Clagett, O. T.: Primary tumors of the ribs and sternum. Surg. Gynecol. Obstet. *104*:390–400, 1957.
98. Poitas, B., Rosenthal, A., and Hall, J. E.: Scoliosis and coarctation of the aorta. J. Pediatr. *86*:476–477, 1975.
99. Pritchard, D. J., Sim, F. H., Ivins, J. C., et al.: Fibrosarcoma of bone and soft tissues of the trunk and extremities. Orthop. Clin. North Am. *8*:869–881, 1977.
100. Probst, F. P.: Chronic multifocal cleido-metaphyseal osteomyelitis of childhood. Acta Radiol. Diagn. *17*:531–537, 1976.
101. Ramsden, R. T., and Barrett, A.: Gorlin's syndrome. J. Laryngol. Otol. *89*:615–629, 1975.
102. Randolph, J. G., Tunnell, W. P., and Morton, D.: Repair of pectus excavatum in children under 3 years of age: a twelve-year experience. Ann. Thorac. Surg. *23*:364–366, 1977.
103. Raney, R. B., Sr., and Brashear, H. R., Jr.: Shand's Handbook of Orthopaedic Surgery. St. Louis, The C. V. Mosby Company, 1971, pp. 293–303.
104. Ravitch, M. M.: The operative treatment of pectus excavatum. Ann. Surg. *129*:429–444, 1949.
105. Ravitch, M. M.: The operative correction of pectus carinatum. Bull. Soc. Int. Chir. *34*(2):117–120, 1975.
106. Reckles, L. N., Peterson, H. A., Bianco, A. J., et al.: The association of scoliosis and congenital heart defects. J. Bone Joint Surg. *57*:449–455, 1975.
107. Reed, J. C., Hallet, K. K., and Feigin, D. S.: Neural tumors of the thorax: Subject review from the AFIP. Radiology *126*:6–19, 1978.
108. Rhodes, K. H.: Antibiotic management of acute osteomyelitis and septic arthritis in children. Orthop. Clin. North. Am. *6*:915–921, 1975.
109. Roberg, O. T.: Chondrosarcoma, the relation of structure and location to the clinical course. Surg. Gynecol. Obstet. *61*:68–82, 1935.
110. Robicsek, F., Daugherty, H. K., Mullen, D. C., et al.: Technical considerations in the surgical management of pectus excavatum and carinatum. Ann. Thorac. Surg. *18*:549–564, 1974.
111. Robbins, P. R., Moe, J. H., and Winter, R. B.: Scoliosis in Marfan's syndrome. J. Bone Joint Surg. *57*:358–368, 1975.
112. Rosenberg, R. F., Rubinstein, B. M., and Messinger, N. H.: Intrathoracic lipomas. Chest *60*:507–509, 1971.
113. Sabiston, D. C., Jr. (ed.):Davis-Christopher Textbook of Surgery. Ed. 11. Philadelphia, W. B. Saunders Company, 1977, p. 2148.
114. Sainsbury, H. S. K.: Congenital funnel chest. Lancet *2*:615–616, 1947.
115. Salmon, J., Shah, P. M., and Heinle, R. A.: Thoracic skeletal abnormalities in idiopathic mitral valve prolapse. Am. J. Cardiol. *36*:32–36, 1975.
116. Schlumberger, H. G.: Fibrous dysplasia of single bones (monostotic fibrous dysplasia). Milit. Surg. *99*:504–527, 1946.
117. Sebes, J. I., Mabry, E. H., and Rabinowitz, J. G.: Lung abscess and osteomyelitis of rib due to yersinia enterocolitica. Chest *69*:546–548, 1976.
118. Seibert, J. J., Rossi, N. P., and McCarthy, E. F.: A primary rib tumor in a newborn. J. Pediatr. Surg. *11*:1031–1032, 1976.

119. Sethi, R. S., Climie, A. R. W., and Tuttle, W. M.: Fibrous dysplasia of the rib with sarcomatous change. J. Bone Joint Surg. 44:183–188, 1962.
120. Shaub, M., Gordonson, J., and Sargent, E. N.: Extrapleural lipoma. West. J. Med. 124:147–149, 1976.
121. Siebold, R. M., Winter, R. B., and Moe, J. H.: The treatment of scoliosis in arthrogryposis multiplex congenita. Clin. Orthop. 103:191–198, 1974.
122. Sinoff, C. L., and Segal, I.: Tuberculous osteomyelitis of the rib. South. Afr. Med. J. 49:865–866, 1975.
123. Smilack, J. D., and Gentry, L. O.: Candida costochondral osteomyelitis. J. Bone Joint Surg. 58:888–890, 1976.
124. Soule, E. H., and Enriquez, P.: Atypical fibrous histiocytoma, malignant fibrous histiocytoma, malignant histiocytoma, and epithelioid sarcoma. Cancer 30:128–143, 1972.
125. Srivastava, K. K., and Kochhar, V. L.: Osteomyelitis of the clavicle. Acta Orthop. Scand. 45:662–667, 1974.
126. Steinberg, I.: Huge osteoma of the eleventh, left rib. J.A.M.A. 170:1921–1923, 1959.
127. Stewart, J. R., Dahlin, D. C., and Pugh, D. G.: The pathology and radiology of solitary benign bone tumors. Semin. Roentgenol. 1:268–292, 1966.
128. Stobbe, G. D., and Dargeon, H. W.: Embryonal rhabdomyosarcoma of head and neck in children and adolescents. Cancer 3:826–836, 1950.
129. Stout, A. P.: Fibrosarcoma. Cancer 1:30–63, 1948.
130. Stout, A. P., and Hill, W. T.: Leiomyosarcoma of the superficial soft tissues. Cancer 11:844–854, 1958.
131. Stout, A. P.: Fibrosarcoma in infants and children. Cancer 15:1028–1040, 1962.
132. Stout, A. P., and Lattes, R.: Tumors of the soft tissues. In Atlas of Tumor Pathology. Series 2, Fascicle 1. Washington, D.C., Armed Forces Institute of Pathology, 1967, pp. 17–186.
133. Sycamore, L. K.: Common congenital anomalies of the bony thorax. Am. J. Roentgenol. 51:593–599, 1944.
134. Tatelman, M., and Drouillard, J. P.: Tuberculosis of the rib. Am. J. Roentgenol. 70:923–935, 1953.
135. Telfer, N.: Nuclear medicine in the management of musculoskeletal tumors. Orthop. Clin. North Am. 8:1011–1021, 1977.
136. Tempo, C. P. B., Rowan, J. A., deLeon, A. C., et al.: Radiographic appearance of the thorax in systolic click–late systolic murmur syndrome. Am. J. Cardiol. 36:27–31, 1975.
137. Ten Eyck, E. A.: Subpleural lipoma. Radiology 74:295–297, 1960.
138. van der Werf-Messing, B., and van Unnik, J. A. M.: Fibrosarcoma of the soft tissues. Cancer 18:1113–1123, 1965.
139. Verska, J. J.: Surgical repair of total cleft sternum. J. Thorac. Cardiovasc. Surg. 69:301–305, 1975.
140. Vieta, J. O., and Maier, H. C.: Tumors of the sternum. Int. Abstr. Surg. 114:513–525, 1962.
141. Waldvogel, F. A., Medoff, G., and Morton, N. S.: Osteomyelitis: a review of clinical features, therapeutic considerations and unusual aspects. Part I. N. Engl. J. Med. 282:198, 1970.
142. Weinstein, R. A., Jones, E. L., Schwarzmann, S. W., et al.: Sternal osteomyelitis and mediastinitis after open-heart operation: pathogenesis and prevention. Ann. Thorac. Surg. 21:442–444, 1976.
143. Weiss, S. W., and Enzinger, F. M.: Myxoid variant of malignant fibrous histiocytoma. Cancer 39:1672–1685, 1977.
144. Welch, K. J.: Satisfactory surgical correction of pectus excavatum deformity in childhood. A limited opportunity. J. Thorac. Surg. 36:697–713, 1958.
145. White, R. I., Jr., Jordan, C. E., Fischer, K. C., et al.: Skeletal changes associated with adolescent congenital heart disease. Am. J. Roentgenol. 116:531–538, 1972.
146. Winham, A. J.: Ewing's tumor of a rib with pulmonary metastasis: report of a case with a ten year survival. Am. J. Roentgenol. 71:445–447, 1954.
147. Wolfel, D. A., and Dennis, J. W.: Multiple myeloma of the chest wall. Am. J. Roentgenol. 89:1241–1245, 1963.
148. Yaghmai, I.: Angiographic features of fibromas and fibrosarcomas. Radiology 124:57–64, 1977.
149. Yaghmai, I.: Angiographic manifestations of soft-tissue and osseous hemangiopericytomas. Radiology 126:653–659, 1977.
150. Zimmer, J. F., Dahlin, C., Pugh, D. G., et al.: Fibrous dysplasia of bone: analysis of 15 cases of surgically verified costal fibrous dysplasia. J. Thorac. Surg. 31:488–496, 1956.

Part XI
Iatrogenic Lesions of the Lungs

WILLIAM J. TUDDENHAM, M.D.

With the development in recent years of increasingly aggressive diagnostic and therapeutic procedures, iatrogenic disease has become an increasingly important consideration in the differential diagnosis of lesions of the chest.

Iatrogenic lesions arising from the mechanical trauma of surgical procedures, including biopsy and various other diagnostic techniques, have been considered in several other chapters of these volumes; they are presented here only in summary form.

PULMONARY LESIONS INDUCED BY DRUG THERAPY

Mechanism of Action

We tend to speak of *the* problem of drug-induced pulmonary disease as if all such lesions shared a common origin. Such, of course, is far from the truth; various drugs induce pulmonary lesions by a variety of mechanisms. Some reactions, exemplified by the cardiotoxic reaction to Adriamycin, are true toxic reactions. They are predictable, dose-related, and reproducible in experimental animals. Others, such as those produced by nitrofurantoin, are apparently idiosyncratic or are hypersensitivity reactions. They are essentially unpredictable, affect only a limited number of people, are not dose-dependent, and are not reproducible in animals.

In explanation of the mechanism of hypersensitivity (allergic) reactions, it is said that many drugs combine with proteins *in vivo* to form antigenic conjugates that induce the formation of antibodies. Antigen and antibody then react in the presence of complement to produce specific lesions. It is this sort of reaction, producing inflammatory lesions in very small vessels, for example, that is thought to give rise to the lupus syndrome, a type of adverse response that is associated with more than a score of drugs.[27]

The unpredictability of idiosyncratic and hypersensitivity reactions and their relative infrequency may be explained by an interesting theory advanced by Peters. He has proposed that the drug itself may be nontoxic but that some genetically determined people possess enzyme systems that convert the nontoxic agent to a lethal one via metabolic pathways normally present in the cell — a process for which Peters has coined the phrase "lethal synthesis."[23] An extension of this concept suggests that cellular response to interaction with drugs or their metabolic products may include cellular adaptation or transformation, including the induced activation of enzyme systems. It is proposed, therefore, that the unpredictability of idiosyncratic and hypersensitivity reactions depends not on the specific drug but rather on the presence or inducibility of enzyme systems capable of metabolizing the drug to a toxic product.[30]

Problems of Diagnosis

Whatever the mechanisms, a host of drugs are known to be capable of inducing pulmonary lesions. Such lesions produce profound morbidity and may be fatal.

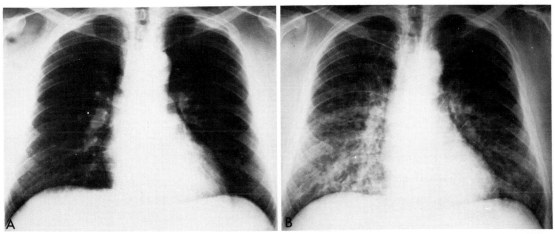

Figure 19–226. Rechallenge to establish drug responsible for adverse reaction. Suspected of a hypersensitivity reaction to one of four drugs prescribed for his hypertension, this patient was admitted to the hospital and challenged successively with each agent individually. *A,* Chest radiograph on admission. *B,* Chest radiograph one hour after a challenge dose of hydrochlorothiazide. (*From* Beaudry, C., and LaPlante, L.: Severe allergic pneumonitis from hydrochlorothiazide. Ann. Intern. Med. *78*:251–253, 1978. Reproduced by permission.)

Diagnosis is exceedingly difficult, however, even if the possibility of a drug-induced lesion is entertained. This is true because the radiologic findings are usually nonspecific and because patients frequently receive a number of medications concurrently, making it difficult to establish which, if any, is the etiologic agent in the event of an adverse reaction (see Fig. 19–235). The only way to establish a diagnosis unequivocally is to challenge the patient with the suspected agent to see whether it produces the lesions ascribed to it. This is usually considered too hazardous to risk. In a hospital setting it can be done with relative safety if it is essential to patient management (Fig. 19–226), but even challenging the patient in this way may not establish the diagnosis with certainty if the onset of the adverse reaction is delayed, as in the case of cyclophosphamide.[28]

Radiographic Manifestations

Drugs known to produce pulmonary or pleural lesions are most often classified by their routes of administration or their primary pharmacologic actions (Table 19–8; see Table 19–9 for equivalent drug name). Since the radiologist is seldom aware of the patient's medications, however, it is more useful from his viewpoint to classify drugs in terms of the radiographic manifestations of the reactions they produce. Accordingly, such a classification is attempted here. It should be noted, however, that this classification serves largely to draw attention to the broad spectrum of abnormalities that may be produced by drug reactions and to encourage the radiologist to consider adverse drug reactions in the differential diagnosis of pulmonary lesions. Few drug reactions produce pathognomonic radiographic changes, and to attempt to identify a lesion as an adverse reaction to a specific drug on the basis of its radiographic appearance alone is hazardous indeed.

CARDIAC ABNORMALITIES. Some drug reactions are manifested primarily as cardiovascular abnormalities. Thus, antithyroid drugs in excess, paraaminosalicylic acid, and even resorcinol (in skin lotions) may by virtue of their antithyroid effect

TABLE 19–8. DRUGS KNOWN TO PRODUCE PULMONARY OR PLEURAL LESIONS*

Antibiotics

Nitrofurantoin	Kanamycin
Sulfonamides	Gentamicin
Penicillin	Polymyxin B
Neomycin	Colistin
Streptomycin	Para-aminosalicylic acid (PAS)

Chemotherapeutic Agents

Cytotoxic	Noncytotoxic
Busulfan	Methotrexate
Cyclophosphamide	Procarbazine
Bleomycin	Melphalan
Acute radiation reaction	

Analgesics (including illicit drugs)

Heroin	Aspirin
Methadone	Indomethacin
Propoxyphene	

Endocrine Agents

Corticosteroids
Oral contraceptives
Pituitary snuff

Inhalants

Oxygen	Cromolyn sodium
Mineral oil	Acetylcysteine
Isoproterenol	Polymyxin B

Neuroactive and Vasoactive Agents

Methylsergide	Hexamethonium, mecamylamine, pentolinium
Diphenylhydantoin	Propranolol

Intravenous Agents

Blood	Hysterographic opaque
Lymphangiographic opaque	Particulate matter

Miscellaneous

Drugs that induce systemic lupus erythematosus	Vitamin D, calcium, inorganic phosphate
Hydrochlorothiazide	Radiation
Chlordiazepoxide	Drugs that induce pulmonary infiltrate with
Anticoagulants	eosinophilia (PIE) syndrome

*Adapted from Rosenow, E. C., III: Drug-induced pulmonary disease. Clin. Notes Respir. Dis. *16*:3–11, 1977.

produce cardiomegaly.[1] Other drugs produce, by a variety of mechanisms, the familiar clinical and radiographic picture of congestive failure with pulmonary edema. Propranolol, used to relieve angina, depresses cardiac contractility and thus may produce congestive failure. Adriamycin and its analog daunomycin, are antileukemic agents that may produce cardiomyopathy, leading to congestive failure and pulmonary edema (Fig. 19–227). The development of cardiomyopathy is related to the cumulative dose of the drug and results in death in a high percentage of cases.[18, 26, 34] Imipramine and monoamine oxidase inhibitors are used in the therapy of depression. Imipramine produces congestive failure by damaging the conduction system of the heart; the monoamine oxidase inhibitors are said to produce hypertensive crises in patients whose dietary amine content is high.[1] Methysergide, used for its antiserotonin effect in the therapy of migraine, produces extensive fibrosis of various sites, including the heart valves. Such valvular lesions may result in congestive failure and sometimes necessitate valve replacement.[21]

TABLE 19–9.   EQUIVALENT NAMES OF DRUGS

Generic Name	Trade Name
bleomycin sulfate	Blenoxane
busulfan	Myleran
chlorambucil	Leukeran
cyclophosphamide	Cytoxan
diphenylhydantoin (see phenytoin)	
daunorubicin (rubidomycin)	Daunomycin*
doxorubicin	Adriamycin
5-fluorouracil	Fluorouracil
hexamethonium**	
hydralazine hydrochloride	Apresazide, Apresoline, Dralserp, Dralzine, Hydrotensin-Plus, Ser-Ap-Es, Serpasil-Apresoline, Unipres
imipramine hydrochloride	Imavate, Janimine, Presamine, SK-Pramine, Tofranil
isoniazid	INH
mecamylamine	Inversine
melphalan	Alkeran
6-mercaptopurine	Purinethol
methadone	Dolophine
methotrexate	Methotrexate
methysergide	Sansert
monoamine oxidase inhibitors	Eutonyl, Eutron, Nardil, Parnate
nitrofurantoin	Furadantin, Macrodantin, Nitrex
para-aminosalicylic acid	
phenylbutazone	Azolid, Butazolidin, Sterazolidin
phenytoin	Dilantin
procainamide hydrochloride	Pronestyl
procarbazine	Matulane
propoxyphene	Darvon, SK-65, Unigesic-A, Wygesic
propranolol hydrochloride	Inderal
resorcinol	Acnomel cream, Bensulfoid lotion, Komed lotion, Rezamid lotion
vincristine	Oncovin

*Experimental drug
**No longer available

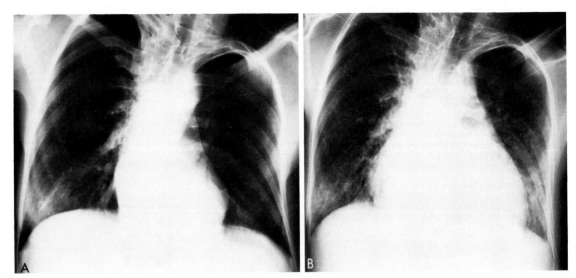

Figure 19–227. Drug-induced cardiomyopathy. Radiographs taken before (*A*) and after (*B*) the administration of Adriamycin showing evidence of congestive failure secondary to drug-induced cardiomyopathy — a life-threatening complication related to total cumulative dose of drug administered. (Courtesy of R. Steiner, M.D.)

LUPUS SYNDROME. The lupus syndrome has been associated with a large number of drugs (Table 19–10), but more than 90 per cent of reported cases have been associated with the administration of procainamide, hydralazine, phenytoin (diphenylhydantoin), or isoniazid. Spontaneous-onset lupus involves the lungs and pleura (Fig. 19–228) less often than drug-induced lupus, whereas drug-induced lupus rarely involves the kidneys.[28]

PLEURAL ABNORMALITY. Pleural effusion is one of the radiologic findings in the lupus syndrome. It may also be seen in the acute form of adverse reaction to nitrofurantoin and is occasionally associated with busulfan lung and pulmonary irradiation.[28]

Methysergide is associated with a pleural abnormality that typically produces bilaterally symmetric areas of "ground-glass" opacity at the lung bases. These shadows have been ascribed by some to pleural fluid, but Rosenow believes that the lesions are largely due to pleural thickening.[28] Such lesions show partial clearing following

TABLE 19–10. DRUGS THAT INDUCE LUPUS*

Aminosalicylic Acid	Oral contraceptives
Digitalis	Penicillin
Ethosuximide	Phenylbutazone
Gold	Phenytoin (diphenylhydantoin)
Griseofulvin	Primidone
Guanozan	Procainamide
Hydralazine	Propylthiouracil
Isoniazid	Reserpine
Isoquinazepon	Streptomycin
Mephenytoin	Sulfonamides
Methyldopa	Tetracycline
Methylthiouracil	Thiazides

*Adapted from Roberts, S. R., Land, W. C., Sewell, C. W., and Nixon, D. W.: Drug-induced pulmonary disease. Weekly Radiol. Sci. Update *48*, 1977.

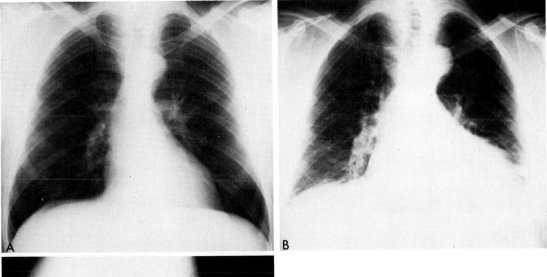

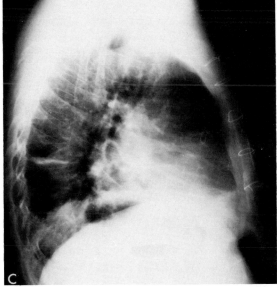

Figure 19–228. Drug-induced lupus syndrome. Radiographs before (*A*) and after (*B* and *C*) the administration of procainamide to control cardiac arrhythmia. Note characteristic findings of hypoinflation, pleural and pericardial effusions, linear atelectasis, and a diffuse pattern of interstitial pneumonitis.

withdrawal of the drug (Fig. 19–229); the lesions are sometimes asymmetric and uncharacteristic in appearance (Fig. 19–230).

MEDIASTINAL WIDENING.   The principal mediastinal abnormality attributable to the administration of drugs is the widening of the superior mediastinal shadow that results from the lipomatosis produced by corticosteroids (Fig. 19–231). The mediastinal fat deposit is part of a generalized pattern of fat deposition, and prominent cardiophrenic fat pads often are a clue to the nature of the mediastinal widening.[1, 27] The absence of tracheal narrowing also helps to distinguish lipomatosis from a true mediastinal mass. Clinically, patients with mediastinal lipomatosis are invariably cushingoid.[28]

HILAR ADENOPATHY.   Hilar adenopathy may occur as part of any generalized hypersensitivity reaction. It is most often seen following the administration of phenytoin, but other anticonvulsants and drugs of other classes that produce hypersensitivity states may also cause hilar adenopathy.[6]

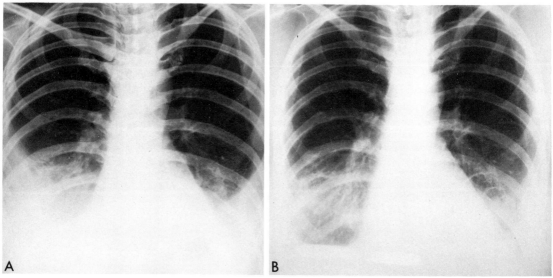

Figure 19–229. Pleural thickening produced by methysergide. *A,* A radiograph taken at the height of reaction shows characteristic bilaterally symmetric "ground-glass" pleural thickening at the bases. *B,* Three years after the withdrawal of the drug, partial resolution of the lesion is seen. (Courtesy of Adele K. Friedman, M.D., Philadelphia, Pennsylvania.)

FOCAL PULMONARY PARENCHYMAL LESIONS. Lesions involving the pulmonary parenchyma are difficult to categorize. A few drugs, however, typically produce focal lesions that may be difficult to distinguish from pneumonic consolidation or neoplasm. For instance, pulmonary infarcts are a well-known hazard in patients using oral contraceptives. The clinical and radiographic manifestations of such lesions do not

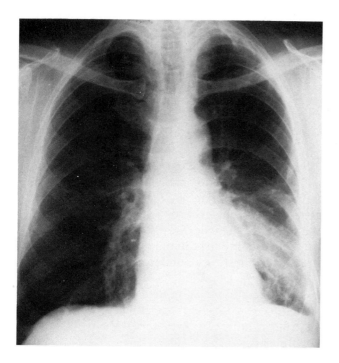

Figure 19–230. Pleural thickening produced by methysergide. A less common, asymmetric, distribution of the lesion is evident.

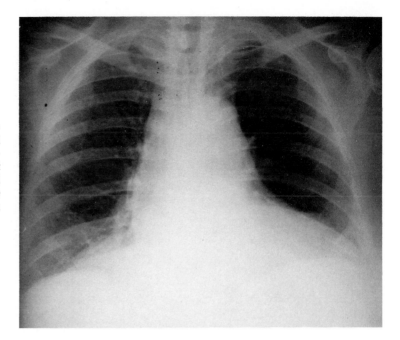

Figure 19–231. Mediastinal lipomatosis produced by prolonged corticosteroid therapy. An innocuous abnormality, the fat deposit does not compress vital structures. (Courtesy of Rolfe Shapiro, M.D. and the American College of Radiology.)

differ from those of pulmonary infarcts of any other source; the diagnosis depends largely on knowledge of the clinical history and on a high index of suspicion.

Lipoid pneumonia secondary to the aspiration of mineral oil or oil-based nose drops may be the most common and most innocuous of the drug-induced lesions.[28] It may take many forms but occasionally produces a focal lesion that is notoriously difficult to distinguish from carcinoma. It is one of only two drug-induced types of pulmonary lesion that can be diagnosed by the pathologist on the basis of sputum cytology (Fig. 19–232).[28]

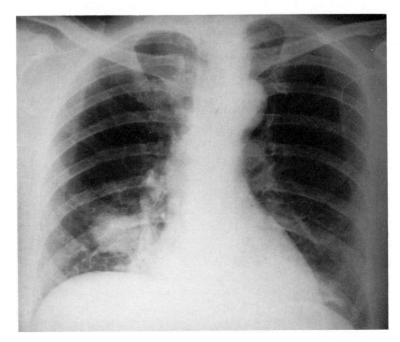

Figure 19–232. Lipoid pneumonia. Focal consolidation such as this is said to be typical of lesions resulting from the instillation of oil-based nose drops. Aspiration of mineral oil by debilitated patients is likely to produce a more widespread aspiration pneumonia.[1] An innocuous lesion, lipoid pneumonia is often resected because its radiographic appearance resembles carcinoma of the lung. The correct diagnosis can be made from sputum cytologic tests if the possibility is considered. (Courtesy of Adele K. Friedman, M.D. and the American College of Radiology.)

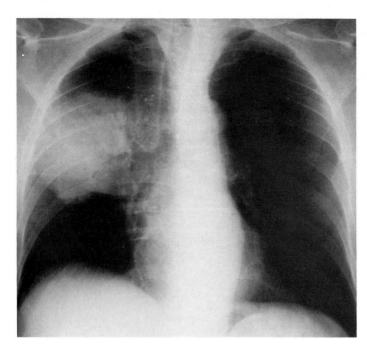

Figure 19–233. Focal parenchymal lesion of infectious etiology. Radiograph showing circumscribed gram-negative pneumonia in a patient on immunosuppressive drug therapy. (Courtesy of Norman Blank, M.D. and the American College of Radiology.)

Other parenchymal lesions that are usually localized, at least initially, and that are in a sense drug-induced are the infectious processes whose rapid development and spread are common problems in patients receiving immunosuppressive or cytotoxic drugs. The reactivation of focal tuberculous lesions, the formation of lung abscesses,[32] and the development of opportunistic infections are well-known complications of these agents (Fig. 19–233).

GENERALIZED PULMONARY PARENCHYMAL LESIONS. Diffuse drug-induced pulmonary parenchymal lesions have been variously characterized as "alveolar," "interstitial," "acinar," "reticular," and "mixed" infiltrates. Such descriptive terms are of little value in the differential diagnosis. The radiographic appearances of drug-induced lesions are nonspecific, and those due to a single agent may vary markedly in appearance from patient to patient (Fig. 19–234). Since the number of such lesions is large, they are subdivided here as a matter of convenience partly on the basis of radiographic appearance (noncardiac edema, interstitial fibrosis) and partly on the basis of associated findings (hypersensitivity state, abnormal cytologic condition of the sputum). This classification does not mean that lesions in one group can be reliably distinguished from those in another by the radiographic appearance alone.

NONCARDIAC PULMONARY EDEMA. Noncardiac pulmonary edema may result from simple fluid overload, a relatively common iatrogenic lesion, or an overdose of heroin. Many drugs (steroids, salicylates, methadone, propoxyphene, and possibly phenylbutazone) cause sodium and water retention and thus induce pulmonary edema.[1, 28] Hexamethonium and mecamylamine, which have been used in the treatment of hypertension, are reported to produce a chronic fibrinous intra-alveolar pulmonary edema.[1, 6]

HYPERSENSITIVITY STATES. Nitrofurantoin is an antimicrobial agent used in urinary tract infections. It is the antibiotic most commonly responsible for drug-induced pulmonary lesions and is associated with three discrete and probably mutually exclusive forms of pulmonary abnormality: (1) diffuse pulmonary infiltrates of acute onset (see Fig. 19–234), (2) a delayed chronic fibrosing lesion indistinguishable

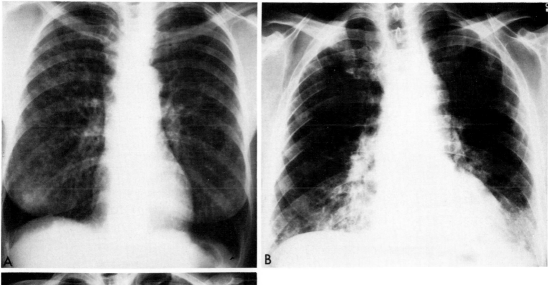

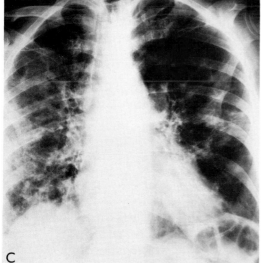

Figure 19–234. Pulmonary lesions produced by nitrofurantoin. Radiographs of three different patients illustrating the nonspecific character of drug-induced pulmonary lesions as well as the wide range of appearances that may be produced by a single agent. *A* and *B,* Acute pulmonary reactions. *C,* Probable chronic fibrosing form of reaction. (*A* Courtesy of Adele K. Friedman, M.D. *B* and *C* courtesy of Robert Steiner, M.D.)

radiologically from Hamman-Rich syndrome, and (3) severe bronchospasm.[28] Ruikka et al. regard the chronic fibrosing lesion as the end-stage of the acute pulmonary lesions.[29] Clinical symptoms in the acute form include chills, fever, myalgia, dyspnea, and nonproductive cough. The acute pulmonary infiltrates probably represent noncardiac edema.[28] They are usually associated with clinical evidence of a generalized hypersensitivity reaction, including lymphadenopathy and eosinophilia. Death has been attributed to both acute and chronic forms of the disease.[10, 17, 29]

The syndrome of pulmonary infiltrates with eosinophilia (PIE syndrome) is typical of adverse reactions to penicillin,[9] occasionally complicates para-aminosalicylic acid therapy, and has been reported in patients receiving isoniazid and sulfonamides.[15]

Thiazides have been reported to produce an acute allergic pneumonitis, but without eosinophilia (see Fig. 19–226).

Methotrexate, used to treat lymphoma; procarbazine, used to treat Hodgkin's disease; and melphalan, used to treat myeloma, all induce acute pulmonary lesions that apparently represent sensitivity reactions (Fig. 19–235). These lesions, too, appear

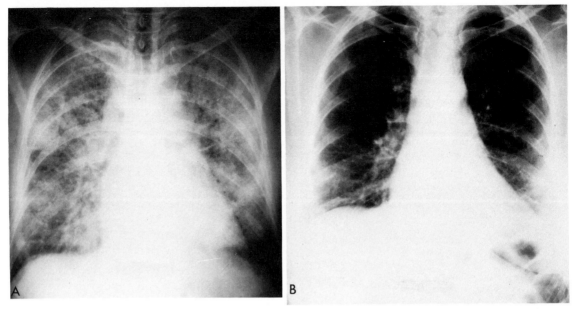

Figure 19–235. Methotrexate lung. *A,* Radiograph illustrating diffuse parenchymal infiltrates, typical of findings ascribed to methotrexate toxicity. *B,* Radiograph showing typical clearing of lesions following withdrawal of all medication. Patient had received multiple drug therapy for acute myelogenous leukemia but was receiving only methotrexate when pulmonary symptoms developed. The diagnosis of "methotrexate lung" was made "by exclusion." Establishing the specific etiology of a drug-induced lesion is often difficult. (*From* Lisbona, A., Schwartz, J., Lachance, C., et al.: Methotrexate-induced pulmonary disease. J. Can. Med. Assoc. *101:*62–65, 1965. Reproduced by permission.)

radiographically as nonspecific pulmonary infiltrates. Histologically, the changes in methotrexate therapy involve primarily the alveolar spaces, with only minimal interstitial involvement. The findings have been described as those of "allergic granulomatous pneumonia."[8]

DIFFUSE "CYTOTOXIC" PULMONARY LESIONS. Busultan, cyclophosphamide, and bleomycin are chemotherapeutic agents that result in the formation of bizarre, atypical type II pneumocytes that can be identified cytologically in the sputum. The onset of symptoms (cough, dyspnea, and fever) and of radiographic abnormalities (Fig. 19–236) does not usually occur until several months after the start of therapy with one of these agents. The lesions may result in a respiratory death,[11] or if the drug is withdrawn, they may regress.[22] In the case of bleomycin, at least, a specific cumulative dosage level (450 mg) has been established, above which the likelihood of pulmonary lesions developing is greatly increased, although fatal reactions have been reported at much lower levels.[13] Critical dosage levels have not yet been established for cyclophosphamide and busulfan.[28] There may be a synergistic effect among drugs of this group and between such drugs and ionizing radiation in the production of pulmonary lesions.[13, 22]

In cases of bleomycin toxicity, the pulmonary lesions are usually "diffuse linear interstitial" opacities.[11, 31]

Pulmonary reactions to 5-fluorouracil, vincristine, 6-mercaptopurine, or Leukeran have not been reported so far (as of 1977).[28]

OXIDANT GASES — OXYGEN TOXICITY. An inspired oxygen fraction in excess of 50 per cent for a period of three days or more produces significant pathologic changes at the level of the alveolocapillary interface. Type I pneumocytes, the epithelial cells that

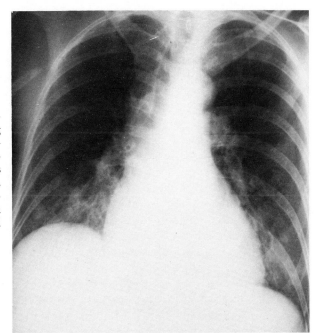

Figure 19–236. Busulfan lung. Since systemically administered drugs reach the lung via the blood stream, the distribution of drug-induced lesions tends to reflect regional differences in pulmonary blood flow. Such lesions usually involve the lung bases predominantly, as seen here, but predominant upper lobe involvement has been reported in a patient with cephalization of blood flow secondary to mitral stenosis.[25]

give rise to the large, exquisitely thin, platelike cytoplasmic extensions that line the alveoli, are particularly sensitive to the toxic effect of oxygen. Capillary endothelial cells are also damaged and often destroyed by oxygen in high concentrations, whereas the type II pneumocyte, a cuboidal cell responsible for the elaboration of surfactant or its precursors, is more resistant. With the death of type I pneumocytes and coincident capillary damage, an exudative lesion develops, characterized by intra-alveolar hemorrhage and hyaline membranes.

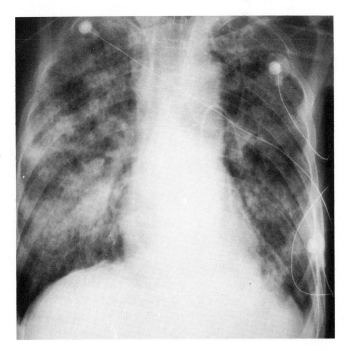

Figure 19–237. Oxygen toxicity. A radiograph exposed shortly before the death of this patient shows diffuse, confluent, bilateral infiltrates typical of advanced oxygen toxicity.

Physiologic repair depends on the proliferation of surviving cells, but type I pneumocytes appear incapable of proliferation; repair, therefore, results in the rapid proliferation of type II pneumocytes, which line the alveoli almost totally within seven days of the initial injury. Thus, the thin cytoplasmic extensions of type I cells are replaced by cuboidal epithelium. This thickening of the barrier between air space and capillary, compounded by fibroplasia, cell debris, and hemorrhage, markedly reduces the efficiency of gas diffusion, producing significant hypoxemia. This in turn results in arteriovenous shunting, which intensifies the hypoxemia and calls for greater concentrations of oxygen in the inspired gas mixture. Thus, a vicious cycle is set up that invariably proves fatal unless interrupted.[2]

The radiologic evidence of oxygen toxicity consists of bilateral patchy areas of opacity, somewhat reminiscent of acute alveolar pulmonary edema, that progress to become confluent and to involve virtually the whole of both lungs (Fig. 19–237).[1, 4] It is important to consider and to suggest the possibility of oxygen toxicity because the vagaries of mixing valves are such that patients may unwittingly and unnecessarily be given dangerously high concentrations of oxygen.[12] With careful monitoring this can be avoided, and with PEEP it is now usually possible to treat pulmonary insufficiency without the use of dangerous concentrations of oxygen. Once thought to progress inexorably to death, oxygen toxicity can be reversed if the concentration of oxygen can be reduced (Fig. 19–238). For this reason it is critically important to recognize evidence of oxygen toxicity in its early stages.

The pathogenesis of the lesions of oxygen toxicity represents, in Weibel's view, the only mechanism by which the lung is able to respond to epithelial damage. Hence one might expect a similar pulmonary reaction to a host of traumatic events and agents. Such a uniform pattern of response does indeed occur, and it is that pattern that has come to be known as the adult respiratory distress syndrome. Also bronchopulmonary dysplasia in infants is probably not the result of the respiratory distress syndrome per se but rather is causally related to the oxygen therapy performed on these infants.[33]

OTHER DIFFUSE PULMONARY LESIONS. Three other patterns of diffuse lung involvement merit comment. First, Brettner et al. state "...there is good documentation

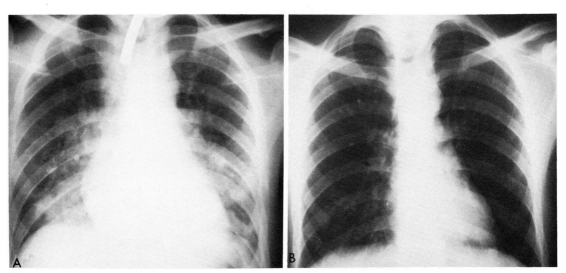

Figure 19–238. Oxygen toxicity. *A*, Radiograph showing early lesion. It was possible to reduce the oxygen concentration in this case. *B*, Complete regression of the lesions is demonstrated. (Courtesy of Adele K. Friedman, M.D.)

that nitrofurantoin, busulfan, hexamethonium, mecamylamine, and methysergide can produce a chronic interstitial pattern on chest radiographs."[6] In the case of nitrofurantoin, this appearance seems to represent a discrete form of adverse reaction unrelated to the acute hypersensitivity reaction. It is probable, however, that two discrete types of reaction do not occur in the case of the other drugs listed. Also, a diffuse pattern of interstitial fibrosis, probably secondary to an allergic alveolitis, has been described in patients who inhale pituitary snuff over long periods.

Second, diffuse pulmonary ossification has been described in busulfan toxicity,[16] and Ansell cites a case of "extensive metastatic calcification" in the lungs, without involvement of other tissues, in a patient receiving large doses of calcium gluconate intravenously together with vitamin D.[1]

Finally, a number of drugs, including acetylsalicylic acid, propranolol, and aerosolized isoproterenol, polymyxin-B, cromolyn sodium, and acetylcysteine, produce bronchospasm,[28] which is manifested radiographically by diffuse pulmonary hyperinflation.

DIFFERENTIAL DIAGNOSTIC CONSIDERATIONS. In hospital practice, it is exceedingly difficult to distinguish pulmonary lesions resulting from adverse drug reactions from pulmonary edema, from aspiration pneumonia, and particularly in the case of patients receiving cytotoxic or immunosuppressive therapy, from opportunistic, nosocomial infections.

The radiologic characteristics of aspiration pneumonia and pulmonary edema are well known; nosocomial and opportunistic infections merit brief comment. The contaminated respirator is a notoriously common source of nosocomial infections, most of which are produced by gram-negative organisms. Of these, *Pseudomonas* is by far the most common (Fig. 19–239). Radiologically, such infections are said to occur as finely nodular interstitial patterns of increased opacity that progress to confluent areas of consolidation and often excavate. Pleural effusion or thickening is seen but is not a prominent feature.[25]

An interesting aspect of the problem of opportunistic infection is the fact that the compromised host, in whom such infections are most common, is susceptible to a

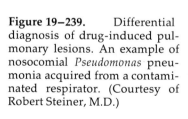

Figure 19–239. Differential diagnosis of drug-induced pulmonary lesions. An example of nosocomial *Pseudomonas* pneumonia acquired from a contaminated respirator. (Courtesy of Robert Steiner, M.D.)

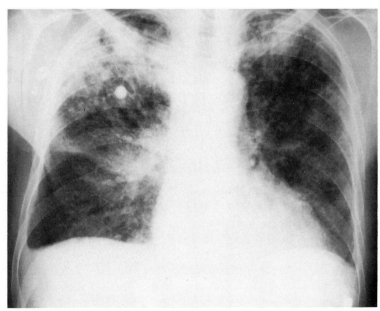

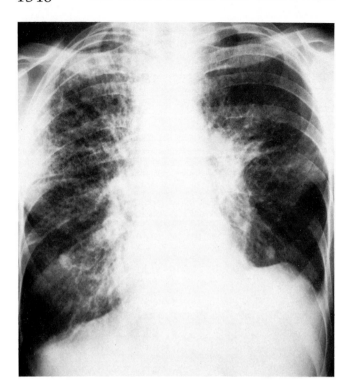

Figure 19–240. Differential diagnosis of drug-induced pulmonary lesions. Opportunistic *Pneumonocystis carinii* infection in a patient receiving radiation therapy for carcinoma of the lung. (Courtesy of Robert Steiner, M.D.)

considerable number of opportunistic invaders including *Pneumocystis carinii* (Fig. 19–240), *Klebsiella,* various anaerobic organisms, and fungi. New infections by new agents may evolve even while the patient is being treated for an initial lesion. In such patients, it is hazardous to assume that a new lesion represents the recurrence of a previous infection. The source of each new lesion must be separately established if appropriate therapy is to be instituted.[4]

Carcinogenic Effects of Drugs

There is yet another aspect to the problem of iatrogenic pulmonary lesions induced by drugs. Many of the immunosuppressive and cytotoxic agents in current use are directly carcinogenic for animals and human beings.[24] The risk of lung carcinoma is increased sevenfold in patients who receive immunosuppressive therapy following renal transplantation; the risk of a second malignancy is increased 23-fold in patients with Hodgkin's disease who receive intensive radiation and chemotherapy.[31]

Effects of Ionizing Radiation

An iatrogenic pulmonary lesion of particular interest to the radiologist is that produced by ionizing radiation. Radiation pneumonitis is generally recognized as an acute exudative process that usually develops within 12 to 16 weeks of the completion of radiation therapy; it is usually, but not always, limited to the portion of the lung that has been irradiated, and it is dose related. (Clinically apparent radiation penumonitis seldom occurs with a dose of less than 1500 rads.) The lesion may regress or go on to dense fibrosis. It is not well known, but radiation pneumonitis occasionally runs a fulminant course, terminating in the patient's death.[5]

Two interrelationships concerning radiation pneumonitis are significant. First, the "sensitizing" effect of actinomycin-D significantly reduces the radiation dose at which acute radiation pneumonitis develops. Braun et al. have suggested that this effect may persist for an extended period (up to at least a year) after the actinomycin-D has been discontinued.[5] Adriamycin may have a similar effect in potentiating and reactivating the effects of irradiation.[20] Second, Castellino et al. have reported the onset of radiation pneumonitis following the administration and abrupt withdrawal of corticosteroids long after the completion of radiation therapy in patients who had previously shown no evidence of radiation pneumonitis. These authors believe that the rapid withdrawal of the steroid in such cases activates occult or subclinical tissue injury resulting from the antecedent radiation therapy (Fig. 19–241).[7]

Therapy

Although the therapy of drug-induced lesions is not truly the province of the radiologist, it should be noted for the sake of completeness that no specific generally applicable therapy is known for drug- and radiation-induced pulmonary lesions. In view of the variety of mechanisms by which they are induced, this is certainly not surprising. In general, patients with such lesions appear to respond well to the withdrawal of the offending drug. The value of steroid administration in the control of radiation pneumonitis appears well established. Steroids have been reported to be helpful in the control of some of the hypersensitivity drug reactions, but in the absence of controlled series it is difficult to assess their true value, and certainly their usefulness is not unequivocally established.

Whereas most drug-induced lesions regress once the responsible agent is withdrawn, some progress inexorably to respiratory failure and death. At the other end of the spectrum, the remission of pulmonary lesions attributed to methotrexate has been reported in the absence of any specific therapy and without withdrawal of the drug.[31]

LESIONS OF THE CHEST PRODUCED BY MINOR DIAGNOSTIC AND THERAPEUTIC PROCEDURES

The complications of major surgical procedures produce extensive morbidity and significant patient mortality; they are widely discussed in the medical literature and are a matter of great concern. The chest complications arising from minor diagnostic and therapeutic procedures are tacitly acknowledged but are infrequently discussed. Endoscopy, biopsy, catheter emplacement, and so forth, are widely regarded as essentially innocuous procedures. In fact, they account for considerable morbidity and some patient mortality. Inasmuch as many of these procedures are discussed in other sections, data concerning them are presented here in abridged form in Table 19–11; only selected procedures are included. Those chosen are judged to be representative of the many minor procedures that have come to be an essential part of medical practice.

Iatrogenic lesions produced through the agency of needles, catheters, tubes, scopes, and the like are usually due to direct mechanical trauma resulting in extrapulmonary gas dissection in the case of injury to the respiratory tract, and in mediastinal, pleural, or intrapulmonary collections of blood in the case of injury to the vascular bed.

Text continued on page 1355

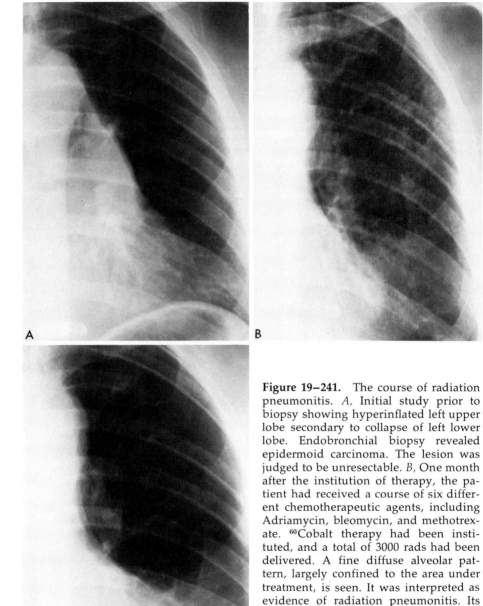

Figure 19–241. The course of radiation pneumonitis. *A,* Initial study prior to biopsy showing hyperinflated left upper lobe secondary to collapse of left lower lobe. Endobronchial biopsy revealed epidermoid carcinoma. The lesion was judged to be unresectable. *B,* One month after the institution of therapy, the patient had received a course of six different chemotherapeutic agents, including Adriamycin, bleomycin, and methotrexate. ^{60}Cobalt therapy had been instituted, and a total of 3000 rads had been delivered. A fine diffuse alveolar pattern, largely confined to the area under treatment, is seen. It was interpreted as evidence of radiation pneumonitis. Its onset was more rapid than usual but may have been accelerated by the sensitizing effect of Adriamycin or possibly by the reported synergism between cytotoxic agents and radiation. *C,* Following interruption of radiation therapy and the administration of prednisone, the alveolar pattern in the left lung has resolved. Such a response would be expected in the case of radiation pneumonitis treated with steroids.

Legend continued on the opposite page

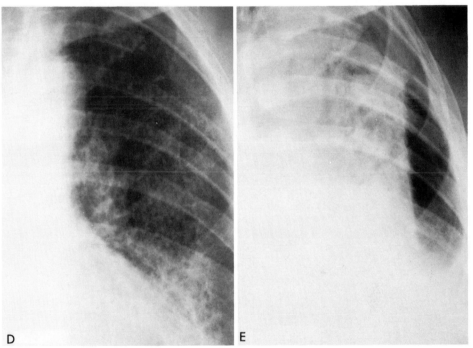

D

E

Figure 19–241 *Continued. D,* Following rapid reduction of the prednisone dosage, the alveolar pattern in the left lung has recurred. This too is consistent with the expected response of radiation pneumonitis. *E,* Twenty-two months after the start of radiation therapy, the lesion in the left lung has progressed to dense fibrosis. This case demonstrates many of the problems of "drug-induced" pulmonary disease, including the difficulty of establishing a precise diagnosis — the diagnosis of radiation fibrosis here is at best presumptive. In addition, this case illustrates the possible effect of Adriamycin in sensitizing the patient to the effects of ionizing radiation; the typical response of radiation pneumonitis to the administration of steroids and to their withdrawal; and the ultimate course of radiation pneumonitis going on to fibrosis.

TABLE 19–11. MINOR DIAGNOSTIC AND THERAPEUTIC PROCEDURES PRODUCING IATROGENIC CHEST LESIONS

Procedure	Reported Complications	Morbidity Rate	Mortality Rate	Source of Data
Fiberoptic bronchoscopy	Hemorrhage* Airway perforation→pneumothorax* Cardiovascular complications (cardiac arrest, arrhythmia) Anesthetic reactions Subglottic edema Bronchospasm Infection	0.3%	0.01–0.03%	Suratt et al., 1976. Review of 48,000 procedures[13] Credle et al., 1974. Review of 24,580 procedures[3]
Mediastinoscopy	Hemorrhage (Fig. 19–242)* Pneumothorax* Vocal cord paralysis* Dissemination of tumor cells Arrhythmia Infection	1.6%	0.1%	Foster et al., 1972. Review of 3742 procedures[5]
Esophagoscopy	Perforation→pneumomediastinum,* pneumothorax,* hydrothorax,* interstitial emphysema,* pneumoperitoneum*	0.4–0.7% with rigid bronchoscope; no data available for flexible bronchoscope	Of those perforated, 0–34% if therapy is prompt; 68 to 75% if therapy is delayed; 26% overall	Quintana et al., 1970[10]
Transbronchial biopsy	Pneumothorax* Hemorrhage*	6.8%	0.2%	Herf et al., 1977. Review of 2628 procedures[6]
Percutaneous lung biopsy	Pneumothorax (1/3 require suction)* (Fig. 19–243)* Subcutaneous emphysema (Fig. 19–243)* Hemorrhage* Air embolism	40%	0.5%	Sargent et al., 1974. Review of 410 procedures[11]
Coronary arteriography	Myocardial infarct Cerebral embolism Arrhythmia Local site complications	3.0% by brachial route 4.0% by femoral route	0.13% by brachial route 0.78% by femoral route. 0.44% overall 0–8.0%	Adams et al., 1973. Survey of 25,000 procedures by each technique[1] Other reported series
Tracheostomy; Endotracheal intubation	Tracheal obstruction Dislocated cuff* Eccentric tip* Endobronchial intubation*	30–49%	3.7% 0–8.0%–range reported	Pemberton, 1972. Compilation of several studies[9]

Procedure	Complications	Incidence		Reference
	emphysema→pneumothorax (may be bilateral) Pneumothorax* Aerophagia* Aspiration (80% with tracheostomy; 20% with endotracheal tube)* Infection Tracheal stenosis (Fig. 19–244)* Hemorrhage* Tracheal dilatation* Tracheal rupture Tracheoesophageal fistula*			
Continuous ventilatory support	Pneumothorax (95% of total with pneumothorax had tension pneumothoraces)*	17% of those on PEEP	16% of those developing pneumothoraces (7% with prompt treatment, 31% with delayed treatment)	Steier et al., 1974[12]
Central venous catheterization	Pneumothorax (may be bilateral if multiple attempts at emplacement)* Catheter embolus (Fig. 19–245)* Air embolus Septicemia (27% on hyperalimentation) Hematoma (Fig. 19–246)* Mediastinal, pericardial, pleural infiltration*	1.2–10%	? 1.4% in a very small series	James, 1974. Study of 3500 procedures[7] Adar and Mozes, 1971[2]
Swan-Ganz catheterization	Pulmonary ischemic lesions Infarction (100% of those left over 72 hours) (Fig. 19–247)* Vascular occlusion Arrhythmia Knotting* Arterial Puncture→hemorrhage Pneumothorax* Infection	7.2%	No data available	Foote et al., 1974. Study of 125 procedures[4]
Transtracheal catheterization	Infection	0.36% (in 1983 procedures)	Rare	Ungar and Moser, 1973[14]
	Subcutaneous emphysema*	5.0% (in 102 procedures)		
	Mediastinal emphysema*	2.0% (in 102 procedures)		

*Radiographically demonstrable

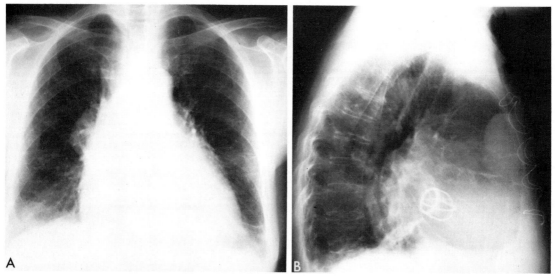

Figure 19–242. *A* and *B*, Posteroanterior and lateral radiographs exposed following mediastinoscopy demonstrate a large anterior mediastinal hematoma secondary to mediastinoscopy. Such lesions, as in this case, are usually better visualized in the lateral than in the frontal view. (Courtesy of Adele K. Friedman, M.D.)

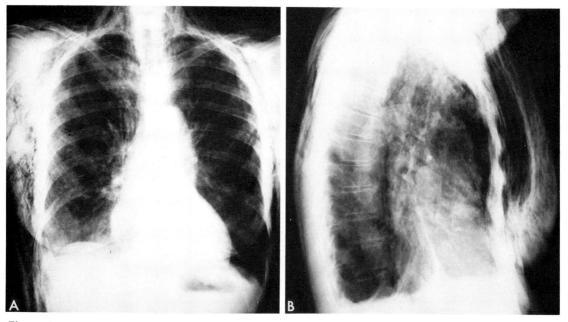

Figure 19–243. *A* and *B*, Posteroanterior and lateral radiographs demonstrating massive subcutaneous and mediastinal emphysema secondary to percutaneous lung biopsy.

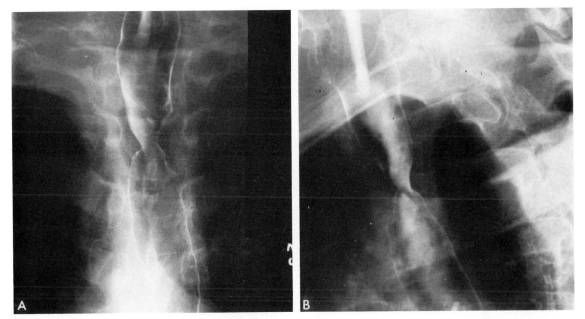

Figure 19–244. *A* and *B,* Two projections of a tracheogram showing tracheal stricture secondary to previous tracheostomy. Multiple dilatations proved unavailing. The lesion was successfully treated by resection and end-to-end anastomosis.

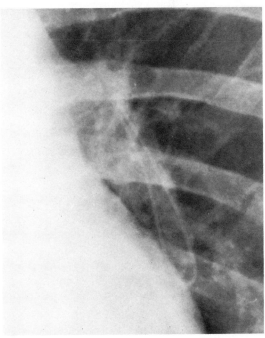

Figure 19–245. Detail of a posteroanterior chest radiograph showing embolized catheter fragment in left pulmonary artery. (Courtesy of Adele K. Friedman, M.D.)

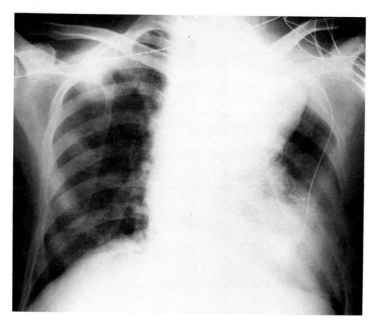

Figure 19–246. Posteroanterior radiograph showing a huge mediastinal hematoma secondary to laceration of the subclavian artery in the course of central venous catheter emplacement. (Courtesy of Adele K. Friedman, M.D.)

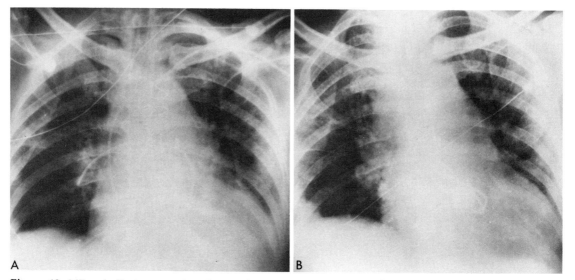

A

B

Figure 19–247. *A,* Posteroanterior chest radiographs showing Swan-Ganz catheter in position in the right lung. *B,* A developing infarct at the right base is seen 48 hours later. (*From* McLond, T. C., and Putnam, C. E.: Radiology of the Swan-Ganz catheter and associated pulmonary complications. Radiology *116*:19–22, 1975. Reproduced by permission.)

Such lesions usually have an immediate onset and, assuming that the radiologist is aware of the antecedent procedure, are easily identified. Representative examples are illustrated in Figures 19–242 to 19–247.

SUMMARY

Iatrogenic lesions due to infection or to the administration of metabolites or medicaments are usually nonspecific and often not temporally related to the precipitating event; for a variety of reasons, the true cause of such lesions may never be established with certainty.

The compromised host — the patient with chronic respiratory insufficiency, the patient on immunosuppressive therapy, the patient with coagulopathy, the neonate — is at greater risk with respect to iatrogenic lesions than the general population.

Because of the increasing incidence of iatrogenic chest lesions, the radiologist's index of suspicion must be heightened, and referring physicians must be reminded that accurate diagnosis depends on the radiologist's knowledge of details of patient management — procedures performed and therapeutic agents administered.

References

Drug-Induced Pulmonary Lesions

1. Ansell, G.: Radiological manifestations of drug-induced disease. Clin. Radiol. 20:133–148, 1969.
2. Bachofen, M., and Weibel, E. R.: Basic patterns of tissue repair in human lungs following nonspecific injury. Chest 65:145–215, 1974.
3. Beaudry, C., and LaPlante, L.: Severe allergic pneumonitis from hydrochlorothiazide. Ann. Intern. Med. 78:251–253, 1978.
4. Blank, N.: Opportunistic fungal infection. *In* Tuddenham, W. J.: Chest Disease (Second Series) Syllabus. Set 8. American College of Radiology Professional Self-Evaluation and Continuing Education Program. New York, Waverly Press, 1975, pp. 308–310.
5. Braun, S. R., Guillermo, A. D., Olson, C. E., et al.: Low-dose radiation pneumonitis. Cancer 35:1322–1324, 1975.
6. Brettner, A., Heitzman, E. R., and Woodin, W. G.: Pulmonary complications of drug therapy. Radiology 96:31–38, 1970.
7. Castellino, R. A., Glatstein, E., Turbow, M. M., et al.: Latent radiation injury of the lungs or heart activated by steroid withdrawal. Medicine 80:593–599, 1974.
8. Clarysse, A. M., Cathey, W. J., Cartwright, G. E., et al.: Pulmonary disease complicating intermittent therapy with methotrexate. J.A.M.A. 209(12):1861–1864, 1959.
9. Geller, M., Kriz, R. J., Zimmerman, S. W., et al.: Penicillin associated pulmonary hypersensitivity reaction and interstitial nephritis. Ann. Allergy 37:183–190, 1976.
10. Geller, M., Dickie, H.A., Kass, D. A., et al.: The histopathology of acute nitrofurantoin associated pneumonitis. Ann. Allergy 37:257–279, 1976.
11. Horowitz, A. L., Friedman, M., Smith, J., et al.: The pulmonary changes of bleomycin toxicity. Radiology 106:65–68, 1973.
12. Hyde, R. W., and Rawson, A. J.: Unintentional iatrogenic oxygen pneumonitis — response to therapy. Ann. Intern. Med. 71:517–531, 1969.
13. Iacovino, J. R., Leitner, J., Abbas, A. K., et al.: Fatal pulmonary reaction from low doses of bleomycin. J.A.M.A. 235(12):1253–1255, 1976.
14. Joffe, N., and Simon, M.: Pulmonary oxygen toxicity in the adult. Radiology 93:460–465, 1969.
15. Jonas, G. R., and Malone, D. N. S.: Sulphasalazine induced lung disease. Thorax 27:715–717, 1972.
16. Kuplic, J. B., Higley, C. S., and Niewoehner, D. E.: Pulmonary ossification associated with long-term busulfan therapy in chronic myeloid leukemia. Am. Rev. Respir. Dis. 106:759–762, 1972.
17. Kursh, E. D., Mostyn, E. M., and Persky, L.: Nitrofurantoin pulmonary complications. J. Urol. 113:392–395, 1975.
18. Kushner, J. P., Hausen, V. L., and Hammar, S. P.: Cardiomyopathy after widely separated courses of Adriamycin exacerbated by actinomycin-D and mithramycin. Cancer 36:1577–1584, 1975.

19. Lisbona, A., Schwartz, J., Lachance, C., et al.: Methotrexate-induced pulmonary disease. J. Can. Med. Assoc. *101*:62–65, 1969.
20. Mc Inerny, D. P., and Bullimore, J.: Reactivation of radiation pneumonitis by Adriamycin. Br. J. Radiol. *50*:224–227, 1977.
21. Munroe, D. S., Allen, P., and Cox, A. R.: Mitral regurgitation occurring during methysergide (Sansert) therapy. Can. Med. Assoc. J. *101*:62–65, 1969.
22. O'Neill, T. J., Kardinal, C. G., and Tierney, L. M.: Reversible interstitial pneumonitis associated with low dose bleomycin. Chest *68*:265–267, 1975.
23. Peters, R. A.: Biochemical Lesions and Lethal Synthesis. New York, MacMillan, Inc., 1963.
24. Podoll, L. N., and Winkler, S. S.: Busulfan lung. Am. J. Roentgenol. *120*:151–155, 1974.
25. Renner, R. R., Coccaro, A. P., Heitzman, E. R., et al.: Pseudomonas pneumonia: a prototype of hospital-based infection. Radiology *105*:555–562, 1972.
26. Rinehart, J. J., Lewis, R. P., and Balcerak, S. P.: Adriamycin cardiotoxicity in man. Ann. Intern. Med. *81*:475–478, 1974.
27. Roberts, S. R., Land, W. C., Sewell, C. W., et al.: Drug-induced pulmonary disease. Weekly Radiology Science Update 48, 1977.
28. Rosenow, E. C., III: Drug-induced pulmonary disease. Clin. Notes Resp. Dis. *16*(1):3–11, 1977.
29. Ruikka, I., Vaissalo, T., and Saarimaa, H.: Progressive pulmonary fibrosis during nitrofurantoin therapy. Scand. J. Respir. Dis. *52*:162–166, 1971.
30. Smuckler, E. A.: Iatrogenic disease, drug metabolism and cell injury: lethal synthesis in man. Fed. Proc. *36*(5):1708–1714, 1977.
31. Sostman, H. D., Matthay, R. A., and Putman, C. E.: Cytotoxic drug-induced lung disease. Am. J. Med. *62*:608–612, 1977.
32. Stein, E. M., Raque, C. J., Harrell, D. D., et al.: Occult lung abscess complicating high-dosage corticosteroid therapy. Postgrad. Med. *51*:97–101, 1972.
33. Tsai, S. H., Anderson, W. R., Strickland, M. B., et al.: Bronchopulmonary dysplasia associated with oxygen therapy in infants with respiratory distress syndrome. Radiology *105*:107–112, 1972.
34. Von Hoff, D. D., Rozencweig, M., Layard, M., et al.: Daunomycin-induced cardiotoxicity in children and adults. Am. J. Med. *62*:200–207, 1977.

Lesions Secondary to Endoscopy, Biopsy and Other Mechanical Procedures

35. Adams, D. F., Fraser, D., and Abrams, H. L.: Hazards of coronary arteriography. Semin. Roentgenol. *7*:357–368, 1972.
36. Adar, R., and Mozes, M.: Fatal complications of central venous catheters. Br. Med. J. *3*:746, 1971.
37. Credle, W. F., Jr., Smiddy, J. F., and Elliott, R. C.: Complications of fiberoptic bronchoscopy. Am. Rev. Respir. Dis. *109*:67–72, 1974.
38. Foote, G. A., Schabel, S. I., and Hodges, M.: Pulmonary complications of the flow-directed balloon-tipped catheter. N. Engl. J. Med. *290*:927–930, 1974.
39. Foster, E. D., Munro, D. D., and Dobell, A. R. C.: Mediastinoscopy. Ann. Thorac. Surg. *13*:273–285, March, 1972.
40. Herf, S. M., Suratt, P. M., and Arora, N. S.: Deaths and complications associated with transbronchial lung biopsy. Am. Rev. Respir. Dis. *115*:708–710, 1977.
41. James, P. M.: Clinical uses of central venous cannulation. Postgrad. Med. *55*:155–160, 1974.
42. McLoud, T. C., and Putman, C. E.: Radiology of the Swan-Ganz catheter and associated pulmonary complications. Radiology *116*:19–22, 1975.
43. Pemberton, L. B.: A comprehensive view of tracheostomy. Am. Surg. *38*:251–256, 1972.
44. Quintana, R., Bartley, T. D., and Wheat, M. W., Jr.: Esophageal perforation — analysis of ten cases. Ann. Thorac. Surg. *10*:45–53, 1970.
45. Sargent, E. N., Turner, A. F., Gordonson, J., et al.: Percutaneous pulmonary needle biopsy — report of 350 patients. Am. J. Roentgenol. *122*:758–768, 1974.
46. Steier, M., Ching, N., Roberts, E. B., et al.: Pneumothorax complicating continuous ventilatory support. J. Thorac. Cardiovasc. Surg. *67*:17–23, 1974.
47. Suratt, P. M., Smiddy, J. F., and Gruber, B.: Deaths and complications associated with fiberoptic bronchoscopy. Chest *69*:747–751, 1976.
48. Unger, K. M., and Moser, K. M.: Fatal complication of transtracheal aspiration. Arch. Intern. Med. *132*:437–439, 1973.

Part XII
Fat Embolism Syndrome

M. SIMON, M.D.
B. A. SACKS, M.D.

Fat embolism is a clinical syndrome usually occurring one to three days after significant trauma, particularly trauma involving fractures of long bones.[1, 3, 4, 6-9] However, pancreatitis, acute fatty cirrhosis in alcoholics, bone infarcts in sickle cell disease, transosseous venography, and lymphography have also been incriminated as occasional etiologic factors.[3, 6] Symptoms occur as a result of fat embolization to the lungs and to systemic organs. Pulmonary symptoms consist of cough, dyspnea, hemoptysis, and pleuritic chest pain. The physical findings may include fever, tachypnea, tachycardia, rales, rhonchi, and a friction rub. Acute cor pulmonale and circulatory shock may result in severe cases. Although all organs are involved in the systemic embolization, the major manifestations are related to the brain (confusion, irritability, stupor, delirium, and coma) and skin (petechiae in the axillae, conjunctivae, and retina).[2] Lipiduria has been used as a diagnostic test, but its value is questionable since it is a common finding in many patients after major trauma. Its absence is probably more significant, effectively excluding the diagnosis of fat embolism.[5]

PATHOPHYSIOLOGIC MECHANISM

After trauma, fat enters the venous blood stream from the marrow space predominantly, a conclusion based upon the finding of other bone marrow particles in the lungs pathologically. Small fat droplets may also pass through the lungs and are then distributed systemically. Theories of the mechanism of lung involvement are twofold: (1) Mechanical occlusion of small vessels, with resultant ischemia, and (2) physicochemical causes. These are summarized in Figure 19–248.

In the Mayo Clinic series 12 of 36 patients died.[2] The most common cause of death is respiratory failure, usually within two weeks after the initial trauma. At autopsy the lungs are heavy and contain bloody secretions in the airways. Histologically, there is extensive intra-alveolar hemorrhage and, to a lesser degree, edema fluid. Alveoli and alveolar capillaries may show fatty vacuoles. If patients survive the pulmonary complications, death may occur from cerebral infarction or hemorrhage, the next most common causes. If death occurs later than a month after the initial event, the histologic evidence of fat embolism will no longer be detectable.

RADIOLOGIC FINDINGS (Fig. 19–249)

Despite clinical symptoms, if the condition is not severe, it may be radiologically undetectable and the chest radiograph may be within normal limits. In the classic presentation, the chest film shows widespread consolidation (due to hemorrhage and edema) with a predominantly peripheral arrangement rather than the central distribution of cardiogenic pulmonary edema. Another differentiating feature is the lack of other signs of left ventricular failure — cardiomegaly, pulmonary vascular redistribution, and interstitial edema. The radiologic findings usually appear about one to two

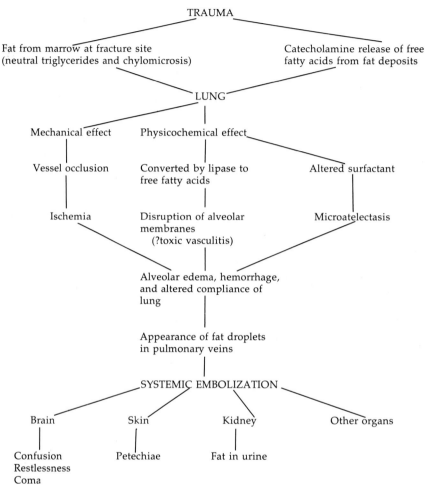

Figure 19–248. Pathophysiologic mechanisms of fat embolism syndrome.

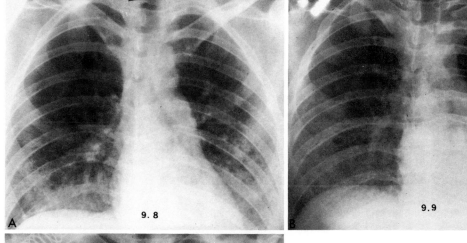

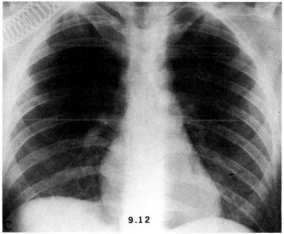

Figure 19–249. Fat embolism. This 23-year-old man developed shortness of breath, hemoptysis, and pleuritic chest pain 48 hours after sustaining multiple fractures in an automobile accident. *A,* Chest x-ray demonstrated peripheral infiltrates in the bases. *B,* These progressed in accord with the symptoms over the next 24 hours. No other cause, such as pneumonia, aspiration, or congestive failure, could be found. Fat globules were found in the urine. *C,* The patient began to improve, and chest x-ray findings cleared. The radiographic and clinical manifestations are characteristic of the fat embolism syndrome.

days after the onset of symptoms and resolve slowly over seven to ten days, although occasionally they may persist up to four weeks.

References

1. Benatar, S. R., Ferguson, A. D., and Goldschmidt, R. B.: Fat embolism — some clinical observations and a review of controversial aspects. Q. J. Med. *41*:85–98, 1972.
2. Burgher, L. W., Dines, D. E., Linschield, R. L., et al.: Fat embolism and the adult respiratory distress syndrome. Mayo Clin. Proc. *49*:107–109, 1974.
3. Editorial: Fat embolism. Lancet *1*:672, 1972.
4. Fraser and Paré: Diagnosis of Diseases of the Chest. Philadelphia, W. B. Saunders Company, 1970.
5. Morton, K. S.: Fat embolism: incidence of urinary fat in trauma. Can. Med. Assoc. J. *74*:441–442, 1956.
6. Moylan, J. A.: Fat embolism syndrome. *In* Sabiston, D. C., Jr. (Ed.): Davis-Christopher Textbook of Surgery. Ed. 11. Philadelphia, W. B. Saunders Company, 1977.
7. Sevitt, S.: Fat embolism in patients with fractured hips. Br. Med. J. *2*:257–262, 1972.
8. Sevitt, S.: The significance and classification of fat embolism. Lancet *2*:825–828, 1960.
9. Weisz, G. M., Steiner, E.: The cause of death in fat embolism. Chest *59*:511, 1971.

20

PULMONARY EMBOLISM

MORRIS SIMON, M.D.
BARRY A. SACKS, M.D.

INTRODUCTION

There are few situations in medicine today in which an incorrect diagnosis, either positive or negative, is more fraught with disaster than pulmonary embolism. There are also few situations in which the diagnostic difficulties and confusion are greater. The risks of inappropriate treatment on the one hand and the denial of needed treatment on the other are substantial. The diagnostic challenge is real, and the radiologist plays a vital role since the major diagnostic modalities are radiologic.

The controversy reflects conflicting viewpoints. On the one hand, Sasahara,[14] Dalen,[5] and others contend that pulmonary embolism is underdiagnosed and undertreated; on the other hand, Robin[13] cautions that it is overdiagnosed and overtreated. Just when we have begun to rely upon noninvasive diagnostic tests, such as the plain chest x-ray and isotopic lung scan,[10] we are warned that without pulmonary angiography we may be taking unjustifiable risks[13] in basing therapeutic action on the simpler tests alone.

The problems are twofold. The first is the confusing nature and varying forms of presentation of pulmonary embolism. It is, in fact, not a disease but a complication of a common complication of a great variety of diseases. The underlying diseases affect many organ systems, and the clinical settings in which pulmonary embolism may be encountered therefore vary tremendously. No two cases are alike. Patients referred to the radiologist come from all clinical services and subspecialties. Some may be hospitalized patients suffering from terminal illnesses, others are being followed in ambulatory clinics, and still others are apparently healthy at the time of a sudden clinical episode. Underlying diseases vary from acute to chronic and embrace a broad clinical spectrum (Table 20–1). They do, however, have in common a tendency to the primary complication of venous thrombosis.

The secondary complication involves detachment of a piece or all of the clot and its migration to the lungs. Not only do the clinical settings differ but the impact of the embolus itself varies greatly according to its size and the medical condition of the

TABLE 20–1. STATES PREDISPOSING TO PULMONARY EMBOLISM

Congestive heart failure
Chronic obstructive pulmonary diseases
Post-traumatic
Postoperative
Postpartum
Thrombophlebitis
Extensive body burns
Carcinoma
"The pill" (hormonal birth control medication)
Diabetes
Obesity, old age, varicose veins, and so forth

patient, particularly the state of the lungs and heart. Such episodes range from trivial and transient to massive and lethal.[14] The clinical severity and form of any particular episode of pulmonary embolism is usually of secondary interest, since the patient has survived it, and the major concern is now the risk of a recurrence, possibly fatal.

The second problem is our still sketchy knowledge of the true incidence, natural history, and effects of treatment. It is clear that the prevalence of venous thrombosis is great. Even though pulmonary embolism occurs in only a small fraction of these cases, it is undoubtedly a major cause of death in any general hospital.[5] The pressure to make a diagnosis is considerable, since venous thrombosis and pulmonary embolism have been shown to be largely preventable and treatable. Therefore, like generals in the field armed with incomplete knowledge of the number, disposition, or plans of enemy forces, we are forced to make decisions that hinge upon assumptions and extrapolations that may prove invalid. One such assumption, recently challenged by Robin, is that all patients with pulmonary embolism can be managed by a single diagnostic and therapeutic protocol.[13] Indeed, it seems likely that patient populations differ greatly and that some may be overdiagnosed and overtreated while others may be underdiagnosed and undertreated. It is probable, for example, that older patients with chronic diseases predisposing to thrombosis may have a higher recurrence rate than those with acute episodes. Further, embolism causes greater damage if there is pre-existing heart or lung disease than if these vital organs are intact. Pulmonary embolism thus represents a far more serious risk for some patients than for others. These are important considerations, since the risk of recurrent pulmonary embolism must ultimately be balanced against the risks of aggressive diagnosis and treatment. It is therefore pertinent to review the present situation from a radiologic perspective, distinguishing well-established approaches from those that are still speculative or controversial.

VENOUS THROMBOSIS

The major launching site of emboli is the deep veins of the lower limbs and pelvis. Only rarely do emboli arise from other sites, such as the right heart, upper limb, neck, or head veins. Superficial leg venous thrombosis is also an unlikely source of emboli, perhaps because the veins are too small and too tortuous, or are more likely to be associated with inflammatory changes and firm clot adherence to the vessel wall. The most significant emboli are of large caliber and originate from thrombi in the popliteal-femoral-iliac system. These are thought to form by proximal propagation from their original sites of attachment in the deep calf veins. Such a thrombus may almost fill the lumen of a large vein without further mural attachments. Thrombosis that remains

TABLE 20–2. INCIDENCE OF DEEP VEIN THROMBOSIS USING ^{125}I FIBRINOGEN*

Clinical Setting	Incidence (%)
Myocardial infarction	23–38
Stroke	60
Hip fracture	48–74
Major abdominal surgery	14–33
Thoracic surgery	26–65
Retropubic prostatectomy	24–51
Gynecologic surgery	14–19
Childbirth	3

*After Hirsh, J., and Genton, E.: Physiological Pharmacology. New York, Academic Press, 1974.

confined to the calf area is considered unlikely to cause significant embolism, and anticoagulant treatment may be withheld as long as the thrombosis remains localized.

The pathogenesis of deep vein thrombosis is related to one or more of the classic triad: (1) slowing or stasis of the venous blood flow; (2) intimal injury; and (3) altered blood coagulability. Perusal of the predisposing diseases (see Table 20–1) confirms that many are associated with circulatory slowing, as in heart failure or prolonged bed rest; with direct trauma to the veins of the lower limbs or pelvis, as in injury or surgery; or with altered blood coagulability, as in malignancy, pregnancy, the postoperative state, or contraceptive pill use. There is an extraordinary incidence of deep vein thrombosis after major thoracic, abdominal, pelvic, or hip surgery (Table 20–2). Following hip fractures the incidence may be as high as 60 to 70 per cent, and following myocardial infarction approximately 30 to 40 per cent.

Clinical Findings

It must be emphasized that symptoms and signs of deep vein thrombosis may be absent in more than 50 per cent of patients (Table 20–3). This complicates the diagnosis considerably, and the presence of deep vein thrombosis may be easily overlooked until after pulmonary embolism has occurred. Classically, deep vein thrombosis presents with lower limb swelling and evidence of thrombophlebitis, i.e., tenderness, redness, and heat.

In recent years a number of excellent tests have been developed for evaluation of lower limb venous thrombosis. These have proved of value not only for diagnosis but

TABLE 20–3. POSTOPERATIVE DEEP VEIN THROMBOSIS AND PULMONARY EMBOLI*

	Postoperative	Deep Vein Thrombosis		Pulmonary Emboli
Total Number of Patients (40 years and over)	132			4 (3% of total)
Positive I-125 Fibrinogen		40	(30% of total)	10% of deep vein thrombosis
Transient		14	35%	
Persistent		26	65%	15%
Popliteal-femoral extension		9	35%	44%
Symptomatic		20	50%	

*After Kakkar, V. V., Howe, C. T., Flanc, C., et al.: Natural history of postoperative deep-vein thrombosis. Lancet 2:230–232, 1969.

TABLE 20–4. TESTS FOR DEEP VEIN THROMBOSIS

125-I fibrinogen
Impedance plethysmography
Doppler ultrasound
Venography
Isotope venography
Fibrin split-products assay

also for evaluation of the progression of the thrombosis or the effects of treatment (Table 20–4). Impedance plethysmography and Doppler ultrasound are both noninvasive tests with a high degree of reliability when positive, particularly if there is thrombosis in the thigh veins or those more proximal.[2] They detect mechanical interference with lower limb venous blood return in the presence of occlusion of major venous channels. However, a negative result with either test does not exclude venous thrombosis, particularly in the calf. Radioactive fibrinogen (I-125) given intravenously localizes in areas of developing thrombosis, which present as hot spots. This test is very sensitive, particularly in calf thrombosis, but requires 24 hours from the time of injection for results. It is of great value in surgical cases when given preoperatively in high-risk patients and in cases of established venous thrombosis under observation for propagation. It is inapplicable in the majority of cases of random pulmonary embolism.

Radioisotope venography using technetium-99 MAA to study flow and "hold-up" is an alternative to positive-contrast venography. It is currently undergoing evaluation, and its role is still uncertain. It can be obtained as a by-product of the lung scan if the technetium macroaggregates are injected via a foot vein on the affected side (or bilaterally in patients with clinically normal-appearing legs). Assay of fibrin split-products in the circulating blood seemed promising, but indirect biochemical tests are technically complex and subject to a significant rate of false positive and false negative results.

The gold standard remains lower limb venography. It must be stressed that for maximum reliability the procedure should be performed by the thorough technique of Rabinov and Paulin,[12] with the examined leg non-weight bearing, without tourniquet, and with the use of large volumes of contrast medium to fill the venous bed when the patient is tilted to between 45 and 60 degrees. Fluoroscopy and spot filming or standard films are used. In this way the previously high rate of misinterpretation is avoided. It should be emphasized, however, that all tests designed to detect lower limb venous thrombosis are of value in the diagnosis of pulmonary embolism only on the basis of guilt by association. The value of these tests in the diagnosis of pulmonary embolism is discussed later in the chapter.

PULMONARY EMBOLISM

Detachment of Emboli

Little is known about the circumstances that initiate the journey of the clot. Uneven distribution of fibrinolytic activity along the length of a thrombus, vigorous or sudden movements of the limb housing the thrombus, increased blood flow during exercise, or fortuitous massage of the lower limbs may initiate the detachment. The emboli are not easily broken off, and many angiographers have negotiated angiographic catheters past or even through venous thrombi without dislodging them.

Prevention

Attempts to reduce the incidence of venous thrombosis have received much attention. Prevention is an obvious way to reduce the incidence of pulmonary embolism, particularly in hospitalized patients. Prophylactic measures have included (1) early ambulation and physical activity; (2) leg elevation at bed rest; (3) stocking compression; (4) prophylactic anticoagulation or "miniheparin" therapy in selected cases; (5) treatment of primary conditions, such as congestive failure; and (6) use of intraoperative devices, e.g., pneumatic boots, particularly in prolonged procedures. These are all aimed at overcoming venous stasis or reducing blood coagulability, prime factors in the initiation of the venous thrombotic process.

Autopsy studies have shown a drop in the incidence of venous thrombosis from 53 per cent in controls to 18 per cent in those who were exercised.[3] The difference was less impressive in living patients studied by ^{125}I fibrinogen, which showed an overall incidence of 25 per cent thrombosis for exercised patients and 35 per cent for controls. Among older patients undergoing major surgery there was a very significant difference between the exercised and the control groups: 24 per cent (exercised) versus 61 per cent (nonexercised).

Low-dose or "mini-" heparin involves the use of 5000 units of heparin 2 hours preoperatively followed by 5000 units 8 to 12 hours postoperatively until the patient is ambulatory. Dosages and duration of anticoagulation vary from one institution to another. Many studies have been done to evaluate this prophylactic modality, using I-125 fibrinogen, impedance plethysmography, and venography. Most have shown significant reduction of venous thrombosis.[7] However, despite a multicenter trial involving over 4000 patients, it has still not been possible to demonstrate a comparable significant reduction of postoperative pulmonary embolism.[9]

Size of Embolus

It is highly probable that small emboli occur commonly, and perhaps even normally, during lysis of peripheral venous thrombi but are easily controlled by the inherent thrombolytic activity of the circulating blood and the enhanced thrombolytic mechanisms of the lung. This may account for transient areas of nonperfusion sometimes seen on lung scans in young and apparently normal subjects. Emboli associated with clinical symptoms and signs of pulmonary embolism sufficient to bring to the attention of a physician are usually large.

In the UPET study,[20] the majority of recent emboli seen on initial angiography ranged from 5 to 15 mm in diameter and 15 to 150 mm in length. Clearly, these macroemboli would have a significant hemodynamic impact on the lungs, and their presence would be clinically overt. Our angiographic experience indicates that the symptomatic cases of pulmonary embolism represent only a small fraction of its probable prevalence. Milder episodes of pulmonary embolism are rarely brought to our attention. Perhaps this clinical insensitivity is fortunate, since pursuit of a diagnosis in marginal cases would overwhelm most diagnostic facilities. Furthermore, aggressive therapy in many of these "milder" cases could prove to be inappropriate.

Occasionally a patient may have respiratory or cardiovascular symptoms suggestive of pulmonary embolism but angiographically is found to have unexpectedly small arterial lesions. It is possible that these emboli may have been much larger at the time of the original insult and that substantial fibrinolysis may have occurred prior to the time angiography was performed. We have not seen major symptoms of pulmonary embolism associated with small emboli on angiograms performed within 24 hours of the clinical episode in an untreated patient.

The Effect of a "Significant" Embolus on the Lungs

The pathophysiologic consequences of a large thromboembolus or multiple small emboli reaching the lungs are now reasonably well established in animal experiments and human clinical studies.

MECHANICAL EFFECTS. Each embolus is arrested in the pulmonary artery tree at a level appropriate to its size. This may cause complete or almost complete obstruction of main, lobar, or segmental branches with cessation or marked reduction of blood flow distally (Figs. 20–1C, 20–2B, 20–3 to 20–7, 20–8A, and 20–9). Alternatively, an embolus may lodge at an arterial bifurcation as a "saddle," with relatively little reduction of blood flow (Fig. 20–10). There are immediate vessel caliber changes. Beyond the emboli the pulmonary vessels become smaller, probably reflecting the absent or reduced blood flow and lowered pressure. At the site of the embolus the vessel may become locally distended by impaction of the clot owing to the water-hammer effect of the beating right ventricle (see Fig. 20–5A).

REGIONAL VENTILATION-PERFUSION IMBALANCE. Despite the impairment of perfusion produced by an embolus, the lung tissues in that region generally remain viable and air enters and leaves normally (see Fig. 20–3, Fig. 20–11). However, since no gas exchange can occur with the circulating blood this simply represents an increase in the functional dead space. The tissues beyond the embolus remain viable because (a) the lung parenchyma can exchange oxygen and carbon dioxide directly with the air spaces; (2) the bronchial circulation provides a collateral blood supply; and (3) the obstruction is usually not absolute and some blood flows around or through the interstices of the embolus. The nutritional demands of the lung itself are very small.

VOLUME LOSS. There is a reduction in volume of the affected regions of the lung (see Fig. 20–5, Figs. 20–12 and 20–13). The explanation is still unclear but appears to be multifactorial. A local surfactant deficiency is manifest within hours. Surfactant is required to maintain alveolar patency, and its deficiency results in alveolar collapse at a microscopic level. This probably accounts for the loss of lung volume as well as the decreased compliance of the affected region. Additionally, areas of segmental or subsegmental atelectasis are found in the vicinity of an embolus, probably also an effect of surfactant deficiency. Bronchoconstriction may be another factor in the loss of lung volume. This may result from local release of serotonin or histamine from platelets on the surface of the emboli or may result from local hypocapnia due to the sudden cutoff of the blood circulation.

The gross effect of a focal loss of volume is to produce spatial rearrangement of the adjacent lung structures, the interlobar fissures, the diaphragm, and the mediastinum to accommodate to the reduced volume of the affected portion of the lung (see Figs. 20–5, 20–12, and 20–13).

HYPOXEMIA. This mysterious pathophysiologic effect is encountered in about 90 per cent of patients with significant pulmonary embolism and is most severe in patients with massive embolism. The finding implies that some areas of the lung are being well perfused but poorly ventilated, in diametric opposition to the expected V/Q disturbance of pulmonary embolism. This represents physiologic shunting of blood and will produce an increased alveolar-arterial oxygen gradient. It has not been possible to demonstrate gross regions of lung with impaired ventilation and with normal or increased perfusion. In fact, the diagnosis of pulmonary embolism by ventilation and

Text continued on page 1375

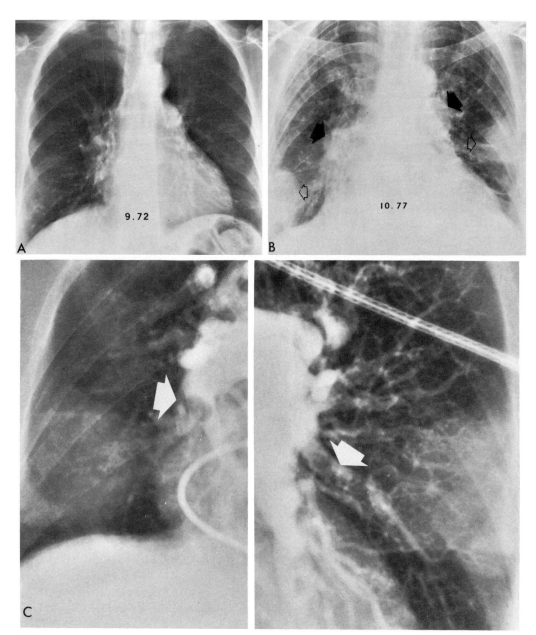

Figure 20–1. Pulmonary infarcts. *A,* A baseline routine chest radiograph in September 1972 shows slight prominence of the main pulmonary artery of unknown significance. *B,* Chest radiograph in October 1977 at the time of presentation with pulmonary embolism shows distention of the right and left proximal pulmonary arteries (dark arrows). Bilateral "Hampton's humps" (open arrows) are visualized peripherally, indicating infarcts. *C,* Confirmatory angiography demonstrates bilateral emboli (arrows) proximal to each infarct.

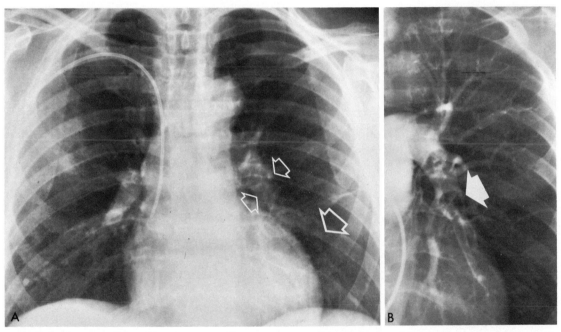

Figure 20–2. Westermark's sign. *A,* Chest x-ray reveals a prominent left main pulmonary artery (small open arrows). There is constriction of pulmonary vessels in the lateral aspect of the left lower lobe (large arrow), and a small plate atelectasis is present laterally. *B,* Arteriographic correlation demonstrates the intraluminal thrombus (arrow) with a ghost outline of the vessel serving this area. There is absent distal perfusion in the lateral lower lung field.

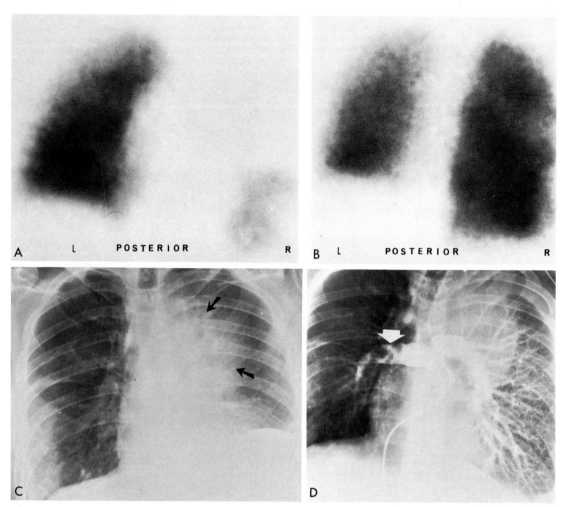

Figure 20–3. This patient with known carcinoma of the left lung and mediastinum (*C*, arrows) developed sudden shortness of breath, severe hypoxemia, and right chest pain. Lung scan shows virtually no perfusion of the right lung (*A*) with normal ventilation (*B*) (V/Q mismatch, greater than lobar). Arteriography (*D*) was performed because there was a possibility of tumor invasion or compression of the right pulmonary artery. This demonstrated a large embolus in the right intermediate artery. Under normal circumstances the combination of lobar perfusion defect with normal ventilation would represent a high probability (94%+) for pulmonary embolism, and arteriography would not be essential.

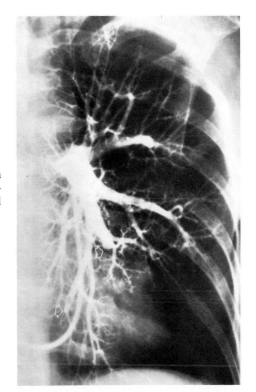

Figure 20–4. Cutoff. Two sharp arterial "cutoffs" (open arrows) indicate pulmonary emboli. Distal perfusion is reduced beyond the more medial cutoff (lower arrow) and absent distal to the more proximal vessel occlusion (upper arrow).

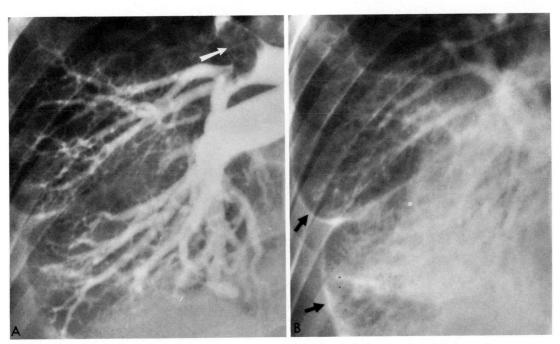

Figure 20–5. Parenchymal stain and distention of vessel by embolus. *A,* Arterial phase demonstrates emboli in the right upper lobe (arrow). The upper lobe vessel is distended by the thrombus, and there is crowding of the lower lobe vessels. A moderate-sized effusion is seen laterally. *B,* A later film in the series shows a dense rim peripherally (arrows), due to compressed subpleural parenchyma, and a dense blush in the atelectatic lower lobe.

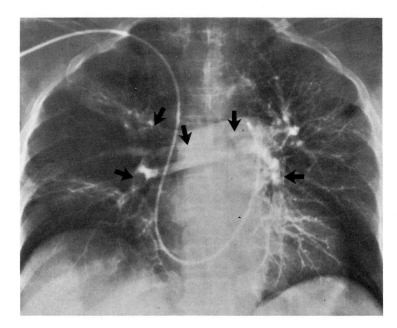

Figure 20–6. Saddle embolus. An extremely large saddle embolus (central two arrows) extends across the right lung to the left. More distally, the major lower lobe branches are involved bilaterally (lower arrows), and another embolus is present in the right upper lobe (upper arrow).

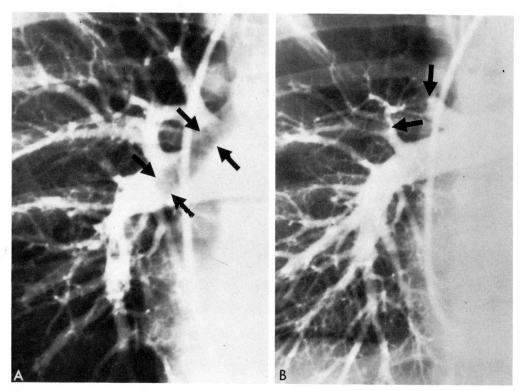

Figure 20–7. Fragmentation. *A,* A large proximal embolus (arrows) is noted in the right main pulmonary artery. Distal perfusion of the right upper lobe is relatively normal. *B,* Forty-eight hours later, fragmentation of the proximal embolus has occurred, and smaller fragments have dispersed peripherally. As a result, perfusion in the right upper lobe has significantly diminished (arrows).

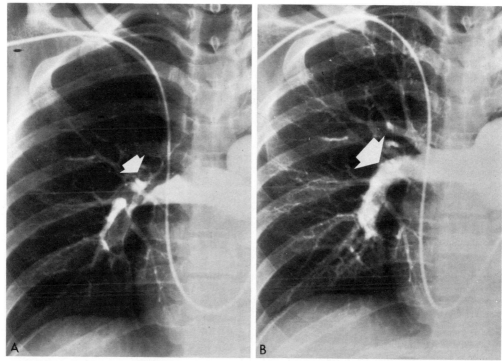

Figure 20–8. Clot lysis. *A,* A large embolus is present in the right pulmonary artery (arrow). *B,* Twenty-four hours following urokinase therapy, the embolus is no longer visualized and the distal perfusion is markedly improved.

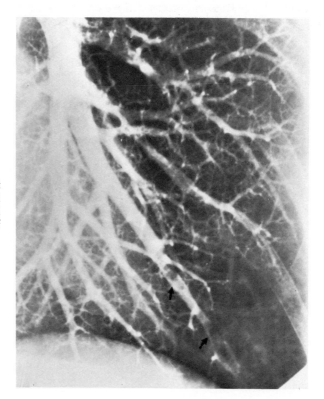

Figure 20–9. Peripheral emboli. Excellent magnification study demonstrating small emboli (arrows) not appreciated on the initial main pulmonary artery injection. (Courtesy of Constantin Cope, M.D.)

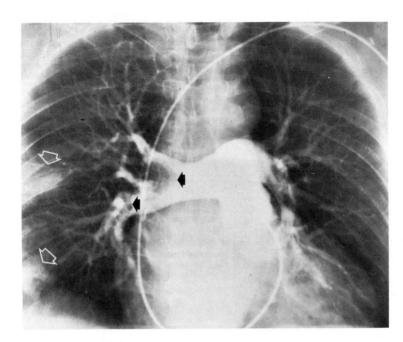

Figure 20–10. Proximal emboli with distal infarcts. Large proximal pulmonary emboli are present (black arrows), while the infarcts (open white arrows) are small and peripherally situated.

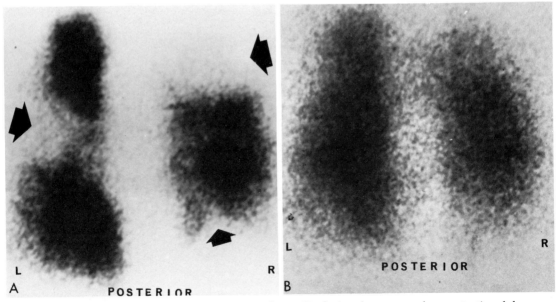

Figure 20–11. Classic lung scan, V/Q mismatch. *A,* Perfusion lung scan demonstrating lobar segmental and subsegmental defects (arrows). *B,* Ventilation scan, first breath. All nonperfused areas ventilate normally.

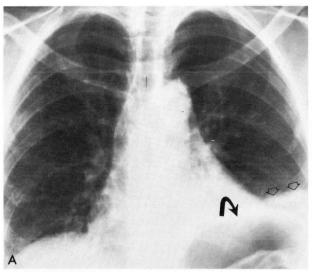

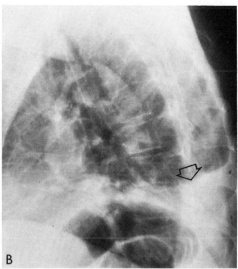

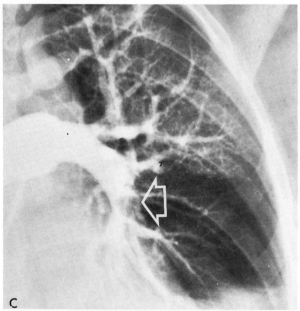

Figure 20–12. Atelectasis with pulmonary embolism. *A,* Chest radiograph reveals left lower lobe consolidation and atelectasis in the retrocardiac region, with elevation of the left hemidiaphragm (curved arrows). The open arrows show a peripheral consolidation. *B,* Lateral view shows left costophrenic angle blunting due to a small effusion. *C,* Arteriography demonstrates an embolus in the lower lobe artery with crowding of the medial lower lobe branches. The obstructed lateral basal segment branch (arrow) is associated with a small peripheral infarct corresponding to the area of consolidation in *A.*

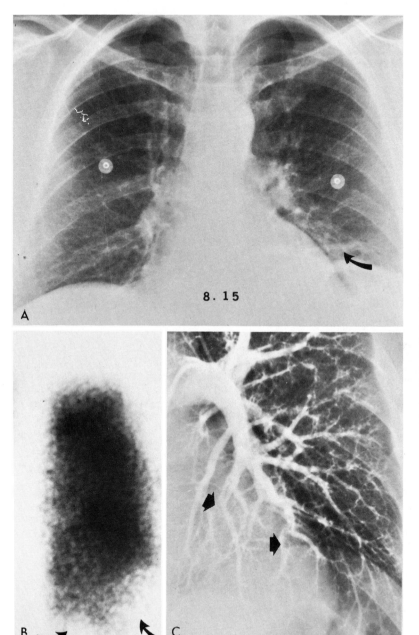

8.15

A

B

C

Figure 20–13. Patient with sudden left pleuritic chest pain on August 15th. *A*, Chest radiograph reveals subsegmental atelectases at the left base (arrow) with elevation of the diaphragm. *B*, The perfusion lung scan shows small subsegmental defects (arrows). *C*, Selective arteriography confirms small emboli (arrows) in segmental branches of the left lower lobe.

perfusion lung scans depends upon the demonstration of the opposite combination, absent perfusion in areas of "normal" ventilation.

It is probable that the shunting occurs at the microscopic level, well below the resolution of the isotope scanning systems, and reflects regional patchy alveolar collapse secondary to surfactant deficiency. Other less acceptable explanations have been proposed, for example, large atelectases that remain well perfused; associated heart failure causing an increase of right-to-left shunting; overperfusion of the remaining normal lung region, and opening up of true intrapulmonary precapillary arteriovenous shunts. It has been suggested that hypoxemia in the recovery phase could reflect reperfusion of previously nonperfused and nonventilated areas of "hemorrhagic alveolar congestion."

PULMONARY HYPERTENSION. Slight pulmonary artery pressure elevation is found fairly commonly in pulmonary embolism, but moderate or severe pulmonary hypertension is seen only in the presence of massive pulmonary embolism (Fig. 20–14) or in patients with prior cardiopulmonary disability and reduced pulmonary reserve capacity.[14] This is probably a direct effect of the mechanical resistance of the emboli, possibly aggravated by reflex vasoconstriction due to release of serotonin or other humoral factors. Patients with a history of heart failure or emphysema, conditions that reduce the pulmonary reserve capacity, tend to develop severe pulmonary hypertension. In such patients, even moderate embolism may be lethal. There is some suggestion that the degree of hypertension may be greater with emboli from recent thrombosis than with aged emboli, but this is controversial.

Rarely, acute cor pulmonale may be encountered in unexpected circumstances with

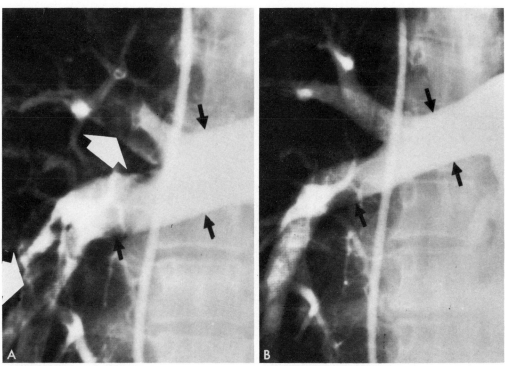

Figure 20–14. Acute pulmonary hypertension. *A,* Patient with massive pulmonary emboli (white arrows). There is marked distention of the main and intermediate pulmonary arteries (black arrows), indicating acute pulmonary hypertension. *B,* After 24 hours the patient has improved clinically. The pulmonary artery size is now within normal limits (black arrows).

submassive embolism, for example, postpartum in previously healthy subjects. No clear explanation is available, although massive vasoconstriction on a humoral basis has been suggested. It has been estimated that at least 50 per cent of the vascular bed must be obstructed for significant pulmonary arterial hypertension to occur.

CARDIAC FAILURE. Acute right ventricular failure (acute cor pulmonale) is a relatively rare event in pulmonary embolism owing to the remarkable reserve capacity of the normal lung, although it is still a popular expectation among clinicians. It is most often encountered in patients with severe cardiopulmonary diseases, usually as the terminal event. Left ventricular failure, on the other hand, is very frequently associated with pulmonary embolism, usually in older patients. The most likely explanation is the sensitivity to hypoxemia of the left ventricular myocardium of those patients with previously marginally compensated coronary artery disease. The alternative sequence of left ventricular failure leading to venous thrombosis and pulmonary embolism is also common, since such patients are often bedridden and have poor peripheral circulation. The appearance of pulmonary edema following pulmonary embolism is almost always on the basis of left ventricular failure.

INFARCTION. The term "infarction" is derived from the Latin word meaning "to stuff into." In Laennec's original description in 1819, it was applied to the filling of the air spaces of the lung beyond an embolus by blood and edema fluid (see Figs. 20–1B and 20–10). Only later was tissue necrosis added to the definition. In fact, the great majority of pulmonary consolidations beyond an embolus are of the hemorrhagic type and are completely reversible. A small minority of the lesions proceed to necrosis and, if the patient recovers, fibrotic scarring (Fig. 20–15). For this reason the term "infarct" should encompass both hemorrhagic and necrotic lesions, particularly as they are indistin-

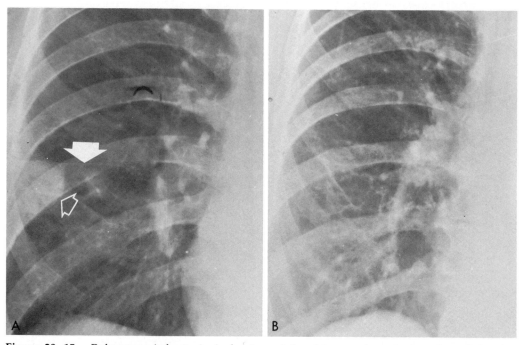

Figure 20–15. Pulmonary infarct. *A,* A classic peripheral hump-shaped parenchymal density (open arrow) is noted abutting the minor fissure (solid white arrow). Notice the constriction of vessels in the middle lobe region and the prominence of the proximal right pulmonary. *B,* Follow-up study shows resolution of the parenchymal density with residual streaks of fibrosis. Larger peripheral pulmonary vessels can now be visualized.

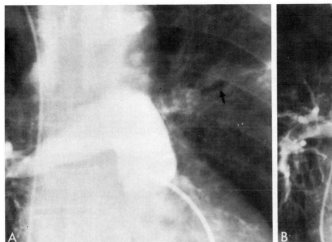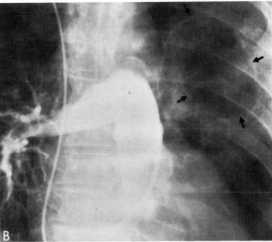

Figure 20–16. Infarct cavitation with development of pneumatocele. *A,* Arteriography reveals complete occlusion of the left pulmonary artery and air within an area of ill-defined consolidation, possibly an infarct (arrow). *B,* Forty-eight hours later, a large pneumatocele has developed (arrows). There is no significant change in the arteriographic findings.

guishable in living subjects except by hindsight. Somewhat less than 40 per cent of patients with pulmonary embolism have a hemorrhagic lesion, and probably less than 5 per cent show evidence of associated necrosis (Fig. 20–16). The conditions necessary for hemorrhagic infarction appear to be (a) complete obstruction of a segmental or larger-sized pulmonary artery; (b) impairment of bronchial collateral circulation, as in congestive heart failure, or (c) chronic airways disease, as in chronic bronchitis and emphysema.

Occasionally an infarct may develop for no apparent reason, for example, in the postpartum period, and other factors, e.g., bronchoconstriction, are presumed to have damaged the capillary and alveolar linings. The hemorrhagic "infarct" will regress and disappear within days or weeks, and the terms "incomplete infarction," "transient infarction," or "hemorrhagic congestion" are therefore preferred by some. The lesions are presumed to result from loss of surfactant and ischemia, which leads to rupture of the normally impermeable capillary-alveolar membranes and results in alveolar hemorrhage.

INFECTION. The infarct serves as a good culture medium, and frequently the general medical condition of the patient is poor. The area of the infarct may become infected within a few days, probably more commonly than is recognized, since fever and high white blood cell count are accepted as signs of infarction even without infection. Infection may be a factor in the development of necrosis and subsequent lung scarring.

EFFUSION. In patients with infarction the incidence of associated pleural effusion is very high (see Fig. 20–1, Fig. 20–17). An infarct without effusion is extremely rare. In general, the larger the infarct the larger the associated effusion, but this is not an invariable rule. On occasion, relatively small infarcts may be associated with large effusions and vice versa. Infrequently, effusion occurs in pulmonary embolism without overt evidence of infarction (see Fig. 20–12). The effusion implies damage to the visceral pleura at the site of an infarction. Its pathogenesis without an infarct is obscure, although associated heart failure may be a contributory factor.

DISRUPTION OF LUNG PARENCHYMA. The lung is a unique organ in that it is continually subjected to distracting forces of ventilation that tend to pull the tissues apart. This is normally resisted by the elastic recoil of the lung parenchyma. Lung tissue

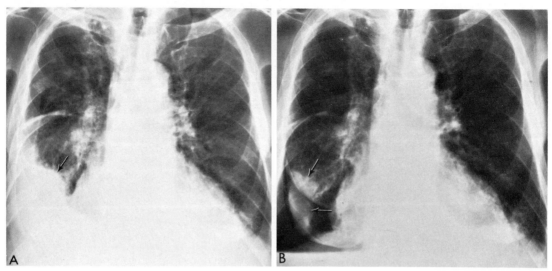

Figure 20–17. Pulmonary infarction with effusion. *A,* The initial chest radiograph reveals a hump-shaped opacity (arrow) in the right lower lobe with an associated effusion. Note the plump right hilus and constricted intermediate vessels. *B,* Following thoracentesis and introduction of a small amount of air, the characteristic infarcts are seen in subpleural locations (arrows) in the partially collapsed lower and middle lobes.

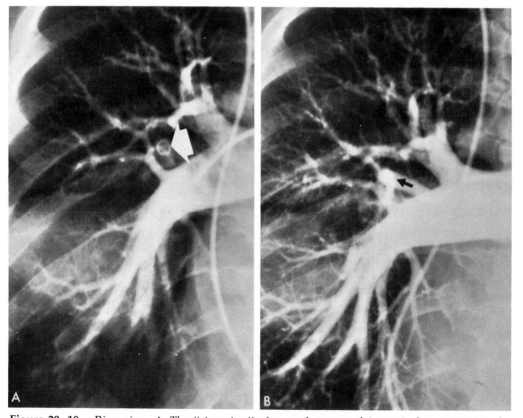

Figure 20–18. Ring sign. *A,* The "ring sign" of an end-on vessel (arrow), demonstrating the embolus outlined by a rim of contrast. *B,* A film taken 24 hours later shows lysis of the embolus and filling of the previously almost occluded vessel (arrow).

weakened by embolic ischemia, infarction, or infection may be torn apart by the negative pressures of breathing. This can result in cavitation or pneumatocele formation (see Fig. 20–16), focal "emphysema," or if the pleura is involved, pneumothorax. These are, however, relatively rare complications of pulmonary embolism.

Fate of Emboli

The patency of pulmonary arteries is almost always restored following nonfatal thromboembolism (see Figs. 20–7 and 20–14; Fig. 20–18). However, the time ranges from days to weeks or even months. The mechanisms involved in this process are as follows.

THROMBOLYSIS. This is particularly effective in the lungs, since in addition to the circulating fibrinolysins there are endothelial fibrinolysins secreted from the lining of the pulmonary arteries. The net effect is more rapid dissolution of the thrombus in the lungs than in a systemic vein. Large clots may disappear in 24 to 48 hours, particularly if they are "fresh," i.e., complicating acute venous thrombosis.

DISPERSAL TO PERIPHERY OF LUNG. In the course of thrombolysis an embolus may disintegrate, and the fragments may be dispersed to small peripheral pulmonary arteries. This restores patency of the large central vessel and improves perfusion of the

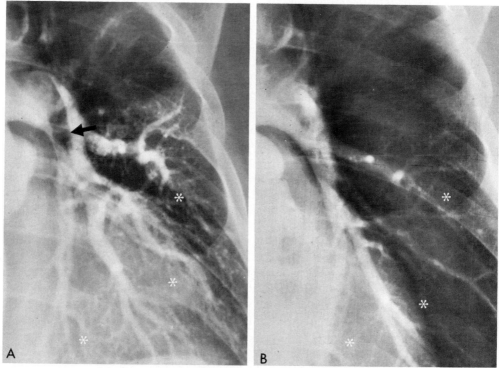

Figure 20–19. Fragmentation of emboli. *A,* Initial arteriogram shows a large proximal left pulmonary artery embolus (arrow) with absent flow into the left upper lobe but good perfusion of the lingula and lower lobe (asterisks). *B,* Forty-eight hours later, the proximal embolus is still seen but is significantly smaller. However, the peripheral perfusion in the lingula and lower lobe is now worsened (asterisks). This is due to fragmentation and dispersion of the emboli peripherally. Such a new perfusion defect on a lung scan could easily be misinterpreted as recurrent, or "breakthrough," embolism.

region beyond. Sometimes an embolus causing incomplete obstruction of a larger branch may fragment and cause total occlusion of multiple smaller branches, so that perfusion may actually worsen peripherally (see Fig. 20–7, Fig. 20–19). Peripheral dispersion may also account for the pruning effect seen on angiograms, although vasospasm may be a factor.

ORGANIZATION. The process of organization of emboli, usually involving those derived from thrombi that have aged for days or weeks in a systemic vein, involves cellular and capillary invasion of the embolus. It results in varying patterns of recanalization and formation of residual intimal plaques, webs, or bridges. Only rarely is there permanent obstruction due to fibrotic stenosis.

All three mechanisms may be involved to a varying degree in restoring patency of the blood vessels. The variations in time, ranging from one or two days to months, reflect the age of the embolus, the size and number of emboli, and the cardiopulmonary and fibrinolytic status of the patient.

Incidence of Pulmonary Embolism

There is general agreement that pulmonary embolism is a very common disorder in any general hospital. However, exact numbers are difficult to derive.

AUTOPSY STUDIES. Routine autopsy examinations, comprising a highly selective patient sample, show a 20 to 30 per cent incidence of pulmonary embolism as the terminal event. Freiman was able to demonstrate that with a meticulous examination technique there was evidence of pulmonary embolism, either recent or old, in 64 per cent of all autopsies in a general teaching hospital.[7a] It is clear from these impressive numbers that the incidence of pulmonary embolism is indeed very high, since the majority of emboli resolve. In fact, it is tempting to conclude that a normal function of the lung is to serve as a "blood filter" to remove particulate by-products of venous thrombosis from the circulation.

IN VIVO STUDIES. The nonspecificity of many of the diagnostic tests for pulmonary embolism other than pulmonary angiography makes it difficult to determine the true clinical incidence of this entity. There is no justification for angiography on epidemiologic grounds. However, Sasahara was able to demonstrate an incidence of pulmonary embolism in 23 of 1000 inpatient admissions at the Veterans' Administration Hospital in West Roxbury, Massachusetts.[14] These patients were selected on the basis of a clinical suspicion of pulmonary embolism supported by positive lung scan, and all were followed by angiography.

If the population of this hospital is considered representative, the numbers can be extrapolated to 630,000 nonfatal and about 200,000 fatal cases of pulmonary embolism per year in the United States. These numbers closely correlate with an independent study by Dalen and Alpert (Table 20–5).[4] The fatal cases (200,000 per year) can be further subdivided into about 50,000 in which the embolism is the primary cause and 150,000 in which it is a contributory factor. To bring these numbers into clearer perspective, a 500-bed hospital admitting 15,000 in-patients per year should encounter 345 cases of pulmonary embolism per year or almost one patient per day. Of these, about 220 will remain undiagnosed.

On this basis, Sasahara argues persuasively that the condition is greatly under-diagnosed, even in teaching hospitals.[14] It should be pointed out, however, that many of the patients in Veterans' Hospitals have chronic heart and lung disease and are particularly vulnerable to this complication. Robin argues on the contrary that in the subpopulation of previously normal patients the incidence of pulmonary embolism

TABLE 20–5. INCIDENCE OF PULMONARY EMBOLISM IN THE UNITED STATES*

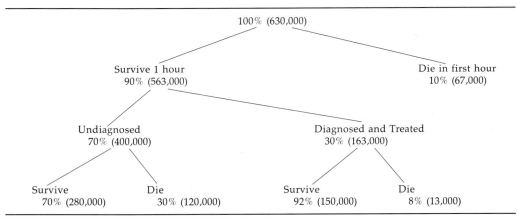

*Adapted from Dalen, J. E., and Alpert, J. S.: Natural history of pulmonary embolism. Prog. Cardiovasc. Dis. *17*(4):259–270, 1975.

must be substantially lower, the recurrence rate lower, and the clinical effects less.[13] In this group we would be guilty of gross overdiagnosis and overtreatment, at great human cost, unless pulmonary angiography was routinely performed.

Mortality Rate

The mortality of pulmonary embolism is radically affected by prophylactic therapy with anticoagulants or venous interruption. In a number of early studies the mortality rate without treatment was 30 per cent. In recent studies of diagnosed and treated patients the mortality has dropped to about 8 per cent (UPET).[18] It is probable, however, that the great majority (at least two thirds) of patients with pulmonary embolism are still not being recognized.[5]

Recurrence Rate

Once pulmonary embolism is diagnosed, what is the risk of a recurrent and possibly fatal episode? Data extrapolated from clinical observation in hospitalized patients give us crude approximations at best. Mortality figures are slightly more helpful. Without treatment, the mortality of pulmonary embolism is 30 per cent; with treatment it is 8 per cent.[18] Treatment is largely prophylactic and succeeds by minimizing the rate of recurrence. The difference in mortality of 22 per cent thus reflects the lethal recurrence rate of untreated embolism. Since less than one third of patients with pulmonary embolism die, the overall recurrence rate in the untreated may exceed 60 per cent.

This very high number is not surprising in view of the nature of the embolic process. If one piece of a long thrombus that is freed into the blood stream breaks off and embolizes, it seems likely that the same separation process will be repeated and other emboli will be released. This is supported by the angiographic observation that pulmonary emboli are almost always multiple, although this could also reflect fragmentation in the right heart. A solitary embolus is rare (7 per cent). The clinical recurrence rate after vena caval interruption averaged 7.3 per cent in a series of studies, with fatal recurrence of less than 2 per cent.[2a] It is clear that IVC interruption is an effective method of preventing pulmonary embolism.

The Clinical Effects of Pulmonary Embolism

The variability and nonspecificity of the clinical findings in pulmonary embolism are well documented in a number of studies. We have learned from experience that the absence of clinical evidence of pulmonary embolism does not exclude its presence. The "classic" presentation (clinical signs of thrombophlebitis, sudden shortness of breath, chest pain and hemoptysis, a normal-appearing chest film, and a perfusion lung scan with multiple segmental or larger defects) is rarely encountered. More commonly, the patient has chronic heart or lung disease or is recovering from recent surgery or trauma (see Table 20–1). The symptoms and signs of the underlying disease, for example, dyspnea, cough, hemoptysis, and tachycardia, overlap and obscure those of pulmonary embolism. Sudden and unexpected changes in severity of symptoms should alert the physician to the possibility of pulmonary embolism. Particularly susceptible are the patient with chronic cardiac disease who suddenly decompensates or develops atrial fibrillation, the patient with chronic pulmonary disease whose dyspnea and cyanosis suddenly become worse, and the immobilized patient who suddenly experiences dizziness or syncope.

The variety of symptoms include, in descending order of frequency, dyspnea, apprehension, cough, pleuritic pain, and hemoptysis. The equally nonspecific physical signs include tachycardia, tachypnea, fever, accentuated P_2, pleural rub, S3 gallop, cyanosis, and hypotension. There may also be signs of thrombophlebitis. These clinical findings vary greatly in their presence, severity, and combinations. The differential diagnosis in these circumstances includes a number of common and rare conditions, notably myocardial infarction, pneumonia, aspiration pneumonia, dissecting aneurysm, pneumothorax, pleurisy, and asthma.

LABORATORY DIAGNOSIS

There is no effective laboratory test for pulmonary embolism. The white blood cell count is normal or moderately elevated, and the sedimentation rate varies widely. Electrocardiographic or vector cardiographic changes are common, although variable and nonspecific. The classic S1-Q3-T3 pattern of acute cor pulmonale is found in only about 10 per cent of patients. Enzyme tests have proved disappointing. The initial suggestion that elevation of LDH and serum bilirubin in the presence of a normal SGOT was diagnostic has been rejected.

The arterial oxygen saturation is a popular test. It is of some value when positive (below 90 mm Hg) only in the relatively young and previously normal person. Unfortunately, hypoxemia occurs in a variety of acute lung diseases, such as viral pneumonia and acute bronchitis. In patients with some cardiorespiratory problem, a Po_2 value above 90 mm Hg would reduce the probability of pulmonary embolism to about 8 per cent. Measurement of fibrin degradation products in the circulating blood also seemed promising but has not proved practical or reliable.

Some of the tests for deep vein thrombosis in the lower limbs may help tilt the scales of probability toward pulmonary embolism in clinically suspicious cases. Caution must be exercised in basing the diagnosis of pulmonary embolism on the association of deep vein thrombosis and respiratory findings. This association is often coincidental, since deep vein thrombosis, pulmonary infections, and cardiac failure are all common problems of hospitalized patients.

RADIOLOGIC DIAGNOSIS

Radiologic studies constitute the most effective approach to the diagnosis of pulmonary embolism.[15] These include the plain chest radiograph, the perfusion and ventilation lung scan, and pulmonary angiography. Lower limb venography has a limited and indirect role.[12] It is the interplay between these tests that concerns the radiologist. The only absolutely certain way of establishing the diagnosis is by pulmonary angiography. However, the use of the less invasive methods in appropriate clinical settings may provide sufficient certainty of pulmonary embolism to justify anticoagulant therapy without angiography. The most valuable noninvasive combination has proved to be the plain chest film and the isotope lung scan (perfusion and ventilation). When positive in patients with a suggestive clinical presentation, this combination has resulted in significantly reduced use of pulmonary angiography. Of all patients diagnosed and treated for pulmonary embolism at our hospital, approximately 25 per cent have had pulmonary angiography. This figure varies from 10 to 70 per cent at different centers, reflecting a wide range of attitudes and practices regarding the degree of certainty necessary for the diagnosis of pulmonary embolism before treatment is instituted.

The Plain Chest Radiograph

The plain film of the chest shows abnormalities in 40 to 60 per cent of patients with pulmonary embolism, all nonspecific findings. On rare occasions, a combination of plain film findings in an appropriate clinical situation may be strongly suggestive of a pulmonary embolism. For example, a peripheral hump-shaped opacity associated with ipsilateral pleural effusion, elevation of diaphragm, regional hilar plumpness, and peripheral vasoconstriction can hardly be explained on any other basis (Figs. 20–1, 20–15, and 20–17).

Despite the great contributions of Fleischner and others, plain film analysis has not proved as helpful as was hoped. Greenspan has challenged the diagnostic value of plain film findings taken in isolation and has emphasized their nonspecificity. However, the plain film findings become more meaningful when they are interpreted in conjunction with the lung scan and when the clinical options are limited. Once the question of pulmonary embolism is raised on clinical grounds, the chest film and perfusion lung scan become obligatory not only in evaluating the possibility of pulmonary embolism but also in diagnosing other diseases with similar presentations (Fig. 20–20).

The plain film findings reflect the pathophysiologic changes of pulmonary embolism that were noted earlier. The appearances fall broadly into three categories: (1) pulmonary embolism without infarction; (2) pulmonary embolism with infarction; and (3) pulmonary embolism complicating pre-existing cardiac or pulmonary disease. The frequency of the findings varies widely with the patient population.

PULMONARY EMBOLISM WITHOUT INFARCTION

"NORMAL" APPEARANCE. The plain chest film may appear to be within normal limits in the presence of multiple small or large emboli. This is particularly true if no recent baseline films are available for the evaluation of subtle changes. The normal

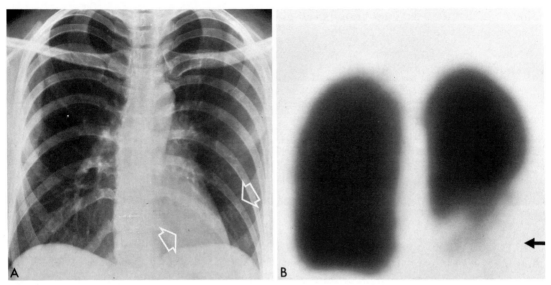

Figure 20–20.   Classic Westermark sign. *A,* Chest x-ray reveals constricted vessels (arrows) to the left lower lobe. No infiltrates, atelectasis, effusion, or proximal pulmonary arterial prominence are noted. *B,* Lung scan reveals no perfusion to the left lower lobe (arrow). As this young and previously healthy patient had a classic clinical presentation of pulmonary embolism, treatment was instituted on the basis of these two confirmatory studies without an arteriogram.

appearance reflects the facts that ventilation remains grossly unimpaired and the viability of the lung parenchyma does not depend entirely on the pulmonary circulation. If a comparison film is available, slight changes in vascular caliber may be detectable. The "normal" chest radiograph is valuable if there is clearly no parenchymal abnormality in regions shown to be underperfused on the perfusion scan. This may be the basis for the diagnosis of pulmonary embolism without angiography in many cases.

VASCULAR CHANGES.   Focal vasoconstriction of pulmonary vessels distal to an embolus (the Westermark sign) is a common plain film finding in pulmonary embolism, occurring in about two thirds of cases, particularly if the changes are unilateral and basal (see Figs. 20–2 and 20–20) and if previous films are available for comparison. According to Greenspan, these changes are often so subtle that they are recognized only in retrospect.[8] Decreased vessel caliber and the resulting local hyperlucency are most readily appreciated at the lung bases, since in the standard upright film the lower zone vessels are normally much more prominent than those in the upper zone (see Figs. 20–2A and 20–20A). An additional supine view may be useful in assessing vascular constriction in the upper zones. The vessels will fail to distend despite the altered posture and the increased blood volume if there is an upper lobe embolus. The size of the oligemic region may range from a single segment to an entire lung.

Focal oligemia must be distinguished from focal emphysema, in which there is separation and bowing of the narrowed vessels, from bullae that are circumscribed and avascular, and also from the bibasilar vasoconstriction of left ventricular failure, which tends to be symmetric and is associated with left ventricular enlargement and sometimes with interstitial edema.

Local distention of the artery at the site of impaction of an embolus may be recognized as a plumpness of a lobar or larger hilar vessel. This contrasts sharply with the constricted distal branches of the same region (see Figs. 20–2, 20–14, and 20–17).

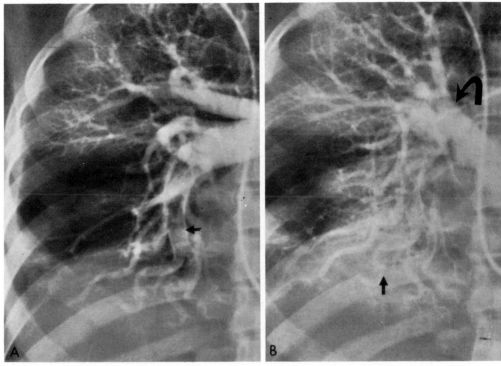

Figure 20–21. Delayed flow. *A,* A large embolus is present as a filling defect in the right lower lobe pulmonary artery (arrow), which appears as a ghost outline. *B,* Marked delay in blood flow is noted in the lower lobe (straight arrow). The upper lobe shows the contrast already well into the venous phase (curved arrow), while arteriolar filling is still present in the lower lobe. The vessels in the right lower lobe also show tortuosity.

The finding is generally unilateral and thus should not be misinterpreted as evidence of pulmonary arterial hypertension.

The plain film findings of acute pulmonary arterial hypertension or acute cor pulmonale are rarely seen (less than 10 per cent of the time) (see Fig. 20–14*A*). These are distinguished from hilar plumpness due to an impacted embolus by their bilateral and symmetric configuration, by their involvement of the main pulmonary artery trunk, and associated generalized peripheral pulmonary vasoconstriction. As the patient recovers, the degree of central arterial dilatation diminishes (see Fig. 20–14*B*). The development of chronic cor pulmonale with persistent vascular changes is extremely rare and usually results from the cumulative effects of recurrent pulmonary embolism, in which individual episodes may be clinically unimpressive. This is accompanied by right ventricular enlargement and subsequent failure.

Loss of Lung Volume. The most common manifestation of regional volume loss associated with pulmonary embolism is unilateral elevation of the diaphragm. This finding is encountered in almost 60 per cent of patients and is best recognized by comparison with a previous film (see Figs. 20–12 and 20–13), since there is a wide normal variation of diaphragm position. On fluoroscopy, the elevated diaphragm is found to move freely in phase with respiration, and there is no evidence to suggest protective "splinting." Other associated spatial rearrangements, such as displacement of a fissure, a hilus, adjacent pulmonary vessels, or the mediastinum, are less obvious but are found occasionally.

Atelectasis. Platelike atelectases are commonly seen as linear shadows in the region of an embolus with or without infarction. Occasionally, typical wedge-shaped opacities of collapsed segmental or larger lung regions are observed in or adjacent to the embolized area. These probably result from airway obstruction by secretions or blood (see Figs. 20–2, 20–12, and 20–13). They must not be confused with infarcts. An infarct never presents as a linear or triangular opacity, although the latter is a common textbook misconception (see Figs. 20–10, 20–15, and 20–17).

PULMONARY EMBOLISM WITH INFARCTION. The radiologic use of the term "pulmonary infarction" embraces the completely reversible lesion of hemorrhagic congestion (35 per cent) as well as the much less frequent hemorrhagic infarction with necrosis (less than 5 per cent), since these are indistinguishable except at autopsy or, in survivors, only after a long period of time. The classic infarct, seen in profile, is a pleural-based, shallow, hump-shaped lesion about 2 cm to 5 cm deep and 5 cm to 10 cm along its pleural surface (see Figs. 20–10, 20–15, and 20–17). It may be seen along a fissure, at the lung periphery, or at a costophrenic angle. Although the pleural margin is sharp, the pulmonary profile of the hump is ill-defined. When seen *en face*, the infarct appears as a faint, ill-defined, and generally rounded opacity simulating a patchy pneumonia or an area of edema (see Fig. 20–10). In such cases, fluoroscopy is recommended to rotate the suspicious area into profile. On rare occasions the infarct may be deep-seated in the lung parenchyma and fail to reach a pleural surface.

An infarct is almost always associated with pleural effusion, and this may modify its appearance on the chest film (see Figs. 20–15 and 20–18A). The infarct also tends to occur more commonly in patients with left ventricular failure or chronic lung disease, so that it may be partly obscured by pulmonary edema, large pleural effusions, or pre-existing parenchymal lesions.

The rate of evolution of an infarct is very variable. It tends to resolve within a few days or weeks depending upon its size, the age and rate of lysis of the embolus, and the cardiopulmonary status of the patient. It usually regresses from its periphery toward its center, as opposed to a resolving pneumonia, which disappears downward toward its most dependent border under the influence of gravity. Some patients in whom there has been necrosis of tissue will have a permanent fibrotic scar in the area, visible as a small irregular opacity (see Fig. 20–15B).

PLEURAL EFFUSION. Pleural effusion, as expected, accompanies infarction in the great majority of patients with pulmonary embolism. It is generally unilateral but if bilateral tends to be asymmetric. There is a rough correlation between the size of the effusion and the size of the infarct, but occasionally a large infarct may exist with little effusion and vice versa. Small effusions are best detected in the posterior costophrenic sulcus on the lateral film or on lateral decubitus views. An effusion may occur without evidence of infarction, although this is uncommon and difficult to explain (see Fig. 20–12). The effusions may also be due to coincident cardiac failure and occasionally to infection, injury, or some other cause. The classic plain film appearance of embolism with infarction and effusion is a convex hump between two concave pleural fluid reflections — a hill between two valleys (see Fig. 20–17A).

PULMONARY EMBOLISM ASSOCIATED WITH CARDIAC OR PULMONARY DISEASE. The well-known plain film manifestations of left ventricular failure, particularly when accompanied by bilateral pleural effusion and pulmonary edema, may largely obscure the findings of pulmonary embolism with or without infarction. The common association of these entities should always be kept in mind, particularly if no other clear-cut cause of acute failure has been determined. An infarct may be recognized only as a persistent opacity after the edema clears in response to treatment for cardiac failure. If right ventricular failure is also present, the pleural effusions may be very large and the changes due to embolism almost impossible to detect.

Concurrent cardiac and pulmonary disease also complicate the picture and greatly reduce the value of both the plain chest radiograph and the lung scan. The presence of background emphysema, interstitial fibrosis, multifocal pneumonitis, the adult respiratory distress syndrome, and other conditions should precipitate an early decision to perform pulmonary angiography if embolism is in question (see Fig. 20–3).

The Isotope Lung Scan

The major controversy in the diagnosis of pulmonary embolism is related to the value and reliability of isotope lung scans. In his recent critical review, Robin concludes that perfusion scans are useful in excluding the diagnosis of pulmonary embolism only if they are completely normal.[13] He states:

The prevalence of false-positive scans is so high that diagnoses based on them are unreliable and the degree of unreliability increases with the presence of preexisting lung disease . . . Ventilation scans may show matching defects in patients with pulmonary embolism and may be normal in areas of parenchymal disease sufficient to produce perfusion defects in the absence of pulmonary embolism.

He therefore argues that because of the danger of overdiagnosis and overtreatment as well as expense, ventilation scans should not be part of the routine evaluation. A further argument by Novelline[11] is that lung scans are unreliable because of substantial inter- and intraobserver disagreement. These investigators recommend pulmonary angiography as the primary method of validation of pulmonary embolism and state that it should be used before treatment is undertaken, particularly in previously healthy patients, in whom the error rate is greatest.

The case for the reliability of lung scans as a diagnostic tool for pulmonary embolism is presented persuasively by McNeil and others.[1, 10] By carefully analyzing the scan appearances and judiciously complementing the perfusion scans with ventilation scans, it is possible to define those circumstances in which the lung scans become very effective diagnostic tools for justifying treatment, greatly reducing the need for pulmonary angiography.

We perceive the current status to be as follows (Table 20–6):

1. The perfusion scan is an exquisitely sensitive but nonspecific test for the

TABLE 20–6. CURRENT STATUS OF ISOTOPE LUNG SCANS

Radiographic Findings	Probability of Pulmonary Embolism*		
Normal perfusion	0%		
Perfusion defects alone (McNeil)	15–40%		
	Multiple SS	9%	
	S	50%	
	L	81%	
Perfusion defects, negative chest x-ray	SS	(?9–50)	
	S	(?50–100)	
	L	(?81–94)	
Perfusion and matching ventilation defects	<5%		
Perfusion defects, normal ventilation (McNeil)	80–85%		
	Multiple SS	50%	
	S	100%	
	L	94%	

*SS = subsegmental; S = segmental; L = lobar.

detection of abnormal distribution of blood flow due to any cause. Therefore, a negative perfusion scan effectively rules out pulmonary embolism. This fact alone justifies its routine use. However, it must be a technically perfect four-view study, and in some instances oblique views may be needed as well.

2. A positive perfusion scan on its own has an overall probability of detecting pulmonary embolism ranging from 10 per cent to 40 per cent, depending on the patient population and clinical selection. However, by limiting the cases to those with multiple filling defects, which constitute the great majority of pulmonary embolism patients, and by subdividing these cases into those in which the largest defects are (a) subsegmental, (b) segmental, and (c) lobar or whole lung, McNeil was able to achieve an 81 per cent probability of pulmonary embolism in the lobar or whole-lung group (see Fig. 20–11A). However, a one-in-five chance of mistreatment is probably still unacceptable. This situation would perhaps be improved slightly if the shape of the defect and its changing pattern over short periods of time were taken into account, but this awaits statistical analysis.

3. The combination of a positive scan with multiple defects (of which the largest is greater than a segment) and a plain chest radiograph that shows the region of a major defect to be clearly free of disease improves the 81 per cent figure for the scan alone. In many ways this approach is analogous to the combination of perfusion and ventilation scans. The plain film eliminates errors due to pneumonic consolidation, neoplastic infiltration, atelectasis, pleural effusions, focal emphysema, bullae, and other disease states; the combination offers a promising but as yet untested approach. The ventilation scan is clearly more sensitive in detecting mild underlying chronic lung changes (e.g., mild obstructive pulmonary disease, focal areas of emphysema, and bullae) even if the chest x-ray appears to be within normal limits.

4. The combination of a positive perfusion scan and a corresponding defect on ventilation scan makes the diagnosis of pulmonary embolism most unlikely, but as many as 10 per cent of such patients may still have a pulmonary embolism. To identify these individuals one must review the total clinical constellation of findings and proceed to angiography if reasonable doubt persists.

5. The combination of a positive perfusion scan in a patient with multiple defects (segmental or larger) and a normal ventilation scan in those areas represents the most exciting and valuable nuclear imaging contribution to the diagnosis of pulmonary embolism. When the largest defects are segmental the probability of pulmonary embolism approaches 100 per cent (see Fig. 20–11). When the largest defects are lobar or total lung the probability is 94 per cent (see Fig. 20–3). If the multiple defects are subsegmental, the results are poor (about 50 per cent). Single lesions also have poor probability correlations. Of course, not all patients with large pulmonary emboli can cooperate well enough to have a ventilation scan. For this reason it is important to re-emphasize the value of the plain chest film as the poor man's ventilation scan, recognizing its limitations.

Pulmonary Angiography

Pulmonary angiography remains the ultimate and only direct method of establishing an absolute diagnosis of pulmonary embolism.[15] All the other tests are indirect, although in combination they may support a sufficient probability of the diagnosis to either negate treatment or warrant one or another form of therapy without angiography.

A positive angiogram makes treatment obligatory; a negative study, performed early, effectively rules out the diagnosis. In a sense, angiography is the end of the line. Yet there must be a small but undefined incidence of false negative and a smaller incidence of false positive results. Emboli may be too small to be identified, may be obscured by contrast medium, may be missed by the observer, or may be unrecognizable because of suboptimal technique or patient motion. False negative diagnosis may result from misinterpretation of composite vascular or airway shadows. However, these difficulties usually apply to very small emboli. Large emboli are nearly always obvious. The interobserver error is small.[18] Autopsy data have shown a diagnostic correlation with angiography of close to 100 per cent. The clinical accuracy of negative angiographic procedures has been demonstrated by Novelline.[11]

The technique of pulmonary angiography is well established. Most hospitals in the United States are adequately equipped for the procedure and have an angiography staff with the necessary skills. The procedure has been shown to be reasonably safe, with a mortality rate of below 0.5 per cent despite the critical clinical condition of some of the patients.

INDICATIONS FOR ANGIOGRAPHY. The indications for angiography are as follows.

1. The primary indication is persistent diagnostic doubt. This usually implies an indeterminate chest x-ray and lung scan. Examples include (a) a single perfusion scan defect of any size; (b) multiple segmental or subsegmental lesions with matching radiographic opacities; (c) multiple segmental or subsegmental defects without radiographic opacities — but in a patient in whom a ventilation study is not possible and (d) mixed perfusion-ventilation defects, some matching, some nonmatching.

2. The presence of extensive prior pulmonary disease, which would interfere with all tests.

3. The possibility of massive embolism for which embolectomy or at least a vena caval interruption procedure is contemplated.

4. Clinical conditions in which the use of anticoagulants represents a particularly high risk, for example, internal injuries, stroke, peptic ulceration, or previous gastrointestinal bleeding.

5. Previously healthy young patients, in whom recurrence and morbidity could be expected to be low.

THE ANGIOGRAPHIC PROCEDURE. Pulmonary angiography should be performed within 48 hours of a defined clinical episode to ensure maximum accuracy. The normal thrombolytic process will not have had sufficient time to dissolve and disintegrate the clot. Beyond this time negative angiography, however well performed, cannot completely rule out the diagnosis. This time frame permits the strategy of temporary short-term heparinization, making it possible for the procedure to be performed on an urgent but elective basis rather than as an emergency, for example, on the morning following the night-time decision to perform the study. An emergency examination is justified only if there is a contraindication to use of anticoagulants and if the angiography is to be followed immediately by vena caval interruption or by embolectomy.

To ensure optimal film quality, the contrast agent, 60 to 80 ml of diatrizoate meglumine and sodium or a similar medium (e.g., Renografin 76), should be injected directly into the pulmonary artery trunk at the rate of 20 to 25 ml per second through a number 7 or 8 French pigtail or Grollman catheter with side holes. The transfemoral or transbrachial routes are equally acceptable. On occasion it may be expedient to deliver a larger injection into the vena cava or right atrium. The arterial, capillary, and venous phases of the angiographic procedure are displayed by exposure of films at the rate of two or three per second for four seconds and one per second for a further four to six seconds. The diagnosis is usually made on a single anteroposterior series. Occasionally, a second injection is required using half the amount of contrast medium delivered selectively to one lung, with the patient in a steep posterior oblique position to the same side. Only rarely is a superselective injection required, with the catheter advanced into a more peripheral branch. The advantages of the superselective magnification technique[11] remain questionable (see Fig. 20–9).

The pressure in the pulmonary artery must be measured before the contrast agent is injected. If there is significant pulmonary arterial hypertension, one performs, as the initial step, a selective study using smaller amounts of contrast medium on the side under greater suspicion.

ANGIOGRAPHIC FINDINGS. A definitive diagnosis of pulmonary embolism is made only by demonstrating clear-cut filling defects or abrupt obstructions of the arterial tree or both (see Figs. 20–1 to 20–10, 20–12, 20–13, 20–14 to 20–16, 20–18, 20–19, and 20–21). These are usually multiple and may be found at any level ranging from the main pulmonary artery to a subsegmental branch. Often a small amount of contrast medium percolates around an obstructing embolus to produce a ghost outline of the embolus (see Fig. 20–2, Fig. 20–21). When seen end-on it may appear as a ring shadow with a contrast rim, the embolus forming the lucent center (see Fig. 20–18). Filling defects vary greatly in number, size, and shape, but if seen early they tend to be surprisingly large, i.e., 8 to 12 mm in diameter and many centimeters in length. They may present as straight, convoluted, or amorphous defects. Later they may appear as eccentric plaques causing irregular narrowing of the lumen. They are frequently hooked over a bifurcation as a "saddle embolus" (see Figs. 20–6, 20–10, and 20–14). For example, they may arise between the upper lobe and the intermediate arteries, in

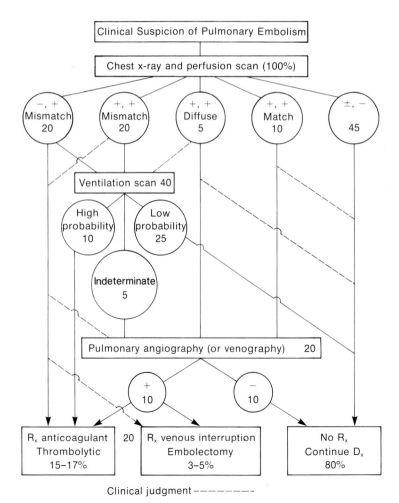

Figure 20–22. The decision tree reflects a typical investigation and treatment protocol for patients suspected of having pulmonary embolism. It assumes that all subjects will have a routine chest radiograph and perfusion lung scan. Some patients will require ventilation scans or angiography or both. Typical outcome probabilities are noted at each step, but these percentages will vary with patient populations and local practices. The solid lines represent the usual pathway, the broken lines an alternative option depending upon the specific clinical circumstances.

which case there may be relatively little perfusion deficit. Contrast medium may linger in the cul-de-sac above an obstruction on successive films well into the venous phase (Fig. 20–21). If there is an infarct it will be located well beyond the point of impaction of the embolus (see Fig. 20–10).

If the examination is delayed beyond 48 hours the emboli may be much smaller and therefore difficult to identify. In the Urokinase Pulmonary Embolism Trial, many emboli showed dramatic reduction in size and restoration of lumen patency within 24 hours, particularly when thrombolytic drugs were used (see Fig. 20–8).[18]

The secondary angiographic signs of pulmonary embolism are not diagnostic but serve merely to localize the areas of suspicion. A search for filling defects or obstructions can be made in such areas, or additional selective studies can be performed.[11] These secondary signs include focal flow retardation, with delayed filling and delayed emptying of the affected vessels; absent or reduced filling of a lung zone; regional tortuosity of vessel branches; pruning of small branches; and rapid tapering of a vessel lumen. Areas of partial atelectasis may appear as a dense blush during the capillary phase. In the presence of pleural effusion the rim of the underlying lung may also show deep opacification due to compression of the superficial alveoli (see Fig. 20–5). These dense "stains" clear more slowly than the parenchyma elsewhere.

The angiographic appearances are more complicated, of course, in the presence of chronic obstructive pulmonary disease, left ventricular failure, or mitral valve disease. These also cause vasoconstriction changes, randomly in emphysema, bibasilar in pulmonary hypertension. The secondary angiographic findings are then of little value, and the diagnosis must hinge upon finding a clear-cut obstruction or filling defect.

Lower Limb Venography (See also Chapter 23)

The role of lower limb venography in the diagnosis of pulmonary embolism is controversial. When the patient develops acute respiratory signs or symptoms and plain film or isotope scan changes are consistent with pulmonary embolism, the demonstration of deep vein thrombosis, with or without leg symptoms, may tilt the scales of probability strongly in favor of the diagnosis of pulmonary embolism. This is particularly true if the leading ends of the thrombi are shown to be floating in the blood stream ready for launching.

It has been argued that lower limb venography is a simpler procedure than pulmonary angiography, requiring less sophisticated equipment, less expense and involving less risk to the patient. It is recommended in situations in which lung scans are without value and pulmonary angiography is risky, for example, in the presence of severe emphysema or pulmonary fibrosis, especially if complicated by pulmonary hypertension. Furthermore, deep vein thrombosis itself warrants anticoagulant treatment and vena caval interruption also be justifiable in some circumstances, even without absolute proof of pulmonary embolism.

Negative venography does not exclude pulmonary embolism, particularly from an atypical source, such as the deep pelvic veins or even the right side of the heart.

CONCLUSION

The step-by-step decision tree that we currently use is summarized in Figure 20–22.

It is apparent that the diagnosis of pulmonary embolism depends heavily upon the radiologist, who may be called upon to perform and interpret a challenging and complicated series of tests starting with the plain chest film, proceeding to the perfusion and ventilation lung scans, and often ending with pulmonary angiography or occasionally lower limb venography. Each patient is unique, and decisions must be made on an individual basis at each step. The penalties of an error in diagnosis are great and may cost the patient's life. The radiologist therefore has an obligation to know as much as possible about the natural history of pulmonary embolism, the value and limitations of each test, the specific findings to look for, and the criteria necessary to establish or exclude the diagnosis. The radiologist's involvement may extend to assist in treatment by insertion of a Mobin-Uddin umbrella, a Kimray-Greenfield filter, or other transvenous device via an internal jugular or femoral venotomy under fluoroscopic control. Newer devices that can be introduced through ordinary angiographic catheters are still in the experimental stages[16] and may become available for patient use. This will simplify the decision to use caval interruption. A device for transvenous embolectomy has also been developed,[6] again requiring the collaboration of the radiologist to locate and withdraw the embolus. These interventional procedures will remain a challenge to the skills and ingenuity of the radiologist for a long time to come.

References

1. Adelstein, S. J., and McNeil, B. J.: A new diagnostic test for pulmonary embolism: how good and how costly? N. Engl. J. Med. *399*(6):305–307, 1978.
2. Benedict, K. T., Wheeler, B., and Patwardhan, N. A.: Impedence plethysmography: correlation with contrast venography. Radiology *125*:695–699, 1977.
2a. Bernstein, E. F.: The role of operative inferior vena caval interruption in the management of venous thromboembolism. World J. Surg. *2*:61–71, 1978.
3. Camishion, R. C., Pierucci, L. J., Fishman, N. H., et al.: Pulmonary embolectomy without cardiopulmonary bypass. Am. J. Surg. *111*:723–727, 1966.
4. Coon, W. W.: The spectrum of pulmonary embolism. Arch. Surg. *3*:398–402, 1976.
5. Dalen, J. E., and Alpert, J. S.: Natural history of pulmonary embolism. Prog. Cardiovasc. Dis. *17*(4):259–270, 1975.
6. Greenfield, L. J.: Pulmonary embolism: diagnosis and management. Chicago, Year Book Medical Publishers, 1976.
7. Fratantoni, J., and Wessler, S.: Prophylactic Therapy of Deep Venous Thrombosis and Pulmonary Embolism. DHEW Publication (NIH) 75-886, 1975.
7a. Freiman, D. G., Suyemoto, J., and Wessler, S.: Frequency of pulmonary thromboembolism in man. N. Engl. J. Med. *272*:1278, 1965.
8. Greenspan, H., and Steiner, R. E.: The radiologic diagnosis of pulmonary embolism. *In* Simon, M., Potchen, E. J., and LeMay, M. (eds.): Frontiers of Pulmonary Radiology. New York, Grune & Stratton, 1969.
9. Kakkar, V. V., et al.: Prevention of fatal postoperative pulmonary embolism by low doses of heparin. An international multicenter trial. Lancet *2*:45, 1975.
10. McNeil, B. J.: A diagnostic strategy using ventilation-perfusion studies in patients suspect for pulmonary embolism. J. Nucl. Med. *17*:613–616, 1976.
11. Novelline, R., Baltarowich, O. H., et al.: The clinical course of patients with suspected pulmonary embolism and a negative pulmonary arteriogram. Radiology *126*:561–567, 1978.
12. Rabinov, K., and Paulin, S.: Roentgen diagnosis of venous thrombosis in the leg. Arch. Surg. *10*:134–144, 1972.
13. Robin, E. D.: Overdiagnosis and overtreatment of pulmonary embolism. The emperor may have no clothes. Ann. Intern. Med. *87*:775–781, 1977.
14. Sharma, G. V. R. K., Tow, D. E., Parisi, A. F., and Sasahara, A. A.: Diagnosis of pulmonary embolism. Ann. Rev. Med. *28*:159–166, 1977.
15. Simon, M.: Plain film and angiographic aspects of pulmonary embolism. *In* Moser, E., and Stein, M., (eds.): Pulmonary Thromboembolism. Chicago, Year Book Medical Publishers, 1973 pp. 197–215.
16. Simon, M., Kaplow, R., Salzman, E., et al.: A vena cava filter using thermal shape memory alloy. Experimental aspects. Radiology *125*(1):87–94, 1977.
17. Tow, D. E., and Simon, A. L.: Comparison of lung scanning and pulmonary angiography in the detection and follow up of pulmonary embolism: the Urokinase-Pulmonary Embolism Trial Experience. Prog. Cardiovasc. Dis. *17* (4):239–245, 1975.
18. Pulmonary angiography. *In* The Urokinase Pulmonary Embolism Trial: Circulation (Suppl. II) *47* (4):38–45, 1973.

21

THE MEDIASTINUM

RONALD GRAHAM GRAINGER, M.D.,
F.R.C.P., F.R.C.R., F.A.C.R. (Hon.),
F.R.A.C.R., (Hon.)

The mediastinum is that irregular space lying extrapleurally between the two lungs in the midsagittal plane of the thorax. It is bounded anteriorly by the sternum, posteriorly by the bodies of the thoracic vertebrae, and laterally by the parietal pleura covering the medial aspects of the right and left lungs. On the transverse cross section of the body, best displayed in life by computerized tomography (CT), the mediastinum is seen to be of irregular biconvex lenticular shape, having narrow (even pointed) anterior and posterior limits, where the pleura of the two lungs come into contact with each other and with the sternum and the vertebral bodies, respectively.

The bony anterior and posterior limits of the mediastinum are fixed and rigid, but the lateral convex walls, being formed by pleura covering the lungs, are flexible. A mediastinal space-occupying lesion may readily bulge these lateral walls still farther into the soft and compressible lung tissue. This almost uninhibited displacement of the lateral walls of the mediastinum explains the frequent absence or paucity of symptoms in the presence of even a large mediastinal mass.

By convention, the mediastinal space is divided into a superior mediastinum, between the thoracic inlet and a plane connecting the sternal angle to the disc between the fourth and fifth dorsal vertebrae, and a lower mediastinum, which is below this plane. The lower mediastinum is divided into anterior, middle, and posterior mediastinal compartments by the anterior and posterior surfaces of the pericardium. The plane separating the superior from the inferior mediastinum is purely arbitrary, for several major structures in the three compartments of the lower mediastinum extend into or through the superior compartment.

In this text, masses within the superior mediastinum are considered to be in the anterior, middle, or posterior compartments, according to their position in the sagittal plane. Nevertheless, the concept of a superior mediastinal compartment is convenient, since some abnormal masses have a strong predilection for this region (p. 1434).[11, 19, 20]

1393

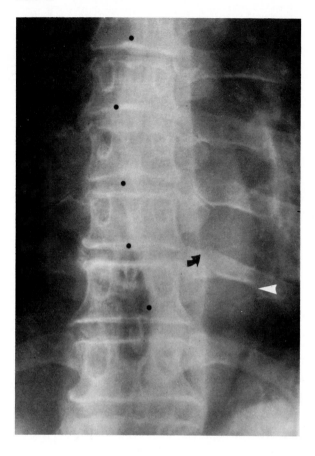

Figure 21–1. Some pleural reflection lines in the lower mediastinum. Medial reflection of the azygoesophageal recess (dots), • • • •, left paraspinal line of pleural reflection (black arrow), and left border of the descending aorta (white arrowhead).

RADIOGRAPHIC TECHNIQUE

Posteroanterior and lateral chest radiographs form the basis of radiographic technique for assessment of the mediastinum. The posteroanterior or frontal film should be well penetrated, preferably by the use of high kilovoltage technique (more than 130 kvp) with a fine-line grid or an air gap. If "conventional" low kilovoltage (70 to 90 kvp) chest radiography with high milliampere second exposure is used, then a second, overpenetrated, posteroanterior film with an absorption grid (either moving Potter Bucky diaphragm or fine-line grid) must be available for assessment of the mediastinum.

It is essential that the important anatomic landmarks within the mediastinum be recognized — the trachea, the carina, and the main bronchi; the aortic arch and the descending thoracic aorta; the azygos vein; and the posterior paravertebral (or paraspinal) lines, where the mediastinal pleura becomes reflected, to become the vertebrocostal pleura. Below the aortic arch, the left paravertebral line (Fig. 21–1) is readily identified and lies farther from the midline than the right paravertebral line. The left paraspinal line is due to the reflection of the pleura from the posterior aspect of the descending thoracic aorta onto the anterior aspect of the vertebral bodies, but it does not usually follow the line of a tortuous aorta.

Some (or all) of the more recently recognized lines of pleural reflection may also be identified on the high kilovoltage frontal radiograph. The anterior mediastinal stripe is the line of contact behind the manubrium sternum between the anterior mediastinal pleura of the two lungs, which separate slightly as they approach the apices. The superior posterior pleural line (thicker and extending higher than the anterior mediastinal stripe) represents the line of contact of the upper posterior mediastinal pleura of the two upper lobes and incorporates the upper thoracic esophagus. This line is sometimes called the right paraesophageal line or the esophagopleural stripe, and it is interrupted by the azygos vein arch over the right main bronchus. Below this level the posterior mediastinal line is continuous with the left border of the azygoesophageal recess, which is a tongue of lung tissue protruding from the medial surface of the right lung in front of the vertebral portion of the azygos vein making contact with the right border of the middle and lower thoracic esophagus approximately at the midline (see Fig. 21–1).

These mediastinal pleural reflection lines, or stripes, are often difficult to identify, even in good quality high kilovoltage frontal radiographs. Rarely can one identify more than two or three of these lines on a single radiograph. The posterior paraspinal lines are the more important radiographic features and are often noticeably deformed in cases of spinal or posterior mediastinal lesions (Figs. 21–2 and 21–3). The other stripes, although of considerable anatomic and radiologic interest, rarely make a major diagnostic contribution.

Two closely related radiographic signs — the silhouette and overlay signs, named by Felson[10] — are of extreme importance in localizing the plane of an opacity detected on conventional radiographs, particularly on the frontal film. The silhouette sign is an outline border seen on a radiograph only when there is physical contact of two structures of considerably different radiodensity, for example, the heart and the lung. If this (heart) border is not seen on an appropriately exposed frontal film, then the anatomic structure must be in contact with, and therefore on, the same sagittal plane as a structure of similar radiodensity (Figs. 21–4 and 21–5).

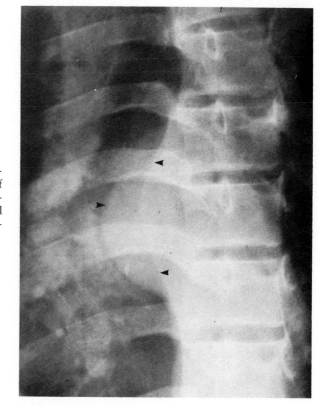

Figure 21–2. Neurofibroma. Note the localized displacement of the right paraspinal line of parietal pleura (right arrowheads) from its normal position closer to the spine. The spherical neurofibroma is easily identifiable (left arrowhead).

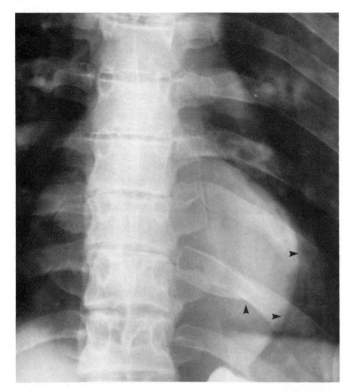

Figure 21–3. Ganglioneuroma. A convex mass at the posterior left vertebrocostaldiaphragmatic angle is demonstrated. Note the localized loss of the normal left paraspinal line, which now forms the outer border of the mass (horizontal arrowhead). Note the localized pressure indentation on the ribs (vertical arrowhead). The medial part of the left diaphragm is visible through the tumor. All of these features indicate that the mass lies posteriorly in the chest. On an underpenetrated frontal chest radiograph, the mass may be completely obscured by the heart in front of it.

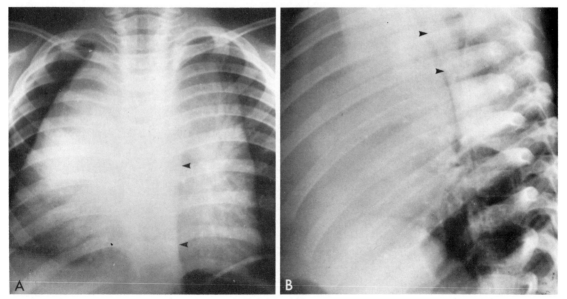

Figure 21–4. Massive thymic lymphosarcoma. The patient is a nine-month-old male child with marked dyspnea and stridor. A, Massive tumor obliterating the cardiac outline, extending down to the diaphragm, and approaching the lateral chest walls is demonstrated. Note the clarity of the descending aorta (arrowheads), indicating the probable lack of involvement of the posterior mediastinum. Note the visibility of the markings of left lung through the mass. B, Lateral radiograph demonstrates the complete loss of the normal retrosternal air space. There is marked backward displacement, bowing, and narrowing of the trachea (arrowheads). The complete lack of visibility of the heart borders on the frontal and lateral radiographs indicates the marked extension of tumor into the middle mediastinum. The child died from asphyxia. At autopsy, massive lymphosarcoma, apparently originating in the thymus and infiltrating widely throughout the anterior and middle mediastinum, was discovered.

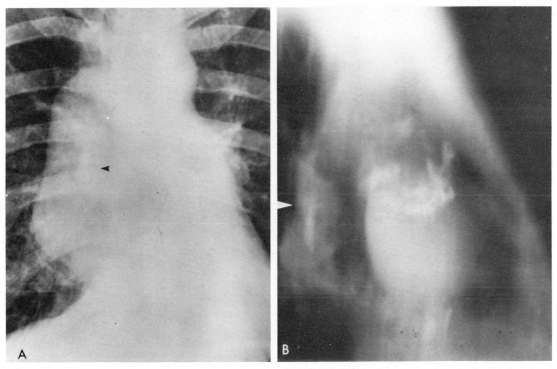

Figure 21–5. Large calcified teratodermoid cyst. *A,* Large lobulated mass is seen bulging the right mediastinal border. Note the loss of visibility of the right heart border, suggesting that the mass is in contact with this border. Note the faint visibility of right hilum (arrowhead), which suggests that the mass does not involve the hilum. *B,* Lateral tomography demonstrates marked, irregular calcification within the mass, which is situated mainly in the plane of the heart extending into the anterior mediastinum. The right hilum (arrowhead) lies well behind the mass.

If the heart outline can still be seen through a tumor radiodensity, then the tumor must be in front of or behind the heart (Figs. 21–6 and 21–7; see Figs. 21–3 and 21–4). This is an example of the overlay sign. When normally visible structures (for example, the heart or the pulmonary vessels) remain visible through an abnormal opacity on the frontal radiograph (overlay sign), then the abnormal lesion must lie in a different sagittal plane (Fig. 21–8, see Fig. 21–4). Both silhouette and overlay signs can, of course, be identified on projections other than frontal radiographs.

The lateral chest radiograph must also be well penetrated and taken with an absorption grid. The superior mediastinum may be almost "blacked out" if conventional low kilovoltage technique is used, and a mass within it, especially if it contains fat (as does a thymoma), may be almost invisible. Therefore, if a superoanterior mediastinal mass is suspected (as in the case of myasthenia gravis), it is important to take an additional coned lateral view of lower radiographic density. The patient's arms must be pulled well back and down (or vertically upward), so that they do not obscure this region.

Additional useful radiographic techniques for mediastinal assessment include tomography (Fig. 21–10), which is invaluable for the improvement of visualization, the detection of possible cavitation or calcific content, and the localization of a mediastinal lesion.

Fluoroscopy is often useful in localizing a mediastinal mass through the observation of its movement during rotation of the patient and during respiration. Expansile pulsation indicates a mass involving a major vascular structure, such as the aorta, but it

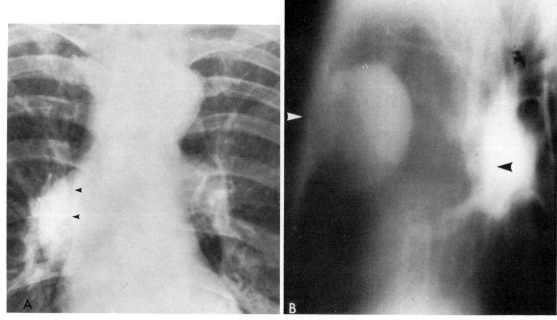

Figure 21–6. Thymoma. *A,* Note the unusual rounded contour of the apparent right "hilar" opacity. On the original film, the hilar vessels could be seen "through" the opacity; note the clarity of the right border of the ascending aorta (arrowheads), and the right atrium, indicating that the mass does not lie in the plane of the hilum or the heart. *B,* Lateral tomogram demonstrates the classic position of a thymic mass, which is well in front of the hilum (right black arrowhead) and immediately behind the sternum (left white arrowhead). (A thymic tumor with lymphocytic invasion was removed. Despite the invasion of the capsule, there was no recurrence seven years after excision.)

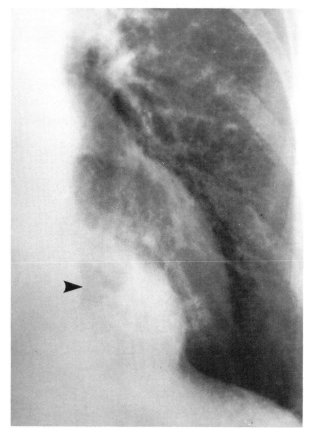

Figure 21–7. Diaphragmatic hiatus hernia. Note the convex mass containing an air bubble at the left vertebrodiaphragmatic angle (arrowhead). The mass would be obscured by the cardiac opacity on an underexposed radiograph.

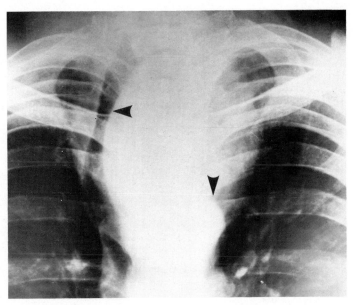

Figure 21–8. Retrosternal goiter. The patient is a male, aged 50 years, who presented with superior mediastinal obstruction. There is a large mass with convex lateral borders. Note the marked narrowing of the trachea, which is displaced and bowed to the right (left arrowhead). The aortic knuckle is visible (right arrowhead) and not displaced.

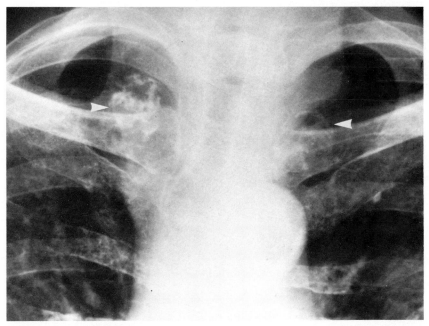

Figure 21–9. Calcified thyroid nodule. This is a relatively small cervical goiter with a heavily calcified nodule (left arrowhead) and a much fainter calcification of a left nodule (right arrowhead).

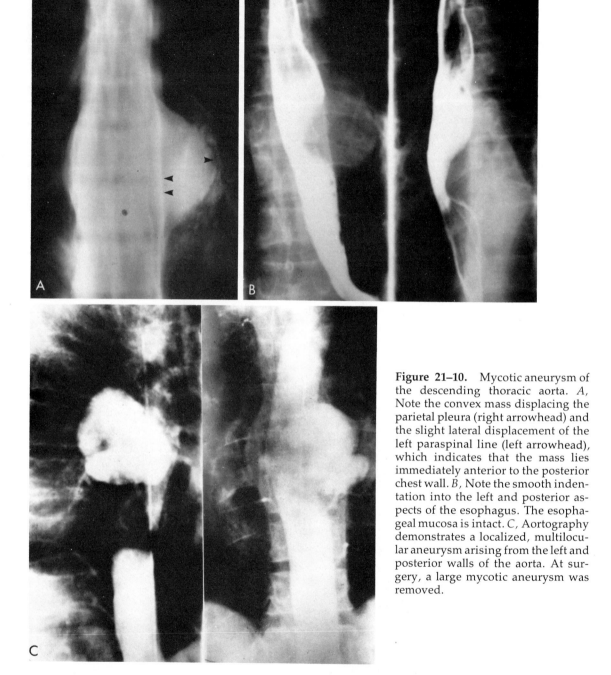

Figure 21–10. Mycotic aneurysm of the descending thoracic aorta. *A,* Note the convex mass displacing the parietal pleura (right arrowhead) and the slight lateral displacement of the left paraspinal line (left arrowhead), which indicates that the mass lies immediately anterior to the posterior chest wall. *B,* Note the smooth indentation into the left and posterior aspects of the esophagus. The esophageal mucosa is intact. *C,* Aortography demonstrates a localized, multilocular aneurysm arising from the left and posterior walls of the aorta. At surgery, a large mycotic aneurysm was removed.

may be impossible to distinguish this from transmitted pulsation in structures adjacent to the major cardiovascular organs.

Barium examination of the esophagus is essential for the study of the posterior or middle mediastinum, for the esophagus runs throughout the length of the posterior mediastinum and lies immediately behind the trachea (Fig. 21–11), carina, carinal glands, and left atrium. Primary diseases of the esophagus, such as achalasia or carcinoma, are readily diagnosed by barium swallow (Fig. 21–12). The displacement or

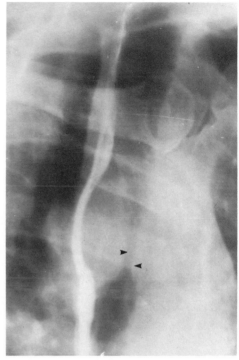

Figure 21–11. Tracheal neoplasm. The patient is a 59-year-old male with a 3-month history of dyspnea and productive cough. The frontal and lateral chest radiographs are normal. R.A.O. barium swallow demonstrates a mass between the trachea and the esophagus, which are separated from each other and narrowed. Note the severe narrowing of the trachea (arrows), which is reduced to about 25 per cent of its normal caliber. A bronchoscopic biopsy reveals squamous cell carcinoma extending from the lower trachea into the origin of the right main bronchus.

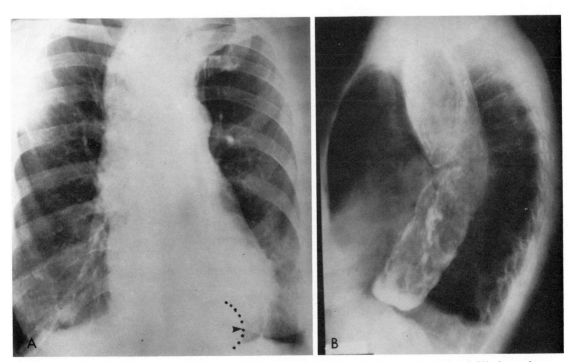

Figure 21–12. Achalasia. The unusual right mediastinal border is the result of a food-filled esophagus. The curved opacity at the left vertebrodiaphragmatic angle (*A,* dotted line) is caused by the terminal horizontal section of the elongated esophagus.

involvement of the esophagus is a valuable indicator of paraesophageal lesions (see Fig. 21–10).

Interventional cardiovascular studies, such as aortography, venacavography, azygos venography, and angiocardiography, are occasionally useful, particularly in the investigation of lesions arising within or involving these vascular structures or in juxtaposition to them. Myelography may occasionally be necessary in the study of para- or prespinal lesions: It provides definitive differentiation of dumbbell neurofibroma from thoracic meningoceles.

Pneumomediastinography is occasionally useful, particularly in demonstrating thymic tumors by lateral tomography, but it is now rarely practiced, especially since CT scanning is becoming more readily available.

Computerized Tomography

The introduction of computerized tomography (CT), devised by Hounsfield, has provided a completely new radiologic method for the assessment of the normal and abnormal regions of the body, including the mediastinum. Heitzman and his colleagues have made a major contribution by analyzing the visibility of the details of normal mediastinal structures on both conventional radiographs and CT scans.[3, 17] They have demonstrated that CT is of real value in the detection and evaluation of mediastinal lesions partially or completely invisible on conventional radiographs, and in the evaluation of the mediastinum and the hila when they seem to be abnormal on conventional radiographs. The determination of the extent and localization of tumor masses, particularly lymphoma and carcinoma of the bronchus, is greatly facilitated and leads to more accurate radiotherapy. Repeated CT scanning permits a noninterventional assessment of the response to treatment and the management of subsequent therapy.

The greatly increased sensitivity of CT scanning (when compared with film-screen combinations) in the assessment of radiodensity is a major diagnostic advance. The attenuation coefficient provided by CT permits confident diagnosis of fat deposits (lipomas [Figs. 21–13 and 21–14], thymolipomas, pads of fat, and lipomatosis of the mediastinum), clear fluid (pericardial cysts), blood (especially when accentuated by contrast medium), and minor deposits of calcium.

Ultrasound

Ultrasound often distinguishes fluid from solid lesions in the chest (Fig. 21–15), but only when the lesion is up against a chest wall or diaphragm.

MEDIASTINAL MASSES[11, 19, 20]

Thirty to fifty per cent of mediastinal tumors do not produce symptoms and are discovered on a radiograph of the chest taken for other reasons, such as during occupational or insurance examination. The ease with which the mediastinal pleura is deformed and indented into the adjacent compressible aerated lungs explains the paucity of symptoms. Malignant masses usually produce symptoms, but the majority of benign masses are first detected incidentally on a chest film. In many cases, however, even with an extensive radiologic assessment, no definitive diagnosis can be established without histologic examination.

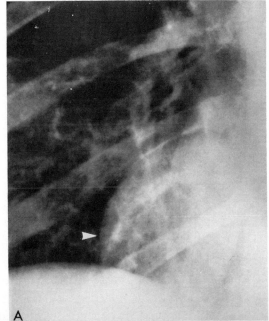

Figure 21–13. Pericardial lipoma. *A,* Convex mass (arrowhead) of low radiopacity at the right anterior cardiophrenic angle is well seen on this right posterior oblique radiograph. *B,* CAT scan shows a well-defined mass (arrowhead) situated at the right anterior cardiac aspect, in contact with the sternum. The attenuation coefficient is −169, indicating a lipoma and not a pericardial cyst. (Courtesy of R. E. Heitzman, M.D. Syracuse, New York.)

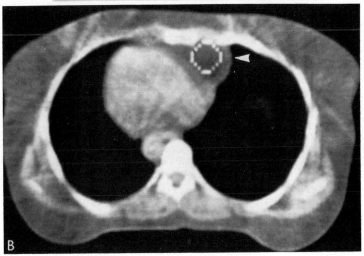

The relative incidence of the various mediastinal masses is difficult to assess because many series of published cases exclude some or all of the following: retrosternal goiter, aortic aneurysm, dilated esophagus, metastatic tumor, and inflammatory and parasitic masses. Excluding all of these lesions, an analysis of papers reporting a cumulative total of 2200 patients with radiologically evident mediastinal masses reveals the following approximate incidences: neurogenic tumors, 25 per cent; thymic tumors and cysts, 15 per cent; teratodermoid tumors, 15 per cent; lymphatic masses, 15 per cent; and bronchogenic, enterogenous, and pericardiac cysts, 15 per cent.

The most important features in the radiologic study of a mediastinal mass are its *content,* which is determined by its radiodensity, and its *position* in the sagittal plane of the chest (Fig. 21–16). Computerized tomography is making a completely new and

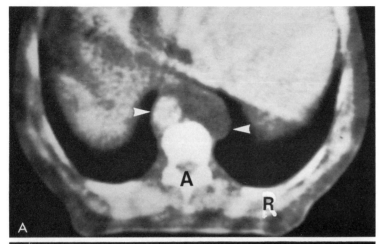

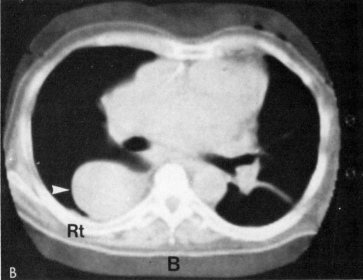

Figure 21–14. *A,* Prespinal and paraspinal lipoma. Note the low-density mass (right arrowhead) to the right of aorta (left arrowhead) on this CT scan. The attenuation coefficient of the mass was −129, which indicates its fat content. (Courtesy of E. R. Heitzman, M.D., Syracuse, New York.)

B, Posterior costovertebral pleural effusion. A convex mass (arrowhead) is seen on this CT scan to displace the pleura and project from the right mediastinal border. (Courtesy of A. M. McIlrath, M.D., Belfast, Ireland.)

specific contribution to the assessment of radiopacity, but the less sensitive conventional radiography also provides useful information about the contents of a mediastinal mass.

Mediastinal tumors tend to arise in predictable positions in the sagittal plane; it is therefore logical to consider them in the context of the conventional mediastinal compartments. It must, however, be clearly understood that this compartmentalization is by no means infallible. Teratodermoid tumors are almost always in the anterior mediastinum, but some have been seen in the middle and even the posterior mediastinum. Some mediastinal masses involve more than one compartment; for example, aneurysm of the aortic arch region may involve the anterior, middle, posterior, and superior mediastinum. Lymphomas or thymomas often cause massive tissue enlargement in the anterior, superior, and middle mediastinum (Fig. 21–17; see Fig. 21–4). Despite these exceptions, the determination of sagittal compartmental position of mediastinal masses is a useful basis for assessment (see Fig. 21–16).

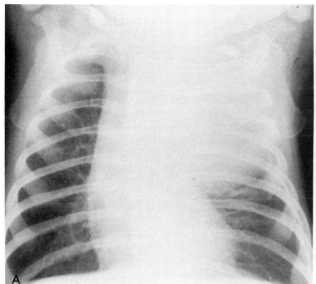

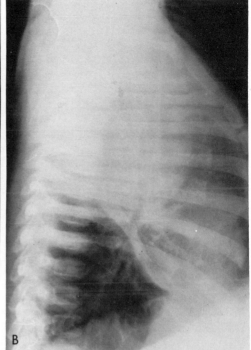

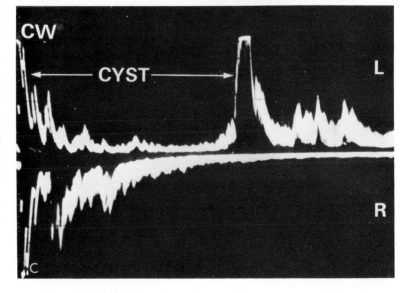

Figure 21–15. Neuroenteric cyst. *A* and *B,* Large mass occupies the upper left chest posteriorly. *C,* Ultrasound "A" scan of the upper part of the chest of a prone patient demonstrating a transsonic cyst in the left posterior chest. CW = chest wall; L = tracing from the left side of the chest; R = normal inverted tracing from the right side of the chest. At surgery, a large neuroenteric cyst was removed. It was situated posterior to the parietal pleura of the left lung and contained blood from a bleeding peptic ulcer on the medial wall, which contained gastric mucosa. The ulcer had penetrated the left subclavian artery, which had to be ligated. (*From* Sweet, D. M.: *In* Forfar, J. D., and Arneil, G. C. (eds.): Textbook of Paediatrics. Edinburgh, Churchill Livingstone, 1978. Reproduced by permission.)

The determination of the position of the mass in the coronal plane (that is, its laterality) is generally of much less value, except in the evaluation of unilateral structures, such as the aortic knuckle, or in main pulmonary arterial lesions.

Contents of Mediastinal Mass Lesions

The contents of mediastinal mass lesions may be demonstrated by careful conventional radiography, especially on well-coned films of optimal radiodensity, and

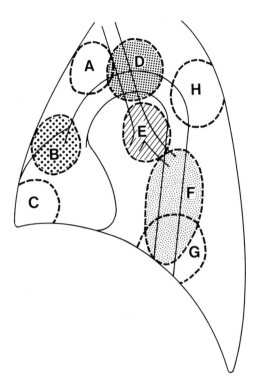

Figure 21–16. Sagittal position of mediastinal masses. Most masses of the mediastinum occur in predictable positions in the sagittal plane, as illustrated here. Tumors may occur in unusual situations, however, and the zones in this figure overlap. Zone A is the location of thyroid tumors (retrosternal), thymic tumors and cysts, parathyroid tumors, lymphangiomas, hemangiomas, and reticuloses. Teratodermoid tumors and cysts, and aneurysms of the sinus of Valsalva are commonly situated in Zone B. C is the usual site of pericardial pads of fat, pericardiac cysts, humps on the diaphragm, and hernias of Morgagni. In Zone D, aneurysms of the aortic arch and brachiocephalic arteries, tortuosity of the innominate artery, pseudocoarctation or congenital kinking of the arch, right aortic arches, aortic rings, systemic-pulmonary arterial connections, dilatation of superior vena cavae, and dilatation of azygos veins commonly occur. E is the usual location of paratracheal and hilar lymphadenopathy, sarcoidosis, lymphomatous diseases, carcinomas of the bronchus and trachea, and bronchogenic cysts. Dilatation of the esophagus (achalasia), aneurysms of the descending aorta, para-aortic and paraesophageal masses, and neuroenteric cysts are generally situated in Zone F. Hiatal hernias, hernias of Bochdalek, and ruptures of the diaphragm occur in Zone G. Zone H is the common site of neurogenic tumors (and meningoceles), spinal tumors and infections, paraspinal tumors and infections, paraspinal lipomatosis, and extramedullary hematopoiesis.

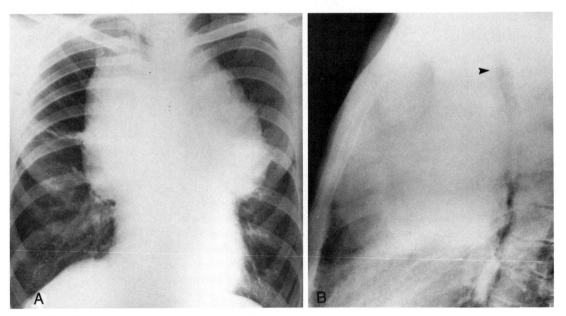

Figure 21–17. Mediastinal lymphosarcoma. The patient, a 48-year-old male, presented with superior vena caval obstruction. A, Posteroanterior radiograph shows a large mass in both the superior and the inferior compartments of the mediastinum extending deeply into both lung fields. B, Lateral radiograph demonstrates the extension of the mediastinal mass into the superior, anterior, and middle mediastinum. Note the loss of normal air radiolucency behind the manubrium and the upper sternum. There is marked backward displacement of the trachea (arrowhead).

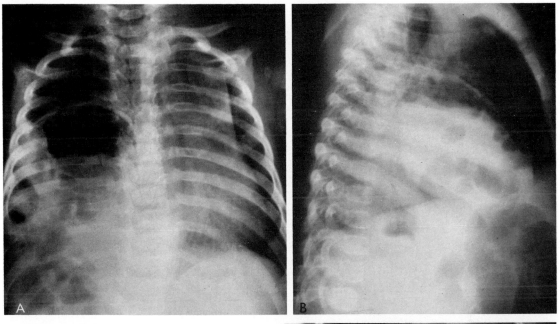

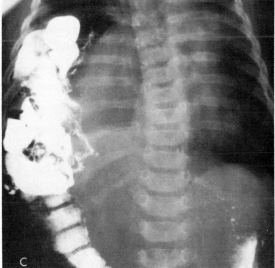

Figure 21–18. Hernia of Morgagni. *A,* Note the bowel with gas content in the right lower chest displacing the heart to the left. *B,* Lateral radiograph shows the herniated bowel to lie anteriorly. *C,* Barium meal follow-through demonstrates the herniation of the hepatic flexure of the colon into the right chest. On operation, deficiency of the right diaphragm anteriorly and a well-marked hernial sac containing the right lobe of liver and small and large bowel were found.

tomography. Gas, fat, calcium, and soft tissue (water, blood, muscle, and all cellular tissues produce soft tissue density) are the only radiographic densities that may be recognizable on conventional radiographs. A much more sensitive and specific method for the determination of the tissue content of a lesion is computerized tomography.

The demonstration of gas is of major importance in the diagnosis of a mediastinal mass lesion. It is most commonly seen in diaphragmatic hernias (for example, gastric hiatal [Fig. 21–7] or Morgagni [colonic] hernias [Fig. 21–18]). Gas, usually mixed with food, is often seen in a dilated esophagus (for example, in cases of achalasia [see Fig. 21–12]) or occasionally in a diverticulum or a communicating duplication cyst. Occasionally, a bronchogenic cyst or a mediastinal abscess may communicate with the airways and thereby acquire an air content. Gas in the mediastinal tissue planes is the

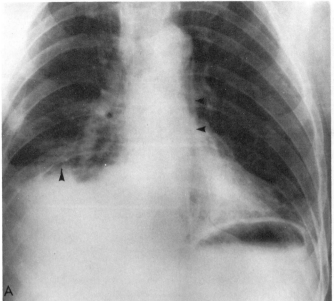

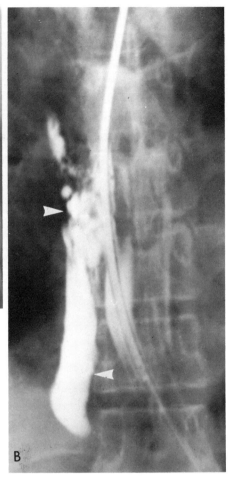

Figure 21–19. Boerhaave's syndrome. Spontaneous perforation of the esophagus during vomiting. *A,* Pneumomediastinum is best seen by the air (right arrowheads) separating the parietal pleura from the left aspect of the descending aorta. Note the horizontal fluid level (left arrowhead) due to a right pneumothorax. *B,* Injection of contrast medium via a tube into the lower esophagus demonstrates the tear in the esophagus (upper arrowhead) leading into the right extrapleural space (lower arrowhead).

diagnostic radiologic feature of mediastinal emphysema from any cause (Figs. 21–19 to 21–21).

Fat is of low radiographic density, but its presence in intrathoracic lesions may be difficult to identify by conventional radiography; it is particularly well detected by CT scanning (see Figs. 21–13 and 21–14). Abnormal accumulations of fat occur in the pericardium, mediastinal lipomas, cases of diffuse mediastinal lipomatosis, and thymolipomas. CT scanning usually provides a positive tissue diagnosis (see Figs. 21–13 and 21–14), because of the low attenuation coefficient of fat.

Calcium is an important constitutent of mediastinal lesions. It is best identified by CT scanning but is often well demonstrated by conventional tomography or even on plain radiographs. Calcifications may be found in thyroid tumors (central or eccentric nodular calcifications [see Fig. 21–9]), in aortic aneurysms (curvilinear calcifications [Fig. 21–22]) and in teratodermoid cysts (peripheral rim [Fig. 21–23], central calcifications [see Fig. 21–5], or dental fragments). Thymomas may also show peripheral rim calcification or central spots of calcium, usually of low radiographic density. Lymph gland masses may demonstrate calcification, especially granulomas, such as tuberculous lesions (Fig. 21–24), sarcoidosis (Fig. 21–25), or silicosis (eggshell or pebble

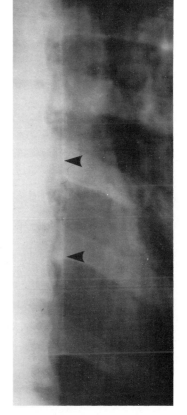

Figure 21–20. Mediastinal emphysema. Status asthmaticus. Note the left paraspinal parietal pleura (arrowheads) displaced by air from its normal position much closer to the spine.

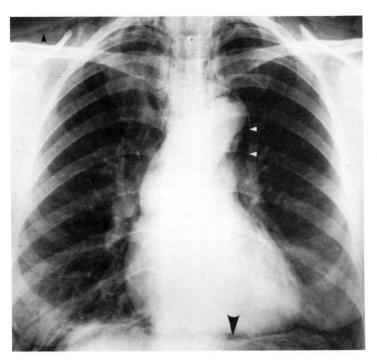

Figure 21–21. Mediastinal and subcutaneous emphysema following a biopsy of the rectal mucosa. Note the separation of the left parietal pleura from the aortic knuckle by gas (white arrowheads). Note the air (lower black arrowhead) separating the diaphragm from the parietal pericardium. Stripes of gas are evident in the soft tissues of neck (upper black arrowhead).

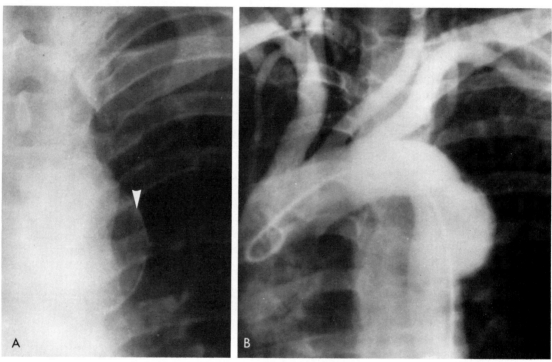

Figure 21–22. Traumatic dissecting aneurysm of the aortic arch. The patient is an asymptomatic young male who had been in a motorcycle accident. *A,* Curvilinear calcification (arrowhead) is visible just below the aortic arch. *B,* Arch aortogram reveals a localized aneurysm of the upper descending aorta.

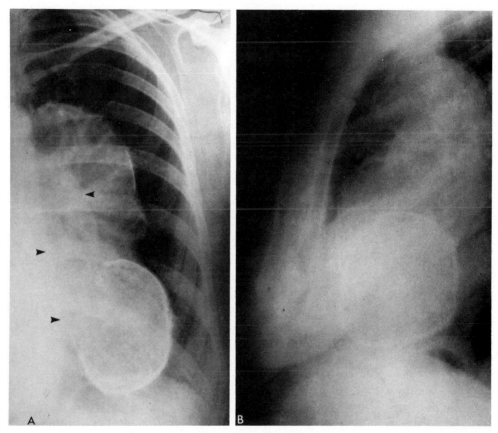

Figure 21–23. Large calcified teratodermoid cyst. *A,* Large lobulated mass in left mediastinum exhibits well-marked curvilinear calcification. Note the clarity of the left border of the descending aorta (left arrowheads) and the left hilum (right arrowhead), which indicates that the mass does not involve these structures. *B,* Lateral view shows the anterior position of the mass, which is especially well identified by its large lower calcified loculus.

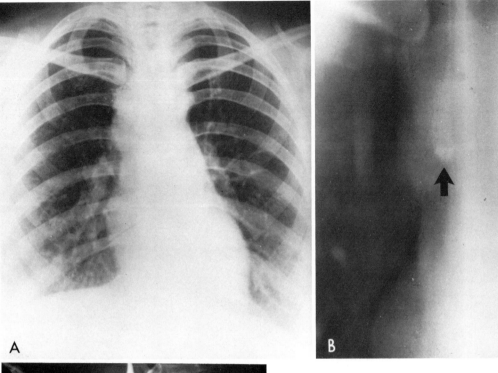

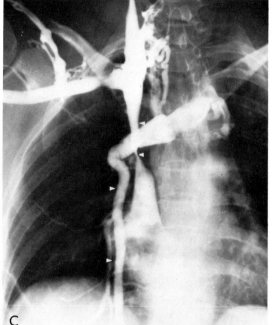

Figure 21–24. Chronic fibrosing mediastinitis. The patient is a female, aged 20, with superior vena caval obstruction. At thoracotomy, tuberculous granulation tissue was found. *A,* Lobulated prominence of the right upper mediastinum is visible. *B,* Frontal tomogram demonstrates calcification (arrow) within the mass. *C,* Right subclavian venogram demonstrates marked narrowing at the upper end of the superior vena cava (right arrowheads). There is marked retrograde opacification of the right internal mammary vein (left arrowheads). The lateral radiograph also demonstrated faint retrograde opacifications of the azygos vein.

calcification), and occasionally in Hodgkin's disease that has been treated by radiotherapy (Fig. 21–26). Uncommon mediastinal masses, such as hemangiomas (phleboliths) or neuroblastomas, may exhibit calcification, and rarely, the wall of a bronchial cyst may become calcified.

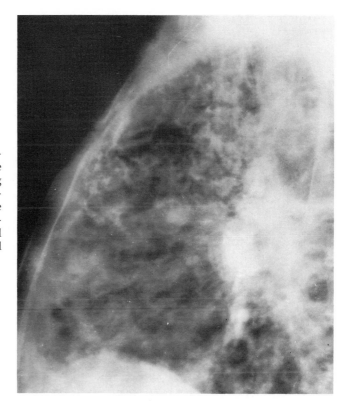

Figure 21–25. Mediastinal glandular calcification in a case of sarcoidosis. Extensive calcification of eggshell pattern affecting sarcoid glands in anterior, middle, and superior mediastinum. The 48-year-old male patient was first diagnosed as having sarcoidosis 14 years earlier and later acquired extensive pulmonary fibrosis. He died from spontaneous pneumothorax.

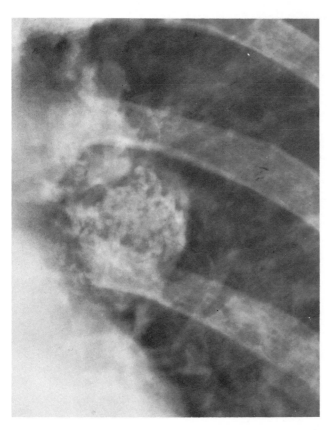

Figure 21–26. Calcified Hodgkin's lymph gland after radiotherapy. A well-documented but uncommon result of radiotherapy for lymphadenoma is calcification of the glands.

Anterior Mediastinal Masses

RETROSTERNAL THYROID. Although often not included in the term "mediastinal tumors," an enlarged thyroid is in fact the most common abnormal mass in the mediastinum. The patient is often a middle-aged female without compression symptoms and without thyrotoxicosis. The slowly growing thyroid tissue usually derives from the lower part of a normally situated cervical thyroid gland (which is often enlarged), and over a period of many years it sinks into the anterior mediastinum immediately behind the manubrium. Its slow growth and benign nature as well as lack of invasion of neighboring tissues usually delay the development of symptoms that might have been expected owing to the rigid bony confines of the thoracic inlet. In some patients, however, the trachea is severely compressed and displaced, causing stridor, dyspnea, and hoarseness (see Fig. 21–8); occasionally dysphagia is caused by esophageal compression (Fig. 21–27) and, rarely, superior vena caval obstruction develops (Fig. 21–28).

On the frontal radiograph, the retrosternal goiter is usually shaped like a truncated cone, base uppermost, with well-defined convex, occasionally lobulated, lateral borders. It usually has a homogeneous density, but nodular calcification within it is a reasonably common diagnostic feature (see Fig. 21–9). The mass is usually moderate in size but may become very large (see Fig. 21–27).

About 80 per cent of retrosternal goiters are situated in front of the trachea, which may be considerably narrowed from front to back, and displaced backward, away from the sternum. The other 20 per cent of retrosternal goiters lie between the trachea, in

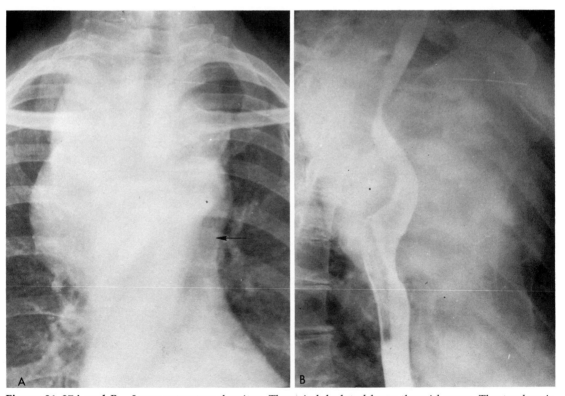

Figure 21–27A and B. Large retrosternal goiter. There is lobulated large thyroid mass. The trachea is displaced backward. The esophagus is shown to be markedly indented and deformed on the right anterior oblique radiograph. Note the absence of displacement of the aortic knuckle.

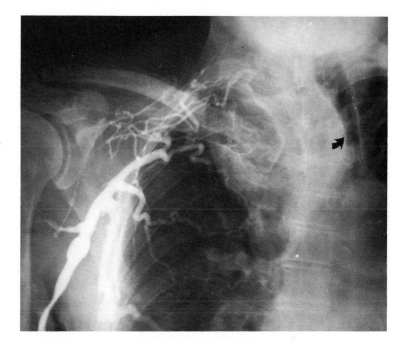

Figure 21–28. Retrosternal goiter with superior vena caval obstruction. A large retrosternal goiter is displacing and bowing the narrowed trachea to the left (arrow). The right arm venogram demonstrates complete obstruction of the right subclavian vein.

front, and the esophagus, behind; both of these structures are usually compressed, narrowed, deformed, and separated from each other by the thyroid mass, which in these rare cases is usually predominantly right-sided. The more frequent anterior retrosternal goiters lie eccentrically on both sides of the trachea, which is usually considerably compressed and deformed in the coronal plane and displaced in a convex bowline to either side (see Figs. 21–8 and 21–28), returning toward the midline below. The relationship of the goiter to the trachea may be so close that the goiter may be seen on fluoroscopy to move upward on swallowing.

The brachiocephalic vessels, aortic arch, and superior vena cava are often displaced by retrosternal goiter; occasionally the veins may be sufficiently compressed to produce a superior vena caval compression syndrome (see Fig. 21–28).

If the goiter contains functioning tissue, it takes up radioactive iodine isotope, thereby aiding in diagnosis.

Radiographs must include well-penetrated grid frontal and lateral (arms pulled backward and downward) views of the thoracic inlet. A barium swallow examination may also be performed; occasionally, venography or aortography may be necessary to differentiate retrosternal goiter from vascular masses.

THYMIC TUMOR. The normal thymus of an infant occasionally causes an extensive radiographic opacity in the anterosuperior mediastinum, which may be disturbing to the inexperienced clinician. The opacity is well defined, usually with a straight or convex right lateral border and a horizontal lower border, resembling a sail billowing in the breeze (Fig. 21–29). It is usually more prominent on the right but may protrude on the left, particularly if the infant is in a slight left anterior position. The thymic opacity is much more prominent during expiration and during slight rotation. Instead of further radiographs, fluoroscopy should be performed for a few seconds, with any rotation corrected; the almost total disappearance of the opacity should result on deep inspiration.

Thymic tumors are usually solid and of soft consistency, but they may be cystic, a differentiation that may be made by CT scanning. These tumors usually contain much

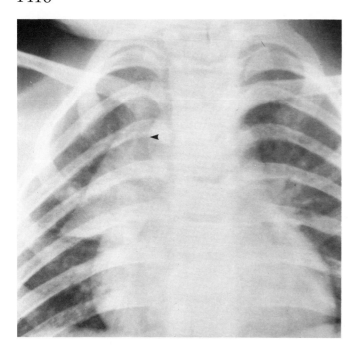

Figure 21–29. Normal thymus in an infant. The infant is slightly rotated to the right as demonstrated by the visible right edge of the manubrium (arrowhead). This rotation increases the prominence of the typical sail-like opacity extending from the right upper mediastinum. The opacity has a characteristic horizontal lower border.

fat (and are therefore of low radiographic density), with lymphoid tissue and some Hassall's corpuscles; they occasionally calcify, either as a peripheral rim or as a faint nodular central calcification. A thymolipoma has a specific histologic structure, with a capsule of thymic tissue and a central tumor mass of fat. It is a benign tumor but may grow to an enormous size (a 6-kg tumor has been reported). No relationship between thymolipoma and myasthenia gravis has been reported.

Thymic tumors are usually benign but may be aggressively and widely invasive and malignant, with disseminated metastases. One type of malignant thymic tumor is a seminoma, occurring in young males and histologically identical to testicular seminoma.

About 20 per cent of patients with myasthenia gravis have either a benign or a malignant thymic tumor. About 50 per cent of patients with a thymic tumor have myasthenia gravis. Surprisingly, the excision of a normal-sized thymus results in improvement in about 80 per cent of myasthenics, particularly young people with recent onset of myasthenia. The excision of a thymic tumor is also beneficial for patients with myasthenia, but their prognosis is worse than that of patients who have had a normal-sized thymus excised.

Thymic tumors tend to be small (less than 5 cm in diameter), and since they usually lie in the midline in the anterior mediastinum behind the manubrium, they may be completely hidden by the normal mediastinal opacity on the frontal radiograph. Low kilovoltage, well-coned lateral tomography of the upper anterior mediastinum, with the arms pulled downward and backward, is essential for their demonstration (see Fig. 21–6). A careful examination must always be made of patients with myasthenia gravis. CT scanning is considerably more effective than lateral tomography and will indicate the high fat content of thymic tumors.

Thymic tumors are usually spherical or ovoid but may be layered like plaques on the aortic arch and its brachiocephalic branches. As the tumors enlarge, they protrude from one or both sides of the mediastinum as well-defined convex or lobulated lateral borders (see Fig. 21–4). Occasionally, massive tumors may touch the lateral chest walls and the diaphragm. Since the tumors are often of low radiographic density and usually less deep sagittally than coronally, normal lung markings are usually visible through even a massive thymic tumor on correctly exposed frontal radiographs (see Fig. 21–4). Such a massive tumor may displace the trachea and vascular structures backward, but it rarely causes major compression until the terminal stages, since its pliable consistency usually allows it to fill the anterior mediastinum and bulge extensively into the anterior medial portion of the lungs. The extremely soft consistency of many fatty tumors (including thymolipomas) may permit marked change in the shape and position of the tumors with variation of posture or respiration. On erect radiographs, a thymolipoma may have teardrop shape, indicating its plasticity. The anterior rib ends may indent these soft tumors.

Occasionally, faint linear or spotty calcification may develop circumferentially. This is best demonstrated by CT scanning but may also be shown by lateral tomography. CT scanning has virtually replaced pneumomediastinography which, in conjunction with lateral tomography, occasionally helped to demonstrate a small thymic mass. CT scanning is essential before a small thymic tumor can be excluded.

TERATODERMOID TUMORS. These intriguing masses are derived from multipotential embryonic germ cells and may be solid or cystic. If ectodermal (skin) elements strongly predominate, the masses are regarded as dermoids. Teratomas contain significant amounts of ectodermal, mesodermal, and endodermal tissues, the last being the most likely to become malignant. The considerable majority (about 70 per cent) of teratodermoid tumors are benign and are usually discovered incidentally on chest radiographs of asymptomatic young adults.[6, 11, 16, 19, 20]

Radiologically, teratodermoid tumors are usually smooth and spherical or ovoid in shape (Fig. 21–30), but they may be gently lobulated (see Figs. 21–5 and 21–23). They

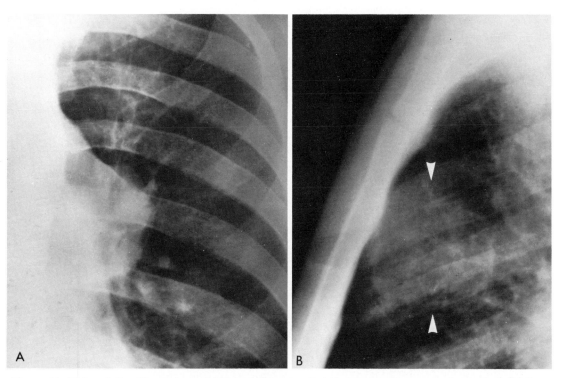

Figure 21–30A and B. Teratodermoid tumor. Spheric, slightly lobulated mass overlying the left hilum, is seen on the lateral view (arrows) to lie immediately behind the sternum. A dermoid cyst was removed from the asymptomatic 26-year-old patient.

usually protrude into only one lung, indenting both lungs only when the tumor becomes massive. The tumors are well defined, and the adjacent lung is usually normal unless sepsis, malignancy, or perforation develops.

The location of teratodermoid tumors is characteristically in the anterior mediastinum, frequently in front of the origin of the great vessels from the heart, which may be displaced backward. The sternum is occasionally bowed forward. Very rarely, a teratodermoid tumor may be in the middle or posterior mediastinum.

The contents of teratodermoid tumors often give the main diagnostic clue. Calcium is frequently present, as part of the well-calcified rim (see Fig. 21–23) or situated within the mass (see Fig. 21–5) as bone, cartilage, or dental fragments. It is best demonstrated by tomography (see Fig. 21–5) or CT scanning, which may also reveal radiolucent fat content as well as providing information of its anatomical relationships.

Teratodermoids are usually slow growing but occasionally grow rapidly owing to hemorrhage, sepsis, or malignancy, each of which may be complicated by perforation into the pericardium, pleura, or mediastinal tissues.

Mediastinal malignant teratodermoid tumors are uncommon, accounting for 20 to 30 per cent of chest teratomas, but they may be highly invasive, particularly the endodermal sinus, or yolk sac, tumor which may secrete α fetoprotein, the blood level of which can be used to assess the response to radiation or chemotherapy. Unfortunately, these tumors are almost invariably rapidly fatal. A pleural or pericardial effusion (especially if bloody) associated with a mediastinal tumor should always raise the possibility of malignancy.

LIPOMAS AND LIPOMATOSIS. Tumors of fat in the mediastinum are most common in the upper anterior compartment but may occur in any mediastinal location (see Fig. 21–14). They are almost always benign and consist of soft, pliable fat, which rarely causes significant compression of vital adjacent organs, so that even large tumors may not cause symptoms. They range widely in size and may become massive, even touching the lateral chest walls and diaphragm.[2, 11, 19, 20] The fatty tumors have low radiopacity, so that, as in the case of thymic tumors, the lung tissue can usually be seen through the mass, even on normal-penetration radiographs. Mediastinal lipomas or thymolipomas may be so pliant that they may change considerably in shape or position when there is a change in posture and respiration. They often have an undulating lobulated outline sometimes produced by indentation from the ribs.

Lipomatosis is usually iatrogenic, secondary to corticosteroid therapy, which mobilizes fat and deposits it in the mediastinum. Both the anterior and the middle portions of the mediastinum are involved, with fat collecting around the thymus, the great vessels, the pericardium, and the cardiophrenic angles. The mediastinal contours tend to be enlarged, featureless, and smooth, but either cardiomegaly or a true mediastinal mass may be simulated. Comparison of current with previous radiographs and a history of corticosteroid therapy usually suggest the diagnosis, and CT scanning confirms it. CT diagnoses not only the position but also the content of the lesion.

The confident diagnosis of lipoma by its low attenuation coefficient on CT scans is a major advance in patient management, for only about 3 per cent of mediastinal fat masses become malignant. As lipomas seldom cause symptoms, the usual management is observation by yearly radiography rather than surgical excision.

HERNIA OF MORGAGNI. This hernia is due to a congenital deficiency anteriorly between the sternal and the costal attachments of the diaphragm. In this condition, which is much more frequent on the right side, the abdominal contents (usually liver, omentum, or colon) herniate into the chest. If liver or omentum is the content, then a homogeneous soft tissue density convex mass projects into the lung field from the right cardiophrenic angle. The definitive diagnosis may be established (if necessary) by

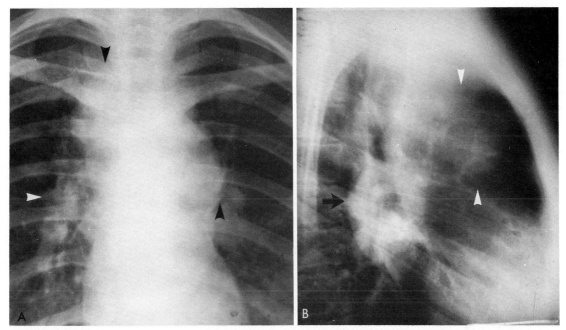

Figure 21–31A and B. Lymphadenopathy in the anterior-superior mediastinum (sarcoid). Note the mass of enlarged lymph glands in the anterior mediastinum involving both superior (downward-pointing arrowhead) and inferior (upward-pointing arrowhead) paratracheal compartments. There is also hilar gland enlargement (horizontal arrowhead). This appearance is much more typical of reticulosis but mediastinoscopy, biopsy, and the clinical examination of the patient revealed typical sarcoidosis.

inducing an artificial pneumoperitoneum and then obtaining erect radiographs, which show the injected air rising above the hernial contents to outline the upper border of the hernial sac. If there is bowel (usually transverse colon) in the hernia, the diagnosis is more easily made on conventional chest radiographs (particularly the lateral projection) because of the recognizable pattern of colonic gas (see Fig. 21–18). This diagnosis can readily be confirmed by barium enema.

A hernia of Morgagni is usually asymptomatic and discovered on a chest radiograph taken for other reasons, but rarely the hernial contents may strangulate, producing an acute thoracoabdominal crisis.

LYMPHADENOPATHY. The enlargement of the lymph glands in the anterior mediastinum is usually evident in the superior compartment and is often associated with the involvement of the thymus and paratracheal lymph glands: The combination is usually due to lymphomatous disease (see Fig. 21–17) but may be due to sarcoidosis (Fig. 21–31).

Occasionally, the lymph glands in the internal mammary chain are enlarged and may be visible behind the costal cartilage on lateral tomographs. They are much better visualized by CT, the use of which has revealed their frequent involvement by lymphoma (see also Middle Mediastinum, p. 1420).

HEMANGIOMA. This is an unusual mediastinal tumor that has been seen most frequently in the anterior superior compartment. It is usually benign but may occasionally become sarcomatous. Its only distinguishing radiologic features are the occasional presence of phleboliths and, rarely, rib or vertebral changes (pressure defect, erosion, or hypertrophy).

LYMPHANGIOMA (HYGROMA). This is also an unusual mediastinal mass, more frequent in children, usually found in the upper anterior compartment. It consists of multilocular lymphatic cysts or loculi and may extend into the neck as a soft, fluctuant, compliant mass. In the superior mediastinum it is seen as a lobulated, clearly defined, usually bilateral mass and may be associated with a chylothorax. Pressure symptoms are unusual.

Middle Mediastinal Masses

The heart is the principal organ in the middle mediastinum and is considered in another chapter (see The Heart). In most cases, the enlargement of a cardiac chamber can be readily identified as being of cardiac origin, but occasionally an aneurysm of the left ventricle or the central pulmonary arteries may protrude eccentrically and resemble a mediastinal mass, thus requiring angiography or CT for definitive diagnosis.

LYMPHADENOPATHY. One of the most frequent causes of a mediastinal mass is enlargement of the lymph glands of the middle mediastinum. The paratracheal, carinal, tracheobronchial, and bronchopulmonary (hilar) groups are often involved, and the pathologic condition is usually reticulosis or bronchial neoplasm. Inflammatory disease and sarcoidosis usually (but not always) cause less marked glandular enlargement, often dominant at the hila.

LYMPHOMATOUS DISEASES. Hodgkin's disease is the most frequent lymphomatous disease to affect the mediastinum. Lymphosarcoma, reticulum cell sarcoma, and giant follicular lymphoma are less frequent; leukemia may have an identical radiologic appearance. The histologic type can be established only by microscopic examination of tissue.

The enlargement of one or more of the paratracheal lymph glands is frequently the most obvious feature and may be the sole apparent radiologic abnormality (Fig. 21–32). The enlarged right or left paratracheal glands may protrude laterally, as may a well-

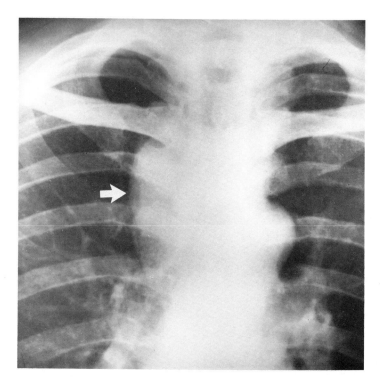

Figure 21–32. Right paratracheal lymphadenopathy. The patient is a middle-aged male with a six-week history of retrosternal discomfort. There is a clearly defined, elongated mass with a convex outer border (arrow) lying in the paratracheal position above and opposite the aortic knuckle. This appearance is indistinguishable from that in Figure 21–34. A scalene-node biopsy demonstrated malignant lymphoma.

defined convex mass, sometimes lobulated, situated above the hilum (see Fig. 21–32). When the enlargement is massive, it is usually bilateral and also involves the anterior superior mediastinum (see Fig. 21–17). The thymus is often involved in the lymphomatous diseases (see Fig. 21–4), and the normal air space between the sternum and trachea may be completely eliminated.

The hilar lymph nodes (which are outside the mediastinum) may be involved, usually in association with more extensive involvement of the glands higher up. Isolated symmetric hilar glandular enlargement is unusual in lymphomatous diseases and is much more suggestive of sarcoidosis. Occasionally, sarcoid lymphadenopathy (see Fig. 21–31) may be extensive and may closely simulate a lymphoma.

Mediastinal lymphadenopathy may be sufficiently massive to cause compressive symptoms, especially of the superior vena cava, but occasionally of the trachea or bronchi. Lymphomatous infiltration may involve the important mediastinal nerves — the phrenic (diaphragmatic paralysis), the recurrent laryngeal (hoarseness), and the sympathetic (Horner's syndrome).

The radiosensitivity of mediastinal lymphadenopathy is a variable feature. Some patients respond dramatically to radiotherapy, which may rapidly "melt" away a massive mediastinal mass and produce a normal chest radiograph. Unfortunately, the tumor frequently recurs.

One distinctive histologic variety of lymphoma is sclerosing nodular Hodgkin's disease, which tends to affect young people. It nearly always causes a well-defined mass involving the thymus and the anterosuperior mediastinal lymph glands, is frequently associated with cervical lymphadenopathy, tends to remain localized, and has a more favorable prognosis.

MALIGNANT GLANDS. Metastatic lymph glands in the mediastinum are usually secondary to carcinoma of the bronchus, but the primary tumor may be outside the thorax. In carcinoma of the bronchus, the mediastinal metastases may be large and may be the dominant radiologic feature. Mediastinal enlargement from metastatic nodes is more often unilateral, less massive and less radiosensitive than that from reticulosis, and it tends to occur in older patients. There is often radiologic evidence of a primary malignant pulmonary or bronchial lesion. A full investigation, including sputum cytologic screening, tomography, bronchoscopy, lung biopsy, scalene-node biopsy, and mediastinoscopy, usually confirms the diagnosis of carcinoma of the bronchus with mediastinal lymphadenopathy.

CALCIFICATION. The calcification of mediastinal lymph glands is most frequent in cases of chronic inflammatory granulomatous disease (for example, tuberculosis [see Fig. 21–24] or coccidioidomycosis). Eggshell or pebblelike calcification may, however, occur in cases of hypercalcemic sarcoidosis (see Fig. 21–25) and pneumoconiosis. Lymphomatous glands do not calcify except occasionally after radiotherapy in patients with Hodgkin's disease (see Fig. 21–26).

BRONCHOGENIC CYSTS.[6, 11, 16, 19, 20] These embryonic cysts are usually found in asymptomatic patients in the second or third decade of life as an incidental finding on a frontal chest radiograph. They are usually lined by respiratory-type epithelium, may have cartilage in their wall, and contain a unilocular cavity filled with milky or brown mucoid fluid. Rarely, the walls of these cysts may calcify, or they may communicate with a bronchus, producing an air-fluid level on erect radiographs.

Bronchogenic cysts are almost always situated close to the trachea or main bronchi, typically in the region of the carina (Fig. 21–33), but occasionally at another level in the mediastinum or the hilum (Figs. 21–34 and 21–35). The cyst presents radiologically as a smooth, ovoid, rarely lobulated, homogeneous opacity projecting from the mediastinum; it is almost always solitary and unilateral. CT scanning demonstrates a low attenu-

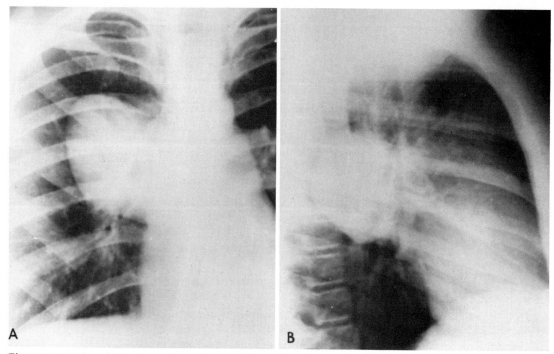

Figure 21–33A and B. Bronchogenic cyst. The patient is an asymptomatic girl of ten years. A well-defined, homogeneous mass with smooth, convex borders projects backward and to the right from behind the right tracheobronchial junction. A bronchogenic cyst was removed.

ation factor, indicating the fluid content. The cyst rarely causes compression symptoms but may displace neighboring soft structures, such as vessels (see Fig. 21–34) or the esophagus (see Fig. 21–35).

PERICARDIAL CYSTS.[6, 11] Pericardial cysts are single-cavity cysts containing clear

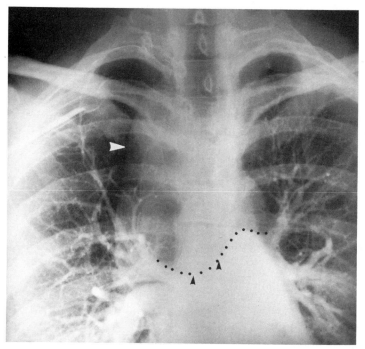

Figure 21–34. Bronchogenic cyst deforming the right pulmonary artery. The patient is an asymptomatic woman of 36 years. There is a well-defined mass in the right paratracheal region with a clear, convex right lateral border (white arrowhead). Note the deep, concave indentation into the upper border (black arrowheads) of the right pulmonary artery, outlining the inferior border of the cyst. The appearance is indistinguishable from that of Figure 21–32. A bronchogenic cyst lined by ciliated epithelium and containing fat, muscle, vessels, and nerves was removed.

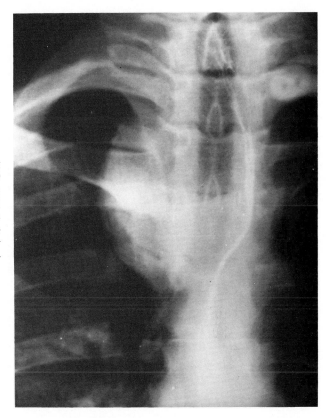

Figure 21–35. Bronchogenic cyst displacing the esophagus. The patient is a male of 30 years with a two-week history of tightness in the throat after influenza. A right paratracheal mass with a smooth convex border displaces the barium-filled esophagus to the left. The trachea is not displaced. A cyst lined by respiratory-type epithelium containing "purulent" fluid was removed.

watery fluid and sometimes connected to the main pericardiac cavity. They are usually situated at the anterior cardiophrenic angle (more commonly on the right), from which they project as smooth, ovoid, conical, or teardrop, soft tissue homogeneous densities (Fig. 21–36). They usually blend continuously into the cardiac opacity but may

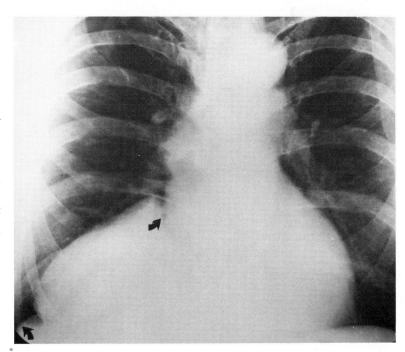

Figure 21–36. Pericardial cyst. The patient is a male, aged 53 years, with unrelated symptoms. A large, smooth, well-defined opacity with a convex right margin is situated at the right anterior cardiophrenic angle. Note the sharp angles at its junctions with the right heart border (right arrow) and the right diaphragm (left arrow).

occasionally be separated from the heart by a line of pericardial fat. Their walls do not often calcify. CT scanning clearly differentiates the fluid content of bronchial or pericardial cysts from solid structures.[3]

TRACHEAL NEOPLASMS (See also under Chapter 19, Part VII).   Tracheal neoplasms are uncommon, and they usually remain undiagnosed until late in the disease process. The tumors are usually malignant but are occasionally benign (for example, fibroma and chondroma). They are usually mucosal and intraluminal, encroaching on the tracheal lumen, which becomes progressively occluded (Fig. 21–37; see Fig. 21–11). The conventional frontal chest radiograph may be entirely normal, and even on well-penetrated films the endotracheal lesion may not be evident. Lateral radiographs and, especially, lateral tomography usually reveal the irregular mucosal growth narrowing the tracheal lumen (see Fig. 21–37). There may also be an extramural mass (usually small), which may separate the trachea from the esophagus; this mass is also best seen in oblique or lateral films or tomography (see Fig. 21–11) or on CT scanning, which also reveals the intraluminal lesion.

Clinically, there may be stridor, wheezing, or dyspnea with cough and hemoptysis, despite a normal frontal radiograph. Obstructive emphysema, with poor deflation of the lungs on expiration, may be clinically or fluoroscopically evident. If the tracheal mass encroaches on the carina, one lung only may be obstructed in expiration, causing unilateral obstructive emphysema (Fig. 21–38).

Primary tumors of the right or left main bronchi are nearly always carcinomas but, rarely, may be benign (for example, carcinoid, fibroma, neurofibroma, myoma, and chondroma) (see Fig. 21–38). They may be evident radiologically as either an exo-

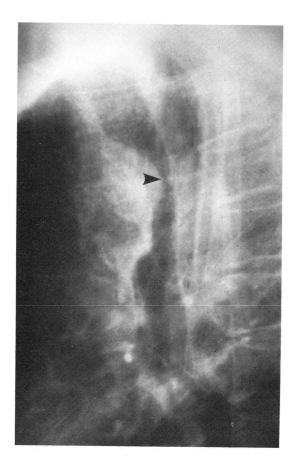

Figure 21–37.   Tracheal neoplasm. The patient is a 48-year-old male with a two-month history of stridor, cough, hoarseness, and slight hemoptysis. The frontal chest radiograph is normal. An irregular mass involves the anterior wall of the trachea, which is severely narrowed (arrowhead). A bronchoscopic biopsy revealed a highly malignant undifferentiated carcinoma.

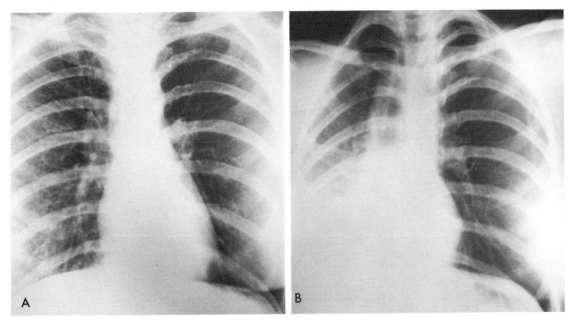

Figure 21–38. Leiomyoma of the left main bronchus. The patient is a woman of 43 years with a short history of dyspnea and wheezing. *A,* Inspiratory frontal radiograph shows an overinflated left lung with widely separated ribs; poor vascularity and increased radiolucency of the left lung are evident. *B,* Expiratory frontal radiograph demonstrates marked air trapping in the left lung, which is virtually unchanged from the inspiratory film (owing to endobronchial obstruction of the left main bronchus). The tumor was removed at thoracotomy, after which both lungs functioned normally with normal inspiratory expansion and expiratory deflation.

bronchial mass at the hilum or the distal effect of bronchostenosis (that is, obstructive emphysema [Fig. 21–38], collapse, and consolidation). Obstructive emphysema will probably be missed without fluoroscopy or an expiratory film (see Fig. 21–38).

ENLARGED MEDIASTINAL VESSELS IN MIDDLE MEDIASTINUM. The main arteries or veins of the mediastinum may become enlarged and project from the normal mediastinal contours, simulating a mass lesion. Unless the radiologic appearance is understood, an unnecessary (and perhaps dangerous) thoracotomy may be performed.

TORTUOSITY OF THE BRACHIOCEPHALIC ARTERIES. Tortuosity of the head and arm arteries, especially the innominate artery, is frequent in elderly, sthenic people. The affected arteries are buckled rather than dilated, and the tortuous innominate artery may cause a considerable convex mass to project from the right upper mediastinal border and obscure the medial part of the apex of the right lung. The tortuous innominate artery is the most frequent cause of this appearance, particularly if the aortic arch is unduly prominent and bowed. Angiography is rarely necessary for confirmation.

ANEURYSM OF ASCENDING AORTA AND AORTIC ARCH (See also Chapter 22, Part I). This may cause bulging and distortion of the normal contours of the mediastinum. The aneurysms are usually fusiform rather than saccular. Intrapericardiac aneurysms of the ascending aorta are often contained within the normal heart contours, but aneurysms arising elsewhere in the aorta cause a mediastinal mass. The clinical features (possibly including Marfan's syndrome, a syphilitic condition, or aortic valve disease) and the suggestive radiologic (including barium swallow) appearances usually indicate the diagnosis, but aortography may be necessary, particularly for preoperative assessment.

SYSTEMIC-PULMONARY ARTERIAL COMMUNICATIONS. In cyanotic patients with severe pulmonary arterial stenosis (such as severe tetralogy of Fallot), there may exist large branches, usually from the upper descending aorta or the subclavian arteries, that run to the lung hila. These abnormal arteries may be large enough to deform the upper mediastinal contours on the frontal radiograph. They may indent the esophagus and occasionally simulate a small mass lesion. These arteries convey systemic blood to the ischemic lungs; thus, they are beneficial anastomoses. The diagnosis is readily confirmed by aortography.

CONFLUENCE OF VEINS. The confluence of the veins of the right lung may cause a discrete opacity near the right border of the left atrium, sometimes resembling an abnormal mediastinal mass. The cardiovascular system may be normal, but in some patients, pulmonary arterial plethora (left-to-right shunt), or pulmonary venous congestion (mitral stenosis) may be the cause of the enlargement of the venous confluences.

SUPERIOR VENA CAVAE. The right (and occasionally a persistent left) superior vena cava may become so dilated that it simulates an upper mediastinal mass lesion. The most usual cause of this condition is supracardiac total anomalous pulmonary venous drainage, in which pulmonary venous blood is conveyed to the right atrium via the dilated superior vena cavae, rather than to the left atrium by the pulmonary veins. Pulmonary plethora or hypertension or both are usually present. The enlarged heart, surmounted by the dilated right and left superior vena cavae, gives rise to the "cottage loaf," "snowman," or "figure 8" radiologic cardiac appearance. The diagnosis is readily confirmed by cardiac catheterization and angiocardiography (Fig. 21–39).

VENA AZYGOS ENLARGEMENT.[1, 10] This condition may project as a convex mass above the right hilum, opposite the aortic knuckle. It is much more prominent when the patient is supine rather than erect. The usual cause of such a large azygos vein is the congenital interruption of the inferior vena cava, in which condition venous blood from the abdomen and legs is returned via the dilated ascending azygos veins, which termi-

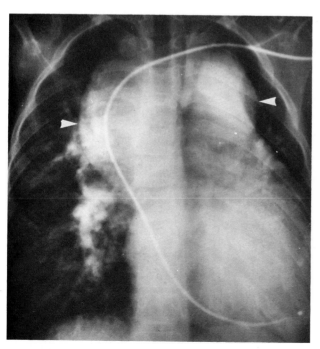

Figure 21–39. Gross enlargement of the superior vena cavae. Supracardiac total anomalous pulmonary venous drainage is evident. Contrast medium has been injected into the right ventricle. The pulmonary veins drain into the dilated right (left arrowhead) and left (right arrowhead) superior vena cavae, which return pulmonary venous blood to the right atrium. In this frame the superior vena cavae are opacified with contrast medium.

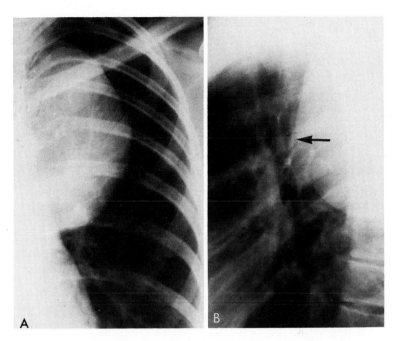

Figure 21–40A and B. Neurofibroma. A well-defined ovoid homogeneous opacity occupies the left posterior vertebrocostal gutter. Note the convex anterior surface (arrow) on lateral view. No bone change is apparent.

nate where the dilated right azygos arch enters the back of the superior vena cava. There is usually an associated left-to-right intracardiac shunt. Superior or inferior vena caval thrombosis and cirrhosis of the liver are other causes of marked enlargement of the azygos vein.[1, 11]

Posterior Mediastinal Masses

NEUROGENIC TUMORS. Neurogenic tumors account for three of four posterior "true" mediastinal tumors, and of all mediastinal masses they are second in incidence only to retrosternal goiter.[5, 11] Histologically, these tumors vary and include neurofibroma (from the nerve sheath), neurilemmoma (from the sheath of Schwann), sympathetic ganglia (benign ganglioneuroma), ganglioneuroblastoma (usually malignant), neuroblastoma (highly malignant), paragangliomic tumors (pheochromocytoma and chemodectoma).[11] Radiologic examination does not usually permit the identification of the specific cell type, but the sympathetic ganglia tumors may have a longer mediastinal attachment, and neuroblastomas may show extensive bone destruction and spotty calcification.

Posterior neurogenic mediastinal tumors arise from the intercostal nerves and the sympathetic chain. They usually occupy the angle between the vertebral body and the posterior end of the ribs and are not in the mediastinum proper but lie in the posterior costovertebral gutter (Fig. 21–40). Since they protrude laterally from the normal mediastinal opacity on frontal chest radiographs, they are conventionally regarded as posterior mediastinal masses.

Radiologically, the neurogenic tumors project as smooth, usually nonlobulated, spherical or ovoid masses from the costovertebral gutter, displacing the pleura anterolaterally (see Fig. 21–40). The mass is usually of homogeneous soft tissue (muscle or water) density on conventional radiographs, but CT scanning shows the mass to have a high attenuation factor owing to the compactness of its cellular structure. Spotty calcification may be seen in the malignant neuroblastoma on tomograms and CT scans and is therefore a sign of considerable diagnostic importance; pheochromocytomas may exhibit peripheral rim calcification, but they are uncommon in the chest.

Neurogenic mediastinal tumors are almost always in contact with the posterior ends of the ribs or the adjacent thoracic vertebrae or both. The associated bone changes are of major importance in suggesting the diagnosis. The adjacent ribs may be separated by the mass (Fig. 21–41), which may cause a smooth, corticated pressure indentation, usually on the lower margin of the rib (see Fig. 21–3). The ribs may be twisted or distorted (see Fig. 21–3) but do not show destructive changes, except in the rare malignant varieties (for example, neuroblastoma).

In the contiguous vertebrae, smooth indentations of the pedicles, transverse processes, or posterolateral aspects of the vertebral bodies may result from the more frequent benign tumors, and erosive bone destruction of these parts may be due to the uncommon malignant neurogenic tumors. The characteristic myelographic appearance of dumbbell neurofibroma arising from the emerging spinal nerve includes the enlargement of the exit intervertebral foramen; a smooth, curved indentation on the posterolateral aspect of the vertebral body; and an extradural intraspinal mass displacing the spinal cord. The bone changes may be well seen on coned frontal, lateral, and oblique radiographic projections but are always better demonstrated by tomography and CT scanning.

Neurogenic tumors, especially neurofibroma and neurilemmoma, usually occur in young adults. Malignant neuroblastomas and ganglioneuromas tend to occur in young children (Fig. 21–42). These latter tumors may secrete catecholamines, causing diarrhea, flushing, sweating, and hypertension; degradation products, such as vanillylmandelic acid, are excreted in the urine. There is a histologic spectrum of neurologic tumors, and the malignant neuroblastoma may mature into a benign ganglioneuroma, and a benign tumor may become malignant.[5]

Benign neurogenic tumors are slow-growing but in rare cases may enlarge rapidly, owing to hemorrhage, cystic degeneration, or malignant change. They are usually asymptomatic but may cause considerable bone and chest wall pain, particularly if the

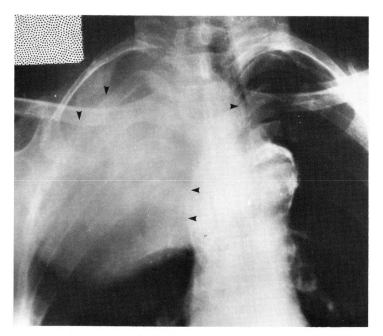

Figure 21–41. Large neurofibroma. A large neurofibroma is seen separating the first and second right (downward-pointing arrowheads) ribs posteriorly. This feature, the visibility of the ascending aorta (leftward-pointing arrowheads), and the extension of the mass well above the right clavicle indicate that the tumor lies posteriorly, although it indents the trachea and displaces it to the left (rightward-pointing arrowhead).

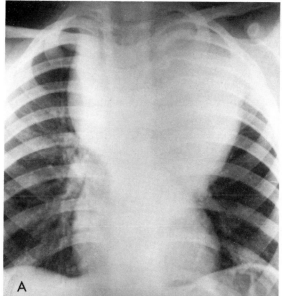

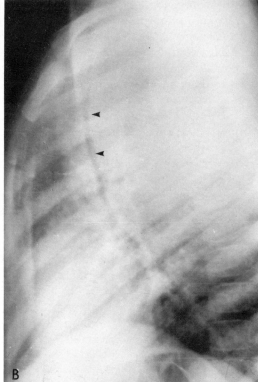

Figure 21–42A and B. Huge ganglioneuroma. The patient is five-year-old girl with diarrhea and excessive sweating. There are high vanillylmandelic acid levels in the urine. The large tumor in the upper posterior mediastinum is displacing and bowing the trachea forward (arrowheads). The trachea is narrowed. A large ganglioneuroma (secreting catecholamines) was removed, resulting in the disappearance of symptoms.

bones are eroded by pressure or by invasion. Puncture of neurogenic tumors (during fluoroscopic needle biopsy) causes severe pain.

An unusual posterior mediastinal neurogenic tumor is the anterior thoracic meningocele, which is always associated with congenital malformations of the cervical or thoracic vertebral bodies (butterfly or hemivertebra, spina bifida, or vertebral fusion). The diagnosis is suggested on radiographs of the spine, preferably tomograms, and confirmed by myelography performed with the patient in the prone position. Anterior thoracic meningocele is almost always associated with neurofibromatosis, but with this condition, neurogenic solid tumors of any cell type are more frequent.

Another variety of thoracic meningocele occurring in neurofibromatosis is positioned laterally, projecting through and enlarging an intervertebral foramen. It protrudes as a convex mass from the lateral mediastinal border in the posterior costovertebral sulcus and resembles an intercostal dumbbell-type neurofibroma, having similar bone changes. However, it fills with contrast medium on myelography, and CT scanning indicates a fluid-containing lesion with a low attenuation factor.

NEUROENTERIC CYSTS. These cysts were previously regarded as enteric cysts but are now known to contain neurogenic elements and are frequently associated with deformities of the dorsal (or cervical) spine of the type seen in cases of anterior thoracic meningocele. They are usually found in infants and may assume a considerable size (see Fig. 21–15), causing symptoms by the compression of intrathoracic structures, such as the lungs and esophagus.

Neuroenteric cysts are seen radiographically as spherical, ovoid, or elongated masses in the posterior mediastinum (see Fig. 21–15), usually displacing and deforming the esophagus. Ultrasound may confirm their cystic nature. Occasionally, these cysts communicate with the esophagus, contain air (or food or both), and may be opacified by swallowed barium. On other occasions, they may communicate with the spinal subarachnoid space and be filled by contrast medium during prone myelography. This spinal communication is a dangerous one and may result in meningitis. Peptic ulceration may occur in ectopic gastric mucosa within the cyst.

ESOPHAGUS.   Disorders of the esophagus may cause a space-occupying lesion in the posterior mediastinum; radiology plays the major role in the assessment.

ACHALASIA.   The esophagus is more dilated in advanced achalasia than in any other condition. It may become extremely dilated, displacing the mediastinal pleura from the posterior compartment and thus indenting and displacing the medial surface of the right lung. The patient may have no symptoms, and the diagnosis may be first suggested by the frontal chest radiograph. More frequently, the patient has a long history of dysphagia and sometimes of recurrent respiratory infection; even after successful surgical treatment and eradication of symptoms, the esophagus always remains dilated.

Radiologically, advanced achalasia may be responsible for an elongated opacity, convex and often gently undulating, to the right of the heart border (which can often be seen "through" the abnormal opacity — the overlay sign), extending from the thoracic inlet to the diaphragm (Fig. 21–43; see Fig. 21–12). The esophagus in achalasia elongates as well as dilates; the upper and middle esophagus bow to the right, but the lower segment tends to turn horizontally to the left to reach the esophageal hiatus. It may cause a convex radiologic opacity on the left at the spinal-diaphragmatic angle seen through the cardiac opacity (see Fig. 21–12).

A characteristic radiologic feature is the mottled appearance of the opacity resulting

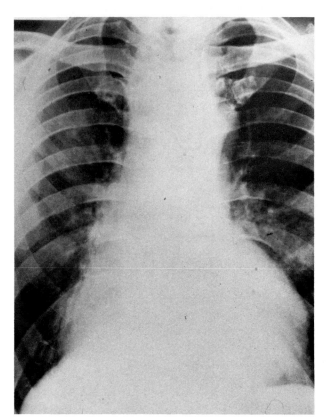

Figure 21–43.   Achalasia. The unusual right mediastinal border is not formed by the heart but by the dilated esophagus, full of food. Note the loss of the normal gas bubble in the stomach.

from retained food and air; occasionally a fluid level is seen in the esophagus. There is usually no gas in the fundus of the stomach. A lateral radiograph demonstrates that the opacity lies posteriorly behind the heart and often bows the trachea anteriorly. Once achalasia is considered as a possible cause of the mediastinal "mass," the diagnosis is readily confirmed by barium swallow, which demonstrates the dilated esophagus, its retained food content, and its tapered, smooth, parrot-beak lower end, at which there is considerable delay before the barium enters the stomach (see Fig. 21–12).

Occasionally, achalasia is complicated by carcinoma, which is demonstrable radiologically as a fixed defect within the esophagus. Carcinoma and stricture of the esophagus usually do not cause sufficient proximal esophageal dilatation to suggest a mediastinal mass.

BENIGN TUMORS. Benign tumors of the esophagus are uncommon. They are usually leiomyomas derived from the muscle wall and may be large enough and may project sufficiently from the outer surface of the esophagus to cause a considerable spherical or ovoid posterior mediastinal mass closely related to and smoothly indenting the esophagus, usually without mucosal invasion and often without marked deformity of its lumen.

ENTEROGENOUS DUPLICATION CYSTS. These are thick-walled fluid-containing cysts, which usually contain both digestive tract and neural elements and are therefore best described as "neuroenteric cysts." They usually occur in infants as large, elongated posterior mediastinal masses (see Fig. 21–15), which may cause compression symptoms. They are closely related to the esophagus, with which they may communicate. They may also communicate with the spinal subarachnoid space, in which case they fill with contrast medium during prone myelography. Complications include peptic ulceration in the ectopic gastric mucosa lining the cysts (see Fig. 21–15); rupture into the esophagus, mediastinum, or pleura; and infection, possibly spreading to the meninges as well as to other neighboring tissues. There are usually developmental defects in the cervical or dorsal vertebrae.

ESOPHAGEAL DIVERTICULA. The upper esophageal or pharyngeal (Zenker's) diverticulum projects through the posterior wall through the dehiscence between the oblique and transverse fibers of the inferior constrictor muscle of the pharynx. Although usually small (but causing troublesome dysphagia), the diverticulum may occasionally grow to several centimeters in diameter and may pass from the neck into the posterior mediastinum to form a radiologically evident, smooth, ovoid mass, which may contain a fluid level. The diverticulum descends behind the upper esophagus, which is displaced forward. During barium swallow, the barium enters the diverticulum first and then spills over into the anteriorly displaced esophagus.

Diverticula of the esophagus may occur in the middle or lower esophagus and are probably minor forms of intestinal duplication. Rarely, a diverticulum may become large enough to cause a space-occupying lesion in the posterior mediastinum. During barium swallow the diagnosis is readily confirmed by the filling of the lumen of the "mass" from the esophagus.

Barium examination of the esophagus is an essential part of the radiologic investigation of the middle and posterior mediastinum; it must never be omitted.

DIAPHRAGMATIC HERNIATION

HIATUS HERNIA. This is by far the most frequent type of diaphragmatic hernia. In the case of a "fixed" hiatus hernia, a loculus of the stomach is herniated permanently into the chest through the esophageal hiatus, often without symptoms. It causes a rounded opacity, which is seen through the cardiac opacity at the left costovertebral angle on a well-penetrated chest radiograph. A diagnostic feature is the demonstration on an erect radiograph of gas or a fluid level within the opacity (see Fig. 21–7). A lateral film reveals that the mass lies behind the heart. A barium examination readily confirms the diagnosis and is another example of the necessity of routine barium swallow, which prevents an occasional complete misinterpretation of plain radiographs.

POSTERIOR DIAPHRAGMATIC HERNIA. This condition is usually due to a deficiency of fusion of the posteromedial spinal and the costal portions of the diaphragm (foramen of Bochdalek or pleuroperitoneal canal). The hernia may be massive and cause respiratory distress in infants, or it may be found incidentally on routine chest radiographs of adults. Radiography reveals the hernial contents lying in the chest behind the heart, usually on the left side. If the hernia contains bowel, it is readily diagnosed by its gas content, but the smaller hernias may contain only solid viscera, such as portions of the liver, kidney, or spleen. Conventional radiology confirms the position of the opacity in the costovertebral recess just above the diaphragm, but it is usually not possible to make a confident diagnosis of herniation unless gas-containing bowel is in the sac. Barium studies confirm the presence of bowel, but the induction of a pneumoperitoneum may be necessary for the diagnosis to be confirmed if no bowel is present in the hernia. Sometimes there is no hernial sac, but there is a free communication existing between the peritoneal and pleural cavities (persistent pleuroperitoneal canal); in this case, the induced pneumoperitoneum results in a pneumothorax.

DESCENDING AORTA AND AORTIC ARCH

ANEURYSMAL DILATATION OF THE AORTIC ARCH. This causes a well-defined convex opacity that projects from the mediastinum to the left and upward in place of the normal, smoothly curved aortic knuckle. It may have a peripheral rim of calcification and usually exhibits marked pulsation; it displaces the trachea and the esophagus, which is easily demonstrated by barium swallow.

ANEURYSMAL DILATATION OF THE DESCENDING THORACIC AORTA. This is usually fusiform but may be localized and saccular (see Fig. 21–10), especially in the uncommon event of mycotic aneurysm. The left lateral border of the descending aorta is always well demonstrated on penetrated frontal radiographs and is seen to bulge and bow laterally and posteriorly as the aorta dilates and elongates. The esophagus usually also bows to the left, parallel to the dilated aorta, and it becomes indented by any localized aortic dilatation (see Fig. 21–10). Fluoroscopy may reveal intrinsic pulsation in the aneurysm, but para-aortic masses frequently exhibit considerable transmitted pulsation and the thick-walled, partly clotted aneurysms may not pulsate. It may occasionally be impossible to distinguish on conventional films between an aneurysm of the aorta and a para-aortic mass, but aortography (or CT scans) are decisive (see Fig. 21–10).

MARKED BOWING OF THE DESCENDING AORTA. This may occur in elderly patients and may bulge extensively, usually to the left, in the midthorax, or sometimes to the right, just above the diaphragm. The tortuosity may cause a well-defined knuckle that simulates a mediastinal mass, but the diagnosis can usually be readily established by well-exposed frontal and lateral radiographs, fluoroscopy, and barium swallow, which demonstrate that the esophagus usually closely follows the dorsal aorta even when it is in an unusual position.

CONGENITAL KINKING OF THE AORTIC ARCH (PSEUDOCOARCTATION). This is an unusual malformation in which the descending limb of the aortic arch is pulled sharply forward at the attachment of the ligamentum arteriosum.[4] The aortic arch above the kink is abnormally high and prominent and may closely resemble an upper posterior mediastinal tumor. Several such cases have been explored for mediastinal tumor, but knowledge of the condition, careful inspection of frontal and lateral penetrated radiographs, and barium swallow (which reveals a prominent dual abnormal indentation) often confirm the diagnosis.[4] Aortography may be necessary. Coarctation of the aorta may occasionally produce an identical appearance to congenital kinking of the aortic arch. Wtih coarctation, there is a hemodynamic stenosis with rib notching and reduced femoral pulses, but there is no stenosis, rib notching, or pulse deficit with pseudocoarctation.

TRAUMATIC DISSECTING ANEURYSM OF THE DISTAL LIMB OF THE AORTIC ARCH. This usually causes a well-defined convex opacity (sometimes rimmed by calcification) to project from the left border of the upper posterior mediastinum (see Fig. 21–22). Patients with this condition usually were involved in a severe automobile accident several years before, that resulted in sternal compression. Aortography readily confirms the diagnosis and is a prerequisite for surgery (see Fig. 21–22).

THE SPINE. Abnormalities of the dorsal spine, for example, fractures, tumors, myeloma, osteomyelitis (including tuberculosis), and paravertebral abscess, may so deform one or both of the paraspinal lines of pleural reflection that on frontal radiographs they may simulate primary posterior mediastinal space-occupying lesions. Radiographs of the dorsal spine, assisted by tomography if necessary, readily confirm the presence of a primary spinal lesion.

PARAVERTEBRAL LESIONS. Thickening of the tissues between the dorsal spine and the paraspinal lines of pleural reflection causes lateral bulging of the paraspinal lines, which may be undulating and considerably separated from the lateral vertebral margins. One important cause is extramedullary hematopoiesis, usually secondary to a severe chronic hemolytic anemia (for example, Cooley's anemia [Fig. 21–44] or leukemia).[7] Tomography confirms the presence of paravertebral thickening, the normality of the

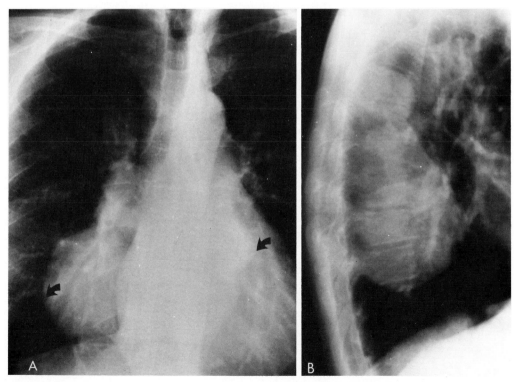

Figure 21–44A and B. Paraspinal extramedullary erythropoiesis. A large, lobulated mass is seen extending into both lung fields and lying on each side of (arrows) and anterior to the dorsal spine. The patient was of Mediterranean origin and had severe Cooley's anemia. This is an extreme example of extramedullary erythropoiesis (Courtesy of R. O. Hill, M.D., Montreal, Canada.)

dorsal spine, and the absence of calcification. Occasionally, one or more localized spherical masses of hemopoietic tissue occur in the posterior mediastinum, instead of the more common elongated paraspinal tissue thickening (Fig. 21–44).[7] The liver and spleen are usually enlarged, and a chronic anemic state is usually present, features that suggest the correct diagnosis — paravertebral hematopoiesis.

Soft tissue tumors, such as lipomas, fibromas, and hemangiomas, may occur adjacent to the dorsal vertebra, causing lateral bulging of the paraspinal line. CT scanning enables the exact localization of these paraspinal lesions and yields valuable information about their contents (see Fig. 21–14A), particularly if they are lipomas, with their characteristic low attenuation coefficients.

A loculated pleural effusion may cause some difficulty in diagnosis, but conventional radiographs, sometimes aided by CT scanning, are usually decisive (see Fig. 21–14B). Aspiration by needle puncture confirms the diagnosis.

Masses in the Superior Mediastinum

Masses frequently seen in the superior mediastinum are retrosternal thyroid, thymoma, lipoma, lymphatic cyst, hemangioma, tortuous innominate artery, aneurysm of the aortic arch, dissecting aneurysm of the aortic arch, congenital kinking of the aortic arch, abnormal systemic arteries supplying the lung in cyanotic congenital heart disease, and dilatation of the superior vena cavae or azygos vein.

Other masses, such as bronchogenic cysts, neuroenteric cysts, and neurogenic tumors, frequently develop in or extend into the superior mediastinum but do not show the strong predilection for this location as do the previously mentioned lesions.

Acute Mediastinitis

The mediastinum is rarely the site of primary hematogenous infection, but occasionally acute mediastinitis is caused by the rupture of the esophagus or, less commonly, the tracheobronchial tree, or by the extension of infection from neighboring tissue planes in the neck or abdomen.

The rupture or perforation of the esophagus is usually a complication of instrumentation (esophagoscopy or bouginage) and, less commonly, of the impaction of a foreign body or the ulceration of esophageal carcinoma. A distinctive clinical picture results from a spontaneous tear of the lower esophagus during vomiting or retching (Boerhaave's syndrome or Mallory-Weiss). The patient presents with acute central thoracoabdominal pain and often with a sensation of choking; the patient may be in shock, presenting as an acute emergency.

Radiology plays the major diagnostic role. The frontal chest radiograph may demonstrate the widening and loss of the normal contours of the upper mediastinum, within which there may be streaks of air separating the mediastinal pleura from the aorta and the heart owing to pneumomediastinum (see Fig. 21–19). The investigation of the esophagus is best performed by gently passing a soft tube into the stomach and slowly injecting water-soluble contrast medium as the tube is withdrawn. The esophageal tear, which is usually vertical and situated immediately above the diaphragm, is demonstrated by the escape of contrast medium into the mediastinal tissues or into the pleural cavity (see Fig. 21–19).

There is frequently unilateral or bilateral pleural effusion or hydropneumothorax (see Fig. 21–19). Escape of air into the neck and chest wall produces the characteristic radiologic appearance of surgical emphysema.

Chronic Fibrosing Mediastinitis

This is also an uncommon condition, usually resulting from a marked fibrotic reaction secondary to chronic granulomatous mediastinal lymphadenitis (usually, but not always, tuberculosis or histoplasmosis).[9] The patient presents with swelling of the head, neck, and eyes resulting from superior vena caval obstruction. Occasionally, the esophagus or tracheobronchial tree may be obstructed by extrinsic pressure.

One variety of chronic fibrosing mediastinitis is of unknown origin and may be associated with chronic fibrosis of other tissues, particularly retroperitoneal, thyroid, and orbit. Some of these patients have a history of methysergide therapy for migraine, although retroperitoneal fibrosis with ureteric obstruction is a more frequent complication than fibrosing mediastinitis.

The frontal radiograph usually shows slight widening of the superior mediastinum, with a localized bulge of the right paratracheal glands, which may show calcification on tomography (see Fig. 21–24). Venography confirms superior vena caval obstruction, which is usually localized and tapering (see Fig. 21–24) and situated at the entry of the azygos vein. The principal differential diagnosis is from carcinoma or other malignancy of the mediastinum, which usually causes a larger, more localized mediastinal mass producing major indentations into and occlusions of the vena cava and innominate veins. It may, however, prove impossible to differentiate malignancy from mediastinitis even at surgery, for there may be an extensive, infiltrating, dense, white fibrotic mass in cases of chronic mediastinitis that closely simulates malignancy. Histologic examination usually establishes the diagnosis of granulomatous mediastinitis, but the causative organism is identified only in a minority of cases.[9]

The natural history of the condition also distinguishes the inflammatory from the malignant condition: In the case of fibrosing mediastinitis the vena caval obstruction tends to improve as collateral venous channels open, whereas malignant caval obstruction is nearly always progressive and unremittent.

Pneumomediastinum or Mediastinal Emphysema

Gas in the mediastinal tissues has several possible origins — the lungs, tracheobronchial tree, esophagus, stomach, small or large bowel, or external air.[8, 11] The most common cause is the rupture of alveoli in neonates and infants due to aspiration and bronchial obstruction. The air escapes from the alveoli into the lung tissue, causing interstitial pulmonary emphysema, which tracks to the hilum, thereby entering the mediastinal tissues along the great vessels and bronchi. There is frequently an associated pneumothorax resulting from pleural rupture.

Pneumomediastinum may complicate an asthmatic attack; (whooping) cough; respiratory infection; strenuous exercise, labor; or resuscitation attempts with intubation, cardiac massage, and artificial respiration. Perforation of the esophagus (due to vomiting, intubation, or a foreign body) or trachea (due to a foreign body, intubation, or trauma) also causes pneumomediastinum. Retroperitoneal gas, either injected for diagnostic purposes or resulting from retroperitoneal perforation of the gut, may spread into the mediastinum and thence into the neck.

Clinically, there may be no symptoms if only a small amount of gas has entered the mediastinal tissues, but a large amount of gas may cause severe distress with chest pain, dyspnea, and venous obstruction, resulting in a swollen, engorged neck.

Radiologically, there is usually lateral displacement of the fine "white" line of mediastinal pleura by radiolucent "dark" stripes of air (see Fig. 21–20). This feature is diagnostic and best seen adjacent to the aortic arch and left border of the heart on the frontal radiograph (see Fig. 21–21). Air may also be seen between the lower surface of the heart and the diaphragm.[8, 11]

Pneumomediastinum may resemble pneumopericardium or pneumothorax, but in the latter conditions the gas is strictly confined to the pericardial or pleural spaces and is mobile within these cavities according to the position of the patient. Gas (or fluid) in the mediastinal tissues does not shift with change in posture. Gas in the mediastinum often spreads into the tissues of the neck and chest wall, where it can be readily appreciated both clinically and radiologically (see Fig. 21–21). Gas in the pericardium or pleural space remains confined and does not spread into these planes.

The lateral chest radiograph is also useful in the diagnosis of mediastinal emphysema, for the gas tends to separate the anterior surface of the pericardium from the sternum, particularly in infants and children (Fig. 21–45).[8, 11]

Mediastinal Hemorrhage

Most patients with severe mediastinal hemorrhage have been involved in an automobile accident that resulted in severe chest injury, often from the steering wheel. Rupture of a heart chamber, aorta, vena cavae or their main branches can result in torrential bleeding into the mediastinum, causing immediate shock, mediastinal tamponade, and frequently rapid death.

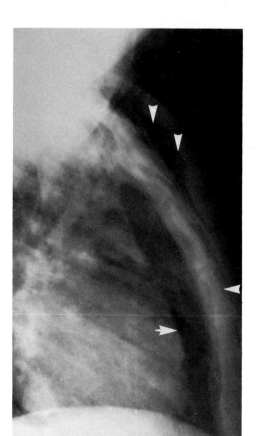

Figure 21–45. Mediastinal emphysema. The lateral radiograph demonstrates gas between the mediastinum (lower left arrowhead) and the sternum (lower right arrowhead). Note the subcutaneous emphysema (upper arrowheads).

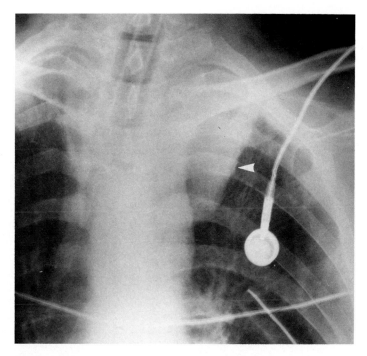

Figure 21–46. Mediastinal bleeding. Bleeding into the upper posterior mediastinum strips the parietal pleura (arrowhead) from its normal position. An aneurysm has been excised from the middle descending aorta.

More often, the bleeding is less severe and may, in fact, cause no thoracic symptoms. Moderate bleeding causes widening and loss of normal contours, particularly of the upper mediastinum (Fig. 21–46). The aortic knuckle, descending aorta, and paraspinal lines of pleural reflection may be displaced laterally. Localized lateral bulging of the paraspinal lines may suggest vertebral injury and hematoma.

Postoperative Mediastinum

The mediastinal tissues are usually drained by a tube after surgical exploration. Bleeding and chylous and serous fluid may collect within the mediastinum, however, and cause important radiologic changes.

If the fluid remains localized, it may cause a space-occupying opacity bulging from the mediastinal contours (Fig. 21–46). More frequently the fluid tracks through the mediastinum and may extend into the extrapleural tissue spaces with which the mediastinum is continuous. This produces a radiologic appearance similar to that of intrapleural fluid, but if the fluid lies in the extrapleural space it does not move so freely with change in posture and is therefore not so gravitationally dependent (Fig. 21–47B). Indeed, the fluid may be so localized that in some radiologic projections it may resemble a mass.

Air enters the mediastinal tissues at surgery, particularly when a large mediastinal mass has been removed. This may produce pneumomediastinum and surgical emphysema or, if more localized and associated with fluid, may cause a postoperative mediastinal fluid level (Fig. 21–48) or extrapleural fluid level (see Fig. 21–47A).

The radiologic appearances after surgery of specific mediastinal organs, such as the heart or esophagus, are dealt with in the appropriate sections. Of particular importance is the recognition of a mass density resembling a tumor due to aneurysm formation following the complicated ligature or division of a patent ductus (Fig. 21–49). These postoperative aneurysms may calcify. Localized collections of

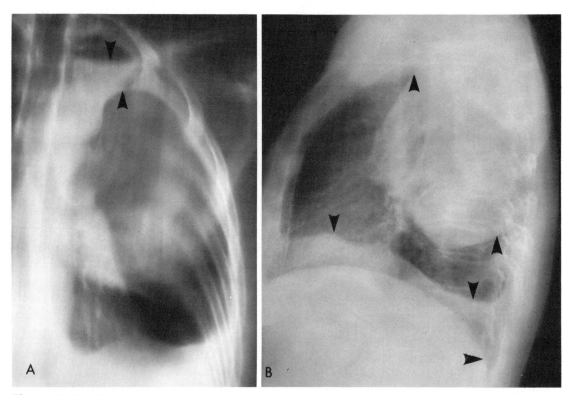

Figure 21–47. Mediastinal hemorrhage. Following cervical sympathectomy for Raynaud's syndrome, an extensive opacity appeared in the upper left chest. Aspiration revealed almost pure blood. *A,* Erect radiograph demonstrating an air-fluid level (upper arrowhead) in the left extrapleural space above the apex of the left lung (lower arrowhead), which has been stripped downward. *B,* Lateral radiograph demonstrates considerable stripping of the pleura. Note the acute angles (upward-pointing arrowheads) where the pleura meets with the chest wall, suggesting that the mass lies extrapleurally. A little intrapleural fluid is visible above left diaphragm (downward-pointing arrowheads) contrasting with the acute right posterior costophrenic angle (horizontal arrowhead).

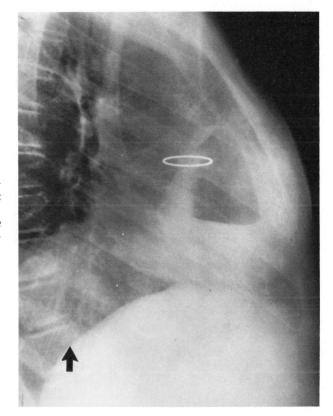

Figure 21–48. Mediastinal hydropneumothorax. Fluid and air are present in the right anterior mediastinum following surgery. Only the left diaphragm (arrow) is clear; the right diaphragm is obscured by a pleural effusion.

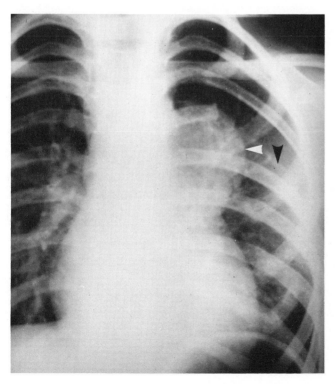

Figure 21–49. Pseudoaneurysm after the ligature of the patent ductus. A large left mediastinal mass (white arrowhead) is evident following a difficult ligature of a patent ductus arteriosus. Note the rib resection (black arrowhead). At a second thoracotomy, a large false aneurysm was found; surgery was so difficult that a left pneumonectomy was performed.

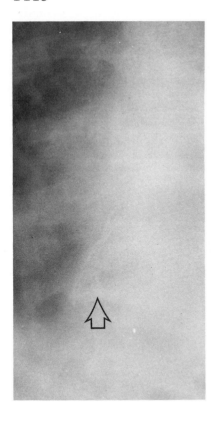

Figure 21–50. Swab in the mediastinum. Note the faint metal strip in the surgical swab (arrow) left in the mediastinum. All surgical swabs must have radiopaque markers.

Figure 21–51. Esophageal perforation (postoperative). Following total gastrectomy, there is a major leak from the anastomosis (lowest arrowhead). The left paraspinal line (middle arrowhead) is displaced owing to paraesophageal swelling. Note the partial collapse and consolidation of the left lower lobe, with a marked air bronchogram (uppermost arrowhead).

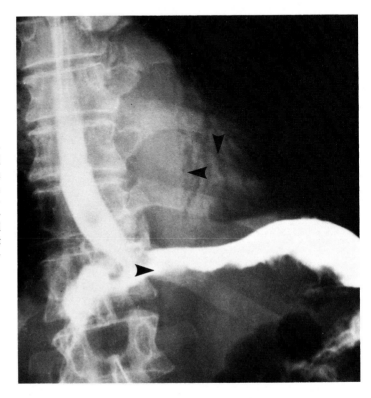

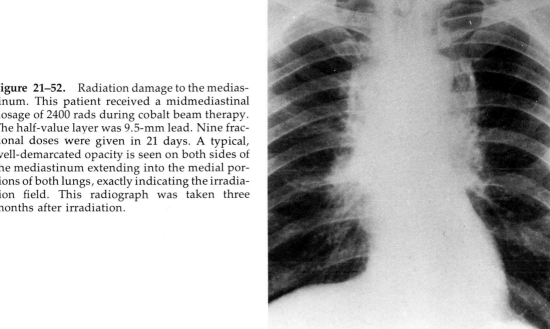

Figure 21–52. Radiation damage to the mediastinum. This patient received a midmediastinal dosage of 2400 rads during cobalt beam therapy. The half-value layer was 9.5-mm lead. Nine fractional doses were given in 21 days. A typical, well-demarcated opacity is seen on both sides of the mediastinum extending into the medial portions of both lungs, exactly indicating the irradiation field. This radiograph was taken three months after irradiation.

pericardial fluid may considerably deform the cardiac contour, as may postincisional ventricular aneurysms. Figure 21–50 illustrates a swab, inadvertently left in the mediastinum.

Following esophageal excision and replacement by bowel, a characteristic radiologic appearance is produced by the bowel gas pattern. The bowel may be implanted within the mediastinum proper or subcutaneously anterior to the sternum. Esophageal surgery may be complicated by leaks and paraesophageal bleeding and edema (Fig. 21–51). Tubes (which may be radiopaque) are often implanted in the esophagus in cases of obstructing carcinoma.

Irradiation of Mediastinum

Mediastinal irradiation may result in a characteristic radiologic appearance owing to fibrosis within the mediastinum and neighbouring pleura and lung. If supervoltage therapy is used, there may be sharp delineation of the affected tissue, indicating the exact field of irradiation (Fig. 21–52). The normal mediastinal contours may be lost and replaced by featureless, slightly ragged, laterally displaced borders; sometimes the normal mediastinum may be faintly seen through the paramediastinal postirradiation opacity.

References

1. Castellino, R. A., Blank, N., and Adams, D. F.: Dilated azygos and hemi-azygos veins presenting as paravertebral intrathoracic masses. N. Engl. J. Med. *278*:1087–1091, 1968.
2. Cicciarelli, F. E., Soule, E. H., and McGoon, D. C.: Lipoma and liposarcoma of the mediastinum. J. Thorac. Cardiovasc. Surg. *47*:411–429, 1964.

3. Goldwin, R. L., Heitzman, E. R., and Proto, A. V.: Computed tomography of the mediastinum. Radiology 124:235–241, 1977.
4. Grainger, R. G., and Pattinson, J. N.: Congenital kinking of the aortic arch. Br. Heart J. 21:555–561, 1959.
5. Greenfield, L. J., and Shelley, W. M.: The spectrum of neurogenic tumours of the sympathetic nervous system. Maturation and adrenergic function. J. Natl. Cancer Inst. 32:215–226, 1965.
6. Oschner, J. L., and Oschner, S. F.: Congenital cysts of the mediastinum. 42 cases. Ann. Surg. 163:909–920, 1966.
7. Papavasiliou, C. G.: Tumor simulating intrathoracic extramedullary hematopoiesis. Clinical and roentgenologic considerations. Am. J. Roentgenol. 93:695–702, 1965.
8. Rudhe, U., and Ozonoff, M. B.: Pneumomediastinum and pneumothorax in the newborn. Acta Radiol. Diagn. 4:193–205, 1966.
9. Schowengerdt, C. G., Suyemoto, R., and Main, F. B.: Granulomatous and fibrous mediastinitis — a review of 180 cases. J. Thorac. Cardiovasc. Surg. 57:365–379, 1969.

General Radiology of the Chest

10. Felson, B.: Chest Roentgenology. Philadelphia, W. B. Saunders Company, 1973.
11. Fraser, R. G., and Paré, J. A. P.: Diagnosis of Disease of the Chest. Ed. 2. Philadelphia, W. B. Saunders Company, 1977.
12. Heitzman, E. R.: The Lung. Roentgenologic-Pathologic Correlations. St. Louis, The C. V. Mosby Company, 1973.
13. Shanks, S. C., and Kerley, P. J. (eds.): A Textbook of X-Ray Diagnosis by British Authors. Ed. 4. Vol. 3. London, H. K. Lewis & Company, Ltd., 1973.
14. Simon, G.: Principles of Chest X-Ray Diagnosis. Ed. 4. London, Butterworth, 1978.
15. Sutton, D., and Grainger, R. G. (eds.): Text-book of Radiology. Ed. 2. Edinburgh, Churchill-Livingstone, 1974.

General Radiologic and Pathologic Features of the Mediastinum

16. Burkell, C. C., Cross, J. M., Kent, H. P., et al.: Mass Lesions of the Mediastinum. Chicago, Year Book Medical Publishers, Inc., 1969.
17. Heitzman, E. R.: The Mediastinum: Radiological Correlations with Anatomy and Pathology. St. Louis, The C. V Mosby Company, 1977.
18. Leigh, T. F., and Weens, H. S.: The Mediastinum. Springfield, Illinois, Charles C Thomas, Publisher, 1959.
19. Leigh, T. F.: Mass lesions of the mediastinum. Radiol. Clin. North Am. 1:377–394, 1963.
20. Schlumberger, H. G.: Tumours of the mediastinum. In Atlas of Tumor Pathology. Section 5. Fascicle 18. Washington, D. C., Armed Forces Institute of Pathology, 1951.
21. The mediastinum. Semin. Roentgenol. 4:1–101, 1969.

22

THE ARTERIAL SYSTEM

Part I

Aneurysms of the Chest and Neck

ERICH K. LANG, M.D.

Advances in medical diagnosis and treatment, prevention of predisposing conditions, changes in dietary habits, and particularly, increased exposure to trauma are responsible for the changed incidence of aneurysms of various causes. About 70 per cent of all aneurysms are of arteriosclerotic origin.[29] While luetic aneurysms accounted for 30 per cent of all thoracic aneurysms in earlier reports, they are responsible for only about 5 per cent in current series.[29, 30] Nonsyphilitic mycotic aneurysms are estimated to constitute approximately 2.5 per cent of all thoracic aneurysms.[18, 19, 29, 57]

Traumatic aneurysms are rapidly increasing in incidence and account for 15 to 25 per cent of all aneurysms of the thoracic aorta.[7, 20, 25, 29] The remaining aneurysms — a numerically small group — are attributable to a variety of conditions, such as cystic degeneration of the media found with Marfan's syndrome, Erdheim's syndrome, Ehlers-Danlos syndrome, Turner's syndrome, giant cell arteritis, relapsing polychondritis, pregnancy-related disorders, and congenital aortic or subaortic stenosis.[1, 5, 31, 34-36, 49]

Certain morphologic patterns are almost specific for determining etiology (Table 22–1). Arteriosclerosis, for example, most frequently produces a fusiform aneurysm.[29] Medial necrosis predisposes to dissecting aneurysm.[1, 3, 16, 26, 34-36, 39, 49] Mycotic, luetic, and traumatic causes most often produce a saccular aneurysm.[6-8, 18, 19, 30, 32, 48, 57] However, because of the preponderance of arteriosclerotic aneurysms, most fusiform as well as most saccular and dissecting aneurysms are of arteriosclerotic origin (Table 22–1, Fig. 22–1).

The location, etiology, and relationship of an aneurysm to the aortic root and brachiocephalic vessels influence prognosis.[1, 16, 49] Age, severity of hypertension, duration of acute symptoms, and type of surgical or medical management are other important factors affecting survival and curability.[1, 16, 29]

1443

TABLE 22–1. INCIDENCE OF ANEURYSMS OF THE THORACIC AORTA*

	Morphologic Appearance				
Etiology	*Saccular*	*Fusiform*	*Dissecting*	*False*	*Sinus of Valsalva*
Arteriosclerosis	+++✓✓	+++✓✓✓	(+)++✓(✓)		+✓
Medial necrosis		+✓	+++✓✓✓		+✓✓
Mycotic (TB)	++✓✓✓			++✓✓	
Luetic	++✓✓✓	++✓✓	+✓		+✓✓
Traumatic	++✓✓✓	++✓✓	+✓	++✓✓	+✓

*Frequency of incidence.

Overall occurrence	For this etiology only
Most common: +++	Most common: ✓✓✓
Common: ++	Common: ✓✓
Relatively rare: +	Relatively rare: ✓

The predominant symptoms of thoracic aneurysms are pain, dyspnea, and dysphagia. Dry cough and hoarseness are also frequent.[29] Hypertension, neurologic deficits, and decreased femoral pulses are most commonly found with dissecting aneurysms.[11, 16, 23, 26, 28, 33-36, 49] Valvular insufficiency is most often caused by a dissecting aneurysm involving the sinus of Valsalva or a luetic aneurysm involving the aortic root.[16, 28, 30, 31, 37, 39, 41, 42]

Aortography is recommended to differentiate aneurysms from other mediastinal

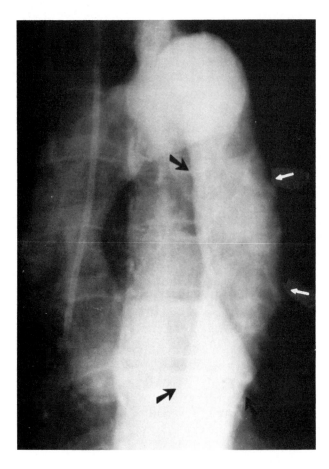

Figure 22–1. Fusiform aneurysm. An aortogram performed via a transbrachial approach demonstrates a fusiform aneurysm involving the descending thoracic aorta (arrows). This is the characteristic appearance of an arteriosclerotic aneurysm.

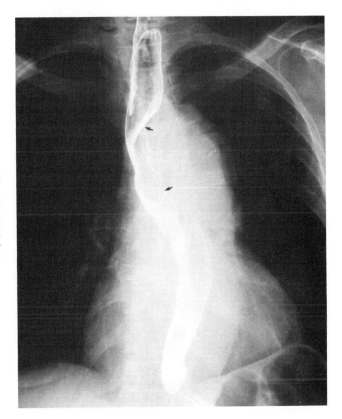

Figure 22–2. Aneurysm of descending aorta. Widening of the mid-mediastinum and an irregular contour margin of the descending thoracic aorta suggest the presence of an aneurysm. Effacement and displacement of the midportion of the esophagus (arrows) are caused by this mass.

mass lesions, to evaluate the relationship of the aneurysm to other vessels, to ascertain the presence of dissection, and to identify associated conditions, such as coarctation, aortic insufficiency, and pathologic conditions of the aortic wall.

The propensity for progression results in high mortality for untreated thoracic aneurysms and makes imperative the earliest possible diagnosis and appropriate surgical or medical management.

On chest films the most common findings are widening of the mediastinum by a mass or localized widening of a segment of the aortic shadow. Displacement and compression of the esophagus and trachea are frequent. Large aneurysms arising from the upper ascending aorta or anterior arch displace the trachea and esophagus to the left and posteriorly. If the aneurysm originates in the knob or descending aorta, displacement is usually to the right and often anteriorly.[28] Linear calcification of the wall of the aneurysm is frequent (Figs. 22–2 to 22–4).

While a dissecting aneurysm may be associated with a somewhat blurred edge of the aortic knob,[29] in general the border of an aneurysm is sharp and distinct. An associated pleural effusion raises the possibility of leakage from the aneurysm, especially in left-sided lesions.[28, 48]

Infrequently, erosion of a vertebral body or posterior rib results from a large pulsatile aneurysm of the ascending aorta.

THORACIC AORTA ANEURYSMS

Nondissecting aneurysms of the thoracic aorta are of arteriosclerotic, syphilitic, traumatic, or congenital origin. In the past, syphilitic aneurysms accounted for up to 20

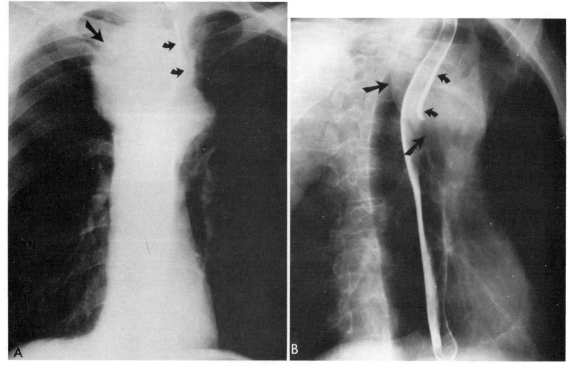

Figure 22–3. Aneurysm of aortic arch. *A,* A large mass (long arrow) is seen in the superior mediastinum projecting to the right. Note displacement of the tracheal air shadow and esophagus to the left (short arrows). The mass, which is contiguous with the ascending aorta and the aortic arch, is caused by an aneurysm originating from the arch and involving the innominate artery. *B,* A left anterior oblique projection demonstrates the contiguous nature of this mass extending from the aortic arch onto the innominate artery (long arrows). Note the characteristic effacement of the esophagus (short arrows).

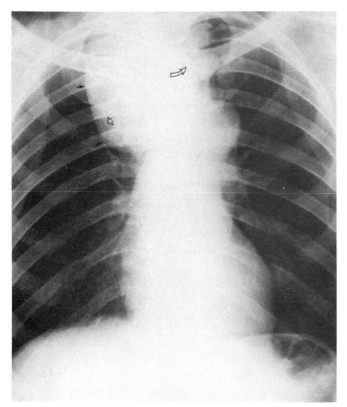

Figure 22–4. Aortic aneurysm. A posteroanterior chest roentgenogram demonstrates a mass in the superior mediastinum projecting to the right. Note the displacement of the tracheal air shadow to the left (curved arrow) and the faint shell-like calcifications attributable to calcifications of the intima of the aneurysm (open arrowhead).

1446

per cent of all thoracic aneurysms. Current statistics, however, suggest a luetic cause in only 5 per cent. About 78 per cent of thoracic aneurysms are attributable to arteriosclerotic disease, 15 per cent to trauma, and 2 per cent to congenital causes.[29] Aneurysms of the thoracic aorta occur with a male preponderance of three to one.

The average age at diagnosis is 60 years. However, depending on the etiology, a wide age range is noted. Traumatic aneurysms occur more frequently in the younger age group and do not show a marked male preponderance. Arteriosclerotic aneurysms occur more commonly in the older age group, predominantly in males.[29]

The descending thoracic aorta is the most common location (45 per cent), the arch and the ascending aorta are next most frequent. Involvement of the entire aorta by a nondissecting aneurysm is relatively rare.[29]

The fusiform aneurysm from arteriosclerosis is the most common morphologic type (78 per cent). Saccular aneurysms represent less than 20 per cent of the total.

Clinical Signs and Symptoms

At the time of diagnosis only 25 per cent of patients have symptoms referable to aneurysms.[29] In the symptomatic group, pain is the predominant symptom, occurring in 65 per cent. Dyspnea is present in less than 30 per cent, followed by hoarseness, dysphasia, and cough, in descending order of frequency.

Mediastinal widening and demonstration of an irregular contour of the aorta on routine chest roentgenograms are the signs most often responsible for the discovery of a thoracic aortic aneurysm (Figs. 22–2 to 22–4). Although evidence of erosion of thoracic vertebrae and posterior rib may be noted on roentgenograms, only one-third of these patients have symptoms of back pain.[29] Hypertension is found in more than one-third

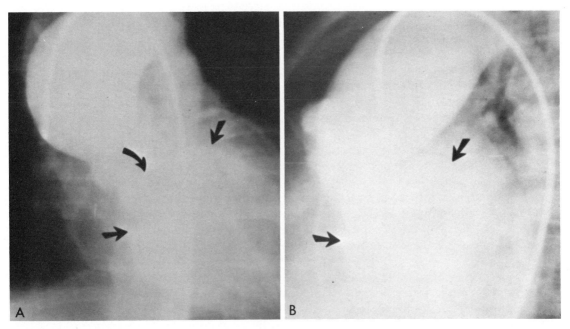

Figure 22–5. Aneurysm of ascending aorta. *A,* An aortogram in anteroposterior projection demonstrates massive aneurysmal dilatation of the ascending thoracic aorta. Note regurgitation of contrast medium into the left ventricle (arrows), proving resultant aortic insufficiency. *B,* A lateral projection confirms regurgitation (arrows), and the narrowing at the distal portion of the aneurysm suggests a coarctation of the descending thoracic aorta at the point of attachment of the ligamentum arteriosum.

of patients with thoracic aneurysms, while associated cardiovascular disease is present in less than one-third.

Roentgenographic and Angiographic Findings

Widening of the aortic shadow is the most common roentgenographic finding indicating the presence of aneurysm of the thoracic aorta.[29, 41] Depending on the location and size of the aneurysm, this may result in shift of the trachea to the right, displacement of the esophagus anteriorly and to the right, and widening of the paraspinal shadow (see Figs. 22–2 and 22–3A). The presence of a left pleural effusion indicates leakage from an aneurysm (see Fig. 22–14). Left ventricular enlargement and dilatation of the aortic root suggest aortic insufficiency, involvement of the sinus of Valsalva or both.[31] Disappearance of the incisura between the ascending aorta and the right atrium may result from marked dilatation of the aortic root.[31]

Calcifications are commonly demonstrated in aneurysms of arteriosclerotic origin and may identify dissection on the basis of abnormal widening of the space between the intimal calcification and the outer soft tissue contour of the aorta.

Aortography is the principal diagnostic modality for demonstrating aneurysms of the thoracic aorta (see Fig. 22–1; Fig. 22–5). CT scanning during contrast infusion can readily identify an aneurysm. Echocardiography and radionuclide angiography are also sometimes helpful in diagnosis.[41]

DISSECTING ANEURYSMS

Dissecting aortic aneurysms are the consequence of forceful penetration of blood through a tear of the aortic wall, resulting in dissection of the layers of the aorta and development of a false channel.[49] In general, this false channel forms between the inner two-thirds and the outer third of the media.[49] However, dissection may occasionally occur between the adventitia and the media, causing a subadventitial hematoma.[29]

Ten to twenty-five per cent of all thoracic aortic aneurysms are dissecting lesions.[26] An overall preponderance of male patients has been established, although under age 40 there is nearly equal distribution between the sexes, with many of the dissecting aneurysms occurring in women during pregnancy.[1, 36]

Pathogenesis

A number of mechanisms for the development of dissection have been proposed. Intimal tears leading to false channels occur predominantly at two sites. One is the supravalvular area of the aorta just above the attachment of the pericardium. The other is the point of attachment of the ligamentum arteriosum in the descending thoracic aorta.

Pre-existing disease other than arteriosclerosis can weaken the media, as in medial necrosis of Erdheim's syndrome, Marfan's syndrome, Ehlers-Danlos syndrome, giant cell arteritis, or relapsing polychondritis. This facilitates dissection once blood has gained entry through the intima.[20] Although the histopathologic appearance may be vastly different (Marfan's syndrome is characterized by fragmentation of the elastic components of the media, whereas Erdheim's medial necrosis causes separation of elastic fibers by interposed pools of mucoid material), both conditions weaken the media and predispose to dissection.[31] However, an added insult, such as trauma, is necessary to cause a tear of the intima and allow access of blood to the media. Moreover, the shearing force of a deceleration injury can also sever vasa vasorum and, owing to traumatic thrombosis, set the stage for medial necrosis.[20] An increased incidence of medial necrosis observed in patients who sustained and survived aortic injury for more than 12 hours supports this supposition.[47]

In general, intimal dehiscence at the level of the ligamentum arteriosum is associated with trauma, whereas intimal tears in the supravalvular area of the ascending aorta are more frequently found in the presence of predisposing conditions such as arteriosclerosis, Erdheim's syndrome, Marfan's syndrome, Ehlers-Danlos syndrome, or relapsing polychondritis and giant cell aortitis.[6, 20, 21, 25, 26, 28, 34, 35, 47] Subadventitial dissection is almost exclusively caused by blunt chest trauma.[20]

Classification

Although several classifications have been proposed, the one introduced by DeBakey based on the origin and extent of the dissection seems best suited to categorization, prognostication, and selection of appropriate therapy.[15, 49]

Dissections are grouped into three categories.

Type 1: The dissection involves the entire aorta, extending from the ascending aorta to the arch and beyond. This is the most common type, accounting for 60 per cent of all dissecting aneurysms.

Type 2: The dissection is limited to the ascending aorta. This is the rarest type, and Marfan's syndrome is the most common etiology.

Type 3: The dissection originates distal to the subclavian artery, usually at the point of fixation by the ligamentum arteriosum, and may or may not be confined to the thoracic aorta. It is usually the result of trauma.[1]

Clinical Features

Severe chest pain radiating to the back is the most common symptom.[1] Neurologic deficits, paraparesis, and transient paralysis are other frequent findings.[28] Hypertension and unequal or absent pulses in the limbs are ominous findings suggesting a dissecting aneurysm, particularly in young pregnant patients.[1, 36] Unilateral distention of the neck veins may herald an expanding mediastinal hematoma.[1] Exertional dyspnea is a common symptom of aortic root aneurysm or dissection extending into the sinus of Valsalva or both.[31]

Roentgenographic Findings

A common but not pathognomonic roentgenographic finding is widening of the mediastinum and the aortic shadow (see Fig. 22–2). Observation of progressive widening of the aortic shadow on sequential films is highly suggestive. Blurring of the outer border of the aortic knob may indicate involvement of the arch and therefore a probable type 1 dissecting aneurysm.[28] Widening of the ascending aorta suggests a type 1 or type 2 dissecting aneurysm. Shift of the trachea to the right, displacement of the esophagus anteriorly and to the right, and widening of the paraspinal shadow are frequent findings. The presence of a left pleural effusion (or an extrapleural density surrounding a lung apex) are indicative of possible leakage from a dissecting aneurysm (see Fig. 22–3B). An increased space between intimal calcification and the outer aortic soft tissue contour is highly suggestive of dissection. Left ventricular enlargement and dilatation of the aortic root may indicate the presence of aortic insufficiency secondary to retrograde dissection and involvement of the sinus of Valsalva.[31] Progressive dilatation of the aortic root causes disappearance of the incisura between the ascending aorta and the right atrium, a bulging contour margin representing the composite shadows of right atrium and contiguous aortic root may result. Progressive displacement of a nasogastric tube to the right indicates an expanding mediastinal hematoma.[52]

ECHOCARDIOGRAPHY. The presence of a dissecting flap of an aortic aneurysm is suggested by a regularly oscillating echo elicited from the intimal flap in the false lumen (Fig. 22–6).[14, 42] Echocardiographic evidence of enlargement of the aortic root, widening of the components of the aortic wall, and demonstration of abnormal opening of the aortic leaflets are other criteria of aortic dissection.[37, 41, 42]

COMPUTED TOMOGRAPHY. When this noninvasive study is performed during intravenous contrast infusion, identification of a simple or dissecting aortic aneurysm usually can be made (see Fig. 22–17). Thrombi, intimal calcifications, the intimal flap, and the true and false lumens can be appreciated in most cases of dissection. Currently, the CT scan is the study of choice prior to arteriography when an aneurysm is clinically suspected.

AORTOGRAPHY. Aortography is the definitive method used to establish the diagnosis of a dissecting aneurysm and to demonstrate the location of the intimal tear, the extent of dissection or false channel, the deformity of the true channel with resultant embarrassment or involvement of branch arteries, and the presence and degree of aortic insufficiency.[1, 16, 20, 24, 26, 28, 47, 49] A hemopericardium and clinical evidence of shock are contraindications for aortography in types 1 and 2 dissecting aneurysm of the thoracic aorta.[49]

TECHNIQUE. Catheterization can be carried out via a transfemoral or a transaxillary approach. Prior to pressure injection of large volumes of contrast medium, the location of the catheter within the true aortic lumen must be verified.[49]

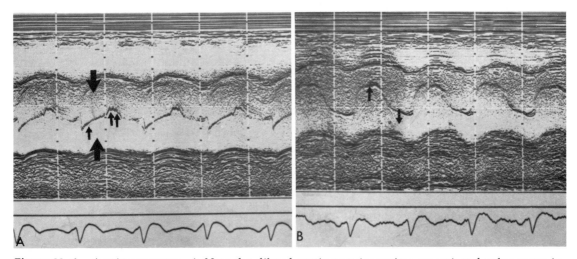

Figure 22–6. Aortic aneurysm. *A,* Note the dilated aortic root (opposing arrows) and valve cusps in systole (upward arrow) and diastole (double arrows). *B,* The m mode echocardiogram demonstrates classic anterior motion of the flap in systole (upward arrow) and posterior motion in diastole (downward arrow).

Legend continued on the opposite page

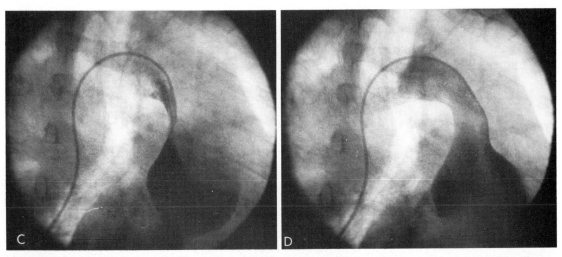

Figure 22–6 *Continued. C*, A cineangiogram recording a supravalvular injection in diastole shows posterior movement of the flap. *D*, The cineangiographic recording demonstrates anterior movement of the flap in systole. (*From* Curati, W. L., Peticlerc, R., Dyrda, I., et al.: Echographic demonstration of mobility of the dissecting flap of an aortic aneurysm. Radiology *123*:173–174, 1977. Reproduced by permission.)

ANGIOGRAPHIC CRITERIA OF DISSECTING ANEURYSMS. The intimal tear is demonstrable on aortograms as a radiolucent line (Fig. 22–7A). In types 1 and 2 dissecting aneurysm, the intimal tear is located in the supravalvular region of the ascending aorta. In type 3, it is distal to the left subclavian artery in the descending thoracic aorta at the level of the ligamentum arteriosum.

Injection of contrast medium proximal to the intimal tear may result in opacification of both the true and the false channels (Fig. 22–6B). A linear lucency representing the intimal flap may delineate the border between the true and the false channels.[1, 16, 49] Frequently there is a difference in flow rate. Opacification as well as washout of contrast medium from the false channel may be delayed (Fig. 22–8).[28, 49] The false channel is usually located to the right and posteriorly along the ascending aorta and to the left and posteriorly along the descending aorta (Fig. 22–9).[49]

On rare occasions, the aortogram may demonstrate merely a deformity of the true channel — the result of a solid blood clot occluding the false channel.[16] Failure of the false channel to opacify may occur if the tear is located far from the site of injection, and the existing communication may go undetected. In a few cases the intimal tear may never be found. The most likely cause, however, is thrombosis of the false channel and sealing of the proximal end of the dissection by a thrombus (Fig. 22–9).[16]

A distance in excess of 3 mm between the contrast medium column and the lateral soft tissue margin raises the question of a nonopacified false channel. However, fat abutting the aorta may erroneously create an impression of increased wall thickness (Fig. 22–10).[44]

In exceptional cases, the false lumen may become the main conduit and may then demonstrate a more rapid blood flow (see Figure 22–7A).[28] Opacification of the false lumen is possible only if the false channel is located within layers of the media; subadventitial dissections do not opacify with contrast medium (Fig. 22–11).[20]

In types 1 and 2 dissecting aneurysms, aortic insufficiency may occur, and its recognition is surgically important. Angiograms may show dilatation, deformity, and a lower than usual position of the sinus of Valsalva. Contrast medium may reflux into the left ventricle. The degree of aortic insufficiency is indicated by the degree and speed of

Text continued on page 1455

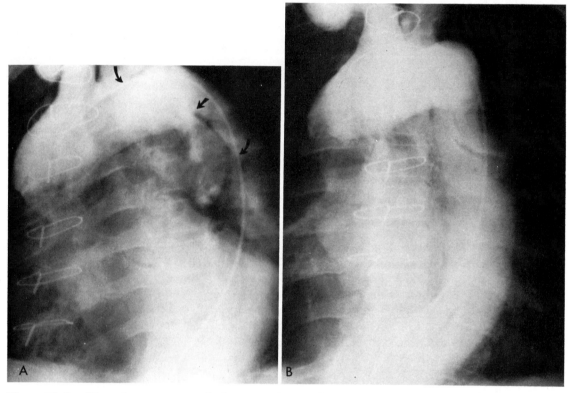

Figure 22–7. Dissecting aneurysm. *A,* A retrograde transfemoral aortogram demonstrates opacification of the aortic arch and the false channel. Note the linear lucency, representing the intimal flap, delineating the border between the true and false channel (arrows). The intimal tear occurred at the point fixed by the ligamentum arteriosum, characteristic of deceleration injury. During injection, the catheter has moved close to the centrifugal wall of the aorta (curved arrow). A location of the dissecting aneurysm distal to the left subclavian artery identifies this as a type 3 dissecting aneurysm. *B,* The delayed film shows beginning washout from the false channel and opacification of the true channel in the descending thoracic aorta. This is an unusual pattern—accelerated flow in the false channel and delayed filling and emptying of the true channel.

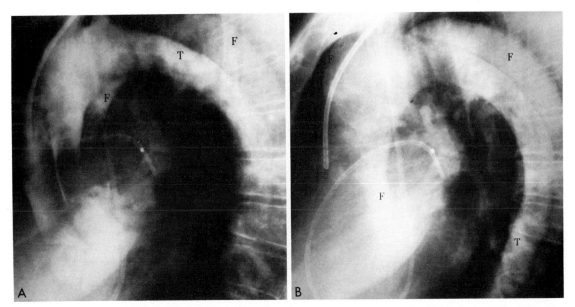

Figure 22–8. Dissecting aneurysm. *A,* An early-phase aortogram demonstrates opacification of a narrowed and a deformed true channel (T) of the aorta. *B,* A later-phase aortogram demonstrates opacification of both the true and the false (F) channels separated by a linear lucency representing the intimal flap. (*From* Soto, B., Harman, M. A., Ceballos, R., et al.: Angiographic diagnosis of dissecting aneurysms of the aorta. Am. J. Roentgenol. *116*:146–154, 1972. Reproduced by permission.)

Figure 22–9. Dissection. Note the marked encroachment upon the true channel by a huge nonopacified false channel (arrows). As usual, the false channel is located to the left and posteriorly along the descending thoracic aorta. Injection at the supravalvular level of the ascending aorta failed to opacify the false channel because of a more proximal location of the entry tear.

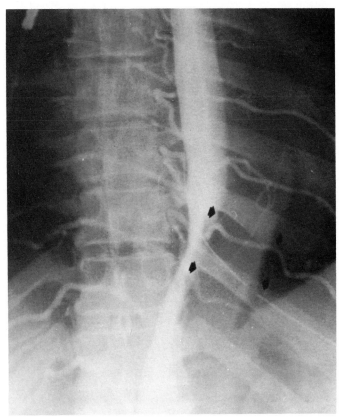

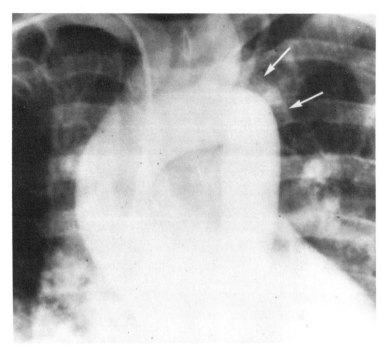

Figure 22–10. Fat in aortic wall. There is an increase in the apparent aortic wall thickness best seen in the region of the proximal descending thoracic aorta (arrows). This increase in wall thickness proved to be fat. (*From* Price, J. E., Jr., Gray, R. K., and Grollman, J. H.: Aortic wall thickness as an unreliable sign in the diagnosis of dissecting aneurysm of the thoracic aorta. Am. J. Roentgenol. *113*:710–712, 1971. Reproduced by permission.)

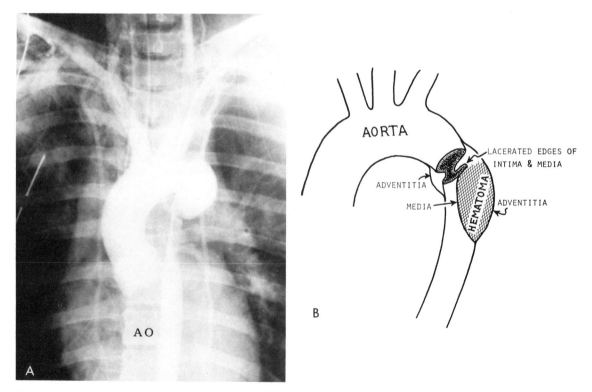

Figure 22–11. Subadventitial dissection. *A,* A transaxillary aortogram demonstrates infolding of the intimal and medial flap. A subadventitial dissection and hematoma have formed, presenting as a bulge but characteristically failing to opacify. Marked narrowing of the aortic lumen results. *B,* Schematic drawing of laceration infolding of intimal and medial edges and subadventitial hematoma. (*From* Faraci, R. M., and Westcott, J. L.: Dissecting hematoma of the aorta secondary to blunt chest trauma. Radiology *123*:569–574, 1977. Reproduced by permission.)

opacification of the left ventricle.[47] Echocardiography may document prolapse of aortic leaflets.[41, 42]

The dissection may extend into branches of the aorta. Occlusion of coronary or renal arteries may result from embarrassment by concentric compression by a dissecting false channel.[47] In some instances, the false channel may opacify late and communicate with the true lumen of branch vessels (see Fig. 22–15).[50] The dissection may also extend in a retrograde fashion and rupture into the right atrium or pericardium. Contrast in the aortic root will then spread into and opacify the pericardial space or the right atrium.[39]

Prognosis

Location, extent of dissection, underlying disease of the aorta, and duration of dissection are critical factors influencing survival.[16] If left untreated, 30 per cent of all dissecting aneurysms will prove fatal within 24 hours after onset of symptoms. Sixty per cent will die within the first three weeks, and 80 per cent in the first three months.[23] The highest survival is seen in patients with type 3 dissecting aneurysms restricted to the descending thoracic aorta. The surgical mortality for this group is about 12 per cent.[15] However, patients treated medically also have a fair prognosis. Type 2 dissecting aneurysms involving only the ascending aorta have a surgical mortality of about 29 per cent.[15] This may be partly due to a frequent association with Marfan's syndrome.

Angiographic documentation of thrombosis of the false channel is a favorable prognostic sign (see Fig. 22–9). Dinsmore reported a 90 per cent survival rate in patients without demonstrable communication between the aortic lumen and the false channel.[16] Poor survival statistics of patients treated by surgical fenestration to create reentry into the true lumen support Dinsmore's findings.[3]

TRAUMATIC ANEURYSMS

The increase in automobile accidents has resulted in a corresponding rise in deceleration injuries to the thoracic aorta. Traumatic aneurysms are responsible for 16 per cent of all fatalities attributable to vehicular accidents[32] and account for 25 per cent of all thoracic aneurysms.[8] Aneurysms caused by penetrating injury are uncommon, since this type of injury generally results in immediately fatal hemorrhage.[8]

Mechanism of Injury

Variability in the fixation of different segments of the thoracic aorta has been postulated as a mechanism for deceleration injury. Rapid deceleration will result in "whipping" of the relatively unfixed segment against the point of fixation.[8, 32, 48] Fixation of the descending thoracic aorta by the ligamentum arteriosum makes this a favored site for this type of injury.

Axial rotation of the heart during rapid deceleration causes stress between the supravalvular segment of the ascending aorta and the segment fixed by the origin of the great vessels. Rotation of the neck at the time of deceleration produces a shearing force vector at the point of fixation of the aortic arch by the origin of the great vessels and may therefore result in avulsion of the great vessels.[24]

Site and Type of Injury

Eighty per cent of all deceleration injuries to the thoracic aorta occur at the isthmus segment fixed by the ligamentum arteriosum distal to the origin of the left subclavian artery (see Fig. 22–7A).[8, 32, 48] The second most common site of injury (15 per cent) is above the aortic valve.[6]

A transverse intimal tear results from a lesser force. Greater trauma causes stellate and spiral intimal tears involving both intima and media, with complete transection of all layers of the aorta. Since the adventitia provides the tensile strength of the aorta, this tissue layer is capable of absorbing greater stress. Survival of patients in the first few hours is usually dependent upon an intact adventitia (Fig. 22–11). Chronic traumatic or false aneurysms are rare because untreated victims are unlikely to survive (Figs. 22–12 and 22–13; see Fig. 22–17).[8]

Clinical Presentation

The frequent coexistence of aortic rupture and other major injuries may confuse the clinical picture. Evidence of major thoracic injury, with or without shock, should alert the clinician to this possibility. Progressive decrease in or absence of femoral pulses with hypertension in the upper extremities is a particularly ominous sign suggesting

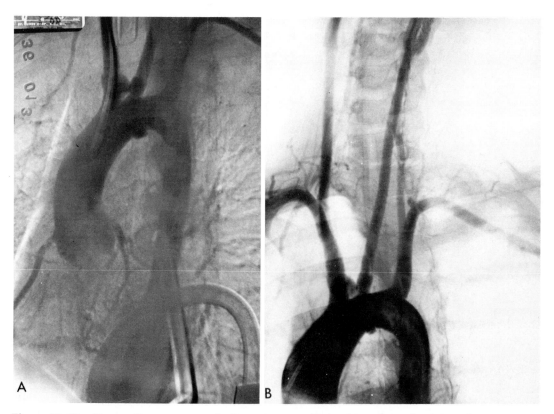

Figure 22–12. Traumatic aneurysms. *A,* An aortogram obtained two days after injury demonstrates pseudoaneurysms of the innominate artery, the left carotid, and the aorta. *B,* An aortogram obtained 15 months after injury shows an identical appearance of the pseudoaneurysms of the aorta and great vessels. (*From* Koury, W. C., and Davidson, K. C.: Multiple chronic traumatic pseudoaneurysms of the aorta and great vessels. Radiology *116*:23–24, 1975. Reproduced by permission.)

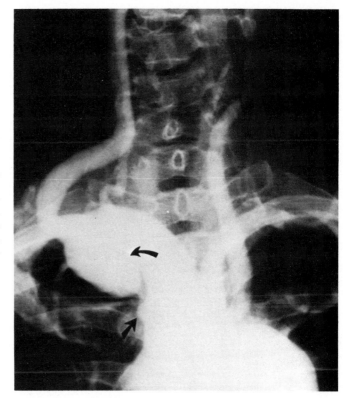

Figure 22–13. Traumatic aneurysms. An aortogram demonstrates traumatic pseudoaneurysms of the innominate artery. The lucent line separating the large pseudoaneurysm from the opacified main channel of the innominate artery (curved arrow) represents the wall of the pseudoaneurysm. A second smaller traumatic aneurysm is seen near the point of origin of the innominate artery (arrow).

aortic injury.[21] Severe interscapular pain, tachypnea, and dysphagia are other common presenting symptoms of traumatic aortic injury in patients who survive the initial insult.

Roentgenographic Findings

As with dissecting aneurysms, widening of the mediastinum is the most frequent finding on chest roentgenograms. Deviation of the trachea to the right, depression of the left mainstem bronchus, widening of the left mediastinum, and loss of definition or irregular bulging of the aortic outline are further evidence of a mediastinal hematoma, possibly caused by dehiscence of the aorta.[20, 21, 48] All these findings can occur in mediastinal hematomas caused by severance of lesser arteries, such as the internal mammary or subcostal arteries, or even by bleeding from venous channels.[24, 48] Conversely, progressive deviation of a nasogastric tube to the right and increasing extrapleural extension of a mediastinal bleed on sequential roentgenograms implicate the aorta as the source of bleeding (Fig. 22–14).

AORTOGRAPHY. This procedure is considered mandatory if bleeding into the mediastinum is suggested on plain roentgenograms. As with dissecting aneurysms, there is controversy as to whether antegrade or retrograde aortography is preferable. Since a large number of traumatic ruptures involve the isthmus segment of the aorta distal to the origin of the left subclavian artery, antegrade aortography via a right axillary approach is probably the safest method. Cautious advancement of a J-shaped guide wire under fluoroscopic and tactile guidance introduced via a femoral entry site has also proved safe for catheterization of the ascending aorta. Intraluminal position of the

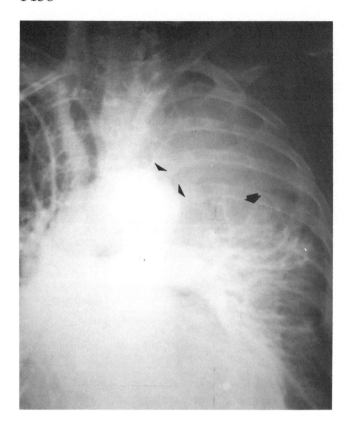

Figure 22–14. Bleeding dissecting aneurysm. A forward aortogram (via injection into the right ventricle outflow tract) demonstrates depression of all branches of the left upper pulmonary artery (arrow). The left upper pleural spaces are homogeneously opacified by an enormous extrapleural hematoma. A traumatic dissecting aneurysm of the descending thoracic aorta is identified (arrowheads).

advancing guide wire should show a characteristic pulsatile excursion. Proper intraluminal position of the catheter can be confirmed by fluoroscopic monitoring of small test injections of contrast medium. For definitive diagnosis, pressure injection of a bolus of 50 to 60 ml of contrast medium and simultaneous recording in either anteroposterior and cross-table lateral projections or right posterior oblique and appropriate right-angle projections are recommended. Despite rupture or near-dehiscence of all layers of the aortic wall, adverse effects of pressure injection have not been reported. This reflects the relatively minor rise in aortic pressure (less than 10 per cent over baseline pressure) attending pressure injections into the ascending aorta.

The angiographic appearance of traumatic aortic aneurysms ranges from a transverse radiolucent line of variable size, indicating an intimal tear, to a fusiform widening of the aortic isthmus segment or an obvious false saccular aneurysm (see Figs. 22–7A, 22–12A, and 22–13).[49] A sharply defined linear defect at either the proximal or the distal margin of an aneurysm reflects protrusion of the transected intima, media, and possibly even adventitia (see Fig. 22–11.)[4, 49] Frank extravasation of contrast medium into the periaortic space is an uncommon finding, since most patients with this condition do not reach the treatment facility alive. Associated contiguous or separate injury of brachiocephalic vessels is likewise demonstrable on aortogram (see Fig. 22–12; Fig. 22–15).[32]

The most common angiographic manifestation of traumatic aneurysm is a bamboo deformity of both outer contour and inner lumen, delineated by the contrast medium. This angiographic picture suggests a circumferential tear involving intima and media with an intact adventitia. The width of the "bamboo ring" reflects the degree of separation of the intimal and medial layers.

Demonstration of marked narrowing of the true aortic lumen and lack of opacifica-

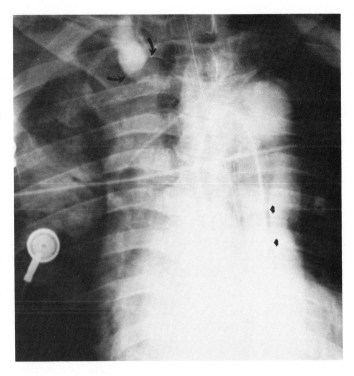

Figure 22–15. Dissecting aneurysm. A late-phase film aortogram demonstrates filling of both the true and the false channels of a traumatic dissecting aneurysm in the region of the descending thoracic aorta. A radiolucent line identifies the intimal flap separating the two channels (arrows). Contrast medium has washed out from the true channel of the ascending thoracic aorta; however, the distal segment of the innominate artery is now well opacified (arrow). This indicates extension of the dissection from the ascending aorta (false channel, right and posteriorly) onto the first segment of the innominate artery and resultant compression. The false channel communicates with and re-enters the main channel at the level of the bifurcation of the subclavian and carotid arteries (curved arrow).

tion of branch vessels arising from this segment suggest dissection with either severance or compression of branch vessels (see Fig. 22–15). A soft tissue bulge at the distal end of the dissection indicates a subadventitial hematoma (see Fig. 22–11).[20]

Chronic post-traumatic aneurysms usually present as a soft-tissue mass on routine chest roentgenograms. On angiograms, the saccular type opacifies promptly, but large false aneurysms show markedly delayed or absent opacification (see Figs. 22–13 and 22–17).

Prognosis

Eighty to ninety per cent of patients sustaining traumatic aortic transection die immediately of exsanguination. Some 10 to 20 per cent survive the immediate injury, the hemorrhage being temporarily controlled by an intact adventitia or confined by the parietal pleura. However, even if the patient survives the immediate injury, rupture with exsanguinating hemorrhage is the common outcome unless the aneurysm is surgically corrected.[8] Despite the ominous implications, there does not appear to be an appreciable difference in early survival of patients sustaining partial as opposed to circumferential tear of intimal or intimal and medial layers of the aorta.[8]

MYCOTIC ANEURYSMS

A mycotic aneurysm is caused by bacterial invasion of an arterial wall, excluding *Treponema pallidum* infection. Mycotic aneurysms of the aorta are relatively rare (2.5 per cent of all aneurysms).[7] With the use of antibiotics, the incidence of mycotic aneurysms has fallen steadily, with the notable exception of premature infants, in whom a marked increase has been reported.[19, 57]

Mycotic aneurysms can be primary or secondary. Primary aneurysms are thought to result from implantation of bacteria on intimal plaques or via vasa vasorum during bacteremia. Secondary mycotic aneurysms occur from direct extension of an inflammatory process. The major mechanisms are: (1) septic emboli, (2) contiguous extension of an adjacent suppurative process into the aorta, (3) contiguous lymphogenous spread, (4) extension of bacterial endocarditis, and (5) traumatic injury of the intima predisposing to subsequent infection (e.g., an indwelling umbilical artery catheter in premature infants).

Primary mycotic aneurysms occur most commonly in patients with arteriosclerosis. Secondary mycotic aneurysms are usually related to subacute bacterial endocarditis and septic emboli.

Contiguous involvement of the aorta by a suppurative process is usually due to a resistant anaerobic infection or to tuberculosis. Tubercular mediastinal nodes in particular may become adherent to the outer wall of the aorta, and a fistula may result between the lumen of the aorta and the suppurated lymph nodes (Fig. 22–16).[18]

Greater use of indwelling umbilical artery catheters has caused an increasing number of mycotic aortic aneurysms in premature infants.[19, 57] Mechanical irritation of the aorta, hypoxia-related changes of the aortic wall induced by mechanical pressure of a catheter, and introduction of bacteria through a catheter are postulated as causes.

Coarctation of the aorta, Marfan's syndrome, cystic medial necrosis, vascular

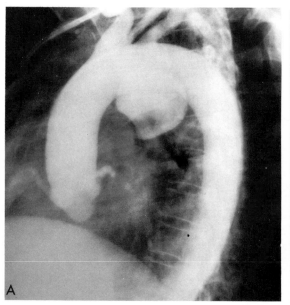

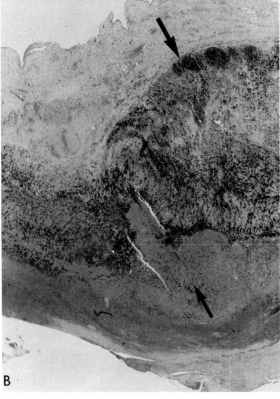

Figure 22–16. Mycotic aneurysm. *A,* The oblique projection of the thoracic aortogram demonstrates a saccular aneurysm of the aortic arch with a crescentic defect in the base. *B,* A photomicrograph of the aneurysm wall demonstrates necrotizing granulomatous inflammation of the aortic wall (small arrow) and anthracotic pigment in an attached lymph node with caseation necrosis. This establishes the diagnosis of a mycotic aneurysm secondary to contiguous extension of an adjacent suppurative process (tuberculosis). (*From* Efremidis, S. C., Lakshmanan, S., and Hsu, J. T.: Tuberculous aortitis: A rare cause of mycotic aneurysm of the aorta. Am. J. Roentgenol. *127:*859–861, 1976. Reproduced by permission.)

dysplasia, and trauma are other predisposing factors in mycotic aneurysms.[7] Abbott reported 14 mycotic aneurysms occurring just distal to a coarcted segment in about 200 patients with coarctation of the aorta.[19]

Clinical Presentation

The clinical presentation is nonspecific, and the aneurysm may be asymptomatic until rupture occurs.[7, 19] The sudden appearance and rapid enlargement of a mediastinal or abdominal mass should alert the clinician to the possibility of mycotic aneurysm.

Diagnostic Imaging Examinations

Ultrasonography and computed tomography are invaluable for differentiating aneurysmal aortic dilatation from extension of an adjacent mass into the wall of the aorta (Fig. 22–17).[4, 19] Gallium scintiscanograms may help identify the suppurative inflammatory process and in conjunction with radionuclide flow studies using [99]m-technetium pertechnetate may establish the diagnosis of mycotic aneurysm by delineating the abnormal anatomy of the aortic aneurysm and the associated contiguous inflammatory mass.

AORTOGRAPHY. Aortograms readily demonstrate a saccular aneurysm but usually cannot disclose the etiology (see Fig. 22–16A). A particularly shaggy appearance of the aneurysm wall, demonstration of inflammatory neovascularity in the rim of the aneurysm, and crescentic defects caused by an associated mediastinal mass should suggest the diagnosis of mycotic aneurysm. The shaggy appearance results from coagulation necrosis of the aortic wall and formation of a false wall, with the aortic lumen extending into the abscess cavity. The inflammatory neovascularity in the rim of the mass is a convincing finding for an inflammatory process. The neovascularity is limited to the rim, since the center has undergone coagulation necrosis and cavitation. Topographic proximity of an aneurysm and prominent mediastinal and carinal nodes, which may cause crescentic defects in the aneurysm, should raise the question of a mycotic aneurysm caused by direct extension of a suppurative process in adjacent lymph nodes.

These criteria are also demonstrable on contrast-enhanced computed tomograms. Furthermore, the topographic relationship of disease spread is better assessed on these cross-sectional anatomic studies (Fig. 22–17).[4]

In general, the diagnosis of mycotic aneurysm should be considered in the presence of a rapidly enlarging mass and a clinical picture compatible with an active inflammatory process.

ANEURYSMS OF THE SINUS OF VALSALVA

Aneurysms of the sinus of Valsalva may be congenital or acquired; isolated lesions are usually congenital.[46] Acquired aneurysms may be traumatic, luetic, tuberculous, or endocarditic.

Weakness or defect of the elastic tissue of the media of the aorta extending to the annulus fibrosus of the aortic valve ring predisposes to the formation of such aneurysms.

Location

The central location of the sinus of Valsalva explains possible rupture of these aneurysms into virtually every cardiac chamber and the pericardium. By far the most common congenital aneurysm of the sinus of Valsalva involves the right coronary sinus and projects into the right ventricular outflow tract; it is associated with a high

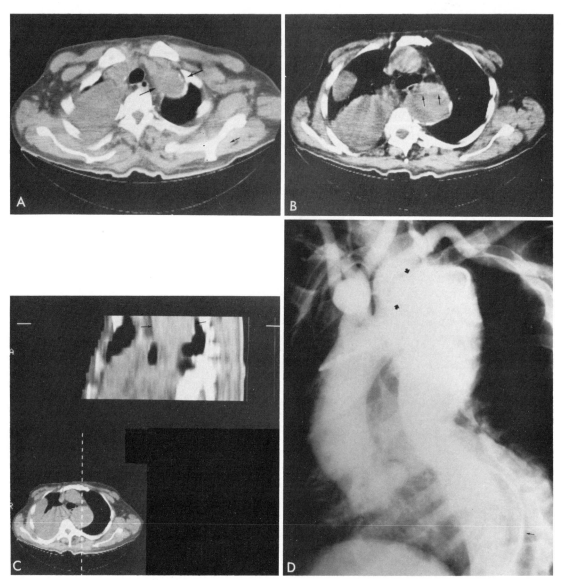

Figure 22–17. *A,* A computed tomogram through the middle of the thoracic outlet demonstrates an aneurysm projecting superiorly from the aortic arch (arrows). *B,* A computed tomogram in the mid-thoracic area clearly identifies the false channel of a huge dissecting aneurysm defined by linear intimal calcifications (arrows) and a difference in the attenuation coefficient established for the false and true lumen of the aorta. Note the collection of blood in the right extrapleural space. *C,* A sagittal reconstruction of computed tomograms graphically demonstrates the extent of the aortic aneurysm involving the descending thoracic aorta (arrows). *D,* A transfemoral aortogram in right posterior oblique projection confirms the findings of the computed tomogram and demonstrates a saccular aneurysm involving the aortic arch just distal to the point of origin of the left subclavian artery and projecting cephalad (arrows) as well as a huge dissecting aneurysm involving the descending thoracic aorta. The catheter is identified in the nonopacified false lumen.

ventricular septal defect,[46] which in turn is attributable to a specific developmental defect.[46]

The frequent association of aneurysm of the sinus of Valsalva and coarctation of the aorta may result from the effect of high aortic pressure and an inherently weak point in the aortic wall.

Aneurysms from the right coronary sinus extending into the right atrium are the second most common type. Aneurysms originating from the posterior portion of the left coronary sinus may protrude or rupture into the pericardial cavity.[46]

Symptomatology

Prior to rupture, aneurysms of the sinus of Valsalva are usually asymptomatic. After rupture, a harsh to-and-fro murmur is associated with sudden onset of dyspnea and weakness.

Roentgenographic Findings

Conventional chest roentgenograms are usually normal. However, high-kilovoltage anteroposterior or left anterior oblique films may demonstrate a striking dilatation of the supravalvular segment of the ascending aorta. Lateral roentgenograms may disclose an unusually prominent pulmonary artery segment displaced anteriorly by the dilated intrapericardial portion of the aorta.[54]

AORTOGRAMS. Intact aneurysms show a characteristic dilatation and deformity of the sinus of Valsalva on aortograms. Insufficiency of the valves from dilatation of the

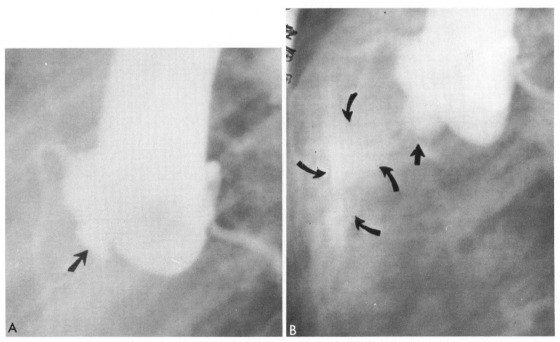

Figure 22–18. Aneurysm of sinus of Valsalva. *A,* The injection into the ascending thoracic aorta recorded in lateral projection demonstrates a typical aneurysm of the right coronary sinus (arrow). *B,* A later-phase film demonstrates contrast medium in the right ventricle (arrows), indicating rupture of the aneurysm of the sinus of Valsalva.

supravalvular segment may cause regurgitation into the left ventricle. The magnitude of opacification of the left ventricle following injection into the supravalvular segment of the aorta is a gross indicator of the degree of insufficiency (Fig. 22–18).

Opacification of the right ventricle, the right atrium, or possibly the pericardial space from an injection of contrast medium into the supravalvular segment of the aorta indicates rupture of an aneurysm of the sinus of Valsalva.[39]

ECHOCARDIOGRAPHY. The echocardiogram offers a noninvasive technique for diagnosing intact and ruptured aneurysms of the sinus of Valsalva as well as associated ventricular septal defects.[5, 37, 39, 41, 42, 58] Standard echocardiograms of the aortic root recorded near the left sternal border in the third intercostal space will demonstrate an aneurysm of the sinus of Valsalva as well as the presence of an interventricular septal defect (see Fig. 22–6).

A significant difference in the mean distance between echoes elicited from the anterior and posterior aortic walls and those elicited from the sinuses of Valsalva indicates the presence and approximate size of the aneurysm (see Fig. 22–6).[37, 39, 41] Disappearance of the echo normally elicited from the anterior aortic wall in diastole indicates a supracristal ventricular septal defect. The cephalad shift of the base of the heart in diastole moves the interventricular septum through the ultrasound beam, and a defect or absence of the septum causes disappearance of the echo normally produced by the contiguous anterior aortic wall and the intact septum.[37]

M-MODE SCANS. M-mode echocardiography is particularly useful for demonstrating the variable degree of herniation of the aneurysm wall into another cardiac chamber. Discontinuity of the echo between the anterior aortic wall and the interventricular septum indicates an interventricular septal defect.[37]

TWO-DIMENSIONAL ECHOCARDIOGRAPHY. Echocardiography in a horizontal plane is helpful in visualizing both the degree of prolapse of the sinus of Valsalva into the right ventricular outflow tract and a supracristal ventricular septal defect. Sections in the rear of the long axis of the heart are best suited to show protrusion of an aneurysm wall into the right ventricular outflow tract and to identify its rupture, which is heralded by a disruption of the echo elicited by the aneurysm wall.[37]

CAROTID BODY TUMORS

Carotid body tumors belong to the group of chemodectomas or nonchromaffin paragangliomas. They arise from chemoreceptor tissue located in the carotid body at the bifurcation of the common carotid artery. Chemoreceptor tissue is also found in other locations in the head and neck, particularly in the glomus jugulare, located at the jugular bulb, in the glomus tympanicum, arising from the tympanic branch of the glossopharyngeal (Jacobson's) nerve, in the ciliary ganglion, and around the superior ganglion.[38] Like other chemoreceptor organs, the carotid body is sensitive to changes in blood pH, CO_2, Po_2, and temperature. Normally, its physiologic activity is mediated through the ninth and tenth cranial nerves.[38]

Clinical Presentation

Carotid body tumors frequently present as a palpable mass at the angle of the mandible. Characteristically, they are freely movable in a lateral direction but immobile in a vertical direction.[10] A loud bruit may be heard and a palpable thrill felt over the mass. Ipsilateral retro-orbital headaches are a common presenting symptom.[10, 12]

Roentgenographic Findings

Soft tissue roentgenograms may demonstrate a mass at the carotid bifurcation, which on rare occasion may contain dystrophic calcifications indicating necrosis within the tumor. Because of the location, carotid body tumors do not cause osseous erosions.

ARTERIOGRAPHY. This is the best study for demonstrating carotid body tumors.[10, 12] The blood supply of these tumors is derived almost exclusively from branches of the external carotid artery.[10] The tumor consists of a network of meandering, small-caliber, tortuous vessels, usually well demarcated in relation to the carotid bifurcation (Fig. 22–19A). An intense tumor blush tends to persist for several seconds, after which the tumor drains into large dilated tortuous veins (Fig. 22–19B). Because of their location, carotid body tumors cause a characteristic lateral and posterior displacement of the internal carotid artery, and an anterior lateral or anterior medial displacement of the external carotid (Fig. 22–19A). This displacement is best appreciated on the lateral projection.[10, 12]

Direct tumor invasion of major vessels, most often the internal carotid artery, can be shown on angiograms. Demonstration of parasitic vascular supply to the tumor from the thyrocervical trunk is suggestive of malignancy. Approximately 5 per cent of all chemodectomas show malignant changes.[38]

Because of the propensity of chemodectomas for multifocal occurrence, both the

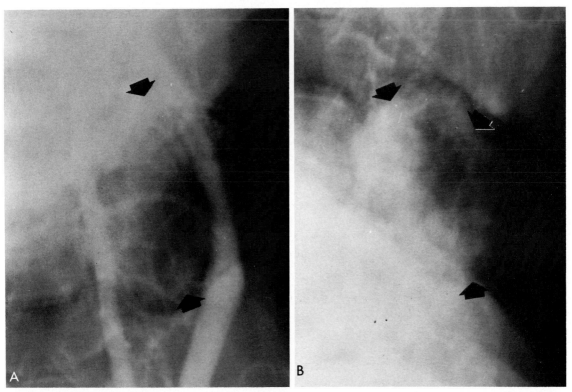

Figure 22–19. Chemodectoma. A, Note the characteristic lateral displacement of the internal carotid artery by a highly vascular tumor (arrows) deriving its supply from the external carotid. The external carotid is likewise displaced laterally. B, Late-phase arteriograms demonstrate an intense doughnut-shaped tumor blush (arrows) that persisted for several seconds. Note the beginning opacification of large dilated tortuous veins. The doughnut-shaped blush with central lucency is felt to be characteristic of chemodectomas. The location identifies this chemodectoma as a carotid body tumor.

carotids and the ipsilateral thyrocervical trunk should be studied. This is best accomplished by selective catheterization via a transfemoral approach. Retrograde jugular venography is recommended for detailed assessment of possible coexisting glomus jugulare tumors.

Management and Prognosis

Surgical resection is the procedure of choice.[10, 12] Bilateral carotid angiography is necessary to identify (1) the precise vascular supply of the tumor, (2) possible tumor invasion of the internal carotid artery, and (3) the status of the intracerebral circulation and the circle of Willis.[12] Since repair or resection of a segment of the internal carotid artery may be necessary, it is imperative to ascertain collateral flow via the circle of Willis in order to establish tolerance limits for the disruption of flow in one carotid artery.[12] Despite apparently complete surgical resection, local recurrence is reported in about 10 per cent of patients.[10, 12, 38]

ANEURYSMS OF THE CAROTID ARTERY

Depending on their location in the intracranial compartment or the neck, aneurysms of the carotid artery require vastly different management. The diagnostic investigation must be designed to provide information about the vascular lesion and factors influencing management. Computed tomograms and radionuclide brain scans are recommended as triage procedures. Cerebral angiography serves for finite preoperative evaluation of intracerebral aneurysms.

Since the cervical segment of the carotid is readily accessible, preoperative assessment is limited to the aneurysm of the carotid itself and to potential collateral flow via the circle of Willis in order to establish the feasibility and tolerance for temporary disruption of flow in one carotid.

Etiology

Most intracerebral aneurysms are congenital, while extracranial carotid aneurysms are due to a variety of causes, such as trauma, pre-existing disease of the media, and infection.[2, 11, 51, 54] Blunt or penetrating trauma to the carotid artery may cause a dissecting aneurysm, a true post-traumatic aneurysm, or a false traumatic aneurysm (see Fig. 22–12).[51] Small dissecting aneurysms of the internal or common carotid artery are a not uncommon complication of percutaneous needle puncture for carotid angiography (Fig. 22–20).[13, 50]

The most common blunt traumatic injury of the carotid artery results from a sudden forceful stretching over the upper cervical spine during a cervical hyperextension injury. The resulting intimal laceration may be the starting point for a dissecting aneurysm and the source for cerebral emboli from a thrombus forming at this point.[51] Laceration of both intima and media may cause a true post-traumatic aneurysm. Laceration of intima, media, and adventitia can result in a traumatic pseudoaneurysm.[32]

Cystic medial necrosis, arteriosclerosis, and hypertension are important predisposing factors in spontaneous dissecting aneurysms of the carotid artery.[11, 27] Unrecognized intramural dissecting aneurysms, which may be the basis for subsequent

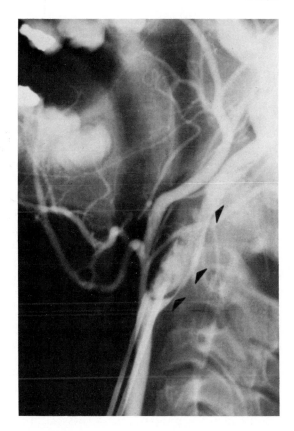

Figure 22–20. Dissecting aneurysm. A small iatrogenic dissecting aneurysm (arrowheads) has resulted from percutaneous carotid needle angiography.

thrombotic occlusion of arteriosclerotic arteries,[11] are the most common serious complication of percutaneous carotid needle angiography.[13, 50] Fibromuscular dysplasia may produce "microaneurysms," which in fact are small sacculations of the arterial wall.[27]

Mycotic aneurysms were a feared fatal complication of peritonsilar infections in the pre-antibiotic era[2] but have since become exceedingly rare. These aneurysms are caused by contiguous extension of an infection from the tonsilar fossa, and consistently involve the segment of the internal carotid artery above the angle of the mandible. This space is bounded posteriorly by the cervical vertebrae, and laterally by the styloid process, a dense aponeurotic fascia, the ramus of the mandible, and the digastric and stylohyoid muscles. Consequently, the aneurysm follows the path of least resistance and expands into the soft tissues of the lateral pharynx and tonsilar fossa. Because of this location and the ensuing symptoms of dysphagia and dyspnea, such mycotic aneurysms are frequently confused with peritonsilar abscess, peritonsilar neoplasm, or even chemodectomas.[2]

Clinical Symptoms

Symptoms of cerebral embolization are the most common clinical findings. Depending on the location of the aneurysm, a pulsatile mass may be palpated, although redundancy and tortuosity of arteriosclerotic carotid arteries may mimic these findings.[51] A bruit is not pathognomonic for an aneurysm, more frequently being due to arteriosclerosis and plaques.[2]

Arteriography

Transfemoral four-vessel catheter arteriography is favored for assessment of aneurysms of the carotid artery. Selective engagement of the origin of the common carotid arteries allows demonstration of the entire length of the common, internal, and external carotids. Moreover, catheter angiography permits free motion of the neck and thus facilitates positioning for oblique projections (see Fig. 22–12).

Four-vessel angiography is undertaken to identify (1) the location and extent of the lesion; (2) complicating factors, such as dissection and intraluminal thrombosis; (3) underlying predisposing conditions, such as medial necrosis, fibromuscular dysplasia, and arteriosclerotic plaques; and (4) the presence and effectiveness of intracerebral collateral pathways (circle of Willis). In dissecting carotid aneurysms the arteriogram is invaluable for demonstrating injuries that may alter surgical management, such as (1) a valvelike flap of intima projecting into the lumen of the artery, indicating the precise location and degree of the tear; (2) formation of a thrombus at the site of intimal injury, a common source of cerebral embolization; (3) opacified double channels identifying the site of reentry of the false channel; and (4) an apparent narrowed true channel, suggesting thrombosis of the false lumen.[11]

Management

The arteriographic findings are of paramount importance in the selection of the surgical procedure or the decision for conservative management. If conservative management is elected, repeat arteriography is useful to monitor such aneurysms and to identify progression of dissection, thrombosis, or formation of post-traumatic saccular aneurysms. Radionuclide angiograms may be substituted for postsurgical follow-up and for repeated assessment of physiologic data.

The development of transducers offering highly detailed ultrasonographic resolution of morphologic abnormalities of blood vessels, combined with physiologic data available from radionuclide angiogram, may make invasive arteriography obsolete.

COMPLICATIONS OF SURGICAL REPAIR OF ANEURYSMS OF THE THORACIC AORTA

Despite the risk of complications, surgery remains the preferred management for all types of aneurysms involving the thoracic aorta, since it offers the best chance for survival.[56] The underlying disorder and the type of surgical procedure, such as excision of the aneurysm, obliteration of the false channel, end-to-end anastomosis after resection, and replacement of a diseased segment by a woven Dacron graft predispose to specific complications.

Complications can be early or late. Hemorrhage, edema, thrombosis, and infection are the most common early complications.[22, 40, 43] Occlusion of the graft and aneurysm formation are common late complications.

Technically imperfect vascular reconstruction predisposes to thrombosis and hemorrhage. Meticulous operative monitoring with plethysmography, electromagnetic flow probes, and Doppler ultrasonography can detect changes in arterial flow and thus suggest the presence of technical complications at the time of surgery. Angiography during surgery can usually identify the cause of incipient complications that might jeopardize the results of reconstruction.[40] Immediate correction obviates reoperation with its significantly increased morbidity and mortality.

Ultrasonography and computed tomography are particularly useful in the identification of hemorrhage and abscess formation complicating graft infection in the early postoperative period.[17, 22] Retroperitoneal hematoma is most often attributable to improper technique of the primary repair or inadequate control of nonanastomotic diffuse bleeding from the surgical bed and is readily demonstrable on ultrasonograms and computed tomograms.[22, 39]

The dread complication of infection with a gas-forming organism, a specific hazard of employing bovine and woven grafts, is readily detected on computed tomograms.[22] Demonstration of extraluminal gas collections located posteriorly in the aortic bed strongly suggests infection by a gas-forming organism; gas in the anterior para-aortic region is usually attributable to residual air trapped in the tissues following the surgical procedure (Fig. 22–21).[22]

The presence of a non–gas forming abscess is shown on ultrasonograms or computed tomograms as an enlarging mass around the graft; sonographically it is characterized by low echogenicity. Percutaneous needle aspiration under ultrasound or CT guidance can corroborate this diagnosis and furnish substrate for identification and culture of the offending organism.

Early thrombosis of the graft, most often caused by improper surgical technique, is detectable by Doppler ultrasonography and antegrade arteriography. Antegrade arteriography, best performed via a transaxillary route, offers detailed information of the precise site and possible cause of thrombosis and the presence of collateral flow reconstituting the distal run-off.[40]

Delayed graft failures most commonly result from (1) complications of healing; (2) technical errors in surgery; (3) progression of the underlying disease; (4) deterioration of the anastomotic suture material; (5) deterioration of the prosthesis; and (6) infection.[55] Graft occlusion and aneurysm formation are the usual results.[43] The formation of false aneurysms, usually at the site of anastomosis of the Dacron prosthesis, is probably caused by a combination of factors, including deterioration of anastomotic suture material and prosthesis, technical errors at the time of surgery, and insult by the unabated thrust transmitted to the reflecting structures of the anastomosis from the noncompliant fabric tube.[9, 17] The presence of varicosities of the venous allografts at the

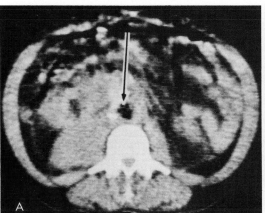 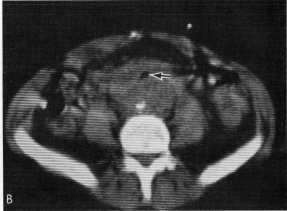

Figure 22–21. Graft infection. *A,* A computerized tomogram shows a small gas pocket (arrow) posteriorly within the area of the aortic graft. Although the diagnosis of graft infection with gas-forming organisms was not accepted initially because of the patient's stable condition, removal of an infected graft and a resection of an aorticoduodenal fistula three months later confirmed the initial diagnosis. *B,* A CT scan seven days after surgery for aneurysm repair shows gas in a location anterior to the aortic bed. The anterior location of the gas suggests residual postoperative air (arrow). (*From* Haaga, J., Baldwin, G. N., Reich, N. E., et al.: CT detection of infected synthetic grafts, preliminary report of a new sign. Am. J. Roentgenol. *131*:317–320, 1978. Reproduced by permission.)

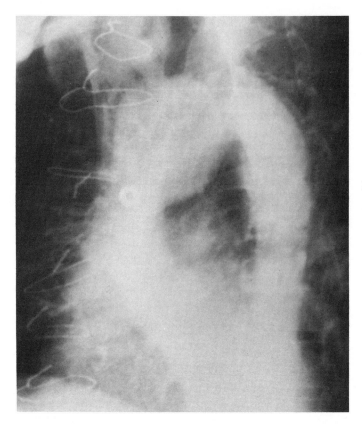

Figure 22-22. Saccular aneurysm. A right posterior oblique view of a thoracic aortogram demonstrates a saccular aneurysm involving the cephalad end of an aortic homograft.

time of acquisition predisposes to the formation of aneurysms.[43] Mycotic aneurysms may be the consequence of a smoldering infection at the suture line, which is often suppressed by prolonged antibiotic therapy.

Sequential sonograms offer the earliest diagnosis of a developing false or true aneurysm; Doppler ultrasonography offers early criteria for imminent graft occlusion. However, the definitive assessment for corrective surgical intervention rests on antegrade arteriograms, again best performed via a transbrachial route (Fig. 22–22).[53]

References

1. Anagnostopoulos, C. E., Prabhakar, M. J. S., and Kittle, C. S.: Aortic dissections and dissecting aneurysms. Am J. Cardiol. 30:263–273, 1972.
2. Anderson, R. D., Liebeskind, A., Zingesser, L. H., et al.: Aneurysms of the cervical internal carotid artery. Am. J. Roentgenol. 116:31–36, 1972.
3. Austen, W. G., and DeSanctis, R. W.: Surgical treatment of dissecting aneurysm of the thoracic aorta. N. Engl. J. Med. 272:1314–1317, 1965.
4. Axelbaum, S. P., Schellinger, D., Gomes, M. N., et al.: Computed tomographic evaluation of the aortic aneurysms. Am. J. Roentgenol. 127:75–78, 1976.
5. Barnes, R. J.: Rupture of the sinus of Valsalva. Br. Med. J. 1:683, 1968.
6. Beal, A. C., Jr., Arbegast, N. R., Ripepi, A. C., et al.: Aortic laceration due to rapid deceleration. Arch. Surg. 98:595–601, 1969.
7. Bennett, D. E.: Primary mycotic aneurysms of the aorta: report of cases and review of the literature. Arch. Surg. 94:758–765, 1967.
8. Bennett, D. E., and Cherry, J. K: The natural history of traumatic aneurysms of the aorta. Surgery 61:516–523, 1967.
9. Berroya, R., Aleman, J., and Mannix, E.: A longterm failure of prosthetic graft in coarctation. J. Cardiovasc. Surg. 11:329–332, 1970.

10. Bosniack, M. A., Seidenberg, B., Rubin, I. C., et al.: Angiographic demonstration of bilateral carotid body tumors. Am. J. Roentgenol. *92*:850–854, 1964.
11. Brown, O. L., and Armitage, J. L.: Spontaneous dissecting aneurysms of the cervical internal carotid artery. Am. J. Roentgenol. *118*:648–653, 1973.
12. Cordell, A. R., Myers, R. T., and Hightower, F.: Carotid body tumors. Ann. Surg. *165*(3):880–887, 1967.
13. Crawford, T.: The pathological effects of cerebral arteriography. J. Neurol. Neurosurg. Psychiatry. *19*:217–221, 1956.
14. Curati, W. L., Peticlerc, R., Dyrda, I., et al.: Echographic demonstration of mobility of the dissecting flap of an aortic aneurysm. Radiology *123*:173–174, 1977.
15. DeBakey, M. E., Henley, W. S., Cooley, D. A., et al.: Surgical management of dissecting aneurysm involving ascending aorta. J. Cardiovasc. Surg. *5*:200–211, 1964.
16. Dinsmore, R. E., Willerson, J. T., and Buckley, M. J.: Dissecting aneurysms of the aorta (aortographic features affecting prognosis). Radiology *105*:567–572, 1972.
17. Eastcott, H. H. G.: An appraisal of the use and function of vascular grafts in England. *In* Sawyer, P. N., and Kaplitt, M. J. (eds.): Vascular Grafts. New York, Appleton-Century-Crofts, 1978, pp. 220–225.
18. Efremidis, S. C., Lakshmanan, S., and Hsu, J. T.: Tuberculous aortitis: a rare cause of mycotic aneurysm of the aorta. Am. J. Roentgenol. *127*:859–861, 1976.
19. Faer, M. J., and Taybi, H.: Mycotic aortic aneurysm in premature infants. Radiology *125*:177–180, 1977.
20. Faraci, R. M., and Westcott, J. L.: Dissecting hematoma of the aorta secondary to blunt chest trauma. Radiology *123*:569–574, 1977.
21. Freed, T. A., Neal, M. P., Jr., and Vinik, M.: Roentgenographic findings in extracardiac injuries secondary to blunt chest automobile trauma. Am. J. Roentgenol. *104*:424–432, 1968.
22. Haaga, J. R., Baldwin, G. M., Reich, N. E., et al.: CT detection of infected synthetic grafts: preliminary report of a new sign. Am. J. Roentgenol. *130*:317–320, 1978.
23. Harris, P. D., Maln, J. R., Bigger, J. T., Jr., et al.: Follow-up studies of acute dissecting aortic aneurysms managed with antihypertensive agents. Circulation *35*:183–187, 1967.
24. Hermanutz, K. D., and Buecheler, E.: Traumatic non-perforating lesions of the thoracic aorta and the intra-thoracic aortic arch branches. Fortschritte Rontgenstrahlen *120*:156–163, 1974.
25. Higgins, C. B., Silverman, N. R., Harris, R. D., et al.: Localized aneurysms of the descending thoracic aorta. Clin. Radiol. *26*:475–482, 1975.
26. Hirst, A. E., Johns, V. J., and Kime, S. W.: Dissecting aneurysm of the aorta: a review of five hundred and five cases. Medicine *37*:217–279, 1958.
27. Houser, O. W., and Baker, H. L., Jr.: Fibromuscular dysplasia and other uncommon diseases of cervical carotid artery: angiographic aspects. Am. J. Roentgenol. *104*:201–212, 1968.
28. Itzchak, Y., Rosenthal, T., Adar, R., et al.: Dissecting aneurysm of the thoracic aorta: reappraisal of radiologic diagnosis. Am. J. Roentgenol. *125*:559–569, 1975.
29. Joyce, J. W., Fairbairn, J. F. II, Kincaid, O. W., et al.: Aneurysms of the thoracic aorta: a clinical study with special reference to prognosis. Circulation *29*:176–181, 1964.
30. Kampmeier, R. H.: The Late Manifestations of Syphilis: Skeletal, Visceral, and Cardiovascular. Medical Clinics of North America *48*(3):667–697, 1964.
31. Keene, R. J., Steiner, R. E., Olson, E. J., et al.: Aortic root aneurysm — radiographic and pathologic features. Clin. Radiol. *22*:330–340, 1971.
32. Koury, W. C., and Davidson, K. C.: Multiple chronic traumatic pseudoaneurysms of the aorta and great vessels, a case report. Radiology *116*:23–24, 1975.
33. Lindsay, J., Jr., and Hurst, J. W.: Clinical features in prognosis in dissecting aneurysm of the aorta: a re-appraisal. Circulation *35*:880–888, 1967.
34. McKusick, V. A.: The cardiovascular aspects of Marfan's syndrome: a heritable disorder of connective tissue. Circulation *11*:321–342, 1955.
35. Magarey, F. R.: Dissecting aneurysm due to the giant cell aortitis. J. Pathol. Bacteriol. *62*:445–446, 1950.
36. Mandel, W., Evans, E. W., and Walford, R. L.: Dissecting aortic aneurysm during pregnancy. N. Engl. J. Med. *251*:1059–1061, 1954.
37. Matsumoto, M., Matsuo, H., Beppu, S., et al.: Echocardiographic diagnosis of ruptured aneurysm of sinus of Valsalva: report of two cases. Circulation *53*(2):382–389, 1976.
38. Medellin, H., and Wallace, S.: Angiography in neoplasms of the head and neck. Radiol. Clin. North Am. *8*(3):307–321, 1970.
39. Millward, D. K., Robinson, N. J., and Craige, E.: Dissecting aortic aneurysm diagnosed by echocardiography in a patient with rupture of the aneurysm of the right atrium. Am. J. Cardiol. *30*:427–431, 1972.
40. Mulherin, J. L., Jr., Allen, T. R., Edwards, W. H., et al.: Management of early postoperative complications of arterial repair. Arch. Surg. *112*:1371–1374, 1977.
41. Nanda, N. C.: Echocardiography of the aortic root. Am. J. Med. *62*:836–842, 1977.
42. Nicholson, W. J., and Cobbs, B. W., Jr.: Echocardiographic oscillating flap in aortic root dissecting aneurysm. Chest. *70*:305–307, 1976.
43. Piccone, V. A., Jr.: Preserved allografts of dilated saphenous vein for vascular access in hemodialysis: a three-year experience. *In* Sawyer, N., and Kaplitt, M. J. (eds.): Vascular Grafts. New York, Appleton-Century-Crofts, 1978, pp. 328–334.

44. Price, J. E., Jr., Gray, R. K., and Grollman, J. H.: Aortic wall thickness as an unreliable sign in the diagnosis of dissecting aneurysm of the thoracic aorta. Am. J. Roentgenol. 113:710–712, 1971.
45. Rao, P. B., and Narayanan, P. S.: Carotid body tumour. J. Laryngol. Otol. 83:837–842, 1969.
46. Sakakibara, S., and Konnom, S.: Congenital aneurysm of the sinus of Valsalva: anatomy and classification. Am. Heart J. 63(3):405–424, 1962.
47. Sandborn, J. C., Heitzman, E. R., and Markarian, B.: Traumatic rupture of the thoracic aorta. Radiology 95:293–298, 1970.
48. Simeone, J. F., Minagi, H., and Putman, C. E.: Traumatic disruption of the thoracic aorta: significance of the left apical extrapleural cap. Radiology 117:265–268, 1975.
49. Soto, B., Ceballos, H. R., and Barcia, A.: Angiographic diagnosis of dissecting aneurysms of the aorta. Am. J. Roentgenol. 116:146–154, 1972.
50. Spudis, E. V., Scharyj, M., Alexander, E., et al.: Dissecting aneurysms in neck and head. Neurology 12:867–875, 1962.
51. Sullivan, H. G., Vines, F. S., and Becker, D. P.: Sequelae of indirect internal carotid injury. Radiology 109:91–98, 1973.
52. Tisnado, J., Tsai, F. Y., Als, A., et al.: A new radiographic sign of acute traumatic rupture of the thoracic aorta: displacement of the nasogastric tube to the right. Radiology 125:603–608, 1977.
53. Unger, E. L., and Massoni, R. E., Ruptured aneurysms twenty years after surgery for coarctation of the aorta. Am. J. Roentgenol. 129:329–330, 1977.
54. Waga, S., Matsuda, M., and Handa, H.: Bilateral giant aneurysms of the internal carotid artery. Am. J. Roentgenol. 116:23–30, 1972.
55. Wesolowski, S. A.: Discussion. In Sawyer, P. N., and Kaplitt, M. J. (eds.): Vascular Grafts. New York, Appleton-Century-Crofts, 1978, pp. 226–230.
56. Wheat, M. W., Jr.: Dissecting aneurysms of the aorta. In Sabiston, D. C., Jr. (ed.): Davis-Christopher Textbook of Surgery. Philadelphia, W. B. Saunders Co., 1977, pp. 1882–1892.
57. Wood, B. P., Young, L. W., and Elbadawi, N. A.: Primary mycotic aortic aneurysm in infancy and childhood. Am. J. Roentgenol. 118:109–115, 1973.
58. Yuste, P., Aza, V., Minguez, I., et al.: Dissecting aortic aneurysm diagnosed by echocardiography: a pre- & postoperative study. Br. Heart J. 36:111–113, 1974.

Part II

Aneurysms of the Abdominal Aorta, Visceral Branches, and Arteries of the Lower Extremities

MANUEL VIAMONTE, JR., M.D.

SHELDON A. ROEN, M.D.

MICHAEL S. LEVINE, M.D.

The normal aorta has a diameter of 2 to 3 cm and a wall thickness of 0.3 to 0.6 cm. There is a tapering effect of the abdominal aorta, so that its infrarenal portion is smaller in caliber than its suprarenal segment. The distance of the posterior wall of the abdominal aorta from the vertebrae should never exceed 1 cm. In adults older than 45 years the incidence of calcification is reported to be 60 to 70 per cent.

Less than 10 per cent of abdominal aortic aneurysms begin above the renal arteries.[28] According to Fomon, when aneurysms of the abdominal aorta are smaller than 5 cm in diameter the incidence of rupture is 1.9 per cent. When they measure 5 to 10 cm the incidence of rupture is 25 per cent, and when they exceed 10 cm in diameter the incidence of rupture is 70 per cent. Darling has stated that the incidence of rupture of aneurysms of the abdominal aorta 4 cm in diameter or smaller is 9.5 per cent. When they measure from 4.1 to 5 cm in diameter, it is 23.4 per cent; 5.1 to 7 cm, 25.3 per cent; 7.1 to 10 cm, 45.6 per cent; and more than 10.1 cm, 60.5 per cent.[2, 4, 9, 10, 12, 13, 25]

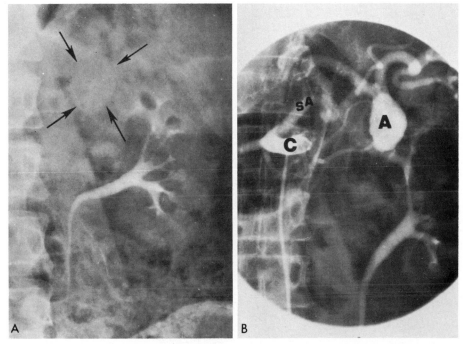

Figure 22–23. Splenic artery aneurysm. *A,* Closeup of the left upper quadrant showing a calcified aneurysms (arrows) medial and superior to the left kidney. *B,* Selective celiac arteriogram. C = celiac trunk; SA = splenic artery; A = aneurysm.

The size of aneurysms of the visceral branches also appears to have a direct relationship to the incidence of rupture. Aneurysms of the splenic artery are considered to be surgical lesions when the patients are less than 50 years of age and symptomatic,[2, 29] when the aneurysms are noncalcified (as in cases of pancreatitis), and when larger than 3 cm in diameter (Figs. 22–23 to 22–25). Hepatic artery aneurysms (rare

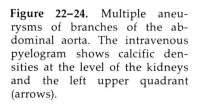

Figure 22–24. Multiple aneurysms of branches of the abdominal aorta. The intravenous pyelogram shows calcific densities at the level of the kidneys and the left upper quadrant (arrows).

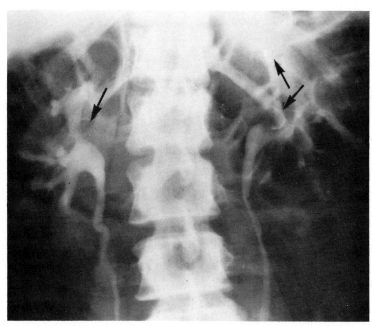

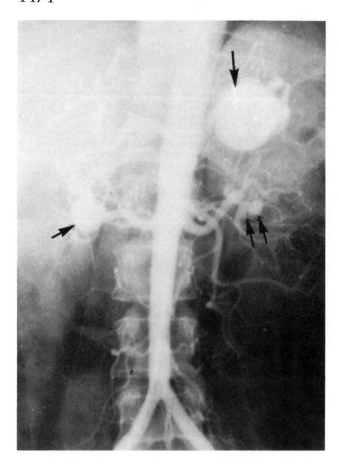

Figure 22–25. The same patient as in Figure 22–24. The patient is asymptomatic. The abdominal aortogram shows aneurysm of the splenic artery (upper arrow), both renal arteries (lower arrows), and hypogastric arteries.

lesions) are single in 80 per cent of cases and are usually extrahepatic.[21, 22] If untreated, they often rupture. Sixty per cent of ruptures occur into the biliary ducts, causing hemobilia.[16] The remainder rupture into the peritoneal cavity (Figs. 22–26 and 22–27). Aneurysms of the visceral branches of the abdominal aorta[6, 27, 31] have been classified as saccular or dissecting. Saccular aneurysms may be congenital; secondary to arteriosclerosis, bacterial infection,[19, 26] or trauma (see Fig. 22–39), or neoplastic.[36] Dissecting hematomas most often involve the renal arteries and must be distinguished from through-and-through perforation of the artery. They are classified as primary or as secondary to the extension of a dissecting hematoma of the thoracic or abdominal aorta.

The radiologic evaluation of aneurysms of the abdominal aorta, of its visceral branches, and of the arteries of the lower extremities consists of two steps: (1) noninvasive diagnostic imaging and (2) the performance of definitive diagnostic tests (angiography).

NONINVASIVE IMAGING TECHNIQUES

Conventional radiographic examination of the abdomen with frontal, lateral, and often oblique projections (Fig. 22–28) is used to demonstrate the size and position of an abdominal aortic aneurysm and to assess pelvic arteries. Calcification of the intima of the aorta, iliac, and visceral arteries may be detected. The displacement of abdominal viscera may also suggest the location of the aneurysm. Sometimes there is a clinical-

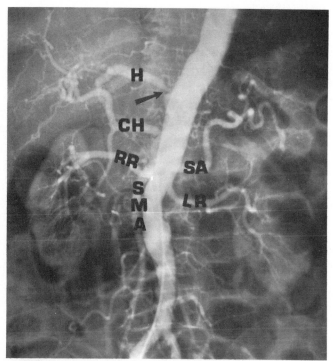

Figure 22–26. Dissecting hematoma of the hepatic artery. The abdominal aortogram shows narrowing at the origin of left hepatic artery (H) (arrow). CH = common hepatic artery; RR = right renal artery; SA = splenic artery; LR = left renal artery; SMA = superior mesenteric artery.

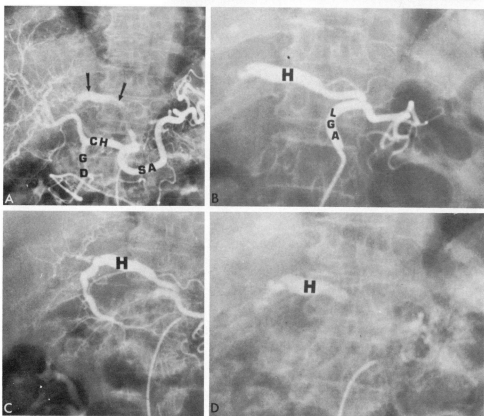

Figure 22–27. A selective study of the celiac trunk and left gastric artery of the same patient as in Figure 22–26. A, Celiac trunk injection. Contrast is retained in the enlarged left hepatic artery (arrows). CH = common hepatic artery; GD = gastroduodenal artery; SA = splenic artery. B, Selective injection of the left gastric artery (LGA). Note the slight narrowing at the origin of the left hepatic artery (H). C and D, Late films of selective left gastric artery injection. Note the stasis of contrast in the left hepatic artery at the site of traumatic dissection.

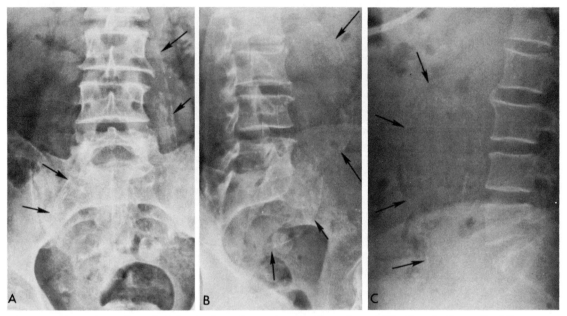

Figure 22–28. Plain film of abdominal aortic aneurysm. Note the calcification in the wall of the aneurysm (arrows). *A,* Anterior view. *B,* Posterior oblique view. *C,* Lateral view.

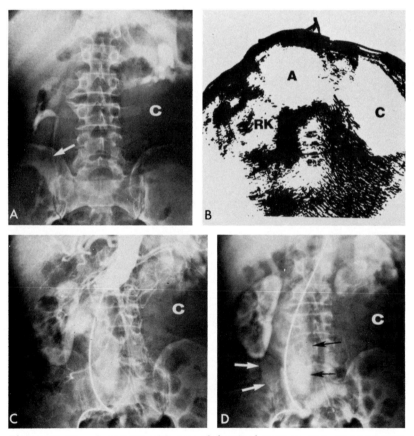

Figure 22–29. A patient with two abdominal masses, one, an aneurysm of the abdominal aorta (A) and the other, a left renal cyst (C). *A,* Film from an intravenous pyelogram showing the displacement of the right ureter (arrow) and a low-density mass arising in the lower pole of the left kidney (C). *B,* Abdominal echogram, transverse section. Note right kidney (RK), aneurysm (A), and cyst (C). *C* and *D,* Catheter aortogram showing an aneurysm to the right of the midline. A large mural thrombus is outlined by two white arrows in *D.* Note the left renal cyst (C).

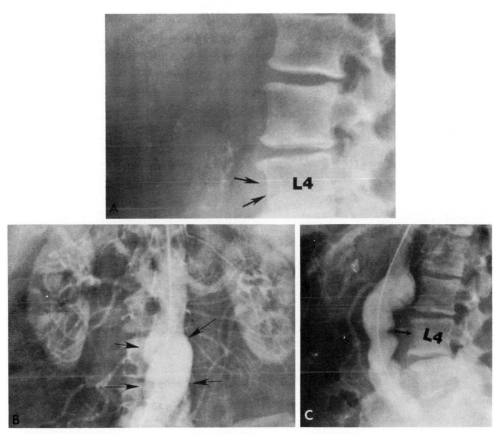

Figure 22–30. Aneurysm of the abdominal aorta causing the erosion of L_4. *A,* Lateral abdominal roentgenogram. Note the erosion of the anterior portion of L_4 (arrows). *B* and *C,* Abdominal aortograms. Note the aneurysm in the intrarenal portion of the abdominal aorta (arrowheads).

radiologic discordance when aneurysms are palpable but do not appear calcified. Overlapping bowel contents may obscure the presence of an abdominal aortic aneurysm. Intravenous pyelography often reveals abnormalities, such as the displacement of the ureters (Fig. 22–29). The destruction of vertebral bodies may occasionally be observed (Figs. 22–29 to 22–32).

Echography (Ultrasonography)[18, 20, 34]

A pulsatile abdominal mass may be related to a normal aorta (in a thin patient), a tortuous abdominal aorta, or an abdominal aortic aneurysm, or such a mass may be proximal to the abdominal aorta, transmitting its pulsation. Ultrasonography is the method of choice to establish the presence of an abdominal aortic aneurysm and to differentiate it from a juxta-aortic mass (Figs. 22–29*A* and 22–33). Echography can accurately measure the diameter of the abdominal aorta and the wall thickness and can detect the presence of a mural thrombus, hematoma or focal thickening of its wall, which is seen with dissecting hematomas. The displacement of the abdominal aorta and of adjacent structures can be discerned by echography. The extension of the aneurysm into the iliac arteries may also be evaluated. The involvement of the renal arteries can

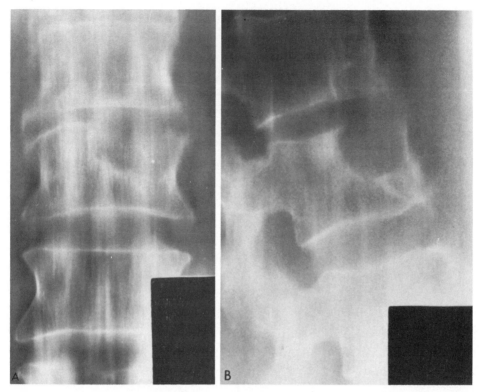

Figure 22–31. Aneurysm causing bone involvement. *A* and *B,* Tomograms of a patient with back pain and destroyed anterior aspect of two vertebral bodies.

rarely be determined. Surgical correction of an abdominal aortic aneurysm does not seem to be adversely affected when there is no knowledge of renal artery involvement prior to laparotomy. However, presurgical evaluation with angiography is requested frequently by vascular surgeons.

Radionuclide Angiography

If echography is not definitive or is technically impossible, or offers inconclusive results, radionuclide investigation is the next logical step. The radionuclide angiogram assesses the patency of the abdominal aorta and flow to the iliac vessels (Fig. 22–34).

The supine patient is studied with a gamma camera positioned over the abdomen. Approximately 10 to 20 mc of sodium pertechnetate ([99m]technetium) are administered intravenously, and sequential images are obtained at two-second intervals. Renal blood flow can also be gauged. As with a conventional angiogram, the maximal diameter of the aorta may be underestimated because of mural thrombus, but this radionuclide study has the advantages of speed and noninvasiveness.

Computer-Assisted Tomography

The cross-sectional evaluation of the abdominal aorta can be accurately made using this technique (see Fig. 22–32). The calcium in the walls of the aorta and the surrounding fat allow an accurate demonstration of this vessel. The presence of obesity,

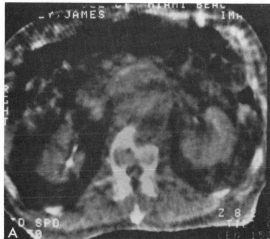

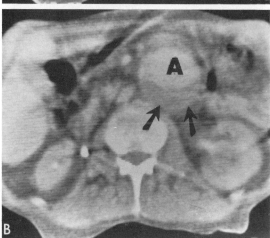

Figure 22–32. CT scan of the same patient as in Figure 22–29. *A,* Note the vertebral destruction. *B,* The aortic aneurysm (A) has a large mural thrombus (arrows).

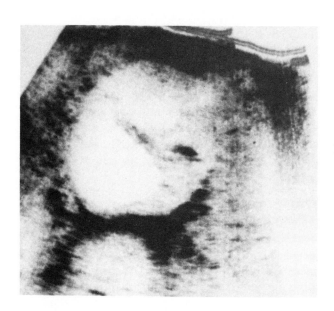

Figure 22–33. Abdominal echogram, transverse section. Note the aneurysm, with internal echoes secondary to mural thrombi.

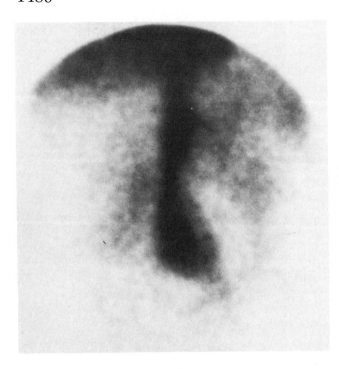

Figure 22–34. Isotopic aortogram. Note the aneurysm involving the infrarenal portion of the abdominal aorta. There is delayed flow in the right common iliac artery.

overlapping, bones, and considerable intestinal gas do not interfere with the study, as they do with ultrasonography. Mural thrombus, dissection, and periaortic hematoma are detectable, particularly when contrast media are injected to enhance the examination. The radiation exposure is 2 to 3 rads, and this examination is more costly than ultrasonography.

INVASIVE IMAGING TECHNIQUES

Abdominal Aortography

Abdominal aortography is used to confirm the presence of an abdominal aortic aneurysm suggested by other studies (echography, radionuclide angiography, or CT). It has been stated that 11 per cent of clinical examinations yield false positive findings. Abdominal aortography is also employed to determine the presence of suprarenal extension of the aortic aneurysm, which occurs in approximately 5 to 10 per cent of patients. Another important use of this method is the demonstration of associated stenotic lesions. One or both renal arteries may appear involved (in 17 per cent and 5 per cent of cases, respectively). The celiac trunk or the superior mesenteric artery may be involved in 11 per cent of cases (Fig. 22–35), and both of these arteries in 1 per cent.

The discovery of occlusive lesions in peripheral and brachiocephalic arteries is another contribution of aortography (Figs. 22–36 to 22–42). Occlusive disease has been found in the iliacs in 24 per cent of cases and the femoral popliteal arteries in 24 per cent. The occlusion of the brachiocephalic arteries has been reported in about 5 per cent of patients with abdominal aortic aneurysms. The angiographic assessment of different vascular territories depends upon individual clinical circumstances. The inferior mesenteric artery is the most commonly involved vessel. Abdominal aortography also can

Text continued on page 1487

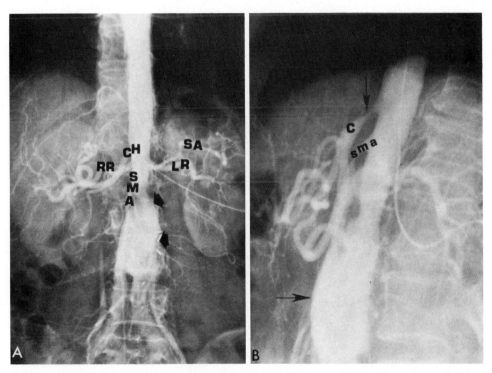

Figure 22–35. Biplane examination of the abdominal aorta. Note the aneurysm below the origin of the renal arteries (RR and LR). The superior mesenteric artery courses over and to the right of the aneurysm (SMA). CH = common hepatic artery; SA = splenic artery. The arrows indicate the aneurysm. *B* is a lateral aortogram. Note the symmetric narrowing (arrow) of the celiac trunk (C). The superior mesenteric artery (sma) is uninvolved.

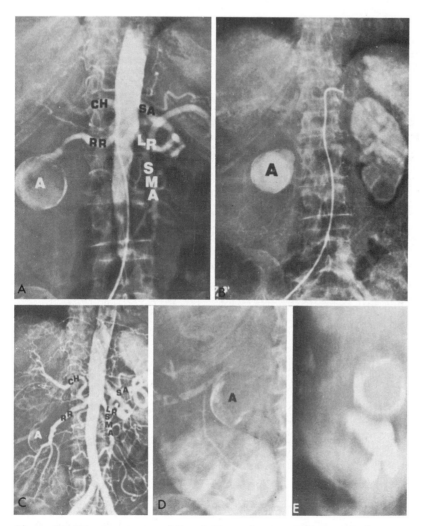

Figure 22–36. Aneurysm of the right renal artery before and after surgery. *A,* Midstream aortogram (top left) showing aneurysm of the right renal artery (A). RR = right renal artery; CH = common hepatic artery; LR = left renal artery; SMA = superior mesenteric artery; SA = splenic artery. *B,* Late phase of the abdominal aortogram. Note the retained contrast in the right renal artery aneurysm (A). Note the absent function of the right kidney. *C, D,* and *E,* Postoperative studies. Note the exclusion of the aneurysm from the path of the right renal artery (RR). The lower half of the right kidney is now functioning. A = aneurysm. The upper half of the right kidney was infarcted.

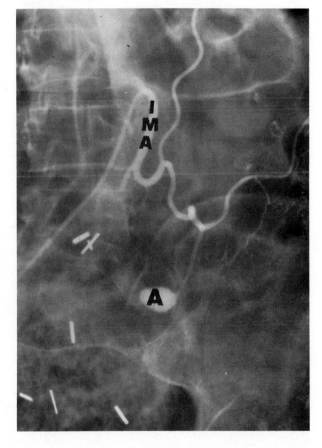

Figure 22–37. Traumatic aneurysm of the superior rectal artery. The patient had an abdominal perineal resection, followed by massive bleeding. The catheterization of the inferior mesenteric artery (IMA) shows the aneurysm (A) arising from the superior rectal artery. The patient was reoperated, and the aneurysm was successfully resected.

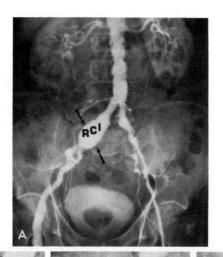

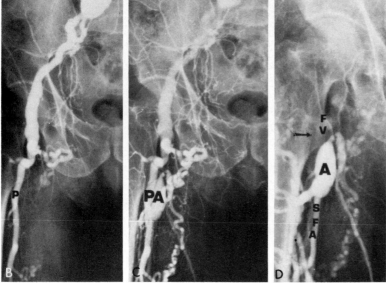

Figure 22–38. Aneurysm of the right superficial femoral artery associated with an aneurysm of the right common iliac artery. *A,* Abdominal aortogram shows a fusiform aneurysm of the right common iliac artery (RCI). *B, C,* and *D,* Arteriosclerotic ectasia of the right external and common femoral arteries is demonstrated. Note the obstruction at the origin of the superficial femoral artery. The aneurysm fills from collaterals. A = aneurysm; SFA = superficial femoral artery. P = profunda femoral (PA identifies two structures: P = profunda femoral and A = aneurysm); FV = femoral vein.

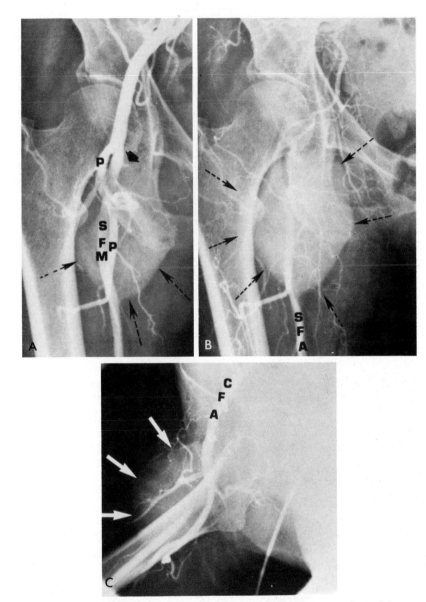

Figure 22–39.   Aneurysm of the right common femoral artery (CFA) following a stab wound of the proximal thigh. *A* and *B,* Note the right superficial femoral artery (SFM) and the filling of aneurysm from the profunda (P). *C,* Lateral view shows the common femoral artery displaced dorsally by the aneurysm (see arrows Fig. 22–38).

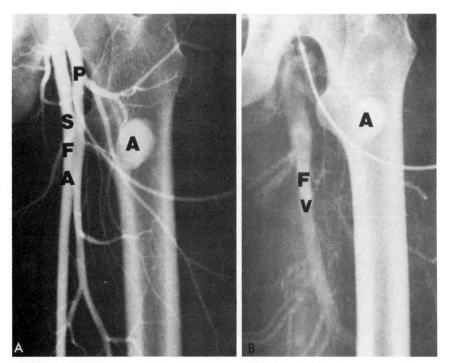

Figure 22–40. Aneurysm of a branch of the profunda. *A,* Normal-appearing superficial femoral artery (SFA) and profunda femoris (P). The aneurysm (A) fills from the lateral circumflex branch of the profunda femoris. *B,* Note the early opacification of femoral vein (FV).

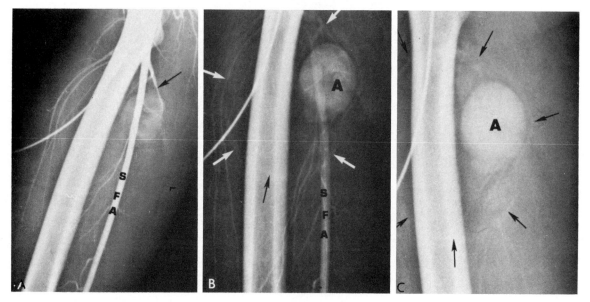

Figure 22–41. *A* to *C,* Traumatic aneurysm of right superficial femoral artery. In this right femoral arteriogram, the aneurysm (A) fills from the superior medial branch of the superficial femoral artery (SFA). Arrows outline a hematoma surrounding the aneurysm.

rule out the presence of other aneurysms, such as those affecting the iliac (41 per cent) and the hypogastric and femoral popliteal arteries (15 per cent). The recognition of multiple renal arteries (17 per cent of cases, 45 per cent of these with stenosis) is of value to the surgeon. In addition, a mural thrombus is usually present in the large aneurysm (Fig. 22–43).

TECHNIQUE. After the clinical examination of the patient and the review of conventional abdominal roentgenograms, a decision is made to use either a translumbar or a catheter approach. The latter is via the femoral or brachioaxillary arteries (Fig. 22–44). The radiologist should palpate the abdomen, the groin, and the peripheral arteries. The lower and upper extremity pulses are palpated, and the intensities are recorded. The femoral pulses should be palpated simultaneously to detect a slight disparity, which may indicate a severe stenosis in a pelvic artery. With this information the appropriate angiographic approach can be determined.

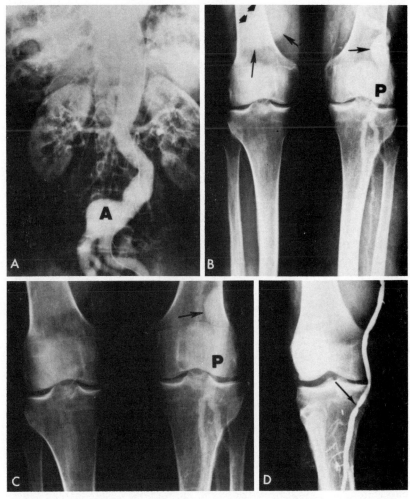

Figure 22–42. Bilateral popliteal artery aneurysms and a small aneurysm of the distal abdominal aorta. A, Small saccular aneurysm of the distal abdominal aorta (A). B and C, Saccular aneurysms of both popliteal arteries (P = left popliteal artery). D, Femoropopliteal bypass graft showing the patency of the branches of the right popliteal artery. Slight narrowing is noted at the anastomotic site (arrow).

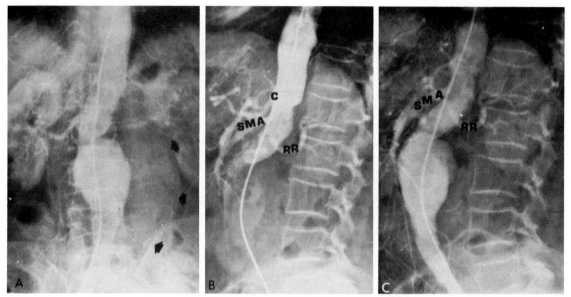

Figure 22–43. Biplane study of the abdominal aorta showing a large mural thrombus. *A,* Frontal view showing the large aneurysm and the mural thrombus (arrows). *B* and *C,* Lateral aortograms showing narrowing at the origin of the celiac trunk (C), with an uninvolved superior mesenteric artery (SMA) and right renal artery (RR).

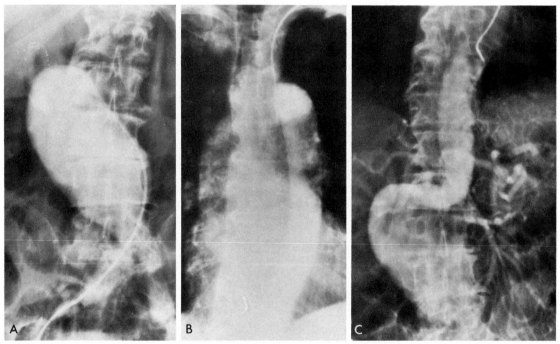

Figure 22–44. Aneurysm of the abdominal aorta studied by the two-catheter technique. *A,* Catheter passes from the right femoral artery into the aneurysm. Note that the superior portion of the abdominal aorta is not opacified. *B* and *C,* Catheter approach to the thoracic and abdominal aorta from a high left brachial artery puncture. In film *B,* the catheter is left beyond the origin of the left subclavian artery. Note the unremarkable appearance of the descending aorta. Film *C* shows the second injection of the tip of the catheter into the lower descending aorta. Note the upper abdominal aorta and the aneurysm below the origin of the renal arteries. A sharp turn of the abdominal aorta made the catheterization of the abdominal aorta from the femoral artery approach technically difficult.

The right common femoral artery is the preferential puncture site when the femoral pulses are equal bilaterally, since aneurysms usually present to the left of the spine, which tends to straighten the course of the right iliac artery and make the left iliac artery tortuous. The occasional aneurysm that presents to the right of the midline requires a left femoral approach. If there is a disparity in the pulsation of the femoral arteries, the more prominent pulsatile vessel is used. The percutaneous technique of Seldinger, familiar to the angiographer, is employed.

Initially, a J-curve guide wire with movable mandarin is used. This guide wire has a curved, floppy end that can be adjusted and lengthened by partially withdrawing the mandarin. The wire facilitates the subsequent advancement of a catheter into atheromatous vessels, minimizing trauma to the artery. When resistance is encountered owing to stenosis, extreme tortuosity, or inability to traverse the proximal opening of the aneurysm, an Amplatz guide wire is used.* The Amplatz guide wire has a long, floppy end that can be manipulated by fixing the wire in the palm of the hand with the fourth and fifth fingers and moving the outer coiled wire over the mandarin with the thumb and index finger. A number 6 or 7 French catheter with multiple side holes is advanced to the level of the diaphragm (T_{11} to T_{12}). If the aneurysm is large, a Straub end-hole occluder is used to give rigidity to the catheter to prevent its recoiling into the aneurysm, which could result in perforation.

When the femoral pulses are inadequate for catheterization, a high translumbar percutaneous approach is the procedure of choice (Fig. 22–45). An 8-inch, 19-gauge needle with an 18-gauge Teflon sleeve is used for the translumbar approach. A J-guide wire is used, since a straight or single-curved wire at times goes caudal rather than cephalad. Injections of up to 18 ml per second can be safely performed. Because of possible puncture, aneurysms that appear to extend above the renal artery should not be evaluated by the translumbar route. The high brachial or brachial artery should then be catheterized.

A high brachial (approximately 4 to 5 cm distal to the axillary fold) or a low brachial approach is a less desirable method because of potential complications. The success of both approaches depends greatly upon the training and experience of the angiographer. If patients have severe atheromatous disease involving the lower and upper extremities, hypertension (diastolic reading above 110 mm of mercury), or other contraindications to arterial catheterization, femoral vein catheterization with a large bolus of contrast injected into the proximal inferior vena cava may yield an adequate abdominal aortogram on the levophase (Fig. 22–46). When the upper extremity approach is employed, tortuosity of the brachiocephalic arteries may pose technical difficulties in advancing the catheter into the descending aorta. The use of guide wires and, occasionally, of a deflector assembly facilitates the advancement of the catheter into the descending aorta. We have substituted a high brachial approach for the classic axillary puncture. The axillary artery is surrounded by the brachial plexus, which may be damaged at the time of puncture or by the development of a hematoma.

COMPLICATIONS OF ANEURYSM. Possible complications of an abdominal aortic aneurysm are the occlusion of visceral branches of the aorta, rupture with intraperitoneal[5, 7, 14, 32, 33, 35] or retroperitoneal hemorrhage, peripheral embolization, and aortocaval fistula. The last may occur in elderly patients, who usually have a history of arteriosclerosis, syphilis, Marfan's syndrome, or cystic medial necrosis.

Hypotension resulting from retroperitoneal hemorrhage is characterized by back or abdominal pain, a tender pulsatile mass, and often, shock. Systemic arterial insufficiency involving the central nervous system is characterized by confusion, syncope,

---

*Amplatz flexible 6-mm T-fixed cord (0.9 mm) USCI.

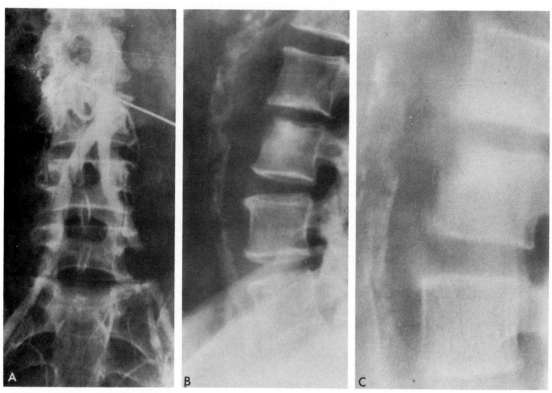

Figure 22–45. Complication of translumbar aortography. *A,* Infrarenal puncture of the abdominal aorta with the extravasation of contrast medium to the right of the aorta. *B* and *C,* Lateral roentgenograms taken three months later. The patient complained of back pain and low-grade fever. Note the anterior displacement of the heavily calcified abdominal aorta and destructive changes involving the anterior superior aspect of L_3. Osteomyelitis developed at this site.

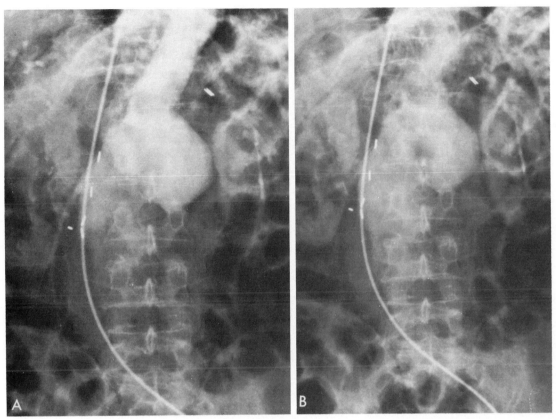

Figure 22–46.   *A* and *B,* Intravenous abdominal aortogram by catheter technique. The patient had severe occlusive arterial disease of the upper and lower extremities. A catheter was passed from the left femoral vein into the inferior vena cava. Contrast was injected at that level. Note the aneurysm of the midabdominal aorta, with considerable flow retardation.

and coma. Shock, oliguria or anuria, weakened femoral pulses, and intermittent claudication are other manifestations of arterial insufficiency. Venous hypertension leads to edema of the lower extremities, hepatomegaly, ascites, hematuria, rectal bleeding, and pulsatile veins in the perineum and lower abdominal wall or lower extremities. Anterior displacement of the aorta, blunting of the psoas margin in cases of retroperitoneal hemorrhage, and abnormal calcifications are often found on conventional films of the abdomen. Acquired aortocaval fistula in younger patients is usually secondary to penetrating wounds, surgery (particularly vertebral disc surgery) or external trauma.[22, 29] Aortocaval fistulas are often manifested clinically by high-output heart failure, cardiomegaly, diastolic gallop, a palpable mass, and a continuous bruit in the abdomen. Prompt surgical treatment of aortocaval fistula is essential to save the patient's life. Surgical mortality is approximately 50 per cent, and the most common cause of death during or after surgery is cardiac arrest or pulmonary embolism.

COMPLICATIONS OF SURGICAL TREATMENT[15]

The incidence of complications from arterial repairs is reported to be 0.7 per cent.[24, 38] The most frequent complications of vascular surgery are thrombosis and hemorrhage. Hemorrhage usually occurs in the early postoperative period. Most patients are re-explored within 12 hours. Although most frequent at the arterial anastomosis, hemorrhage may occur in other locations. Capsular lacerations of the spleen, for example, can cause hemorrhage. Often, no bleeding site is detected, in spite of the presence of large retroperitoneal hematomas. In most instances, there is no need to perform angiographic examination.

Following intestinal surgery, however, postoperative hemorrhage of unknown location and cause may be assessed by arteriography. Stress ulcers of the stomach, traumatic aneurysms, and unrelated gastrointestinal disease can be causes of bleeding. When a traumatic aneurysm is detected, the surgeon can readily treat this complication.

The most frequent complication requiring reoperation following vascular surgery is thrombosis. The thrombosis can occur at the site of vascular anastomosis or in the distal arterial bed. Its occurrence in the latter location may be the result of atheromatous emboli. At the time of surgery, the use of various intraoperative monitoring devices, such as digital and segmental plethysmography, electromagnetic flow probes, and Doppler ultrasound, have been helpful to confirm early obstruction to the run-off. When peripheral vascular surgery becomes necessary, intraoperative arteriography is valuable. The routine reversal of systemic heparinization with protamine sulphate, the maintenance of blood pressure at normal levels, and the rapid control of hypertension in the early postoperative period have minimized the incidence of postoperative hemorrhage.

Frequent inspection, palpation of the pulses, and blood pressure determination with the use of a Doppler probe may detect early occlusive arterial disease. It is extremely important to discover these common complications within 48 hours postoperatively. Craver has indicated that when bleeding occurs later than 48 hours postoperatively, sepsis is often involved and local repair is likely to fail.[8] (For graft infection, see p. 1469 and Fig. 22–21.)

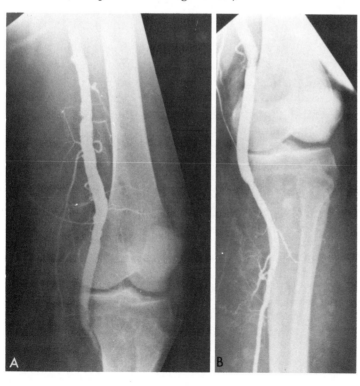

Figure 22–47. Left femoral arteriogram following resection of left popliteal artery aneurysm in the same patient as in Figure 22–40. Note the patency of the distal femoral and popliteal arteries and of the posterior tibial artery.

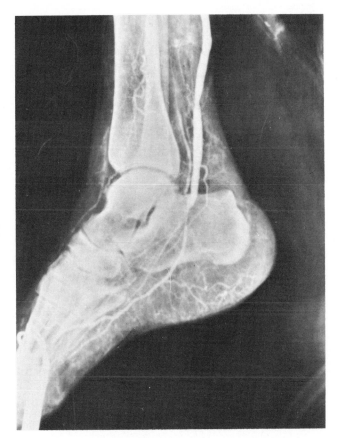

Figure 22–48. Operative arteriogram following a femoroposterior tibial bypass. Note the patent peroneal, posterior tibial and plantar arteries.

Femoral exploration is usually successful when femoral occlusion occurs after aortoiliac femoral bypass.[11] Thrombectomies; the inspection of the anastomotic site (for the detection of stenosis, rough edges, or intimal dissection); and the determination of the caliber, quality, and position of the vein grafts are most valuable maneuvers at the time of reoperation. Most vascular surgeons perform operative arteriography at the time of re-exploration (Figs. 22–47 and 22–48).

SUMMARY

There are several techniques available for the evaluation of abdominal aortic aneurysms. Each has its place and its limitations. Conventional abdominal roentgenograms show calcifications of the abdominal aortic aneurysm in 55 to 85 per cent of patients. In some patients, there is sufficient calcification to determine the maximal diameter of the aneurysm. Low back pain may be related to a noncalcified abdominal aortic aneurysm, however, and therefore the examination should not be limited to a lumbosacral spine study.

Contrast angiography is the classic method of defining the abdominal aorta and its branches. Because it is an invasive study, its use may be contraindicated in cases of shock or renal failure, in the presence of hemorrhagic diathesis, and occasionally, in cases of hypersensitivity to contrast media. The few false negative studies that occur are usually due to the presence of a mural thrombus. With aortography, the luminal size is easily measured; if no calcifications are present, however, the greatest external aortic diameter can only be estimated.

Of the three newer noninvasive imaging methods described (echography, radionuclide angiography, and computed tomography), ultrasound appears to be the best. It is rapid, noninvasive, and does not expose the patient to radiation. It can easily determine the external diameter of an aneurysm and has the unique capability of demonstrating the aorta in both the longitudinal and the cross-sectional planes. The course of a tortuous aorta can be followed easily, since scanning can be done from any angle. Frequently, however, the involvement of the renal arteries is not demonstrable.

The radionuclide angiographic examination is rapid and noninvasive. It gives a good temporal-dynamic relationship and can demonstrate flow to the iliac and renal arteries. It cannot show mesenteric flow, as does contrast angiography, and may yield false negative results.

Computer-assisted tomography provides cross-sectional evaluation of the abdominal structures and the aorta. This is a costly technique, however, and exposes the patient to radiation; thus, it should be considered only when ultrasound examinations fail to provide the necessary information. The computed tomograms provide images that are more esthetically pleasing, and the study requires less skill to perform and interpret.

References

1. Baker, W.H., Sharzer, L.A., and Ehrenhaft, J.L.: Aortocaval fistula as a complication of abdominal aortic aneurysms. Surgery 72:933–938, 1972.
2. Benetti, E.J., DeMeletti, B.N., Busnelli, L.F., et al.: Aneurisma de aorta abdominal en la infancia, de origen arterioscleroso. A proposito de un caso. Angiology 29:65–67, 1977.
3. Brewster, D.C., Retana, A., Waltman, A.C., et al.: Angiography in the management of aneurysms of the abdominal aorta. N. Engl. J. Med. 292:822–825, 1975.
4. Brewster, D.C., Darling, R.C., Raines, J.K., et al.: Assessment of abdominal aortic aneurysm size. Circulation 56:11-164–11-169, 1977.
5. Case Records of the Massachusetts General Hospital (Case 21-1974). N. Engl. J. Med. 290:1248–1253, 1974.
6. Case Records of the Massachusetts General Hospital (Case 19-1975). N. Engl. J. Med. 292:1068–1073, 1975.
7. Case Records of the Massachusetts General Hospital (Case 41-1977). N. Engl. J. Med. 297:828–834, 1977.
8. Craver, J.M., Ottinger, L.W., Darling, R.C., et al.: Hemorrhage and thrombosis as early complications of femoropopliteal bypass grafts; causes, treatment, and prognostic implications. Surgery 74:839–845, 1973.
9. Darling, R.C., Messina, C.R., Brewster, D.C., et al.: Autopsy study of unoperated abdominal aortic aneurysms. Circulation 56:11-161–11-164, 1977.
10. David, J.P., Marks, C., and Bonneval, M.: A ten year institutional experience with abdominal aneurysms. Surg. Gynecol. Obstet. 138:591–594, 1974.
11. Dhall, D.P., and Mavor, G.E.: Long term behavior of reversed saphenous vein grafts for advanced femoropopliteal disease. Surg. Gynecol. Obstet. 146:241–243, 1978.
12. DiGiovanni, R., Nicholas, G., Volpetti, G., et al.: Twenty-one years' experience with ruptured abdominal aortic aneurysms. Surg. Gynecol. Obstet. 141:859–862, 1975.
13. Fomon, J.: Personal communication.
14. Geary, S.R., and Walworth, E.Z.: Aortoduodental fistula secondary to metastatic carcinoma. Angiographic demonstration. J.A.M.A. 235:2520–2521, 1976.
15. Guilmet, D., Goudot, B., Bachet, J., et al.: Tratamiento quirurgico de los aneurismas toraco-abdominales: a proposito de siete observaciones. J. Sciences Med. de Lille 94:269, 1976.
16. Hill, D.E., Lobell, M., and Edwards, J.E.: Primary dissecting aneurysm of the hepatic artery. Arch. Intern. Med. 133:471–474, 1974.
17. Jones, J.G.: An unusual case of back pain. Proc. R. Soc. Med. 69:499–501, 1976.
18. Leopold, G.R., Goldberger, I.E., and Bernstein, E.F.: Ultrasonic detection and evaluation of abdominal aortic aneurysms. Surgery 72:939–945, 1972.
19. Liotta, D., Donato, F.O., and Bertolozzi, E.: Staphylococcal aortic pseudoaneurysm. Chest 72:243–245, 1977.
20. Maloney, J.D., Pairolero, P.C., Smith, B.F., et al.: Ultrasound evaluation of abdominal aortic aneurysms. Circulation 46:11-80–11-85, 1977.

21. Mays, E.T.: The hepatic artery. Surg. Gynecol. Obstet. *139*:595–596, 1974.
22. Mays, E.T., and Wheeler, C.S.: Demonstration of collateral arterial flow after interruption of hepatic arteries in man. N. Engl. J. Med. *290*:993–996, 1974.
23. Mohr, L. L., and Smith, L. L.: Arteriovenous fistula from rupture of abdominal aortic aneurysm. Arch. Surg. *110*:806–812, 1975.
24. Mulherin, J.L., Allen, T.R., Edwards, W.H., et al.: Management of early postoperative complications of arterial repairs. Arch. Surg. *112*:1371–1374, 1977.
25. Ottinger, L.W.: Ruptured arteriosclerotic aneurysms of the abdominal aorta. J.A.M.A. *233*:147–150, 1975.
26. Patel, S., and Johnston, K.W.: Classification and management of mycotic aneurysms. Surg. Gynecol. Obstet. *144*:691–694, 1977.
27. Pond, G.D., Ovitt, T.W., Witte, C.I., et al.: Aneurysm of the superior hemorrhoidal artery: an unusual cause of massive rectal bleeding. J. Can. Assoc. Radiol. *28*:144–145, 1977.
28. Rodin, A.E.: The significance of William Osler's museum specimens of aortic aneurysms. Chest *72*:508–511, 1977.
29. Saw, E.C., Arbegast, N.R., Schmalhorst, W.R., et al.: Splenic artery aneurysms. Arch. Surg. *106*:660–662, 1973.
30. Schapiro, R.L., and Hahn, F.J.Y.: Primary aortoduodenal fistula. J.A.M.A. *236*:2541–2542, 1976.
31. Scheflan, M., Kadir, S., Athanasoulis, C.A., et al.: Pancreaticoduodenal artery aneurysm simulating carcinoma of the head of the pancreas. Arch. Surg. *112*:1201–1203, 1977.
32. Scribner, R.G., Baker, M.S., Tawes, R.L., et al.: Recurrent aortoduodenal fistula. Arch. Surg. *112*:1265, 1977.
33. Shaigany, A., Gillespie, L., Mock, J.P., et al.: Aortoenteric fistula. Arch. Intern. Med. *136*:930–932, 1976.
34. Shawker, T.H., and Stinefeld, A.D.: Ultrasonic evaluation of pulsatile abdominal masses. J.A.M.A. *239*:419–422, 1978.
35. Smiley, K.: Aortoduodenal fistula a complication of synthetic grafts. J. Florida MA *62*:24–26, 1975.
36. Steffelaar, J.W., van der Heul, R.O., Blackstone, E., et al.: Primary sarcoma of the aorta. Arch. Pathol. *99*:139–142, 1975.
37. Stephenson, H.E., Jr., and Lockhart, C.G.: Treatment of the ruptured abdominal aorta. Surg. Gynecol. Obstet. *144*:855–861, 1977.
38. Volpetti, G., Barker, C.F., Berkowitz, H., et al.: A twenty-two year review of elective resection of abdominal aortic aneurysms. Surg. Gynecol. Obstet. *142*:321–324, 1976.

Part III

Leriche Syndrome: Aortoiliac Ischemic Disease

KLAUS M. BRON, M.D.

INTRODUCTION

The preoperative assessment of aortoiliac–femoral ischemic disease requires both accurate anatomic delineation and objective functional evaluation. The location, extent, and severity of the obstructive process involving the arterial lumen may be readily and safely determined by arteriography. The patient's clinical symptoms, physical findings, and arteriographic findings form the diagnostic triad of lower-extremity thromboblit-erative disease. However, because the extent of disease encountered at surgery may be more severe than had been delineated on the arteriogram, functional impairment should also be quantified. This has been investigated by pressure measurements, pulse wave recordings, and plethysmography, but the results are controversial.

THROMBOTIC AORTOILIAC OBSTRUCTION

In 1940, Leriche described a group of patients with a symptom complex caused by chronic obstruction of the distal aorta and the proximal iliac arteries.[14] These patients were entirely different from those with an acute aortic occlusion due to a saddle embolus.[15] Patients with chronic aortic or iliac obstruction typically complain of severe fatigue in both lower extremities and have atrophy of the limbs, pallor of the legs and feet, and no trophic changes of the skin or nails. In males, the most distressing symptom may be impotence, especially since aortoiliac lesions are encountered in relatively young men. Our experience coincides with that reported in the literature,[8, 17, 33] and in our series of 38 patients there was a 2:1 male preponderance. The males ranged in age from 45 to 71 years, with the peak incidence in the 45 to 49 year group. In women, the range was identical, but the peak incidence occurred in the sixth and seventh decades. In addition to the primary form of progressive thrombotic aortic occlusion due to arteriosclerosis (Figs. 22–49A and 22–50A), there is a secondary type that results from aortic bypass surgery, blunt trauma,[18] or even intentional aortic ligation. The last may be necessary to manage a mycotic aneurysm.

Diagnosis of primary arteriosclerotic thrombosis of the distal aorta is largely based on its clinical presentation, which is generally characteristic. The symptoms were initially described by Leriche, but it is now evident that intermittent claudication may also be significant.[26] The purpose of arteriography[9] is: (1) to confirm the clinical impression; (2) to demonstrate the proximal site and extent of occlusion; (3) to indicate the collateral circulation and distal site of arterial reconstitution; and (4) to identify any arterial obstruction in the thighs or distal run-off vessels (Figs. 22–49 A to D, 22–50 A to D, and 22–51 A to D). This information helps the surgeon to plan the most suitable type of graft procedure.

The proximal site of aortic occlusion is most often at the infrarenal artery level (see Fig. 22–49 A) and, less frequently, below the inferior mesenteric artery (see Fig. 22–50 A

Text continued on page 1501

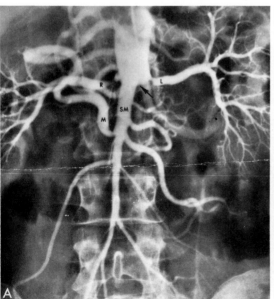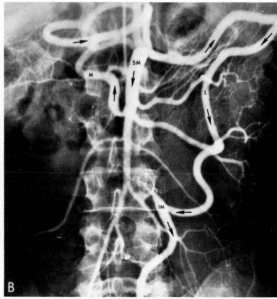

Figure 22–49. A 50-year-old man presented with a long history of progressive hip and thigh weakness, intermittent calf claudication, impotence, and absent femoral pulses. *A,* The abdominal aorta is occluded at the infrarenal level (arrow). Bilaterally, the renal arteries (R and L) are stenosed at their origin. *B,* The principal collateral circulation is via the viscerosystemic system. The arrows indicate the direction of blood flow through the collaterals, starting at the superior mesenteric artery (SM), to the middle colic artery (M), to the left colic artery (L), and then to the inferior mesenteric artery (IM).

Legend continued on the opposite page

Figure 22–49 *Continued. C,* In the pelvis (early phase), the visceral collaterals continue via the superior hemorrhoidal artery (S) to the middle and inferior hemorrhoidal branches of the internal iliac arteries on each side (I). *D,* In the pelvis (late phase), the systemic arteries reconstituted are the external iliac vessels on each side (E). The common iliac arteries are occluded. *(From* Bron, K. M.: Thrombic occlusion of the abdominal aorta. Am. J. Roentgenol. *96*: 887, 1966. Reproduced by permission.)

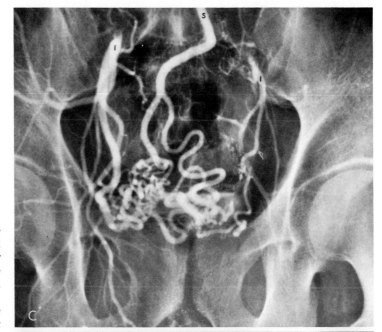

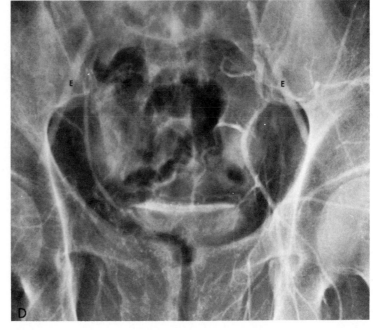

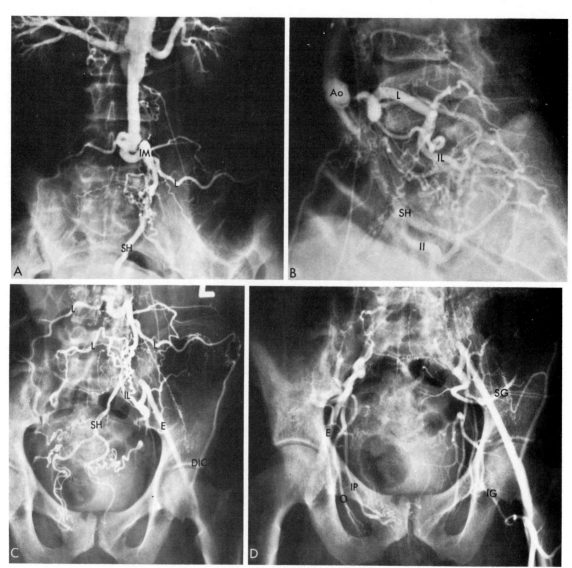

Figure 22–50. A 52-year-old man with classic symptoms of Leriche syndrome. *A,* The aortogram, via the axillary artery, reveals atherosclerotic narrowing of the infrarenal aorta and complete occlusion below the inferior mesenteric artery (IM). The collateral circulation to the pelvis consists of the inferior mesenteric (IM), superior hemorrhoidal (SH), and lumbar (L) arteries. These are components of the viscero-systemic and systemic-systemic collateral circulations. *B,* The lateral aortogram demonstrates the occluded aorta (Ao) and the collateral circulation in the presacral area of the pelvis. The dilated collaterals are the lumbar (L), superior hemorrhoidal (SH), iliolumbar (IL), and an internal iliac branch (II). *C,* In the pelvis during the early phase, the left external iliac artery (E) reconstitutes. The deep iliac circumflex (DIC) arises from the left lower lumbar artery (L). The iliolumbar (IL) and superior hemorrhoidal (SH) arteries are dilated as well as a few right lumbar (L) branches. *D,* The pelvis (late phase), shows that the right internal pudendal (IP) and obturator (O) arteries are patent as is the external iliac artery (E). The common iliac arteries are occluded. The left superior (SG) and inferior gluteal (IG) arteries are partially filled with contrast.

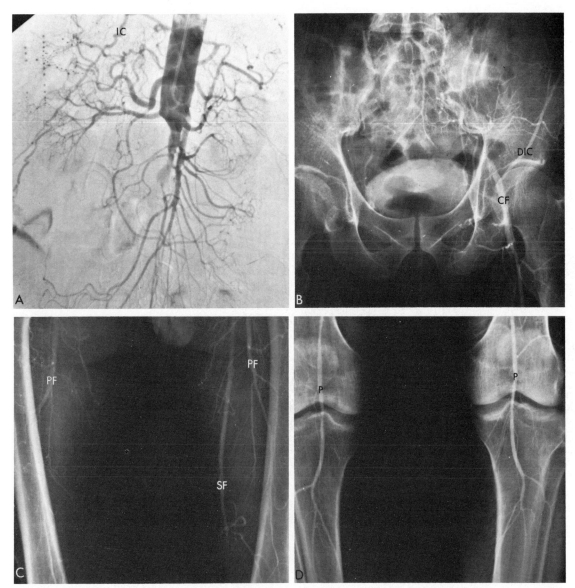

Figure 22–51. A 59-year-old man with progressive symptoms of obliterative aortoiliac disease. *A,* The abdominal aortogram (early phase, subtraction film) shows infrarenal aortic occlusion. The collateral circulation to the pelvis and lower extremities consists of intercostal arteries (IC), part of the systemic-systemic collaterals. *B,* In the pelvis, the only systemic artery noted to reconstitute is the left common femoral artery (CF). The deep circumflex iliac artery (DIC), a systemic collateral, is responsible for the reconstitution. *C,* In the thigh, the left superficial femoral artery (SF) is segmentally occluded distally, at the adductor canal. The left profunda femoris (PF) is patent. The right superficial femoral artery is totally occluded, and only the profunda femoris artery (PF) is patent. *D,* At the knee, both the popliteal (P) and the distal runoff arteries are patent. Both popliteal arteries were reconstituted via profunda femoris collaterals.

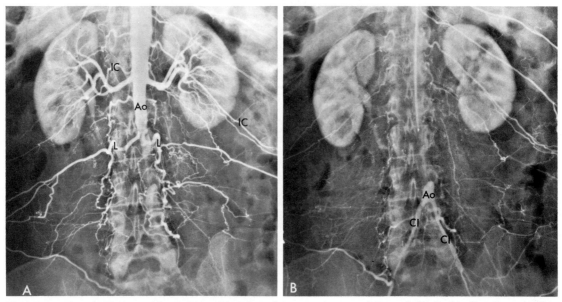

Figure 22–52. A 58-year-old woman with a long history of severe hip and thigh claudication. *A,* The infrarenal aorta (early phase, Ao) is segmentally occluded at L_2 but subsequently reconstitutes below the inferior mesenteric artery. The collateral circulation is mainly via the dilated lumbar (L) and intercostal (IC) arteries. *B,* The distal aorta (late phase, Ao) reconstitutes via collateral circulation, as do the common iliac arteries (CI).

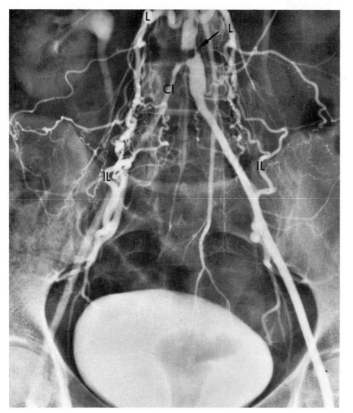

Figure 22–53. A 48-year-old woman complained of increasing hip and thigh heaviness and associated weakness of the same parts. The distal abdominal aorta is severely stenosed at the bifurcation (arrow). The right common iliac artery (CI) is stenosed at its origin, whereas the left is aneurysmally dilated. The lower lumbar arteries (L), bilaterally, are dilated and form the iliolumbar collaterals (IL) on each side. The remaining pelvic, thigh, and distal runoff arteries are all normal.

and *B*). Rarely, segmental occlusion of the aorta develops between the level of the renal and inferior mesenteric arteries (Fig. 22–52 *A* and *B*). The Leriche syndrome may also occur with severe stenosis without complete occlusion (Fig. 22–53).

The site of distal artery reconstitution is variable and is determined by the patency of the distal vessels and the available collateral circulation. Usually, the common iliac arteries are occluded in association with the aorta, and the external iliac arteries may be reconstituted (see Figs. 22–49 *D* and 22–50 *C* and *D*). Reconstitution also occurs more distally at the superficial or profunda femoris artery level (see Fig. 22–51 *B* and *C*). The reconstitution pattern may differ on each side.

COLLATERAL CIRCULATION

When chronic aortoiliac occlusion occurs, the body spontaneously attempts to re-establish continuity of circulation to the lower extremities via collateral ves-

Figure 22–54. *A,* Components of the viscero-systemic (visceral) collateral circulation. These collaterals may develop when the infrarenal aorta and proximal iliac arteries are obstructed. The collateral vessels originate from the superior mesenteric artery (SMA) and terminate in the common iliac arteries. The arrows indicate the direction of blood flow. The shaded area indicates the obstructed infrarenal aorta and common iliac vessels. *B,* Components of the systemic-systemic (parietal) collateral circulation. Various of these collaterals may develop in response to obstruction of the infrarenal aorta and proximal iliac arteries. The main components are the intercostal and lumbar artery branches of the aorta on each side. These may terminate in the internal iliac or external iliac arteries on their respective side. The arrows and shaded area refer to the same regions as *A*. (*From* Bron, K. M.: Thrombic occlusion of the abdominal aorta. Am. J. Roentgenol. *96*:887, 1966. Reproduced by permission.)

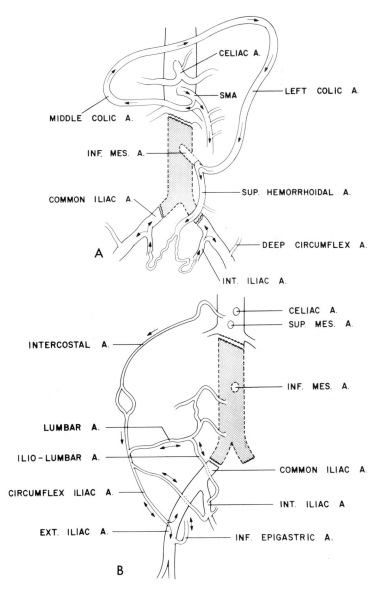

sels.[3, 10, 13, 22, 27] These vessels are components of two collateral systems that anatomically are classified as the viscero-systemic (visceral) and systemic-systemic (parietal) circulations (Fig. 22–54 A and B). Various combinations of the two systems are possible; these collaterals reconstitute the remaining patent pelvic and leg arteries in order to support function of the limbs.

Viscero-Systemic (V-S) or Visceral Collateral Arteries

These collaterals arise from the visceral circulation and eventually terminate in the systemic arteries of the pelvis (Fig. 22–54A), or, if these are occluded, in the thigh. The three principal V-S collateral components are the superior and inferior mesenteric arteries (Figs. 22–49 B and 22–51 A and B) and the pelvic visceral branches of the internal iliac arteries (see Fig. 22–49 C; Fig. 22–55 A and B). These V-S branches anastomose to both sides of the pelvis. The level of aortic occlusion, whether at the renal or the inferior mesenteric artery, determines the origin of the collateral circulation. If the aortic occlusion extends to the infrarenal level, the V-S collateral circulation begins at the superior mesenteric artery (see Fig. 22–49 A).

Anatomically, the main V-S collateral tributary (see Figs. 22–49 B and 22–54 A) arises as the middle colic branch of the superior mesenteric artery and continues as the transverse colic branch toward the splenic flexure. In the splenic flexure area, the transverse branch anastomoses with the left colic branch of the inferior mesenteric

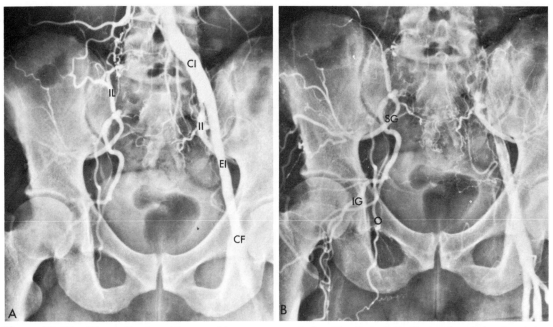

Figure 22–55. The patient, a 44-year-old man, presented with clinical findings of unilateral pelvic and lower extremity occlusive disease. A, The early-phase pelvic arteriogram shows occlusion of the right common and external iliac and common femoral arteries. A few right internal iliac branches reconstitute via the iliolumbar collateral (IL). The left pelvic arteries, the common iliac (CI), the external iliac (EI), the internal iliac (II), and the common femoral (CF) are patent. B, The midphase pelvic arteriogram demonstrates that the major reconstituted arteries are the superior gluteal (SG), the inferior gluteal (IG), and the obturator (O). These collaterals reconstitute the profunda femoris artery in C.

Legend continued on the opposite page

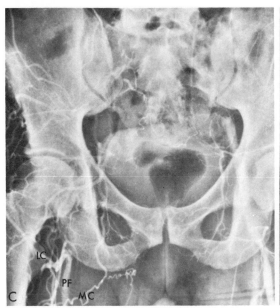 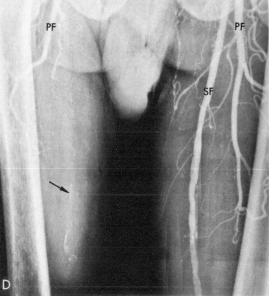

Figure 22–55 *Continued.* *C,* The late phase shows the reconstituted profunda femoris artery (PF). The collaterals reconstitute the PF via its lateral (LC) and medial circumflex (MC) branches. *D,* In the thigh the right PF is patent, but the superficial femoral artery is occluded. The left PF and superficial femoral (SF) arteries are patent. Intimal arteriosclerotic calcification is present in the wall of the right SF artery (arrow).

artery. The main inferior mesenteric artery is usually a short trunk, on the average about 2 cm in length, and it continues into the pelvis as the superior hemorrhoidal artery. The left colic branch continues to anastomose with the superior hemorrhoidal branch, even when the main trunk of the inferior mesenteric artery is occluded (see Fig. 22–49 *B*). This is important, since the main trunk of the inferior mesenteric artery is frequently occluded. The superior hemorrhoidal artery descends into the pelvis anteriorly along the sacrum (see Fig. 22–50 *B*), terminating in a fine tortuous network of vessels that anastomose with the middle and inferior hemorrhoidal branches of the internal iliac artery (see Fig. 22–49 *C*). The inferior hemorrhoidal branches are actually branches of the internal pudendal arteries, which originate from the internal iliac arteries.[32] As the blood flow passes retrograde to the origin of the internal iliac artery, it then can proceed antegrade in the systemic external iliac artery if this vessel is patent (see Figs. 22–49 *C* and *D* and 22–54 *A*). If the external iliac and common femoral arteries are occluded, then the obturator and internal pudendal branches of the internal iliac arteries may anastomose with the medial iliac circumflex branch of the profunda femoris artery and reconstitute the systemic thigh vessels (see Figs. 22–55 *A* to *D* and 22–59 *B*). In the pelvis, the visceral collaterals include the vesical artery and, in females, the uterine and vaginal branches of the anterior trunk of the internal iliac arteries. These pelvic branches form an extensive network of V-S collaterals that circumvent arterial occlusions of the aorta, common iliac, or internal iliac arteries.

Systemic-Systemic (S-S) or Parietal Collateral Arteries

The other major network of collateral vessels is the systemic-systemic or parietal system of arteries. Together, the V-S and S-S collaterals bridge occlusions of the aorta and proximal iliac arteries. The systemic collateral branches arise posteriorly from the aorta and consist of the intercostal, lumbar, and middle sacral arteries (see Fig. 22–54 B). These vessels anastomose with each other and with pelvic branches on the side of the occlusion they circumvent. Unlike the V-S collaterals, the S-S collaterals do not anastomose with their contralateral equivalents.

The intercostal and lumbar arteries are paired vessels, one on each side of the body. In instances of infrarenal aortic or common iliac artery occlusion they may anastomose with branches of the internal iliac artery, namely, the iliolumbar and superior gluteal vessels (see Figs. 22–50 C, 22–52 A and B, 22–54, and 22–55 A). The intercostal and lumbar arteries also frequently collateralize with the deep iliac circumflex artery, especially when the hypogastric branches are occluded (see Figs. 22–50 C, 22–51 B, and 22–54 B). The middle sacral branch of the aorta may anastomose with the iliolumbar artery or the lateral sacral branches of the internal iliac artery.

Another vital component in the S-S collateral circulation is the branches of the internal iliac artery; three each from the anterior and posterior trunks of this vessel. The posterior branches are the iliolumbar, lateral sacral (presacral), and superior gluteal (see Fig. 22–55 B). The anterior branches are the inferior gluteal, obturator, and internal pudendal (see Figs. 22–50 D, 22–55 B, and 22–56). Generally, the posterior branches are the most important as collaterals, but numerous variations are possible and essentially unpredictable.

The external iliac artery has two branches that form important collaterals in the S-S network (see Fig. 22–54 B). One is the deep iliac circumflex branch, which anastomoses with the intercostal, lumbar, iliolumbar, and superior gluteal arteries (see Fig. 22–51 C

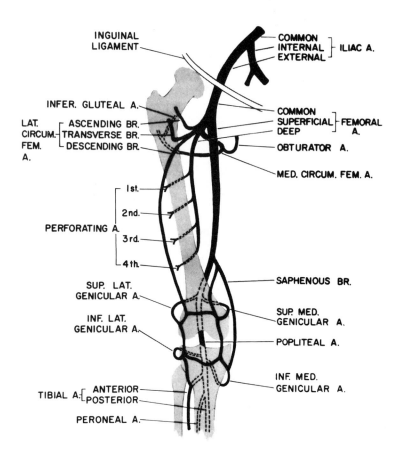

Figure 22–56. The normal lower extremity arteries and the potential collateral circulation via the deep femoral artery (profunda femoris) branches when the superficial femoral artery is obstructed. Also indicated is the potential collateral circulation around the knee when the popliteal artery is obstructed. (*From* Abrams, H. L.: Angiography. Ed. 2. Boston, Little Brown and Company, 1971. Reproduced by permission.)

and *D*). This vessel is particularly important when the internal iliac branches are unavailable to serve as collateral channels. The other external iliac branch is the inferior epigastric artery. It anastomoses with the internal mammary and superior epigastric arteries in the chest and abdomen, respectively. This source of collateral circulation can be demonstrated by injection of the aortic arch or of the internal mammary artery on the same side as the pelvic artery occlusion. The inferior epigastric artery also communicates with the obturator branch of the internal iliac artery. Although this usually is not significant, this potential collateral pathway may occasionally become important.[27]

Leg Collaterals

The common femoral artery is the link between the external iliac artery of the pelvis and the superficial and profunda femoris arteries of the thigh (see Fig. 22–56). The profunda femoris artery is the deep branch formed when the common femoral artery bifurcates; the superficial femoral artery is the continuation of the common femoral artery in the thigh.

The profunda femoris artery is a very important branch because of its direct connections with the pelvic collaterals; hence, it functions as the principal collateral in the thigh to the distal run-off when the superficial femoral artery is occluded (see Figs. 22–55 *B* to *D* and 22–66 *B*).[11] The medial and lateral femoral circumflex arteries are the branches of the profunda femoris that anastomose with the pelvic vessels. Generally, these vessels arise very close to the origin of the profunda femoris. Anatomic variations may cause one or both femoral circumflex branches to arise from the common femoral artery.[27]

The medial femoral circumflex artery may collateralize with the obturator, pudendal, and inferior gluteal branches of the internal iliac artery. It also may join in an arcade with the lateral femoral circumflex artery around the upper femur in the region of the femoral neck (see Figs. 22–55 *C*, 22–56, and 22–59 *B*). The lateral femoral circumflex artery divides into the ascending, transverse, and descending branches. In turn, these branches communicate with the superior and inferior gluteal branches of the internal iliac artery, the deep iliac circumflex, the inferior epigastric branches of the external iliac artery, and the first perforating branches of the profunda femoris (see Fig. 22–56). The profunda femoris, through its muscular and perforating branches, is instrumental in reconstituting the distal superficial femoral and popliteal arteries when the proximal portions are occluded (see Fig. 22–66 *B*). The descending branch of the lateral femoral circumflex is especially important in this regard, since it anastomoses with the superior geniculate, lower profunda perforating, and geniculate branches of the popliteal artery near the adductor canal (see Fig. 22–56).

REVASCULARIZATION

The principle of surgical management for ischemic disease of the lower extremity is to attempt restoration of the blood flow. This can be accomplished either by endarterectomy or bypass grafting.[1, 7, 24] Endarterectomy is generally confined to limited segmental occlusions of the aorta and iliac arteries, but occasionally may be used for short occlusions of the superficial femoral and proximal popliteal arteries. When this technique is used for the repair of aortic occlusion, extreme care must be taken to avoid the potential hazard of embolizing arteriosclerotic debris into the renal arteries.[29]

Most often, aortoiliac occlusion is a chronic clinical problem with a long history of hip and thigh, or even calf, claudication and absent femoral pulses. The arteriogram confirms the clinical diagnosis and establishes the anatomic limits of the obstruction. The preferred therapeutic procedure in most instances of aortoiliac occlusion is bypass surgery using a prosthetic Dacron graft,[12] rather than endarterectomy. In unilateral aortoiliac occlusive disease, it has been shown that unilateral aortofemoral, iliofemoral, or femorofemoral crossover grafts are not as effective as bilateral aortobifurcation grafts. A recent study revealed that 52 per cent of unilateral grafts remained patent for 5 years, whereas 78 per cent of the bilateral bifurcation grafts remained patent.[16] The principal reasons for graft failure are progression of the arteriosclerotic process distal to the graft (Fig. 22–57), problems at the anastomosis (false aneurysm, stricture, or infection) (Figs. 22–58 and 22–59 B), and problems with the graft itself (incorrect caliber and length, or kinks).[4, 28] The late failure rate, for both unilateral and bilateral aortobifurcation grafts, ranges from 10 to 28 per cent.[19, 21]

Extra-anatomic grafts, such as femorofemoral crossover (Fig. 22–60) and axillofemoral bypasses, are used primarily for patients with occlusion of one limb of an aortobifurcation graft.[2, 5, 23] The crossover femorofemoral bypass was originally described for poor surgical risk patients with unilateral iliac obstructive disease (see Fig. 22–57 A), since the procedure carries a low operative risk.[31] It is now the procedure of choice when one limb of an aortobifurcation graft is occluded, because of its technical simplicity, low operative risk, and high rate of graft patency.[6, 30] Because this is an

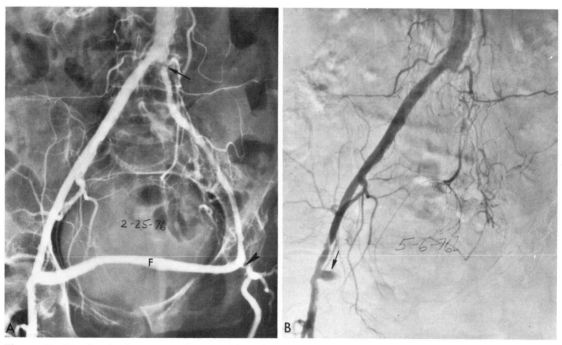

Figure 22–57. In this 72-year-old arteriosclerotic woman, a femorofemoral crossover graft had been performed to circumvent the left iliac stenosis, because the patient's associated medical problems precluded aortic bypass surgery. A, The examination of February 25, 1976 showed a patent femoro-femoral crossover graft (F), from the right to left side. The left proximal common iliac artery is severely stenosed (arrow). Distal to the graft anastomosis, on the left side, the common femoral artery is markedly stenosed (arrowhead). B, On May 6, 1976 the pelvic subtraction film shows the crossover graft and left pelvic arteries to be thrombosed. A small sac-like projection (arrow) is all that remains of the graft. The graft presumably occluded because of disease progression distal to the graft and the stricture at the distal anastomosis.

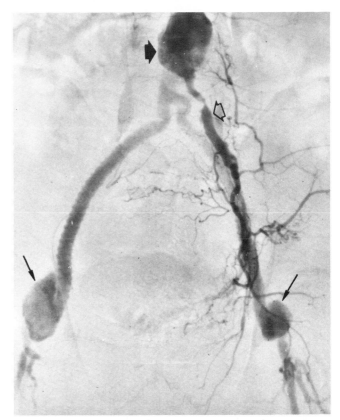

Figure 22–58. A florid example of multiple anastomotic aneurysms, a complication of bypass grafts. The subtraction film of the pelvic arteriogram, demonstrates an anastomotic aneurysm at the proximal (arrowhead) and distal graft (arrow) sites of the aortobifemoral bypass graft. Note the typical serrated margin of a prosthetic graft in the right limb. A few of the original left pelvic arteries are visualized (open arrowhead).

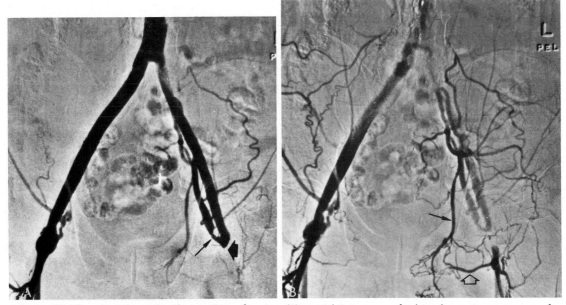

Figure 22–59. Anastomotic obstruction, due to either stricture or occlusion, is a common cause for subsequent graft failure in aortobifurcation grafts. *A,* The pelvic subtraction film reveals that the left limb of the aortobifurcation graft is occluded at the distal anastomosis (arrowhead). The left external iliac artery is stenosed (arrow) at its junction with the graft, secondary to fibrosis at the anastomosis. Retrograde filling of the left external iliac artery and a few internal iliac artery collateral branches occurs. Note the anastomotic aneurysm at the right distal graft site. *B,* In the later arterial phase, the anastomotic occlusion is shown to be segmental. The profunda femoris artery is reconstituted via the obturator (arrow) and medial femoral circumflex (arrowhead) arteries.

1507

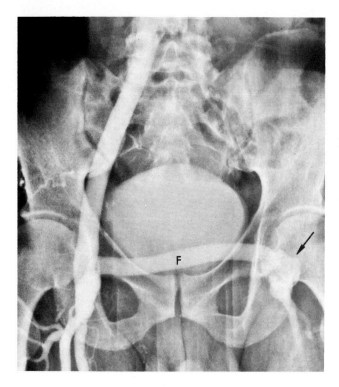

Figure 22–60. One month after an aortobifemoral graft was inserted for pelvic artery occlusion, unilateral left graft limb occlusion occurred. A femorofemoral crossover graft (F) was constructed to provide adequate circulation to the left lower extremity. An anastomotic aneurysm (arrow) is present at the distal anastomosis.

extra-abdominal procedure, it can be performed under local anesthesia. It has been shown that a "steal phenomenon" may occur in the donor limb after a femorofemoral bypass when a significant stenosis is present in the proximal iliac artery of the donor limb.[30]

Various catheter techniques have recently received attention and are discussed in Chapter 43.

References

1. Bell, J. W.: Surgical treatment of chronic occlusion of the terminal aorta. Am. Surg. *38*:481–485, 1972.
2. Brief, D. K., Alpert, J., and Parsonnet, V.: Crossover femoro-femoral grafts. Arch. Surg. *105*:889–894, 1972.
3. Bron, K. M.: Thrombotic occlusion of the abdominal aorta. Am. J. Roentgenol. *96*:887–895, 1966.
4. Christensen, R. D., and Bernatz, P. E.: Anastomotic aneurysms involving the femoral artery. Mayo Clin. Proc. 47:313–317, 1972.
5. Crawford, F. A., Sethi, G. K., Scott, S. M., et al.: Femorofemoral grafts for unilateral occlusion of aortic bifurcation grafts. Surgery *77*:150–155, 1975.
6. Davis, R. C., O'Hara, E. T., Mannick, J. A., et al.: Broadened indications for femorofemoral grafts. Surgery 72:990–994, 1972.
7. DeBakey, M. E., Crawford, E. S., Cooley, D. A., et al.: Surgical considerations of occlusive disease of the abdominal aorta and iliac and femoral arteries: analysis of 803 cases. Ann. Surg. *148*:306–324, 1958.
8. Downs, A. R.: Aorto-iliac occlusive disease. Surg. Clin. North Am. *54*:195–212, 1974.
9. Foster, J.: Arteriography. Arch. Surg. *109*:605–611, 1974.
10. Friedenberg, M. J., and Perez, C. A.: Collateral circulation in aorto-iliac femoral occlusive disease — as demonstrated by a unilateral percutaneous common femoral artery needle injection. Am. J. Roentgenol. *94*:145–158, 1965.
11. Haimovici, H., and Escher, D. J.: Aortoiliac stenosis — diagnostic significance of vascular hemodynamics. Arch. Surg. 72:107–117, 1956.
12. Hobson, R. W., Rich, N. M., and Fedde, C. W.: Surgical management of high aortoiliac occlusion. Am. Surg. *41*:271–280, 1975.

13. Krahl, E., Pratt, G. H., Rousselot, L. M., et al.: The collateral circulation in the arterial occlusive disease of the lower extremity. Surg. Gynecol. Obstet. 98:324–330, 1954.

14. Leriche, R.: De la resection du carrefour aortico-iliaque avec double sympathectomie lombaire pour thrombose arteritique de l'aorte. Le syndrome de l'obliteration termino-aortique par arterite. Presse Med. 54–55:601–604, 1940.

15. Leriche, R., and Morel, A.: The syndrome of thrombotic obliteration of the aortic bifurcation. Ann. Surg. 127:193–206, 1948.

16. Levinson, S. A., Levinson, H. J., Halloran, L. G., et al.: Limited indications for unilateral aortofemoral or iliofemoral vascular grafts. Arch. Surg. 107:791–796, 1973.

17. Liddicoat, J. E., Bekassy, S. M., Dang, M. H., et al.: Complete occlusion of the infrarenal abdominal aorta: management and results in 64 patients. Surgery 77:467–472, 1975.

18. Matolo, N. M., Cheung, L., Albo, D., Jr., et al.: Acute occlusion of the infrarenal aorta. Am. J. Surg. 126:788–793, 1973.

19. Minken, S. L., DeWeese, J. A., Southgate, W. A., et al.: Aortoiliac reconstruction for atherosclerotic occlusive disease. Surg. Gynecol. Obstet. 126:1056–1060, 1968.

20. Morris, G. C., Edwards, W., Cooley, D. A., et al.: Surgical importance of profunda femoris artery. Arch. Surg. 82:32–37, 1961.

21. Mozersky, D. J., Sumner, D. S., and Strandness, D. E.: Long-term results of reconstructive aortoiliac surgery. Am. J. Surg. 123:503–509, 1972.

22. Muller, R. F., and Figley, M. M.: The arteries of the abdomen, pelvis, and thigh. Am. J. Roentgenol. 77:296–311, 1957.

23. Plecha, F. R., and Pories, W. J.: Extra-anatomic bypasses for aortoiliac disease in high-risk patients. Surgery 80:480–487, 1976.

24. Rob, C. G., and Downs, A. R.: Chronic occlusive disease of the aorta and iliac arteries. J. Cardiovasc. Surg. 1:57–64, 1960.

25. Rockwell, E. G., Jr.: Aorto-iliac disease. Minn. Med. 55:430–474, 1972.

26. Staple, T. W.: The solitary aortoiliac lesion. Surgery 64:569–576, 1968.

27. Strandness, D. E., Jr.: Collateral Circulation in Clinical Surgery. Philadelphia, W. B. Saunders Company, 1969.

28. Szilagyi, D. E., Smith, R. F., Elliot, J. P., et al.: Anastomotic aneurysms after vascular reconstruction: problems of incidence, etiology, and treatment. Surgery 78:800–816, 1975.

29. Thurlbeck, W. M., and Castleman, B.: Atheromatous emboli to the kidneys after aortic surgery. N. Engl. J. Med. 257:442–447, 1957.

30. Trimble, I. R., Stonesifer, G. L., Jr., Wilgis, E. F., et al.: Criteria for femorofemoral bypass from clinical and hemodynamic studies. Ann. Surg. 175:985–993, 1972.

31. Vetto, R. M.: The treatment of unilateral iliac artery obstruction with a transabdominal, subcutaneous, femorofemoral graft. Surgery 52:342–345, 1962.

32. Warwick, R., and Williams, P.: Gray's Anatomy. Philadelphia, W. B. Saunders Company, 1973.

33. Weston, T. S.: Thrombosis of the lower aorta. Australas. Radiol. 17:313–315, 1973.

Part IV

Femoral Bypass

KLAUS M. BRON, M.D.

DIAGNOSTIC CONSIDERATIONS

Arteriosclerosis obliterans is a diffuse process, in many instances involving the cerebral, coronary, and peripheral circulations. Despite the widespread involvement, arteriographic studies indicate that the occlusive process in this disease is mainly segmental.[2] The segmental feature of the disease has provided the stimulus for endarterectomy and bypass grafting. Surgical management depends on diagnostic arteriography to accurately define the anatomic limits of these lesions.[1, 3, 7]

Arteriosclerosis obliterans in the legs, as elsewhere, involves either the intimal or the medial arterial coat.[6] The intimal lesion consists of atheromatous plaques, randomly deposited along the vessel surface. Growth of these plaques causes gradual encroachment on the lumen, with resultant stenosis and eventual occlusion. There may be

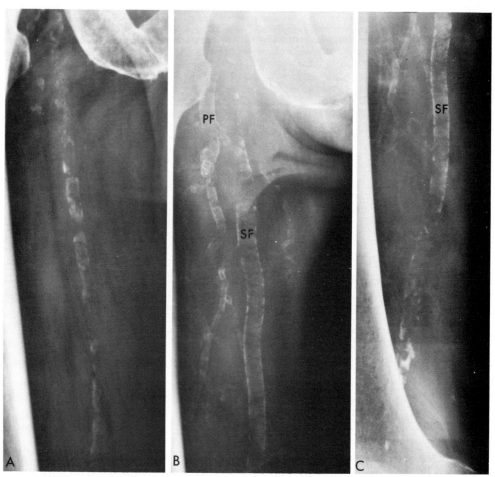

Figure 22–61. A comparison of intimal and medial types of arteriosclerotic calcification. *A,* Intimal calcification is identified by an amorphous, diffuse, and irregular pattern. This is the most common type of arteriosclerotic calcification and may be present in the wall of the aorta, pelvic, and lower extremity arteries. *B,* Medial calcification (arrows) is character-ized by a regular, linear, parallel track appearance. This type of calcification is noted mainly in the extremity arteries as opposed to the aorta or pelvic vessels. Medial calcification occurs much less frequently than intimal calcification. Note the extensive involvement of both the superficial femoral (SF) and the profunda femoris (PF) arteries by both types. *C,* This is the same patient as in *B.* In the adductor canal region of the superficial femoral artery (SF), the calcification changes in character from the medial to the intimal type (arrow).

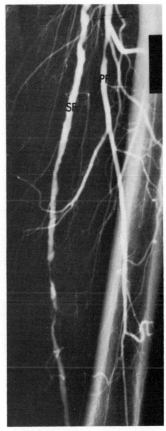

Figure 22–62. The patient had symptoms of severe peripheral vascular disease and a history of adult-onset diabetes mellitus. The superficial femoral artery (SF) shows diffuse arteriosclerotic changes of the wall. The vessel lumen demonstrates typical varying degrees of obstruction. The narrowest focal stenosis is accompanied by vessel calcification in the adductor canal region. A focal stenosis is present in a profunda femoris branch (PF); this change in the profunda femoris is usually associated with diabetes mellitus.

associated calcification in the subintimal base of the plaque. This calcification (Fig. 22–16A) is irregularly distributed and involves only a portion of the vessel wall, in comparison with medial calcification.[2] Intimal arteriosclerotic lesions may cause thrombosis on their intraluminal surface, leading to progressive obstruction and eventual obliteration of the lumen (Fig. 22–62). Intimal arteriosclerotic lesions are more common than medial lesions.

Medial or Mönckeberg's arteriosclerosis is identified on radiographs by uniformly distributed linear calcific deposits that resemble parallel tracks (see Fig. 22–61B and C). The deposits are fine-grained and usually encompass the entire vessel circumference. Occlusion of the lumen is not generally associated with this lesion; on the contrary, the lumen may be dilated.

SITE OF OBSTRUCTION AND OTHER FACTORS

In the lower extremities, the vessel that is most frequently involved initially by arteriosclerosis obliterans is the superficial femoral artery in the region of the adductor canal (Fig. 22–63). Correlative roentgenologic-pathologic studies[5, 6] indicate that intimal thickening is first most pronounced at the adductor foramen. It has been speculated that the location of this lesion is due to a stress factor as the artery passes through the unyielding aponeurotic tunnel.[2] This lesion may first manifest as a severe stenosis, then advance to a segmental occlusion of varying length, and finally progress retrograde to occlude the entire superficial femoral artery. Only rarely does the occlusion propagate

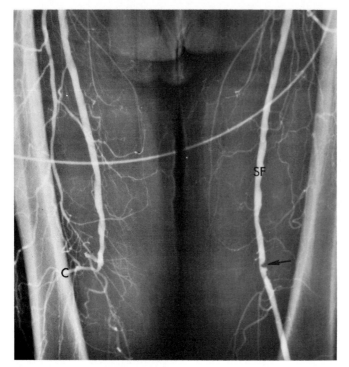

Figure 22–63. Symptoms of progressively severe claudication of the right leg are present, with recent development of similar symptoms on the left. The left superficial femoral artery (SF) shows a severe focal stenosis in the adductor canal portion of the vessel (arrow). This location is typical for the onset of obstructive arteriosclerosis in the superficial femoral artery. On the right side, the process has progressed to complete occlusion at this location, with collateral vessels (C) reconstituting the popliteal artery.

Figure 22–64. The proximal popliteal artery is a frequent site of initial obstruction in the lower extremity arteries. There is severe segmental stenosis of the right proximal popliteal artery (arrow). The left proximal popliteal artery is occluded, together with the distal superficial femoral artery. The left distal popliteal artery (P) reconstitutes via collateral vessels.

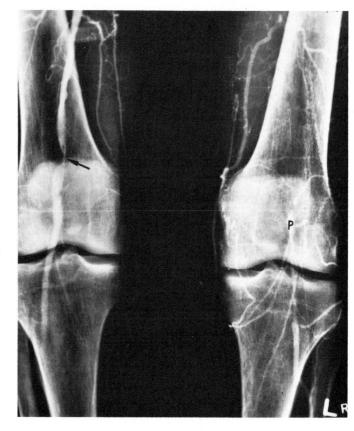

distally into the popliteal artery, probably because of the extensive collateral circulation entering the superificial femoral artery just distal to the adductor canal.

The second most common site for initial occlusion is the popliteal artery immediately proximal to the knee joint (Fig. 22–64).[2, 6] Like the adductor canal region, it is a zone of mechanical stress, which may account for occlusion at this site. Stretching and bending motions of the knee joint may be a cause of trauma to the popliteal artery as it runs posteriorly along the femur. Initial occlusive lesions may also occur in the distal run-off arteries; such lesions usually appear in patients over 60 years of age.

In a study of the relative incidence of lesions in the femoropopliteal arteries, the location of the lesions was classified into nine different patterns.[2] In approximately 50 per cent of the 137 limbs studied, the occlusive lesion was confined to an area in the superficial femoral or proximal popliteal artery. The profunda femoris artery was rarely occluded and served as the most important collateral when the superficial femoral artery was segmentally or entirely occluded (see Fig. 22–66B). Stenosis and occlusion of the profunda femoris artery are possible but occur almost exclusively in diabetic patients (see Fig. 22–61B).

Diabetes mellitus affects the pattern of arteriosclerosis obliterans in the lower extremities. In a study of the run-off arteries, in nondiabetic and diabetic arteriosclerotic patients, the latter had a higher incidence of lesions in the distal arteries with more severe obstruction.[2] Also, when simultaneous or combined lesions of the femoral, popliteal, and distal arteries were evaluated, about two thirds of these occurred in patients with diabetes (Figs. 22–65A and B).

Occlusive disease of the femoropopliteal–tibial arteries most often does not occur as isolated lesions. In a study of 321 extremities, 74 per cent of the occlusions were combined lesions, whereas only 26 per cent were isolated lesions involving single leg

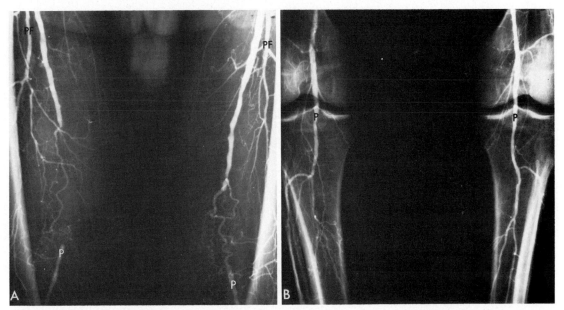

Figure 22–65. Simultaneous obstructive lesions of the femoral, popliteal, and runoff arteries are common in elderly diabetic patients such as this 60-year-old man. *A,* The superficial femoral arteries are segmentally occluded in their distal portions. Collateral circulation from the profunda femoris arteries (PF) reconstitutes the popliteal arteries (P). The superficial femoral arteries proximal to the occlusion show moderately severe arteriosclerotic changes. *B,* Both popliteal arteries (P) are patent but show evidence of arteriosclerotic changes of the walls. The occluded runoff arteries are the right posterior tibial and peroneal, and the left anterior tibial beyond its proximal portion.

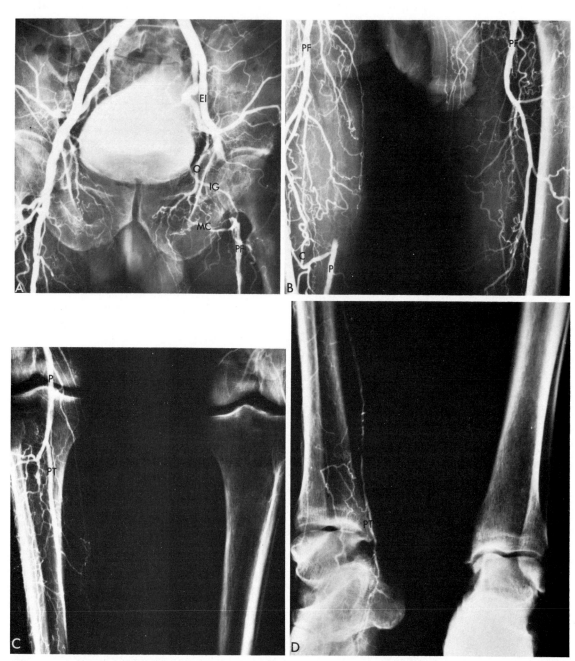

Figure 22–66. The association of pelvic vessel "inflow" obstruction and distal femoropopliteal run-off disease, is common in lower extremity arteriosclerosis obliterans. *A,* The pelvic left external iliac artery (EI) is partially occluded, and the common femoral artery is totally occluded. The left profunda femoris artery (PF) reconstitutes via the obturator (O), inferior gluteal (IG), and medial circumflex (MC) collaterals. *B,* In the thighs, both superfical femoral arteries are occluded, but the profunda femoris arteries (PF) are patent and dilated. The right popliteal (P) reconstitutes via the dilated PF collaterals (C). *C,* At the knee, the right popliteal (P) is patent, but the left is occluded. The right run-off arteries consist of a patent posterior tibial (PT) and occluded anterior tibial and peroneal arteries. On the left side, the popliteal and run-off arteries below the knee are occluded. *D,* At the ankle, only the right posterior tibial artery is patent. The remaining right and left run-off arteries never reconstitute via collateral vessels. The knee and run-off vessel examination was performed using enhanced circulation by ischemic exercise.

arteries.[3] In 27 per cent of femoropopliteal–tibial occlusions, there was associated aortoiliac disease in the form of stenosis, occlusion, or aneurysm (Fig. 22–66). Aortoiliac stenosis was the most prevalent associated lesion, followed by iliac occlusion and aortoiliac aneurysms. The association of aortoiliac and femoropopliteal–tibial occlusive disease is an important consideration when surgical management of femoropopliteal lesions is contemplated.[7] The "inflow" obstruction in the iliac vessels may substantially affect the results of distal endarterectomy or bypass grafting.

REVASCULARIZATION

Femoropopliteal and more distal bypass grafts—femorotibial or femoroperoneal—are employed to manage ischemic lower limbs when occlusive disease is present

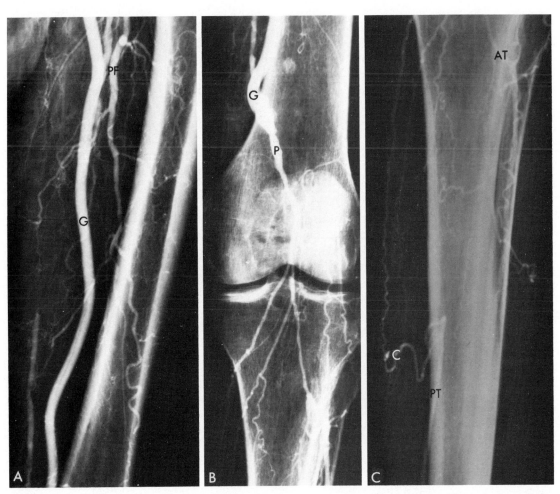

Figure 22–67. A femoropopliteal bypass graft was performed in this patient with occlusion of the superficial femoral artery, in an effort to revascularize the lower limb. *A,* In the thigh, the femoropopliteal graft (G) is patent and tortuous. The original superficial femoral artery, medial to the graft, is occluded down to the distal third, where it reconstitutes via profunda femoris (PF) collaterals. *B,* At the knee, the graft (G) is anastomosed to the proximal popliteal artery (P). The remainder of the popliteal artery is severely narrowed secondary to arteriosclerosis. *C,* In the lower leg, the anterior tibial artery (AT) is patent. The proximal posterior tibial artery (PT) is occluded, but it reconstitutes distally via a dilated tortuous collateral (C).

in the superficial femoral, popliteal, or more distal arteries.[11] A femoropopliteal graft (Fig 22–67) is the most popular procedure for lower extremity revascularization, because it carries a lower complication rate than the other types of distal graft procedures.[4, 11] The indications for bypass grafting are: (1) limb salvage as an alternative to amputation for rest pain or gangrenous ulceration; (2) intermittent claudication interfering with occupation; and (3) claudication severely limiting activities of the elderly.[9] The selection of a femoropopliteal bypass graft depends on patency of the popliteal artery and at least one distal branch, preferably a tibial artery.[4]

Femorotibial and femoroperoneal bypass grafts are performed when the popliteal artery is occluded or severely obstructed, and only if a patent tibial or peroneal artery is demonstrated by arteriography. Diabetic patients have a higher incidence of occluded distal run-off arteries (tibial and peroneal). In all instances of leg grafts, autologous vein rather than synthetic material offers the best hope for maintaining graft patency.

When the results of femoropopliteal and femorotibial bypass grafts were compared in a recent series of 73 patients, patency was achieved in 49 per cent of the popliteal and 51 per cent of the tibial grafts.[4] However, in the same series, complications requiring reoperation occurred in 4 of 39 popliteal grafts, and in 16 of 34 tibial grafts. In another series, femoropopliteal grafts were performed in 62 per cent (224 of 364) patients, whereas a femorotibial or peroneal bypass was required in 39 per cent (140 of 364) patients.[11] The initial patency and limb salvage rate for popliteal grafts was 81 per cent; for tibial grafts the rate was 72 per cent. The late results in surviving patients, after a 1- to 11-year follow-up, were a limb salvage rate of 45 per cent (76 of 167) for popliteal grafts and 52 per cent (45 of 86) for tibial grafts. The late occlusion rate, during the same time span, was 25 per cent for popliteal grafts and 17 per cent for tibial grafts. The evidence that bypass grafts to the small-caliber arteries below the knee does preserve limb function and does offer an alternative to amputation should stimulate the angiographer to adequately visualize the distal run-off vessels to the ankle.

Currently, considerable success has been obtained in selected cases by catheter balloon dilatation (Gruntzig technique) of focal strictures. The full import of this non-surgical technique awaits the accumulation of results of success rate and duration of vascular patency (see Chapter 43).

References

1. Foster, J.: Arteriography. Arch. Surg. *109*:605–611, 1974.
2. Haimovici, H., Shapiro, J. H., and Jacobson, H.: Serial femoral arteriography in occlusive disease. Am. J. Roentgenol. *84*:1042–1062, 1960.
3. Haimovici, H., and Steinman, C.: Aortoiliac angiographic patterns associated with femoropopliteal occlusive disease: significance in reconstructive arterial surgery. Surgery *65*:232–240, 1969.
4. Hallin, R. W.: Femoropopliteal versus femorotibial bypass grafting for lower extremity revascularization. Am. Surg. *42*:522–526, 1976.
5. Lindbom, A.: Arteriosclerosis and arterial thrombosis in the lower limb: a roentgenological study. Acta Radiol. (Suppl.) *80*:1–80, 1950.
6. Mavor, G. E.: The pattern of occlusion in atheroma of the lower limb arteries. The correlation of clinical and arteriographic findings. Br. J. Surg. *43*:352–364, 1956.
7. Milanes, B., Perez-Stable, E., Casanova, R., et al.: Chronic arterial occlusions of the lower extremities. Radiology *60*:394–400, 1953.
8. Perdue, G. D., Long, W. D., and Smith, R. B.: Perspective concerning aorto-femoral arterial reconstruction. Trans. South. Surg. Assoc. *82*:330–334, 1970.
9. Reichle, F. A., and Tyson, R. R.: Bypasses to tibial or popliteal arteries in severely ischemic lower extremities. Ann. Surg. *176*:315–320, 1972.
10. Reichle, F. A., and Tyson, R. R.: Femoroperoneal bypass: evaluation of potential for revascularization of the severely ischemic lower extremity. Ann. Surg. *181*:182–185, 1975.
11. Reichle, F. A., and Tyson, R. R.: Comparison of long-term results of 364 femoropopliteal or femorotibial bypasses for revascularization of severely ischemic lower extremities. Ann. Surg. *182*:449–455, 1975.

Part V
Arterial Injuries

KLAUS M. BRON, M.D.

PELVIC ARTERIAL INJURY

Acute traumatic arterial injury in the pelvis and lower extremities, unless promptly recognized and treated, has a high risk of death or loss of limb from hemorrhage or ischemia.[6] Fracture of the pelvis is the most common type of civilian trauma causing massive extraperitoneal hemorrhage; gunshot and stab wounds may also injure major vessels. Clinically, it is generally impossible to distinguish between venous and arterial bleeding,[19, 22] although the latter is less responsive to massive blood and fluid replacement. Massive extraperitoneal hemorrhage is the principal cause of death following pelvic fracture, because the bleeding site cannot be identified.[5, 20, 26] Surgical exploration, the traditional method for localizing the bleeding source, is generally unsuccessful because of the massive accumulation of blood.[28] In addition, surgical exploration may disturb the tamponading effect of a hematoma and further contribute to intraperitoneal rupture and exsanguinating hemorrhage.[19] Even if bleeding is controlled by surgery, subsequent sepsis may develop. However, the accepted treatment for massive pelvic hemorrhage has been ligation of the internal iliac artery, whether or not the bleeding site is identified.[6, 10, 31] Because the proximal arterial

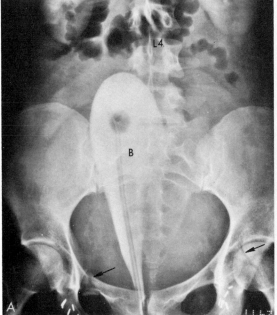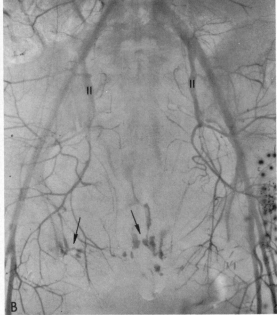

Figure 22–68. Pelvic trauma may cause severe and often fatal hemorrhage unless the bleeding site is promptly located, as in this 32-year-old car accident victim. *A,* Extensive pelvic hemorrhage in the form of a soft tissue mass is present. The contrast-filled bladder (B) is distorted by the mass which extends to the level of the L_4 vertebral body. The air-filled loops of bowel are pushed out of the pelvis by the mass. Note the fracture of the right superior pubic ramus and left acetabulum (arrows). *B,* A subtraction film of the pelvis, in the late arterial phase, demonstrates multiple areas of punctate contrast extravasation (arrows) in the midline and along the right pubic ramus. The blood supply to these areas comes from several branches of both internal iliac arteries (II).

ligation has no effect on the extensive pelvic collaterals, this form of therapy has had variable results.[23, 29]

The diagnosis and location of the bleeding site in pelvic trauma are the decisive factors in the management of these injuries. Arteriography (Fig. 22–68) used early in the management of these patients can reduce the rate of mortality and the complications of prolonged and massive hemorrhage.[19, 27, 30] If arteriography identifies a bleeding site, a nonsurgical alternative may be available for controlling the hemorrhage. Utilizing transcatheter embolization,[19] or an intra-arterial balloon catheter,[30] it may be possible to occlude the traumatized vessel responsible for the bleeding.

The type of pelvic fracture may correlate with the location of arterial injury. A fracture of the ilium or separation of the sacroiliac joint is associated with injury to the common or external iliac vessels.[32] A fracture of the pubic rami may cause a laceration of the obturator and internal pudendal arteries.[30] A fracture of the posterior pelvis is associated with laceration of the superior gluteal arteries.[22] The obturator and superior gluteal branches of the internal iliac artery are the principal vessels involved in massive bleeding associated with pelvic fractures. An occasional late complication is the development of a false aneurysm at the site of arterial injury. Bilateral fractures are common in traumatic pelvic injuries and were noted in four of six cases in a recent report.[30] Bilateral bleeding sites were demonstrated in three of the six cases, indicating the importance of a careful scrutiny of the branches of both internal iliac arteries. This is best accomplished by selective arteriography of each internal iliac artery; in many instances, aortography at the aortic bifurcation may be adequate.

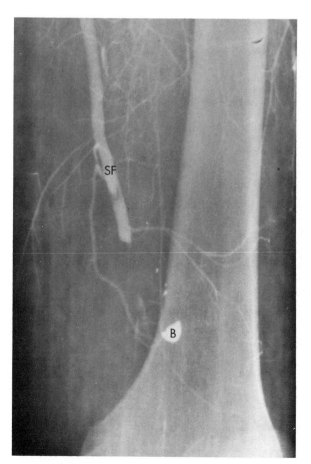

Figure 22–69. Traumatic arterial obstruction may result from penetrating injury, such as that caused by a bullet. The superficial femoral artery (SF) occlusion is secondary to the dense radiopaque metallic fragment of bullet (B).

THIGH, POPLITEAL, AND DISTAL RUN-OFF ARTERY INJURY

Prior to the Korean War, severe peripheral arterial trauma was treated by ligation of the bleeding vessel and limb amputation.[8] The intent was to salvage life even if the extremity had to be sacrificed. Extensive arterial reconstruction was first utilized in the Korean War, and the reports of this procedure indicated its efficacy and its superiority to earlier techniques.[1, 12, 14] The wartime experience with arterial reconstruction was soon applied to civilian injuries for both penetrating and blunt vascular trauma.[4, 7, 11, 18, 25]

Traumatic arterial injury of the lower extremity is the result of either penetrating or blunt injury (Fig. 22–69). The artery is most easily injured where it is close to the surface, adjacent to a bone, or held fixed in position by a muscle.[17] In the lower extremity, the superficial femoral artery is most vulnerable in its distal third, where it is held in position close to the bone as it passes through Hunter's canal. A fracture of the distal femur is likely to injure the artery at this location (Fig. 22–70). Another site of injury is where the popliteal artery passes along the posterior capsule of the knee joint (Fig. 22–71). Here the artery is held fixed in position by the muscles; thus, a posterior dislocation of the knee tends to cause arterial injury. The anterior tibial artery is easily injured as it passes anteriorly through the interosseous membrane in fractures of the proximal tibia (Fig. 22–72). The anterior tibial artery is also frequently damaged by fractures of the distal tibia (Fig. 22–73). However, it has been pointed out that in

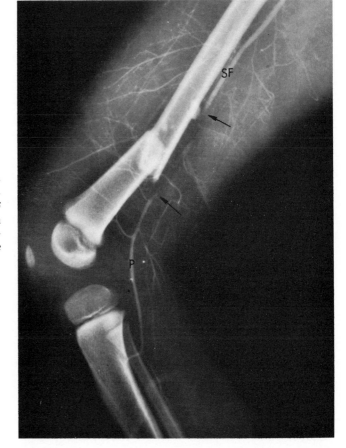

Figure 22–70. The distal superficial femoral artery (SF) is a frequent site of occlusion in fractures of the femur. The SF artery is segmentally occluded between the arrows. The popliteal artery (P) reconstitutes via collateral circulation, and the proximal distal run-off vessels are patent.

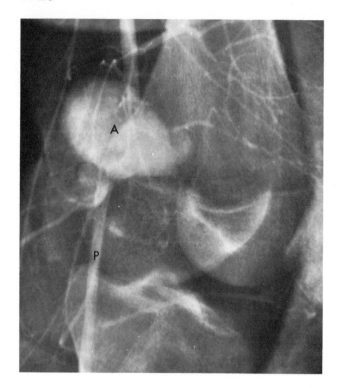

Figure 22–71.   The popliteal artery segment posterior to the knee joint is easily injured. Iatrogenic trauma to the vessel, secondary to meniscectomy, was responsible for this false aneurysm (A), which presented as a mass. The false aneurysm consists of an irregular-shaped contrast-filled mass. It is important to verify the patency of the popliteal artery (P) distal to the aneurysm.

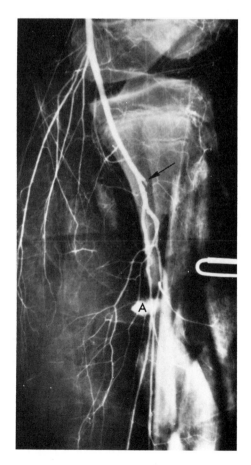

Figure 22–72.   The anterior tibial artery (arrow) is occluded where it passes anteriorly through the interosseous membrane. The artery sustained injury from compound fractures of the tibia and fibula. There is also contrast extravasation in a false aneurysm (A).

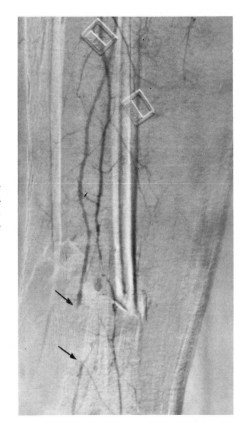

Figure 22–73. The anterior tibial artery is segmentally occluded between the arrows. The vessel was injured by the displaced fracture of the distal tibia and fibula. The segmental nature of the vessel injury was clearly visualized only in the subtraction film.

fractures of the femoral shaft, the incidence of superficial femoral artery injury is not high.[3, 33] Multiple extremity fractures should always be evaluated by arteriography if there is any clinical suspicion of vascular obstruction (Fig. 22–74).

Traumatic injury of the popliteal artery is similar in most respects to injury of the superficial femoral artery. The vessels are comparable in the cause and mechanism of injury, the clinical features, the need for rapid arterial reconstruction, and the techniques of surgical repair. They differ, however, in the results of surgical repair, with amputation being required more frequently after popliteal artery injury.[7] Since the type of injury affects the outcome of popliteal artery trauma, penetrating injury has a better salvage rate than blunt injury.[7]

DIAGNOSIS AND MECHANISM OF INJURY

The clinical signs of arterial injury are those of acute ischemia distal to the site of injury, namely, pain, blanched skin, coldness to touch, loss of cutaneous sensation, absence of motor function, and faint or absent arterial pulsations. These clinical findings are frequently sufficient to establish the diagnosis. Any doubt about the diagnosis or the location of the lesion is an indication for an arteriogram. Actually, an arteriogram is probably warranted in every case of suspected arterial injury if it can be readily accomplished and not delay the surgical repair of the lesion. The suggested mechanisms of lower-extremity arterial injury due to trauma are: (1) overstretching without transection, and (2) transection. Experimental work has shown that the intima

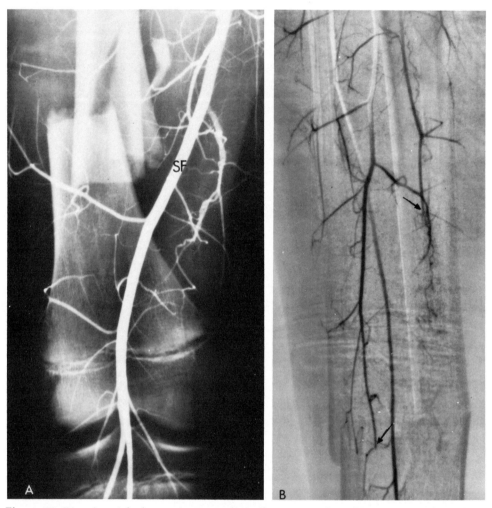

Figure 22–74. Arterial obstruction was clinically suspected in this 13-year-old accident victim, who had sustained multiple fractures. *A,* The distal femoral shaft is fractured, but the superficial femoral artery, although displaced is intact. The location of this fracture is typical of the type that may cause injury to the superficial femoral artery (SF). *B,* A subtraction film of the distal run-off shows occlusion of the posterior tibial artery in the mid-third (arrow) and of the peroneal artery distally (arrow). Observe the fractures of the tibia and fibula distally.

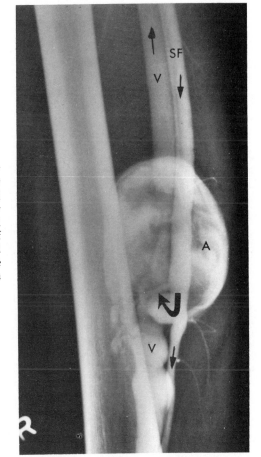

Figure 22–75. Several weeks after a knife wound injury of the thigh, a mass and thrill were palpable. The early arterial phase demonstrates an arteriovenous fistula and false aneurysm. The proximal superficial femoral artery (SF) is markedly dilated compared with the portion distal to the aneurysm (A). The arrows indicate the direction of blood flow. The draining vein (V) both in its proximal and distal portions is dilated. The vein segment distal to the aneurysm is prominently lobulated. The false aneurysm is 6 cm in diameter and sharply marginated.

ruptures before the other coats of the arterial wall.[2] The artery without transecting may become contused and form an intramural hematoma, or the intima may dissect and form a flap. Transection of the wall may result from penetration by an external object or a fractured bone fragment. Spasm of the artery is not a clinical or arteriographic diagnosis but must be established by surgical exploration.[24] Arterial obstruction may be the result of acute injury, but trauma can also cause late complications, namely, arteriovenous fistulas and false aneurysms (Fig. 22–75).

THERAPY

The elapsed time before definitive repair of the arterial injury is attempted is referred to as the ischemic time. It is generally acknowledged that the longer the delay before arterial reconstruction, the greater the chance of a poor result, necessitating amputation or leading to contracture or atrophy.[21] Ischemic times of no longer than 6 to 12 hours have been cited as critical.[8, 16, 21] Probably the time delay is relative rather than absolute, since additional factors, such as the degree of associated soft tissue damage and the extent of collateral circulation, influence the ultimate result.[13] The surgical techniques of arterial repair include primary end-to-end anastomosis, patch grafts, and replacement grafts.[9]

References

1. Beall, A. C., Diethrich, E. B., Morris, G. C., et al.: Surgical management of vascular trauma. Surg. Clin. North Am. 46:1001–1011, 1966.
2. Bergan, F.: Traumatic intimal rupture of the popliteal artery with acute ischemia of the limb in cases with supracondylar fractures of the femur. J. Cardiovasc. Surg. 4:300–302, 1963.
3. Blichert-Toft, M., and Hammer, A.: Treatment of fractures of the femoral shaft. Acta Orthop. Scand. 41:341–353, 1970.
4. Bradham, R., Buxton, J. T., and Stallworth, J. M.: Arterial injury of the lower extremity. Surg. Gynecol. Obstet. 118:995–1000, 1964.
5. Braunstein, P. W., Skudder, P. A., McCarroll, J. R., et al.: Concealed hemorrhage due to pelvic fracture. J. Trauma 4:832–838, 1964.
6. Bystrom, J., Dencker, H., Jaderling, J., et al.: Ligation of the internal iliac artery to arrest massive haemorrhage following pelvic fracture. Acta Chir. Scand. 134:199–202, 1968.
7. Conkle, D. M., Richie, R. E., Sawyers, J. L., et al.: Surgical treatment of popliteal artery injuries. Arch. Surg. 110:1351–1354, 1975.
8. DeBakey, M. E., and Simeone, F. A.: Battle injuries of the arteries in World War II: An analysis of 2471 cases. Ann. Surg. 123:534–579, 1946.
9. Hardy, J. D., Raju, S., Neely, W. A., et al.: Aortic and other arterial injuries. Ann. Surg. 181:640–652, 1975.
10. Hauser, C. W., and Perry, J. F., Jr.: Control of massive hemorrhage from pelvic fractures by hypogastric artery ligation. Surg. Gynecol. Obstet. 121:313–315, 1965.
11. Hershey, F. B., and Spencer, A. D.: Surgical repair in civilian arterial injuries. Arch. Surg. 80:953–962, 1960.
12. Hughes, C. W.: Acute vascular trauma in Korean War casualties: An analysis of 180 cases. Surg. Gynecol. Obstet. 99:91–100, 1954.
13. Inui, F. K., Shannon, J., and Howard, J. M.: Arterial injuries in the Korean Conflict: experiences with 111 consecutive injuries. Surgery 37:850–857, 1955.
14. Jahnke, E. J., Jr., and Seeley, S. F.: Acute vascular injuries in the Korean War: an analysis of 77 consecutive cases. Ann. Surg. 138:158–177, 1953.
15. Kelly, G. L., and Eiseman, B.: Civilian vascular injuries. J. Trauma 15:507–514, 1975.
16. Kirkup, J. R.: Major arterial injury complicating fracture of the femoral shaft. J. Bone Joint Surg. 45B:337–343, 1963.
17. Klingensmith, W., Oles, P., and Martinez, H.: Fractures with associated blood vessel injury. Am. J. Surg. 110:849–852, 1965.
18. Kootstra, G., Schipper, J. J., Boontje, A. H., et al.: Femoral shaft fracture with injury of the superficial femoral artery in civilian accidents. Surg. Gynecol. Obstet. 142:399–403, 1976.
19. Margolies, M. N., Ring, E. J., Waltman, A. C., et al.: Arteriography in the management of hemorrhage from pelvic fractures. N. Engl. J. Med. 287:317–321, 1972.
20. McCarroll, J. R., Braunstein, P. W., Cooper, W., et al.: Fatal pedestrian automotive accidents. J.A.M.A. 180:127–133, 1962.
21. Miller, H. H., and Welch, C. S.: Quantitative studies on the time factor in arterial injuries. Ann. Surg. 130:428–438, 1949.
22. Miller, W. E.: Massive hemorrhage in fractures of the pelvis. South. Med. J. 56:933–938, 1963.
23. Motsay, G. J., Manlove, C., and Perry, J. F.: Major venous injury with pelvic fracture J. Trauma 9:343–346, 1969.
24. Nolan, B., and McQuillan, W. M.: Acute traumatic limb ischaemia. Br. J. Surg. 52:559–565, 1965.
25. Owens, J. C.: The management of arterial trauma. Surg. Clin. North Am. 43:371–385, 1963.
26. Peltier, L. F.: Complications associated with fractures of the pelvis. J. Bone Joint Surg. 47A:1060–1069, 1965.
27. Pradhan, D. J., Juanteguy, J. M., Wilder, R. J., et al.: Arterial injuries of the extremities associated with fractures. Arch. Surg. 105:582–585, 1972.
28. Quinby, W. C., Jr.: Pelvic fractures with hemorrhage. N. Engl. J. Med. 28:668–669, 1971.
29. Ravitch, M. M.: Hypogastric artery ligation in acute pelvic trauma. Surgery 56:601–602, 1964.
30. Ring, E. J., Athanasoulis, C., Waltman, A. C., et al.: Arteriographic management of hemorrhage following pelvic fracture. Radiology 109:65–70, 1973.
31. Seavers, R., Lynch, J., Ballard, R., et al.: Hypogastric artery ligation for uncontrollable hemorrhage in acute pelvic trauma. Surgery 55:516–519, 1964.
32. Stone, H. H., Rutledge, B. A., and Martin, J. D., Jr.: Massive crushing pelvic injuries. Am. Surg. 34:869–878, 1968.
33. Suiter, R. D., and Bianco, A. J., Jr.: Fractures of the femoral shaft. J. Trauma, 11:238–247, 1971.

Part VI
Acute Arterial Occlusion

KLAUS M. BRON, M.D.

Emboli are a common cause of acute arterial occlusion of the lower extremities and therefore share the clinical features of traumatic occlusions.[2, 9] The incidence of emboli may be increasing as a result of improved cardiac care, an aging population, and more extensive use of prosthetic heart valves. Newer therapeutic techniques for managing emboli have increased the limb salvage rate and decreased the need for amputation. The mortality rate remains high because of the seriousness of the underlying cardiac disease that is nearly always present.[8]

DIAGNOSIS

The clinical diagnosis of a peripheral arterial embolus is usually quite apparent because of the sudden onset of pain or a feeling of limb heaviness, followed by pallor,

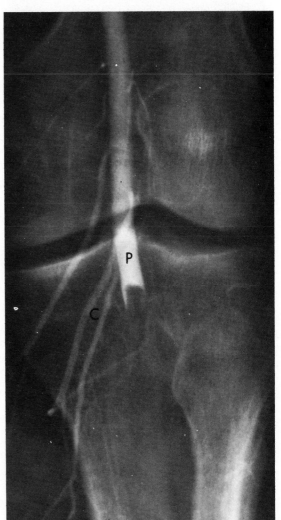

Figure 22–76. Popliteal artery embolus. This patient had an atypical clinical history for an embolus, but typical arteriographic findings. The distal popliteal artery (P) is occluded, with a concave intraluminal filling defect typical of an embolus. A few sural collaterals (C) are present.

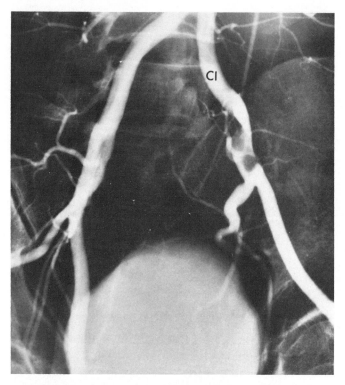

Figure 22–77. Embolus in iliac artery. The patient's symptoms were those of sudden ischemia of the lower extremity. Arteriosclerotic thrombosis or an acute embolus was considered the most likely possibility. The pelvic arteriogram demonstrates the intravascular filling defect causing partial occlusion of the left distal common iliac artery (CI), The filling defect is smooth and distinctly marginated, which is characteristic of an embolus. Note the absence of arteriosclerotic plaques in the pelvic arteries.

coldness, numbness, and absent pulses distal to the site of obstruction. These clinical features are invariably associated with a history of cardiac disease, proximal aneurysms, or recent cardiovascular surgery. If the clinical onset is insidious rather than acute, then embolism must be differentiated from arterial thrombosis and deep vein thrombophlebitis. Angiography can be helpful in distinguishing these possibilities (Figs. 22–76 and 22–77). A less frequent cause of arterial emboli is intravascular ulcerated atheromatous plaques; these may shower cholesterol or atheromatous debris into the smaller vessels of the foot, causing occlusion.[1]

In a recent series of 203 arterial embolectomies, 76 per cent of the emboli had lodged in the leg arteries, and of these 42 per cent were located in the femoral artery.[8] Then in descending order of frequency, emboli were located in the following arteries: iliac, 19 per cent; popliteal, 14 per cent; posterior tibial, 1 per cent; and anterior tibial, 0.5 per cent. The emboli in this series were overwhelmingly cardiac in origin; 78 per cent of cases were due to myocardial infarction, atrial fibrillation, and atherosclerosis without fibrillation or infarction. The second most frequent cause of peripheral arterial emboli was cardiovascular surgery, but this accounted for only 7 per cent of cases. In 10 per cent of the cases no etiology was established. In another series of 300 balloon-catheter embolectomies, similar statistics of anatomic location and etiology were reported.[4]

THERAPY

As with acute occlusion from other causes, the success of therapy in embolic occlusion depends on rapid clinical recognition and location of the obstruction. The location of the occlusion and the patency of the vessels distal to this site are quickly evaluated by arteriography. In reports concerned with the management of emboli it has been stressed that embolectomy should be performed as soon as possible (Fig. 22–78).[5-7]

Limb amputation rate is proportional to the increase in the lag time between the acute occlusion and embolectomy. Different time delays have been cited by various authors, but according to two recent reports, when embolectomy was performed within 24 hours the amputation rate ranged between 0.1 per cent and 4.4 per cent, whereas the amputation rate after a 24-hour delay ranged between 4.3 per cent and 19.4 per cent.[4, 8] It has been further suggested that the time delay after the acute episode increases the chances of secondary thrombosis distal to the primary site of acute embolic occlusion.[6] This enhances the ischemic changes in the distal portion of the extremity. Even when an extended time delay occurs and amputation is imminent, it is still worthwhile to perform an embolectomy, since this may permit a more distal amputation and improve vascularization of the stump.

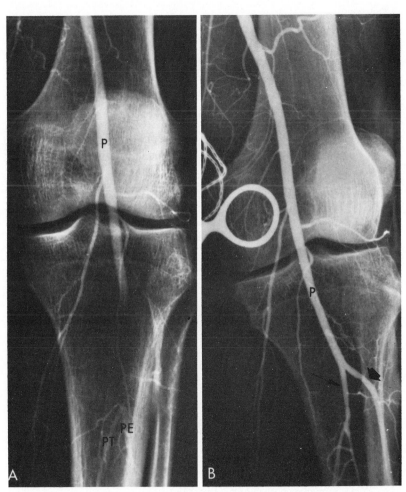

Figure 22–78. Arteriographic evaluation pre- and postembolectomy of a patient with acute symptoms of lower leg ischemia, demonstrating the site of occlusion and the distal vessels. *A,* The pre-embolectomy study shows occlusion of the distal popliteal artery (P) and origin of the anterior tibial artery. At the point of occlusion there is gradual fading of the intraluminal contrast material. This is another arteriographic presentation of embolic occlusion. The vessels distal to the occlusion, the posterior tibial (PT) and peroneal arteries (PE), are faintly visualized, having reconstituted via collateral circulation. *B,* An intraoperative arteriogram after a Fogarty balloon embolectomy. The popliteal (P), common posterior tibial (arrow), and anterior tibial (arrowhead) arteries are all patent.

The limb salvage rate following embolectomy has been reported to be as high as 93 per cent and 95 per cent, in two series of 163 and 300 patients, respectively.[4, 8] The operative mortality rate in these two series was 15 and 16 per cent; more than 50 per cent of these deaths were due to cardiac causes, consistent with the origins of the emboli. Some of the deaths resulted from pulmonary emboli; it has been postulated that microemboli are released into the venous system at the time of arterial embolectomy.[7]

Since 1963, when Fogarty described the instrumentation and technique of balloon-catheter embolectomy, this has become the universally accepted method for the management of arterial emboli.[3] The attractions of this procedure are its simplicity and effectiveness. The balloon catheter is introduced into the femoral artery and successively directed into the proximal and distal vessels, clearing them of embolic and thrombotic debris. The procedure can be performed under local anesthesia, a significant advantage when dealing with patients who are poor surgical risks because of their debilitating cardiovascular disease. Usually, embolectomy is performed without definitive arterial reconstruction, but in patients whose general condition is good the latter is occasionally attempted.

References

1. Crane, C.: Atherothrombotic embolism to lower extremities in arteriosclerosis. Arch. Surg. 94:96–101, 1967.
2. Darling, R. C., Austen, W. G., and Linton, R.: Arterial embolism. Surg. Gynecol. Obstet. 124:106–114, 1967.
3. Fogarty, T. J., Cranley, J. J., Krause, R. J., et al.: A method for extraction of arterial emboli and thrombi. Surg. Gynecol. Obstet. 116:241–244, 1963.
4. Fogarty, T. J., Daily, P. O., Shumway, N. E., et al.: Experience with balloon catheter technic for arterial embolectomy. Am. J. Surg. 122:231–237, 1971.
5. Levy, J. F., and Butcher, H. R., Jr.: Arterial emboli: an analysis of 125 patients. Surgery 68:968–973, 1970.
6. Linton, R. R.: Peripheral arterial embolism: a discussion of the postembolic vascular changes and their relation to the restoration of circulation in peripheral embolism. N. Engl. J. Med. 224:189–194, 1941.
7. Stallone, M. D., Blaisdell, M. D., Cafferata, H. T., et al.: Analysis of morbidity and mortality from arterial embolectomy. Surgery 65:207–217, 1969.
8. Thompson, J. E., Sigler, L., Raut, P. S., et al.: Arterial embolectomy: a 20 year experience with 163 cases. Surgery 67:212–220, 1970.
9. Weston, T. S.: Arterial embolism of the lower limbs. Australas. Radiol., 11:354–358, 1967.

Part VII
Arteriovenous Fistula

KLAUS M. BRON, M.D.

Arteriovenous malformations (fistulas) have long fascinated clinicians because of their pathophysiologic behavior. These malformations have defied various forms of therapy and have been difficult to treat. There are two types of arteriovenous fistulas, the acquired and the congenital.

ACQUIRED FISTULAS

Acquired arteriovenous fistulas almost always result from penetrating trauma that causes vascular injury to an adjacent artery and vein. Gunshot and stab wounds (see Fig. 22–75) account for more than 50 per cent of the lesions in most series of civilian injuries.[3, 11] Less common causes are steel or glass splinters, iatrogenic injury in pelvic surgery,[8, 20] intervertebral disc resection, balloon thrombectomy,[7, 19] and percutaneous arterial catheterization.[23] Rarely have arteriovenous fistulas been reported following rupture of a mycotic aneurysm or a traumatic false aneurysm. Military traumatic arteriovenous fistulas have most commonly followed shrapnel injuries secondary to low-velocity fragments from artillery shells, mortars, and land mines.[10] In the Vietnam War, vascular injuries due to Claymore mines were a significant cause of these fistulas.

As might be anticipated from their etiology, most acquired arteriovenous fistulas involve the extremities. In the extremities, adjacent arteries and veins are relatively close to the surface and thus vulnerable to penetrating injury. In most series of acquired arteriovenous fistulas,[3, 10, 11] whether due to civilian or wartime vascular injuries, the lower extremities are most often involved; the femoral artery is the single vessel most often affected (see Fig. 22–75).

CONGENITAL FISTULAS

Although congenital arteriovenous fistulas may occur at any site and in any organ, the majority occur in the extremities,[24] followed by the brain, kidney, and lung. The origin of congenital fistulas is uncertain, but the embryologic and histologic studies of Woollard[26] suggest that developmental arrest at an early stage in the formation of arteries and veins is responsible. He described certain stages of vessel development, such as the capillary or cavernous and the retiform. During early development, there are many complex stages in which future arteries and veins are poorly differentiated and communicating. Persistence of these communications probably results in the clinical varieties of arteriovenous fistulas designated as cirsoid aneurysms, arteriovenous malformations, and cavernous hemangiomas. The anomalous types of more mature vascular arteriovenous fistulas probably result from maturation arrest in the later or more differentiated stage of development. Thus, congenital fistulas may be multiple and may be associated with multiple vessels supplying blood to a localized lesion. This is in contrast to the acquired fistula, in which there is generally a single lesion supplied by a single dominant artery. However, in acquired vascular injuries caused by multiple pellets, multiple fistulas may be encountered initially, or may occur at another site after surgical ligation (Fig. 22–79).[3]

DIAGNOSIS

The diagnosis of an arteriovenous fistula, regardless of type, is usually simple and depends on the physical findings of an audible bruit and palpable thrill. Associated findings are a swollen mass that may pulsate, venous distention or varices, and superficial ulceration with possible hemorrhage. Congenital fistulas may be associated with unilateral limb elongation if the lesion antedates epiphyseal closure of the long bones.[15] In chronic fistulas, severe limb edema and pain may be present.

To confirm the location and extent of the lesion, selective arteriography is mandatory, especially if surgical intervention is contemplated. Arteriography determines (1) the size and number of the feeding arteries; (2) the extent of the arterial collateral circulation; (3) the possible presence of an aneurysm; (4) the extent of the venous dilatation and collateral circulation; and (5) the state of the arterial circulation distal to the fistula. There has been recent interest in the diagnostic possibilities of radioisotopic studies and ultrasound for the evaluation of arteriovenous fistulas.[9, 22]

PATHOPHYSIOLOGY

The pathophysiology of arteriovenous fistulas has been most fully investigated and described by Holman.[12-14] The presence of a fistula causes a drop in the arterial blood pressure and a rise in the pulse rate. Cardiac output increases concomitantly because

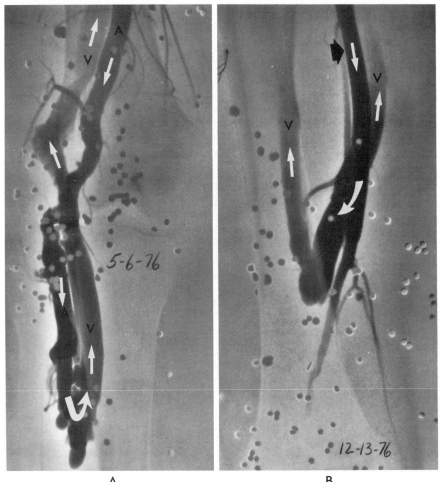

A   B

Figure 22–79. A shotgun pellet vascular injury may initially cause multiple arteriovenous fistulas, or recurrences after surgical ligation. *A,* The initial examination on May 6, 1976 (subtraction film) shows an arteriovenous fistula between a dilated artery (A) and vein (V) below the knee joint. The arrows indicate the direction of the blood flow in the markedly dilated artery and vein. No distal run-off arteries are visualized. Multiple metallic pellets are present in the soft tissues. At surgery the fistula was ligated, and no other abnormal connection was noted. *B,* On December 13, 1976 the patient was re-examined because of recurrent symptoms. A subtraction film of the early arterial phase reveals another fistulous connection at a more proximal site than previously. The arrows indicate the direction of blood flow between the superficial femoral artery (arrowhead) and draining veins (V).

more blood returns to the heart, being short-circuited through the low-resistance venous circulation. There is also an increase in the total blood volume, and compensatory generalized vasoconstriction in order to reduce the size of the circulatory bed. When an arteriovenous fistula is closed, these findings are reversed. The blood no

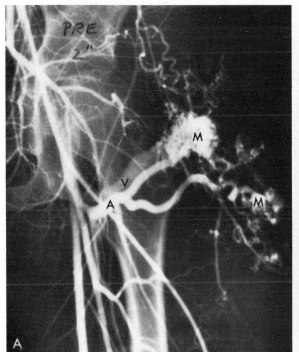

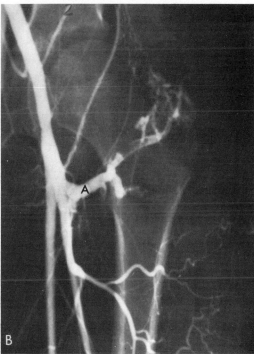

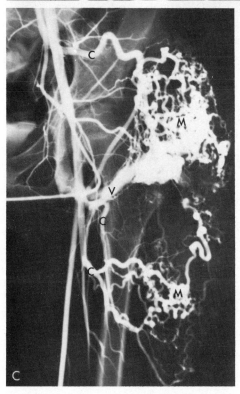

Figure 22–80. Congenital arteriovenous malformations are difficult management problems. This patient initially had been treated by surgical ligation and extirpation, but the lesion recurred. Intentional intra-arterial embolization with cyanoacrylate was tried, but collateral circulation caused recurrence. *A,* The pre-embolization study of March 7, 1972, at 2 seconds, shows an arteriovenous malformation and fistula of the hip and thigh. The malformation (M) consists of fine tortuous vessels concentrated over the greater trochanter and thigh. The lesion is supplied primarily by a dilated lateral circumflex branch of the profunda femoris artery (A), and drained by an accompanying vein (V). *B,* The post-embolization film after the infusion of cyanoacrylate on the same date shows almost complete obliteration of the malformation. The dilated feeding arteries (A) are partially occluded by clot. No early draining vein is seen. *C,* The hip mass recurred about three years later, and another examination was performed on February 3, 1975. The malformation (M) and fistula had recurred and were now supplied by collateral branches (C) from the internal iliac and profunda femoris arteries. The malformation has increased in size. A single dilated vein (V) is noted to drain the malformation.

longer circulates through a low-resistance vascular bed, and there is an immediate rise in the arterial blood pressure. The pulse rate slows, initiated by a vagal response to the increased distention of the aorta and cerebral arteries. The cardiac output decreases, and a temporary but prompt generalized vasodilation occurs. Within a few days the circulatory blood volume contracts to normal levels.

The dramatic slowing of the pulse rate when a fistula is closed is a useful diagnostic finding. Temporary digital compression of the fistula elicits this clinical response, which is known as Branham's sign.[1] The increased cardiac output from an arteriovenous fistula may cause cardiac dilation and congestive heart failure, depending on the size and location of the fistula and the velocity of blood flow. Thus, aortovenacaval and iliac-venacaval fistulas are more apt to lead to congestive heart failure.

THERAPY

The management of arteriovenous fistulas has been primarily surgical. Successful surgery resulting in an intact functioning extremity has been mainly limited to acquired fistulas.[3-5, 11, 18, 25] The majority of acute acquired fistulas have a single arterial blood supply, which may be either ligated or repaired. In chronic acquired and congenital fistulas, ligation of the feeding arteries is generally ineffective, because alternative collaterals develop (Fig. 22–80). In these patients, even multiple attempts to eradicate the lesion by successive ligations of the feeding arteries usually are unsuccessful. Amputation of the affected digit, hand, foot, or entire extremity is often the final result. There have been some successful ligations and extirpations of these fistulas, but most often a poorly functioning limb results. A technique that has proved helpful is the use of hypothermia and circulatory arrest during surgery, thus obtaining a relatively bloodless field for excision of the fistulous mass.[2]

Alternatives to surgery for managing arteriovenous fistulas have been mainly experimental and utilize transcatheter intravascular embolization[27] and electrocoagulation.[6] In an experimental animal study[27] using a tissue adhesive (cyanoacrylate) for transcatheter embolization, it was demonstrated that aneurysms and arteriovenous fistulas could be occluded. This same material was utilized to successfully occlude a renal arteriovenous fistula in one patient.[16] In another report, Gelfoam was used successfully to occlude two arteriovenous fistulas, an acquired and a congenital lesion.[21] In both patients, previous surgical attempts had been unsuccessful. One of the patients developed a pulmonary embolus following the intravascular embolization. In another experimental animal study, arteriovenous fistulas were successfully occluded by intra-arterial transcatheter electrocoagulation.[17] The drawback to this procedure is the time required to produce occlusion of a fistula. Nevertheless, the enthusiasm and interest shown in attempts to find alternatives to surgery for the management of arteriovenous fistulas offer hope for improved results in the treatment of these difficult lesions.

References

1. Branham, H. H.: Aneurismal varix of the femoral artery and vein following a gunshot wound. Int. J. Surg. 3:250, 1890.
2. Brickman, R. D., Yates, A. J., Crisler, C., et al.: Circulatory arrest during profound hypothermia. Arch. Surg. 103:259–264, 1971.
3. Dry, L. R., Conn, J. H., Chavez, C. M., et al.: Arteriovenous fistula: An analysis of fifty-eight cases. Am. Surg. 38:154–160, 1972.

4. Fraser, G. A.: Traumatic aneurysms and arterio-venous fistulae. Vasc. Surg. 4:258–268, 1970.
5. Fry, W. J.: Surgical considerations in congenital arteriovenous fistula. Surg. Clin. North Am. 54:165–174, 1974.
6. Gardner, A. M. N., and Stewart, I. A.: Treatment of arteriovenous malformation by endarterial electrocoagulation. Br. J. Surg. 59:146–148, 1972.
7. Gaspard, D. J., and Gaspar, M. R.: Arteriovenus fistula after Fogarty catheter thrombectomy. Arch. Surg. 105:90–92, 1972.
8. Gaylis, H., Levine, E. Van Dongen, L. G. R., et al.: Arteriovenous fistulas after gynecologic operations. Surg. Gynecol. Obstet. 137:655–658, 1973.
9. Handa, J., Handa, H., Torizuka, K., et al.: Radioisotopic study of arteriovenous anomalies. Am. J. Roentgenol., 115:751–759, 1972.
10. Hewitt, R. L., and Collins, D. J.: Acute arteriovenous fistulas in war injuries. Ann. Surg. 169:447–449, 1969.
11. Hewitt, R. L., Smith, A. D., and Drapanas, T.: Acute traumatic arteriovenous fistulas. J. Trauma 13:901–906, 1973.
12. Holman, E.: The physiology of an arteriovenous fistula. Arch. Surg. 7:64–82, 1923.
13. Holman, E.: Abnormal Arteriovenous Communications: Peripheral and Intracardiac; Acquired and Congenital. Springfield, Illinois, Charles C Thomas, Publisher, 1968.
14. Holman, E.: Reflections on arteriovenous fistulas. Ann. Thorac. Surg. 11:176–186, 1971.
15. Janes, J. M., and Musgrove, J. E.: Effect of arteriovenous fistula on growth of bone. Surg. Clin. North Am. 30:1191–1200, 1950.
16. Kerber, C. W., Freeny, P. C., Cromwell, L., et al.: Cyanoacrylate occlusion of a renal arteriovenous fistula. Am. J. Roentgenol. 128:663–665, 1977.
17. Phillips, J. F., Robinson, A. E., Johnsrude, I. S., et al.: Experimental closure of arteriovenous fistula by transcatheter electrocoagulation. Radiology 115:319–321, 1975.
18. Raskind, R., and Weiss, S. R.: Arteriovenous malformations: follow-up in 68 cases. Vasc. Surg. 5:30–35, 1971.
19. Rob, C., and Battle, S.: Arteriovenous fistula following the use of the Fogarty balloon catheter. Arch. Surg. 102:144–145, 1971.
20. Saunders, W. G., and Ellis, R.: Acquired pelvic arteriovenous fistula: case report and literature review. Milit. Med. 137:308–310, 1972.
21. Stanley, R. J., and Cubillo, E.: Nonsurgical treatment of arteriovenous malformations of the trunk and limb by transcatheter arterial embolization. Radiology 115:609–612, 1975.
22. Stephenson, H. E., Jr., and Lichti, E. L.: Application of the Doppler Ultrasonic Flowmeter in the surgical treatment of arteriovenous fistula. Am. Surg. 38:537–538, 1972.
23. Thadani, U., and Pratt, A. E.: Profunda femoral arteriovenous fistula after percutaneous arterial and venous catheterization. Br. Heart J. 33:803–805, 1971.
24. Tice, D. A., Clauss, R. H., Keirle, A. M., et al.: Congenital arteriovenous fistulae of the extremities. Arch. Surg. 86:130–135, 1963.
25. Treiman, R. L., Cohen, J. L., Gaspard, D. J., et al.: Early surgical repair of acute post-traumatic arteriovenous fistulas. Arch. Surg. 102:559–561, 1971.
26. Woollard, H. H.: The development of the principal arterial stems in the forelimbs of the pig. Contrib. Embryol. 14:141–154, 1922.
27. Zannetti, P. H., and Sherman, F. E.: Experimental evaluation of a tissue adhesive as an agent for the treatment of aneurysms and arteriovenous anomalies. J. Neurosurg. 36:72–79, 1972.

Part VIII
Carotid Occlusive Disease

GUSTAVE FORMANEK, M.D.

KURT AMPLATZ, M.D.

Ischemic cerebrovascular disease was first described by Hippocrates, who also coined the term "apoplexy."[5] Extracranial vascular lesions were not recognized as a cause of cerebral ischemia or infarction until this century, however.

Based on a study of 70 autopsies, Chiari offered the first description, in 1905, of the relative frequency of cerebral embolization arising from the common carotid artery bifurcation secondary to atherosclerosis ("endarteritis chronica deformans").[3] Fisher stressed in 1951 and 1954 that stenosis of the carotid artery and cerebral embolization play an important role in the pathogenesis of cerebrovascular disease.[6, 7] These reports led to surgical treatment of carotid artery lesions.[4] It is now well accepted that transient ischemic attacks and strokes may be caused by extracranial as well as intracranial vascular disease. Only the extracranial lesions are considered here.

If cerebral ischemia is suspected, angiography must include the visualization of the brachiocephalic vessels in their entire course. At least two right-angle projections of the carotid bifurcations should be obtained.[13] The origins of the neck vessels should be demonstrated either by aortography or by selective injections. After the neck vessels have been satisfactorily visualized, an intracranial study of the affected side may be indicated.

The most frequent surgically accessible arteriosclerotic lesions (34 per cent of cases) are at the level of the carotid bifurcations (both the right and the left sides).[9] Isolated lesions in the proximal internal carotid arteries are rare. With arch aortography, only oblique films of the neck can be obtained. Since the great majority of the lesions are on the posterior wall of the carotid bifurcations,[16] a selective study with a true lateral projection is preferable. The second most common surgically accessible atherosclerotic lesions are the extraspinal portions of the vertebral arteries (18 per cent are on the right side, 22 per cent on the left).[9]

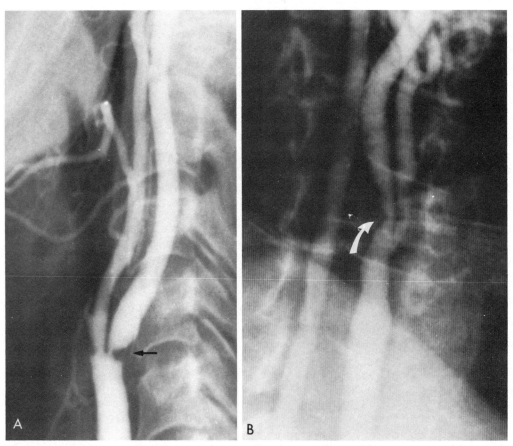

Figure 22–81. *A,* Eccentric plaques of internal and external carotid artery encroaching upon the carotid bifurcation posteriorly (arrow). *B,* Left posterior oblique projection shows a more extensive lesion (arrow) involving a longer segment.

Legend continued on the opposite page

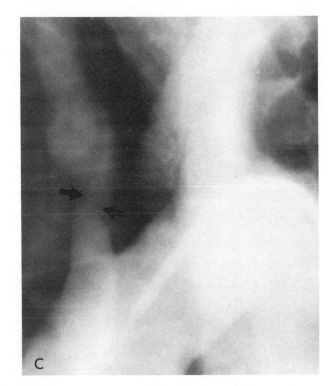

Figure 22–81 *Continued.* Concentric circumferential stenosis (arrows) in the proximal right innominate artery.

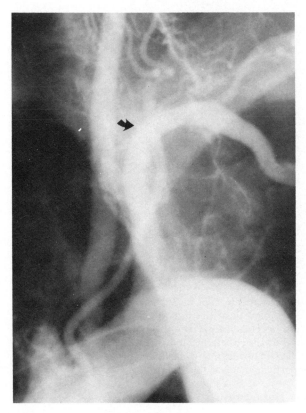

Figure 22–82. Complete occlusion of the right innominate artery 1 cm distal to its origin. The diffusely diseased left subclavian artery and occlusion of the left vertebral artery at its origin (arrow) are seen.

When transient ischemic attacks occur, visualization of the intracranial circulation may reveal mass lesions stimulating cerebral ischemia[11] and emboli secondary to ulcerated plaques. Today computerized tomography offers a more precise and noninvasive way to diagnose cerebral mass lesions and infarction.

The preferred technique for four-vessel angiography is catheterization of the femoral or the axillary arteries. Direct carotid angiography may be more dangerous, particulary if a high puncture is made. Even minor local trauma to the cervical carotid bifurcation can precipitate embolism from atheromatous plaques.[8, 10, 15]

The arteriosclerotic lesions in the brachiocephalic vessels are similar to the lesions in the ileofemoral system. Usually the plaques are eccentric (Figs. 22–81A and B; see Fig. 22–84), but they may also be concentric and circumferential (Fig. 22–81C).

It is important to realize that only severe stenoses are hemodynamically significant. According to Brice et al., a significant pressure gradient across a carotid artery stenosis occurs only in a cross-sectional area smaller than 5 square mm, with a corresponding

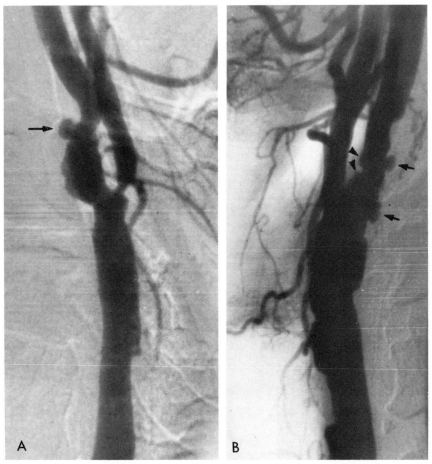

A   B

Figure 22–83. Arteriosclerotic ulcers. *A,* Excellent demonstration of an ulcerating atheroma (arrow) located typically on the posterior wall of the proximal internal carotid artery. The ulcer base is smooth, with a typical neck. The ulcer seems to protrude beyond the confines of the artery but is actually located in a large plaque of the bulbous portion of the artery. *B,* Several ulcers (arrows) along the posterior wall of the right internal carotid artery. The lesions on the anterior wall (arrowheads) may be either small ulcers or several small plaques in close proximity. Note also the disease in both common carotid arteries.

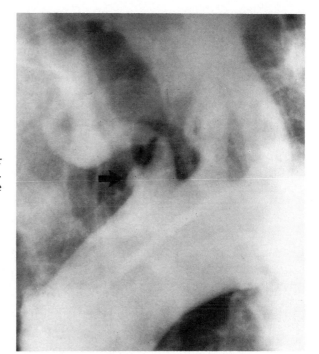

Figure 22–84. Classic arteriosclerotic ulcer niche in the right innominate artery (arrow). Subtotal occlusion distal to the ulcer by a large eccentric atheroma is seen.

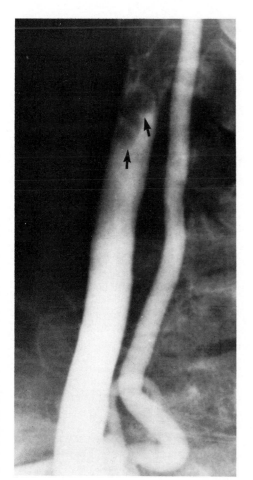

Figure 22–85. Typical thrombus characterized by a smooth, round filling defect (arrows) protruding into the common carotid artery and causing occlusion of the internal and external carotid arteries.

diameter of the stenotic segment of 2 mm or less. Whether such severe stenoses cause clinical symptoms depends greatly on the size of the communicating arteries of the circle of Willis and the status of the remaining brachiocephalic vessels.

Complete obstruction of the neck vessels occurs not only at the bifurcation but also at their origin (Fig. 22–82). Such an occlusion of carotid bifurcation has no clinical sequelae in 15 per cent of the patients.[1] Owing to the frequent involvement of the proximal left subclavian artery (12 per cent of cases)[9] a subclavian steal syndrome is common in patients with arteriosclerotic occlusive disease.

Softened atherosclerotic material may embolize, leaving an area of ulceration that can be readily recognized by angiography. The ulcer cavity resembles an ulcer niche in the barium-filled stomach, but it does not protrude beyond the confines of the vessel (Fig. 22–83). The base of the ulcer is usually smooth; if it is irregular a diagnosis of

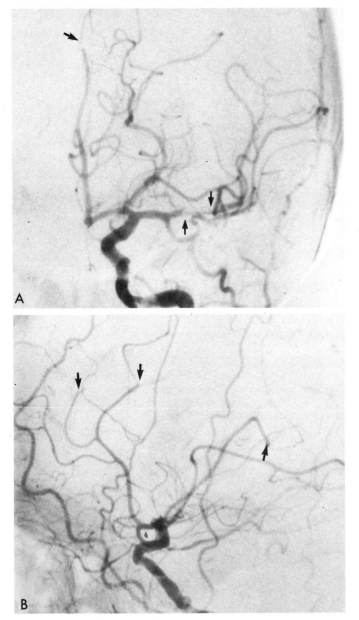

Figure 22–86. Anteroposterior (A) and lateral (B) projections of a left carotid angiogram. Numerous filling defects (arrows) in several branches indicate showers of emboli. Note the typical convex borders, usually not seen in atherosclerotic lesions.

incomplete evacuation or superimposed thrombus may be postulated. Numerous small ulcers are difficult to differentiate from a series of atherosclerotic plaques.[16] Ulcerations occur most commonly at the carotid bifurcation and are rarely seen in the proximal neck vessels (Fig. 22–84).

Superimposed thrombi secondary to carotid artery atherosclerosis are another source of emboli. They occur in approximately 10 per cent of patients with severe carotid artery stenosis.[14] Thrombi appear as smooth, round, intraluminal filling defects (Fig. 22–85).

If angiography is performed immediately after an embolic episode, the emboli can commonly be demonstrated intracerebrally.[12] The round or longitudinal intraluminal filling defects with convex borders are characteristic of emboli (Fig. 22–86).

References

1. Altemus, L. R.: Angiographic demonstration of critical arteriosclerotic lesions of the carotid bifurcation. J. Maine Assoc. 66:314–318, 1975.
2. Brice, J. G., Dowsett, D. J., and Lowe, R. D.: The effect of constriction of carotid blood flow and pressure gradient. Lancet 1:84–85, 1964.
3. Chiari, H.: Ueber das Verhalten des Teilungswinkels der Carotis communis bei der Endarteritis chronica deformans. Verhandl. Deutsch. Pathol. Ges. 9:326–330, 1905.
4. Fields, W. S., Maslenikov, V., Meyer, J. S., et al.: Joint study of extracranial arterial occlusion. V. J.A.M.A. 211:1993–2003, 1970.
5. Fields, W. S.: Aortocranial occlusive vascular disease (stroke). Clin. Symp. 26:4, 1976.
6. Fisher, C. M.: Occlusion of the internal carotid artery. Arch. Neurol. Psychiatr. 65:346–377, 1951.
7. Fisher, C. M.: Occlusion of the carotid arteries: further experiences. Arch. Neurol. Psychiatr. 72:187–206, 1954.
8. Gore, I., and Collins, D. P.: Spontaneous atheromatous embolization. Am. J. Clin. Pathol. 33:416–426, 1960.
9. Hass, W. K., Fields, W. J., North, R. R., et al.: Joint study of extracranial arterial occlusion. II. J.A.M.A. 203:961–968, 1968.
10. Hollenhorst, R. W.: Significance of bright plaques in the retinal arterioles. J.A.M.A. 178:23–29, 1961.
11. Houser, O. W., Sundt, T. M., Jr., Holman, C. B., et al.: Atheromatous disease of the carotid artery: correlation of angiographic, clinical, and surgical findings. J. Neurosurg. 41:321–331, 1974.
12. Kishore, P. R. S., Chase, N. D., and Kricheff, I. I.: Carotid stenosis and intracranial emboli. Radiology 100:351–356, 1971.
13. Maddison, F. E., and Moore, W. S.: Ulcerated atheroma of the carotid artery: arteriographic appearance. Am. J. Roentgenol. 107:530–534, 1969.
14. Roberson, G. H., Scott, W. R., and Rosenbaum, A. E.: Thrombi at the site of carotid stenosis. Radiology 109:353–356, 1973.
15. Witmer, R., and Schmid, A.: Cholesterinkristall als retinaler arterieller Embolus. Ophthalmologica 135:432–433, 1958.
16. Wood, E. H., and Correll, J. W.: Atheromatous ulceration in major neck vessels as a cause of cerebral embolism. Acta Radiol. 9:520–536, 1969.

Part IX
Subclavian Steal Syndrome

GUSTAVE FORMANEK, M.D.

KURT AMPLATZ, M.D.

The reversal of the blood flow in the vertebral artery secondary to subclavian artery occlusion was first described by Contorni in 1960.[2] The hemodynamic explanation of the syndrome was given by Reivich et al.[8] At the same time, the appropriate term "subclavian steal syndrome" was used in an editorial.[7]

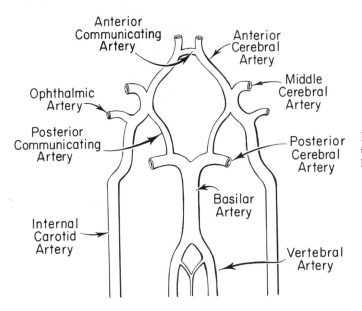

Figure 22–87. Schematic drawing of the circle of Willis with the vertebral basilar system.

Normally the blood flow occurs toward the brain in all four vessels, which communicate with each other by the circle of Willis and basilar artery (Fig. 22–87). Under normal hemodynamic conditions there is no significant flow through the circle from one artery to the other, since no pressure gradient exists. It was shown by Reivich that a small pressure imbalance in the circle may cause flow toward the low-pressure system.[8] Thus, decreased pressure in either subclavian artery causes a compensatory

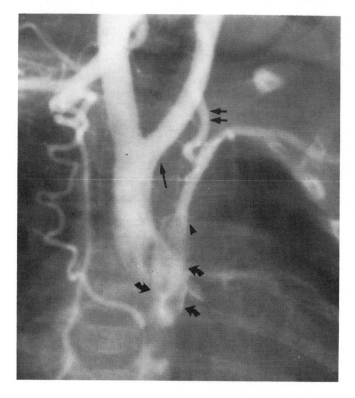

Figure 22–88. Right brachial retrograde aortogram of a seven-week-old infant. The aortic arch is interrupted just distal to the left common carotid artery (arrow). The left subclavian artery (arrowhead) originates from the proximal descending aorta (low-pressure system) and is opacified from the left vertebral artery (double arrow), indicating a steal. Even the descending aorta (small arrows) is relatively well opacified via the vertebral-subclavian arterial collateral.

flow reversal in the corresponding vertebral artery. The reversal of blood flow in the vertebral artery is thought to "steal blood" from the cerebral circulation, causing signs of cerebrovascular insufficiency. The clinical symptoms of these patients are usually aggravated by vasodilatation secondary to upper extremity activity, a fact that confirms this hemodynamic hypothesis.

The two most common pathologic entities causing this syndrome are arteriosclerotic occlusive disease and Takayasu's arteritis, which commonly affect the subclavian arteries.[4-6] The congenital causes of subclavian steal syndrome are isthmic coarctation; interruption of the aortic arch, with the left subclavian artery originating distal to the obstruction or interruption;[7, 9] and supravalvular aortic stenosis that involves the origin of the subclavian arteries.

A definite diagnosis of subclavian steal syndrome can be made by angiography. Not only is the exact anatomic basis for the altered circulation demonstrated but also the abnormal hemodynamics.

In many cases, the diagnosis can be made by simple arch aortography (Fig. 22–88). Selective injections of the contralateral vertebral artery yield better results, however. It is important to keep in mind that a direct injection of contrast medium into the

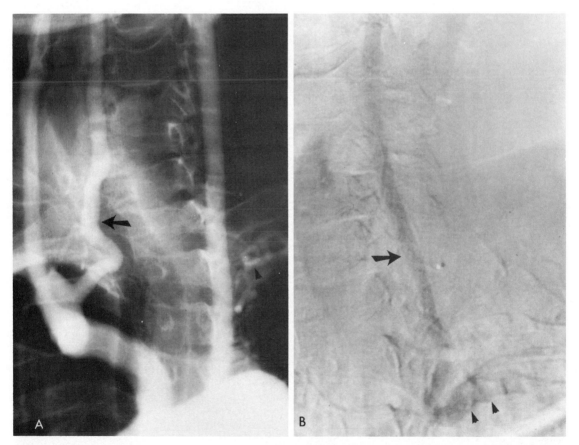

Figure 22–89. The late and reversed filling of the left vertebral artery (*B*, arrow) in an arch aortogram is characteristic of a subclavian steal syndrome. Also, the subclavian artery (arrowheads) is faintly visualized. Note the enlarged right vertebral artery (*A*, arrow) secondary to increased blood flow. The tortuous, dilated first intercostal artery (*A*, arrowhead) serves as a collateral vessel between the aorta and occluded left subclavian artery. For the diagnosis of subclavian steal syndrome, selective arteriographic studies demonstrate the delayed opacification of the vessels better than thoracic aortograms.

vertebral artery may cause flow reversal in the contralateral vertebral artery without subclavian stenosis. In the absence of a subclavian artery obstruction, this angiographic artifact ceases at the end of the injection, and the contrast material clears in a normal cephalad direction.

Reversal of vertebral artery flow without subclavian artery stenosis may even occur with injection into the subclavian artery because of a side hole close to the opposite vertebral artery ostium.[10] Therefore, a definite angiographic diagnosis of the subclavian steal syndrome can be made only if the reversal of blood flow in the vertebral artery and a significant stenosis of the subclavian artery are demonstrated.

The arch aortogram (made either via the axillary artery or via the femoral artery) is best performed in left anterior oblique projections, which demonstrate the origin of the brachiocephalic vessels. Delayed imaging (five to seven seconds) is mandatory. In normal patients, the three large brachiocephalic vessels opacify almost simultaneously. In a subclavian steal syndrome the vertebral artery with reversed blood flow opacifies and clears later than the other brachiocephalic vessels (Fig. 22–89). This flow phenomenon is much better shown on selective contralateral vertebral arteriograms, which may also demonstrate the distal stump of an occluded subclavian artery (Fig. 22–90).

In a rare form of subclavian steal syndrome, shown Fig. 22–91, the collateral blood flow toward the occluded subclavian artery occurs via enlarged muscular branches

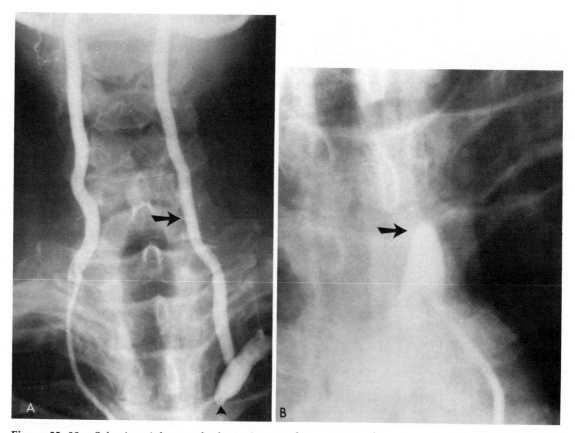

Figure 22–90. Selective right vertebral arteriogram demonstrates the retrograde filling (fifth frame of the angiographic series) of the opposite vertebral artery and left subclavian artery (arrow). *A,* The distal stump of the occluded subclavian artery is well seen (arrowhead). *B,* The proximal stump of the occluded left subclavian artery is visualized by selective injection (arrow).

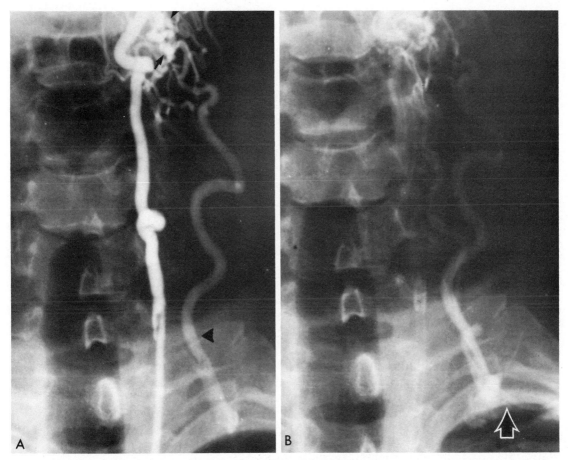

Figure 22–91.   *A,* Left vertebral arteriogram shows the vertebral artery arising directly from the aortic arch. A rich network of collaterals connects the muscular branches of the vertebral artery (arrows) with the large, tortuous ascending cervical artery (arrowhead), filling in a retrograde fashion. *B,* The next frame of the angiogram shows good filling of the left subclavian artery (arrow) via the large ascending cervical branch. This variant of the subclavian steal syndrome can occur only in patients with origination of the left vertebral artery from the aorta and occlusion of the ipsilateral subclavian artery proximal to the thyrocervical trunk.

rather than the vertebral artery itself because it arises directly from the aortic arch (a relatively common variant). In this case, the blood flow through the vertebral artery is not reversed, but a steal phenomenon nevertheless occurs because of loss of blood through vertebral collaterals. A similar collateral pattern was described in a patient with congenital isthmic coarctation of the aorta and congenital aplasia of both proximal subclavian arteries.[1]

References

1. Bosniak, M. A.: Cervical arterial pathways associated with brachiocephalic occlusive disease. Am. J. Roentgenol. *91*:1232–1244, 1964.
2. Contorni, L.: Il circolo collaterale vertebrovertebrale nella obliterazione dell' arteria succlavia alla sue origine. Minerva Chir. *15*:268, 1960.
3. Hachiya, J.: Current concepts of Takayasu's arteritis. Semin. Roentgenol. *5*:245–259, 1970.
4. Hass, W. K. Fields, W. S., North, R. R., et al.: Joint study of extracranial arterial occlusion. II. J.A.M.A. *203*:961–968, 1968.

5. Killen, D. A., Foster, J. H., Gobbel, W. G., Jr., et. al.: The subclavian steal syndrome. J. Thorac. Cardiovasc. Surg. 51:539–560, 1966.
6. Midgley, F. M., and McCleuathan, J. E.: Subclavian steal syndrome in the pediatric age group. Ann. Thorac. Surg. 74:252–257, 1977.
7. A new vascular syndrome: "the subclavian steal." Editorial. N. Engl. J. Med. 265:912–913, 1961.
8. Reivich, M., Holling, H. E., Roberts, B., et al.: Reversal of blood flow through the vertebral artery and its effect on cerebral circulation. N. Engl. J. Med. 265:878–885, 1961.
9. Shaher, R. M., Patterston, P., Stranahan, A., et al.: Congenital pulmonary and subclavian arteries steal syndrome. Am. Heart J. 84:103–109, 1972.
10. Shockman, A. T.: Retrograde vertebral artery flow as in artifact of technique. Am. J. Roentgenol. 91:1258–1262, 1964.

Part X

Takayasu's Arteritis

GUSTAVE FORMANEK, M.D.
KURT AMPLATZ, M.D.

Until recently, Takayasu's arteritis[1, 10, 19] was a confusing entity indicated by numerous synonyms: aortoarteritis,[24] pulseless disease,[27] young female arteritis,[26] aortitis syndrome,[28] thromboangiitis obliterans subclavia-carotica,[20] atypical coarctation,[12] and elongate coarctation.[18] In 1908 Takayasu described unique anastomosis of arterioles and venules in the eyes of a young female.[11] At the same time, two other Japanese investigators described decreased peripheral pulses in patients who had similar eye manifestations.[11] Because the original descriptions came from Japan, it was commonly believed that the disease was prevalent among Orientals. Numerous reports from all over the world, however, demonstrated that the disease is distributed worldwide.[1, 3, 16, 21, 22] In a recent cooperative study of the International Arteriosclerotic Project, it was estimated that the incidence of Takayasu's arteritis is approximately 0.11 per cent in the United States.[25] The study also pointed out that the disease may often occur without clinical symptoms. The manifestation of clinical symptoms in cases of Takayasu's arteritis is more common in females in the second and third decades of life.[19]

The pathologic process of Takayasu's arteritis is characterized by chronic arteritis involving the entire arterial wall, which is thickened and hardened.[8, 20] The arteries tend to be affected segmentally. The underlying process is a granulomatous or diffuse productive arteritis complicated by early secondary arteriosclerosis.[20] The disease may involve the entire aorta and may extend into any of its branches, leading to stenoses or complete occlusions. Involvement of the main pulmonary artery and its large branches has been reported.[10, 13]

The cause of Takayasu's arteritis is not known, but one recent theory suggests an autoimmune mechanism.[6, 19, 29]

CLINICAL MANIFESTATIONS

Takayasu's arteritis manifests itself in two stages.[10, 14, 19] At the onset, there may be fever, myalgia, arthralgia, nausea, night sweats, weight loss, chest and abdominal pain, and skin rash. All these symptoms are nonspecific, and therefore the correct diagnosis may be overlooked. The second stage, which may follow many months later,[10, 28] is characterized by arterial stenoses or occlusions. Depending on the vascular bed involved, there may be ocular or cerebral manifestations, upper- and lower-extremity ischemia, renovascular hypertension, hypertension identical to coarctation, angina pectoris, or myocardial infarction due to coronary ostial stenosis. Involvement of the visceral arteries is usually asymptomatic because of excellent collaterals.

RADIOLOGIC FINDINGS

Sometimes Takayasu's arteritis can be suggested on chest roentgenograms, but angiography is required for a definitive diagnosis. Rib notching involving the lower ribs (ninth and lower) is typical of long-standing stenosis or occlusion of the low thoracic or upper abdominal aorta (Fig. 22–92, see Fig. 22–101). Caliber changes in the aortic arch or the descending aorta (Fig. 22–93) or segmental calcifications in a woman of middle age[15] may suggest the diagnosis of Takayasu's arteritis. Sparseness of pulmonary vasculature suggests involvement of the pulmonary arterial tree (see Fig. 22–93).

Angiography

Aortography may be more specific than laboratory tests. Opacification of the arterial tree via catheter is superior to translumbar aortography, which may be difficult or impossible owing to the frequent involvement of the abdominal aorta. The angiographic features of Takayasu's arteritis are (1) aortic and arterial stenoses or occlusions; (2) less commonly, diffuse dilatations or fusiform aneurysms; (3) a combination of the first two features; and (4) segmental involvement.[4, 12, 14, 15]

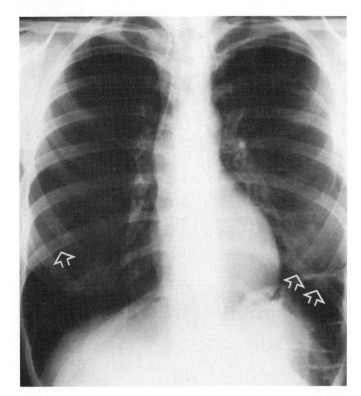

Figure 22–92. Typical rib notching of the lower ribs (arrows). The patient was explored for isthmic coarctation, which was not found; the fifth left rib was removed. The posterior left ninth rib is missing owing to surgery for abdominal coarctation. The rib notching (collateral flow through enlarged intercostal arteries) of the lower ribs is typical of abdominal coarctation in Takayasu's arteritis.

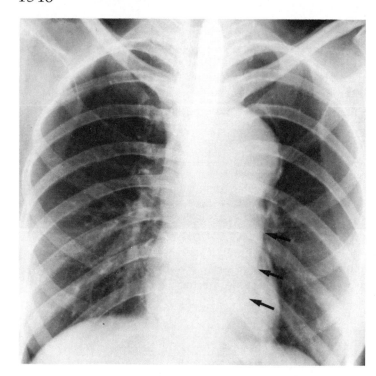

Figure 22–93. Markedly dilated aortic knob in a 22-year-old Vietnamese female. The descending aorta shows a wavy, irregular contour (arrows). The decreased pulmonary vasculature in the left lower lobe suggests pulmonary involvement.

Figure 22–94. Lateral abdominal aortogram in an 18-year-old female with hypertension and an abdominal bruit. Sudden narrowing of the aorta at the L_1 level and complete occlusion below the renal arteries are apparent. There is severe stenosis at the origin of the superior mesenteric artery (arrow). The lower intercostal arteries (arrowhead) are markedly dilated and tortuous. The first lumbar artery originating from the stenotic segment of the aorta is not a collateral and is therefore of normal size (small arrow).

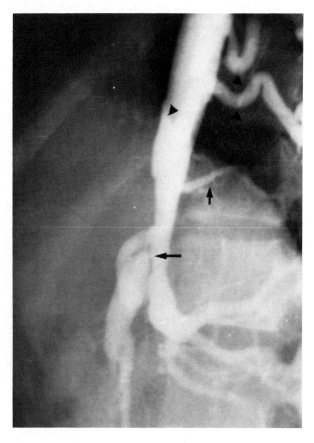

The transition from arterial disease to arterial normal tends to be abrupt. Classically, the involved segments are either stenotic or dilated, and they appear smooth unless there is superimposed atherosclerosis. Stenotic areas in the aorta are commonly located in the vicinity of the diaphragm, but they may occur anywhere distal to the left subclavian artery. Stenotic lesions do not occur in the ascending aorta.[4] Involvement of the abdominal aorta is usually diffuse, wtih concomitant branch stenoses (Figs. 22–94 and 22–95). The formation of aneurysms is due to the destruction of the arterial wall and its replacement by deficient fibrotic tissue. The cause of these aneurysms can be suggested by the patient's age and sex and by the demonstration of a thick arterial wall, skip areas, and stenoses of other arteries (Fig. 22–96).

Arterial branch stenoses commonly involve the subclavian arteries. Both the distal (Fig. 22–97) and the proximal subclavian arteries (Fig. 22–98) may be affected.

Takayasu's arteritis usually involves the proximal carotid arteries (see Fig. 22–96B). In the case of occlusion, the stump may show a peculiar "flame" shape (see Fig. 22–98), which is characteristic of Takayasu's arteritis.[4, 15] Sometimes the brachiocephalic vessels are involved without angiographic evidence of aortic disease.[6, 19] In these cases, the typical location of the lesion and a careful history may confirm the diagnosis of Takayasu's arteritis (see Fig. 22–97).

Significant stenosis or occlusion of the renal arteries is a common feature in abdominal forms of Takayasu's arteritis. The extent of the arterial involvement may vary, from localized ostial to long, tubular narrowing or complete occlusion (see Fig. 22–95, Fig. 22–99). A typical finding in cases of Takayasu's arteritis is the development

Text continued on page 1551

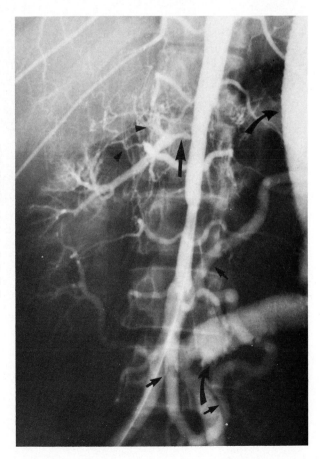

Figure 22–95.   Long, tubular narrowing of the abdominal aorta (from L_1 to L_4). The opaque contour is slightly wavy but smooth. The left kidney has been removed. The upper proximal right segmental renal artery is severely stenosed (large straight arrow). There is a rich network of retroperitoneal collaterals (arrowheads) to the right kidney. The inferior mesenteric artery is enlarged (small arrows) because it serves as a collateral for the occluded superior mesenteric artery and celiac axis. There is a large Dacron graft bypassing the stenotic segment of the aorta (curved arrows).

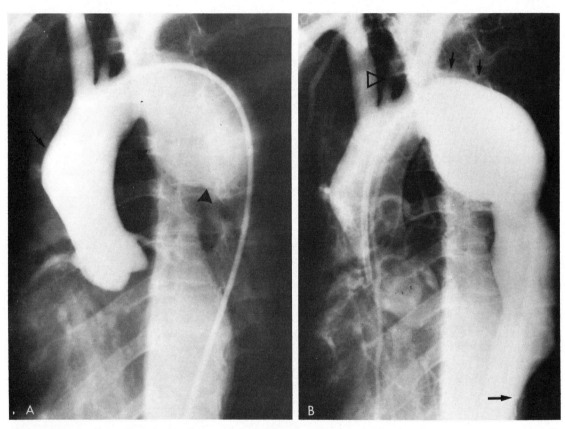

Figure 22–96.   Same patient as in Figure 22–93. *A,* Left anterior oblique aortogram shows a normal proximal ascending aorta. Mild dilatation of the distal ascending aorta (arrow) and frank aneurysm of the distal aortic arch (arrowhead) are evident. *B,* Abnormal dilatation extends almost to the level of the diaphragm, where there is an abrupt transition (arrow) to the normal aortic size. Tapering stenosis of the left common carotid artery helps support the diagnosis of Takayasu's arteritis (arrowhead). Note also a thick aortic wall (small arrows).

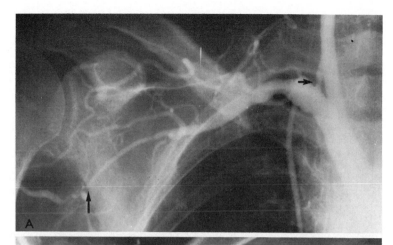

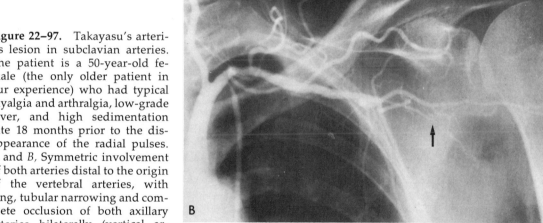

Figure 22–97. Takayasu's arteritis lesion in subclavian arteries. The patient is a 50-year-old female (the only older patient in our experience) who had typical myalgia and arthralgia, low-grade fever, and high sedimentation rate 18 months prior to the disappearance of the radial pulses. *A* and *B*, Symmetric involvement of both arteries distal to the origin of the vertebral arteries, with long, tubular narrowing and complete occlusion of both axillary arteries bilaterally (vertical arrows) at exactly the same location. There is a mild stenosis at the origin of the right vertebral artery (horizontal small arrow). *C,* Aortogram shows only minimal irregularities of the descending aorta.

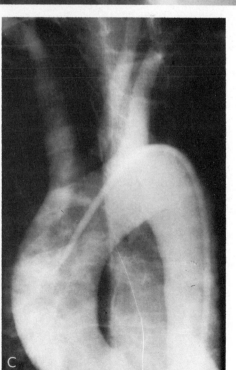

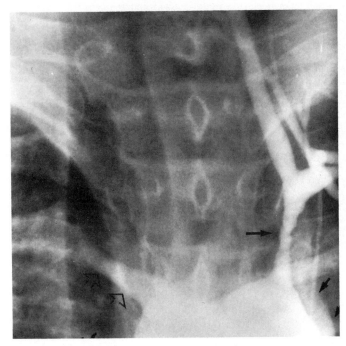

Figure 22–98. Diffuse narrowing of the left subclavian artery (arrows) proximal to large vertebral artery, which is the only patent artery supplying the brain. A typical flame-shaped occlusion of the innominate artery (open arrow) is seen. The wall of the distal aortic arch (small arrows) is significantly thickened. The patient is a 35-year-old male with a visual disturbance.

Figure 22–99. Excellent demonstration of extensive collaterals (arrowheads) to two segmental renal arteries (arrows) occluded in a case of Takayasu's arteritis.

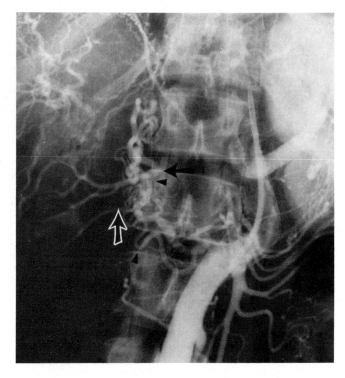

of unusually abundant collateral circulation.[14] This fact explains the absence of symptoms in many patients with complete occlusions of large arteries (see Figs. 22–95 and 22–99).

Takayasu's arteritis must be differentiated from atherosclerosis and syphilis. Arteriosclerosis is rare in young females, affecting most commonly the abdominal aorta below the renal arteries. Takayasu's arteritis typically involves the thoracic and upper abdominal aorta. The aortic wall in Takayasu's arteritis is much thicker than it is in arteriosclerosis, which shows pronounced intimal irregularities. The most common atherosclerotic lesions are at the carotid bifurcations, at the distal abdominal aorta, and in the iliofemoral-popliteal system. The pelvic and lower-extremity arteries are not affected by Takayasu's arteritis. Today syphilitic aortitis is rare. It involves predominantly the thoracic aorta (89 per cent of cases), particularly the ascending portion.[7] It is most common in men older than 40. Syphilitic aneurysms may be saccular or fusiform and are invariably associated with extensive secondary atherosclerosis. Aortic regurgitation is common.[2] Extensive intimal calcifications are usually caused by syphilis. If intimal calcifications involve the ascending aorta and aortic sinuses, the diagnosis of syphilitic aortitis is strongly suggested.[17] Giant cell arteritis occurs predominantly in patients older than 60 years of age,[20] and it is only rarely associated with aortic arch syndrome.[5, 23] The commonly associated temporal arteritis and the

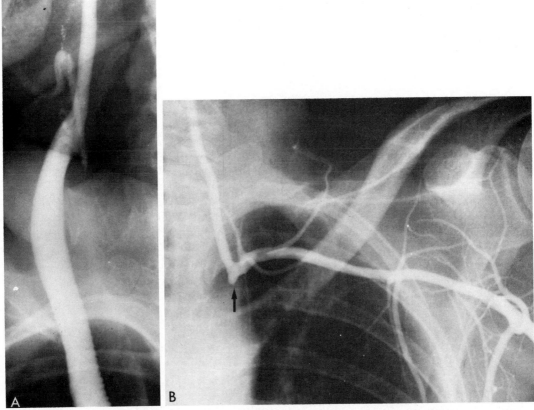

Figure 22–100. Same patient as in Figure 22–98. *A,* Well-functioning Dacron graft from ascending aorta to the right internal carotid artery is seen. *B,* Owing to improved intracranial blood pressure after grafting the stenosed left subclavian artery became occluded (arrow). (The previously patent artery is shown in Figure 22–98.)

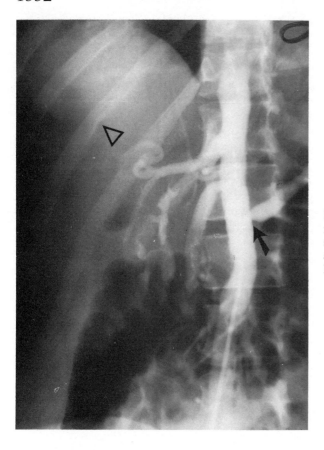

Figure 22–101. The left renal artery after the re-anastomosis to the abdominal Dacron graft shows the stenosis at its origin (arrow). Note also the notching of the tenth right rib (arrowhead).

involvement of the smaller arterial branches[4] help differentiate this entity from other types of arteritis.[9]

Therapy is indicated in both phases of Takayasu's arteritis. Corticosteroids markedly alleviate the symptoms of the first stage, normalize the erythrocyte sedimentation rate, and decrease the level of serum C-reactive protein and globulins.[8, 29] In some cases, there is improvement of the diminished peripheral pulses.[10, 19, 28]

Surgical bypass should be reserved for the obstructive stage (Fig. 22–100). On occasion, an originally diseased but currently patent artery may become completely occluded after bypass surgery because of a lack of flow (Fig. 22–100B).

Frequent stenosis of the renal arteries, causing hypertension, is best treated by a bypass graft, autotransplantation, or attachment of the renal arteries to the abdominal bypass graft. Occasionally the renovascular hypertension may persist if the stenotic origin of the renal artery is not surgically excised (Fig. 22–101).

References

1. Ask-Upmark, E., and Fajers, C. M.: Further observations on Takayasu's syndrome. Acta Med. Scand. *155*:275–291, 1956.
2. Dinsmore, R. E., and Yang, G. C.: Roentgen diagnosis of aortic disease. Prog. Cardiovasc. Dis. *16*:151–185, 1973.
3. Edling, N. P., Nystrom, B., and Seldinger, S. I.: Branchial arteritis in the aortic arch syndrome. Acta Radiol. *55*:417–432, 1961.
4. Hachiya, J.: Current concepts of Takayasu's arteritis. Semin. Roentgenol. *5*:245–259, 1970.

5. Hamrin, B., Jonsson, N., and Landberg, T.: Involvement of large vessels in polymyalgia arteritica. Lancet 1:1193–1196, 1965.
6. Harrell, J. E., and Manion, W. C.: Sclerosing aortitis and arteritis. Semin. Roentgenol. 5:261–266, 1970.
7. Heberer, G., Rau, G., and Löhr, H. H.: Aorta and Grosse Arterien. Berlin, Springer-Verlag, 1966.
8. Hirsch, M. S., Aikat, B. K., and Basu, A. K.: Takayasu's arteritis. Report of five cases with immunologic studies. Bull. Johns Hopkins Hosp. 115:29–64, 1964.
9. Hunder, G. G., Ward, L. E., and Burbank, M. K.: Giant cell arteritis producing an aortic arch syndrome. Ann. Intern. Med. 66:578–582, 1967.
10. Ishikawa, K.: Natural history and classification of occlusive thromboaortopathy (Takayasu's disease). Circulation 57:27–35, 1978.
11. Judge, R. D., Currier, R. D., Gracie, W. A., et al.: Takayasu's arteritis and the aortic arch syndrome. Am. J. Med. 32:379–392, 1962.
12. Kozuka, T., Nosaki, T., Sato, K., et al.: Roentgenologic diagnosis of atypical coarctation of the aorta. Acta Radiol. 4:497–507, 1966.
13. Kozuka, T., Nosaki, T., Sato, K., et al.: Aortitis syndrome with special reference to pulmonary vascular changes. Acta Radiol. 7:25–32, 1968.
14. Lande, A., and Gross, A.: Total aortography in the diagnosis of Takayasu's arteritis. Am. J. Roentgenol. 116:165–178, 1972.
15. Lande, A., and Rossi, P.: The value of total aortography in the diagnosis of Takayasu's arteritis. Radiology 114:287–297, 1975.
16. McKusick, V. A.: A form of vascular disease relatively frequent in the Orient. Am. Heart J. 63:57–64, 1962.
17. Merten, C. W., Finby, N., and Steinberg, I.: The antemortem diagnosis of syphilitic aneurysm of the aortic sinuses. Report of nine cases. Am. J. Med. 20:345–360, 1956.
18. Milloy, F., and Fell, E. H.: Elongate coarctation of the aorta. Arch. Surg. 78:759–765, 1959.
19. Nakao, K., Ikeda, M., Kimata, S. I., et al.: Takayasu's arteritis. Clinical report of eighty-four cases and immunological studies of seven cases. Circulation 35:1141–1155, 1967.
20. Nasu, T.: Pathology of pulseless disease. A systematic study and critical review of twenty-one autopsy cases reported in Japan. Angiology 4:225–242, 1963.
21. Paloheimo, J. A.: Obstructive arteritis of Takayasu's type. Clinical, roentgenological and laboratory studies on 36 patients. Acta Med. Scand. (Suppl.) 468:1–45, 1967.
22. Penn, I.: Abdominal aortic aneurysm in the African patient. Br. J. Surg. 50:598–605, 1963.
23. Pollock, M., Blennerhassett, Y. B., and Clarke, A. M.: Giant cell arteritis and the subclavian steal syndrome. Neurology 23:653–675, 1973.
24. Roentgenologic study of aorto-arteritis. II. Chest x-ray findings and their clinical significance. Fu Wai Hospital, Chinese Academy of Medical Sciences. Chinese Med. J. 1:275–282, 1975. (Cited in Radiology 118:243, 1976.)
25. Restrepo, C., Tejeda, C., and Correa, P.: Nonsyphilitic aortitis. Arch. Pathol. 87:1–12, 1969.
26. Ross, R. S., and McKusick, V. A.: Aortic arch syndromes. Diminished or absent pulses in arteries arising from arch of aorta. Arch. Intern. Med. 92:701–740, 1953.
27. Shimizu, K., and Sano, K.: Pulseless disease. J. Neuropathol. Clin. Neurol. 1:37–47, 1951.
28. Ueda, H., Morooka, S., Ito, I., et al.: Clinical observation of 52 cases of aortitis syndrome. Jap. Heart J. 10:277–288, 1969.
29. Ueda, H., Saito, Y., Ito, I., et al.: Immunological studies of aortitis syndrome. Jap. Heart J. 8:4–18, 1967.

Part XI
Buerger's Disease

WILFRIDO R. CASTANEDA-ZUNIGA, M.D.
KURT AMPLATZ, M.D.

Buerger's disease, or thromboangiitis obliterans, is an occlusive peripheral vascular disease that affects the peripheral arteries and veins in a segmental fashion. It occurs almost exclusively in young men between the ages of 20 and 40 years. It may affect the arms, although the lower extremities are most commonly involved. It is characterized by an insidious or fulminant onset.

The clinical course is characterized by remissions and relapses that may be related to tobacco smoking, although a definite etiologic correlation has not been established. The symptoms include superficial migratory thrombophlebitis in 40 per cent of the cases, sometimes preceding the onset of the arterial disease; hyperhydrosis of the involved extremities; intermittent claudication; and coldness of the extremities, usually accompanied by other vasospastic symptoms such as blanching and numbness of the digits, cyanosis, delayed venous filling time, and gangrene. There is usually severe pain, and there may be reduced or absent pulsations in major arteries.

The arteriographic findings are characteristic but may also be found in other peripheral vascular disorders.[1] They include

1. No evidence of atherosclerotic lesions in arteries that are typically affected by atherosclerosis.

2. Occlusion of the ulnar or radial artery or both at or above the level of the wrist (Fig. 22–102).

3. Persistence of the interosseous arteries, giving terminal collaterals to the radial or ulnar arteries (Fig. 22–102).

4. Attenuation of interruption of one or both palmar arches (Fig. 22–102).

5. Multiple areas of obstruction of metacarpal and digital arteries (Fig. 22–103).

6. "Pruning" of digital arteries (see Fig. 22–103).

7. Bilateral symmetric involvement, which tends to be segmental rather than diffuse.

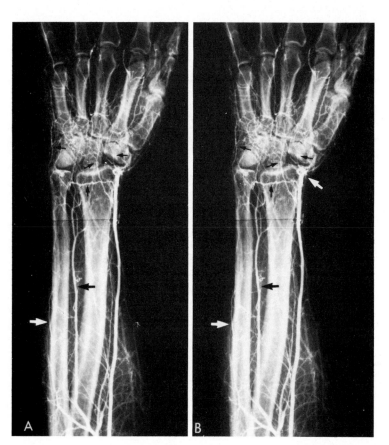

Figure 22–102. *A* and *B,* Brachial angiogram shows a hypoplastic ulnar artery (white arrow), persistence of the interosseous artery (large black arrow), and occlusion of the distal radial artery at the level of the wrist (white arrow), with extensive but small collaterals (small black arrows). There is no reconstruction of the palmar arches. The arterial branches of the palm and fingers are severely narrowed.

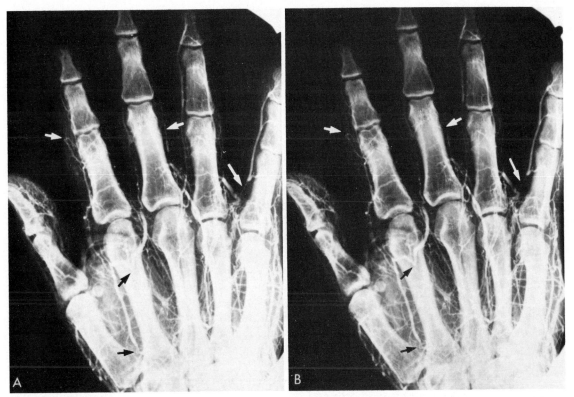

Figure 22–103. *A* and *B,* Absence of both palmar arches, multiple areas of arterial narrowing (large white arrow), obstructions (black arrows), and pruning of digital arteries (small white arrows).

In the lower extremities these changes tend to be less pronounced than similar changes found in the upper extremity. The peroneal artery is less frequently involved than the anterior and posterior tibial arteries.

The histopathologic changes are characteristic of an inflammatory panarteritis, primarily affecting the subintimal layer; no significant changes occur in the arterial wall and subintimal microabscesses.[2]

References

1. McKlusick, F. A., Harris, W. S., Otteson, O. E., et al.: Buerger's disease: a distinct clinical and pathologic entity. J.A.M.A. *181*:93–100, 1972.
2. Walton, J.: Joint discussion no. 5. Section of surgery with section of medicine. Discussion of peripheral vascular lesions. Proc. R. Soc. Med. *37*:621–634, 1944.

Part XII

Raynaud's Syndrome

WILFRIDO R. CASTANEDA-ZUNIGA, M.D.
KURT AMPLATZ, M.D.

This is a vasospastic disorder of unknown origin that is five times more common in women and occurs predominantly between the ages of 15 and 40. The onset is usually gradual, with painful spastic attacks lasting from several minutes to a few hours. Color changes of the digits are typical and include pallor, cyanosis, and rubor. These changes are probably an exaggerated response to various vasospastic stimuli, such as cold or emotional stress. They usually begin in one or two digits, with symmetric involvement of both hands. Unilateral involvement may occur early in the disease. Other affected areas are the toes (50 per cent of cases), the nose, the cheeks, the chin, and the ears. Peripheral pulses are usually normal or slightly diminished. Arterial insufficiency is uncommon, but infrequently these changes may progress and result in symmetric gangrene of the digits. A sense of tingling, burning, or paresthesia may follow the attack. Unlike other vascular disorders causing systemic symptoms, Raynaud's disease is limited to the extremities. Similar vasospastic manifestations (Raynaud's phenomenon) may be secondary to systemic disease, such as scleroderma, lupus erythematosus, and rheumatoid arthritis.

Radiographically, in milder cases, no changes are seen. In severer or prolonged cases, soft tissue atrophy of the tips of the fingers becomes apparent. There may be bone absorption of the tufts of the terminal phalanges, producing tapering and shortening of these phalanges. Discrete calcium deposits may appear in the fingertips, most often when Raynaud's phenomenon is associated with scleroderma (Fig. 22–103A).

The angiographic findings in the hand are indistinguishable from those of Buerger's disease, but classically the radial and ulnar arteries are not involved. In the purely vasospastic form of the syndrome, the vessels may appear normal, but severe

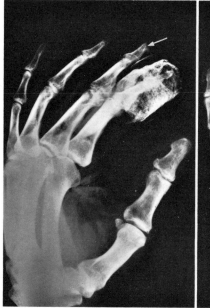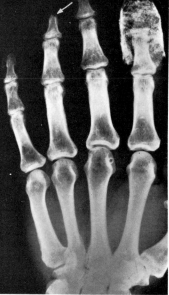

Figure 22–103A. Raynaud's phenomenon. The tufts of the terminal phalanges of the middle and fourth digits have been resorbed (arrows), as often happens in severe cases. (The bandaged finger is infected. Soft tissue atrophy is present but is not apparent in this film.) The Raynaud phenomenon is found in a variety of diseases in which vasoconstriction is inherent, especially scleroderma.

cases, especially when associated with collagen-vascular disease, show permanent occlusion, particularly of the digital arteries.

References

1. Kent, S. J. S., Thomas, M. L., and Browse, N. L.: The value of arteriography of the hand in Raynaud's syndrome. J. Cardiovasc. Surg. 17:72–80, 1976.
2. Porter, J. M., Snider, R. L., et al.: The diagnosis and treatment of Raynaud's phenomenon. Surgery 77:11–21, 1975.

Part XIII

Circulatory Problems of the Upper Extremity

WILFRIDO R. CASTANEDA-ZUNIGA, M.D.

KURT AMPLATZ, M.D.

ARTERIAL INSUFFICIENCY

Atherosclerotic involvement of the arteries of the upper extremities is uncommon. Even with complete atherosclerotic arterial occlusions, symptoms of arterial insufficiency are usually absent because of the presence of an excellent collateral network. Common sites of atherosclerotic involvement are the origins of the subclavian and innominate arteries; atherosclerotic involvement in these areas may result in the "subclavian steal syndrome." Atherosclerotic involvement of the arteries of the forearm and hand is exceedingly rare.

Peripheral embolism in the upper extremities is a common cause of arterial insufficiency causing a sudden onset of arterial occlusion. Emboli may originate in the heart or from an aneurysm secondary to the thoracic outlet syndrome. The angiographic findings are highly suggestive. Emboli tend to lodge at arterial bifurcations. The caliber of the artery is usually reduced owing to secondary spasm. An angiographic diagnosis can be made with a high degree of accuracy if the convex contour (meniscus sign) of the embolus is demonstrated (Fig. 22–104).

The arterial complications of trauma include spasm; extrinsic compression by a hematoma; intimal, medial tears (Fig. 22–105); and complete disruption of all layers (Fig. 22–106). Traumatic or iatrogenic arteriovenous communications may occur (Figs. 22–107 and 22–108).

VENOUS INSUFFICIENCY

Signs of venous insufficiency of the upper extremities are usually related to occlusions of the axillary, subclavian, or innominate vein, or the superior vena cava. The most common cause of occlusion of the central veins is tumor. Sometimes, however, occlusion of the superior vena cava may occur following surgical procedures

Text continued on page 1560

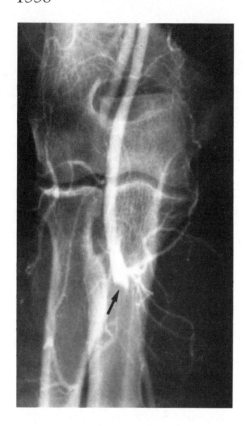

Figure 22–104. Obstruction of the radial artery with a convex contour, the so-called meniscus sign of an embolus (arrow).

Figure 22–105. Radiolucency within an axillary artery representing a probable intimal tear (arrows). Incidentally, there is a fracture of the scapula.

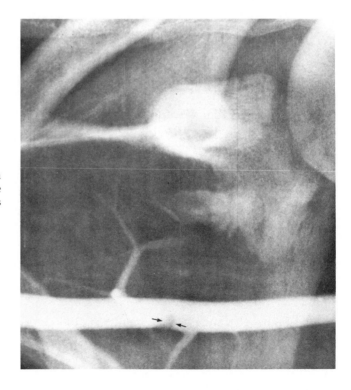

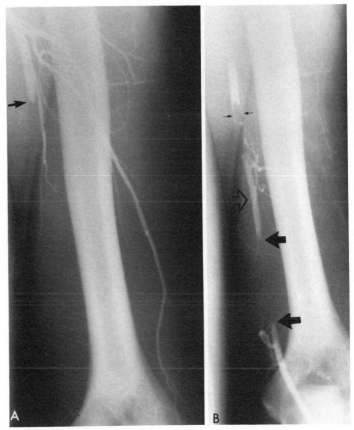

Figure 22–106. *A,* Disruption of the proximal brachial artery (arrow). *B,* Note the superimposed thrombus (small arrow). There is filling of the intermediate segment via collaterals (open arrow), with occlusion of the distal brachial artery by arterial spasm (arrowheads).

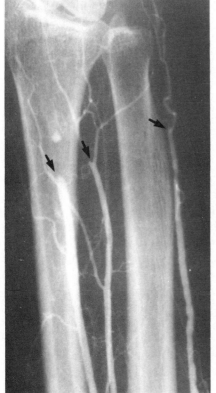

Figure 22–107. Occlusion of radial, ulnar, and interosseous arteries after the surgical creation of arteriovenous fistulas for hemodialysis (arrows).

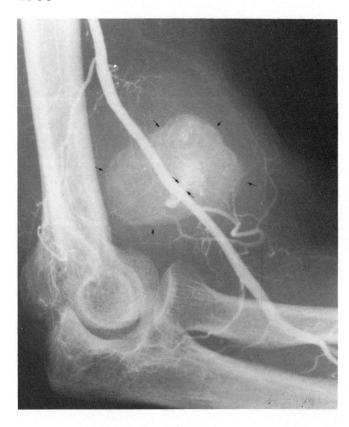

Figure 22–108. Brachial angiogram demonstrating a large pseudoaneurysm (peripheral arrows) occurring after puncture for diagnostic purposes. Note the jet of contrast material (central arrows).

such as Glenn's and Mustard's operations. In recent years, the incidence of venous insufficiency of the upper extremities has increased owing to thromboses of the large veins caused by indwelling catheters (Fig. 22–109) and intravenous pacemakers (Fig. 22–110). A rare cause of superior vena cava syndrome is sclerosing mediastinitis (mediastinal fibrosis). Primary thrombosis of the subclavian vein may be the result of compression by the scalenus anticus when the arms are raised. The angiographic findings of phlebothrombosis are characteristic, and the diagnosis can thus be made with confidence. Filling defects can be readily seen in the veins, and a double-contour effect is commonly created, since contrast medium tends to pass between the thrombus and the venous wall (see Fig. 22–109). This finding is most often seen in new cases of phlebothrombosis. Angiographically, the duration of thrombosis is indicated by the size of the collateral channels. In long-standing cases of phlebothrombosis there are usually large, well-developed collateral channels (Fig. 22–111).

A narrowed, irregular vein is usually indicative of recanalization of a thrombus. Prior to the performance of venography, a clinical diagnosis can be established by measuring the venous pressure. Since the clinical symptoms and increased venous pressure are pathognomonic of venous thrombosis, angiography is usually not necessary.

Primary thrombosis of the subclavian vein or stress thrombosis (effort thrombophlebitis) may be a manifestation of the thoracic outlet syndrome.[10] Other possible causes include primary phlebitis caused by sudden stretching and compression of the veins and endothelial damage caused by axillary venous distention secondary to exaggerated respiratory motion.[6] Patients with primary thrombosis of the subclavian vein or stress thrombosis are usually young and muscular and give an antecedent history of effort or strain occurring with the abduction of the arm. The presence of

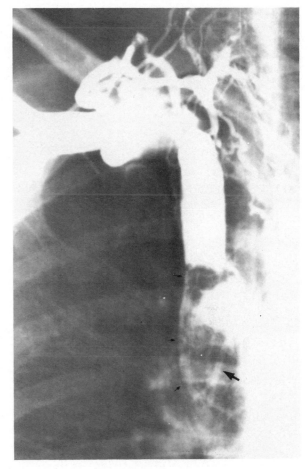

Figure 22–109. Occlusion of the superior vena cava by a large thrombus formed around the tip of an indwelling catheter of a heparin pump (large arrow). Note the double-contour effect (small arrows).

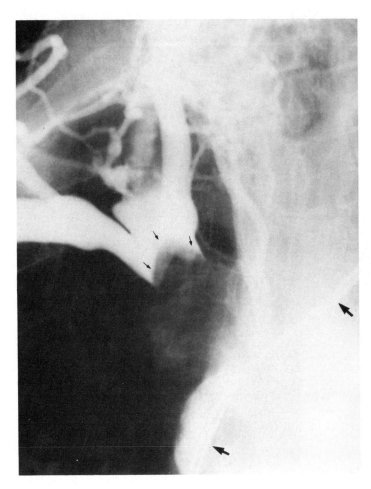

Figure 22–110. Pacemaker wires (large arrows) inserted from the left subclavian vein causing thrombosis of the superior vena cava. Note the concave border of the thrombus (small arrows).

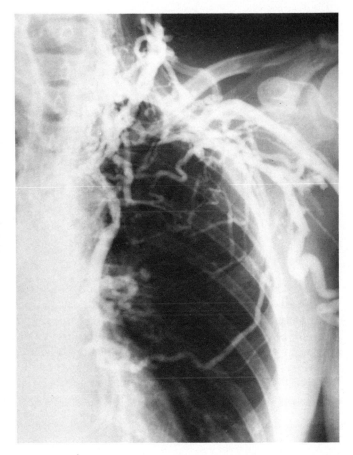

Figure 22–111. Left arm venogram reveals obstruction of the left subclavian vein with unusually well-developed collaterals, suggesting a long-standing process.

venus thrombosis is documented by phlebography. The patient's arms must be abducted in order to determine the source of the obstruction.

ERYTHROMELALGIA

Erythromelalgia is a disease characterized by paroxysmal bilateral vasodilatation. Attacks may last several minutes or hours. Symptoms include burning and pain in the palms and the soles, which later may involve the entire extremity. In typical cases, the peripheral pulses and blood pressure are normal. The attacks seem to be triggered by stimuli causing vasodilatation, such as heat.[1] On physical examination, redness, cyanosis, or a local increase of temperature may be noted. Symptomatic relief may be obtained by the elevation or the cooling of the extremity or by the administration of aspirin. Spontaneous remissions may occur in older patients.[8] In adults, the disease occurs in either a primary, or idiopathic, form or a secondary form, which is occasionally seen in patients with lupus erythematosus, diabetes mellitus, myeloproliferative disease, hypertension, gout, and organic neurologic disorders.[7] The symptoms of erythromelalgia may precede the diagnosis of an underlying systemic disease by as many as 12 years.[2] Men and women are affected equally. The diagnosis is usually made on the basis of the clinical and physical findings. Thermography has become the most useful diagnostic procedure for determining the effect of treatment.[9] The roentgenograms of the feet may be normal (40 per cent of cases) or may show osteoporosis (40 per cent) and hypertrophic osseous changes (20 per cent).[2] Since the clinical picture is so characteristic, angiography is not required for diagnosis.

ACROCYANOSIS

Acrocyanosis is an uncommon benign condition that usually persists throughout life. Since acrocyanosis is always primary, the possibility of systemic disease should not be considered.[4] It may occur at any age, most commonly in women. It is characterized by persistent coldness and marked cyanotic discoloration of the skin of the hands and feet exclusively. The symptoms are usually always present and aggravated by cold. The cause of this condition is unknown, and there is no specific treatment. No characteristic radiographic findings have been described.

SUDECK'S ATROPHY

Post-traumatic reflex atrophy of bone was first described by Sudeck in 1902[12] and usually occurs after minor injury. The disease is manifested by the symptoms and signs of vasomotor hyperactivity, including burning pain, edema, and local increase of temperature. On physical examination there may be cyanosis, soft tissue wasting, and joint stiffness. Distinctive patterns of bone resorption have been described, consisting of trabecular, subchondral, subperiosteal, intracortical, and endosteal bone resorption (Fig. 22–112).[3,5] Severe cases of osteoporosis can show similar roentgen changes, however. A reduction in cortical thickness and bone mineral content of 33 per cent may

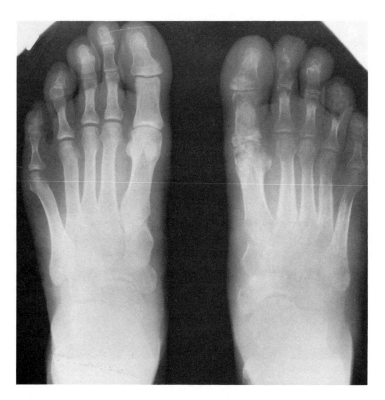

Figure 22–112. Sudeck's atrophy. Comparison views of an unaffected (right) and an affected (left) foot reveal soft tissue swelling and severe diffuse and periarticular demineralization.

be found.[3] If Sudeck's atrophy goes untreated, ankylosis of one or more joints often occurs.

CAUSALGIA

This rare syndrome is characterized by a hyperactive sympathetic nervous system. It may be caused by a minor peripheral nerve injury clinically characterized by burning pain and hyperesthesia. Redness and coldness of the affected extremity is common, and atrophy of the skin and muscle may be present. Limitation of joint movements and permanent disability may develop later. The classic radiographic finding is osteoporosis of bone.[11]

References

1. Allan, E. V., Barker, H. W., and Hines, E. A., Jr. (eds.): Peripheral Vascular Diseases. Philadelphia, W. B. Saunders Company, 1962, p. 1005.
2. Babb, R. R., Alarcon-Segovia, D., and Fairbairn, J. F., II: Erythermalgia. Review of 51 cases. Circulation 29:136–141, 1964.
3. Genant, H. K., Kozin, F., Bekerman, C., et al.: The reflex sympathetic dystrophy syndrome. A comprehensive analysis using fine-detail radiography, photon absorptiometry, and bone and joint scintigraphy. Radiology 117:21–32, 1975.
4. Gifford, R. W.,Jr.: Arteriospastic disorders of extremities. Circulation 27:970–975, 1963.
5. Herrman, L. G., Reineke, H. G., and Caldwell, J. A.: Post-traumatic painful osteoporosis. A clinical and roentgenological entity. Am.J. Radiol. 47:353–361, 1942.
6. Kleinsasser, L. J.: Effort thrombosis of the axillary and subclavian veins: analysis of 16 personal cases and 56 cases collected from the literature. Arch. Surg. 59:258–274, 1949.
7. Mandell, F., Folkman, J., and Matsomoto, S.: Erythromelalgia. Pediatrics 59:45–48, 1977.
8. Mitchell, W. W.: On a rare vasomotor neurosis of the extremities and the maladies with which it may be confounded. Am. J. Med. Sci. 76:2, 1978.
9. Ryan, J.: Thermography. Aust. Radiol. 13:23–25, 1969.
10. Sabiston, D. C., Jr.: Thrombo-obliterative disease of the aorta and its branches. In Sabiston, D. C., Jr., (ed.): Davis-Christopher Textbook of Surgery. Ed. 11. Philadelphia, W. B. Saunders Company, 1977, pp. 1919–1994.
11. Simson, G.: Propranolol for causalgia and Sudeck's atrophy. J.A.M.A. 227:327, 1974.
12. Sudeck, P.: Ueber die akute Trophoneurotische knochenatriophie nach entzundungen und Traumen der extremitaten. Dtsch. Med. Wochenschr. 28:336, 1902.

Part XIV

Visceral Ischemic Syndromes

STEPHEN L. KAUFMAN, M.D.

STANLEY S. SIEGELMAN, M.D.

INTRODUCTION

Increasing attention has been devoted for approximately 20 years to the syndromes of intestinal ischemia. The techniques of visceral angiography have contributed significantly to this awakening of interest since precise anatomic evaluation of these conditions has become practical. Stenosis or occlusion of the major visceral arteries may occur gradually over several years, resulting in a syndrome of chronic progressive ischemia. Alternatively, occlusions of one or more arteries to the bowel may occur acutely, resulting in an abrupt reduction of blood flow, which is usually a catastrophic event demanding immediate diagnosis and treatment.

Knowledge of the normal vascular anatomy of the gastrointestinal tract is necessary for the evaluation of these conditions. The gastrointestinal tract is supplied by three major visceral vessels: the celiac, superior mesenteric, and inferior mesenteric arteries. The celiac artery supplies the stomach and spleen and is usually the major source of blood supply to the liver and pancreas. The superior mesenteric artery supplies all of the small intestine and the ascending and transverse colon, usually to the level of the splenic flexure. The inferior mesenteric artery supplies the descending and sigmoid colon and the rectum. The rectum is also supplied by the middle and inferior hemorrhoidal arteries, which are branches of the hypogastric artery. There are abundant anastomoses normally present between the major visceral arteries, which become important as collateral pathways in the event of occlusion or stenosis of one or two of these vessels. The major anastomosis between the celiac and superior mesenteric arteries occurs via the pancreatoduodenal arcades that course around the head of the pancreas on the medial aspect of the duodenal C-loop (Fig. 22–113). Occasionally an anastomosis exists between the dorsal pancreatic branch of the celiac artery and the superior mesenteric artery or its middle colic branch.[45, 60]

There are two major anastomotic pathways between the superior and inferior mesenteric arteries (Fig. 22–114). The left colic branch of the inferior mesenteric artery, ascending within the transverse mesocolon, anastomoses in the region of the splenic flexure of the colon with the middle colic branch of the superior mesenteric artery.[23, 66] This anastomosis is known as the central anastomotic artery of the colon or the arc of

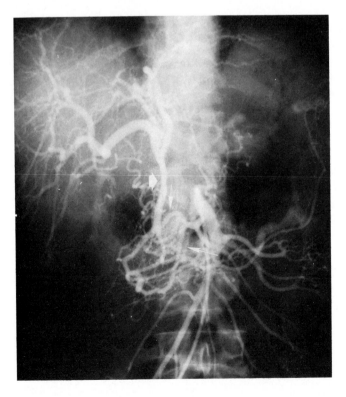

Figure 22–113. Celiac–superior mesenteric artery anastomosis. A superior mesenteric arteriogram of a patient with stenosis of the proximal hepatic artery demonstrates enlarged inferior pancreatoduodenal arcades (small arrow) filling the gastroduodenal (large arrows) and proper hepatic arteries.

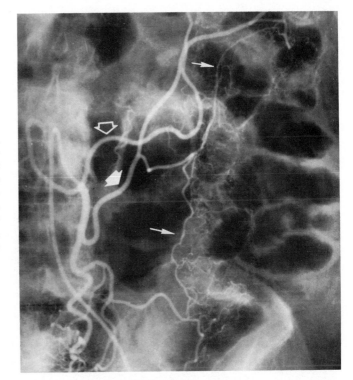

Figure 22–114. Superior mesenteric–inferior mesenteric artery anastomosis. An inferior mesenteric arteriogram demonstrates the anastomosis between the left colic artery (large closed arrow) and the middle colic branch (large open arrow) of the superior mesenteric artery. This is the arc of Riolan. The marginal artery of Drummond (small arrows) is seen adjacent to the mesenteric border of the descending colon.

Riolan.[51, 60] The second anastomotic pathway is the marginal artery of the colon, which runs along the mesenteric border of the entire colon at a distance of 1 to 8 cm from the bowel wall. It receives branches from multiple vessels originating from both the superior and the inferior mesenteric arteries and supplies the terminal arteries to the colon.[23, 66] This marginal artery is often called the marginal artery of Drummond or the peripheral anastomotic artery of the colon.[51, 60] With occlusion or stenosis of one or more of the major visceral vessels, these anastomotic vessels enlarge and provide collateral circulation to the remainder of the bowel.

Angiographic and autopsy studies reveal that stenoses or occlusions of the mesenteric arteries occur commonly in the asymptomatic population, especially in the older age groups. In one autopsy study, 55 per cent of the patients examined had evidence of luminal stenosis of one or more of the visceral vessels.[57] In a second autopsy study, the superior mesenteric artery was stenotic in 35 per cent of cases, and the inferior mesenteric artery was stenotic or occluded in 65 per cent.[19] The inferior mesenteric artery was totally occluded in 6.6 per cent of cases and significantly stenosed in 17 per cent of cases in a series of patients studied by angiography.[31] Stenoses are most frequently at the origins or within the proximal 1 or 2 cm of the major trunks of the mesenteric vessels.[19, 21, 31, 57] These atherosclerotic lesions are commonly associated with atherosclerosis involving the abdominal aorta, coronary arteries, and peripheral vessels.[12, 21, 31, 57] Dilated anastomotic channels are frequently seen in association with stenoses or occlusions of visceral arteries. A prominent network of collateral circulation accounts for the absence of symptoms in the patient with significant visceral artery stenosis. The existence of apparently severe lesions of the mesenteric vessels, often involving significant stenosis or occlusion of two or even three vessels in asymptomatic patients, should always be kept in mind in evaluating patients suspected of having mesenteric ischemia (Fig. 22–115). The clinical situation should always be closely correlated with the anatomic display in each case.

CHRONIC MESENTERIC ISCHEMIA

Multiple Vessel Occusion or Stenosis— The Syndrome of "Intestinal Angina"

The syndrome of intestinal angina is a manifestation of intermittent ischemia of the bowel usually produced by atherosclerotic stenoses or occlusions of the mesenteric

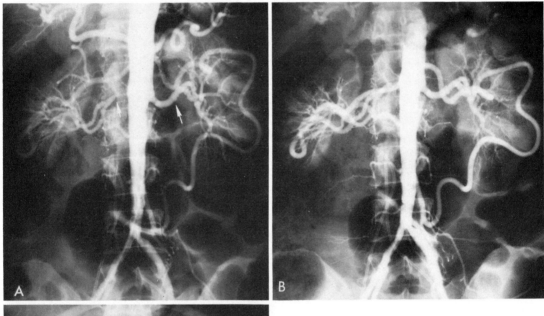

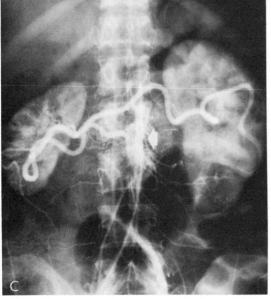

Figure 22–115. Fibromuscular dysplasia involving the superior mesenteric artery in an asymptomatic patient. Early (A), middle (B), and late (C) phases of an abdominal aortogram show evidence of fibromuscular dysplasia involving the renal arteries (small arrows). The superior mesenteric artery was occluded initially but is reconstituted (large arrow) by an enlarged arc of Riolan originating from the inferior mesenteric artery. The patient, a 44-year-old female, was being evaluated for hypertension and had no gastrointestinal symptoms.

vessels.[25, 46, 50] Despite the frequency of mesenteric atherosclerosis, the syndrome is uncommon and occurs less often than manifestations of atherosclerosis in the coronary, cerebral, or lower extremity circulations.[38, 49, 74] This apparent paradox is explained by the rich collateralization within the intestinal circulation.

Intestinal angina is characterized by abdominal pain, usually beginning 15 to 20 minutes after meals and lasting from one to three hours.[6, 25, 28, 46, 49, 50, 70, 74] The pain may be generalized or limited to the epigastrium. Owing to the association of pain with eating, the patient commonly eats small meals or may be reluctant to eat at all. Significant weight loss usually ensues. Malabsorption is present in a minority of cases. A bruit is frequently heard in the epigastrium.

Plain abdominal radiographs and barium studies are usually noncontributory in abdominal angina but are important in excluding other conditions responsible for abdominal pain. Angiography is required for diagnosis. Aortography should be performed in both the anteroposterior and the lateral projections. The lateral projection is necessary for the evaluation of the proximal portions of the superior mesenteric and celiac arteries, which are the most common sites of disease (Figs. 22–116 to 22–118; see Fig. 22–121). Occlusion or significant stenosis (greater than 50 per cent) of two of the three mesenteric trunks is a prerequisite for the diagnosis of intestinal angina (see Fig.

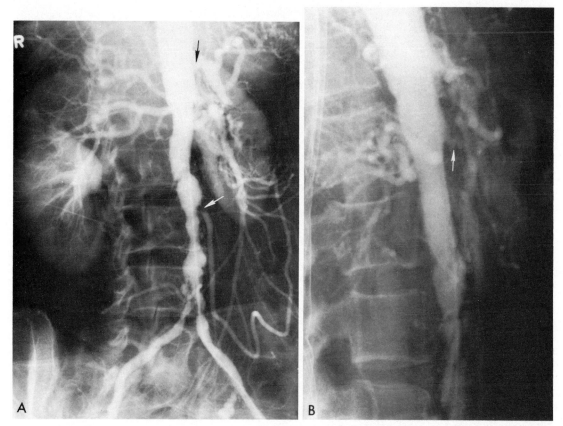

Figure 22–116. Chronic mesenteric ischemia. Left posterior oblique (A) and lateral (B) projections of an abdominal aortogram. The origins of the celiac, superior mesenteric, and inferior mesenteric arteries are stenotic (arrows). There is diffuse atherosclerotic narrowing of the distal abdominal aorta and proximal common iliac arteries. The placement of a distal aortic graft and bypass grafts on the celiac and superior mesenteric arteries relieved the symptoms of claudication and abdominal angina.

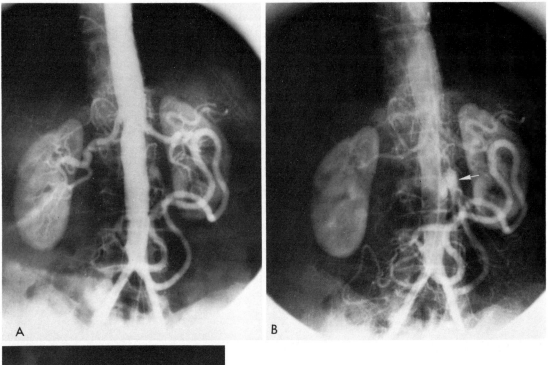

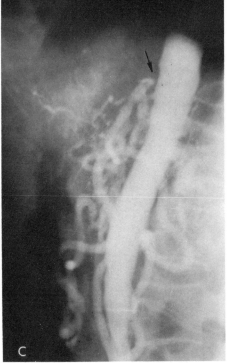

Figure 22–117. Chronic mesenteric ischemia. Occlusion of superior mesenteric artery and marked stenosis of celiac artery are evident. The patient is a 61-year-old female with a five-year history of postprandial abdominal pain. *A,* Mid-arterial phase aortogram shows a large, prominent inferior mesenteric artery. *B,* Late arterial phase aortogram shows the superior mesenteric artery (arrow) being filled in a retrograde fashion by collaterals from the inferior mesenteric artery. It also shows late filling of the hepatic and splenic branches of the celiac artery. *C,* Lateral view shows marked stenosis of the origin of the celiac artery (arrow).

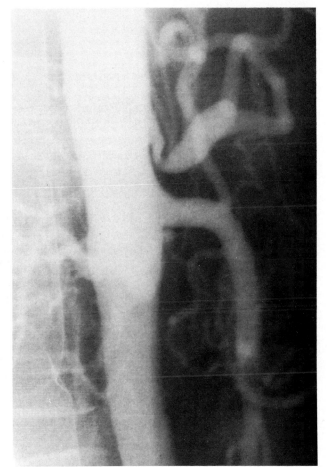

Figure 22–118. Celiac artery compression. This lateral projection of an abdominal aortogram demonstrates extrinsic compression upon the superior aspect of the proximal portion of the celiac axis. There is poststenotic dilatation more distally. The superior mesenteric artery is normal.

22–116).[49, 50, 74] For a definitive diagnosis, all three of the vessels should be significantly involved. The presence of enlarged collateral vessels is often helpful in determining the presence of stenotic lesions of the mesenteric vessels (see Fig. 22–117). Severe atherosclerosis of the abdominal aorta and other vessels is also frequently present.[6, 70] Since stenosis or occlusions of visceral vessels, often with enlarged collaterals, may be seen in asymptomatic patients, the angiographic appearance must be closely correlated with the clinical presentation of the patient. Other conditions, especially carcinoma of the pancreas, should be carefully excluded in the differential diagnosis.

Patients with the classic clinical presentation and corresponding angiographic abnormalities may then be considered to have chronic intestinal ischemia. Therapy in intestinal angina is directed toward both the relief of symptoms and the prevention of acute mesenteric thrombosis and necrosis of bowel. In several series, 50 per cent of the patients presenting with acute intestinal ischemia resulting from thrombosis of the superior mesenteric artery had previous symptoms suggesting chronic mesenteric ischemia.[3, 25, 42, 49, 70] Bypass grafting from the aorta to the patent mesenteric artery is the surgical procedure of choice.[28, 49, 50, 70, 74] Since the mesenteric vessel distal to the proximal 1 or 2 cm is usually free of disease, this form of therapy is usually successful and results in relief of symptoms and weight gain. Although atherosclerosis is the most common origin of chronic intestinal ischemia, impairment of the mesenteric circulation may also occur from fibromuscular dysplasia (see Fig. 22–115), retroperitoneal fibrosis, vasculitis, or occlusion of mesenteric vessels by aneurysms or dissecting hematomas.[16, 27, 74]

Celiac Artery Compression Syndrome

The existence of the celiac artery compression syndrome has been the subject of considerable controversy. As originally described, this syndrome consists of abdominal pain associated with a loud epigastric bruit; it occurs most frequently in young females.[24, 35, 36] The pain is variable in location, usually nonspecific in character, and related to food intake in less than 50 per cent of cases.[26, 35, 67] It is less severe than the pain of intestinal angina. Weight loss, which is occasionally present, is mild. Abdominal aortography in the lateral projection typically demonstrates extrinsic compression of the superior aspect of the proximal celiac artery, frequently with evidence of poststenotic dilatation (Fig. 22–118).[2, 15, 24, 35, 36] The superior and inferior mesenteric arteries are normal, and there is usually no evidence of atherosclerosis.[15, 35] Enlarged collaterals to the celiac axis via the pancreatoduodenal arcades are inconsistently present.[15, 67]

This celiac artery defect has been shown to be due to compression of the celiac axis by fibers of the median arcuate ligament of the diaphragm and the celiac plexus, a collection of sympathetic and parasympathetic neurons surrounding the proximal celiac axis.[34] Surgery, consisting of interruption of the median arcuate ligament fibers, results in immediate relief of symptoms in most cases.[24, 26, 36] The epigastric bruit usually also disappears.

The pathophysiologic mechanisms responsible for this syndrome are not well understood. The origin of the pain is usually attributed to ischemia secondary to compression of the celiac axis.[24, 35] The possibility of a neuritic origin of the abdominal pain has also been considered, and relief of symptoms is attributed to the fact that the celiac plexus is usually interrupted at the time of surgery.[2]

There are several reasons why the existence of this syndrome has been questioned. It is generally accepted that in order for intestinal ischemia to be present at least two of the three major mesenteric vessels must be significantly narrowed.[49, 50, 74] Invariably, patients said to have the celiac artery compression syndrome are found to have a normal superior and inferior mesenteric circulation.[15, 35] Also, the syndrome's symptoms are vague and are clearly postprandial only in the minority of the patients.[26, 67] Significant pressure gradients across the area of celiac artery compression are usually not found, a fact that decreases the likelihood of an ischemic origin of this syndrome.[22, 24]

Extrinsic celiac artery compression is also frequently seen in asymptomatic patients. Angiographic studies have shown extrinsic narrowing of the celiac axis attributable to compression by the median arcuate ligament of the diaphragm in 22 per cent to 31 per cent of asymptomatic patients.[14, 43] Epigastric bruits in asymptomatic patients are also most frequently due to extrinsic compression of the celiac artery.[43] Furthermore, although over 80 per cent of the patients with this syndrome obtain relief of symptoms following surgery, long-term follow-up reveals that only about half of these patients remain asymptomatic.[26] On the other hand, 75 per cent of the patients with the syndrome who are not operated upon obtain relief of symptoms by other means.[26] The lack of a rational pathophysiologic mechanism, the presence of similar angiographic findings in asymptomatic patients, and the transient surgical relief of symptoms cast doubt on the existence of the celiac artery compression syndrome. Since celiac artery compression is rarely symptomatic, the diagnosis must be made with considerable caution and a comprehensive search should be made for other causes of pain.

ACUTE MESENTERIC ISCHEMIA

Acute mesenteric ischemia is a medical emergency that has been associated with a mortality rate of between 86 per cent and 100 per cent.[54, 55, 56, 65, 76] This poor prognosis is partially related to the nonspecificity of the clinical signs and symptoms associated with the early stages of this condition, which causes delays in diagnosis until extensive irreversible bowel necrosis has occurred. With prompt diagnosis and therapy, however, many patients with mesenteric infarction may survive.[32]

Sudden occlusion of the superior mesenteric artery results in abrupt cessation of blood flow to the bowel. Collateral circulation is usually not adequate to sustain the bowel owing to the sudden onset of the occlusion. The four major types of acute mesenteric ischemia are (1) superior mesenteric artery embolization, (2) acute superior mesenteric artery thrombosis, (3) nonocclusive mesenteric ischemia, and (4) mesenteric venous occlusion. Rarely, acute mesenteric ischemia is caused by retroperitoneal fibrosis, vasculitis, or occlusion of the visceral vessels by dissecting hematoma.[16, 54] The pathophysiologic mechanism of acute mesenteric ischemia is the same regardless of its origin. The mucosa is the portion of intestine most sensitive to ischemia.[7, 56] Hemorrhagic necrosis of the mucosa appears soon after the onset of ischemia.[39, 74] Loss of plasma into the bowel lumen occurs largely from the venous side, which even after arterial occlusion is subject to portal vein pressure.[38, 40, 56, 74] The loss of large amounts of plasma into the bowel is accompanied by hemoconcentration and decreased blood volume, resulting in diminished cardiac output and a further decrease in mesenteric circulation.[75] A vicious cycle is thus established. The breakdown of the intestinal mucosa also results in the absorption of toxic substances into the general circulation.[38, 56, 74] Severe ischemia eventually results in full-thickness necrosis of the bowel wall and peritonitis.

Clinically, patients with acute mesenteric ischemia present with diffuse, severe abdominal pain.[10, 32, 42, 54-56, 76, 79] The character of the pain is often nonspecific. The distress of the patient is usually disproportionate to the minimal physical findings. Although the abdomen may be tender to palpation, rebound tenderness is not present until peritonitis occurs. Bowel sounds are frequently absent or diminished. It is the nonspecificity of the presentation and the lack of objective physical findings in the early stages of acute mesenteric ischemia that are usually responsible for the delay in diagnosis.[42, 54] The disparity between the patient's severe discomfort and the paucity of physical findings is actually a characteristic feature of this entity.[10]

Superior Mesenteric Artery Embolization

This condition occurs most frequently in patients with pre-existing cardiac disease. The source of the arterial emboli is most often the heart. Left atrial thrombi in patients with atrial fibrillation and rheumatic heart disease, especially mitral stenosis, and left ventricular mural thrombi in patients with recent myocardial infarctions are the most frequent source of emboli to the superior mesenteric artery.[32, 54, 76, 79] Paradoxical embolization to the superior mesenteric artery has also been reported in patients with thrombophlebitis.[32] Mesenteric embolization should, therefore, be strongly suspected in patients presenting with a sudden onset of severe abdominal pain who have coexisting atrial fibrillation, mitral stenosis, or a history of recent myocardial infarction or symptoms of deep venous thrombosis. Approximately 55 per cent of superior mesenteric artery emboli lodge at the level of the middle colic artery; 18 per cent are found within the main trunk of the superior mesenteric artery proximal to this level; the remainder are found in small peripheral branches.[29]

Acute Mesenteric Artery Thrombosis

This is most often seen in association with atherosclerosis of the aorta and the superior mesenteric artery.[54, 74] In distinction to superior mesenteric artery emboli, superior mesenteric artery thrombosis most often occurs in the proximal 1 or 2 cm of the main trunk of the artery.[10, 29] Patients with acute superior mesenteric artery thrombosis frequently have atherosclerotic involvement of other organ systems, and their prognosis is worse than that of patients with mesenteric artery embolism.[3, 54, 74]

In some series, acute mesenteric artery thrombosis is preceded in approximately 50 per cent of patients by symptoms compatible with intestinal angina.[3, 25, 42, 49, 70] Although this association has not been consistently made,[54] it is a strong argument for prophylactic surgical correction in cases of intestinal angina.

Nonocclusive Mesenteric Ischemia

This entity has received increasing recognition in the last few years.[10, 11, 54, 55, 64, 72] The term "nonocclusive" has been employed because ischemic damage to the bowel occurs despite the fact that the major arteries and veins supplying the area of injury remain intact. Patients with nonocclusive mesenteric ischemia are characteristically elderly, with pre-existing cardiac disease. Most patients with clinically manifest nonocclusive mesenteric ischemia are taking digitalis, which is known to produce mesenteric vasoconstriction.[17] An acute precipitating event — arrhythmia, acute myocardial infarction, congestive heart failure, hypovolemia, or shock — usually precedes the onset of nonocclusive mesenteric ischemia. These conditions result in diminished cardiac output, which may cause active mesenteric vasoconstriction.[64] With dwindling cardiac output, constriction of the vascular bed in the gut is an appropriate physiologic mechanism to divert oxygenated blood to the brain, heart, and kidneys. Persistence of this reactive mesenteric vasoconstriction even after resolution of the initial precipitating event is a pathologic phenomenon that results in ischemic damage to the bowel.[64] In two large series of mesenteric ischemia, the nonocclusive variety composed approximately one half of all cases.[54, 55] This diagnosis should always be considered in elderly patients taking digitalis for cardiac disease who present with severe acute abdominal pain following a period of impaired cardiac output.

Mesenteric Venous Occlusion

This is responsible for approximately 10 per cent of all cases of acute mesenteric ischemia.[54, 55, 74] Mesenteric venous occlusion may be secondary to conditions resulting in hypercoagulability (polycythemia vera or oral contraceptive use), conditions resulting in stasis within the portal circulation (cirrhosis or extrinsic compression of the portal vein by tumor), or infections involving the root of the mesentery or retroperitoneum.[41, 52, 69, 74] Mesenteric venous thrombosis may also occur as an isolated event or as a manifestation of migratory thrombophlebitis.[41, 52, 69] Mesenteric venous thrombosis involving the portal vein or the more proximal portions of the superior mesenteric vein usually does not result in intestinal infarction because of the ordinarily abundant venous collateral circulation in the root of the mesentery and retroperitoneum. It is only when venous thrombosis occurs in the most peripheral branches of the mesenteric veins that mesenteric ischemia occurs, owing to the lack of collateral venous outflow.[52, 59]

The clinical picture in mesenteric venous thrombosis is apt to be less dramatic than in the arterial forms of mesenteric ischemia. Ill-defined, mild abdominal pain, associated with anorexia, nausea, and a change in bowel habits, may occur gradually over a period of several days to weeks.[41, 52, 69] Symptoms are progressive, however, and eventually dehydration and circulatory compromise occur, secondary to loss of fluid into the lumen of the gut and peritoneal cavity. The prognosis for patients with mesenteric venous occlusion is better than that for patients with acute arterial insufficiency. With surgery, a survival rate of 40 to 70 per cent has been reported. The nonoperative mortality rate approaches 100 per cent, however.[41, 52, 69]

Abdominal Radiography

Plain abdominal radiographs are indicated for the patient with possible acute mesenteric ischemia. Unfortunately, most patients have nonspecific mild distention of the bowel (see Fig. 22–122A). Specific findings for acute mesenteric infarction consist primarily of bowel wall thickening and mucosal irregularities due to submucosal edema and hemorrhage (Fig. 22–119).[53, 62, 68] Involved segments of the bowel may appear rigid with a narrowed straight lumen or may be normal or dilated in caliber. Signs of wall and mucosal thickening may be mimicked by intramural hemorrhage into the bowel wall secondary to various forms of clotting dysfunction[68] and must therefore be correlated with the clinical presentation of the patient. Gas within the bowel wall or the distal intrahepatic portions of the portal vein indicates that intestinal necrosis has occurred.[59, 62, 68] Several nonspecific findings, such as a pattern simulating small intestinal obstruction or gaseous dilatation of the colon to the level of the splenic flexure, may also be present.

Positive specific findings on plain abdominal radiographs occurred in 10 per cent to 60 per cent of cases of mesenteric infarction.[53, 62, 68] Patients with venous occlusion had a relatively higher incidence of positive findings than did those with arterial occlusions. The incidence of these findings, however, is directly related to the extent of the mesenteric infarction present,[62] and these suggestive signs are not seen in the early stages of mesenteric ischemia. Therefore, the diagnosis of mesenteric infarction cannot be excluded even in the presence of a normal or nonspecific plain abdominal radiograph (Fig. 22–120A). The plain abdominal radiograph, however, may reveal other conditions that are the cause of the diffuse abdominal pain, such as free intraperitoneal air due to perforated ulcer. Barium examination of the small bowel demonstrates the findings of intestinal mucosal edema.[30, 62, 76] It has not been found to help in the evaluation of the extent or reversibility of ischemic damage[30] and generally should not be performed in suspected cases, since residual barium may interfere with the accurate interpretation of angiographic studies.

Angiography

Angiography is capable of definitively making the diagnosis of acute mesenteric ischemia and establishing the likely cause.[1, 10, 76] Angiography must be performed early in the course of the disease, when the condition is initially suspected and before extensive irreversible bowel necrosis has occurred.[32] This emphasizes the need for careful examination of patients with a constellation of symptoms and signs suggestive of mesenteric ischemia. Aortography in both the anteroposterior and the lateral projections should be carried out initially, the lateral projection being the most

Text continued on page 1578

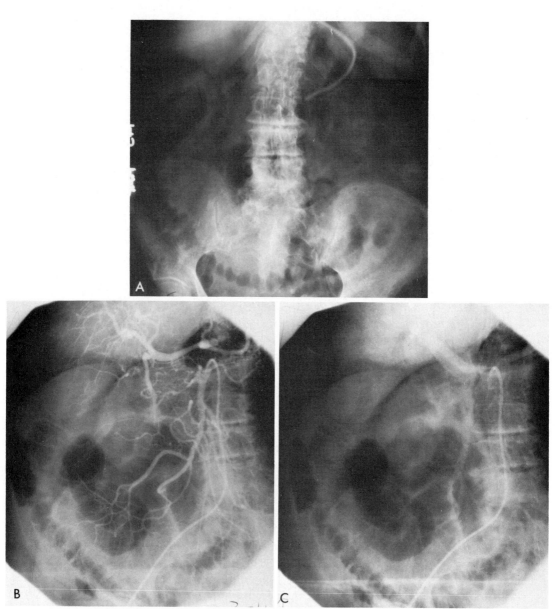

Figure 22–119. Positive plain films with mesenteric ischemia. An 88-year-old female experienced congestive heart failure following a prolonged period of rapid atrial fibrillation. The patient responded after three days of treatment with digitalis and diuretics. Following the control of cardiac arrhythmia, the patient complained of abdominal pain and distention. *A,* The plain film shows a single loop of bowel in the right lower quadrant, which has diffuse submucosal edema strongly suggestive of vascular compromise. *B,* The arterial phase of superior mesenteric arteriogram shows no evidence of an occlusion. All of the arteries are patent. *C,* The venous phase shows all the veins are patent. This is an example of bowel infarction with nonocclusive mesenteric ischemia. The single 6-foot loop of infarcted bowel was successfully resected. (*From* Siegelman, S. S., Sprayregen, S., and Boley, S. J.: Angiographic diagnosis of mesenteric arteriovasoconstriction. Radiology *112:*533–542, 1974. Reproduced by permission.)

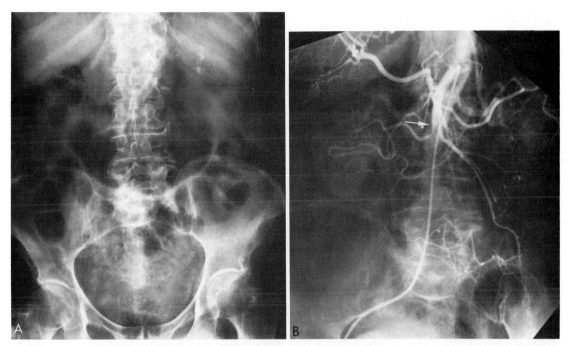

Figure 22–120. Superior mesenteric artery embolus. The patient is a 75-year-old female with a known history of arteriosclerotic heart disease and an earlier embolization to the left iliac artery. The patient experienced a sudden onset of severe abdominal pain. *A,* The plain film shows no definite abnormality. There is a normal distribution of gas in the stomach and small bowel. *B,* A superior mesenteric arteriogram performed immediately after the plain films shows a filling defect in the main portion of the superior mesenteric artery, which indicates an embolus (arrow).

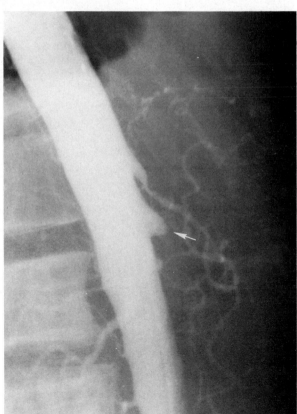

Figure 22–121. Acute superior mesenteric artery thrombosis. The patient is a 72-year-old male with an acute onset of severe abdominal pain, lower gastrointestinal bleeding, and shock. The lateral projection of the abdominal aortogram shows occlusion of the superior mesenteric artery (arrow) within the first centimeter of its origin. There is intense vasoconstriction of the celiac and renal arteries.

valuable for evaluating the proximal superior mesenteric artery. Selective superior mesenteric arteriography should then be performed if the extent of the occlusion of the superior mesenteric artery is not completely defined on the aortogram.

In cases of superior mesenteric artery emboli, there is angiographic evidence of occlusions of the superior mesenteric artery, usually at the level of the middle colic or early jejunal branches (see Fig. 22–120).[29, 32] Emboli in other aortic branches are also frequently seen. Superior mesenteric artery thrombosis, on the other hand, usually occurs in the most proximal portion of the superior mesenteric artery (Fig. 22–121)[10, 29] and is frequently associated with atherosclerosis of the aorta and other vessels.[54, 74] In patients with nonocclusive mesenteric ischemia, angiography reveals mesenteric arterial vasoconstriction, with spasm at the origins of multiple branches of the superior mesenteric artery, slowed flow, and diminished visualization of the intestinal arcades (Figs. 22–122 and 22–123).[1, 11, 64, 76] Vasoconstriction should be at least partially reversed

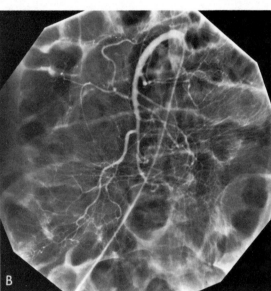

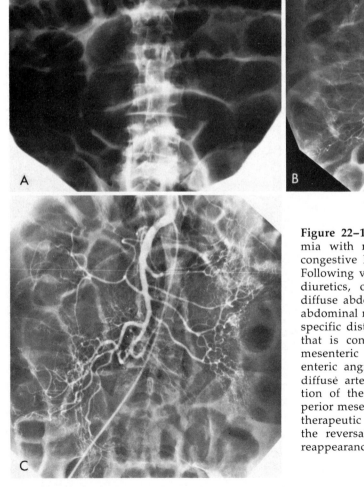

Figure 22–122. Nonocclusive mesenteric ischemia with reversal. This 74-year-old man had congestive heart failure and pulmonary edema. Following vigorous treatment with digitalis and diuretics, on the fourth day he experienced diffuse abdominal pain and distention. *A,* Plain abdominal radiograph shows the pattern of nonspecific distention of the colon and small bowel that is consistent with but not diagnostic of mesenteric ischemia. *B,* Selective superior mesenteric angiogram, arterial phase, demonstrates diffuse arterial spasm with impaired visualization of the intestinal arcades. *C,* Selective superior mesenteric angiogram following a 16-hour therapeutic papaverine infusion demonstrates the reversal of the vasoconstriction, with the reappearance of the intestinal arcades.

Legend continued on the opposite page

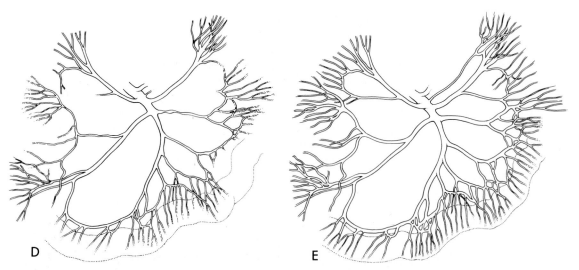

Figure 22–122 *Continued.* D and E, Diagrammatic representation of intestinal vasoconstriction before (D) and after (E) reversal.

Figure 22–123. Generalized irreversible nonocclusive mesenteric ischemia. A 57-year-old male hospitalized with acute myocardial infarction experienced congestive heart failure, pulmonary edema, and oliguria; he was treated with digitalis and diuretics. On his fifth day in the hospital, he had diffuse abdominal pain. The selective superior mesenteric angiogram shows (1) narrowing at the origin of the ileocolic artery (arrow), (2) diffuse spasm and narrowing of jejunal and ilial arteries, and (3) obliteration of the vascular arcades in the small intestine. The vasoconstriction was not reversed by intra-arterial papaverine infusion. A laparotomy performed immediately after this procedure showed extensive intestinal infarction. (*From* Siegelman, S. S., Sprayregen, S., and Boley, S. J.: Angiographic diagnosis of mesenteric vasoconstriction. Radiology *112*:533–542, 1974. Reproduced by permission.)

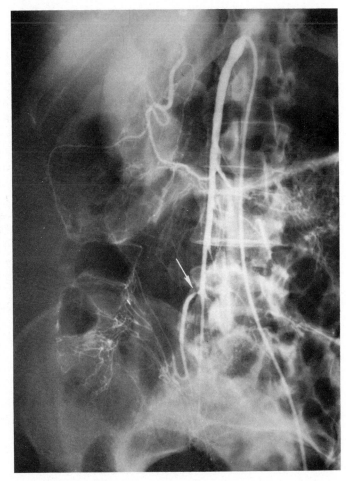

following a test infusion of a vasodilator into the superior mesenteric artery.[64] This angiographic appearance is characteristic of nonocclusive mesenteric ischemia in patients with a typical clinical history, but reactive vasoconstriction can also be anticipated when angiography is performed following administration of vasoconstrictor drugs or in patients with hemorrhagic shock or hypotension associated with peritonitis or sepsis. Mesenteric arterial vasoconstriction has been described in a patient with pancreatic abscess.[76] Angiographic findings in cases of mesenteric venous occlusion are prolongation of the arterial phase, opacification of thickened bowel wall, and failure of the portal venous system to opacify.[74]

Therapy

The therapy for acute mesenteric ischemia due to superior mesenteric artery embolism, thrombosis, or venous occlusion is surgical. Embolectomy is the procedure of choice for emboli located proximal to the origin of the ileocolic artery.[10, 79] Patients with smaller, more distal emboli probably do not require immediate surgery,[32, 33] unless there is clinical evidence of peritonitis.[10] It is often not possible, at the time of embolectomy, to accurately predict the complete extent of nonviable bowel. Re-exploration 24 to 48 hours later, with resection of any necrotic bowel, has been recommended.[10, 40, 79] Prompt diagnosis and therapy of mesenteric embolization has been associated with a mortality rate of only 9 per cent, attributable to intestinal infarction.[32] For thrombosis, surgical therapy includes a bypass graft and resection of necrotic bowel. The prognosis for patients with thrombosis is generally worse than for those with embolization, since the former usually are elderly and have associated diseases.[3, 74]

Therapy for mesenteric venous occlusion consists of resection of necrotic bowel and areas of mesentery involved by thrombosis; anticoagulation therapy has been found to improve the prognosis.[41, 52, 69, 74] Surgery may not be required in patients with nonocclusive ischemia, if reactive vasoconstriction can be reversed before necrosis of the bowel and peritonitis develop.[72] The elimination of the precipitating condition, fluid replacement, and improvement of cardiac function,[72] along with infusion of vasodilators into the superior mesenteric artery for a period of from 16 to 24 hours to reverse mesenteric artery vasoconstriction, are recommended (Fig. 22–122C).[64] Papaverine has been shown to be an effective vasodilating agent in patients with this condition.[64] In experimental studies, prostaglandin E_1 is also effective and has the advantage of being rapidly removed from the circulation by the liver, obviating systemic vasodilation.[18] If infarcted bowel is present, surgical resection is required.[72] The indications for surgical intervention include rebound tenderness or other objective evidence of peritonitis. Severe arterial vasoconstriction visualized by angiography that is not reversed by intra-arterial vasodilators is also an indication of infarcted bowel (see Fig. 22–123).[64]

ISCHEMIC COLITIS

Ischemic colitis is a syndrome produced by diminished blood flow to the colon. Although occasionally seen in younger patients,[48] ischemic colitis is largely confined to those older than 50.[8, 13, 39, 73, 77] Colonic ischemia may be due to a variety of factors, which include reduced cardiac output, use of digitalis, and colonic distention. It is rarely seen following ligation of the inferior mesenteric artery during surgery for resection of abdominal aortic aneurysm or colonic carcinoma.[4, 5, 63, 78] Normally, the inferior mesenteric artery may be safely ligated owing to collateralization from the middle colic branch of the superior mesenteric artery and the hemorrhoidal branches of the hypogastric arteries. With significant atherosclerotic disease of these other mesenteric vessels, however, or with congenital absence of adequate collateralization, ischemia may result. Most frequently, however, ischemic colitis occurs spontaneously without an obvious precipitating event.[71, 77] Ten per cent of cases of spontaneous colonic ischemia are associated with a carcinoma of the colon distal to the ischemic area.[61]

The colonic mucosa is most sensitive to ischemia and consequently is the earliest layer affected by diminution in blood flow.[7, 20, 37] Milder degrees of colonic ischemia are accompanied by mucosal necrosis with submucosal hemorrhage, edema, and inflammation. When ischemia subsides, the submucosal hemorrhages are resorbed or emptied into the bowel lumen. Superficial ulceration may appear, but eventually the mucosa regenerates to normality. With more severe colonic ischemia the muscular and serosal layers may also be affected. If blood flow is not sufficiently reduced to produce full-thickness necrosis of the bowel wall, healing occurs but with resultant fibrosis and areas of colonic narrowing. Very severe colonic ischemia results in gangrene of the entire bowel wall and peritonitis.

These pathologic changes are reflected in the clinical and radiographic findings of ischemic colitis. Patients generally present with mild to moderate lower abdominal pain accompanied by bloody diarrhea or bright red rectal bleeding.[8, 13, 39, 73, 77] Patients presenting with spontaneous colonic ischemia generally have no acute precipitating event, such as arrhythmia or congestive heart failure. Plain abdominal roentgenograms may reveal thickening of the haustral markings and the bowel wall of the involved segments of the colon.[37, 77] The barium enema is diagnostic. The mucosal folds are thickened, and multiple smooth, rounded indentations, frequently termed thumbprints, are seen protruding into the bowel lumen (Fig. 22–124).[37, 39, 73, 77] These thumbprints correspond to areas of submucosal hemorrhage and edema. The splenic flexure and adjacent areas of the transverse and descending colon are most frequently involved.[37, 39, 73] Sigmoid colon involvement is not uncommon. Other areas of the colon, including the rectum, may occasionally be involved by ischemic colitis, however.[8, 37, 77]

In the majority of cases, spontaneously occurring ischemic colitis is self-limited. Symptoms regress in 24 to 48 hours.[8, 73] Follow-up barium enema examinations in one to two weeks usually reveal disappearance of the thumbprinting.[39, 73] Occasionally, superficial ulcerations are seen at this time.[13, 73] Complete healing usually occurs within one month.[37]

With greater degrees of colonic ischemia, fibrosis associated with healing results in the formation of strictures. Ischemic strictures are usually several inches in length, smooth, concentric, and tapered, without the abrupt overhanging edges characteristic of carcinoma of the colon.[37] Since approximately 10 per cent of cases of ischemic colitis are associated with colonic carcinoma, however, this should be excluded by careful barium enema examination.[61] A minority of patients with colonic ischemia may progress to frank gangrene of the colon.[47] Consequently, patients with ischemic colitis should be monitored for signs of clinical deterioration and peritonitis. This may lead to colonic dilatation with air-fluid levels resembling those of toxic megacolon radiographically.[47] Since most cases of colonic ischemia are reversible, conservative management is followed. Surgery is required only in the uncommon cases associated with gangrene of the colon.[73]

Angiography has occasionally been performed in cases of spontaneously occurring ischemic colitis. Although acute occlusion of branches of the inferior mesenteric artery

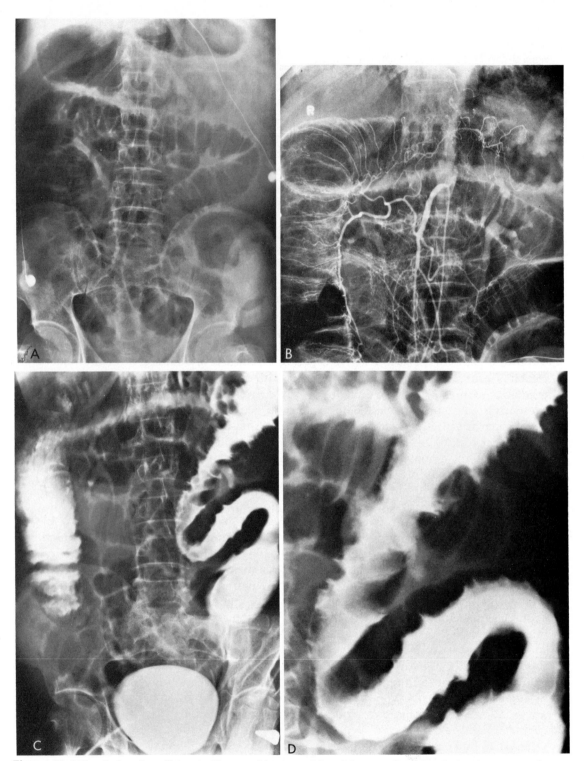

Figure 22–124. Ischemic colitis. A 60-year-old man with a history of myocardial infarction and carcinoma of the colon was hospitalized with weakness, hypotension, and chest pain. Serial studies did not show a myocardial infarction, but on his second day in the hospital the patient also began to experience diffuse abdominal pain. *A,* A plain film of the abdomen shows distended loops of small bowel and some gas in the stomach and right colon. *B,* An emergency superior mesenteric angiogram shows no evidence of vasoconstriction. The arcades in the right colon are prominent. *C* and *D,* A barium enema performed at this point shows extensive submucosal edema of the descending colon to the splenic flexure, manifested by thumbprinting; this is diagnostic of ischemic colitis. The patient was treated conservatively with intravenous fluids and antibiotics. His abdominal pain, tenderness, and fever disappeared over a seven-day period. A follow-up barium enema showed no abnormality.

has been encountered in a few instances,[58, 71] in the majority no occlusions are seen.[73, 77] In a detailed study of the vascularization of the colon at the splenic flexure, Meyers noted that in over 50 per cent of cases there is a congenitally absent or tenuous anastomosis between the ascending left colic–middle colic artery and the marginal artery of the colon at the splenic flexure.[44] He postulates that these patients with poor or absent collateralization at this point may have an increased tendency to acquire colonic ischemia. A combination of poor collateralization at the splenic flexure, low-grade stenosis at the origins of the superior or inferior mesenteric artery, and a low flow state of any variety may result in ischemic colitis.[44] This explanation is consistent with the frequency of involvement of the splenic flexure in spontaneous ischemic colitis. The nature of the low flow state is not well understood. Usually there is no precipitating episode, such as is seen in patients with nonocclusive mesenteric ischemia.

Ischemic colitis proximal to obstructing carcinomas of the colon can be explained by the fact that increased intraluminal pressure causes a decrease in arterial blood flow and a preferential decrease in flow to the intestinal mucosa.[9] It has been postulated that the low flow state in spontaneous ischemic colitis not associated with carcinoma of the colon may also be secondary to a transient elevation in intraluminal pressure.[9] In general, angiography has not been helpful in cases of ischemic colitis.[13, 77] A normal inferior mesenteric artery does not exclude the possibility of ischemic colitis,[39] and although irreversible colitis has been found to occur more frequently with the occlusive variety, the presence or absence of occlusions does not always predict whether gangrene of the colon will eventually occur.[71]

References

1. Aakhus, T., and Brabrand, G.: Angiography in acute superior mesenteric arterial insufficiency. Acta Radiol. 6:1–12, 1967.
2. Barakat, M., Mahmoud, J., and Bentlif, P. S.: Celiac-axis compression syndrome. Am. J. Dig. Dis. 17:373–377, 1972.
3. Bergan, J. J., Dean, R. H., Conn, J., Jr., et al.: Revascularization in treatment of mesenteric infarction. Ann. Surg. 182:430–438, 1975.
4. Bernstein, W. C., and Bernstein, E. F.: Ischemic ulcerative colitis following inferior mesenteric arterial ligation. Dis. Colon Rectum 6:54–61, 1963.
5. Bicks, R. O., Bale, G. F., Howard, H., et al.: Acute and delayed colon ischemia after aortic aneurysm surgery. Arch. Intern. Med. 122:249–253, 1968.
6. Bircher, J., Bartholomew, L. G., Cain, J. C., et al.: Syndrome of intestinal arterial insufficiency ("abdominal angina"). Arch. Intern. Med. 117:632–638, 1966.
7. Boley, S. J., Schwartz, S., Lash, J., et al.: Reversible vascular occlusion of the colon. Surg. Gynecol. Obstet. 116:53–60, 1963.
8. Boley, S. J., and Schwartz, S. S.: Colonic ischemia: reversible ischemic lesions. In Boley, S. J. (ed.): Vascular Disorders of the Intestine. New York, Appleton-Century-Crofts, 1971, pp. 579–596.
9. Boley, S. J., and Veith, F. J.: Effects of bowel distension on intestinal blood flow. In Boley, S. J. (ed.): Vascular Disorders of the Intestine. New York, Appleton-Century-Crofts, 1971, pp. 429–440.
10. Boley, S. J., Sprayregen, S., Veith, F. J., et al.: An aggressive roentgenological and surgical approach to acute mesenteric ischemia. In Nyhus, L. M. (ed.): Surgery Annual. Vol. 5. New York, Appleton-Century-Crofts, 1973, pp. 355–378.
11. Britt, L. G., and Cheek, R. C.: Nonocclusive mesenteric vascular disease: clinical and experimental observations. Ann. Surg. 169:704–711, 1969.
12. Bron, K. M., and Redman, H. C.: Splanchnic artery stenosis and occlusion. Incidence, arteriographic and clinical manifestations. Radiology 92:323–328, 1969.
13. Byrd, B. F., Jr., Sawyers, J. L., Bomar, R. L., et al.: Reversible vascular occlusion of the colon. Ann. Surg. 167:901–908, 1968.
14. Colapinto, R. F., McLoughlin, M. J., and Weisbrod, G. L.: The routine lateral aortogram and the celiac compression syndrome. Radiology 103:557–563, 1972.
15. Cornell, S. H.: Severe stenosis of the celiac artery. Radiology 99:311–316, 1971.
16. Crummy, A. B., Whittaker, W. B., Morrissey, J. F., et al.: Intestinal infarction secondary to retroperitoneal fibrosis. N. Engl. J. Med. 285:28–29, 1971.
17. Danford, R. O.: The splanchnic vasoconstrictive effect of digoxin and its reversal by glucagon. In Boley, S. J. (ed.): Vascular Disorders of the Intestine. New York, Appleton-Century-Crofts, 1971, pp. 421–428.

18. Davis, L. J., Anderson, J., Wallace, S., et al.: Experimental use of prostaglandin E in nonocclusive mesenteric ischemia. Am. J. Roentgenol. *125*:99–110, 1975.
19. Demos, N. J., Bahuth, J. J., and Vines, P. D.: Comparative study of arteriosclerosis in the inferior and superior mesenteric arteries. Ann. Surg. *155*:599–605, 1962.
20. DeVilliers, D. R.: Ischaemia of the colon: an experimental study. Br. J. Surg. *53*:497–503, 1966.
21. Dick, A. P., Graff, R., Gregg, D. McC., et al.: An arteriographic study of mesenteric arterial disease. I. Large vessel changes. Gut *8*:206–220, 1967.
22. Drapanas, T., and Bron, K. M.: Stenosis of the celiac artery. Editorial. Ann. Surg. *164*:1085–1088, 1966.
23. Drummond, H.: Some points relating to the surgical anatomy of the arterial supply of the large intestine. Proc. R. Soc. Med. (Sect. Proct.) *7*:185–193, 1914.
24. Dunbar, J. D., Molnar, W., Beman, F., et al.: Compression of the celiac trunk and abdominal angina. Am. J. Roentgenol. *95*:731–744, 1965.
25. Dunphy, J. E.: Abdominal pain of vascular origin. Am. J. Med. Sci. *192*:109–113, 1936.
26. Evans, W. E.: Long term evaluation of the celiac band syndrome. Surgery *76*:867–871, 1974.
27. Feller, E., Rickert, R., and Spiro, H. M.: Small vessel disease of the gut. In Boley, S. J. (ed.): Vascular Disorders of the Intestine. New York, Appleton-Century-Crofts, 1971, pp. 483–508.
28. Heard, G., Jefferies, J. D., and Peters, D. K.: Chronic intestinal ischemia. Lancet *2*:975–978, 1963.
29. Jackson, B. B.: Occlusion of the Superior Mesenteric Artery. Springfield, Illinois, Charles C Thomas, Publisher, 1963.
30. Joffe, N., Goldman, H., and Antonioli, D. A.: Barium studies in small-bowel infarction. Radiology *123*:303–309, 1977.
31. Kahn, P., and Abrams, H. L.: Inferior mesenteric arterial patterns. An angiographic study. Radiology *82*:429–441, 1964.
32. Kaufman, S. L., Harrington, D. P., and Siegelman, S. S.: Superior mesenteric artery embolization: An angiographic emergency. Radiology *124*:625–630, 1977.
33. Lande, A., and Meyers, M. A.: Iatrogenic embolization of the superior mesenteric artery: arteriographic observations and clinical implications. Am. J. Roentgenol. *126*:822–828, 1976.
34. Lindner, H. H., and Kemprud, E.: A clinico-anatomical study of the arcuate ligament of the diaphragm. Arch. Surg. *103*:600–605, 1971.
35. Lord, R. S. A., Stoney, R. J., and Wylie, E. J.: Coeliac-axis compression. Lancet *2*:795–798, 1968.
36. Marable, S. A., Molnar, W., and Beman, F.: Abdominal pain secondary to celiac axis compression. Am. J. Surg. *111*:493–495, 1966.
37. Marshak, R. H., and Lindner, A. E.: Ischemia of the colon. Semin. Roentgenol. *3*:81–93, 1968.
38. Marston, A.: Patterns of intestinal ischemia. Ann. R. Coll. Surg. Engl. *35*:151–181, 1964.
39. Marston, A., Pheils, M. T., Lea-Thomas, M., et al.: Ischaemic colitis. Gut *7*:1–15, 1966.
40. Marston, A.: Acute mesenteric vascular occlusions. In Boley, S. J. (ed.): Vascular Disorders of the Intestine. New York, Appleton-Century-Crofts, 1971, pp. 509–518.
41. Mathews, J. E., and White, R. R.: Primary mesenteric venous occlusive disease. Am. J. Surg. *122*:579–583, 1971.
42. Mavor, G. E., Lyall, A. D., Chrystal, K. M. R., et al.: Mesenteric infarction as a vascular emergency. The clinical problems. Br. J. Surg. *50*:219–225, 1963.
43. McLoughlin, M. J., Colapinto, R. F., and Hobbs, B. B.: Abdominal bruits. Clinical and angiographic correlations. J.A.M.A. *232*:1238–1242, 1975.
44. Meyers, M. A.: Griffiths' point: critical anastomosis at the splenic flexure. Am. J. Roentgenol. *126*:77–94, 1976.
45. Michels, N. A.: Blood supply and anatomy of the upper abdominal organs. Philadelphia, J. B. Lippincott Company, 1955.
46. Mikkelson, W. P.: Intestinal angina. Its surgical significance. Am. J. Surg. *94*:262–269, 1957.
47. Miller, W. T., Scott, J., Rosato, E. F., et al.: Ischemic colitis with gangrene. Radiology *94*:291–297, 1970.
48. Miller, W. T., De Poto, D. W., Scholl, H. W., et al.: Evanescent colitis in the young adult. A new entity? Radiology *100*:71–78, 1971.
49. Morris, G. C., Jr., Crawford, E. S., Cooley, D. A., et al.: Revascularization of the celiac and superior mesenteric arteries. Arch. Surg. *84*:95–107, 1962.
50. Morris, G. C., Jr., De Bakey, M. E., and Bernhard, V.: Abdominal angina. Surg. Clin. North Am. *46*:919–930, 1966.
51. Moskowitz, M., Zimmerman, H., and Felson, B.: The meandering mesenteric artery of the colon. Am. J. Roentgenol. *92*:1088–1099, 1964.
52. Naitove, A., and Weisman, R. E.: Primary mesenteric venous thrombosis. Ann. Surg. *161*:516–523, 1965.
53. Nelson, S. W., and Eggleston, W.: Findings on plain roentgenograms of the abdomen associated with mesenteric vascular occlusion with a possible new sign of mesenteric venous thrombosis. Am. J. Roentgenol. *83*:886–894, 1960.
54. Ottinger, L. W., and Austen, W. G.: A study of 136 patients with mesenteric infarction. Surg. Gynecol. Obstet. *124*:251–261, 1967.
55. Pierce, G. E., and Brockenbrough, E. C.: The spectrum of mesenteric infarction. Am. J. Surg. *119*:233–239, 1970.
56. Price, W. E., Rohrer, G. V., and Jacobson, E. D.: Mesenteric vascular disease. Editorial. Gastroenterology *57*:599–604, 1969.

57. Reiner, L., Jimenez, F. A., and Rodriguez, F. L.: Atherosclerosis in the mesenteric circulation. Observations and correlations with aortic and coronary atherosclerosis. Am. Heart J. 66:200–209, 1963.
58. Reuter, S. R., Kanter, I. E., and Redman, H. C.: Angiography in reversible colonic ischemia. Radiology 97:371–375, 1970.
59. Rigler, L. G., and Pogue, W. L.: Roentgen signs of intestinal necrosis. Am. J. Roentgenol. 94:402–409, 1965.
60. Ruzicka, F. F., and Rossi, P.: Normal vascular anatomy of the abdominal viscera. Radiol. Clin. North Am. 8:3–29, 1970.
61. Schwartz, S. S., and Boley, S. J.: Ischemic origin of ulcerative colitis associated with potentially obstructing lesions of the colon. Radiology 102:249–252, 1972.
62. Scott, S. R., Miller, W. T., Urso, M., et al.: Acute mesenteric infarction. Am. J. Roentgenol. 113:269–279, 1971.
63. Shaw, R. S., and Green, T. H.: Massive mesenteric infarction following inferior mesenteric artery ligation in resection of colon for carcinoma. N. Engl. J. Med. 248:890–891, 1953.
64. Siegelman, S. S., Sprayregen, S., and Boley, S. J.: Angiographic diagnosis of mesenteric arterial vasoconstriction. Radiology 112:533–542, 1974.
65. Solheim, K.: Acute intestinal infarction. Acute mesenteric vascular occlusion. Acta Chir. Scand. 126:133–143, 1963.
66. Steward, J. A., and Rankin, F. W.: Blood supply of the large intestine: its surgical considerations. Arch. Surg. 26:843–891, 1933.
67. Szilagyi, D. E., Rian, R. L., Elliott, J. P., et al.: The celiac artery compression syndrome: Does it exist? Surgery 72:849–863, 1972.
68. Tomchick, F. S., Wittenberg, J., and Ottinger, L. W.: The roentgenographic spectrum of bowel infarction. Radiology 96:249–260, 1970.
69. Trinkle, J. K., Rush, B. F., Fullmer, M. A., et al.: The operative management of idiopathic mesenteric venous thrombosis with intestinal infarction. Am. Surg. 35:338–341, 1969.
70. Watt, J. K., Watson, W. C., and Haase, S.: Chronic intestinal ischemia. Br. Med. J. 3:199–202, 1967.
71. Wescott, J. L.: Angiographic demonstration of arterial occlusion in ischemic colitis. Gastroenterology 63:486–490, 1972.
72. Williams, L. F., Jr., Anastasia, L. F., Hasiotis, C. A., et al.: Nonocclusive mesenteric infarction. Am. J. Surg. 114:376–387, 1967.
73. Williams, L. F., Jr., Bosniak, M. A., Wittenberg, J., et al.: Ischemic colitis. Am. J. Surg. 117:255–264, 1959.
74. Williams, L. F., Jr.: Vascular insufficiency of the intestines. Gastroenterology 61:757–777, 1971.
75. Williams, L. F., Jr., and Kim, J-P.: Nonocclusive mesenteric ischemia. In Boley, S. J. (ed.): Vascular Disorders of the Intestine. New York, Appleton-Century-Crofts, 1971, pp. 519–530.
76. Wittenberg, J., Athanasoulis, C. A., Shapiro, J. H., et al.: A radiologic approach to the patient with acute, extensive bowel ischemia. Radiology 106:13–24, 1973.
77. Wittenberg, J., Athanasoulis, C. A., Williams, L. F., Jr., et al.: Ischemic colitis. Radiology and pathophysiology. Am. J. Roentgenol. 123:287–300, 1975.
78. Young, J. R., Humphries, A. W., De Wolfe, U. G., et al.: Complications of abdominal aortic surgery. II. intestinal ischemia. Arch. Surg. 86:51–57, 1963.
79. Zuidema, G. D., Reed, D., Turcotte, J. G., et al.: Superior mesenteric artery embolectomy. Ann. Surg. 159:548–553, 1964.

Part XV

Surgical Renovascular Hypertension

ERICH K. LANG, M.D.

JORGEN U. SCHLEGEL, M.D.

ALAN LIST, M.D.

Reports by Goldblatt and Page identifying a relationship between hypertension and impairment of renal circulation greatly stimulated interest in correctible forms of renal hypertension.[8, 30] Although the term "renovascular hypertension" implies an unequivocal cause-and-effect relationship, renal artery stenosis does not always result in elevation of systemic blood pressure, nor does its surgical correction always relieve associated hypertension.[14] Disillusionment with early surgical results prompted a closer look at the role of the kidney in hypertension. This eventually led to the recognition of the renin-angiotensin system and subsequently to the development of laboratory tests to quantitate its actions, allowing sophisticated assessment of the pathophysiologic cause-and-effect mechanism.[13, 26]

Although definitive data on the prevalence of renovascular hypertension have never been established, most investigators doubt that a renovascular mechanism is responsible for more than 5 per cent of all hypertensive patients.[3, 28] However, despite the low incidence of renovascular hypertension and the complexity of diagnostic investigations necessary to establish this relationship, diagnostic pursuit is justified because of the feasibility of ameliorating or totally relieving such hypertension.

The investigation of renovascular hypertension must include arteriographic documentation of the morphology of a renal artery lesion and physiologic proof of a cause-and-effect relationship between the arterial lesion and the existing hypertension. It must also assess the probability of ameliorating or relieving the hypertension by surgical or medical treatment.[1, 13, 14, 26]

To assure a cost-effective diagnostic approach, patients are selected for a complete work-up by certain clinical and historical criteria, and the investigation is pursued along a sequential protocolized approach.

A diastolic pressure greater than 110 mm of mercury; a clinical history of acute hypertension in patients under 30 or over 60 years of age; a history of accelerated or malignant hypertension; the sudden acceleration of chronic hypertension; hypertension developing after hematuria, acute flank pain, or both, or diastolic hypertension complicated by progressive loss of renal reserve are considered pertinent clinical and historical features justifying investigation of renovascular hypertension.[13] A family history of hypertension is not useful for identifying patients who might benefit from investigation, since such history can be elicited in about 80 per cent of patients with primary hypertension and in about one third of those with renovascular hypertension.[1, 13]

The protocol of sequential diagnostic approach advocates an intravenous urogram, then a detailed study for demonstrating the morphology of the arterial lesion (renal arteriography) and finally physiologic studies to determine the functional significance of the demonstrated lesion and the probability of amelioration by surgical or medical management.[1, 26, 28] Renal vein renin assays have today largely replaced renal function studies as the principal physiologic examination.[26]

The computerized radionuclide urogram is considered a hybrid in this scheme, since it provides both a noninvasive triage examination and definitive physiologic data measuring glomerular filtration rate (GFR), renal plasma flow, (ERPS), and ejection fraction (LVEF) (see references 11, 21, and 23 in the section on the renal urogram, p. 1608).

EXCRETORY UROGRAPHY

The rapid-sequence excretory urogram, performed without the use of abdominal compression but augmented by tomograms, is the recommended screening examination for renovascular hypertension.

Renovascular hypertension may result in the following urographic abnormalities: (1) disparity in renal size, (2) disparity in appearance time of contrast medium, (3) disparity in concentration of contrast medium, (4) prolonged nephrographic stain, (5) disparity in the size of the pyelocalyceal structures of the right and left kidney, and (6) notching of the ureters or pelvis (Figs. 22–125 to 22–127).

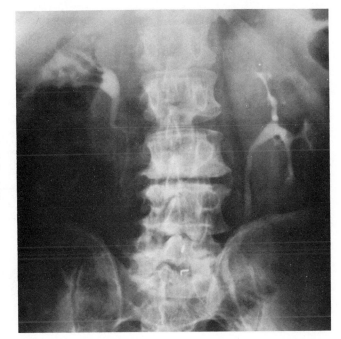

Figure 22–125. RVH. Intravenous pyelogram. Note the disparity in renal size and size of the pyelocalyceal structures. A low urine flow in the ischemic kidney is probably responsible for the small size of the pyelocalyceal structures.

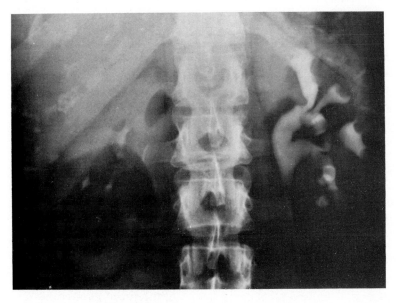

Figure 22–126. RVH. Intravenous pyelogram. The two-minute film of a rapid-sequence excretory urogram demonstrates a marked disparity in the time of appearance of contrast medium. The right kidney is smaller, and the small size of the pyelocalyceal structures reflects a low flow rate.

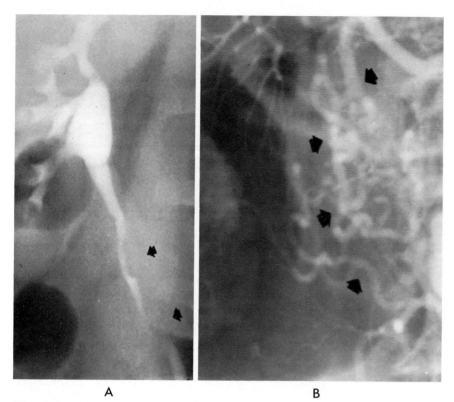

A   B

Figure 22–127. RVH. Intravenous pyelogram and arteriogram. *A,* Note the characteristic notching of the ureter (arrows) indicating the presence of prominent ureteric artery collaterals. *B,* A flush arteriogram demonstrates the extensive collateral network feeding from lumbar arteries via the ureteric artery into the renal artery (arrows). A stenosis at the origin of the renal artery caused the development of this collateral supply. (*From* Lang, E. K.: The arteriographic diagnosis of primary and secondary tumors of the ureter or ureter and renal pelvis. Radiology *93:*799–805, 1969. Reproduced by permission.)

Diminished renal blood flow will eventually cause ischemic atrophy and hence a disparity in renal size. A disparity of 1½ cm or greater in pole-to-pole dimension of the kidneys is generally considered significant. This disparity in size may be expected in about 50 per cent of patients with renovascular hypertension from atheromatous disease and in 80 per cent of those whose condition is due to fibromuscular dysplasia.[13] Significant segmental renal infarction will cause segmental cortical thinning (Fig. 22–128B).[18, 37]

For optimal documentation of disparity in appearance and clearance of contrast medium from the pyelocalyceal system, rapid-sequence filming techniques are advocated. Roentgenograms should be obtained at thirty seconds and at one, two, three, five, ten, fifteen, and thirty minutes after injection of contrast medium; oblique projections are obtained at ten minutes.

Decreased renal blood flow results in a decreased glomerular filtration rate, and hence a delayed appearance of contrast medium on the afflicted side. This is best appreciated on the early-phase roentgenograms (see Fig. 22–125). The nephrographic stain may be prolonged, reflecting decreased renal blood flow, with reduced glomerular filtration rate. Hyperconcentration of contrast medium on later-phase roentgenograms, particularly 15- and 30-minute films, reflects the physiologic response of an ischemic

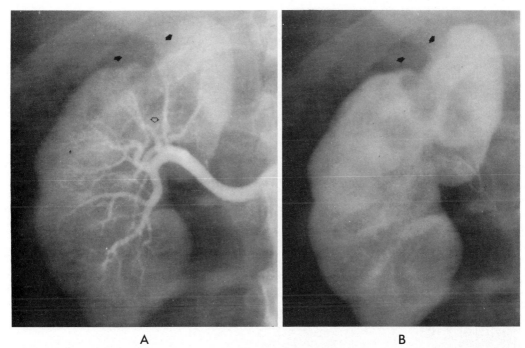

A   B

Figure 22–128.   Renal infarct. *A,* A selective renal arteriogram demonstrates amputation of an interlobar vessel (open arrow). A typical cortical defect has resulted (solid arrows). *B,* The parenchymal phase radiograph demonstrates the classic "bite deformity" of a cortical infarct (solid arrows). (*From* Lang, E. K., Mertz, H. O., and Nourse, M.: Renal arteriography in the assessment of renal infarct. J. Urol. *99:*506–512, 1968. Reproduced by permission.)

kidney to increase sodium and water reabsorption (Howard phenomenon). Retention of contrast medium in the unobstructed pyelocalyceal system is best demonstrated on late-phase roentgenograms (30- and 60-minute films), again indicating a decreased urine flow rate. The often small and spastic appearance of the pyelocalyceal structures is likewise a consequence of greatly reduced flow of urine in the affected kidney (see Fig. 22–126).

The retention of contrast medium in unobstructed pyelocalyceal structures of the afflicted kidney can be enhanced by intravenous infusion of urea or other hypertonic solutions to provoke diuresis. Although the normal kidney responds readily to this stimulus, the ischemic kidney cannot and hence retains more contrast medium in the pyelocalyceal structures (Fig. 22–129).

Notching of the ureter or pelvis reflects the development of arterial collaterals from the ureteral and pelvic vessels (see Fig. 22–127).

The usefulness of the excretory urogram as screening examination for renovascular hypertension was affirmed by the National Cooperative Study.[28] The three major urographic findings, singly or in combination, were present in 78 per cent of the patients with renovascular hypertension versus 11.4 per cent of those with essential hypertension.[1] Delayed appearance time of contrast medium was the most common discriminating abnormality. It was present in 59 per cent of the patients with renovascular hypertension but in only 2 per cent of those with essential hypertension. Disparity in renal length was a finding in 38.6 per cent of patients with renovascular disease versus 5.6 per cent of the patients with essential hypertension.

Notching of the ureter or pelvis was most commonly found with renovascular hypertension secondary to fibromuscular dysplasia.

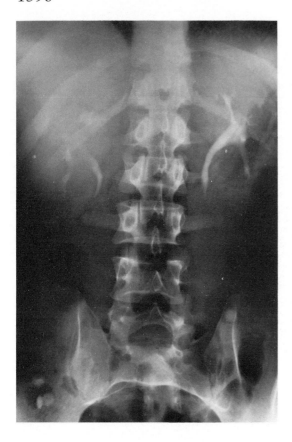

Figure 22–129. Urea washout test. A roentgenogram obtained ten minutes after infusion of urea further accentuates the retention of contrast medium in an otherwise unobstructed pyelocalyceal system of the ischemic kidney.

AORTOGRAPHY AND RENAL ARTERIOGRAPHY

If a renal artery lesion is suspected on the basis of abnormalities on the urogram or computerized radionuclide renogram, arteriography is performed.

Renal hypertension may be caused by a variety of renovascular lesions. Arteriosclerotic lesions are the most common cause (60 per cent of cases).[35] Fibromuscular dysplastic lesions are responsible for about 35 per cent. Renal artery aneurysm, periarteritis nodosa, Takayasu's arteritis, arteriovenous fistula, traumatic arterial occlusion, ureteral obstruction, subcapsular hematoma, and metastatic tumors are less frequent causes of renovascular hypertension.[5, 6, 12, 16, 29–32]

ATHEROSCLEROSIS

Atherosclerotic lesions occur mainly in older patients. Atheromatous disease characteristically involves the proximal third of the renal artery, its orifice, and the aorta itself (Fig. 22–130). Plain films of the abdomen frequently demonstrate calcification in atheromatous plaques of the aorta, but calcifications in plaques in major renal vessels are extremely uncommon. Oblique projections of the aortogram are often necessary to visualize the origin of the renal arteries and to demonstrate encroachment by plaques extending from the aorta into the renal arteries (Fig. 22–131). Selective renal arteriograms show atheromatous plaques as a narrowed segment of the proximal third of the renal artery. Poststenotic dilatation indicates a hemodynamically significant lesion. The

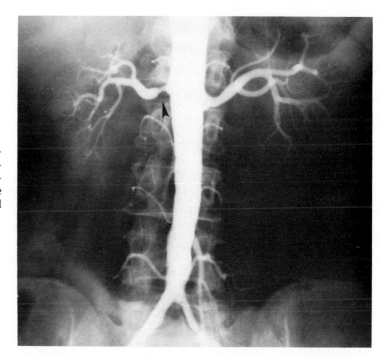

Figure 22–130. RVH. Atherosclerosis. A flush aortogram demonstrates a characteristic arteriosclerotic lesion (arrow) involving the proximal third of the right renal artery.

dilatation is caused by the pressure vector of turbulent flow against a vessel wall, often weakened by degeneration of elastic lamella of its media.

Ninety-five per cent of all atheromatous lesions involve the orifice or the proximal third of the renal arteries or both. Only 5 per cent involve the middle or distal third of the renal artery.

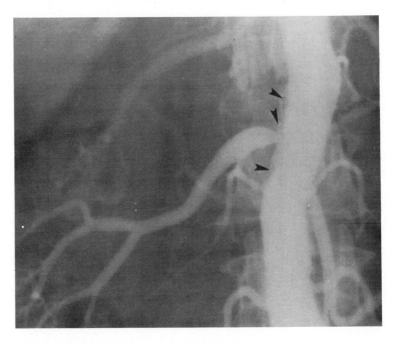

Figure 22–131. RVH. Atherosclerotic plaque. The oblique projection of a flush aortogram best demonstrates a contiguous plaque (arrowheads) extending from the aorta to the renal artery.

Atheromatous disease of the renal arteries progresses in half of the patients. The choice of treatment depends on the age of the patient, the degree of symptomatic cardiovascular disease, and the ability to control hypertension medically.[13]

FIBROMUSCULAR DYSPLASIA

The precise cause of fibromuscular dysplasia remains obscure. Trauma, immunologic injury, and hypermobility of the kidney have been postulated as predisposing factors.[4]

Histologically distinct types of fibromuscular dysplasia have been identified, characterized by involvement of the intima, media, or adventitia. The histologic type can be accurately predicted on the basis of characteristic angiographic criteria (Table 22–2.[11] Most forms of fibromuscular dysplasia show roentgenographic progression.[34] Unlike atheromatous disease, fibromuscular dysplasia predominantly involves the distal two thirds of the main renal artery and less commonly the segmental branches.

Intimal fibroplasia is a rare form characterized pathologically by fibrous proliferation of the intima, which causes a segmental stenotic lesion of the renal artery or its main branches or both.[11] Concentric narrowing of the renal artery is the typical angiographic finding (see Table 22–2).

Medial fibroplasia is the most common lesion, accounting for 60 per cent of all fibromuscular dysplasias.[11] Pathologically, it is characterized by thickened fibromuscular ridges, resulting from the replacement of arterial wall muscle by collagen. Loss of elasticity leads to the formation of mural aneurysms. The serially arranged pseudoaneurysms produce a typical "string of beads" appearance on angiograms (see Table 22–2; Fig. 22–132).

Perimedial fibroplasia is the second most frequent type (20 per cent of cases). Pathologically, this lesion is characterized by fibroplasia involving the outer half of the

TABLE 22–2. PATHOLOGIC RADIOLOGIC CORRELATION OF FIBROMUSCULAR DYSPLASIA

Location and Type	Incidence	Pathologic Findings	Angiographic Findings
Intimal fibroplasia	1%	Intimal fibrous proliferation	Concentric narrowing of involved artery
Media			
Medial fibroplasia	60%	Multifocal stenosis Thickened fibromuscular ridges with intervening mural aneurysms Replacement of smooth muscle with collagen	"String of beads" pattern of involved artery pseudo-aneurysms
Perimedial fibroplasia	20%	Intense fibroplasia of outer half of media	Irregular stenosing lesion, mildly beaded but not aneurysmal (accordion appearance)
Medial hyperplasia	10%	Hyperplasia of smooth muscle without aneurysm formation	Long segment stenosis without aneurysms
Medial dissection	5%	False channel medial to external elastic membrane; fibroplasia	False channel, dissection, and stenosis
Adventitia			
Periarterial fibroplasia	Less than 1%	Collagen and fibroplasia involving adventitia	Long segment tubular or cylindric narrowing of main artery and branches

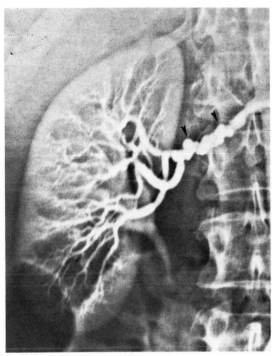

Figure 22–132. RVH. Fibromuscular hyperplasia (medial fibroplasia). The selective arteriogram demonstrates a characteristic "string of beads" appearance of the distal two thirds of the main renal artery (arrowheads). Note such segments of concentric narrowing of subsegmental vessels. The angiographic demonstration of the serially arranged pseudoaneurysms of the distal two thirds of the main renal artery is diagnostic for medial fibroplasia.

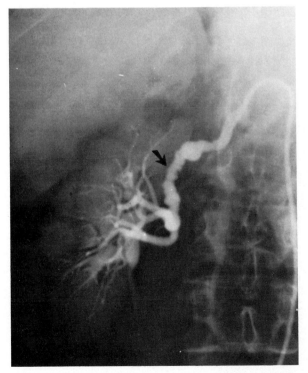

Figure 22–133. RVH. Fibromuscular dysplasia (perimedial fibroplasia). The selective renal arteriogram demonstrates an accordionlike appearance of the distal two thirds of the main renal artery (arrow). The outpouchings are less conspicuous than those associated with medial fibroplasia and no longer suggest aneurysms. The slightly ptotic position of this kidney and the pertinent historical information revealing recent onset of hypertension in this 33-year-old white female establish the diagnosis of perimedial fibroplasia.

media and resulting in an irregular stenosis. Angiographically, this produces an accordion-like appearance of the artery. The outpouchings are less conspicuous than those associated with medial fibroplasia and do not suggest aneurysms (see Table 22–21; Fig. 22–133).

Medial hyperplasia accounts for less than 10 per cent of all fibromuscular dysplasias and histologically appears as a hyperplasia of arterial smooth muscle. On angiograms, this produces a long, smooth stenosis (see Table 22–21; Fig. 22–134).

Medial dissection occurs in about 5 per cent of the fibromuscular dysplasias. A dissecting channel in the outer third of the media but within the external elastic membrane is the characteristic pathologic finding.[11, 36] Fibroplasia of the media predisposes to this complication. Stenosis of a segment of the main renal artery and demonstration of a dissecting aneurysm with a false channel are the angiographic criteria for establishing the diagnosis of medial dissection (see Table 22–21).[11, 31]

Periarterial fibroplasia is a rare lesion involving the adventitia.[11] Fibroplasia and collagen deposits in the periarterial fat and adventitia are the pathologic findings. A tubular stenosis involving a long segment of the main renal artery is seen angiographically.

Aortography and selective renal arteriography are useful to delineate the morphology of a renal artery lesion. If renal vein renin assays and renal function studies confirm the culpability of the arterial lesion, a suitable surgical procedure can be performed.[1, 26] These procedures include prosthetic aortorenal bypass, saphenous vein bypass, patch arterioplasty, endarterectomy, autotransplantation, and in some instances, nephrectomy or heminephrectomy.[13, 15]

Recently,[14a, 25a] successful transluminal dilatation of a narrowed renal artery has been achieved by the use of a Gruntzig catheter. Atherosclerotic stenoses and, occasionally, fibromuscular hyperplasia have responded to this percutaneous catheter technique, with decreased hypertension and fall of renin levels (Fig. 22–135). The permanence of these exciting results has not yet been established.

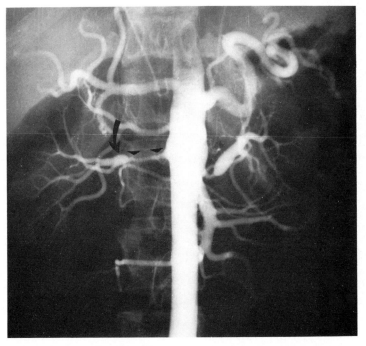

Figure 22–134. RVH. Medial hyperplasia. A flush aortogram demonstrates a characteristic smooth stenosis involving almost the entire main right renal artery (arrowheads). Note a poststenotic dilatation attesting to the hemodynamic significance of this lesion (curved arrow). A similar smooth stenosis, but atypically involving only a short segment, is seen on the left side. Note the normal appearance of the aorta. These angiographic findings suggest medial hyperplasia.

PHARMACOANGIOGRAPHY IN THE ASSESSMENT OF HEMODYNAMICALLY SIGNIFICANT RENAL ARTERY STENOSIS

Recently, criteria for evaluating the hemodynamic significance of renovascular lesions have been developed from pharmacoangiograms.[2] Bookstein proposed intraarterial administration of acetylcholine and epinephrine to manipulate peripheral resistance in the renovascular bed.[2] Redirection of flow in nonparenchymal renal arteries after the reduction of peripheral resistance by acetylcholine has been advocated as a sensitive and specific indication of clinically and hemodynamically significant renal artery stenosis. Conversely, increase of peripheral resistance after the administration of epinephrine will disclose whether there are large collateral vessels capable of providing substantial antegrade collateral blood flow to poststenotic intrarenal vessels (Fig. 22–136).

RENAL ARTERY ANEURYSM

Renal artery aneurysms are responsible for about 2.5 per cent of cases of renovascular hypertension.[36] These aneurysms are discovered during investigation for hypertension.[7, 9]

On the basis of histopathologic criteria, aneurysms can be grouped into true aneurysms, having one or all coats of the arterial wall, and false aneurysms, characterized by a fibrous wall with endothelial lining.

Approximately 17 per cent of renal artery aneurysms are intrarenal and intraparenchymal. Intrarenal aneurysms are of atherosclerotic, traumatic, degenerative, and congenital origin.[24, 32] Polyarteritis nodosa is characterized by a mucoid degeneration of the media of medium-sized arteries, which leads to the formation of multiple, small intrarenal aneurysms.[12, 17]

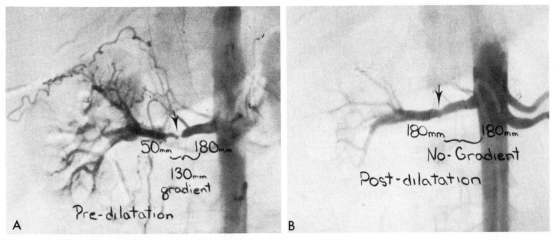

Figure 22–135. Renovascular hypertension: successful catheter dilatation therapy. *A,* Right renal arteriogram of a 48-year-old woman with severe hypertension for eight years shows a severe stenosis (arrow) due to fibromuscular dysplasia. There was a 130 mm Hg gradient across the stenosis. Note the extensive collaterals. *B,* Film made after Grüntzig dilatation shows virtually complete restoration of a normal lumen (arrow), with no gradient. Note the absence of collaterals. The patient became and has remained normotensive. (Courtesy of Audrey R. Wilson, M.D., Philadelphia, Pennsylvania.)

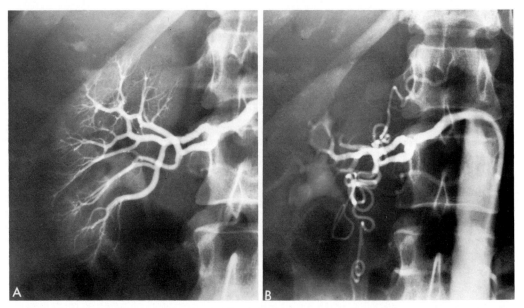

Figure 22–136. RVH. Arteriogram. *A,* The initial arteriogram demonstrates a vague stenosis involving the distal two third of the main renal artery and extending to the subsegmental arteries. *B,* After injection of 3.3 mcg of epinephrine, a large collateral vessel (arrows) is demonstrated, which prior to increasing peripheral resistance in the renovascular bed carried blood to the kidney. (Courtesy of Joseph Bookstein, M.D., San Diego, California.)

Approximately 70 per cent of all renal artery aneurysms are extraparenchymal, located in the main renal artery or at its bifurcation to the segmental vessels. These aneurysms may be degenerative, traumatic, mycotic, or congenital.

Roentgen Diagnosis

The definitive diagnosis of renal artery aneurysm is made by aortography and renal arteriography.

The majority of extraparenchymal renal artery aneurysms show a shell-like calcific shadow on plain films in or near the renal hilus. Urograms obtained in anteroposterior and oblique projections confirm the constant relationship of this crescentic shell-like calcification to the visualized renal pelvis. This finding is helpful in differentiating renal artery aneurysm from calcifications of the splenic, hepatic, or pancreatic arteries, calcified mesenteric nodes or hematomas, calcifications in renal or pancreatic neoplasms and calcifications in old pararenal or tubercular abscesses (Figs. 22–137A and B and 22–138).

The selective renal arteriogram identifies the aneurysm and its morphologic type (saccular or fusiform). Associated changes of the renal artery may give evidence of probable etiology (Fig. 22–137C).

Arteriosclerotic aneurysms are often calcified and saccular. Associated atheromatous disease of the renal arteries is usually demonstrable. Polyarthritis nodosa is characterized by multiple small aneurysms.[12, 17] Aneurysms caused by fibromuscular dysplasias are associated with the other characteristic arteriographic appearance of the latter.[11, 20, 36] These aneurysms are rarely, if ever, calcified.

False aneurysms are most often of traumatic or mycotic origin (Fig. 22–138A). On

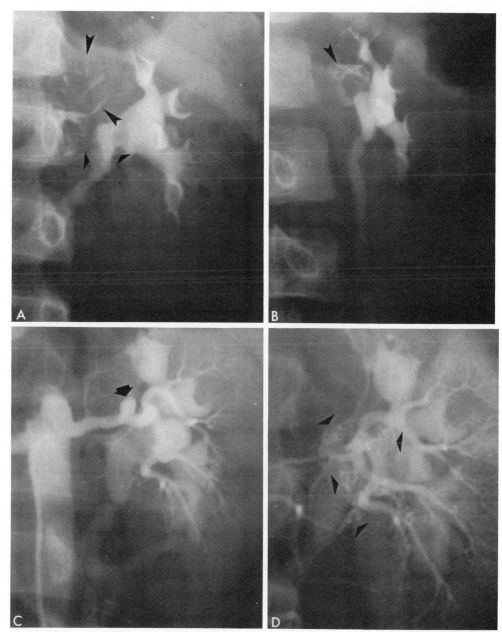

Figure 22–137. Calcified traumatic renal artery aneurysm. A urogram demonstrates shell-like calcifications superior and medial to the kidney pelvis (large arrowhead). Note notching of the pelvis and ureteropelvic junction (small arrowhead). *B,* An oblique projection proves a constant relationship of the crescentic shell-like calcifications (arrowhead) to the visualized renal pelvis in this eight-year-old child. *C,* A selective arteriogram demonstrates a traumatic aneurysm of the main renal artery (arrow). *D,* Late-phase arteriograms demonstrate prominent collaterals causing the previously noted notching of ureteropelvic junction and pelvis (arrowhead). The large, partially thrombosed aneurysm compressed the main renal artery, caused ischemia, and led to the formation of collateral circulation. (Courtesy of J. Schlegel, M.D., and F. Puyau, M.D., New Orleans, Louisiana.)

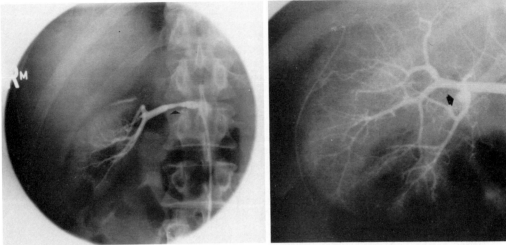

Figure 22–138. *Right,* Aneurysm arising from the subsegmental branch to the lower pole of the right kidney. Note the acute angle formed between the aneurysm sac and the otherwise intact arterial wall. *Left,* Page kidney. The selective arteriogram demonstrates an area of concentric narrowing of the right renal artery, which was caused by an ancient subintimal dissection (arrowhead). A calcific rim within the capsule of the kidney proved to be an ancient calcified subcapsular hematoma. The hypertension is attributed to cortical compression (Page kidney) and to ischemia secondary to the embarrassment of the lumen of the main renal artery.

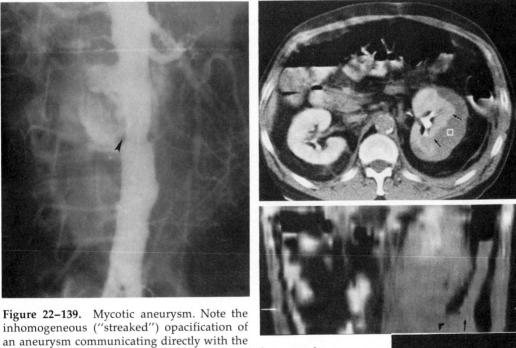

Figure 22–139. Mycotic aneurysm. Note the inhomogeneous ("streaked") opacification of an aneurysm communicating directly with the aorta or the renal artery or both. The acute angle between the aneurysm sac and the arterial lumen (arrowhead) suggests the absence of a true wall and hence a false aneurysm.

Figure 22–139A. *Top,* A computed tomogram demonstrates the extent of a subcapsular hematoma and resultant compression of renal parenchyma (arrows). *Bottom,* A coronal reconstruction of a computed tomogram demonstrates the caudal extension of the hematoma in Gerota's fascia (arrowheads) as well as the extension into the lateral coronal fascial space (long arrows).

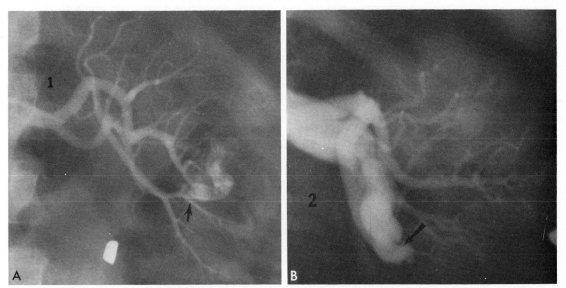

Figure 22–140. RVH. Traumatic pseudoaneurysm. *A,* A selective arteriogram demonstrates the characteristic delayed opacification of a large traumatic pseudoaneurysm (arrow). *B,* The pseudoaneurysm progressed to a huge arteriovenous fistula, (arrow) resulting in renal ischemia and attendant hypertension. (*From* Lang, E. K.: Arteriography in the assessment of renal trauma. J. Trauma *15*:553–566, 1975. Reproduced by permission.)

angiograms they show a characteristic delayed opacification and delayed emptying. Moreover, an acute angle is usually formed by the aneurysm sac and the intact arterial wall (Fig. 22–139).

The hypertension associated with renal artery aneurysm is the result of segmental renal ischemia. This may be caused by compression of a main or segmental renal artery by the aneurysm or compression of parenchyma by a complicating intrarenal or subcapsular hematoma (Fig. 22–139*A*). It may also reflect the hemodynamic disturbance of the renal artery aneurysm itself (Figs. 22–137*D* and 22–140; see Fig. 22–138). Documentation of elevated renal vein renin in samples from the incriminated segmental renal vein proves this cause-and-effect relationship. Demonstration of intrarenal collaterals bypassing the involved segment of artery also indicates the hemodynamic significance of this lesion (see Fig. 22–137*D*).

A calcified saccular aneurysm is less prone to rupture. Parenchymal ischemia and resultant hypertension remain the primary indications for surgical treatment of renal artery aneurysms, rather than the fear of rupture.

RENAL ARTERIOVENOUS FISTULA

Hemodynamically significant arteriovenous fistulas cause ischemia of renal parenchyma by siphoning blood through the fistula and can thus cause hypertension.[22-25]

Renal arteriovenous fistulas can be grouped into congenital, cirsoid, and acquired types. Blunt or penetrating trauma, prior surgery, percutaneous needle biopsy, neoplasia, and rarely, inflammation, are the causes of acquired fistulas.

Clinically significant renal arteriovenous fistulas can produce a classic symptom triad: cardiomegaly, high-output failure resulting in diastolic hypertension, and an abdominal bruit. Diastolic hypertension complicates approximately 50 per cent of all renal arteriovenous fistulas and is due to rerouting of blood flow through the

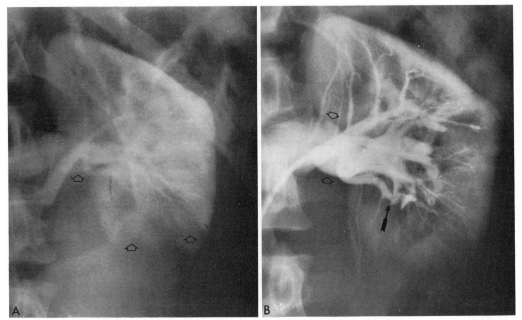

Figure 22–141. RVH. Multiple arteriovenous renal fistulas. *A,* An arteriogram performed hours after a penetrating injury to the lower pole of the left kidney demonstrates lack of parenchymal stain of the lower pole of the left kidney and premature opacification of the renal vein (arrows), indicating the presence of an arteriovenous fistula. *B,* A follow-up arteriogram obtained six weeks later demonstrates multiple traumatic arteriovenous fistulas in the lower pole of the left kidney (small arrow). The marked siphoning effect of the arteriovenous fistula is reflected by decreased staining quality and actual loss of parenchyma of the lower pole of the left kidney. The renal vein is hugely dilated (lucent arrow). Marked hypertension, markedly elevated left renal vein renin levels, and left heart failure attest to the hemodynamic significance of this lesion. (*From* Lang, E. K.: Arteriography in the assessment of renal trauma. J. Trauma 5:553–566, 1975. Reproduced by permission.)

arteriovenous fistula, with attendant reduction of perfusion of renal parenchyma stimulating excess renin release (Fig. 22–141). The resultant ischemic condition of renal parenchyma is also reflected on the radionuclide renogram and causes abnormal divided renal function studies.

Roentgen Diagnosis

The excretory urogram may be normal if the renal arteriovenous fistula is hemodynamically insignificant. A hemodynamically significant arteriovenous fistula results in a poor nephrogram of the afflicted area, occasional delayed appearance of contrast medium, and if long-standing, localized loss of renal parenchyma (Fig. 22–141B).

The renal arteriogram demonstrates premature opacification of the draining vein and, in the presence of a significant shunt, a dilated renal artery and, particularly, a dilated renal vein (see Figs. 22–140B and 22–141B). The volume of parenchyma compromised is indicated by the segment of kidney showing diminished staining quality.[22–25]

A radionuclide renogram can compute the magnitude of the shunt across the arteriovenous fistula.

Small renal arteriovenous fistulas secondary to percutaneous needle biopsy usually close spontaneously.[24, 25]

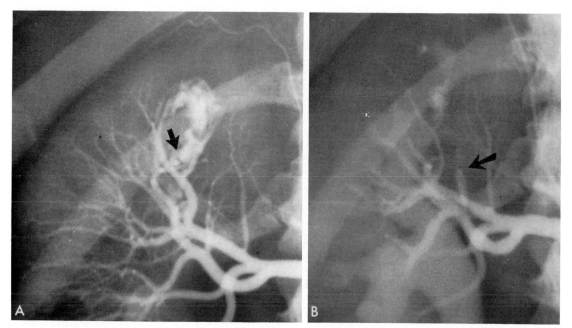

Figure 22–142. Arteriovenous fistula; embolization therapy. *A,* The initial arteriogram demonstrates an arteriovenous fistula in the upper pole of the right kidney (arrow). *B,* The fistula is successfully occluded with Gelfoam (arrow), utilizing a transcatheteral embolization technique. (*From* Lang, E. K.: The role of arteriography in trauma. Radiol. Clin. North Am. *14*:353–370, 1976. Reproduced by permission.)

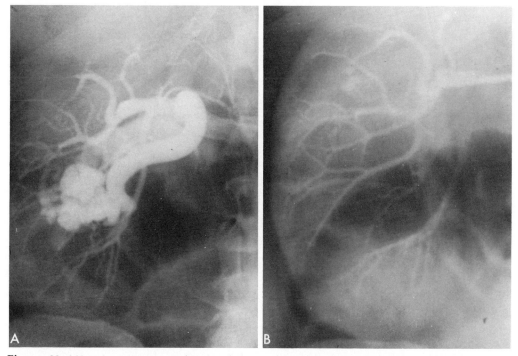

Figure 22–143. Arteriovenous fistula, failure of embolization therapy. *A,* The diagnostic arteriogram demonstrates an enormous arteriovenous fistula in the midportion of the kidney. *B,* Following transcatheter embolization with autologous clot, the fistula is successfully occluded and flow into renal branch vessels and perfusion of renal parenchymal improved.

Selective renal arteriography can serve as a therapeutic procedure, and the arteriovenous fistula can be obliterated by transcatheter embolization.[24, 25] Gelfoam, coiled wire obturators, or autologous muscle are favored as embolic material, since they tend to permanently occlude the arteriovenous fistula (Fig. 22–142).[24, 25] Autologous blood clot temporarily occludes such fistulas, but because of the propensity of lysis of the clot, the fistula may reconstitute within 24 hours (Fig. 22–143). Ligation of the feeding vessel or heminephrectomy are the surgical alternatives.

SEGMENTAL OR MAIN RENAL ARTERY OCCLUSION

Embolic or thrombotic occlusion of a segmental renal artery can produce hypertension, particularly if an ischemic milieu is accentuated by inadequate collateral supply to the segment. Rheumatic heart disease, subacute bacterial endocarditis, myocardial infarction, and cardiac arrhythmias are the most common conditions predisposing to embolization of the renovascular bed.[18]

Subintimal tears of the main or segmental renal arteries secondary to blunt trauma may similarly reduce flow and cause relative ischemia of renal parenchyma (Fig. 22–144, see Fig. 22–138).[22–25]

Clinically, acute occlusion of a branch or of the main renal artery is characterized by sudden, severe flank pain, nausea, fever, leukocytosis, and hematuria. Hypertension develops if some perfusion — antegrade, or collateral — of the compromised renal parenchyma is maintained.

On the intravenous urogram, a segmental ischemic process is reflected by segmental nonfunction or decreased nephrographic stain of the affected segment of the kidney

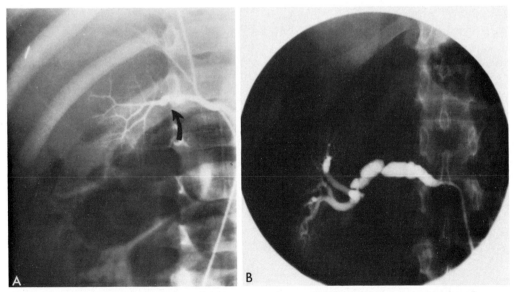

Figure 22–144. Intimal tear; thrombi in two patients. *A,* The selective arteriogram demonstrates the characteristic irregularity of the lumen of the renal artery caused by intimal tear and subintimal clots (arrow). *B,* A selective arteriogram of the right renal artery demonstrates a beaded appearance similar to that seen with medial fibroplasia. In this patient, however, it represents the end stage of traumatic intimal tears and the consequences of healing without surgical repair. Hypertension developed in the six years following the injury.

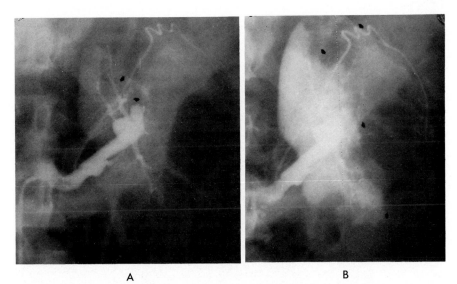

A   B

Figure 22–145. *A,* Only one of the major segmental branches of the left renal artery remains patent; note the fusiform dilatation of the occluded segment of the other main branch (arrowhead), indicating thrombosis. *B,* A later phase film demonstrates staining of viable parenchyma (arrowheads). There is attempt of collateral supply to the cortex via perforating branches from a dilated capsular artery (uppermost arrowhead). This may intensify renin release, since severely ischemic conditions prevail in cortical segments supplied only via these collaterals. (*From* Lang, E. K.: Arteriographic diagnosis of renal infarct. Radiology *88*:1110–1116, 1967. Reproduced by permission.)

and delayed appearance of contrast medium. The retrograde pyelogram is normal. The renal arteriogram can demonstrate the location of the segmental occlusion and, in most instances, differentiate thrombosis from embolization (Fig. 22–145).[19, 24, 25]

Subintimal tears of the artery and attendant thrombosis of segmental renal arteries are readily identified on renal arteriograms (see Fig. 22–144B). Early surgical intervention is indicated, and repair of the intimal tear and evacuation of subintimal clots usually correct this condition.[24, 25]

Segmental renal vein thrombosis can also cause delay in transit of contrast medium and blood through the affected area. This again creates an ischemic condition, which may cause excessive release of renin and consequent hypertension. On renal arteriograms, the delayed transit of contrast medium is reflected by stasis of contrast medium in the intralobar arteries which appear to be stretched and separated by parenchymal edema. A significant decrease in cortical opacification reflects the poor flow through the arcade and intralobular arteries. In the healing phase, the venous circulation is augmented by collateral circulation via the cortical veins to the retroperitoneal veins. The kidney may have sustained parenchymal loss, but at this time, residual parenchyma and vascular supply may be balanced, and hence parenchymal ischemia may no longer exist.

Persistent or increasing renovascular hypertension following apparently successful revascularization procedures is sometimes due to inadvertent occlusion of renal branch vessels. Accessory polar vessels or vessels arising from the main renal artery at an unusual point or angle are particularly vulnerable to inadvertent severance during an attempt to endarterectomize atheromatous plaques in the main renal artery or to establish a prosthetic aorta renal bypass (Fig. 22–146).[21]

Text continued on page 1606

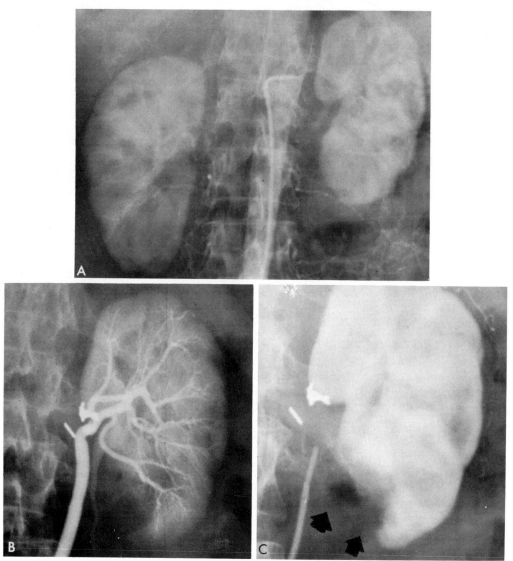

Figure 22–146. Iatrogenic infarction. *A,* The initial flush aortogram demonstrates disparity in the size of the kidneys but otherwise equal parenchymal staining quality. *B,* An area of significantly decreased stain of the medial lower pole of the left kidney is noted on the postoperative selective arteriogram assessing patency of a prosthetic aortorenal bypass. The hypertension intensified several days after the aortorenal bypass procedure. *C,* The parenchymal phase demonstrates a typical area of infarction (arrows) involving the medial lower pole of the left kidney. Inadvertent ligation of a branch supplying this segment of the kidney during the aortorenal bypass procedure caused infarction. (*From* Lang, E. K.: Renal infarction as cause of hypertension developing in patients after corrective surgery for renal artery stenosis. Radiology *92*:984–988, 1969. Reproduced by permission.)

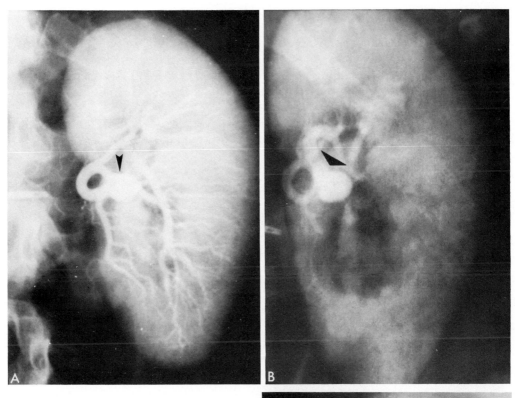

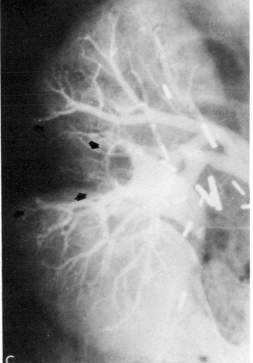

Figure 22–147. Intrarenal aneurysm. *A* and *B,* Selective arteriograms of the left renal artery recorded in the anteroposterior and left posterior oblique projections demonstrate an intrarenal artery aneurysm originating from the branch supplying the posterior upper two thirds of the left kidney (arrowhead). *C,* Postoperative intrarenal aneurysm resection. A postoperative arteriogram demonstrates a small wedged-shaped segment of parenchyma (arrowheads) deprived of perfusion. An intrarenal aneurysm originating from the posterior upper two thirds segmental branch was resected during bench surgery and the kidney reimplanted in the right half of the pelvis. Hypertensive blood pressure levels normalized immediately after surgery.

AORTIC ANEURYSMS INVOLVING THE RENAL ARTERIES

Dissecting aneurysms of the aorta may involve the origin of abdominal vessels and embarrass the blood supply to the respective organs. Dissecting aneurysms of arteriosclerotic, traumatic, and luetic cause can involve the origin of the renal arteries and the dissection may extend into the renal arteries (Fig. 22–147). Resultant compression of the renal arteries and reduction in blood flow cause ischemic conditions of renal parenchyma and attendant hypertension.

Mycotic aneurysms of the aorta or renal arteries may similarly cause ischemia of renal parenchyma and attendant hypertension (see Fig. 22–139).

MISCELLANEOUS ARTERITIDES

Primary arteritis of the aorta, Takayasu's syndrome, and panaortitis are vascular disturbances with a possible autoimmune etiology.[4, 15, 16] Vasculitis following renal transplant can create a stenosis of the main renal artery, causing parenchymal ischemia and hypertension.

NEUROFIBROMATOSIS

Neuroectodermal disorders, such as neurofibromatosis, may involve the abdominal aorta and renal arteries.[10] Resultant stenosis may cause severe hypertension (Fig. 22–148). On arteriograms, this lesion is characterized by high-grade arterial stenosis and large aneurysmal segments.[10]

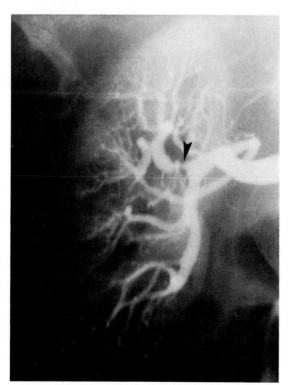

Figure 22–148. Intrarenal artery stenosis. A selective arteriogram demonstrates a classic stenosis of the intrarenal branch supplying the upper posterior two thirds of the right kidney (arrowhead). A poststenotic dilatation suggests the hemodynamic significance of this lesion.

References

1. Bookstein, J. J., Abrams, H. L., Buenger, R. E., et al.: Radiologic aspects of renovascular hypertension. Part 2. The role of urography in unilateral renovascular disease. J.A.M.A. 220:1225–1229, 1972.
2. Bookstein, J. J., Walter, T. F., Stanley, T. C., et al.: Pharmacoangiographic manipulation of renal collateral blood flow. Circulation 54:328–334, 1976.
3. Correa, R. J., Jr., Conway, J., Hoobler, S. W., et al.: Renal-vascular disease as a cause of hypertension: selection of patients for aortographic studies. J. Mich. Med. Soc. 61:1361–1363, 1962.
4. Dornfeld, L., and Kaufman, J. J.: Immunologic considerations in renovascular hypertension. Urol. Clin. North Am. 2:285–300, 1975.
5. Dornfeld, L., Lecky, J. W., and Peter, J. B.: Polyarteritis and intrarenal renal artery aneurysms. J.A.M.A. 215:1950–1952, 1971.
6. Garrett, J., Polse, S. L., and Morrow, J. W.: Ureteral obstruction and hypertension. Am. J. Med. 49:271–273, 1970.
7. Glass, P. M., and Uson, A. C.: Aneurysms of the renal artery. A study of 20 cases. J. Urol. 98:285–292, 1967.
8. Goldblatt, H., Lynch, J., Hanzal, R. F., et al.: Studies on experimental hypertension. I. The production of persistent elevation of systolic blood pressure by means of renal ischemia. J. Exper. Med. 59:347–379, 1934.
9. Grossman, R. E., and Babbitt, D. P.: Renal artery aneurysms: their diagnosis and endocrine implications: a case report in a child. J. Urol. 97:172–175, 1967.
10. Halpern, M., and Currarino, G.: Vascular lesions causing hypertension in neurofibromatosis. N. Engl. J. Med. 273:248–252, 1965.
11. Harrison, E. G., Jr., Hunt, J. C., and Bernatz, P. E.: Morphology of fibromuscular dysplasia of the renal artery in renovascular hypertension. Am. J. Med. 43:97–112, 1967.
12. Horner, B. A., Hunt, J. C., Kincaid, O. W., et al.: Perirenal hematoma secondary to intrarenal microaneurysms of periarteritis nodosa demonstrated radiographically. Mayo Clin. Proc. 41:169–178, 1966.
13. Hunt, J. C., and Strong, C. G.: Renovascular hypertension: mechanisms, natural history and treatment. In Laragh, J. H.: Hypertension Manual: Mechanisms, Methods, Management. New York, Yorke Medical Books, 1974.
14. Kaplan, N. M.: Renin profiles: the unfulfilled promises. J.A.M.A. 238:611–613, 1977.
14a. Katzen, B. T., Chang, J., et al.: Percutaneous transluminal angioplasty for treatment of renovascular hypertension. Radiology 131:53–58, 1979.
15. Kaufman, J. J.: The middle aortic syndrome: report of a case treated by renal autotransplantation. J. Urol. 109:711–715, 1973.
16. Lande, A., and Gross, A.: Total aortography in the diagnosis of Takayasu's arteritis. Am. J. Roentgenol. 116:165–172, 1972.
17. Lang, E. K.: Arteriographic diagnosis of periarteritis nodosa. J. Ind. St. Med. Assoc. 60:928, 1967.
18. Lang, E. K.: Arteriographic diagnosis of renal infarcts. Radiology 88:1110–1116, 1967.
19. Lang, E. K., Mertz, J. H. O., and Nourse, M.: Renal arteriography in the assessment of renal infarct. J. Urol. 99:506–512, 1968.
20. Lang, E. K.: Fibromuscular hyperplasia of the renal artery. J. La. St. Med. Soc. 120:400–401, 1968.
21. Lang, E. K.: Renal infarction as cause of hypertension developing in patients after corrective surgery for renal artery stenosis. Radiology 92:984–988, 1969.
22. Lang, E. K., Trichel, B. E., Turner, R. W., et al.: Renal arteriography in the assessment of renal trauma. Radiology 98:103–112, 1971.
23. Lang, E. K.: Arteriographic assessment of traumatic injury to the kidney: an analysis of 74 patients. J. Urol. 106:1–8, 1971.
24. Lang, E. K.: Arteriography in the assessment of renal trauma. J. Trauma 15:553–566, 1975.
25. Lang, E. K.: The role of arteriography in trauma. Radiol. Clin. North Am. 14:353–370, 1976.
25a. Mahler, F., Krneta, A., et al.: Treatment of renovascular hypertension by transluminal renal artery dilatation. Ann. Intern. Med. 90:56–57, 1979.
26. Marks, L. S., Maxwell, M. H., Varady, P. D., et al.: Renovascular hypertension: Does the renal vein renin ratio predict operative results? J. Urol. 115:365–368, 1976.
27. Massumi, R. A., Andrade, A., and Kramer, N.: Arterial hypertension in traumatic subcapsular perirenal hematoma (Page kidney): evidence for renal ischemia. Am. J. Med. 46:635–639, 1969.
28. Maxwell, M. H., Bleifer, K. H., Franklin, S. S., et al.: Demographic analysis of the study (Cooperative Study of Renovascular Hypertension). J.A.M.A. 220:1195–1204, 1972.
29. O'Dea, M. J., Malek, R. S., Tucker, R. M., et al.: Renal vein thrombosis. J. Urol. 116:410–414, 1976.
30. Page, I. H.: The production of persistent arterial hypertension by cellophane perinephritis. J.A.M.A. 113:2046–2048, 1939.
31. Perry, M. O.: Hypertension and dissecting aneurysm of the renal artery. Arch. Surg. 102:216–217, 1971.
32. Poutasse, E. F.: Renal artery aneurysms. J. Urol. 113:443–449, 1975.
33. Puppel, A. D., and Alyea, E. P.: Hypertension and the surgical kidney. J. Urol. 67:433–440, 1952.

34. Sheps, S. G., Kincaid, O. W., and Hunt, J. C.: Serial renal function and angiographic observations in idiopathic fibrous and fibromuscular stenoses of the renal arteries. Am. J. Cardiol. 30:55–60, 1972.
35. Simon, N., Franklin, S. S., Bleifer, K. H., et al.: Clinical characteristics of renovascular hypertension (Cooperative Study of Renovascular Hypertension). J.A.M.A. 220:1209–1218, 1972.
36. Stanley, J. C., Rhodes, E. L., Gewertz, B. L., et al.: Renal artery aneurysms: significance of macroaneurysms exclusive of dissections and fibrodysplastic mural dilations. Arch. Surg. 110:1327–1333, 1975.
37. Teplick, J. G., and Yarrow, M. W.: Arterial infarction of the kidney. Ann. Int. Med. 42:1041–1051, 1955.

Radionuclide Urogram

The impressive results obtained by surgical therapy in cases of renovascular hypertension make early diagnosis imperative. Patients identified by a simple screening technique are then examined by more invasive diagnostic modalities. Although the cooperative study of renovascular hypertension by the National Heart Institute reported disappointing results for radiorenography, recent technical advances appear to have established the radionuclide urogram as an important screening procedure.[11] Use of the gamma scintillation camera has greatly facilitated quantitation and compartmental analysis and has enhanced the capability of diagnosing segmental renal artery lesions.[2, 23] Wang emphasized the improved correlation between the regional, as opposed to the conventional, renogram and the renal arteriogram.[21]

The 131-iodine–labeled Hippuran renogram and its detailed compartmental analysis form the basis for the radionuclide screening work-up of patients suspected of renovascular hypertension.[3, 14]

THE RADIO-HIPPURAN RENOGRAM

Despite an approximate 13 per cent incidence of false negative results and a 16 per cent rate of false positive results, the radio-Hippuran renogram remains the most suitable noninvasive modality for screening of renovascular hypertension.[8, 12]

Physiologic Basis

The radio-Hippuran renogram examines a complex system reflecting renal function. Hippuran and PAH share the same tubular transport system and are extracted and excreted by the kidney with equal efficiency. The clearance of Hippuran therefore reflects renal functional abnormalities. The disappearance of 131-iodine Hippuran from plasma is attributable to two kinds of compartmental loss, one of which is biliary and urinary excretion and the other, dissipation into the extracellular fluid space.[2] Although instrumentation and the resultant geometry would seem to be of paramount importance in creating a reproducible renogram curve, physiologic factors, such as tubular cell accumulation of Hippuran, glomerular filtration rate, urine concentration, urine flow rate, and renal blood flow, are the major determinants.[20]

The 131-iodo-Hippuran renogram can be divided into three phases.[2, 3, 22–24] The first phase depicts a rapidly rising count rate corresponding largely to the intravascular radioactivity detectable over any region of the body within the first minute following intravenous injection of 131-iodo-Hippuran (Fig. 22–149). Tracing obtained following

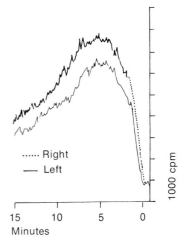

Figure 22–149. A Hippuran renogram recorded by two matched sodium iodide scintillation detectors demonstrates a rapid rise in count rate in the first minute after injection. This corresponds to intravascular radioactivity. The second phase of the renogram shows a more gradual rise in count rate, the peak reached 2.5 to 4.5 minutes after the injection. The segment of declining amplitude represents the third phase of the renogram.

the injection of 131-iodinated albumin in patients with unilateral nephrectomy proved that the deflection of the first phase is almost exclusively due to extrarenovascular radioactivity. In fact, only 16 per cent of the renogram amplitude is assignable to intrarenovascular radioactivity.[22] Even in the first phase of the 131-iodo-Hippuran renogram, 50 per cent of the total count rate caused by intrarenal radioactivity is a consequence of secretion, glomerular filtration, and urinary concentration of 131-iodo-Hippuran.[22, 24]

The second phase of the 131-iodo-Hippuran renogram is characterized by a more gradual rise in the count rate. In a normal well-hydrated subject the peak occurs two and one-half to four and one-half minutes after injection (see Fig. 22–149).[2, 23] While a significant component of the amplitude of the first phase reflects intracellular accumulation of Hippuran, specifically in the cells of the proximal tubules, the radioactivity recorded in the second phase is largely attributable to concentration of 131-iodo-Hippuran within the tubular urine. It is therefore significantly influenced by the rate at which urine is removed from the field of radiation detection.[24]

The segment of declining amplitude is the third phase of the renogram. In normal subjects the third phase levels near the baseline about 20 minutes after the injection.

The count rates achievable during the renogram are a function of the amount of 131-iodo-Hippuran injected and the magnitude of its distribution. The ever-changing blood concentration reflects the equilibration between the extracellular space and the blood, modified by the renal and biliary excretion of Hippuran.[2] The variable nature of the constituents producing the renogram curve defies a precise correlation to physiologic events.[23] However, the propensity for competitive inhibition of tubular transport of Hippuran by massive loading with PAH or nonradioactive Hippuran allows almost selective study of glomerular filtration. The renogram recorded under conditions of competitive blocking of tubular transport functions with nonradioactive Hippuran or PAH indicates the glomerular filtration.[2]

THE RADIO-HIPPURAN RENOGRAM IN RENAL HYPERTENSION

Normal renal function depends upon the maintenance of specific perfusion rates of different zones within the kidney. The ability of the kidney to concentrate urine in turn depends upon the development of a hypertonic medullary interstitium that provides a gradient between the fluid in the collecting ducts and the medulla. Reabsorption of water from the collecting ducts is based upon this gradient.[14] To maintain a hypertonic medullary interstitium the blood flow to this region must be considerably lower per unit of tissue mass than to the renal cortex.[9, 14]

Early hypertensive nephropathy is characterized pathologically by a mild to moderate intimal proliferation or subintimal hyalin deposition associated with medial hypertrophy of arterioles. This causes a reduction in perfusion which is, however, uneven, affecting the cortex more severely than the medulla. Since the glomerular filtration rate is generally lower in outer cortical nephrons than in juxtamedullary nephrons, the glomerular filtration rate is maintained better than the overall renal blood flow, causing an apparent increase in the filtration fraction.[6, 17] Radioactive xenon washout studies document the patchy and uneven cortical perfusion in patients with nephrosclerosis (Fig. 22–150).

Malignant nephrosclerosis is characterized pathologically by a necrotizing arteriolitis with intense and widespread subintimal hyalinization and intimal thickening of arterioles. At this point there is significant reduction in mean blood flow, resulting in a marked reduction in PAH extraction. Reduced renal plasma flow is reflected on the radionuclide urogram by a decreased amplitude of the renogram peak, flattened up-and-down slopes, and delayed peak (Fig. 22–151).[23] Severe decrease of renal function results in a flat curve.

Main or segmental renal artery stenosis of less than 80 per cent reduction in vessel cross section is not likely to cause detectable renogram changes.[2] A significant main renal artery stenosis causes diminution of the initial rise, flattening of the up slope, and a delayed peak of the radionuclide urogram curve similar to the one seen in advanced nephrosclerosis. However, despite the flattening of the up slope, delayed peak, and

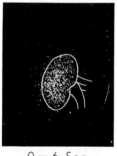

0 — 6 Sec

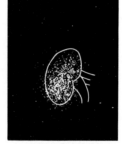

6 — 14 Sec

Figure 22–150. Patchy and uneven cortical washout of radioactive xenon indicates nephrosclerosis.

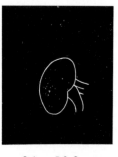

34 — 50 Sec

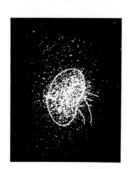

100 — 200 Sec

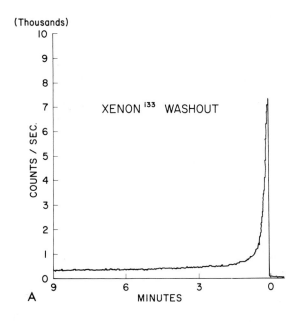

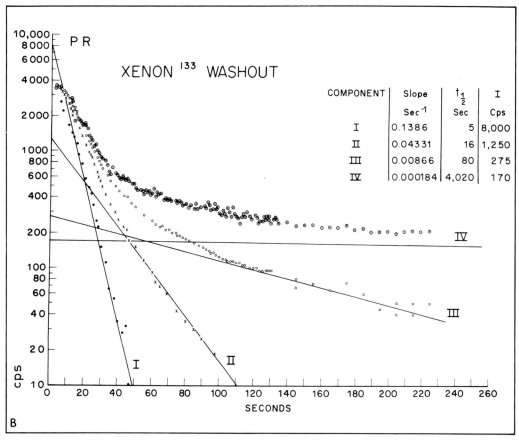

Figure 22–151. *A* and *B,* The radionuclide renogram demonstrates a decreased amplitude of the peak, flattening of the up and down slopes, and a delayed peak. The findings are compatible with the diagnosis of nephrosclerosis.

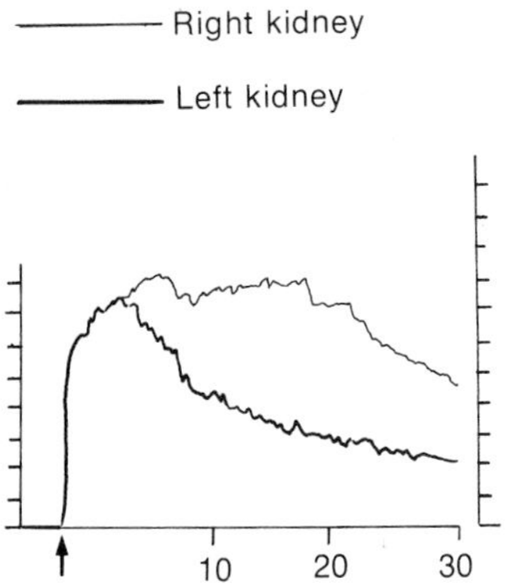

——————— Right kidney

——————— Left kidney

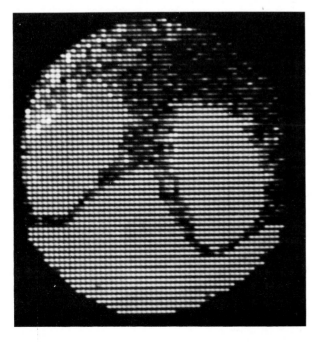

10   20   30

Figure 22–152. Seemingly paradoxic findings of flattening of the up slope—a delayed peak and yet a peak amplitude exceeding that of the normal kidney—is explained by slowed urine flow on the affected side. Increased concentration of the radioactive material is due to water reabsorption and a resulting disproportionately higher count rate over the affected side.

slowed parenchymal clearance, the peak amplitude of the affected side may exceed the peak amplitude of the normal kidney (Fig. 22–152). This seemingly paradoxic response is caused by the increased concentration and slowed urine flow on the affected side, resulting in a disproportionately higher count rate.

Because of the similarity of ^{131}I-Hippuran curves resulting from hemodynamically significant stenotic lesions of the main renal artery and arteriolonephrosclerosis, xenon-133 washout studies may be necessary to differentiate these lesions.

THE COMPUTERIZED RADIONUCLIDE UROGRAM

Data processing of radiotechnetium perfusion studies of the kidney was first advocated by Rosenthall.[14] This technique provided more sensitive criteria than the rapid-sequence hypertensive intravenous urogram and the conventional 131-I Hippuran renogram expressed as a curve and collected via paired external scintillation detectors. Keane and Schlegel have further improved the data handling process, so that

Figure 22–153. Demonstration of electronic tagging one to two minutes following the injection of ^{131}I-Hippuran of both kidneys and background.

effective renal plasma flow, filtration rates, glomerular filtration, and filtration fractions can be determined.[7, 15-17, 19] This sophisticated analysis not only improves the diagnostic accuracy of renovascular hypertensive disease but also introduces criteria that allow the probable outcome of corrective surgery to be predicted.[15, 17]

Technique of the Computerized Radionuclide Urogram

The renal uptake of radio-Hippuran is computed from data gathered during the 1- to 2-minute interval after a rapid injection of 131-iodo-Hippuran. During this interval the bolus of radioactivity will have cleared the liver, spleen, and great vessels, and radioactivity will not yet be present in the urine in the renal pelvis and ureters (Fig. 22–153).

The data are collected by a gamma camera placed under a supine patient. The actual radioactivity present in the kidney is computed by subtraction of the background (counts obtained over the pelvic area) and correction for the depth of the kidney occasioning absorption of radionuclide emissions by interposed tissue and attenuation due to geometric factors.

The computed renal uptake of radio-Hippuran can be equated to renal blood flow by utilizing Norman's regression equation (Fig. 22–154).[13, 16, 19, 20]

$$(13.7 \times \frac{\text{weight}}{\text{height}} + 0.5)$$

Moreover, a linear relationship of radio-Hippuran return to para-aminohippurate clearance has been established.[2, 7] On basis of empirical experience an equation with standard correction factor was developed, permitting computation of a prediction of the excretion of radio-Hippuran in the urine at 30 minutes from the corrected uptake of radio-Hippuran in the kidney at one to two minutes (see Fig. 22–154).[15, 16]

The filtration fraction can be calculated by dividing the uptake of a technetium-labeled compound, presumably handled exclusively by glomerular filtration, by the uptake of 131-iodinated Hippuran.

Criteria of the Computerized Radionuclide Urogram for Diagnosis and Prognostication of Renovascular Hypertension

A delay in the peak as well as a prolonged plateau of high count rates over one kidney are criteria suggesting unilateral renovascular disease responsible for renovascular hypertension. Documentation of a "normal total return" (68 per cent or greater) indicates a normal contralateral kidney that has undergone compensatory hypertrophy

Figure 22–154. The calculation of corrected uptake (Uptake C) is based upon the one to two minute renal count with background subtraction multiplied with the estimated renal depth, which is calculated by the patient's weight and height. This divided by the count of the syringe containing the injected radionuclide times 100 represents the "Uptake C" (see text).

$$\text{UPTAKE } C = \frac{1\text{–}2 \text{ minute kidney count (less background)} \times Y^2}{1 \text{ minute count of radionuclide injected}} \times 100$$

$$Y = \text{Kidney depth in cm} = 13.25 \, x + 0.7$$

$$x = \frac{\text{Weight in kg}}{\text{Height in cm}}$$

Formula for the calculation of renal uptake.

and hence a good probability of favorable response to surgery (Figs. 22–155 and 22–156). Conversely, if the computerized radionuclide urogram identifies a renal artery stenosis on one side but absence of compensatory hypertrophy of the contralateral kidney, parenchymal renal disease or arteriolonephrosclerosis of the "good" kidney must be suspected. In this case, a good prognosis for surgery can no longer be made.[15, 16] The dependence on identifying compensatory hypertrophy of the contralateral kidney for predicting response to surgery militates against the use of the computerized radionuclide urogram in the assessment of bilateral renal artery stenosis. Prediction of prognosis of such patients must rest on combined evaluation of renal vein renin, urine osmolality, and renal angiography.[1]

The computerized radionuclide urogram has been found sensitive for assessment of renovascular hypertension, and in an initial series Keane recorded no false negative results.[7] Although the rate of false positive findings has been reported to be as high as 27 per cent, this does not diminish the screening value of the technique, since further examinations can then be added to confirm the diagnosis.[1, 4, 10, 18]

Although the sensitivity of the computerized 131-iodine Hippuran study in the detection of renovascular hypertension has been reported as excellent, a repeat study

```
NAME: S.T.              DATE:  6/ 21/ 78    AGE: 60     PATIENT NO.      13203
STATE OF HYDRATION:HYDRATED       BLOOD PRESSURE:   150/  100
INJECTED: 131-I HIPPUTOPE(314   UCI)   42543 COUNTS     HEIGHT(CM): 159.00
WEIGHT(KG):  61.60     BSA: 1.6328     TAPE NO.   94


CHANNELS:   R =   286     L =   263     T =   549     B =   317

                 RIGHT                      LEFT
     TIME     COUNTS       %          COUNTS       %

     0 -- 1    1217       47           1331       52
     1 -- 2    2686       52           2421       47
     2 -- 3    2893       51           2728       48
     3 -- 4    2484       45           2951       54
     4 -- 5    2036       38           3294       61
     5 -- 6    1926       34           3611       65
     6 -- 7    2032       35           3772       64
     7 -- 8    1858       31           3960       68
     8 -- 9    1751       31           3877       68
     9 --10    1764       30           3948       69

    15 --16    1336       23           4372       76
    25 --26     704       15           3710       84


TOTAL 1--2 MINUTE COUNTS       5107
RT UPTAKE=       214
LT UPTAKE=       193
TOT UPTAKE=      408

EST RT ERPF=       297
EST LT ERPF=       268
EST TOT ERPF=      565
NORMAL ERPF=       566
NORMAL RETURN= 68%      PREDICTED=        68

TOTAL RETURN AND RESIDUAL URINE
VOIDED      130 ML          RESIDUAL        6 ML
VOIDED      133 UCI          RESIDUAL        7 UCI
VOIDED RET      42 %     RESIDUAL RET        2 %
TOTAL RETURN    45 %
```

Figure 22–155. The "Uptake C" of the right kidney is 214, that of the left is 193, that of both kidneys is 408. The left kidney showed a considerable delay in peak which was reached 26 to 45 minutes after injection, whereas that of the right kidney occurred two to three minutes after injection. These factors suggest a left renal artery stenosis. The normal values obtained from the right kidney indicated a good prognosis from surgery and perhaps the presence of compensatory hypertrophy.

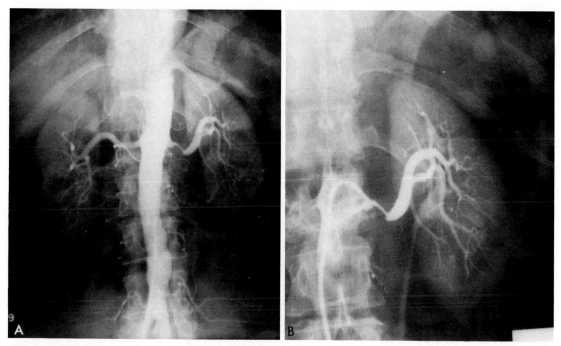

Figure 22–156. *A,* A flush aortogram on the same patient demonstrates a pronounced renal artery stenosis on the left. *B,* A selective left renal arteriogram demonstrates the same lesion, confirming the severity of the renal artery stenosis.

after the patient's blood pressure has been lowered to normotensive levels frequently exaggerates the findings and facilitates recognition of the condition.[10]

References

1. Aguilo-lucia, F., and Serrallach-Mila, N.: The renal blood flow/renal mass relation in renovascular hypertension. Eur. Urol. *4*:81–84, 1978.
2. Blaufox, M. D.: The normal renogram: a compartment analysis of the radiorenogram and kinetics of [131]Hippuran. *In* Blaufox, M. D. (ed.): Progress in Nuclear Medicine. Vol. 2. Baltimore, University Park Press, 1972, pp. 107–124.
3. Brown, N. J. G., and Brittion, K. E.: The theory of renography and analysis of results. *In* Blaufox, M. D., and Funck-Bretano, J.-L. (eds.): Radionuclides in Nephrology, New York, Grune & Stratton, 1972, pp. 315–324.
4. Chisholm, G. C., Short, M. D., and Glass, H. I.: The measurement of individual renal plasma flows using ^{123}I-Hippuran and the gamma camera. Br. J. Urol. *46*:591–600, 1974.
5. Clarke, M. D., Eyler, W. R., Dufault, L. A., et al.: A renogram in hypertension. Radiology *89*:667–675, 1967.
6. Hollenberg, N. K., Epstein, M., Basch, R. I., et al.: No man's land of renal vasculature. An arteriographic and hemodynamic assessment of the interlobar and arcuate arteries in essential and accelerated hypertension. Am. J. Med. *47*:845–854, 1969.
7. Keane, J. M., and Schlegel, J. U.: The use of a scintillation camera system for screening of hypertensive patients. J. Urol. *108*:12–14, 1972.
8. Luke, R. G., Briggs, J. D., Kennedy, A. C., et al.: The radioisotope renogram in the detection and assessment of renal artery stenosis. Q. J. Med. *35*:327–360, 1966.
9. Luke, R. G., Briggs, J. D., Struthers, N. W., et al.: The isotope renogram in renovascular hypertension. *In* Radioisotope in Diagnosis of Diseases of the Kidney, Urinary Tract. Amsterdam, Excerpta Medica Foundation, 1969, pp. 245–248.
10. McAfee, J. G., Thomas, F. D., Grossman, Z., et al.: Diagnosis of angiotensinogenic hypertension: the complementary roles of renal scintigraphy and the saralasin infusion test. J. Nucl. Med. *18*(7):669–675, 1977.

11. Maxwell, M. H.: Cooperative study of renovascular hypertension: current status. Kidney Int. *8*(1975):S-153–S-160.
12. Nordyke, R. A., Gilbert, F. I., and Simmons, E. L.: Screening for kidney disease with radioisotopes. J.A.M.A. *208*:493–496, 1969.
13. Norman, N.: Effective plasma flow of the individual kidney: determination on the basis of the ^{131}I-Hippuran renogram. Scand. J. Clin. Lab. Invest. *30*:395–403, 1972.
14. Rosenthall, L.: The use of intravenous radiopertechnetate angiography as a screening procedure for renovascular hypertension. *In* Blaufox, M. D., and Funck-Bretano, J.-L. (eds.): Radionuclides in Nephrology. New York, Grune & Stratton, 1972, pp. 273–280.
15. Schlegel, J. U.: Radionuclides in urology. *In* Andersson, L. (ed.): Handbuch de Urologie. Band V/1 Supplement. Berlin, Springer-Verlag, 1977, pp. 1–81.
16. Schlegel, J. U., and Hamway, S. A.: Individual renal plasma flow determination in 2 minutes. J. Urol. *116*:282–285, 1976.
17. Schlegel, J. U., Halikiopoulos, H. L., and Prima, R.: Determination of filtration fraction utilizing the gamma scintillation camera. J. Urol. *122*(4):447–450, 1979.
18. Short, M. D., Glass, H. I., Chisholm, C. M., et al.: Gamma camera renography using ^{123}I-Hippuran. Br. J. Radiol. *46*:289–294, 1973.
19. Skripka, C. F., Jr., and Schlegel, J. U.: Accurate determination of renal function by renal histography without collection of blood or urine. II. Correlation of the renal histogram and renal function. J. Urol. *114*:809–812, 1975.
20. Tonnesen, K. H., Munck, O., Hald, T., et al.: Influence on the radiorenogram of variation in skin to kidney distance and the clinical importance thereof. Paper presented at the International Symposium: Radionuclides in Nephrology, Berlin, 1974.
21. Wang, Y.: Regional renogram: a screening test for renal hypertension evaluation. Arch. Intern. Med. *134*:463–466, 1974.
22. Wax, S. H., and MacDonald, D. S.: Analysis of the I[131] sodium O-iodohippurate renogram. J.A.M.A. *179*:140–142, 1962.
23. Wedeen, R. P., and Blaufox, M. D.: The normal renogram. *In* Blaufox, M. D. (ed.): Progress in Nuclear Medicine. Vol. 2. Baltimore, University Park Press, 1972, pp. 107–146.
24. Wedeen, R. P., Goldstein, M. H., and Levitt, M. S.: The radioisotope renogram in normal subject. Am. J. Med. *34*:765–774, 1963.

Renal Vein Renin Assays

To establish the functional significance of a lesion demonstrated by arteriography, separate renal function studies, or renal vein renin assays, must be undertaken. Renal function studies assess the capability of each kidney to excrete urine, to concentrate urine, to reabsorb sodium and water, and to concentrate and clear inulin and para-aminohippuric acid from blood.

Discontinuation of antihypertensive medication is required from two to seven days prior to the study as well as liberal salt intake on the preceding day. Ureteral catheters must be placed cystoscopically at the junction of the lower and middle thirds of the ureters, and care must be taken to collect all urine excreted from the kidneys. Inulin and PAH are infused intravenously in appropriate doses, and after an adequate period of equilibration, urine and blood samples are collected. A difference of urine volume (50 per cent or more), sodium concentration (15 per cent or more), and clearance of inulin and PAH on the side with the renal artery stenosis indicates a hemodynamically significant lesion. The urine osmolality is usually increased on the affected side, as is the concentration of inulin and PAH, by more than 100 per cent. Reabsorption of water and sodium is also markedly greater on the involved side.

Because of the complications of ureteral catheterization, the time-consuming nature of this procedure, and the frequent inaccuracies caused by leakage of urine around the catheters, renal vein renin activity assessment has replaced the separated renal function studies in recent years.

The hemodynamic significance of a renal artery lesion can be determined by assaying various step products of the renin angiotensin mechanism.

An ischemic kidney liberates renin, an acid protease from the juxtaglomerular cells of the afferent arterioles. Renin acts upon the angiotensinogen that has been released by the liver and results in the formation of angiotensin 1. Angiotensin 1 is converted by an enzyme from the pulmonary vascular endothelium into angiotensin 2, an octapeptide. Angiotensin 2 stimulates the zona glomerulosa of the adrenal cortex to secrete aldosterone, which facilitates reabsorption of sodium by the distal tubules. Both angiotensin 1 and angiotensin 2 are potent vasopressors. The ultimate vasopressor effect is directly proportional to the concentration of angiotensin and renin in circulation. Therefore, the hemodynamic significance of a renal artery lesion is once again proportional to levels of renin, angiotensin 1, or angiotensin 2. Radioimmunoassays can identify angiotensin 1, angiotensin 2, and renin. Each part of the system can be tested selectively by blocking other elements, by specific antibodies for renin and angiotensin 1, and by a competitive inhibitor to angiotensin 2, saralasin.

Unfortunately, the estimation of peripheral renin does not accurately reflect renovascular hypertension. High peripheral renin levels are said to be present in renovascular hypertension, whereas essential hypertension is allegedly characterized by low peripheral renin levels. In fact, this may reflect only a stage of disease that has progressed from high renin output.[5] In general, high renin in the presence of a positive sodium balance (a normal renin and suppressed state) seems to be a more accurate indicator of renovascular hypertension.[11]

Definitive proof of the hemodynamic significance of a renal artery lesion, however, relies on a comparison of renal vein renins from both kidneys. A simple mathematical manipulation can reliably predict the success of surgical intervention.[10] False negative results can be a problem but can be minimized by stimulation of renin release in the preparation of the patient prior to sampling.[11, 15]

The method of collection is simple and safe. Specimens are collected from both renal veins and from the inferior vena cava above and below the renal veins with a catheter introduced into the femoral vein. Catheter position, and thus sampling position, can be checked either by injection of small amounts of contrast material or by measurements of oxygen tension changes as the catheter enters the renal vein from the inferior vena cava. Para-aminohippurate extraction percentage has also been used.[3]

Measurement of plasma renin activity is generally done indirectly by measurement of angiotensin 1 or angiotensin 2. Bioassay methods use the pressure elevation in animals and compare this with the effect of a known or standard dose of angiotensin 1 or angiotensin 2. More recently, radioimmunoassay of angiotensin has been used. This has the advantage of greater sensitivity and also permits the processing of large numbers of samples.[13] Chromatographic methods of separation are less accurate and more difficult to process.[1, 13]

Appropriate handling is essential in the collection of samples. All contrast media and flushing solutions must be removed from the catheter prior to the collection of samples. The samples must then be placed in appropriately chilled tubes (usually containing EDTA) and immediately placed in ice. If not processed immediately, the plasma should be frozen. "Collection errors" have been shown to cause greater errors than the assay technique itself, so care is essential at this stage.[4] The addition of EDTA to plasma inhibits the effect of angiotensinases, enzymes that cause the breakdown of angiotensin. Medications must be withdrawn prior to sampling. Hypertensive medications and oral contraceptives should be discontinued three to four weeks prior to sample collection.[13, 16]

A number of methods of stimulating renin release appear to increase the accuracy of the test. Sodium depletion is known to be a stimulant of renin release, and a low-salt diet or salt depletion by diuretics prior to the estimations has been shown to increase the reliability of the examination, especially in decreasing false negative results. Similarly, a change from the supine to the erect position stimulates renin release; having the patient erect prior to sampling increases accuracy.[7, 11, 12, 15]

The aim of renal vein renin activity assay is to accurately predict the outcome of surgery. Interpretation of absolute values is difficult because of wide fluctuation of renin levels secondary to such variables as sodium balance, posture, time of day, diuretic therapy, hormone therapy, and so forth. A ratio of plasma renin activity (PRA) of affected to unaffected side is the most widely accepted method of evaluation. A ratio of 1.5 or greater is generally considered significant.

However, the use of a ratio of affected to unaffected kidney alone can mask bilateral increased secretion of renin. A comparison of plasma renin activity ratios in the affected kidney and the contralateral kidney with the inferior vena cava renin is therefore warranted to exclude increased secretion of renin from both kidneys. A further problem in interpretation is the presence of increased renin excretion from the kidney without renal artery stenosis if affected by more distal vessel changes. In this case, the kidney with the stenosis may in effect be protected from parenchymal hypertensive changes by the main renal artery and therefore excrete less renin at this stage.

Stimulation may also cause rapid fluctuation of renin release.[4] The mere presence of a catheter in the renal artery causes stimulation of renal vein renin release and may be the source of error if the sampling is done soon after renal angiography.[6] In patients with segmental renal artery stenosis, it may be necessary to obtain samples from segmental veins supplying the affected area to adequately evaluate the impact of segmental lesions.[8] Errors due to aberrant renal veins can be avoided by sampling from the inferior vena cava above the renal vein entrance. Thus, if there is an aberrant drainage with high renin, the high inferior vena cava sample will be elevated compared with renal or low inferior vena cava samples. Studies of adrenal venous samples for levels of cortisone, aldosterone, catecholamines, metanephrines, and normetanephrines may be informative for assessment of hypertensive conditions attributable to adrenal hormones.

A plasma renin activity ratio of affected to nonaffected kidney of 1.5 or greater, aided by a comparison ratio of affected kidney to inferior vena cava sample (and nonaffected kidney to inferior vena cava sample to exclude bilaterally increased renin secretion) has been found to be a reliable physiologic test to predict success of surgical intervention for a renal artery lesion.

References

1. Boucher, R., Veyrat, R., de Champlain, J., et al.: New procedures for measurement of human plasma angiotensin and renin activity levels. Can. Med. Assoc. J. 90:194–201, 1964.
2. Ernst, C. B., Bookstein, J. J., Montie, J., et al.: Renal vein renin ratios and collateral vessels in renovascular hypertension. Arch. Surg. 104:496–502, 1972.
3. Hansen, H. J. B., Nielsen, I., Ladefoged, J., et al.: Renal vein renin ratio: predictive value in renal and renovascular hypertension. Acta Chir. Scand. 472:99–102, 1976.
4. Horvath, J. S., Baxter, C. R., Sherbon, K., et al.: An analysis of errors found in renal vein sampling for plasma renin activity. Kidney Int. 11:136–138, 1977.
5. Kaplan, N. M.: Renin profiles: the unfulfilled promises. J.A.M.A. 238:611–613, 1977.
6. Katzberg, R. W., Morris, T. W., Burgener, F. A., et al.: Renal renin and hemodynamic responses to selective renal artery catheterization and angiography. Invest. Radiol. 12:381–388, 1977.
7. Kimura, T., Minai, K., Matsui, K., et al.: Effect of various states of hydration on plasma ADH and renin in man. J. Clin. Endocrinol. Metabol. 42:79–87, 1976.
8. Korobkin, M., Glickman, M. G., and Schambelan, M.: Segmental renal vein sampling for renin. Diagnost. Radiol. 118:307–313, 1976.
9. McAllister, R. G., Jr., Michelakis, A. M., Oates, J. A., et al.: Malignant hypertension due to renal artery stenosis: greater renin release from the nonstenotic kidney. J.A.M.A. 221:865–868, 1972.

10. Marks, L. S., Maxwell, M. H., Varady, P. D., et al.: Renovascular hypertension: Does the renal vein renin ratio predict operative results? J. Urol. *115*:365–368, 1976.
11. Melman, A., Donohue, J. P., Weinberger, W. H., et al.: Improved diagnostic accuracy of renal venous renin ratios with stimulation of renin release. J. Urol. *117*:145–149, 1977.
12. Michelakis, A. M., and Simmons, J.: Effect of posture on renal vein renin activity in hypertension: its implications in the management of patients with renovascular hypertension. J.A.M.A. *208*:659–662, 1969.
13. Sealey, J. E., Gerten-Banes, J., and Laragh, J. H.: The renin system: variations in man measured by radioimmunoassay or bioassay. Kidney Int. *1*:240–253, 1972.
14. Stockigt, J. R., Collins, R. D., Noakes, C. A., et al.: Renal-vein renin in various forms of renal hypertension. Lancet *1*:1194–1198, 1972.
15. Strong, C. G., Hunt, J. C., Sheps, S. G., et al.: Renal venous renin activity: enhancement of sensitivity of lateralization by sodium depletion. Am. J. Cardiol. *27*:602–611, 1971.
16. Vaughan, E. D., Buhler, F. R., Laragh, J. H., et al.: Renovascular hypertension: renin measurements to indicate hypersecretion and contralateral suppression, estimate renal plasma flow, and score for surgical curability. Am. J. Med. *55*:402–414, 1973.
17. Whelton, P. K., Harrington, D. P., Russell, R. P., et al.: Renal vein renin activity: a prospective study of sampling techniques and methods of interpretation. Johns Hopkins Med. J. *141*:112–118, 1977.

Part XVI

Technique of Abdominal-Femoral Arteriography

KLAUS M. BRON, M.D.

A recent review article details the various catheters, techniques, and angiographic equipment that have been developed to examine patients with occlusive aortoiliac femoral run-off disease.[30] Dos Santos was the first to clearly demonstrate that the aorta and its branches could be radiographically studied by direct puncture and injection of radiopaque contrast material.[7] The development of a simple technique for percutaneous catheterization caused an abrupt shift away from translumbar aortography in most major medical centers.[24] Percutaneous catheterization made it easier and safer not only to examine the aorta and its branches but also to explore the lower extremities to their distal terminations.

A significant feature of arteriosclerotic obliterative disease is the generalized nature of the process. There is usually obstructive involvement (stenosis or occlusion) of multiple sites in the aorta, pelvis, thigh, and calf arteries. Combined with obliterative disease of the lower extremities may be obstructive involvement of the visceral (renal, mesenteric, or celiac), coronary, and cerebral vessels. The widespread occurrence of arteriosclerotic obliterative disease requires that the technique of examination adequately assess the arterial circulation from the aorta to the distal run-off vessels.

PREANGIOGRAPHIC CONSIDERATIONS

The radiologist should evaluate the clinical problem and the need for an arteriogram and palpate the peripheral pulses. He or she should also explain the procedure and its potential risk. Mild sedation rather than general anesthesia is usually sufficient for percutaneous retrograde catheterization and arteriography. Premedication usually consists of mild analgesia with Demerol or morphine and a barbiturate appropriate for the patient's size, age, and history of allergies. The renal function should be determined before the procedure is undertaken, especially in diabetic patients, since renal failure may result from injection of radiopaque contrast material.[29] The patient should be well hydrated prior to the procedure in order to diminish any risk of untoward reaction from the renal excretion of the radiopaque contrast material.

Injected radiopaque contrast agents may cause nausea and occasional vomiting, with risk of aspiration. Therefore, four to six hours prior to the examination all solid food is prohibited, but clear liquids are encouraged to prevent dehydration. In diabetic patients requiring insulin or oral hypoglycemics, the dosage of these medications must be adjusted to compensate for possible reduced caloric intake. In patients receiving heparin or coumadin anticoagulation, the clotting and prothrombin times, respectively, should be checked. Vitamin K or protamine may be required to counteract the level of anticoagulation.

PUNCTURE SITE AND CATHETERIZATION

The usual route for catheterization is the transfemoral artery because of its easy accessibility in the inguinal area and its proximity to the aorta and lower-extremity arteries. If both femoral pulses are palpable, the less symptomatic side should be catheterized. This helps to avoid the postangiographic problems of a hematoma at the puncture site, which could interfere with subsequent bypass grafting, or of thrombosis in an already partially occluded vessel. If neither femoral artery pulse is palpable, an alternative peripheral route of catheterization must be found. The axillary artery, especially the left, offers a suitable catheterization site and is particularly useful when aortic occlusion is present.[6, 12] The brachial artery can be used, but this site carries a higher risk of local complications. Translumbar aortography is an alternative when peripheral arterial pulses are absent. This technique can be supplemented by a catheter.[3, 23] However, the transaxillary approach is the method of choice when the femoral arteries are occluded.

When no other catheterization site is available, it may become necessary to directly puncture through a previously inserted prosthetic graft. Although generally considered an undesirable practice, a recent report claims this is a safe procedure[8] and another indicates how to avoid complications.[20]

Frequently, the iliac arteries are tortuous and partially obstructed by arteriosclerotic lesions. This causes difficulty in passing a guide wire from the femoral puncture site into the aorta. A J-guide wire[16] or a J-shaped catheter can then be used.[4] The latter offers an advantage, since a test dose of contrast material may be injected at the site of iliac obstruction and observed fluoroscopically. This will indicate the degree of obstruction and whether or not further retrograde catheterization is feasible.

Varying sizes and types of radiopaque catheter can be used. It is better to use a catheter with the smallest outer diameter, that will withstand the injection of the desired amount of contrast at a predetermined flow rate. Most angiographers use catheters with an outer diameter of 6F to 7F. A recent report suggests that a 5F catheter may be equally effective and possibly safer, because its smaller circumferential diameter causes less obstruction of the catheterized lumen.[19] The catheter can be straight with side holes and a tip occluder,[22] or pigtail-shaped with side holes. In either case there are usually six to eight side holes. The purpose of the tip occluder and the pigtail shape is to reduce the volume of contrast ejected through the end hole. The bulk of the contrast exits via the side holes and is directed into the branches of the aorta. The catheters we have used most often for these studies are the polyethylene Formocath (I.D. .066"-O.D. .095") with six side holes and a tip occluder wire, or the 6F Teflon pigtail catheter with six side holes. The catheter is 100 cm long in order to provide adequate length for the moving table top technique of filming.

SERIAL FILMING EQUIPMENT, FILMING SEQUENCE, AND CONTRAST INJECTION

The purpose of arteriography is to demonstrate the anatomic integrity of the lower extremity circulation, from the aorta to the ankles. In order to follow the normal circulatory progression of the contrast as it travels towards the ankles, various pieces of equipment have been devised. The designs are based on keeping the patient stationary and moving the x-ray tube and films, or on moving the patient and films but keeping the x-ray tube stationary.[30] Originally, the movement of tube and film or patient was performed manually. Film cassettes of varying width and length were changed manually, and the patient was kept stationary. The present changers are automated and can be programmed in various ways. The equipment utilizes a mechanically driven moving table top that sequentially moves the patient over an automatic serial film changer, which is synchronized with automatic exposures of the x-ray tube.[1] The moving table technique allows serial filming of the pelvis and the femoral, popliteal, and run-off circulation with a single injection of contrast.

SEQUENCE OF EXAMINATION

In percutaneous transfemoral catheterization, the catheter tip is first placed at the level of the T_{12}-L_1 intervertebral space for filming the abdominal aorta and its branches. If biplane equipment is available, film series are made in the anteroposterior and lateral positions simultaneously; otherwise the images are obtained successively.[10] From 35 to 50 cc of methylglucamine diatrizoate 76 is injected, depending upon the patient's size. The flow rate is 20 cc per minute to 25 cc per minute, and the entire volume is delivered in approximately 1.5 to 2.0 minutes. The filming rate is three exposures per second for three seconds, one exposure per second for two seconds, and one exposure every two seconds for eight seconds.

The catheter is then withdrawn toward the aortic bifurcation. The tip is positioned about 4 cm above the bifurcation to ensure that the side holes remain above the bifurcation. A single injection of contrast, usually a total of 60 to 70 cc, automatically triggers sequential serial filming of the iliac, femoral, popliteal, and run-off (tibial) arteries. The contrast is injected at a rate of 10 cc per second. The film exposure rate is: pelvis, one per second for four seconds; thigh, one per second for three seconds; knee, one per second for four seconds; and lower leg, one per second for four seconds. Unfortunately, this routine film exposure sequence may fail to adequately demonstrate the obstructive lesions on either side when a large discrepancy due to proximal vessel obstruction exists in the two circulation times. Thus, the portion of the circulation not visualized must be re-examined, with the delayed circulation taken into account.

When the transaxillary route of catheterization is used for the abdominal aorta, the sequence of the examination is reversed; that is, the pelvis and lower extremities are filmed before the aorta. The other technique factors of contrast volume, rate of injection, and film exposure rate are unchanged.

POSITIONING

The principle of obtaining more than one view of a vessel in occlusive disease is well established in cerebral, coronary, and visceral studies but is often omitted in peripheral vascular arteriography. Additional views will furnish a more complete evaluation of the vessel lumen and contour. A lateral view of the abdominal aorta is especially helpful in aneurysms. Obstructive disease of the aorta should be evaluated by both anteroposterior and lateral views. The severity and extent of the lesion may be better portrayed in one view than in the other.[10, 26, 27] A single view may lead to serious underestimation of the degree of arterial constriction (Figs. 22–157 and 22–158). This can have serious consequences if bypass graft surgery is contemplated for a more obvious distal lesion. The severity of the inflow obstruction may go unappreciated, and after a distal bypass graft the patient's symptoms may remain unchanged.

Obstructive disease in the iliac arteries should also be evaluated in several views, since its severity may not be appreciated from only one projection.[25] In the pelvis, an oblique pelvic view is routinely obtained[21] whenever there is suspicion of a focal stenotic lesion in the iliac or common femoral arteries on the anteroposterior view, or if the clinical findings suggest this possibility (Figs. 22–159 and 22–160). The right posterior oblique position clearly demonstrates the bifurcations of the right common iliac and left common femoral arteries, whereas the left posterior oblique position shows the reverse.

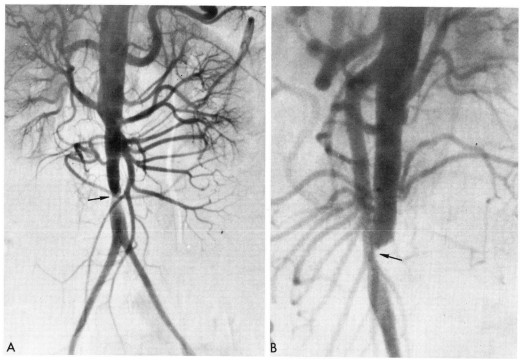

A   B

Figure 22–157. A 42-year-old woman with progressive symptoms of severe buttock and thigh claudication, and nonpalpable femoral pulses. *A,* The anteroposterior view of the abdominal aorta (subtraction film) shows a minimal focal stenosis (arrow). The common iliac and internal iliac arteries are patent. The inferior mesenteric artery is occluded. *B,* The lateral view (subtraction film) demonstrates the marked severity of the focal aortic stenosis (arrow). The degree of lumen narrowing in this view is much greater than that indicated in the anteroposterior view.

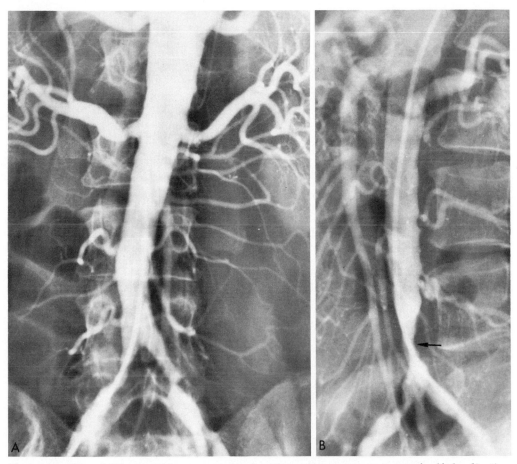

Figure 22–158.   A 53-year-old man presented with progressive symptoms of calf claudication and weakly palpable femoral and popliteal pulses. *A,* The anteroposterior view (AP) of the abdominal aortogram shows no definite focal aortic stenosis and minimal atherosclerosis of the wall. The common iliac and right renal arteries are stenosed. *B,* The lateral view of the abdominal aorta reveals a severe focal stenosis proximal to the aortic bifurcation (arrow). This inflow obstruction is not apparent or even suggested in the anteroposterior view.

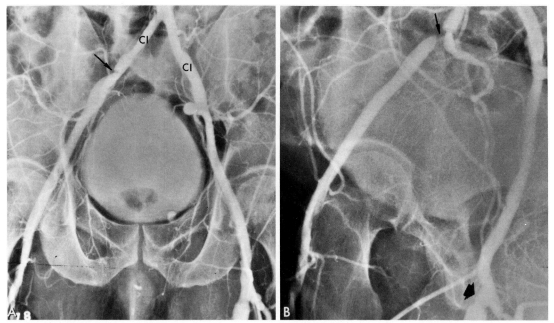

Figure 22–159. The patient, a 56-year-old man, presented with progressive symptoms of intermittent claudication in the right calf. Adult onset of diabetes mellitus had been diagnosed six years earlier; at that time a left femoropopliteal bypass graft was done. *A,* The anteroposterior view of the pelvis suggests possible obstruction of the right common iliac artery at its bifurcation (arrow). This is minimal diffuse atherosclerosis of both common iliac arteries (CI). The origin of the left femoropopliteal bypass graft appears normal. *B,* The right posterior oblique view (RPO) demonstrates severe stenosis at the origin of the external iliac artery and not of the internal iliac artery (arrow). Also, this view reveals that the origin of the left femoropopliteal bypass graft is narrowed (arrowhead).

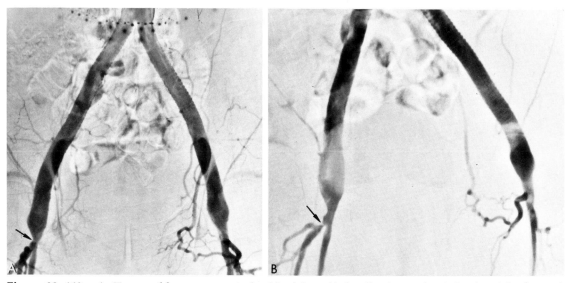

Figure 22–160. A 65-year-old man presented with right calf claudication, a bruit in the right femoral area, a nonpalpable right popliteal pulse, and a previous aortobifemoral bypass graft. *A,* The anteroposterior view of the pelvis (subtraction film) shows narrowing of the right distal graft anastomosis (arrow). The right profunda femoris artery origin is not clearly seen. *B,* In the left posterior oblique view, the right profunda femoris (PF) artery origin is severely stenosed (arrow), which was not apparent in the anteroposterior view. Note the typical serrated edge of the graft. The right superficial femoral artery was subsequently shown to be segmentally occluded; therefore, the anatomic status of the PF artery was very significant.

If a local obstruction is demonstrated on the routine anteroposterior view, the appropriate oblique view is filmed.

In general, the anteroposterior view suffices for evaluation of obstructive lesions of the femoral, popliteal, and distal run-off arteries. Occasionally, a lateral view of a popliteal artery obstruction may be helpful in determining its severity. The distal run-off arteries, at the ankle, are best viewed with the feet in external rotation, a view that separates the arteries.

INTRA-ARTERIAL LIDOCAINE

Varying degrees of pain from the injection of radiopaque contrast are a constant feature of peripheral arteriography. Various efforts have been made to alleviate the problem. General anesthesia is effective but rarely needed for retrograde femoral arteriography. As an alternative, a search for a safe, fast-acting intra-arterial anesthetic has been made. Several recent studies have reported on the use of lidocaine for this purpose. In three reports,[13, 14, 31] 1 to 2 per cent lidocaine was infused intra-arterially immediately prior to, or mixed with, the injected contrast material. There was both subjective and objective evidence of lessened pain perception. This was particularly true when analgesic premedication had been given prior to the infusion of 2 per cent lidocaine. However, another report finds it to be totally ineffective.[9] In fact, in this report of 22 patients without premedication, 12 patients (54.5 per cent) had increased pain from the injected contrast to which lidocaine was added compared with contrast material alone.

The hypertonicity of contrast material appears to be the important factor in the production of pain.[18] An iso-osmotic concentration of Conray has been shown to be painless.[9] Similarly, a new nonionic contrast material, metrizamide, is associated with less pain than Isopaque, an ionic contrast agent.[2]

ENHANCED CONTRAST VISUALIZATION

It has been estimated that in up to 25 per cent of patients studied by routine techniques the popliteal and distal run-off (tibial and peroneal) arteries are not adequately visualized for anatomic evaluation.[17] The poor contrast visualization is the result of delayed blood flow in the lower leg with consequent dilution of the injected contrast material. The problem of delayed circulation is compounded by proximal obstruction in the distal aorta, iliac, or common femoral arteries. Thus, radiopaque contrast may be seen in the distal run-off on one side but not the other, or it may be absent bilaterally.

Anatomic demonstration of the run-off vessels is necessary to determine the feasibility of a femoropopliteal bypass graft or more distal grafts to the tibial or peroneal arteries. In order to obviate the problem of absent or poor run-off visualization, the techniques of reactive hyperemia[5, 28] and pharmacologic vasodilatation[11, 15] have been successfully used. The purpose of both techniques is to increase the blood flow to the popliteal artery and its branches and thus increase the concentration of radiopaque contrast in these vessels. The vasoactive drugs used for this purpose are Priscoline (tolazoline hydrochloride) and bradykinin. However, these vasodilators have not proved as effective as reactive hyperemia.

Reactive hyperemia may result from ischemia alone or from exercise. Ischemia alone is produced by fastening a blood pressure cuff around the thigh and keeping the

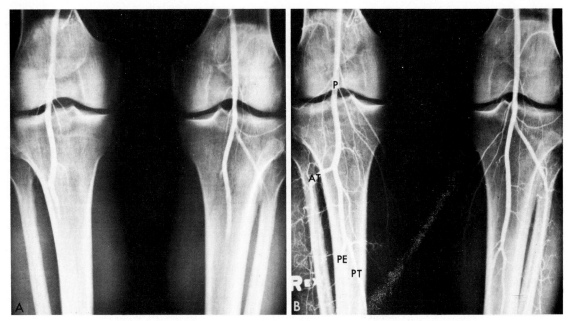

Figure 22–161. A 62-year-old man was readmitted with recurrent bilateral hip and calf claudication. Four years previously, bilateral aortoiliac endarterectomies had been performed. *A,* The unenhanced pre-exercise study at 18 seconds fails to adequately visualize the run-off arteries bilaterally. *B,* The postexercise study at 8 seconds demonstrates good contrast filling of the popliteal (P) and distal run-off vessels. The anterior tibial (AT), posterior tibial (PT), and peroneal (PE) are patent bilaterally. The origin of the anterior tibial arteries is asymmetric between the two sides, an unusual finding.

tourniquet inflated at 150 mmHg for five to seven minutes. The second technique combines the inflated blood pressure cuff with active or passive exercise of the calves and feet. Either method results in increased blood flow into the leg arteries and decreased arteriovenous circulation time. The latter markedly improves visualization of the run-off arteries (Fig. 22–161). In one series,[17] reactive hyperemia achieved excellent filling of the tibial and peroneal arteries in 91 per cent. This enhancement technique is also useful for demonstrating poorly visualized iliac and femoral arteries. The exact mechanisms by which arterial ischemia, either alone or with exercise, produces hyperemia are unknown. Such factors as tissue anoxia; local carbon dioxide and lactic acid accumulation; release of vasoactive polypeptides, such as bradykinin; and, possibly, reduced venous pressure have all been proposed as explanations.[17]

References

1. Agee, O. F., and Kaude, J.: Arteriography of the pelvis and lower extremities with moving table technique. Am. J. Roentgenol. *107*:860–865, 1969.
2. Almen, T., Boijsen, E., and Lindell, S. E.: Metrizamide in angiography. Femoral angiography. Acta Radiol. *18*:33–38, 1977.
3. Amplatz, K.: Translumbar catheterization of the abdominal aorta. Radiology *81*:927–931, 1963.
4. Baum, S., and Abrams, H. L.: A J-shaped catheter for retrograde catheterization of tortuous vessels. Radiology *83*:436–437, 1964.
5. Boijsen, E., and Dahn, I.: Femoral angiography during maximal blood flow. Acta Radiol. *3*:543–553, 1965.
6. Bron, K. M.: Selective visceral and total abdominal arteriography via the left axillary artery in the older age group. Am. J. Roentgenol. *97*:432–437, 1966.

7. Dos Santos, R.: Technique de l'aortographie. J. Int. Chir. 2:609, 1937.
8. Eisenberg, R. L., Mani, R. L., and McDonald, E. J.: The complication rate of catheter angiography by direct puncture through aortofemoral bypass grafts. Am. J. Roentgenol. 126:814–816, 1976.
9. Eisenberg, R. L., Mani, R. L., and Hedgecock, M. W.: Pain associated with peripheral angiography: Is lidocaine effective? Radiology 127:109–111, 1978.
10. Eisenman, J. I., and O'Loughlin, B. J.: Value of lateral abdominal aortography. Am. J. Roentgenol. 112:586–592, 1971.
11. Erikson, U.: Peripheral arteriography during bradykinin induced vasodilation. Acta Radiol. 3:193–201, 1965.
12. Glenn, J. H.: Abdominal aorta catheterization via the left axillary artery. Radiology 115:227–228, 1975.
13. Gordon, I. J., and Westcott, J. L.: Intra-arterial lidocaine: an effective analgesic for peripheral angiography. Radiology 124:43–45, 1977.
14. Guthaner, D. F., Silverman, J. F., Hayden, W. G., et al.: Intraarterial analgesia in peripheral arteriography. Am. J. Roentgenol. 128:737–739, 1977.
15. Jacobs, J. B., and Hanafee, W. N.: The use of priscoline in peripheral arteriography. Radiology 88:957–960, 1967.
16. Judkins, M. P., Kidd, H. J., Friche, L. H., et al.: Lumen-following safety J-guide for catheterization of tortuous vessels. Radiology 88:1127–1130, 1967.
17. Kahn, P. C., Boyer, D. N., Moran, J. M., et al.: Reactive hyperemia in lower extremity arteriography: an evaluation. Radiology 90:975–980, 1968.
18. Lindgren, P., Saltzman, G., and Tornell, G.: Vascular effects of metrizoate compounds, Isopaque Na and Isopaque Na/Ca/Mg. Acta Radiol. 270:44–57, 1967.
19. Mani, R. L., Helms, C. A., and Eisenberg, R. L.: Use of a 5 French catheter with multiple side holes in abdominal aortography. Radiology 123:233–234, 1977.
20. Mani, R. L., and Costin, B. S.: Catheter angiography through aortofemoral grafts: prevention of catheter separation during withdrawal. Am. J. Roentgenol. 128:328–329, 1977.
21. McDonald, E. J., Malone, J. M., Eisenberg, R. L., et al.: Arteriographic evaluation of the femoral bifurcation value of the ipsilateral anterior oblique projection. Am. J. Roentgenol. 127:955–956, 1976.
22. Olin, T.: Studies in angiographic technique. Lund, Hakan Ohlssons Boktryckeri, 1963.
23. Riddervold, H. O., and Seale, D. L.: Translumbar aortography with teflon catheters. Acta Radiol. 12:619–624, 1972.
24. Seldinger, S. I.: Catheter replacement of the needle in percutaneous arteriography. Acta Radiol. 39:368–376, 1953.
25. Sethi, G. K., Scott, S. M., and Takaro, T.: Multiple angiography for more precise evaluation of aortoiliac disease. Surgery 78:154–159, 1975.
26. Simon, H., and Fairbank, J. T.: Biplane translumbar aortography for evaluation of peripheral vascular disease. Am. J. Surg. 133:447–452, 1977.
27. Thomas, M. L., and Andress, M. R.: Value of oblique projections in translumbar aortography. Am. J. Roentgenol. 116:187–193, 1972.
28. Wahren, J., Cronestrand, R., and Juhlin-Dannfelt, A.: Leg blood flow during exercise in patients with occlusion of the iliac artery: pre- and postoperative studies. Scand. J. Clin.Lab. Invest. 32:257–263, 1963.
29. Weinrauch, L. A., Robertson, W. S., and D'Elia, J. A.: Contrast media-induced acute renal failure. J.A.M.A. 239:2018–2019, 1978.
30. Wendth, A. J., Jr.: Peripheral arteriography. An overview of its origin and present status. Crit. Rev. Clin. Radiol. Nucl. Med. 61:369–401, 1975.
31. Widrich, W. C., Singer, R. J., and Robbins, A. H.: The use of intra-arterial lidocaine to control pain due to aortofemoral arteriography. Radiology 124:37–41, 1977.

23

DISORDERS
OF VEINS

ROBERT A. NOVELLINE, M.D.

GROSS ANATOMY OF LOWER EXTREMITY VEINS

The veins of the leg are larger in caliber and more numerous than arteries, and their capacity is greater. There are three anatomically distinguishable groups: the superficial veins, the deep veins, and the perforating (communicating) veins. The superficial, or subcutaneous, veins are located directly beneath the subcutaneous fascia. They have relatively thick muscular walls, and they intercommunicate freely to form a continuous network around each leg. They also communicate with deep veins via the perforating veins. Each lower extremity has two major superficial veins that terminate by penetrating the deep fascia to enter a major deep vein; the lesser saphenous vein drains into the popliteal vein and the greater saphenous vein into the femoral vein (Fig. 23–1A).

The deep veins accompany arteries and are enclosed in the same sheaths as those vessels. The larger arteries, such as the popliteal and superficial femoral arteries, usually have only one accompanying vein. The smaller arteries have paired veins, called venae comitantes, lying on each side of the artery. The paired anterior and posterior tibial veins and the peroneal veins have been referred to as the longitudinal or "stem" veins of the lower leg (Fig. 23–1B). The deep veins have thin walls containing less muscle than the superficial veins. The perforating veins are also thin-walled; they connect the superficial veins with the deep veins.

Venous valves direct blood flow from the distal to the proximal portions of the lower extremities and from the superficial to the deep venous systems. Venous valves consist of two thin-walled cusps attached to a point of vein wall thickening known as the valve ring. There is a dilatation of the vein immediately proximal to the ring known as the valve sinus. Valves are more common in the deep veins and are usually located

---

Figure 23–1. Normal anatomy of the lower extremity veins. *A*, Superficial venous system. *B*, Deep venous system. (Published by Health Sciences Markets Division, Eastman Kodak Company, Rochester, New York.)

See illustration on the opposite page

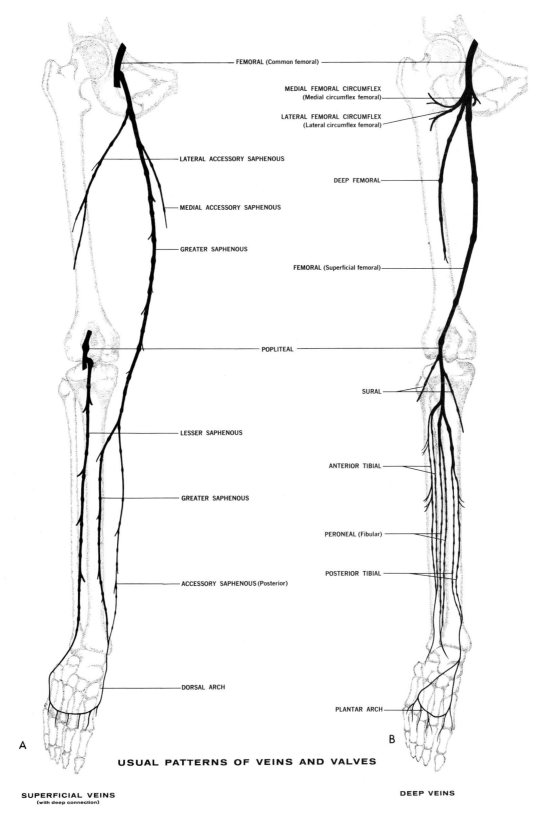

USUAL PATTERNS OF VEINS AND VALVES

SUPERFICIAL VEINS
(with deep connection)

DEEP VEINS

Figure 23–1. *See legend on the opposite page.*

just distal to the site where a tributary vein empties into a main vein. Incompetent valves in lower extremity perforating veins allow filling of the superficial system from the deep system, resulting in the formation of superficial varicosities. In the main deep veins, incompetent valves can cause venous stasis.

Superficial Veins

The greater saphenous vein is the longest vein in the body. It arises on the medial aspect of the foot and ascends along the medial side of the leg, where it receives numerous subcutaneous tributaries. Proximally, it passes through the fossa ovalis and empties into the femoral vein approximately 3 cm below the inguinal ligament.

The lesser saphenous vein begins posterior to the lateral malleolus of the ankle and runs proximally up the middle of the posterior aspect of the lower leg. It perforates the deep fascia of the popliteal fossa and terminates in the popliteal vein between the heads of the gastrocnemius muscle.

Deep Veins

The deep venous system of the leg originates in a network of foot veins. One important group forms the deep plantar venous arch, which accompanies the plantar arterial arch (see Fig. 23–1B). The plantar venous arch is drained by the posterior tibial veins, the venae comitantes of the posterior tibial artery. Consequently, the plantar venous arch is an important landmark on phlebograms for locating the posterior tibial veins. The anterior tibial veins arise from the venae comitantes of the dorsalis pedis artery. They arise anteriorly and ascend laterally, joining the posterior tibial veins to form the popliteal vein. The peroneal veins originate above the ankle joint, ascending along the medial aspect of the fibula; they join with the posterior tibial veins proximally. The soleal veins are muscular veins that drain into the longitudinal deep veins of the calf.

The popliteal vein ascends through the popliteal fossa to the canal of the adductor magnus muscle where it becomes the femoral vein. The long distal segment of the femoral vein is the venous counterpart of the superficial femoral artery, and the proximal segment is the venous counterpart of the common femoral artery. When these segments are discussed individually, they are referred to as the *common* femoral vein and the *superficial* femoral vein. The popliteal vein receives several tributaries corresponding to the branches of the popliteal artery as well as the lesser saphenous vein and muscular veins that drain the gastrocnemius muscle, are called sural veins.

The femoral vein accompanies the superficial femoral artery and receives numerous muscular tributaries. Approximately 3 to 4 cm below the inguinal ligament it is joined by the profunda femoris vein and more proximally by the greater saphenous vein. The profunda femoris vein receives tributaries that correspond to the perforating branches of the profunda femoris artery in addition to the medial and lateral femoral circumflex veins. The femoral vein terminates proximally as the external iliac vein.

Perforating Veins

The perforating veins connect the deep and superficial venous systems as they pass through the deep fascia. They are short, and have an essentially horizontal course. The very proximal portions of the greater and lesser saphenous veins are also perforating veins. Distally, the perforating veins are surrounded only by fat and loose connective tissue. The more proximal perforating veins transversing the calf muscles are known as muscle perforators.

PHYSIOLOGIC FACTORS

Blood flows toward the heart in extremity veins, and the resistance to flow is low. The veins contribute about 10 to 15 per cent of the total resistance to cardiac output. Venous capacity is much greater than arterial capacity, and the cross-sectional area of any individual vein is usually two to three times that of the corresponding artery. Nearly two thirds of the blood volume is contained in the systemic veins. The blood pressure at any point in an extremity vein is the sum of hydraulic pressure, hydrostatic pressure, and transient pressure changes. The hydraulic pressure is produced by the pumping action of the heart and is approximately 15 mmHg at rest. The hydrostatic pressure results from gravity, and at any point in the venous system below the level of the right atrium the pressure is positive and equivalent to the vertical distance from the right atrium. Transient pressure changes are associated with variations in intrathoracic pressure and the action of the "musculovenous pumps."

The intramuscular deep veins of the legs and their surrounding muscles act as reciprocating pumps. Because the musculature of the leg is enclosed by a dense fascia, high intramuscular pressures can be generated during muscle contraction. With contraction the intramuscular veins are compressed and emptied, and the valves in the perforating and deep longitudinal veins direct blood flow proximally. During relaxation the pressure in the intramuscular veins falls, and they refill with blood from the muscle circulation.

Radiographic contrast media injected into a dorsal foot vein of a resting patient placed in an erect or semi-erect position flows into both the deep and the superficial venous systems. Opacification of the deep veins is less satisfactory in the supine position, which has been largely abandoned for ascending phlebography. With the patient supine, the heavier contrast agent layers in the dependent portions of the deep veins, resulting in suboptimal opacification of the lumina, and contrast flows predominantly into and opacifies the dependent veins. The use of a tourniquet is unnecessary during ascending phlebography in the semi-erect position, and in fact the compression produced may result in incomplete filling of portions of both the deep and the superficial venous systems.

RADIOGRAPHIC TECHNIQUES

Phlebography

Phlebography has been in use for many years[6, 7] and is considered the most accurate diagnostic procedure for evaluating the deep and superficial venous systems of the extremities.[4, 32, 40, 46, 50] It is the standard procedure against which other modalities are compared. When properly performed, a negative leg phlebogram excludes a diagnosis of deep vein thrombosis.[4] Several phlebographic techniques are in common use. *Ascending phlebography* is the most popular lower extremity technique. With the patient in the semi-erect position (Fig. 23–2), on a tilting fluoroscope, contrast is injected into a dorsal foot vein and multiple films are obtained of the deep and

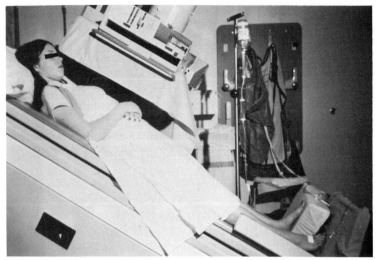

Figure 23–2. Patient position for ascending phlebography. The patient is placed in a semi-upright position approximately 40 degrees from the horizontal on a tilting fluoroscopy table. The opposite leg is placed on a box, so that the extremity being examined is not weight-bearing and can be rotated during the procedure. Contrast medium is injected through a 21-gauge needle, which is inserted percutaneously into an ipsilateral distal dorsal foot vein.

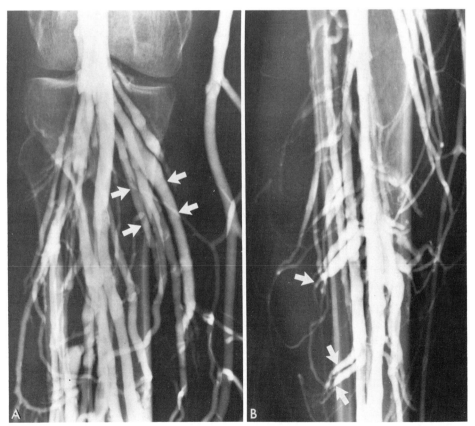

Figure 23–3. Examples of ascending phlebography spot films. *A,* An exposure taken over the proximal tibia shows details of the sural (gastrocnemius) veins (arrows). *B,* This film details the anatomy of perforating veins (arrows) in the calf, which transport blood from the superficial to the deep venous system.

superficial venous systems as contrast ascends.[40] Spot films are taken in the anteroposterior and oblique projections (Fig. 23–3) during injection, and later overhead radiographs are made (Fig. 23–4). About 100 to 150 cc of contrast medium are used for each extremity, and the procedure can be performed in about 20 minutes.

Direct catheterization phlebography is performed in the supine position. This procedure will best opacify the common femoral and iliac veins. A short catheter is inserted directly into the ipsilateral femoral vein. This procedure is done when conventional ascending phlebography inadequately visualizes the proximal femoral vein and iliac veins.

Descending phlebography is a test of competence of the femoral vein and is performed through a catheter in the femoral vein. Contrast is injected while the patient is doing a Valsalva maneuver. If the valves are incompetent, contrast will opacify the distal femoral vein and occasionally the popliteal vein.

Retrograde catheterization phlebography involves the placement of a catheter into the opposite femoral vein, around the confluences of the common iliac veins, and then distally in the involved leg. Contrast medium can then be selectively injected to optimally visualize the femoral vein or profunda femoris vein.

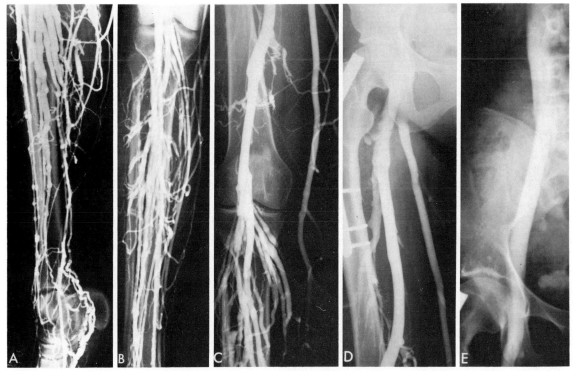

Figure 23–4. Normal ascending phlebography: overhead films. *A,* Oblique projection of the lower leg. The foot is actually in a lateral position, and the plantar venous arch is well seen as are the three paired longitudinal deep veins: the posterior tibial, peroneal, and anterior tibial veins. *B,* Anteroposterior projection of the lower leg. The muscular soleal and sural (gastrocnemius) veins are usually best seen on this view. The longitudinal paired deep veins can also be identified. *C,* Anteroposterior projection taken over the knee area. The popliteal, sural, and greater saphenous veins are all well seen. *D,* Anteroposterior projection of the femoral area showing the femoral and greater saphenous veins. In one half of ascending phlebograms the profunda femoris vein is opacified. *E,* Anteroposterior view of the hemipelvis. For this exposure, the patient is requested to do a Valsalva maneuver, and the involved extremity either is elevated or the calf is compressed by the radiologist to improve opacification of the iliac veins. When properly performed, the external and common iliac veins as well as the distal inferior vena cava can be visualized.

ASCENDING PHLEBOGRAPHY. To circumvent the contrast layering that occurs in the supine position and to obtain optimal opacification of the deep and superficial systems, the procedure is performed with the patient in a semi-upright position on a tilting fluoroscopy table (see Fig. 23–2), according to the method described by Rabinov and Paulin.[40] The procedure room should be equipped with an image-intensifier television system for fluoroscopy, overhead film capability, and 70-mm camera or spot film capability. The table should be positioned approximately 40 degrees from the horizontal; with less than 40 degrees of elevation there is incomplete opacification of veins and less venous distention. The opposite leg is placed on a box approximately 8 inches in height, so that the extremity being examined is not weight bearing and can be easily rotated from the anteroposterior to the oblique position.

The procedure can be painful, and patients may experience severe muscle cramps during contrast medium injection. Oral or parenteral premedication is therefore recommended. The patient is requested to relax the involved extremity during the examination, and all pillows or cushions are removed from beneath the leg so that artifacts will not be produced by external compression. No tourniquets are utilized, since these may occlude both superficial and deep veins and alter the filling of both systems.

Sixty per cent vascular contrast has been used in the past (usually Renografin-60). More recently, 45 per cent contrast has become popular because this concentration reduces patient discomfort; a recent study reports a lower incidence of postphlebography phlebitis with its use.[9] The contrast medium is injected through a number 21 scalp vein needle, which is placed percutaneously in a medial distal dorsal foot vein. The contrast medium is initially injected under careful fluoroscopic control, so that any extravasation will be immediately recognized and the needle can be repositioned in a more satisfactory vein. Local skin complications may occur if extravasation is not recognized and large amounts of contrast are injected subcutaneously.

If no extravasation is seen, contrast medium injection is continued. Fluoroscopic monitoring during injection allows recognition of abnormal flow patterns, intraluminal filling defects, and venous occlusions. The rate and volume of contrast medium injection can be determined by fluoroscopic observation. Spot films (or camera exposures) are taken in both anteroposterior and oblique projections from the foot to the knee and in the anteroposterior projection from the knee to the inferior vena cava (see Fig. 23–3). Multiple spot films are obtained over the proximal femoral vein and the iliac veins.

When spot filming is completed, five overhead radiographs are obtained, including anteroposterior and oblique views of the lower leg, and anteroposterior views of the knee, thigh, and inguinal areas (Fig. 23–4). Between each of the overhead exposures approximately 8 to 10 cc of contrast medium are injected intravenously. To obtain optimal opacification of the proximal femoral vein and iliac veins on the final exposure, the leg is elevated or the calf is compressed while the patient performs a Valsalva maneuver. In some patients, demonstration of the proximal femoral vein and iliac veins may require direct femoral vein catheterization.

In most cases, ascending phlebography of one leg can be accomplished with 100 to 150 cc of contrast medium. Any technical delays require extra contrast medium. After the final overhead film is obtained, the patient is placed in a supine position and the veins are flushed with 100 to 150 cc of normal saline containing 1500 units of heparin. The patient is also asked to exercise the extremity to help pump up residual contrast medium. Care should be taken not to prolong the time that the contrast medium remains in the veins, since contrast medium is hyperosmolar and potentially irritating to the venous endothelium. The entire procedure can be performed in about 20 minutes; the time in which contrast medium opacifies the deep venous system should not exceed four to six minutes.

DIRECT CATHETERIZATION PHLEBOGRAPHY. When the most proximal femoral vein and iliac veins do not adequately visualize on conventional ascending phlebography, or when a defect is seen in these veins that requires further evaluation, direct catheterization phlebography is indicated. With the patient supine, a small no. 5 French single end-hole or multiple side-hole catheter is inserted directly into the involved femoral vein by percutaneous Seldinger technique. Following injection of 20 to 30 cc of 60 per cent contrast medium at 8 to 10 cc per second and serial filming, an excellent examination of the ipsilateral iliac system may be obtained.

DESCENDING PHLEBOGRAPHY. Descending phlebography is a test of venous valve competence; it also is performed with percutaneous femoral vein catheterization. However, the contrast medium is injected while the patient does a Valsalva maneuver. Fluoroscopy and filming are then performed over the entire length of the femoral and popliteal veins.

During straining the intra-abdominal pressure is higher than the venous pressure, and the increased intra-abdominal pressure is transmitted to the iliac veins. The consequent pressure gradient between the iliac and the femoral veins reverses flow in these veins. If the valves of the femoral, profunda femoris, and greater saphenous veins are competent, they will close off to retrograde flow of contrast medium, the proximal veins will dilate, and a pressure equilibrium will be established. If the femoral vein valves are incompetent, contrast medium will be forced distally and may opacify the entire length of the femoral vein and occasionally the popliteal vein. Descending phlebography may be performed in the supine position, although a more physiologic estimate of valve patency is obtained if contrast medium is injected with the patient tilted to the errect position.

RETROGRADE CATHETERIZATION PHLEBOGRAPHY. In order to directly opacify the femoral and profunda femoris veins a selective catheter may be inserted percutaneously from the opposite femoral vein, advanced around the common iliac vein confluence, down the ipsilateral external iliac vein, and selectively into the femoral or profunda femoris veins. Selective retrograde catheterization enables optimal opacification of the femoral and profunda femoris veins so that questionable areas seen on a conventional ascending phlebogram can be further evaluated (Fig. 23–5). This technique has been especially useful in patients who have undergone total hip surgery, in which the incidence of profunda femoris thrombosis is increased.

RADIONUCLIDE PHLEBOGRAPHY. Radionuclide phlebography can be performed as a preliminary to the conventional perfusion lung scan by injecting one half of the ^{99m}Tc macroaggregated albumin in a dorsal vein of each foot simultaneously. With the patient positioned on a floating table top under a scintillation camera, the isotope movement can be monitored on an oscilloscope screen and isotope transit through the venous systems of both legs recorded on video tape for replay. The resulting images demonstrate either patent deep venous pathways or evidence of venous obstruction (Fig. 23–6). Delayed scans (static scans) are taken of the thigh and calf four to five minutes after isotope injection. If any "hot spots" are demonstrated, the static scans are repeated one minute after exercise. Following completion of the radionuclide phlebogram, lung scanning is performed.

Radionuclide phlebography can be a painless, safe technique for detecting deep vein thrombosis in patients with contrast medium allergy or contrast medium contraindication due to renal failure. Its results correlate well with those of ascending phlebography, and its accuracy ranges from 89 to 95 per cent for proximal major deep vein thrombosis.[14, 24, 41, 47]

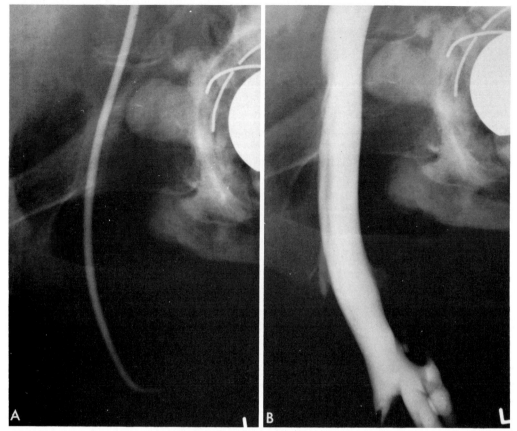

Figure 23–5. Normal retrograde catheterization phlebography. *A,* This plain film shows a catheter oriented in a retrograde direction and terminating in the left (common) femoral vein. The catheter was inserted percutaneously into the right femoral vein, advanced around the confluence of common iliac veins, and then advanced down the left common and external iliac veins. *B,* Excellent opacification of the (common) femoral vein and proximal profunda femoris vein may be obtained when contrast medium is injected into the profunda femoris vein origin.

Cuff Impedance Plethysmography[26, 48, 49]

This procedure is based on the fact that changes in blood volume of the leg alter the electrical resistance (impedance). Electrodes are applied to the calf, and a weak high-frequency alternating current is passed across the leg. The electric impedance between the two electrodes is then measured (Fig. 23–7).

It is a sensitive technique (96 per cent accuracy) for detecting obstruction of the major deep veins in the thigh or pelvis, but it may not detect calf thrombi (Fig. 23–8).

The test is noninvasive and can be performed at bedside. It is a popular procedure for screening patients at high risk for deep venous thrombosis.

[125]I-Fibrinogen Scanning

A diagnosis of venous thrombosis with ^{125}I-fibrinogen leg scanning depends upon the incorporation of previously administered and circulating ^{125}I-labeled fibrinogen

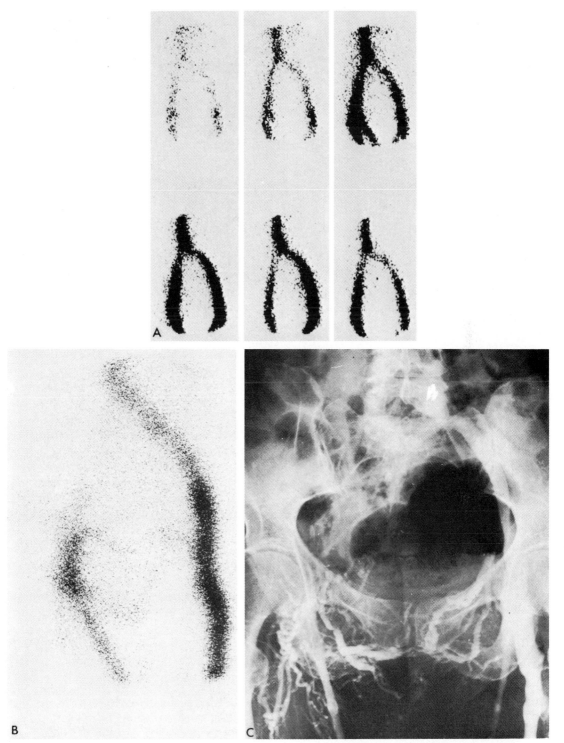

Figure 23–6. Bilateral radionuclide phlebography. *A,* Normal study. *B* and *C,* Occlusion of the right iliofemoral veins, with drainage of the right leg venous blood by the greater saphenous vein and the transpelvic collaterals. (*From* Ennis, J. T., and Elmes, R. J.: Radionuclide venography in the diagnosis of deep vein thrombosis. Radiology *125*(2):441–449, 1977. Reproduced by permission.)

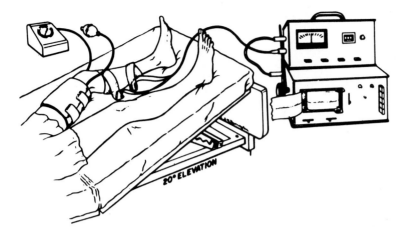

Figure 23–7. Patient position for occlusive impedance plethysmography. A pneumatic cuff is placed around the thigh, and the electrodes are applied to the calf. The leg is elevated, the knee slightly flexed, and the hip externally rotated. (*From* Wheeler, H. B., O'Donnell, J. A., Anderson, F. A., et al.: Occlusive impedance phlebography: a diagnostic procedure of venous thrombosis and pulmonary embolism. Prog. Cardiovasc. Dis. *17*(3):199–205, 1974. Reproduced by permission.)

into a developing thrombus. The thrombus can then be detected by measuring the resulting increase in overlying surface radioactivity with a hand-held rate meter. Since this examination is most effective when the patient has been given labeled fibrinogen before formation of the thrombus, fibrinogen leg scanning is most useful as a screening procedure in patients who do not yet have a thrombus but are at high risk of developing venous thrombosis. At the beginning of the high-risk period, for example, on the day prior to surgery, a patient can be injected intravenously with 100 μCi of ^{125}I-fibrinogen and then can be scanned daily throughout the high-risk period. A single dose of labeled fibrinogen permits scanning for up to eight to ten days; if necessary, this dose may be repeated at eight days for further scanning.

With the exception of the initial isotope injection, fibrinogen leg scanning is painless, easily repeatable, and can be performed at the bedside. Scanning takes approximately 15 minutes. Surface radioactivity is measured over the femoral and popliteal veins and over the calf at 7- to 8-cm intervals. Readings from the rate meter are recorded as a percentage of the surface activity measured over the heart. Venous thrombosis is suspected when there is an increase of more than 20 per cent of heart activity at any point compared with readings over adjacent areas in the same leg, over a corresponding point on the opposite leg, or over the same point on the same leg on the previous day. Venous thrombosis is diagnosed if the increased activity persists for 24 hours or longer.

An advantage over phlebography is that scanning may differentiate new and old deep venous thrombosis when only venous occlusion is demonstrated at phlebogra-

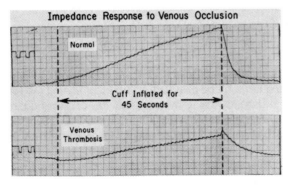

Figure 23–7. Normal and abnormal cuff impedance plethysmography tracings. With obstruction of a major deep vein of the thigh or pelvis, the increase in blood volume with cuff inflation will be reduced, as will the rate of venous outflow when the cuff is deflated. (*From* Benedict, K.: Impedance plethysmography: Correlation with contrast venography. Radiology *125*:695–699, 1977. Reproduced by permission.)

phy. However, leg scanning cannot differentiate superficial and deep venous thrombosis.

In addition, false positive scans may occur over wounds, hematomas, and areas of cellulitis that also incorporate fibrinogen. This is a particular problem in the hip surgery patient, in whom it may not be possible to detect femoral vein thrombus because of the intense radioisotope uptake (blind area) associated with the surgical wound. Also, fibrinogen leg scanning may miss small thrombi that may be detected by phlebography. If phlebography cannot be performed it is recommended that fibrinogen leg scanning be combined with another procedure that has high sensitivity in detecting iliofemoral venous thrombosis, such as cuff impedance plethysmography or Doppler ultrasound.[21, 25, 36] Patients undergoing leg scanning require blocking of iodine uptake by the thyroid prior to isotope injection and do run a slight risk of hepatitis from the injected fibrinogen.

In summary, ^{125}I-fibrinogen leg scanning can be an accurate, sensitive, and easily repeatable bedside screening test for detecting venous thrombosis in high-risk patients. When the scan is positive, phlebography should be performed to confirm findings and to define the extent of thrombosis, especially in the iliofemoral veins. If phlebography is either not available or contraindicated, cuff impedence plethysmography or Doppler ultrasound should be performed.

Doppler Ultrasound

Doppler ultrasound is a noninvasive technique that has been used to diagnose deep venous thrombosis since a report by Strandness in 1972.[3, 5, 8, 28, 33, 35, 45] It is a painless bedside technique that can be easily repeated. The method involves the use of a Doppler ultrasound flow velocity-transducer to determine vein patency. The transducer emits an ultrasonic beam at a frequency of 2 to 15 mH which is directed percutaneously at an underlying vein where it is reflected by the red blood cells. If blood flow is stopped, the frequency of the reflected beam is identical to that of the incident beam and no Doppler sound is emitted. If the blood cells are moving the beam is reflected at a different frequency (Doppler shift), which is proportional to the velocity of blood flow. The difference in frequency between incident and reflected ultrasound beams is amplified into an audible signal, or flow sound.

Doppler flow signals are heard over the femoral, popliteal, and posterior tibial veins. In contrast to arteries, venous flow sounds rise and fall with respiration. After the femoral, popliteal, and posterior tibial veins are located, the changes in Doppler signals are noted on respiration, Valsalva maneuver, and with thigh and calf muscle compression. In the femoral vein, compression of the thigh musculature induces a sudden increase in velocity of femoral vein blood flow.

Deep vein thrombosis is diagnosed when venous signals are absent or when there is greatly impaired flow during muscle compression. The accuracy of Doppler ultrasound in the diagnosis of deep vein thrombosis has been reported to be as high as 72.5 to 93.8 per cent.[3, 5, 8, 28, 33, 35]

However, there are several limitations to this method. Although ultrasound is sensitive to popliteal, femoral, and iliac vein thrombosis, it is relatively insensitive to calf vein thrombosis. Ultrasound cannot differentiate between venous compression and venous thrombosis and has failed to detect small, partially occluding proximal vein thrombi. Also, the interpretation of results is more dependent upon the experience of the examiner than other noninvasive techniques for diagnosing deep venous thrombosis. Although this method undoubtedly will become more refined with time, its exact future role remains uncertain.

Thermography

Associated with venous thrombosis of the lower extremities is an increase in blood flow and an inflammatory reaction causing changes in skin temperature. The temperature may be increased sufficiently to be detected on physical examination, or it may be subclinical. Thermography can detect subclinical temperature changes and has been used to diagnose deep venous thrombosis. The method is noninvasive, requires simple patient cooperation, is easily repeated for follow-up, and can be performed quickly. In a series reported by Bergovist et al., there was a 90.1 per cent correlation between thermography and phlebography in the diagnosis of deep venous thrombosis, although the localization of thrombi was somewhat less accurate.[8]

In normal patients, pretibial and prepatellar areas of cooling are demonstrated by thermography; with deep venous thrombosis, the pretibial and prepatellar cooling is diminished or absent. Occasionally, a thrombus may be seen as a "hot streak" on a thermogram. The thermographic pattern of deep venous thrombosis is rather characteristic. The thermographic picture itself rather than the absolute increase in leg temperature or temperature difference between the legs determines the diagnosis. False positive diagnoses of deep venous thrombosis occur in patients who have increased skin temperature from inflammatory processes and also in patients with superficial phlebitis. Therefore, a positive thermogram should be confirmed by phlebography before treatment is instituted. Thermography cannot identify isolated pelvic vein thrombosis. At the present time, thermography is not in widespread use; its methods of performance and interpretation are still being investigated.

NORMAL ASCENDING PHLEBOGRAM

On a normal ascending phlebogram (see Fig. 23–4) all the major deep and muscular veins are well filled with contrast medium, although there is variable opacification of the superficial venous system and perforating (communicating) veins.

Initially, at fluoroscopy, the foot veins are opacified as the heavier contrast medium begins to replace venous blood. The superficial veins in the lower leg are often visualized before the veins of the deep system. Contrast medium from the deep plantar arch is seen to ascend directly into the posterior tibial veins. The anterior tibial veins drain the veins of the dorsum of the foot. Multiple small tributary veins merge to form the peroneal veins at the level of the ankle. The anterior tibial veins are usually smaller than the peroneal or posterior veins and do not fill with contrast medium in every normal case. Their absence is not necessarily indicative of anterior tibial venous thrombosis. The longitudinal deep veins of the lower leg are recognized by their position, straight course, paired configuration, and numerous valves. Superficial veins that may parallel the course of these deep veins have fewer valves and frequently can be seen to anastomose with other superficial veins.

The muscular veins of the calf fill primarily from below, either from their connections with the deep or superficial venous system, although there may be also some downward filling from above to the most proximal muscle vein valves. The soleal veins may be best demonstrated on films taken in the anteroposterior projection and the gastrocnemius veins in the oblique view. Frequent valves are seen in nearly all muscular veins.

Following opacification of the longitudinal deep veins of the calf there is usually rapid filling of the popliteal and femoral veins. The profunda femoris vein is opacified in only 50 per cent of ascending phlebograms (see Fig. 23–4D). Opacification of this

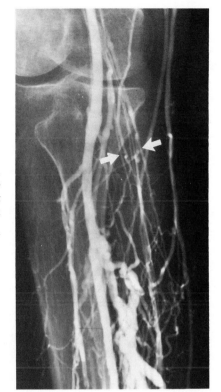

Figure 23–9. Small-caliber muscular veins of inactive patients. The muscular veins of immobilized or bedridden patients are small in caliber and may be difficult to opacify with contrast medium. Note the small sural (gastrocnemius) veins (arrows) in this elderly woman.

vein may be enhanced when the patient does a Valsalva maneuver. If the profunda femoris vein is not visualized, unopacified blood from this vein may be seen to enter the femoral vein, producing a negative flow defect which is an indirect sign of its patency (see Fig. 25–11). The deep veins vary in size and number. Venous duplications are common, these are discussed in later sections. Bedridden patients often have small-caliber deep veins which may be difficult to fill with contrast medium, especially the muscular veins (Fig. 23–9).

The anatomy of the superficial veins varies widely. On ascending phlebograms these veins can be seen to vary in width, distribution, and frequency of valves. In nearly all cases the greater saphenous vein will be opacified with contrast medium, and the lesser saphenous vein can be identified on films of the lower leg taken in the lateral projection.

Spot films and camera exposures may best reproduce the fine details of perforating veins. Ciné radiography or video tape replay can be helpful in determining the direction of blood flow in individual perforating veins in patients with superficial varicosities.

Pitfalls in the Performance and Interpretation of Ascending Phlebography

Errors in technique and interpretation may result in false positive or false negative ascending phlebograms. Below is a list of the common sources of error.

IMPROPER SITE OF CONTRAST MEDIUM INJECTION.   If the needle is positioned too high on the foot, injected contrast medium may not opacify the plantar venous arch or the distal posterior tibial or peroneal veins. The resulting phlebogram should not be falsely interpreted as demonstrating occlusion of the distal portions of these veins. If the needle cannot be positioned more distally, the fluoroscopy table should be tilted at a higher angle; this maneuver alone may improve distal opacification. A tourniquet temporarily placed above the needle may also help. If not, the radiologist should inform the patient's physician that the distal veins cannot be evaluated and that their absence does not necessarily indicate venous thrombosis.

EXTERNAL COMPRESSION DEFECTS. Artifactual filling defects in deep veins may be produced by external compression. For the ascending phlebography technique described in this chapter, tourniquets are not required to drive contrast medium into deep veins and in fact may produce artifactual filling defects in deep veins or fail to opacify them above the level of the tourniquets. A compression artifact may even be produced by a soft pillow placed under the knee for the patient's comfort; it may compress and occlude the popliteal vein (Fig. 23–10).

WEIGHT BEARING. If the involved extremity is weight-bearing during ascending phlebography, contraction of the calf muscles may result in emptying or incomplete filling of the deep veins. Certain deep veins may be completely occluded, and diversion

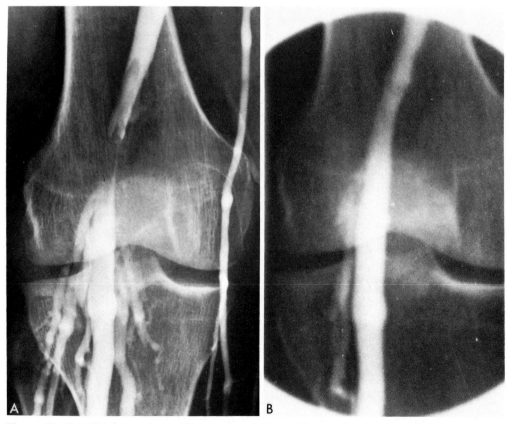

Figure 23–10. Phlebography artifact produced by a pillow under the patient's knee. During ascending phlebography any pillow or cushion placed under the involved extremity for the patient's comfort should be removed so that artifacts will not be produced by external compression. *A,* A compression artifact in the popliteal vein was produced by a small pillow underneath the knee. *B,* A spot film obtained after the pillow was removed showed normal opacification of the popliteal vein.

of contrast medium flow will be demonstrated. The involved extremity should be relaxed throughout the examination, and all the weight should be borne by the opposite leg.

FLOW ARTIFACTS. If the profunda femoris vein does not opacify, unopacified blood may be seen entering the femoral vein, producing flow artifacts that may be incorrectly interpreted as thrombus. Similar flow artifacts may be produced by unopacified blood from other muscular veins that enter the femoral vein. When these defects are identified, the patient should be asked to perform a Valsalva maneuver, which will enhance the opacification of the femoral vein and may be sufficient to eliminate any question of femoral vein thrombus (Fig. 23–11). If a Valsalva maneuver does not clarify the issue, the patient should be examined with retrograde catheterization phlebography (Fig. 23–12).

LAYERING OF CONTRAST MEDIUM. Even in the semi-erect position there may be layering of the heavier contrast medium in the proximal femoral vein, resulting in an apparent narrowing that may be confused with mural thrombus. Improved opacification can be obtained by having the patient perform a Valsalva maneuver or elevating the involved extremity to increase the volume of contrast medium flowing in the proximal femoral vein.

FOOT VEIN THROMBOSIS. Pathologic and radiographic studies have demonstrated isolated foot vein thrombosis,[19] and therefore either spot films or overhead films of the foot should be obtained in every ascending phlebogram so that this diagnosis will not be

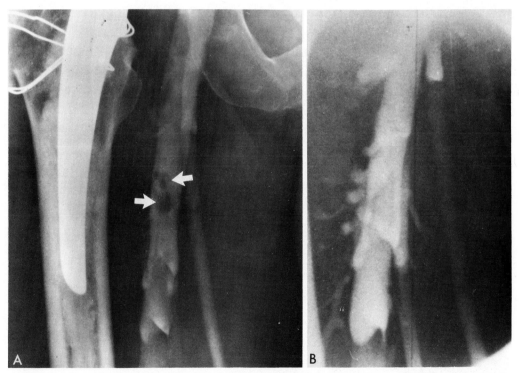

Figure 23–11. Flow artifacts produced in the femoral vein when the profunda femoris vein is not opacified with contrast medium. *A,* Unopacified blood from the profunda femoris and other deep muscular veins may produce flow artifacts (arrows) in the femoral vein that may be difficult to distinguish from venous thrombi. *B,* Often a Valsalva maneuver will improve opacification of the femoral vein and either confirm or disprove a diagnosis of venous thrombosis. If the maneuver is not successful in resolving any questionable areas within the femoral vein, a retrograde catheterization phlebogram should be performed.

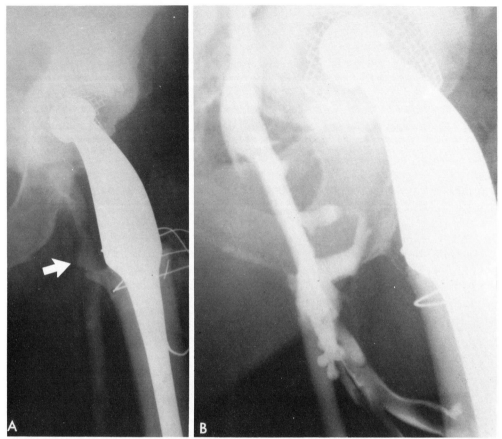

Figure 23–12. Retrograde catheterization phlebography resolves a questionable area on the conventional ascending phlebogram. *A,* An ascending phlebogram following hip surgery suggested a filling defect in the common femoral vein (arrow). However, a diagnosis of venous thrombosis could not be made with certainty. *B,* The retrograde catheterization phlebogram showed a definite thrombus in the (common) femoral vein and also in the profunda femoris vein.

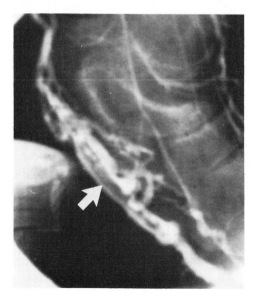

Figure 23–13. Foot vein thrombosis. Isolated foot vein thrombosis (arrow) does occur, and films of the foot should be obtained on all ascending phlebograms so that this diagnosis will not be overlooked.

overlooked (Fig. 23–13). Optimally, the foot should be filmed in the lateral projection to show the plantar arch, where the majority of these thrombi occur.

USE OF SPOT FILMS AND CAMERA EXPOSURES. Because deep vein thrombi may be missed on routine overhead films (Fig. 23–14), it is recommended that multiple spot films or camera exposures be obtained of the entire leg. In the lower leg there is frequent overlap of muscular and longitudinal deep veins, and exposures should be obtained in at least two projections, usually the anteroposterior and oblique.

CONGENITAL ABSENCE OF THE POSTERIOR TIBIAL VEINS. A not uncommon congenital variation of the deep venous system of the leg is congenital absence of the posterior tibial veins (Fig. 23–15). The posterior tibial veins are entirely absent and the plantar arch veins drain into the peroneal veins. The diagonal course of the veins directly connecting the plantar arch and the peroneal veins confirms the diagnosis.

ARTIFACTS PRODUCED BY MUSCULAR CONTRACTION. Ascending phlebography is painful, and patients may experience involuntary muscle contractions and spasms that can result in poor or absent opacification of entire deep veins and venous segments. The radiologist should recognize these events and obtain further exposures when the patient's leg has been relaxed.

NARROWING OF THE POPLITEAL VEIN OWING TO HYPEREXTENSION OF THE KNEE. Hyperextension of the knee may result in apparent narrowing or obstruction of the popliteal vein. Therefore, further spot films should be obtained when the leg is relaxed.

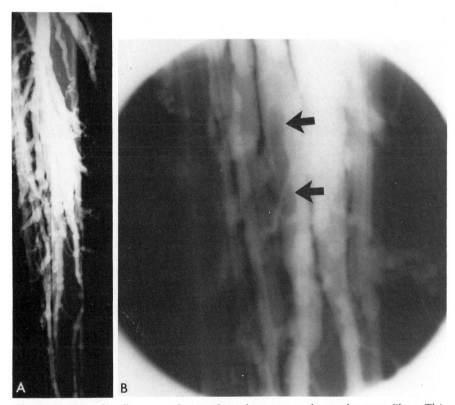

Figure 23–14. Small peroneal vein thrombus seen only on the spot films. This examination showed the value of obtaining multiple spot films during ascending phlebography. *A,* No thrombi were seen on the overhead films, yet a definite peroneal vein thrombosis (arrows) could be identified on several spot films (*B*).

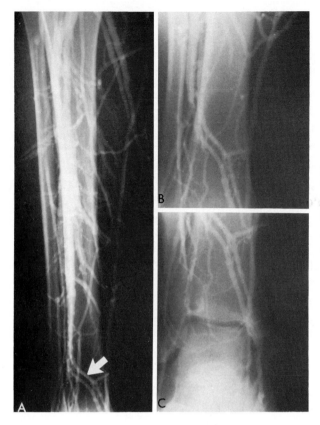

Figure 23–15. Congenital absence of the posterior tibial veins. When the posterior tibial veins are not opacified at ascending phlebography (*A*), they may be congenitally absent. This anomaly is identified when diagonal veins (arrow) are seen connecting the plantar venous arch with the peroneal veins (*B* and *C*).

CONFUSION OF OLD OCCLUSIONS WITH ACUTE DEEP VENOUS THROMBOSIS. If the ascending phlebogram shows only venous occlusion with no evidence of fresh thrombus outlined by contrast medium, then prior phlebograms, if available should be reviewed. If they show the same occlusions and no change, acute deep venous thrombosis can be ruled out. If earlier phlebograms were not performed or are not available, especially if there is a history of prior deep venous thrombosis, the possibility that the venous occlusions are old should be brought to the attention of the referring physician.

SUPERFICIAL PHLEBITIS. The superficial venous system is not entirely opacified during routine ascending phlebography. Therefore, this procedure cannot rule out the presence of acute superficial venous thrombosis even if no superficial thrombi are seen.

Side Effects and Complications of Ascending Phlebography

Most patients complain of discomfort during ascending phlebography, usually a cramping or a painful distended sensation in the calf. It lasts only for the duration of contrast medium injection and is relieved when the patient is placed supine and the venous system is flushed with heparinized saline. Reducing the concentration of contrast medium from 60 per cent to 45 per cent has reduced patient discomfort significantly. In the future, new contrast agents may allow more comfortable phlebography.

The systemic side effects of intravenous administration of contrast media in phlebography are no greater than those seen when similar agents are injected intravenously at other sites for various radiologic procedures.[4] Occasionally, patients experience nausea and vomiting or have minor allergic reactions, such as urticaria. Hypotension and bronchoconstriction are rare and are treated aggressively. There have been no fatalities from ascending phlebography at the Massachusetts General Hospital. Patients with pre-existing renal disease do not tolerate contrast medium as well as those with normal renal function; elevations in blood urea nitrogen and serum creatinine levels have been reported as well as incidents of transient oliguria.[38]

Contrast medium extravasation at the injection site can be minimized by careful fluoroscopic monitoring of the needle during the initial phase of injection as well as fluoroscopic checking of the injection site if the patient inadvertently moves the affected foot during the procedure. With fluoroscopic control, as little as 2 to 3 cc of contrast medium extravasation can be identified. Skin necrosis may occur with large-volume contrast medium extravasation,[43] and skin grafting may be required. Extravasation is especially dangerous in patients with atherosclerotic peripheral vascular disease.

Postphlebography phlebitis is a condition manifested by painful, erythematous limb swelling occurring 2 to 12 hours after phlebography. It has been reported in up to 10 per cent of patients undergoing phlebography, and it may be associated with actual deep venous thrombosis.[2, 9] At the Massachusetts General Hospital, clinical signs of postphlebography phlebitis were noted in 10 out of a series of 220 limbs studied with 60 per cent contrast medium.[4] In six of these ten limbs, repeat phlebography showed venous thrombosis that had presumably been precipitated by the first phlebogram. The incidence of postphlebography phlebitis and venous thrombosis has been reduced by using a more diluted concentration of contrast medium.[9]

CONGENITAL AND DEVELOPMENTAL ANOMALIES

The most common congenital anomaly of lower extremity veins is venous duplication. It occurs in both the deep and the superficial venous systems. Figure 23–16 illustrates duplicated popliteal and femoral veins. Occasionally, duplication of the greater saphenous vein is seen as well as triplication of the femoral or popliteal veins.

There are no clinical syndromes associated with duplication and triplication, although an awareness of their existence is important in the diagnostic work-up of suspected deep venous thrombosis. A patient having one part of a duplication filled with thrombus and the other part patent may have negative cuff impedance plethysmography, Doppler ultrasound, and radionuclide phlebography in the presence of acute major deep vein thrombosis (Fig. 23–17).

Congenital absence of individual deep veins also occurs, most commonly absence of the posterior tibial veins, which was described earlier (see Fig. 23–15). It is important to recognize this entity so that the absent posterior tibial vein opacification at ascending phlebography is not misinterpreted as posterior tibial vein thrombosis.

Congenitally absent or congenitally hypoplastic valves have been recognized in the deep and superficial venous systems unilaterally and bilaterally. When there is extensive involvement of the deep venous system, venous stasis results. This is referred to as primary deep venous insufficiency. The diagnosis should be considered when ever older children or teenagers present with chronic leg swelling or varicosities either unilaterally or bilaterally. The findings at phlebography vary from total absence of the

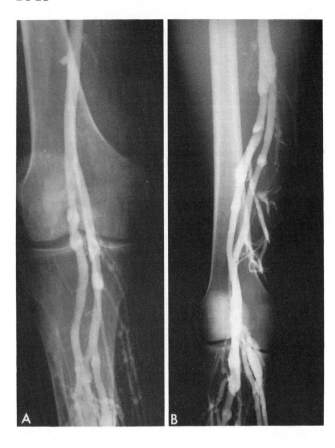

Figure 23–16. Congenital deep vein duplications. Congenital duplications of deep veins are common. *A,* Duplication of the popliteal vein. *B,* Duplication of the femoral vein.

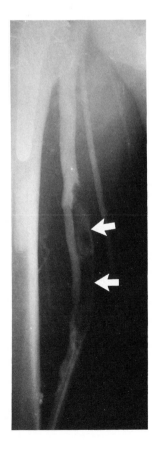

Figure 23–17. Venous thrombosis in a duplicated segment of femoral vein. There is a large fresh thrombus in a duplicated segment of the femoral vein (arrows). Since blood can ascend freely through the patent portion of the duplication, a patient with this condition can have normal cuff impedence plethysmography as well as normal Doppler ultrasound and radioisotope phlebography in the presence of acute femoral vein thrombosis.

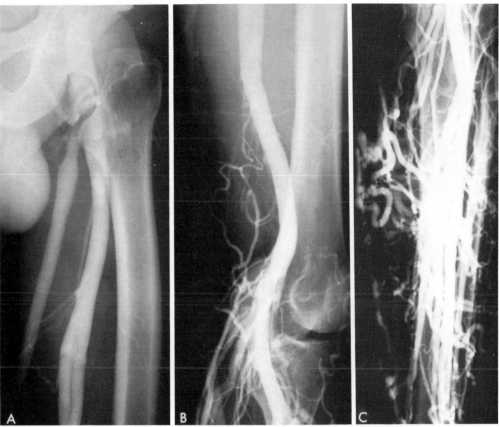

Figure 23–18. *A* to *C,* Primary deep venous insufficiency with varicosities. This young man presented with venous stasis and varicosities. An ascending phlebogram identified hypoplastic venous valves. Note the absence of normal-appearing valve leaflets and sinuses in the popliteal and femoral veins. In addition, superficial calf varicosities and a large-caliber greater saphenous vein can be identified.

femoral, popliteal, and other deep venous valves to valve hypoplasia (Fig. 23–18). Retrograde phlebography during a Valsalva maneuver will show a reverse flow of contrast medium far down into the femoral and popliteal veins and sometimes also into the tibial and peroneal veins. Varicosities, enlargement of the greater saphenous vein, and postphlebitic changes may be seen in conjunction with primary deep venous insufficiency.

Congenital arteriovenous malformations vary in the composition of arterial and venous elements. Some are nearly entirely venous, characterized by masses of enlarged, distended, and tortuous venous channels (Fig. 23–19). They lack the prominent arterial elements seen in other types of arteriovenous malformations, and often arteriograms, with the exception of the venous phase, are normal. Also lacking is the rapid arteriovenous shunting seen in other forms of arteriovenous malformations. The clinical manifestations include soft tissue swelling, limb enlargement, distended superficial venous complexes, venous auscultatory sounds, tenderness, and spontaneous bleeding. Systemic hemodynamic changes are rare. Femoral arteriography and phlebography are useful for diagnosis and planning of therapy. Those malformations with prominent feeding arteries may improve with transcatheter arterial embolization, although these are usually absent in the purely venous type. Phlebography can delineate the anatomic features and the extent of venous lesions when surgical extirpation is being considered.

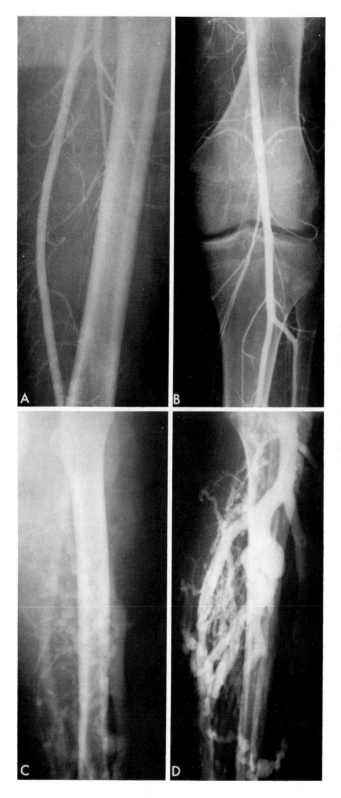

Figure 23–19. Large venous hemangioma. This 17-year-old male presented with a large vascular lesion that involved nearly the entire left leg. Initially he was considered to be a candidate for arterial embolization therapy and was referred for vascular radiology. A femoral arteriogram (*A* and *B*) and an ascending phlebogram (*C* and *D*) showed that the lesion was entirely venous, and therefore the patient could not benefit from arterial embolization.

The iliac compression syndrome is a condition in which left-leg venous congestion is produced by compression of the left common iliac vein by the anteriorly crossing right common iliac artery. The syndrome primarily affects young females.[29] The clinical manifestations include mild to moderate left-leg swelling and an increased incidence of left-leg deep venous thrombosis, especially in women taking birth control pills. Simultaneous aortography and venography show the relationship between the compressed vein and the crossing artery. A pressure gradient can usually be measured above and below the compressed venous segment. Rarely, right-leg venous congestion results from compression of the right common iliac vein by the right common iliac artery. Several patients have been successfully treated with surgery.

VENOUS THROMBOSIS

Venous thrombosis is a frequent complication in hospitalized patients that may lead to significant morbidity and mortality. Detachment of a thrombus from a lower extremity deep vein is the cause of pulmonary embolism in nearly all cases.[12, 42] Venous thrombosis can also cause deep vein occlusion, resulting in significant postphlebitic disability. In the past, venous thrombosis was difficult to establish because of the inaccuracy of clinical diagnosis. One half of patients with deep venous thrombosis have no clinical signs,[31] and in one half of patients with a positive clinical diagnosis, the deep veins are normal.[20, 37]

Today, with the widespread availability of ascending phlebography and the introduction of cuff impedance plethysmography, ^{125}I-fibrinogen scanning, Doppler ultrasound, and other noninvasive studies, the accuracy of diagnosis has significantly improved. It is now important to identify those patients who are at high risk of developing deep venous thrombosis so that noninvasive screening procedures may be performed and those with positive noninvasive examinations can be referred for phlebography. Likewise, phlebography should be performed in those patients with positive clinical signs and symptoms in order to avoid unnecessary treatment in patients who do not have venous thrombosis.

The etiology of venous thrombosis is not entirely clear. It is thought to result from some combination of reduced venous blood flow, hypercoagulability, and endothelial damage. Venous thrombosis may involve the superficial veins, the deep veins, or both. Superficial venous thrombosis is rarely a cause of pulmonary embolism and is associated with significantly less morbidity and mortality than deep venous thrombosis. Superficial venous thrombosis is usually accompanied by a vigorous inflammatory reaction, and consequently the thrombi become adherent to the vein walls. However, the process may extend into the deep system via the perforating veins. Phlebography is useful in ruling out underlying deep venous thrombosis in patients with clinically diagnosed superficial phlebitis. In the absence of deep vein involvement, superficial venous thrombosis can be treated conservatively without anticoagulation measures.

Deep venous thrombosis is common in hospitalized patients, and the incidence increases with age. Surgical patients, especially those undergoing orthopedic procedures, are at high risk. There is a greater than 50 per cent incidence of deep vein thrombosis[15] and a 28 per cent incidence of proximal vein thrombosis[22] in patients who undergo hip surgery. Trauma patients are also at increased risk. Tibial fractures treated nonsurgically with cast immobilization are associated with an incidence of venous thrombosis of up to 45 per cent. Cancer patients, those immobilized for stroke and other neurologic problems, those with congestive heart failure, a history of deep venous thrombosis, varicose veins, obesity, or pregnancy, and those taking oral contraceptives are all at increased risk of developing deep venous thrombosis.[16]

Although clinical findings are absent in 50 per cent of patients with deep venous thrombosis, when present they include pain, swelling, heat, redness, and tenderness. The differential diagnosis of acute deep venous thrombosis includes postphlebitic stasis syndromes, symptomatic varicose veins, congestive heart failure presenting with leg edema, leg trauma, lymphatic obstruction from malignancy, cellulitis, lymphangitis, arthritis, and ruptured Baker's cyst. In both males and females the incidence of deep venous thrombosis is slightly greater in the left leg than in the right, and this is probably related to the increased stasis in the left leg caused by compression of the left common iliac vein by the anteriorly crossing right common iliac artery.

When deep venous thrombosis occurs it involves the calf veins in nearly 90 per cent of cases. In approximately 65 per cent, the process involves veins above the calf. It is unclear whether calf thrombi originate in the venous sinuses of muscular soleal veins or on the valve cusps of the longitudinal deep veins of the lower legs (posterior tibial, anterior tibial, and peroneal veins). Calf vein thrombosis may extend into the popliteal, femoral, and iliac veins. Although uncommon, proximal vein thrombosis may originate independently of calf vein thrombosis, especially in patients who have undergone surgery or trauma to the hip or proximal leg.[23]

Pulmonary embolism may occur at any stage in the proximal progression of deep venous thrombosis, although it is more common in those patients with proximal vein thrombosis involving the deep veins above the knee (iliofemoral venous thrombosis). Nearly all patients with pulmonary embolism at autopsy also have deep venous thrombosis of the lower extremities.[27, 34, 42] Large emboli usually originate in the iliofemoral veins. In living patients, phlebography has demonstrated deep venous thrombosis in 50 to 72 per cent of patients who present clinically with pulmonary embolism.[10, 12] Although isolated calf vein thrombi do not cause significant pulmonary embolism, untreated small thrombi may extend proximally if not treated, resulting in major pulmonary embolism.

Phlebography is the most accurate method of diagnosing deep venous thrombosis, and it is the standard for other modalities. A negative leg phlebogram excludes a diagnosis of deep venous thrombosis.[4] When positive, phlebography not only confirms the diagnosis but also provides details about the exact site and extent of thrombosis.

There are several reliable phlebographic signs of venous thrombosis. Because a thrombus displaces contrast medium it may appear as a constant, sharply delineated filling defect surrounded by contrast medium (Fig. 23–20). Small early thrombi involving only valve cusps may be identified at phlebography (Fig. 23–21). Frequently, thrombi are attached to the vein wall and may be eccentrically located within the vein lumen (Fig. 23–22).

If the entire circumference of the thrombus is adherent to the vein wall, no contrast medium will flow around it and only venous occlusion will be seen on the phlebogram. A short segment or the entire vein may be occluded, with abrupt termination of the opaque column above or below the site of occlusion (Fig. 23–23).

In certain cases the entire deep venous system is occluded, and only the superficial venous system is opacified (Fig. 23–24). However, the deep system normally is opacified above the proximal extent of thrombosis. Figure 23–25 illustrates the proximal extent of thrombus in a patient with thrombosis of the entire deep venous system of the right extremity; the leading edge of thrombus is seen in the proximal femoral vein.

The most reliable sign of acute deep venous thrombosis is demonstration of a thrombus outlined by contrast medium. When only venous occlusion is shown on the phlebogram, it cannot be determined whether the occlusion is new or old. In this situation, comparison with an old phlebogram as well as fibrinogen leg scanning is helpful. If the area where the venous occlusion was identified becomes positive on

Text continued on page 1657

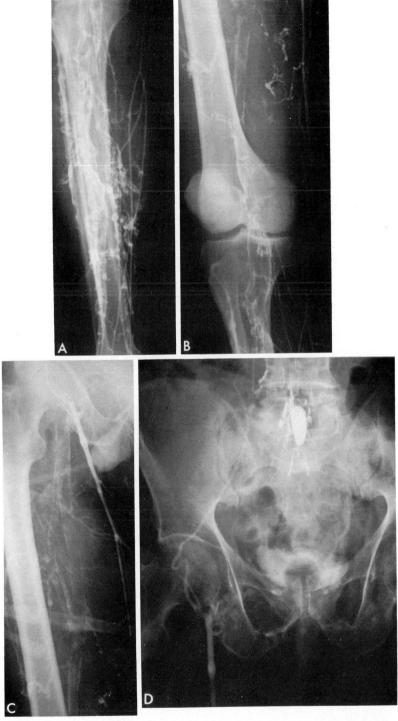

Figure 23–20. Acute iliofemoral deep venous thrombosis. The ascending phlebogram of this patient with acute swelling of the right leg showed thrombus throughout the deep venous system. A small amount of contrast medium can be seen ascending in a narrow space between the blood clot and the vein intima, outlining the extent of thrombosis. The ipsilateral external iliac and common iliac veins are completely occluded. The patent greater saphenous vein is drained by abdominal wall and transpelvic collateral veins. (An incidental finding is residual contrast medium from a previous myelogram seen overlying the spine.)

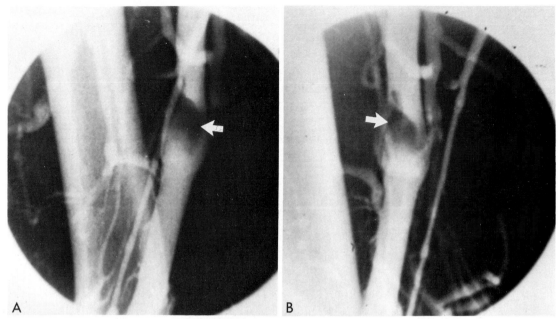

Figure 23–21. Thrombi involving valve cusps. Thrombi often form on or about valve cusps. *A* and *B*, Spot films of a patient with this earliest form of deep venous thrombosis (arrows) following hip surgery.

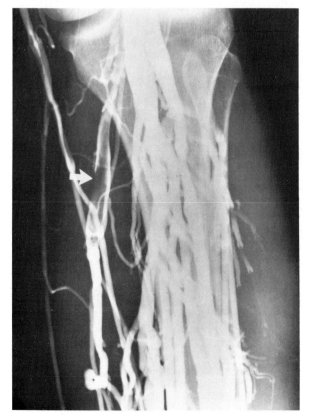

Figure 23–22. Acute venous thrombosis involving a sural (gastrocnemius) vein. This patient developed calf tenderness following hip surgery. The phlebogram showed a thrombus only in a sural (gastrocnemius) vein (arrow). The remainder of the deep and superficial venous systems were normal. If this thrombus had not been detected and proper therapy instituted, the natural history would have been an extension of the thrombotic process.

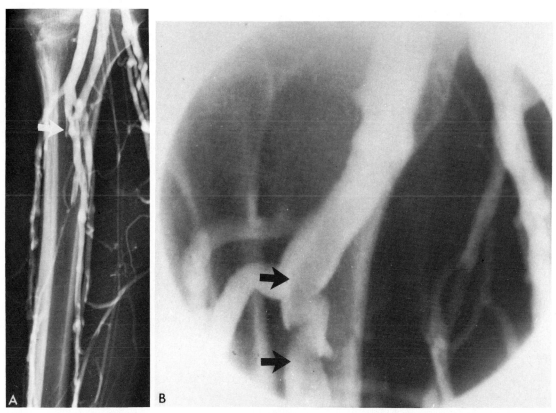

Figure 23–23. Occlusion of the peroneal veins with venous thrombus. The peroneal veins are totally occluded. The anterior and posterior tibial veins are patent. The proximal extent of peroneal vein thrombus (arrows) can be seen extending into the duplicated popliteal veins on both the overhead (*A*) and spot (*B*) films.

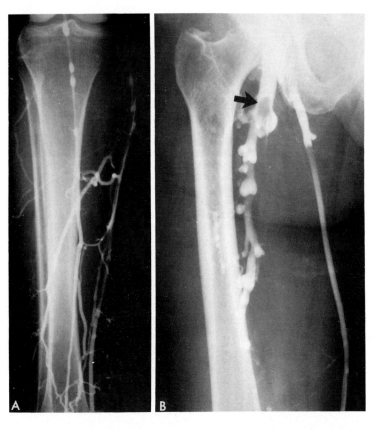

Figure 23–24. Acute venous thrombosis occluding nearly the entire deep venous system of the right leg. In this postoperative patient with new edema of the entire right leg an ascending phlebogram demonstrated occlusion of nearly the entire deep venous system. *A,* In the lower leg only superficial veins are opacified; the peroneal, tibial, popliteal, and distal femoral veins were occluded with thrombus. *B,* In the upper leg, the leading edge of thrombus can be seen extending into the proximal femoral vein (arrow). The profunda femoris vein, greater saphenous vein, and proximal femoral vein are patent.

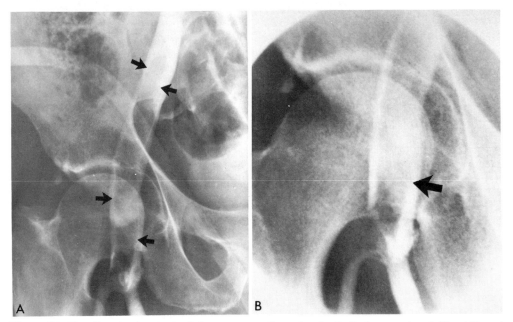

Figure 23–25. Proximal extent of deep venous thrombosis. Both the overhead film (*A*) and the spot film (*B*) show the proximal extent of thrombus in a patient with thrombosis of the entire deep venous system of the right leg. The patient had suffered a femoral fracture, and a portion of the splint is seen overlying the pelvis. The thrombus extends proximally into the (common) femoral vein and distal external iliac vein.

^{125}I-fibrinogen scanning, the occlusion must result from a new thrombus still incorporating fibrinogen. Normally, the posterior tibial and peroneal veins opacify at ascending phlebography. However, opacification of the anterior tibial veins is variable, and absent or poor filling of the anterior tibial veins alone is not indicative of venous occlusion or venous thrombosis. Occlusion of the posterior tibial or peroneal veins, however, definitively indicates new or old venous thrombosis.

Although phlebography is the most accurate test for diagnosing venous thrombosis, it is not a practical examination for screening large numbers of patients who are at high risk but who do not have clinical signs and symptoms of venous thrombosis. In this group, screening with cuff impedance plethysmography, ^{125}I-fibrinogen scanning, and Doppler ultrasound is recommended. If the noninvasive studies are negative, venous thrombosis can be ruled out, although with less accuracy than with phlebography. If positive, the patient should be referred for phlebography before anticoagulation treatment is started or venous interruption is performed. The major contributions of the noninvasive examinations are in screening patients at high risk and following patients who are currently undergoing anticoagulation therapy. Cuff impedance plethysmography and Doppler ultrasound have poor accuracy for detection of calf vein thrombi, and ^{125}I-fibrinogen scanning has poor accuracy for detecting proximal femoral and pelvic vein thrombi. Therefore, when plebography is unavailable or contraindicated, ^{125}I-fibrinogen scanning should be combined with either cuff impedance plethysmography or Doppler ultrasound.

A deep vein occluded with thrombus may remain occluded and bypassed by collaterals. Following a course of anticoagulation therapy, the thrombus may adhere to the vein wall and retract against it, resulting in lumen recanalization. The process of retraction may lead to complete recanalization and a normal-appearing venous system on repeat phlebography, or the vein may become irregular in outline with loss of normal-appearing valves, a pattern referred to as postphlebitic change.

A thrombus remains loose for about a week before the process of adherence begins. Adherence of the thrombosis over its entire circumference results in permanent occlusion, whereas partial adherence results in partial or full recanalization. Retraction starts soon after the first week and the final stages of recanalization several months later.

CHRONIC VENOUS OBSTRUCTION

Occlusion of portions of the deep venous system may result in a variety of chronic venous obstruction syndromes depending upon the anatomic location of the occluded vein and the length of the occluded segment. Iliofemoral venous occlusion produces more marked physiologic changes than tibial vein occlusion, and long segment occlusions have more serious consequences than short occlusions. The significance of the occlusion also depends upon the adequacy of the venous collaterals that develop around the occluded venous segment.

Chronic occlusions of superficial veins are rarely symptomatic. The superficial venous system includes a great number of veins that can act as collaterals, and the perforating veins can bypass occluded superficial segments by draining blood directly into the deep system.

Deep venous thrombosis is the most common cause of chronic venous obstruction, although other processes, such as surgery (Fig. 23–26), trauma, and complications of femoral vein catheterization (Fig. 23–27), may result in venous occlusion. Extrinsic processes may cause venous thrombosis and occlusion by producing venous compres-

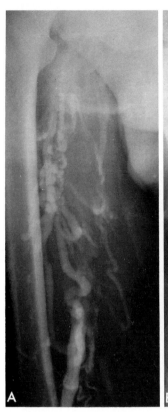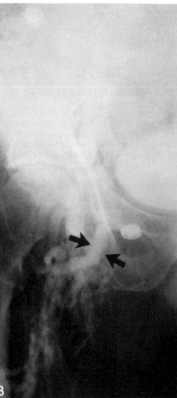

Figure 23–26. *A* and *B*, Chronic venous obstruction resulting from femoral vein ligation. This patient underwent a right femoral vein ligation for deep venous thrombosis that could not be treated with anticoagulation. Following surgery he developed chronic venous obstruction in the right leg. Nearly the entire length of the right femoral vein is occluded. The right leg is drained by collaterals (the arrows point to an enlarged obturator collateral vein) that reconstitute the proximal right femoral vein and right internal and common iliac veins.

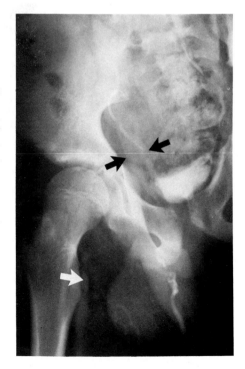

Figure 23–27. Femoral vein occlusion following right heart catheterization. This 12-year-old boy complained of a difference in size between the lower extremities; his right leg had become larger than the left. A history was obtained of a prior right heart catheterization, and an ascending phlebogram was performed. It showed complete occlusion of the right femoral vein (white arrow), with proximal flow of contrast via obturator collaterals to the right hypogastric vein (black arrows). At two weeks of age a cardiac catheterization had been performed via right femoral vein following an episode of cyanosis. The cardiac catheterization procedure was normal; the cyanosis had resulted from an epiglottic lesion that was resected at the time.

sion; these include aneurysms of the femoral and popliteal arteries, abdominal aortic aneurysms, benign and malignant neoplasms in the pelvis and lower extremities, and retroperitoneal fibrosis.

Among the clinical features of chronic venous obstruction are limb swelling, chronic venous outflow obstruction, skin discoloration, and prominence of superficial veins that act as collateral pathways around occluded deep venous segments. Although noninvasive studies, including cuff impedance plethysmography and Doppler ultrasound can confirm the presence of venous obstruction, phlebography is capable of outlining the location and extent of the deep venous occlusions and patterns of postphlebitic changes.

THE POSTPHLEBITIC SYNDROME AND VARICOSE VEINS

When chronic venous obstruction results from prior deep venous thrombosis it is referred to as the postphlebitic syndrome. Deep venous thrombi may cause irreversible damage to deep veins. When recanalization occurs, the newly formed venous lumen may be irregular in outline and the valves damaged or destroyed. At phlebography, the lumen may have a weblike appearance, and sometimes more than one lumen may be identified (Figs. 23–28 and 23–29). The severity of the postphlebitic damage varies with the degree of extension of the primary thrombotic process. The hemodynamic changes vary with the extent of postphlebitic change.

Varicose veins are abnormally dilated and tortuous superficial veins that commonly result from damage to perforating vein valves during episodes of deep venous

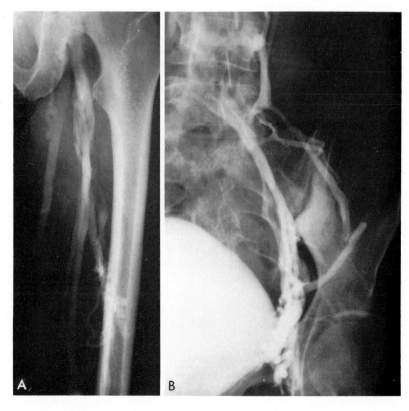

Figure 23–28. Postphlebitic recanalization of the iliofemoral veins. This man presented with chronic left leg edema. Several years earlier he had been treated for acute left iliofemoral venous thrombosis. His current ascending phlebogram (A and B) shows postphlebitic changes in the left femoral and iliac veins. The recanalized venous channels are narrowed and irregular, and no normal valves can be identified. In some areas multiple channels can be seen. These changes are usually associated with damage to the perforating veins, resulting in stasis and dilatation of the superficial venous system. Note the large-caliber greater saphenous vein.

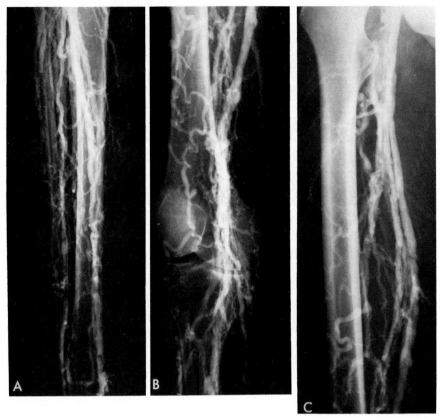

Figure 23–29. Postphlebitic syndrome with extensive superficial varicosities. This patient developed chronic leg edema following an episode of acute deep venous thrombosis. There were prominent superficial varicosities on physical examination. The ascending phlebogram (*A* to *C*) showed postphlebitic changes in the deep veins and extensive superficial varicosities.

thrombosis. The perforating veins become incompetent and, on contraction of the musculovenous pumps, jets of blood from the deep venous system are sent through the perforating veins in reverse direction at high pressure into the superficial veins, resulting in the development of superficial varicosities. In addition, there is usually an associated chronic increase in pressure in the deep venous system owing to valvular damage in the popliteal and femoral veins.

At phlebography, incompetent perforating veins damaged from venous thrombosis are often abnormally wide and tortuous (Fig. 23–29). Usually the valves are absent, although small damaged valve remnants may sometimes be identified. They nearly always empty into enlarged superficial varicosities. Normally, blood flows from the superficial system through perforating veins into the deep venous system; in patients with incompetent perforating veins, blood may be observed to flow in the reverse direction, a process that can be recorded on cine or video tape. Superficial varicosities also have destroyed valves, identifiable by their large caliber and tortuous course. The greater saphenous vein is often enlarged in patients with the postphlebitic syndrome and varicosities, because it functions as a collateral route bypassing the occluded or narrowed deep veins and as a pathway to carry the extra blood flowing into the superficial venous system through incompetent perforating veins.

Fewer than half of patients with post-thrombotic varicose veins have a history of deep venous thrombosis. It appears that clinically silent deep venous thrombosis occurs and is a common cause of varicose veins. The differential diagnosis of post-thrombotic varicose veins includes primary varicose veins resulting from congenital anomalies of the venous valves (see Fig. 23–18), prominence of the superficial veins when they act as pathways around occluded deep venous segments, congenital venous malformations (see Fig. 23–19), and prominent veins associated with traumatic arteriovenous fistulas.

Post-thrombotic superficial varicosities are associated with venous stasis, venous congestion, edema, and an increased incidence of both superficial and deep venous thrombosis. Venous distention itself may be painful. The most disabling sequela is chronic extremity edema associated with stasis dermatitis and stasis ulcers of the skin. In addition, because of the impaired circulation there is an increased vulnerability to trauma.

VENOUS ANEURYSMS

Venous aneurysms are very rare. They have been described in the literature only within the last few years. Occasionally, venous aneurysms are identified as incidental findings at ascending phlebography. They usually are clinically silent. If a venous aneurysm thromboses, a patient may complain of a palpable mass or lump within the soft tissues (Fig. 23–30). In a recent report a thrombosed popliteal vein aneurysm was shown to be the cause of recurrent pulmonary embolism.[13]

VENOUS TRAUMA

Ateriography is the well-accepted procedure for evaluating the vascular system in patients with extremity injuries. In most cases the venous system is opacified at

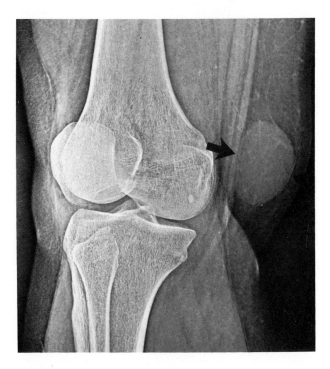

Figure 23–30. Thrombosed venous aneurysm. This obese middle-aged woman complained of a palpable mass adjacent to her right knee. A xerogram showed a well-circumscribed mass within the subcutaneous adipose tissue (arrow). At surgery a thrombosed superficial venous aneurysm was found.

arteriography only when a significant arteriovenous fistula is present. Therefore, several authors have recommended the adjunctive use of phlebography when trauma patients show evidence of impaired extremity circulation. Venous compression and occlusion in an injured extremity may result in nonviability and necessitate amputation.[17] With the venous anatomy outlined preoperatively, venous repair can be performed when there are injuries to major deep venous pathways, or venous ligation can be done at sites of injury when rich collateral networks have been demonstrated phlebographically.

VENOUS THROMBOSIS OF THE UPPER EXTREMITIES

Thrombosis of the deep veins of the upper extremities accounts for less than 2 per cent of all deep venous thromboses. It is a potentially serious condition; in one reported series there was a 12 per cent incidence of pulmonary embolism.[1] Although pulmonary embolism does not occur in the majority of patients, venous thrombosis may cause permanent occlusion of the subclavian or innominate veins, which may result in chronic venous stasis and edema of the involved arm.

Phlebography is the procedure of choice for evaluating upper extremity veins. It is usually performed with the patient in the supine position on a fluoroscopy table, arm positioned at the side (neutral position). Contrast medium is injected through a

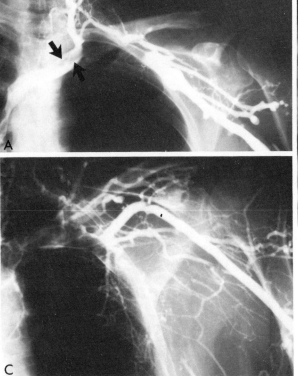
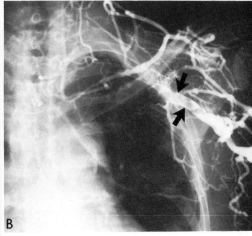

Figure 23–31. Three patients with upper extremity venous thrombosis resulting from indwelling venous catheters. *A,* There is complete occlusion of the left subclavian vein. The axillary vein is patent, and the left innominate vein is reconstituted by collaterals. The leading edge of thrombus can be seen extending into the left innominate vein (arrows). *B,* The left subclavian and left innominate veins are both occluded. Thrombus can be seen within the axillary vein (arrows). The left arm is drained by collaterals to both intercostal and paraspinal veins. *C,* The left axillary, subclavian, and innominate vein are all occluded. Thrombus within these veins is outlined by contrast that ascended via the patent cephallic vein. Extensive collaterals are again identified.

percutaneously placed 19-gauge scalp vein needle. For evaluating the veins of the forearm the venipuncture is done on the dorsum of the hand; for optimal opacification of the upper arm the needle is positioned in an antecubital vein. Usually a hand injection of 50 cc of 45 per cent contrast medium is sufficient. The initial injection is carefully watched fluoroscopically to detect any extravasation. Serial films, spot films, or camera exposures are obtained over the areas of interest. Occasionally, venous catheterization may be required to optimally opacify the subclavian and innominate veins. Patients with a history of recurrent upper extremity venous thrombosis who are suspected of having venous compression at the thoracic outlet should also be studied with the arm abducted and elevated overhead.[18]

In hospitalized patients, upper extremity venous thrombosis is usually associated with the use of central venous pressure catheters, hyperalimentation lines, or transvenous pacing wires. In a recent report, 34 phlebograms were performed in 32 patients 18 months or longer after the placement of transvenous pacing wires; 11 of the phlebograms showed evidence of venous obstruction with collateral circulation.[44] When venous thrombosis occurs with central venous pressure catheters or hyperalimentation lines it usually involves the axillary, subclavian, or innominate veins (Fig. 23–31). As with deep venous thrombosis in the lower extremities, recanalization may occur or permanent venous occlusion may result.

References

1. Adams, J. T., McEvoy, R. K., and Deweese, J.: Primary deep vein thrombosis of upper extremity. Arch. Surg. 91:29–41, 1965.
2. Albrechtsson, U., and Olsson, C. G.: Thrombotic side-effects of lower-limb phlebography. Lancet 1(7962):723–724, 1976.
3. Appleberg, M.: The diagnosis of deep vein thrombosis in the lower limbs by means of the transcutaneous Doppler ultrasound method. S. Afr. Med. J. 50(25):53–55, 1976.
4. Athanasoulis, C. A.: Phlebography for the diagnosis of deep leg vein thrombosis. In Fratantoni, J., and Wessler, S. (eds.): Prophylactic Therapy of Deep Vein Thrombosis and Pulmonary Embolism. Bethesda, Md., National Institutes of Health, 1975, pp. 62–76.
5. Barnes, R. W., Russell, H. E., Wu, K. K., et al.: Accuracy of Doppler ultrasound in clinically suspected venous thrombosis of the calf. Surg. Gynecol. Obstet. 143(3):425–428, 1976.
6. Bauer, A.: A venographic study of thrombo-embolic problems. Acta Chir. Scand. (Suppl. 161) 84:1, 1940.
7. Berberich, J., and Hirsch, S.: Die rontgenologische darstellung der arterien und venen im lebenden menschen. Klin. Wschr. 49:2226, 1923.
8. Bergovist, D., Efsing, H. O., and Hallbook, T.: Thermography: a noninvasive method for diagnosis of deep venous thrombosis. Arch. Surg. 112(5):600–604, 1977.
9. Bettmann, M. A., and Paulin, S.: Leg phlebography: the incidence, nature and modification of undesirable side effects. Radiology 122(1):101–104, 1977.
10. Browse, N. L., and Lea Thomas, M.: Source of non-lethal pulmonary emboli. Lancet 1:258–1974.
11. Carretta, R. F., Denardo, S. J., Denardo, G. L., et al.: Early diagnosis of venous thrombosis using ^{125}I-fibrinogen. J. Nucl. Med. 18(1):5–10, 1977.
12. Corrigan, T. P., Fossard, D. P., Spindler, J., et al.: Phlebography in the management of pulmonary embolism. Br. J. Surg. 61:484–488, 1974.
13. Dahl, J. R., Freed, T. A., and Burke, M. F.: Popliteal vein aneurysm with recurrent pulmonary thromboemboli, J.A.M.A. 236:2531–2532, 1976.
14. Ennis, J. T., and Elmes, R. J.: Radionuclide venography in the diagnosis of deep vein thrombosis. Radiology 125(2):441–449, 1977.
15. Evarts, C. M., and Feil, E. J.: Prevention of thromboembolic disease after elective surgery of the hip. J. Bone Joint Surg. 53:1271–1280, 1971.
16. Gallus, A. S.: Venous thromboembolism: incidence and clinical risk factors. In Madden, J. L., and Hume, M. (eds.): Venous Thromboembolism, Prevention and Treatment. New York, Appleton-Century Crofts, 1976, pp. 1–32.
17. Gerlock, A. J., Thal, E. R., and Snyder, W. H.: Venography in penetrating injuries of the extremities. Am. J. Roentgenol. 126:1023–1027, 1976.
18. Glass, B. A.: The relationship of axillary venous thrombosis to the thoracic outlet compression syndrome. Ann. Thorac. Surg. 19(6):613–621, 1975.

19. Gothlin, J., and Zubriggen, S.: frequency of thrombosis and post-thrombotic conditions of the foot at phlebography. Acta Radiol. Diagn. (*Stockholm*) 16(1):107–112, 1975.
20. Haeger, K.: Problems of acute deep venous thrombosis. 1. The interpretation of signs and symptoms. Angiology 20:219–223, 1969.
21. Harris, W. H., Athanasoulis, C., Waltman, A. C., et al.: Cuff-impedance phlebography and ^{125}I-fibrinogen scanning versus roentgenographic phlebography for diagnosis of thrombophlebitis. J. Bone Joint Surg. 58(7):939–944, 1976.
22. Harris, W. H., Salzman, E. W., Athanasoulis, C. A., et al.: Comparison of warfarin, low-molecular-weight-dextran, aspirin, and subcutaneous heparin in prevention of venous thromboembolism following total hip replacement. J. Bone Joint Surg. 56:1552–1562, 1974.
23. Harris, W. H., Salzman, E. W., Athanasoulis, C., et al.: Comparison of ^{125}I-fibrinogen count scanning with phlebography for detection of venous thrombi after elective hip surgery. N. Engl. J. Med. 292(13):665–667, 1975.
24. Hayt, D. B., Blatt, C. J., and Freeman, L. M.: Radionuclide venography: its place as a modality for the investigation of thromboembolic phenomena. Semin. Nucl. Med. 7(3):263–281, 1977.
25. Hull, R., Hirsch, J., Sackett, D. L., et al.: Combined use of leg scanning and impedance plethysmography in suspected venous thrombosis. An alternative to venography. N. Engl. J. Med. 296(26):1497–1500, 1977.
26. Hull, R., van Aken, W. G., Hirsch, J., et al.: Impedance plethysmography using the occlusive cuff technique in the diagnosis of venous thrombosis. Circulation 53(4):696–700, 1976.
27. Hunter, W. C., Sneeden, V. D., Robertson, T. D., et al.: Thrombosis of the deep veins of the leg. Its clinical significance as exemplifed in three hundred and fifty one autopsies. Arch. Intern. Med. 68:1, 1941.
28. Jaques, P. F., Richey, W. A., Ely, C. A., et al.: Doppler ultrasonic screening prior to venography for deep venous thrombosis. Am. J. Roentgenol. 129(3):451–452, 1977.
29. Johnsson, K., Göthman, B., and Nordstrom, S.: The iliac compression syndrome. Acta Radiol. Diagn. 15: 539–545, 1972.
30. Kakkar, V. V.: The diagnosis of deep vein thrombosis using the ^{125}I-fibrinogen test. Arch. Surg. 104:152–159, 1972.
31. Kakkar, V. V., and Corrigan, T. P.: Detection of deep vein thrombosis: survey and current status. Prog. Cardiovasc. Dis. 17(3):207–217, 1974.
32. Kakkar, V. V., and Flanc, C.: Role of phlebography in deep vein thrombosis. Br. J. Surg. 55:384, 1968.
33. Lindqvist, R.: Ultrasound as a complementary diagnostic method in deep vein thrombosis of the leg. Acta Med. Scand. 201(5):435–438, 1977.
34. McLachlin, J., and Paterson, J. C.: Some basic observations on venous thrombosis and pulmonary embolism. Surg. Gynecol. Obstet. 93:1, 1951.
35. Meadway, J., Nicolaides, A. N., Walker, C. J., et al.: Value of Doppler ultrasound in diagnosis of clinically suspected deep vein thrombosis. Br. Med. J. 4:552–554, 1975.
36. Moser, K. M., Brach, B. B., and Dolan, G. F.: Clinical suspected deep venous thrombosis of the lower extremities: a comparison of venography, impedance plethysmography, and radiolabeled fibrinogen. J.A.M.A. 237(20):2195–2198, 1977.
37. Nicolaides, A. N., Kakkar, V. V., Field, E. S., et al.: The origin of deep vein thrombosis: a venographic study. Br. J. Radiol. 44:653–663, 1971.
38. Older, R. A., Miller, J. P., Jackson, D. C., et al.: Angiographically induced renal failure and its radiographic detection. Am. J. Roentgenol. 126:1039–1045, 1976.
39. Prentice, C. R.: Labelled fibrinogen in the study of deep venous thrombosis. Recent Adv. Clin. Nucl. Med. 1:129–150, 1975.
40. Rabinov, K., and Paulin, S.: Roetgen diagnosis of venous thrombosis in the leg. Arch. Surg. 104(2):134–144, 1972.
41. Ryo, U. Y., Qazi, M., Srikantaswamy, S., et al.: Radionuclide venography: correlation with contrast venography. J. Nucl. Med. 18(1):11–17, 1977.
42. Sevitt, S., and Gallagher, N.: Venous thrombosis and pulmonary embolism: a clinico-pathological study in injured and burned patients. Br. J. Surg. 48:475–489, 1961.
43. Spigos, D. G., Thane, T. T., and Capek, V.: Skin necrosis following extravasation during peripheral phlebography. Radiology 123:605–606, 1977.
44. Stoney, W. S., Addlestone, R. B., Alford, W. C., Jr., et al.: The incidence of venous thrombosis following long-term transvenous pacing. Ann. Thorac. Surg. 22(2):166–170, 1976.
45. Strandness, D. E., and Summer, D. S.: Ultrasonic velocity detector in the diagnosis of thrombophlebitis. Arch. Surg. 104:180– 1972.
46. Thomas, M. A.: Phlebography. Arch. Surg. 104:145, 1972.
47. Vlahos, L., Macdonald, A. F., and Causer, D. A.: Combination of isotope venography and lung scanning. Br. J. Radiol. 49(586):840–851, 1976.
48. Wheeler, H. B., O'Donnell, J. A., Anderson, F. A., et al.: Occlusive impedance phlebography: a diagnostic procedure of venous thrombosis and pulmonary embolism. Prog. Cardiovasc. Dis. 17(3):199–205, 1974.
49. Wheeler, H. B., Pearson, D., O'Connell, D., et al.: Impedance phlebography: technique, interpretation, and results. Arch. Surg. 104(2):164–169, 1972.
50. Williams, W. J.: Venography (editorial). Circulation 47:220, 1973.

24

DISORDERS OF THE LYMPHATIC SYSTEM

SIDNEY WALLACE, M.D.

BAO-SHAN JING, M.D.

Lymphangiography, the radiographic demonstration of the lymphatic system by the injection of contrast material, was introduced as a clinical procedure by Hudack and McMasters.[26] The visualization and eventual clearing of a vital blue dye injected intradermally was interpreted as a manifestation of normal function. Servelle and Deysson injected percutaneously a radiopaque water-based iodine containing contrast material into dilated dermal lymphatic channels in patients with chylous edema. Kinmonth[27] devised lymphangiography in its current form consisting of intradermal injection of a vital blue dye, cannulation of a subcutaneous lymphatic, and intralymphatic injection of a water-based radiopaque contrast material for the evaluation of edema of the lower extremity. Bruun and Engeset[7] introduced an oil-based radiopaque agent into a fistulous tract that was contiguous with the lymphatic system, opacifying the deeper lymphatics and nodes. In 1959, Shanbrom and Zheutlin, by intranodal injection of oil-based radiopaque media, opacified adjacent lymphatics and nodes. Prokopec in 1959, and Hreschyshyn and Sheehan in 1960 employed the intralymphatic injection of an oil-based contrast material, Ethiodol, for the opacification of lymphatic channels and nodes. Wallace et al.[58] further refined this procedure and applied the technique to a wide range of diseases of the lymphatic system.

TECHNIQUE

Pedal Lymphangiography

The method described is a modification of Kinmonth's basic technique. Patent Blue V or Alphazurine 2G, 0.25 to 0.5 ml of a 2.5 per cent solution, is injected intradermally

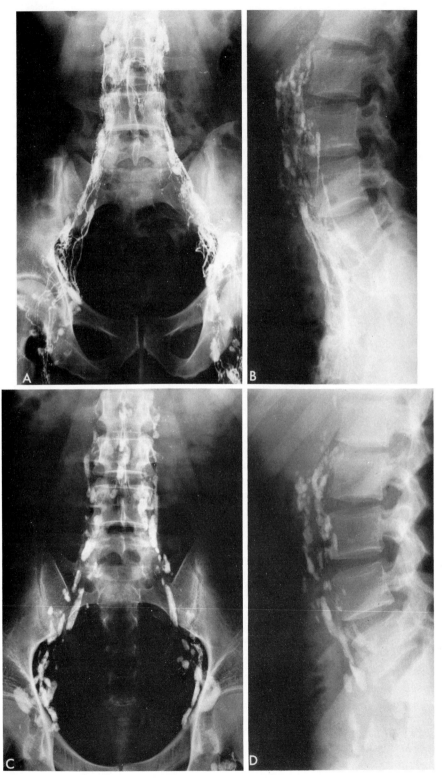

Figure 24–1. Normal lymphangiogram. *A,* Lymphatic phase in anteroposterior projection. *B,* Lymphatic phase in lateral projection. *C,* Nodal phase in anteroposterior projection. *D,* Nodal phase in lateral projection.

in the first interdigital web space on the dorsum of each foot. In the presence of edema, multiple interdigital web spaces are injected. The intradermal dye rapidly enters the intradermal lymphatics and results in almost immediate visualization of these vessels.

The absence of valves in the intradermal lymphatics allows for multidirectional flow with rapid dye opacification of the subcutaneous lymphatics. The centripetal flow in the subcutaneous channels is directed by valves. A small longitudinal incision, 1 cm to 2 cm in length, is made approximately 5 cm proximal to the site of the intradermal injection. When a subcutaneous lymphatic containing the blue dye is visible through the skin, the incision can be made parallel to this vessel. A lymphatic is identified and dissected free of the surrounding tissue. A ligature placed proximally along the lymphatic temporarily occludes the vessel and maximally distends it. The lymphatic is cannulated with a 27- or 30-gauge needle. Ethiodol, an ethyl ester of poppyseed oil containing 37 per cent iodine, is injected under low and constant pressure over approximately one to one and one-half hours.

A similar approach is utilized for the visualization of lymphatics and nodes from the upper extremity, the neck, the testicle, and the penis. Variations in the technique are dictated by the local anatomy.

COMPLICATIONS.   The risks of lymphangiography have been minimal in comparison with the information obtained. Complications can be local or systemic. The local problems include infection, sterile fluid collections, edema, and lymphangitis. Systemic complications are chills, fever, malaise, hypersensitivity (urticaria, asthma, peripheral vascular collapse), blue discoloration, pulmonary embolization, and lymph node lipogranulomas. Tumor dissemination is a potential complication but has not yet been verified.

NORMAL RADIOGRAPHIC LYMPHATIC ANATOMY

Lower Extremity

The cannulation and injection of one lymphatic in each lower extremity opacifies multiple lymphatics and nodes in the inguinal, pelvic, and lumbar areas (Fig. 24–1). The lymphatics of the lower extremity are fine calibered and increase slightly in diameter beyond the inguinal area. The presence of valves is more obvious in the pelvis, producing a beaded appearance. The iliac pathways are formed by three major trunks — medial, middle, and lateral. Internal iliac lymphatics and nodes are inconsistently opacified. At the upper margin of the sacrum, there is intercommunication of the lymphatics from each iliac area making up the para-aortic or lumbar plexus. There are three major trunks, one on each lateral aspect of the vena cava and aorta and one between these vessels.

The thoracic duct, the major collecting channel as described by Bartels,[2, 3] originates from the junction of the lumbar and gastrointestinal trunks to form the cisterna chyli at L_2 to T_{10}. It then traverses the thoracic spine, crossing toward the left at T_5 to empty into the left subclavian vein at the venous angle (Fig. 24–2). This distribution is found in slightly less than 50 per cent of patients. Numerous anatomic variations of the thoracic duct allow for the opacification of mediastinal, hilar, paratracheal, cervical, and axillary lymphatics and nodes. A right-sided lymphatic trunk as a branch of the thoracic duct results in the visualization of hilar, anterior and middle mediastinal, and right supraclavicular nodes as part of the normal distribution. The persistence of a double thoracic duct as well as the many normal variations are explained by the embryologic character of this major collecting trunk.

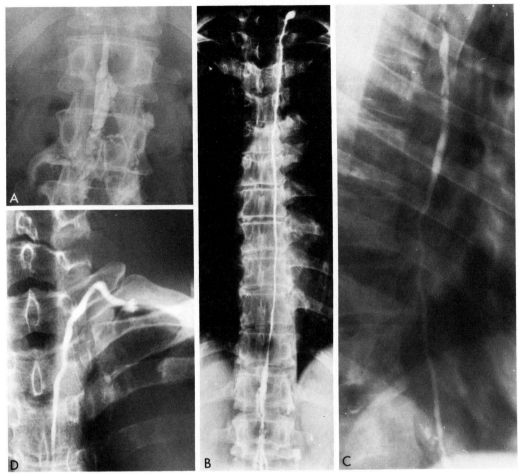

Figure 24–2. Thoracic duct. *A,* Cisterna chyli. *B,* Thoracic duct in anteroposterior view. *C,* Thoracic duct in lateral view. *D,* Terminal portion emptying into the venous angle in the left neck.

Upper Extremity

The normal lymphatics of the upper extremity are of finer caliber than those of the lower limb. The lymphatics that follow the basilic vein, traversing the medial aspect of the arm to the axillary nodes, are usually outlined. In the axilla, the lymphatics branch as they continue through the axillary nodes, frequently opacifying the supraclavicular nodes before reaching the subclavian vein.

LYMPHATIC DYNAMICS

Lymphatic dynamics are governed by the same physiologic principles as those of the blood vascular system, but they function at a decelerated velocity. Abnormalities in any one of the body's fluid compartments precipitate changes in the others in an attempt to maintain homeostasis.

The classic concept of the lymphatic system limits it to the morphologic definition of those endothelium-lined pathways that transport the fluid overload from the blood vascular system centripetally and eventually communicate with the venous system. Acting as a safety valve, they maintain the continuity of the intravascular fluid pool. The lymphatic network is located primarily on the surfaces of the body and viscera. Less numerous endothelium-lined lymphatic pathways, close to the arteries and veins, permeate the parenchyma of the organs and musculoskeletal system.

An essential function of the lymphatic system is the conservation of large particles, primarily proteins, and their restoration to the vascular pool. If this functional definition is accepted, other avenues of fluid transport need to be included in the lymphatic system. The interstitial spaces, the body's potential cavities (pleural, pericardial, and peritoneal), the perivascular and perineural sheaths, and the subserosal and subadventitial spaces can be thought of as the paralymphatic or prelymphatic system. These pathways, probably as extensive as the endothelium-lined lymphatic system but less well defined, supply the necessary avenues for transport from the cellular level to the endothelium-lined lymphatics. This system is analogous to the most primitive mode of fluid transport in invertebrates and plants.

The lymphatic and prelymphatic compartments are probably continuous and eventually drain into the venous system via lymphaticovenous anastomoses. The major site of communication is the junction of the primary collecting trunk, the thoracic duct, and the subclavian vein. Numerous other anastomoses functioning in a reserve capacity are available throughout the body. Lymphaticovenous communications are probably governed by humoral and neurogenic stimuli that regulate the pressure gradients and thus determine directional flow.

DISORDERS OF LYMPHATICS

Interruption of the lymphatic circulation results in the utilization of collateral channels, lymphatic-to-lymphatic, lymphatic-to-prelymphatic, and lymphatic-to-venous, to circumvent the obstruction and re-establish continuity. If these alternate pathways are inadequate there is an accumulation of relatively static fluid.

Edema

Fluid equilibrium at the capillary bed depends upon the arterial supply, the transport at the cellular level, and the outflow via the veins and lymphatics. The accumulation of relatively static fluid results from an upsetting of the balance between these compartments. The major factor in the production of edema is the lymphatic and venous balance. Differentiation of the mechanisms can be made in part by performing both venography and lymphangiography. The purpose of lymphangiography is to establish the diagnosis, to assess lymphatic function, to document the degree of the lymphatic abnormality, and to define change with attempts at therapy.

Lymphedema is classified as (1) primary or idiopathic and (2) secondary to trauma, infection, neoplasm, and so forth.

PRIMARY LYMPHEDEMA. Primary or idiopathic lymphedema may be categorized according to the age at which it occurs, that is, congenital (present at birth); praecox (present before the age of 35 years); and tarda (present after the age of 35). Approximately 10 per cent of cases are believed to be congenital. A small proportion of these is considered to be Milroy's chronic hereditary edema. The majority of patients with primary lymphedema manifest edema from childhood to the third decade, or lymphedema praecox. This form has a three to one female predominance.

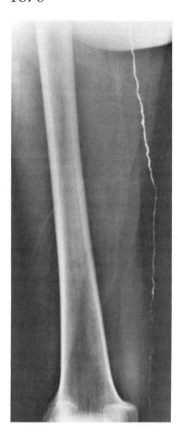

Figure 24–3. Primary lymphedema – hypoplasia.

Primary lymphedema is believed to be related to lymphatic insufficiency at different ages, depending upon the extent of the abnormality and the superimposition of secondary factors. Kinmonth[29] and Eustace and Kinmonth[16] classified idiopathic lymphedema into three major groups:

1. Hypoplasia, the most common, existed in 55 per cent of cases and manifested itself by the opacification of fewer lymphatics that were usually larger in caliber (Fig. 24–3).

2. Hyperplasia, an increase in number and size of lymphatics demonstrated, was found in 24 per cent of cases (Fig. 24–4). Dilated or varicose channels were at times associated with dermal backflow, or the visualization of fine collateral channels in the skin. Dermal backflow alone was the radiographic finding in a still smaller group. The dilated vessels seen in hyperplasia often drained into normal lymphatics without obvious evidence of obstruction. Dilated or varicose lymphatics wth incompetent or absent valves were occasionally associated with lymphangiomatosis, chylous reflux, arterial and venous dysplasias, and capillary angiomas.

3. Aplasia of the lymphatics was diagnosed in 14 per cent of cases after an inability to demonstrate any lymphatics in patients with clinical lymphedema.

SECONDARY LYMPHEDEMA. The etiologic agents include trauma (surgical or otherwise), infection, infestation, and neoplasm. Although the causes are varied, the mechanisms producing edema are similar. Interruption of small lymphatic vessels is usually followed by thrombosis of the transected ends. Fluid is temporarily rerouted through collateral channels. If the transected ends are in close proximity, rapid regeneration and recanalization will establish continuity in a few days. With disruption

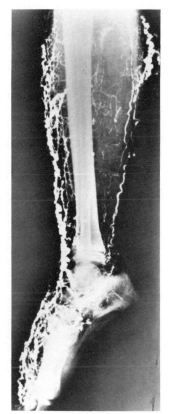

Figure 24–4. Primary lymphedema–hyperplasia.

of larger segments of lymphatic vessels, approximation is impossible and alternate pathways must accommodate the increased fluid load. If these channels are inadequate to circumvent the occlusion, protein accumulates in the interstitial tissues, with resultant edema. The more centrally located the obstruction, the greater is the number of available alternative routes. The compensatory flow patterns depend upon the site and extent of involvement with the utilization of dermal, subcutaneous, and perivascular lymphatics and lymphaticovenous pathways.

The major components in the production of postmastectomy edema are (1) lymphatic obstruction; (2) venous occlusion, both intrinsic or extrinsic; and (3) combined lymphatic and venous disease (Fig. 24–5). Radical mastectomy involves extensive dissection of the regional lymph nodes. The re-establishment of satisfactory lymphatic drainage is dependent upon the existence of the lymphatic vessels that are not resected and upon the development of the collateral lymph channels, with rerouting of lymph flow. The collateral channels may be seen in the anterior chest wall to the internal mammary and mediastinal lymph nodes and, not infrequently, to the opposite axillary nodes. The cephalic (radial) lymphatic trunk is also a major pathway through which the collateral channels drain into the supraclavicular nodes. Collateral channels through the lymphatics in the posterior chest wall to the paravertebral nodes and the opposite axillary nodes may be observed.

LYMPHATIC OBSTRUCTION. The sequelae of lymphatic obstruction have been described previously. Following radical mastectomy and axillary lymph node dissection, the lymphangiographic picture is the one usually seen in cases of lymphatic obstruction. The site of the obstruction is in the axilla. Multiple collateral channels are

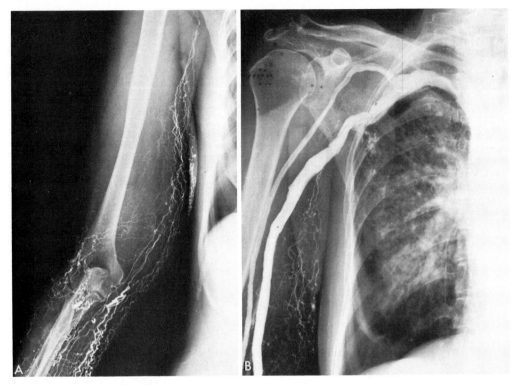

Figure 24–5. Postmastectomy edema. *A,* Lymphatic obstruction. *B,* Normal axillary vein.

seen attempting to circumvent the obstruction. The lymphatics are dilated and tortuous, with associated dermal backflow. The venogram is normal (see Fig. 24–5).

VENOUS OCCLUSION. Venous occlusion may be either intrinsic (thrombophlebitis) or extrinsic (vascular compression) in origin (Fig. 24–6). Chronic thrombophlebitis may be coupled with perivascular lymphangitis. It is postulated that there is stasis in the lymphatics of the extremity, thereby making fewer channels available for active flow. The decrease in caliber may be secondary to the increase in interstitial tissue pressure, stasis, or spasm.

Extrinsic venous disease may be due to enlarged lymph nodes, inflammatory or neoplastic in origin, compressing the veins. It may also be produced by fibrotic or inflammatory changes in the perivascular tissues secondary to surgery or radiation therapy, causing occlusion of the vein (Fig. 24–7).

COMBINED LYMPHATIC AND VENOUS DISEASE. Most frequently encountered is a combination of these two entities. In such situations the vein is involved by either intrinsic or extrinsic disease. Lymphangiograms show lymphatic obstruction. There is usually an associated soft tissue suffusion of contrast material.

Lymphocysts

After injury to larger lymphatics, including the thoracic duct, there may be free egress of lymph. If this lymph is confined, a lymphocyst is formed. The incidence and magnitude of these postoperative complications depend on multiple factors: the caliber

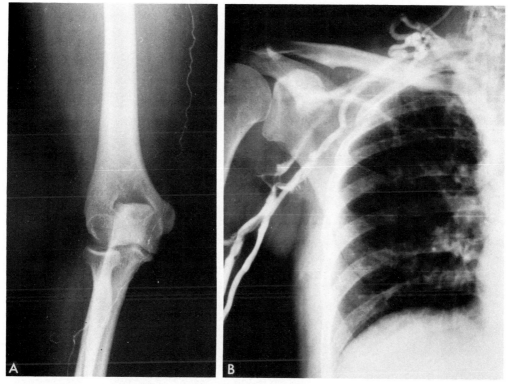

Figure 24–6. Postmastectomy edema — thrombophlebitis. *A,* Decrease in caliber and number of the lymphatics. *B,* Thrombophlebitis of the axillary vein. This patient had carcinoma of the breast, which was treated by radical mastectomy and radical dissection followed by radiation therapy. Postmastectomy edema gradually developed. The venogram (*B*) reveals chronic thrombophlebitis. The lymphangiogram (*A*) shows a decrease in the caliber and number of the lymphatics opacified.

of the transected lymphatics, the intralymphatic pressure, the velocity of lymph flow, the completeness of lymphatic ligation, the availability of residual functioning channels, and the adequacy of collateral pathways. A lymphocyst occurs shortly after surgical intervention, which helps in differentiating it from recurrent disease (Fig. 24–8). The fluid that accumulates in the cyst is not static. Aspiration of this collection is usually followed by fairly rapid reaccumulation, demonstrating this dynamic activity.

Lymphocysts are encountered most frequently as a complication of radical lymph node dissection. If the confined collection is in a strategic position, it causes clinical problems such as distortion and obstruction of the ureter and bladder, the pelvic veins, and even the rectum (Fig. 24–9). When the volume of the confined fluid is great enough it may present as a mass, clinically and radiographically. Ultrasound will show a completely sonolucent mass.

The surgeon is therefore faced with a dilemma when performing a radical node dissection. If all the lymphatics in the area are ligated, obstruction of lymph flow may result in edema below this level. On the other hand, transection and free flow of lymph from the endothelium-lined channels may form a pseudocyst. Incomplete dissection usually results in sufficient channels to maintain flow, bypassing any interruption. Lymphocyst formation therefore depends on the extent of dissection and the thorough ligation of the transected lymphatic channels.

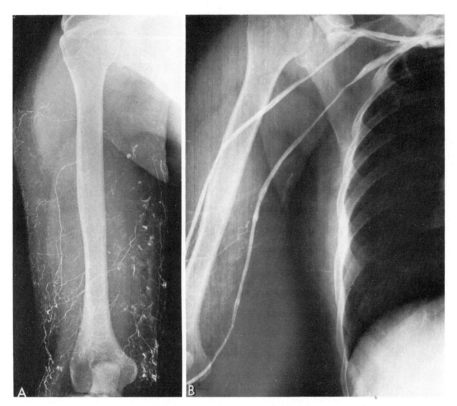

Figure 24–7. Postmastectomy and postradiation edema. *A,* Lymphatic obstruction. *B,* Extrinsic compression of axillary and cephalic veins. Extrinsic venous disease in a patient with a carcinoma of the breast. There was edema of the arm prior to any form of therapy. The lymph nodes compressing the vein proved to be inflammatory.

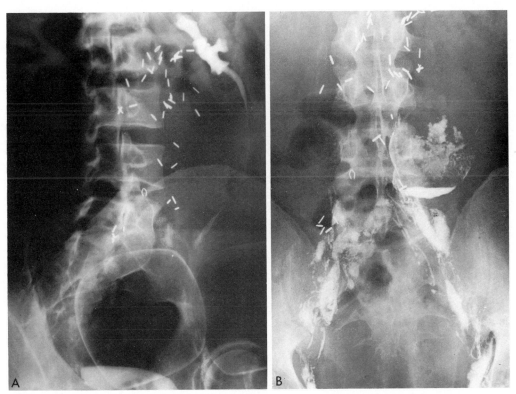

Figure 24–8. Postoperative retroperitoneal lymphocyst. *A,* The left ureter is displaced anteriorly and laterally. *B,* A repeat lymphangiogram opacifies a large retroperitoneal lymphocyst. The fluid-contrast level is obtained by examining the patient in the erect position.

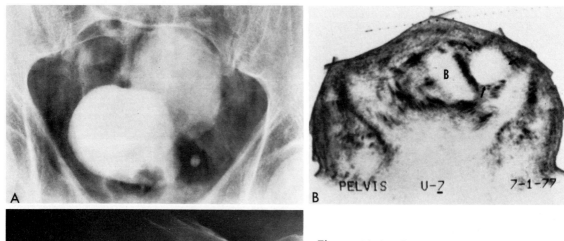

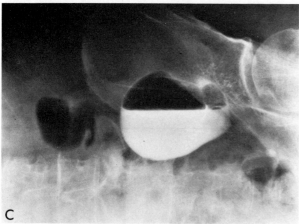

Figure 24–9. Postoperative pelvic lympho-cyst. *A,* The intravenous pyelogram shows a soft tissue mass in the left side of the pelvis, with displacement and deformity of the urinary bladder following resection of soft tissue sarcoma. *B,* A transverse supine sono-gram shows a rounded cystic lesion (arrows) in left side of the pelvis with a pressure defect on the left lateral wall of the bladder (B). *C,* On cystic puncture the cystic lesion proved to be lymphocyst.

Congenital lymphocysts may occasionally be seen in mesenteric or retroperitoneal areas. Those in the mesenteric lymphatics usually do not opacify during pedal lym-phangiography.

Lymphatic Fistulas

The escape of lymph into a potential cavity or viscus or through the skin after transection of the lymphatic channels may cause the formation of a fistulous tract (Fig. 24–10). Considerable circulating fluid may be lost through a lymphatic fistula.

Neoplastic invasion of the lymphatic trunks and, in particular, the thoracic duct may cause the formation of lymphatic fistulas. This may be the result of neoplastic involvement of lymph nodes, as in lymphoma, or direct invasion by a primary neoplasm, such as carcinoma of the pancreas. A persistent pleural effusion (chylotho-rax) can result from a mediastinal neoplasm (Fig. 24–11).

Chylous Reflux

Reflux of chyle from the intestinal lymphatics into the skeletal lymphatic pathways or into the intestinal lumen presents the most dramatic example of altered lymphatic flow. This illustrates both the use of collateral circulation and the production of

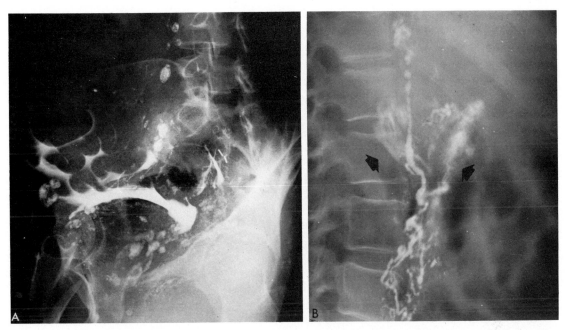

Figure 24–10.   Lymphatic fistulas. *A*, Lymphatic fistula in the pelvic region following a pelvic node dissection. *B*, A lymphatic fistula in the peritoneal cavity, with chylous ascites from invasion of the thoracic duct by a carcinoma of the pancreas, is illustrated by the extravascular contrast material (arrows).

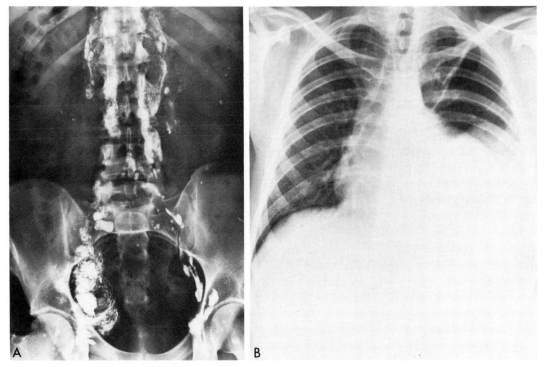

Figure 24–11.   Histiocytic lymphoma with chylothorax. *A*, Lymphomatous lesion involving the lymph nodes in the right side of the pelvic and para-aortic areas. *B*, Pleural effusion in the left lower chest proved to be chylothorax. It is caused by the lymphomatous involvement of the thoracic duct.

fistulous tracts as a means of decompressing the lymphatic system in the face of obstruction.

This phenomenon may result from either congenital or acquired obstruction of the lymphatic system. The congenital incompetence of lymphatic valves, primarily in the thoracic duct, results in stasis and reflux of chyle, a physiologic obstruction with reversal of flow. In children with this condition, the thoracic duct may be visualized in its entirety during lymphangiography. The pressure of injection may overcome the reversal of flow.

The acquired variety of chylous reflux may be associated with any process producing chronic thoracic duct obstruction. Proximal to the point of obstruction there is dilatation of the lymphatics with secondary incompetence of the lymphatic valves, allowing retrograde flow. This picture is dynamically identical to that seen in the congenital type. This results in an increase in the intralymphatic pressure and eventual rupture of these channels, with the production of lymphatic fistulas and an outflow of chyle. Filariasis is the most frequent parasitic agent in the production of chylous reflux. Tuberculosis, neoplasm, trauma, fibrosis, and so forth, may produce the same phenomenon (Fig. 24–12).

Clinical manifestations such as chyluria, chylometria, chylous ascites, and chylous edema depend on the site of obstruction, the anatomic variations of the lymphatic distribution, and the collateral pathways.

CHYLURIA. In chyluria, the kidney is the primary target organ. Chyluria is seen during pregnancy; it may be caused by a mechanical obstruction produced by the enlarging uterus. It may be transient, disappearing after delivery. Even in the absence of pregnancy, chyluria may be intermittent. The exact mechanisms are not totally understood.

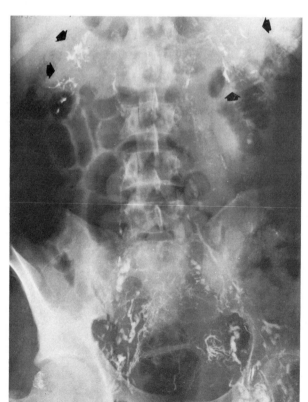

Figure 24–12. Chylous reflux with chyluria. Contrast material is seen in each renal collecting system (arrows) because of retrograde opacification of renal lymphatics secondary to thoracic duct obstruction. (Courtesy of Dr. Henner, Dallas, Texas.)

PROTEIN-LOSING ENTEROPATHY.   The dynamics involved in the production of some forms of protein-losing enteropathy are closely allied to chylous reflux. During lymphangiography, contrast material can be seen entering the small bowel, demonstrating a communication between the lymphatic channels and the visceral lumen (Fig. 24–13).

Lymphangiomatosis

Insufficiency or agenesis of the valves within dysplastic subcutaneous and osseous lymph vessels may lead to lymphatic backflow into the bones similar to dermal backflow (Fig. 24–14). Lymphangiomatosis of bone is probably a congenital malformation of the lymphatic system that is similar to primary lymphedema.

Cirrhosis

The lymphatics of the liver consist of superficial and deep groups. The superficial vessels lie in the subcapsular tissue, and the deeper channels run parallel to the divisions of the portal vein, hepatic artery, and biliary ducts. The vessels join at the porta hepatis where, except for a few superficial channels that pass through the triangular falciform ligaments, all empty via the gastrointestinal and lumbar trunks into the thoracic duct.

In certain disease states it is possible to opacify the hepatic lymphatics by the injection of water-soluble contrast medium into the liver parenchyma. Moreno et al. and Clain and McNulty have shown that dye is rapidly removed from the normal liver by the hepatic veins without visualization of the lymphatics. However, in those intrahepatic diseases characterized by an excessive production of lymph, the lymphatic channels are readily opacified and tend to remain visible after the contrast medium has left the hepatic or portal systems. Visualization of lymphatics is most frequently achieved in various inflammatory states or with acute occlusion of the venous outflow tracts. While this procedure has potential diagnostic value in patients with obscure

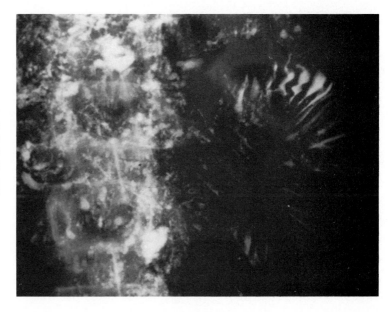

Figure 24–13.   Protein-losing enteropathy. The fistula between the lymphatic system and the small bowel is the probable etiology for the protein-losing enteropathy. (Courtesy of J. P. Desprez-Curely, V. Bismuth, and R. Bourdon, Paris, France.)

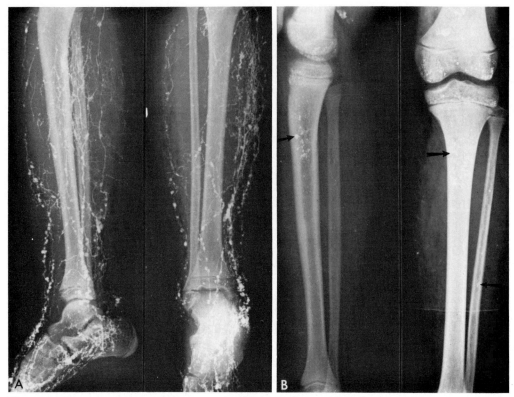

Figure 24–14. Lymphangiomatosis in a child with lower extremity edema. *A,* Numerous dilated tortuous lymphatics in the involved leg. *B,* Opacification of the lacunae in the bone (arrows) suggests communication with skeletal lymphatics.

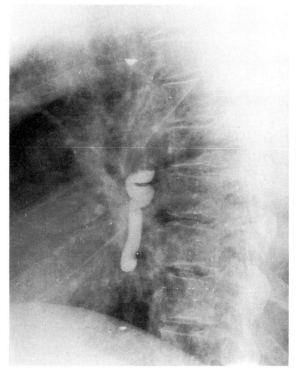

Figure 24–15. Alteration of lymphatic dynamics in cirrhosis. The thoracic duct is markedly dilated.

forms of jaundice, it is particularly useful in the investigation of the pathophysiology of cirrhosis of the liver.

Cirrhosis is characterized by an increased production of lymph. This in turn is reflected in the increased caliber of the thoracic duct (Fig. 24–15). Dumont et al.[15] have found that the flow of thoracic duct lymph is increased three to twelve fold and the diameter of the duct two to four fold in patients with cirrhosis. The normal thoracic duct as demonstrated by lymphangiography measures 2 to 5 mm in diameter; in cirrhotic patients the caliber has consistently been greater. At times the lymph in the thoracic duct in these patients contains blood, presumably representing a reversal of flow from the veins to the lymphatics as the result of increased portal vein pressure.

DISORDERS OF LYMPH NODES

Lymphangiography is the only direct approach to the visualization of the lymphatics and lymph nodes. Of the 1100 patients examined by lymphangiography in 1977 at M. D. Anderson Hospital and Tumor Institute, approximately one half were evaluated to determine the extent of Hodgkin's and non-Hodgkin's lymphoma. The remainder were examined for metastatic disease to pelvic and lumbar lymph nodes, most frequently from carcinomas of the cervix, ovary, testicle, bladder, and prostate. On occasion, patients with melanomas and sarcomas are also studied by lymphangiography. Percutaneous transperitoneal aspiration biopsy of these opacified lymph nodes has further enhanced this approach.

Accuracy in the interpretation depends upon the adherence to rigid criteria. A thorough knowledge of normal lymphatic drainage as well as normal variations is essential. Interpretation depends upon careful scrutiny of both lymphatic and nodal phases. Only positive findings should alter management. Negative studies do not exclude the presence of disease that may be outside the competence of the examination. Doubtful or suspicious findings must be pursued by further study, such as tomography, pyelography, angiography, ultrasonography, computed tomography, percutaneous transabdominal lymph node biopsy, or by a period of watchful waiting. If the diagnosis of metastases is still not established, the study should be considered negative in the management of the patient's disease.

In normal circumstances there is an inverse relationship between the size and the number of nodes. An increase in size is not specific and is found in both benign and malignant conditions.

Normal Lymph Node (Fig. 24–16)

Afferent lymphatics drain into the marginal sinus. The node has a granular or reticular internal architectural pattern. The margin of the node is well defined, with the hilar area demarcated by a smooth indentation. The site of the hilum can be verified by referring to the lymphatic phase, in which the efferent vessels leave the node.

Inflammation (Fig. 24–17)

Acute inflammation is usually indicated by an enlargement of nodes with maintenance of normal architecture. The acute reaction to the lymphangiographic procedure itself may result in a temporary enlargement of the perfused nodes. Local defects

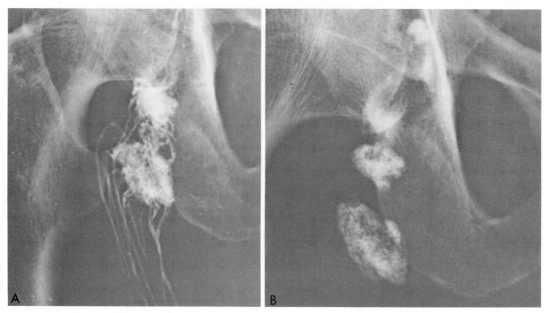

Figure 24–16. Normal lymph nodes. *A,* Lymphatic phase. *B,* Nodal phase.

caused by small abscesses may simulate carcinoma. Chronic inflammatory diseases may lead to confusion in the diagnosis of malignant lesions. The reactive hyperplasia of collagen disease presents a picture not unlike that of leukemia (Fig. 24–17*A*). Granulomatous diseases, such as tuberculosis, sarcoidosis, and syphilis, yield radiographic changes similar to those of Hodgkin's and non-Hodgkin's lymphoma, especially the large cell or histiocytic form. Tuberculosis with cavitation and destruction of a portion of the node may simulate carcinoma (Figs. 24–17 *B* and *C*).

Lymphoma (Fig. 24–18)

Radiographically, diseases of the lymphoid tissue appear as a primary alteration of the nodal architecture. The margin of the node is for the most part intact until the later stages of the disease. Lymphoma produes a foamy or lacy pattern. The nodes are frequently enlarged and increased in number, but neither of these findings is necessarily present. It is impossible to separate radiographically the different types of lymphoma. Nodular sclerosing Hodgkin's disease and large cell (histiocytic) lymphoma are more apt to have discrete filling defects within the nodes. The changes in lymphoma are frequently diffuse, involving many lymph nodes, in contrast to the local changes seen in carcinoma (Figs. 24–19 and 24–20).

Lymphangiography opacifies only a portion of the lymph nodes. In patients with stages I and II Hodgkin's lymphoma with a negative lymphangiogram, staging laparotomy has demonstrated disease in 30 to 35 per cent. Involvement has been found in the spleen, splenic nodes, mesenteric nodes, and liver. These areas are beyond the scope of lymphangiography. However, in only 6 per cent of patients were the retroperitoneal nodes found to be abnormal. Non-Hodgkin's lymphoma has an incidence of 55 to 60 per cent mesenteric node involvement in contrast to the 5 to 6 per cent found in Hodgkin's disease. The mesenteric nodes are not opacified by lymphangiography.

Text continued on page 1687

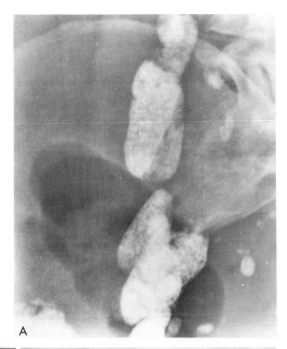

Figure 24–17. Inflammatory nodes. *A,* Reactive lymphoid hyperplasia. The nodes are enlarged, with coarsening of the internal architecture. *B,* Chronic granuloma (sarcoidosis). The changes in sarcoidosis are similar to those in Hodgkin's disease. *C,* Chronic granuloma (tuberculosis). The involved nodes show a crescentic filling defect (arrows) simulating metastatic carcinoma.

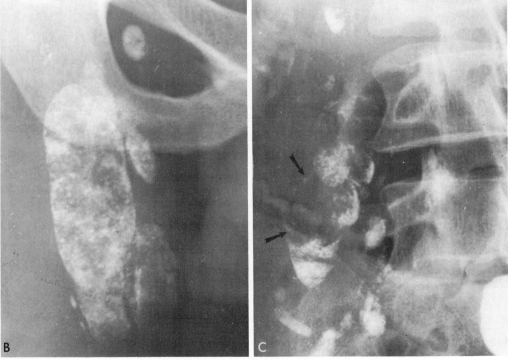

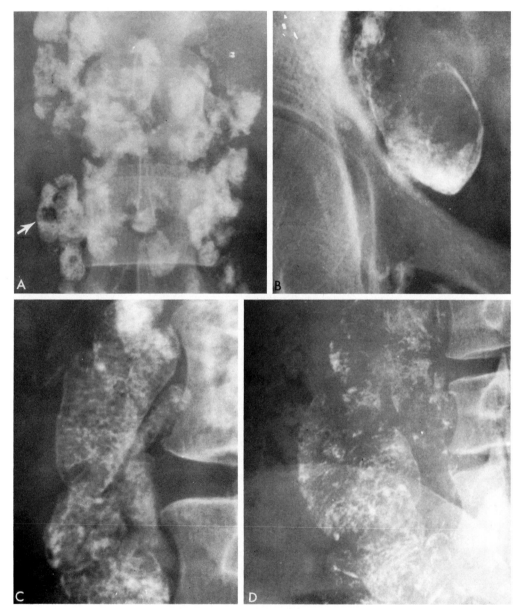

Figure 24–18. Different patterns of malignant lymphoma. *A,* Nodular sclerosing Hodgkin's disease—early appearance. Typical defect in node (arrow). *B,* Nodular sclerosing Hodgkin's disease—late appearance. *C,* Lymphocytic lymphoma—early appearance. *D,* Lymphocytic lymphoma—late appearance.

Legend continued on the opposite page

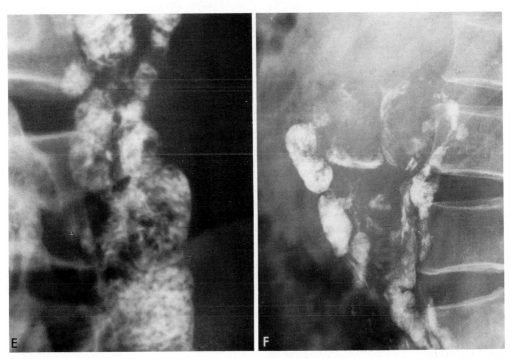

Figure 24–18 *Continued.* E, Histiocytic lymphoma—early appearance. F, Histiocytic lymphoma—late appearance.

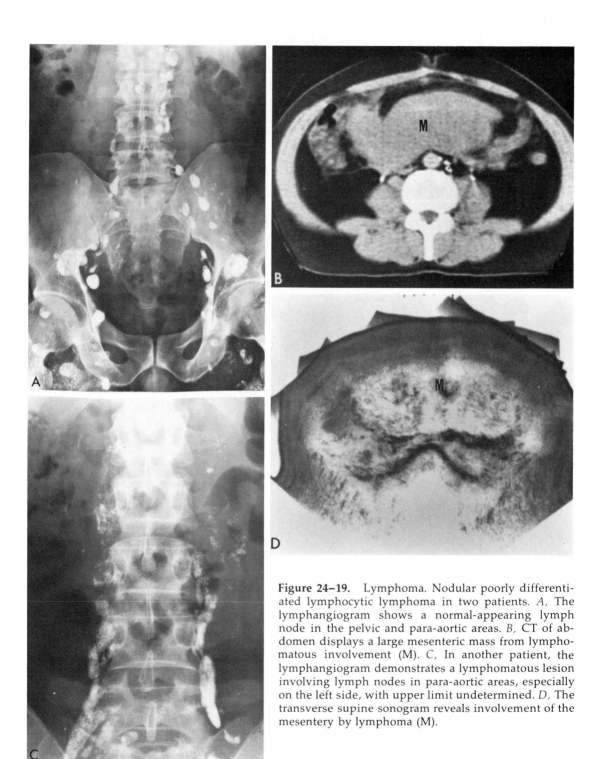

Figure 24–19. Lymphoma. Nodular poorly differenti-ated lymphocytic lymphoma in two patients. *A,* The lymphangiogram shows a normal-appearing lymph node in the pelvic and para-aortic areas. *B,* CT of ab-domen displays a large mesenteric mass from lympho-matous involvement (M). *C,* In another patient, the lymphangiogram demonstrates a lymphomatous lesion involving lymph nodes in para-aortic areas, especially on the left side, with upper limit undetermined. *D,* The transverse supine sonogram reveals involvement of the mesentery by lymphoma (M).

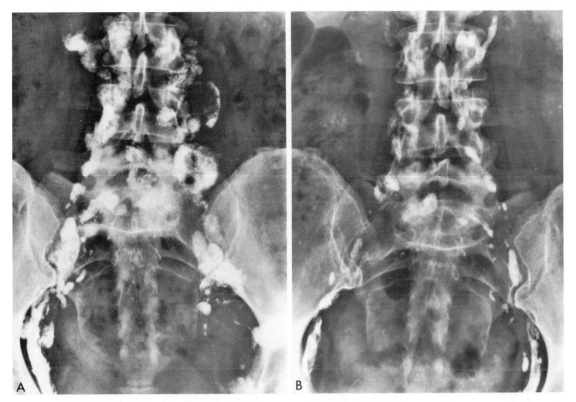

Figure 24–20.   Histiocytic lymphoma. *A,* The preirradiation lymphangiogram shows extensive lymphoma involving the lymph nodes in the pelvic and para-aortic areas on both sides. *B,* The postirradiation lymphangiogram demonstrates complete regression of the lymphomatous lesion without evidence of recurrence.

In view of these statistics, computed tomography, ultrasonography, or both are recommended as complementary procedures to lymphangiography in the initial evaluation of the patient with lymphoma. Although nonspecific, these techniques, especially computed tomography, more completely define the extent of disease. Follow-up evaluation of the residual contrast-filled nodes by a single roentgenogram of the abdomen is more feasible, more rewarding, and financially more acceptable on a three- to six-month basis than is serial computed tomography. Contrast material remains in the nodes, yielding a diagnostically interpretable examination in 75 per cent of patients one year after the initial lymphangiogram.

Carcinoma

The single most reliable criterion for the diagnosis of metastatic carcinoma is a defect in a node not traversed by lymphatics. These defects are caused by tumor emboli, with subsequent growth and destruction of nodal tissue. They are usually peripheral, and the remaining functioning portion of the node is frequently crescent-shaped (rim sign). It is important to note that the lymphatics leading to the defect are disrupted by the destructive process. Therefore, both the lymphatic and the nodal phases of the lymphangiogram must be examined. The appearance described can be simulated by

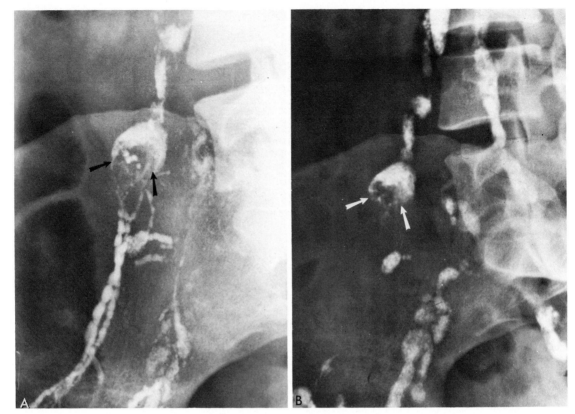

Figure 24–21. Metastatic carcinoma from the uterine cervix. *A,* Lymphatic phase. The lymphatics do not permeate the areas of replacement (arrows) by metastatic carcinoma. *B,* Nodal phase. The defects in the margin of the nodes are areas of tumor deposition (arrows). The remaining functioning portion of the node is opacified, producing a crescentic configuration.

abscess, caseous necrosis, and rarely, fibrosis. In the presence of a primary malignancy, metastasis is most likely to produce the rim sign (Fig. 24–21).

If a node is totally replaced by neoplasm it will not be opacified. However, there may be obstruction or distortion of the lymphatics. When lymphatic channels are obstructed, collateral pathways (lymphatic-to-lymphatic, lymphatic-to-prelymphatic, and lymphatic-to-venous) may be visualized. Interruption of lymphatics may also be caused by the primary neoplasm, surgery, fibrosis, or rarely, infection. Again, in a patient with a known primary malignancy and in the absence of surgery to the nodes, metastatic disease is the most likely etiology (Fig. 24–22).

In patients with carcinoma the accuracy of lymphangiograms interpreted as positive is 90 to 95 per cent. When results are considered negative, approximately 15 to 20 per cent of patients prove to have metastatic disease. False negative results are due to (1) metastases too small to detect and (2) failure of opacification of involved nodes that are either totally replaced or outside of the distribution usually visualized.

PERCUTANEOUS TRANSPERITONEAL LYMPH NODE BIOPSY (Fig. 24–23)

Selective lymphadenectomy in conjunction with lymphangiography for staging prior to therapy has found increasing application. The percutaneous approach to the

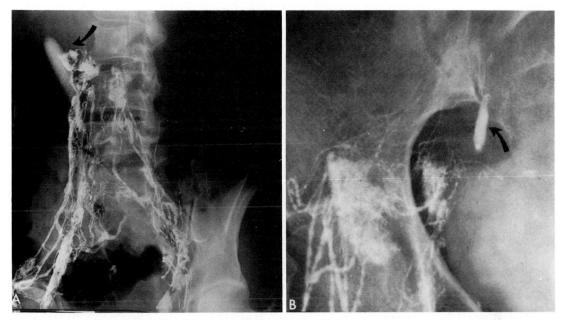

Figure 24–22. Lymphaticovenous anastomoses in patients with metastatic carcinoma. *A,* Lymphatico–inferior vena caval anastomosis. The large collection of contrast material is in the inferior vena cava. The lumbar lymphatics are obstructed by metastases. *B,* Lymphatico–iliac vein anastomosis in the pelvic region. The pelvic lymphatics are obstructed by metastases. A collection of contrast medium is seen in the iliac vein.

retroperitoneal and pelvic lymph nodes with a small-caliber needle is a simple technique to confirm the presence of neoplasm, obviating in selected cases the need for exploratory laparotomy. In view of the relatively anterior position of the para-aortic and pelvic lymph nodes relative to the great vessels, an anterior transperitoneal approach seems most suitable.

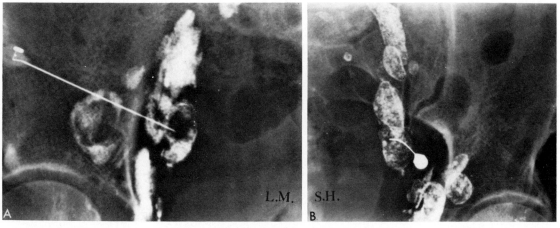

Figure 24–23. Percutaneous lymph node biopsy. *A,* Carcinoma of the cervix. Lymph node biopsy of an external iliac node containing metastatic adenocarcinoma. The site of biopsy is at the filling defect of the lymph node. *B,* Histiocytic lymphoma. Needle aspiration biopsy of an external iliac node in a patient with a concomitant carcinoma of the bladder. Note the relationship of the needle to the opacified node.

With the patient in the supine position, the opacified lymph node is localized by fluoroscopy and the overlying percutaneous puncture site is marked on the skin of the abdomen. The skin is prepared, the area down to the peritoneum is locally anesthetized with 2 per cent xylocaine, and a small incision is made. A thin-walled 23-gauge needle 15 to 20 cm in length; with a 0.6 mm outer diameter, a 0.4 inner diameter, and a 30 degree angle bevel, is utilized. The needle is directed through the abdominal wall into the lymph node. In patients with a thick abdominal wall, a thin-walled 18-gauge needle is passed into the abdominal wall and the 23-gauge needle is threaded through it. Once the needle is in the lymph node, the patient may be rotated into each oblique position to determine the relative relationship. When the node is punctured, synchronous movement of the needle and the lymph node under fluoroscopic control indicates accurate placement. Continuous suction is applied with a 12-cc plastic syringe while the needle is moved through an excursion of approximately 1 cm. After release of the suction the needle is withdrawn. The procedure is repeated two or three times to ensure the collection of sufficient cytologic material. The presence of oil droplets in the aspirate confirms that the node previously opacified during lymphangiography has been punctured. The specimen is fixed in Mucolex solution. The tissue is analyzed by the cytologist in the form of a smear or cell block or both.

The site of biopsy in an opacified lymph node differs according to the histologic type of neoplastic process. The most common lymphangiographic finding in metastatic carcinoma is a defect in a node not transversed by lymphatics. The residual normal functioning portion of the node frequently has a crescentic configuration representing a node partially replaced by neoplasm. Consequently, the biopsy of the node just above the crescentic area would produce the greatest yield. Lymphoma is usually a more diffuse involvement of a lymph node, and the site of biopsy is not as critical.

Percutaneous transperitoneal lymph node biopsy involves the passage of a 23-gauge needle into the peritoneal cavity and through solid and hollow viscera. The potential complications of lymph node biopsy include intra-abdominal bleeding, pancreatitis, and bowel perforation with peritonitis. The possibility of disseminating neoplasm by aspiration biopsy does not seem to present a significant problem, as concluded by laboratory investigation and clinical experience with percutaneous biopsies of lymph nodes and kidney neoplasms using even larger caliber needles.

In over 300 procedures, approximately 80 per cent yielded interpretable biopsy material. Aspiration biopsy of a lymph node in cases of metastatic carcinoma is more successful (85 per cent) than it is in lymphoma (50 per cent). Epithelial metastases, especially those originating in pelvic viscera, are frequently highly cellular, poorly vascularized, and readily distinguishable from the normal lymphocytes of a lymph node. In lymphomas, the diagnosis by fine needle aspiration is more difficult, and the type of lymphoma may be impossible to classify.

References

1. Athey, P. A., Wallace, S., Jing, B. S., et al.: Lymphangiography in ovarian cancer. Am. J. Roentgenol. *123*:106–113, 1975.
2. Bartels, P.: Das Lymphgefaessystem. Jena, 1909.
3. Bartels, P.: Das Lymphgefaessystem. *In* Handbuch d. Anatomie d. Menschen. Jena, G. Fischer, 1909.
4. Bergstrom, J. F., and Navin, J. J.: Luetic lymphadenitis: lymphographic manifestations simulating lymphoma. Report of a case. Radiology *106*:287–288, 1973.
5. Bookstein, J. J., French, A. B., and Pollard, M. H.: Protein-losing gastroenteropathy: concepts derived from lymphangiography. Am. J. Dig. Dis. *10*:573–581, 1965.
6. Buonocore, E., and Young, J. R.: Lymphangiographic evaluation of lymphedema and lymphatic flow. Am. J. Roentgenol. *95*:751–765, 1965.

7. Brunn, S., and Engeset, A.: Lymphadenography. Acta Radiol. 45:389–395, 1956.
8. Castellino, R. A.: Lymphographic-histologic correlation in patients with Hodgkin's disease and non-Hodgkin's lymphoma undergoing staging laparotomy. Lymphology 7:153, 1974.
9. Castellino, R. A., Bellani, F. F., Gasparini, M., et al.: Lymphography in childhood: six years experience with 242 cases. Lymphology 8:74–83, 1975.
10. Castellino, R. A., Billingham, M., and Dorfman, R. F.: Lymphographic accuracy in Hodgkin's disease and malignant lymphoma with a note on the "reactive" lymph node as a cause of most false-positive lymphograms. Invest. Radiol. 9:155–165, 1974.
11. Castellino, R. A., Goffinet, D. R., Blank, N., et al.: The role of radiology in the staging of non-Hodgkin's lymphoma with laparotomy correlation. Radiology 110:329–338, 1974.
12. Choi, J. K., and Weidemer, H. S.: Chyluria: lymphographic study and review of the literature. J. Urol. 92:723–727, 1964.
13. Drinker, C. K., and Yoffey, J. M.: Lymphatics, Lymph and Lymphoid Tissue. Cambridge, Mass., Harvard University Press, 1941.
14. Dumont, A. E.: Lymph flow in the regulation of circulatory congestion and pancreatic interstitial pressure. In Ruttiman, A. (ed.), Progress in Lymphology. New York, Hafner Publishing Co., 1967, p. 91.
15. Dumont, A. E., and Mulholland, J. H.: Alterations in thoracic duct lymph flow in hepatic cirrhosis: significance in portal hypertension. Am. Surg. 156:668–677, 1962.
16. Eustace, P. W., and Kinmonth, J. B.: The normal lymphatic vessels of the inguinal and iliac areas with special emphasis on the efferent inguinal vessels. Lymphology, in press.
17. Feldman, M. G., Kohan, P., and Edelman, S.: Lymphangiographic studies in obstructive lymphedema of the upper extremity. Surgery 59:935–943, 1966.
18. Fraimow, W., Wallace, S., Lewis, P., et al.: Changes in pulmonary function due to lymphangiography. Radiology 85:231, 1966.
19. Fuchs, W. A.: Neoplasms of epithelial origin. In Abrams, H. L. (ed.): Angiography. Ed. 2, Vol. II. Boston, Little, Brown & Company, 1971, p. 1369.
20. Gold, W. M., Youker, J., Anderson, S., et al.: Pulmonary function abnormalities after lymphangiography. N. Engl. J. Med. 273:519–524, 1965.
21. Gruwez, J.: Lymphography, panel discussion. IIA. Complications and accidents. In Progress in Lymphology: Proceedings of the International Symposium on Lymphology. Stuttgart, Georg Thieme Verlag, 1967, p. 322.
22. Hanks, G. E., and Bagshaw, M. A.: Megavoltage radiation therapy and lymphangiography in ovarian cancer. Radiology 93:649–654, 1969.
23. Herman, P. G., Benninghoff, D. L., Nelson, J. H., et al.: Roentgen anatomy of the ilio-pelvic-aortic lymphatic system. Radiology 80:182–193, 1963.
24. Hudack, S., and McMaster, P. D.: The lymphatic participation in human cutaneous phenomenon. A study of the minute lymphatics of the living skin. J. Exp. Med. 57:751, 1933.
25. Janča, K., Popovic, L., and Dimkovic, D.: Lymphography in disease of the penis. Int. Urol. Nephrol. 4:59, 1972.
26. Kaplan, H. S., Dorfman, R. F., Nelsen, T. S., et al.: Staging laparotomy and splenectomy in Hodgkin's disease: analysis of indications and patterns of involvement in 285 consecutive unselected patients. Natl. Cancer Inst. Monogr. 36:291–301, 1973.
27. Kinmonth, J. B.: Lymphangiography in man. Clin. Sci. 11:13–20, 1952.
28. Kinmonth, J. B.: The Lymphatics: Diseases, Lymphography and Surgery. Baltimore, The Williams & Wilkins Company, 1972.
29. Kinmonth, J. B.: Primary lymphedemas: classification and other studies based on oleolymphography and clinical features. J. Cardiovasc. Surg. 1969.
30. Kinmonth, J. B., and Taylor, G. W.: The lymphatic circulation in lymphedema. Ann. Surg. 39:129–136, 1954.
31. Koehler, P. R.: Complications of lymphography. Lymphology 1:116–120, 1968.
32. Kolbenstvedt, A.: Lymphography in the diagnosis of metastases from carcinoma of the uterine cervix stages I and II. Acta Radiol. Diagn. 16:81–97, 1975.
33. Kreel, L.: The EMI whole body scanner in the demonstration of lymph node enlargement. Clin. Radiol. 27:421–429, 1976.
34. Kreel, L., and George, P.: Post-mastectomy lymphangiography: detection of metastases and edema. Ann. Surg. 163:470–477, 1966.
35. Kuisk, H.: Technique of Lymphography and Principles of Interpretation. St. Louis, Warren H. Green, Inc., 1971.
35a. Moreno, A. H., Ruzicka, F. F., and Ronsselot, L. M.: Functional hepatography. Radiology 81:65, 1963.
36. O'Donnell, T. F.: Congenital mixed vascular deformities of the lower limbs: the relevance of lymphatic abnormalities to their diagnosis and treatment. Ann. Surg. 185:162–168, 1977.
37. Olszewski, W.: On the pathomechanism of development of postsurgical lymphedema. Lymphology 6:35–51, 1973.
38. Parker, B. R., Blank, N., and Castellino, R. A.: Lymphographic appearances of benign conditions simulating lymphoma. Radiology 111:267–274, 1974.
39. Reichert, F. L.: The regeneration of lymphatics. Arch. Surg. 13:871, 1926.
40. Renner, R. R., Nelson, D. A., and Lozner, E. L.: Roentgenologic manifestations of primary macroglobulinemia (Waldenström). Am. J. Roentgenol. Radium Ther. Nucl. Med. 113:499–508, 1971.

41. Rouviere, H.: Anatomy of the Human Lymphatic System. A compendium translated from the original by M. J. Tobias. Ann Arbor, Edwards Brothers, Inc., 1938.
42. Rusznyak, I., Foldi, M., and Szabo, G.: Lymphatics and Lymph Circulation. Ed. 2. New York, Pergamon Press, 1967.
43. Rutledge, F., Dodd, G. D., and Kasilag, F. B.: Lymphocysts: a complication of radical pelvic surgery. Am. J. Obstet. Gynecol. 77:1165–1175, 1959.
44. Servelle, M.: A propos de la lymphographie experimentale et clinique. J. Radiol. Electrol. Med. Nucl. 26:165, 1944–1945.
45. Servelle, M.: Pathology of the thoracic duct. J. Cardiovasc. Surg. 4:702–727, 1963.
46. Smedal, M. I., and Evans, J. A.: Cause and treatment of edema of arm following radical mastectomy. Surg. Gynecol. Obstet. 111:29–40, 1960.
47. Steckel, R. J., and Cameron, T. P.: Changes in lymph node size induced by lymphangiography. Radiology 87:753–755, 1966.
48. Threefoot, S. A.: Gross and microscopic anatomy of the lymphatic vessels and lymphaticovenous communications. Cancer Chemother. Rep. 52:1–20, 1968.
49. Threefoot, S. A., Kent, W. T., and Hatchett, B. F.: Lymphaticovenous and lymphaticolymphatic communications demonstrated by plastic corrosion models of rats and by post-mortem lymphangiography in man. J. Lab. Clin. Med. 61:9–22, 1963.
50. Viamonte, J., Jr., Altman, D., Parks, R., et al.: Radiographic-pathologic correlation in the interpretation of lymphangioadenograms. Radiology 80:903–916, 1963.
51. Wallace, S.: Dynamics of normal and abnormal lymphatic systems as studied with contrast media. Cancer Chemother. Rep. 52:31–58, 1968.
52. Wallace, S., Jackson, L., Dodd, G. D., et al.: Lymphatic dynamics in certain abnormal states. Am. J. Roentgenol. Radium. Ther. Nucl. Med. 91:1187–1206, 1964.
53. Wallace, S., Jackson, L., Schaffer, B., et al.: Lymphangiograms: their diagnostic and therapeutic potential. Radiology 76:179–199, 1961.
54. Wallace, S., and Jing, B. S.: Lymphangiography in carcinoma in clinical lymphography. In Clouse, M. E. (ed.): Golden's Diagnostic Radiology. Baltimore, The Williams & Wilkins Company, 1977, pp. 185–273.
55. Walter, J. F., Sodeman, T. M., Cooperstock, M. S., et al.: Lymphangiographic findings in histoplasmosis. Radiology 114:65–66, 1975.
56. Wiljasalo, M., Julkunen, H., and Saluen, I.: Lymphography in rheumatic diseases. Ann. Med. Intern. Fenn. 55:125–128, 1966.
57. Yoffey, J. M., and Courtice, F. C.: Lymphatics, Lymph and Lymphoid Tissue, Cambridge, Harvard University Press, 1956.
58. Zheutlin, N., and Shanbrom, E.: Contrast visualization of lymph nodes. Radiology 71:702, 1958.
59. Zornoza, J., Wallace, S., Goldstein, H. M., et al.: Transperitoneal percutaneous retroperitoneal lymph node aspiration biopsy. Radiology 122:111–115, 1976.

25

THE PERICARDIUM

KENT ELLIS, M.D.
DONALD LATHAM KING, M.D.

INTRODUCTION

In ancient times a "shaggy-haired heart," or pericardium, indicated exceptional valor.[78] Nearly 2000 years ago, Galen successfully drained a case of purulent pericarditis.[76] In 1669, Richard Lower clearly perceived the clinical consequences of cardiac tamponade and constrictive pericarditis. In 1873, Kussmaul described the neck vein distention characteristic of compressive pericardial disorders and the paradoxical decrease and even disappearance of the peripheral pulse with inspiration (despite a beating heart) in acute cardiac tamponade. Pericardial resections were first done in 1913 by Rehn and Sauerbruck, and in 1929 Churchill performed the first successful pericardiectomy in the United States for constrictive pericarditis.[76, 78]

The diagnosis of pericardial disease has many pitfalls. Clinical manifestations may be subtle and are easily misinterpreted. Diagnostic radiology with angiocardiography, computerized tomography, and, especially, echocardiography has much to offer in the clinical detection and evaluation of pericardial disease. The function of the normal pericardium is controversial.[2, 44]

CONGENITAL ANOMALIES OF THE PERICARDIUM

Defects in the Pericardium

COMPLETE ABSENCE OF THE LEFT SIDE. Congenital defects in the pericardium are uncommon. The type most likely to be recognized clinically is complete absence of the left side of the pericardium, and related parietal pleura, so that the residual pericardial cavity is continuous with the left pleural space.[23, 62] The secondary shift of the heart out onto the left diaphragm and the unusually sharp separation of the individual segments of the left heart border may be recognized on a plain chest roentgenogram (Fig. 25–1A and B). Although some patients with this anomaly complain

1693

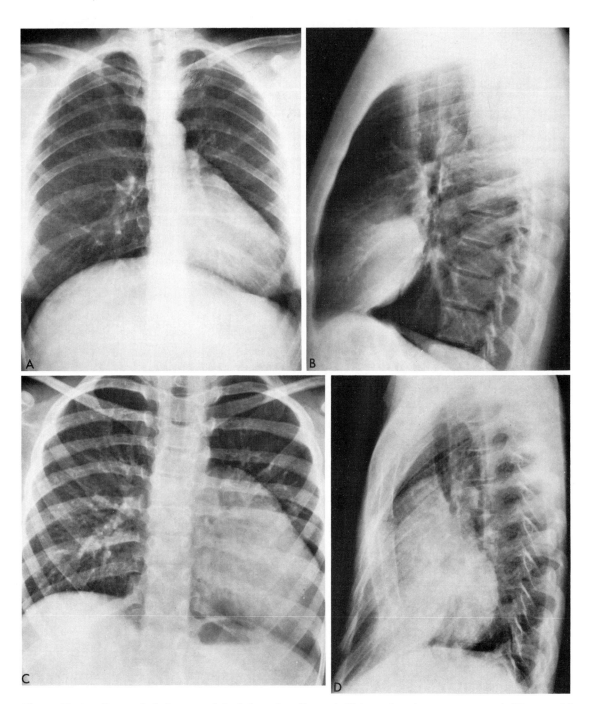

Figure 25–1. Congenital absence of the left pericardium. *A,* This patient is a asymptomatic 25-year-old woman. Note the typical shift of the heart to the left chest and the unusual separation of the aortic arch from the main pulmonary artery in the absence of the left pericardium. *B,* Lateral view. *C,* Frontal projection of a 12-year-old with complete absence of the left pericardium and an ostium primum atrial septal defect. At the time of surgical repair of the atrial septal defect the left side of the pericardium and the corresponding mediastinal pleura were completely absent. *D,* Lateral view showing the not unusual accompanying pectus excavatum deformity.

Legend continued on the opposite page

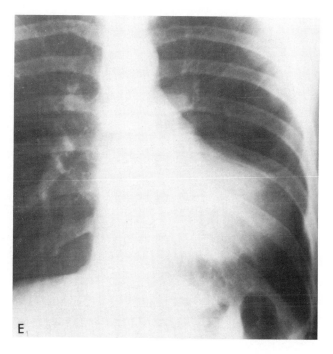

Figure 25–1 *Continued.* *E,* Chronic herniation of the heart through a surgical defect in the left pericardium in a 24-year-old man. This chest roentgenogram shows the heart prolapsed through the pericardial defect into the left chest one year after an emergency left thorocotomy for cardiac tamponade due to stab wound lacerations of the right ventricle. The left pericardium was left open. The cardiac apex became adherent to the left anterior chest wall, but cardiac function seemed normal both clinically and at cardiac catheterization. *(From* Ellis, K., Malm, J. R., Bowman, F. O., Jr., and King, D. L.: Roentgenographic findings after pericardial surgery. Radiol. Clin. North Am. *9:*327–341, 1971.)

of vague and nonspecific chest pains, most have no symptoms. A relatively slow heart rate, electrocardiographic evidence of right axis deviation and right bundle branch block,[19] and pectus excavatum deformity of the chest are frequent associated findings (Fig. 25–1C and D). A similar appearance of the heart can occur after wide surgical incision into or resection of the left pericardium (Fig. 25–1E). The presence of the pericardial defect may be proved by a diagnostic left pneumothorax, although this is not usually necessary.

PARTIAL LEFT-SIDED DEFECTS. Partial defects in the left pericardium are slightly less frequent. Typically, these occur just caudal and anterior to the left hilum, so that the left atrial appendage protrudes through the defect.[64] The resulting masslike deformity of the left heart border on the chest roentgenogram (Fig. 25–2) is easily confused with mediastinal tumor or adenopathy. On fluoroscopy the pulsatile action of the left atrial appendage is very impressive. A diagnostic left pneumothorax may help show the continuity of the left pleural and pericardial spaces. Several deaths have been reported following cardiac strangulation secondary to herniation of the heart through such congenital pericardial defects. Partial strangulation of the left atrial appendage has also been treated surgically.[6] As many as 20 per cent of partial defects are associated with adjacent bronchogenic cysts or sequestrations. Congenital heart disease, especially atrial septal defects, has been present in a few of the cases.

OTHER PERICARDIAL DEFECTS. Congenital defects of the right pericardium occur much less frequently than defects of the left.[59] Defects in the diaphragmatic pericardium may be associated with a *large and/or deformed* cardiac silhouette resulting from herniation of the liver or gastrointestinal tract into the pericardium. Such diaphragmatic pericardial defects may be associated in a syndrome that includes congenital heart disease (often ventricular septal defect and dextroposition of the heart) and defects in the sternum and abdominal wall.[13] Large pericardial defects also accompany more bizarre anomalies, such as ectopia cordis. Post-traumatic tears in the diaphragmatic pericardium may be difficult to distinguish from congenital defects and may be complicated by hernias of the omentum and intestine.

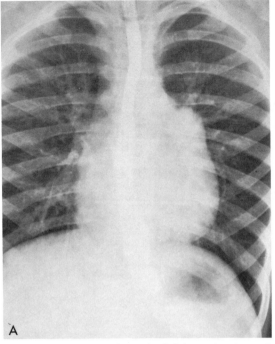

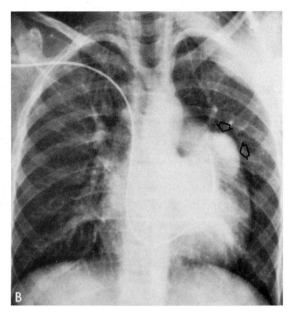

Figure 25–2. Partial absence of left pericardium. *A,* Chest film of a 6-year-old child with partial congenital deficiency of the left pericardium. The abnormal convexity along the left heart border pulsated remarkably at fluoroscopy. *B,* Angiocardiogram showing the left atrial appendage at the site of the local convexity (arrows).

Pericardial Cysts and Diverticula

PERICARDIAL CYSTS. About 70 per cent of these typically asymptomatic masses present in the right anterior cardiophrenic angle, another 15 to 20 per cent present in the left, and the remainder are widely scattered along the margins of the pericardium.[31] Although generally regarded as congenital in origin, some pericardial cysts may be acquired.[65] Usually discovered by chance on a chest roentgenogram, they do not attract attention until they are larger than the fat pads commonly seen in the cardiophrenic angles. Some cysts are pedunculated.[75] The age range is from early childhood to late adult life, but most are discovered in patients 20 to 40 years of age. Although slow-growing, the cysts may become very large and even rupture.[49]

The differential diagnosis of a bulging density in the cardiophrenic angles includes a large fat pad; occasionally, a hernia of the omentum via a foramen of Morgagni; or much more rarely, a teratoma, thymoma, or lymphoma of the anterior mediastinum. Echocardiography (Fig. 25–3A and B) can indicate that the mass is cystic rather than solid.[32] Computerized tomography can clearly identify the fat of a large fat pad or herniated omentum (Fig. 25–3C and D). Once the cystic nature of mass is known, diagnostic or therapeutic needle aspiration may be attempted. Rarely, similar cysts of the epicardium present as large or deformed hearts.[36]

PERICARDIAL DIVERTICULA. Less common than regular pericardial cysts, diverticula tend to be found in older people. Like pericardial cysts, diverticula may arise from congenitally isolated pericardial tissue or be acquired by herniation of the pericardial lining through defects in the fibrous pericardium. Sometimes the diverticula contain part of the heart, for example, the right atrium. Pericardial diverticula may also form by rupture of a cyst into the pericardial cavity.

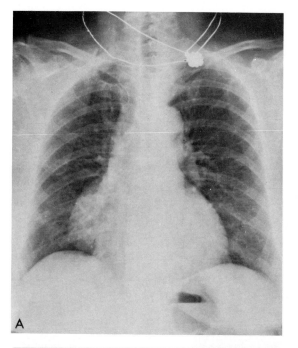

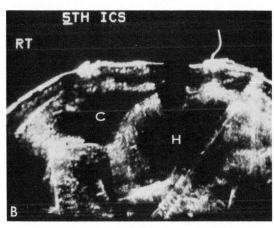

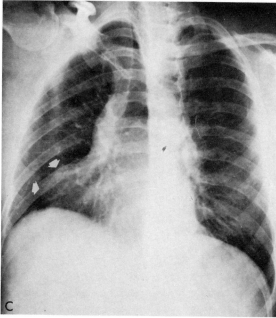

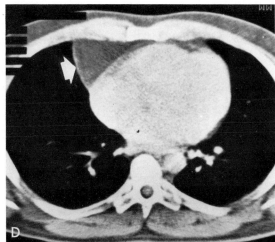

Figure 25–3. Pericardial cyst versus fat pad. *A,* Chest film showing abnormal density just above the right cardiophrenic angle in an asymptomatic 29-year-old woman. *B,* Transverse ultrasonogram demonstrates the mass to be free of internal echoes and therefore a cyst (C) adjacent to the heart (H). RT = right; 5ICS = fifth intercostal space. *C,* Left anterior oblique film in another asymptomatic patient showing a mass (arrows) in the right cardiophrenic angle. *D,* Computerized tomographic transverse chest scan clearly shows that the density of the mass (arrow) shown in *C* is fat (by computer density number), and the mass is a pericardial fat pad.

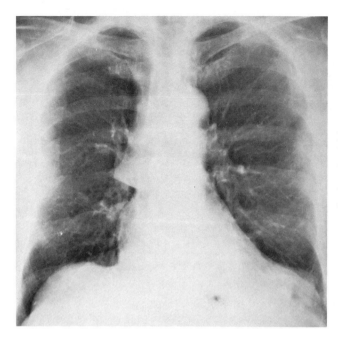

Figure 25–4. Pericardial diverticulum. This mass along the right midheart border completely disappeared at times. At operation it proved to be a pericardial diverticulum in open communication with the pericardial cavity.

The most striking feature of some pericardial diverticula is an ability to change in size in response to posture, respiration, or heart failure — the mass collapsing as fluid is withdrawn into the main pericardial cavity (Fig. 25–4). Such changes may occur very rapidly or very slowly, depending upon the size of the communication. The sudden appearance of a paracardiac mass associated with pleuritic pain, low-grade fever, leukocytosis, and a normal electrocardiogram should raise the suspicion of pericardial fat necrosis.[91]

PERICARDIAL TUMORS

Primary Tumors of the Pericardium

BENIGN TUMORS.   Benign tumors within the pericardial cavity are quite rare but are important, since they are surgically treatable.[14, 54, 93] The most common primary pericardial tumor in the infant or child is a teratoma (about 35 have been reported). Pedunculated in the pericardial cavity and typically attached to the root of the aorta, this tumor usually presents as marked cardiomegaly with or without pericardial effusion and tamponade in early infancy (Fig. 25–5). Surgical excision is curative.

Closely related tumors are found in older children[88] and adults, and some are called intrapericardial bronchogenic cysts.

In adults, a few benign fibromas, lipomas, amyloid tumors, and hemangiomas have been encountered.[92] Some of these tumors produce local symptoms, whereas others are discovered by chance or because of secondary cardiomegaly (Fig. 25–6).[61] Angiocardiography with selective coronary arteriography is usually required for diagnosis. Echocardiography, computerized tomography, and radionuclide imaging are also proving to be useful.

PRIMARY MALIGNANT TUMORS.   Mesothelioma is the primary malignant tumor of the pericardium, but it is very rare. Typically, the tumor presents with large, intractable pericardial effusions and tamponade. Diagnosis may be made by cytologic

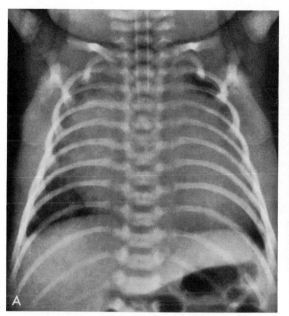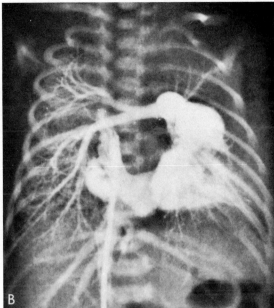

Figure 25–5. Intrapericardial teratoma. *A,* Chest film taken one day after the birth of this infant with respiratory distress shows a huge cardiomediastinal shadow. *B,* Angiocardiography reveals no shunts, but leftward displacement of the right ventricle and separation of it from the superior vena cava and body of the right atrium is evident. The ascending aorta is normal in size and does not account for this large separation. The findings are characteristic of a intrapericardial teratoma, which usually arises via a stalk from the aortic root. Such a teratoma was found at operation. Pathologically it was a benign cystic teratoma.

tests from pericardiocentesis, although surgical exploration of the pericardium is usually required. Partial replacement of aspirated pericardial fluid with gas (carbon dioxide, oxygen, or air) enables radiologic demonstration of the thickness of the fibrous pericardium (Fig. 25–7) and masses within the pericardial space.

Secondary Tumors of the Pericardium

Secondary malignant tumors of the pericardium are much more common than primary ones.[37] The great majority of these are either clinically silent or part of a widespread terminal illness. Some, however, present as pericarditis or pericardial effusion with or without tamponade. Tumors metastatic to the pericardium can arise from primary tumors of the lung and breast, melanoma, lymphoma, and leukemia.

PERICARDIAL EFFUSION AND TAMPONADE

Pericardial effusion is the major gross manifestation of diseases affecting the pericardium. Pericardial fluid formation is mainly from the visceral pericardium and depends upon the relative hydrostatic and osmotic pressures between the pericardial capillaries and the pericardial cavity fluid, the permeability of the barrier between these spaces, and the adequacy of lymphatic drainage.[58] Although physical signs of large heart, friction rub, paradoxical pulse, and distant heart sounds, together with low voltage and typical ST- and T-wave electrocardiographic changes, are very important in diagnosis, radiologic and echocardiographic studies[26, 30] have much to offer.

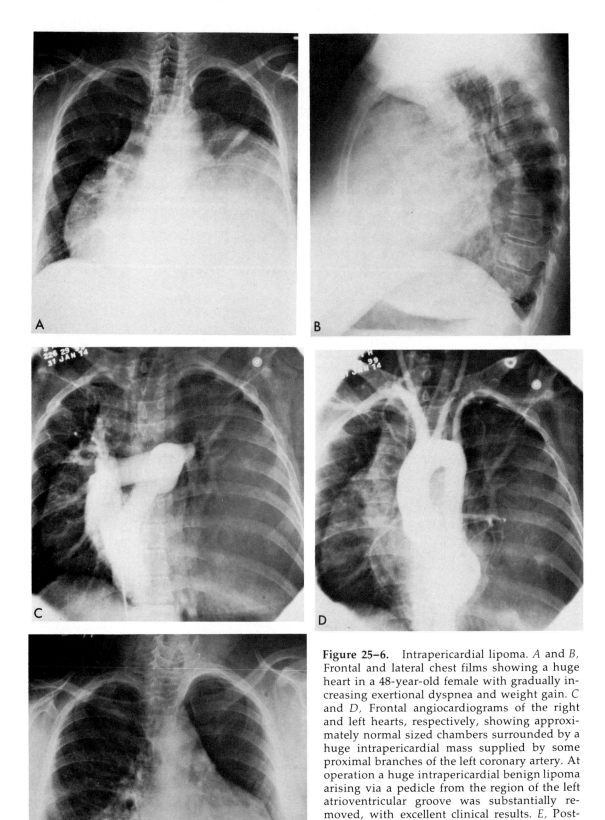

Figure 25–6. Intrapericardial lipoma. *A* and *B,* Frontal and lateral chest films showing a huge heart in a 48-year-old female with gradually increasing exertional dyspnea and weight gain. *C* and *D,* Frontal angiocardiograms of the right and left hearts, respectively, showing approximately normal sized chambers surrounded by a huge intrapericardial mass supplied by some proximal branches of the left coronary artery. At operation a huge intrapericardial benign lipoma arising via a pedicle from the region of the left atrioventricular groove was substantially removed, with excellent clinical results. *E,* Postoperative chest roentgenogram. (Reprinted by permission from the New York State Journal of Medicine. Moulton, A. L., Jaretzki, A. III, Bowman, F. O., Jr., et al.: Massive lipoma of heart. New York State J. Med. 76:1820–1825, 1976.)

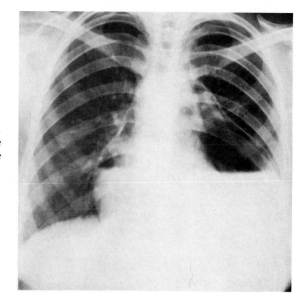

Figure 25–7. Mesothelioma of the pericardium. Following pericardiocentesis, air and fluid are seen in the pericardium. The cause proved to be primary mesothelioma of pericardium.

Plain Chest Roentgenograms

Plain chest roentgenograms document the heart size, the status of the lung vasculature, and the course of the illness. Chronic pericardial effusions generally cause symmetric, nonspecific, flasklike cardiomegaly, with the greatest enlargement in dependent regions (Fig. 25–8A). Encroachment on the retrosternal space (Fig. 25–9A and B) and overlap of the lung hilar regions are characteristic features. Infrequently, loculation of pericardial fluid or asymmetric compliance of the pericardium (for example, after unilateral irradiation)[41] may produce lobulated bizarre pericardial configurations (Fig. 25–10). Typically, the lung fields are clear; that is, they exhibit no signs of elevated pulmonary capillary pressure.

An abrupt change in heart size, especially in the absence of signs of left heart failure, always suggests the possibility of a pericardial effusion. Tamponade is suggested when the lungs are exceptionally clear and the pulmonary vasculature is normal or diminished in prominence despite impressive cardiomegaly and clinical symptoms. Since acute tamponade can be produced by small (200-ml) pericardial effusions, relatively small increases in heart size can be significant (Fig. 25–11).

In the lateral chest roentgenogram particularly, the radiolucency produced by subepicardial fat and that of the adjacent anterior mediastinum often permits visualization of an intervening thin (up to 2 mm wide) "pericardial stripe" (Fig. 25–12A). Thickening of this stripe may be a valuable indicator of pericardial disease and effusion[26, 79] (Fig. 25–12B). Visualization of the subepicardial fat tangential to the tip of a transvenous electrode permits an accurate estimate of the relation of the electrode to the myocardium and of the possibility of perforation.

Fluoroscopy

A large, quiet heart seen fluoroscopically sometimes suggests the presence of pericardial effusion, but this finding is more commonly the consequence of advanced cardiac dilatation resulting from myocardial failure. Vigorous motion of cardiac

Text continued on page 1705

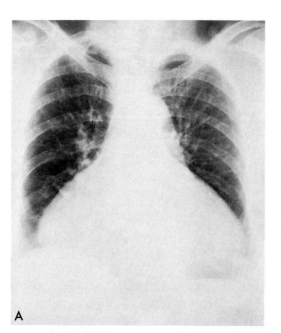

A

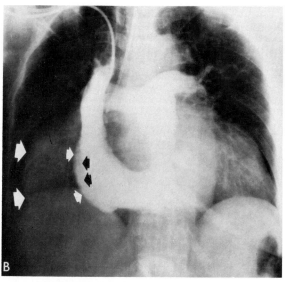

B

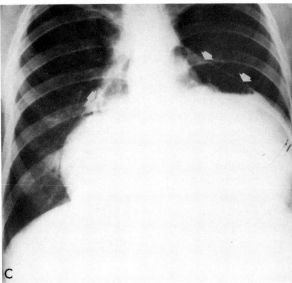

C

Figure 25–8. Large pericardial effusion. *A,* Frontal chest roentgenogram showing massive cardiomegaly and exceptionally clear lungs. *B,* Right heart angiocardiogram showing a large distance (50 mm) from the contrast material in the right atrium to the right lung (large white arrows). Note the double contour of the right atrial border resulting from the superimposed dorsal (black arrows) smooth-walled portion of the atrium and the more ventral (white arrows) component of the right atrium. This right atrium is not compressed by the effusion as it is in frank tamponade (see Fig. 25–12C). *C,* Hydropneumopericardium in another case following intestinal introduction of air into the pericardium after removal of part of a huge effusion secondary to chronic heart failure. Note extension of the normally thin pericardium (arrows) to cephalad portion of ascending aorta. The distended pericardium overlaps and obscures the hilar shadows. (*From* Ellis, K., and King, D. L.: Pericarditis and pericardial effusions. Radiologic and echocardiographic diagnosis. Radiol. Clin. North Am. *11*:393–413, 1973.)

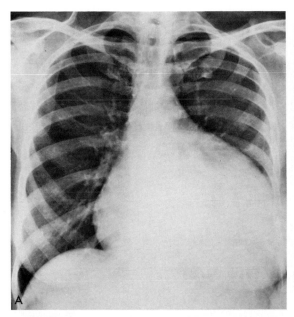

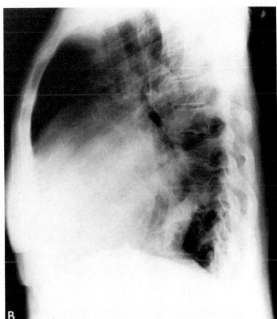

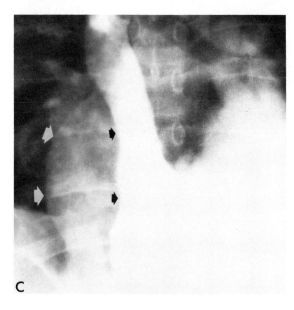

Figure 25–9. Pericardial tamponade in tuberculous effusion. *A,* Frontal roentgenogram shows a huge heart and exceptionally clear lungs. *B,* Lateral view shows massive cardiomegaly with typical encroachment on the retrosternal space. *C,* Frontal angiocardiogram shows the right atrium (black arrows) markedly compressed by a huge effusion. The right lung–pericardial margin is shown by white arrows. Contrast this with the noncompressed right atrium in Figure 25–8*B*. (*From* Ellis, K., and King, D. L.: Pericarditis and pericardial effusions. Radiologic and echocardiographic diagnosis. Radiol. Clin. North Am. *11*:393–413, 1973.)

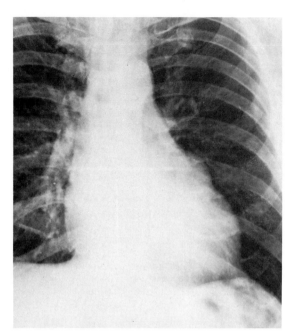

Figure 25–10. Lobulation of the left heart border. Rarely, unusual cardiac configurations are produced by loculation of pericardial effusions. Constrictive pericarditis is likely to be present, as was true in this case. (*From* Ellis, K., and King, D. L.: Pericarditis and pericardial effusions. Radiologic and echocardiographic diagnosis. Radiol. Clin. North Am. *11*:393–413, 1973.)

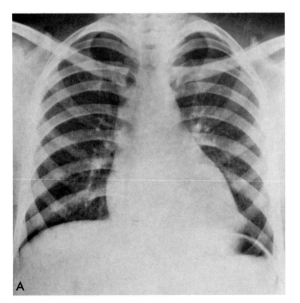
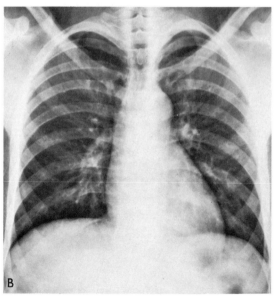

Figure 25–11. Acute pericardial tamponade. *A,* Portable frontal chest roentgenogram showing only modest cardiomegaly but very clearly underperfused lungs in a 21-year-old man obtunded by severe acute cardiac tamponade following a stab wound. *B,* Normal chest film taken two years earlier.

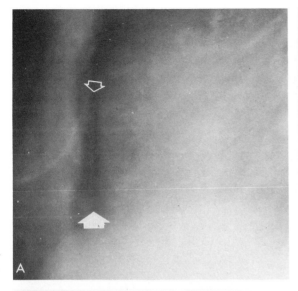

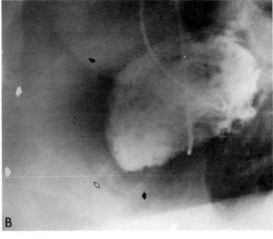

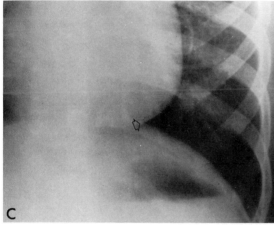

Figure 25–12. Subepicardial fat and pericardial thickening or effusion. *A*, Lateral chest roentgenogram showing a normal retrosternal pericardial stripe (arrows) contrasted against the more lucent (blacker) adjacent fat of the epicardium (behind) and of the anterior mediastinum (in front). *B*, Lucent epicardial fat band (black arrows) in another patient is widely separated from the fat of the retrosternal region (white arrows) because of a large pericardial effusion. This film was an early-phase lateral view during a contrast ventriculogram. *C*, Lucent band in another patient along the lower left heart border due to the subepicardial fat separating pericardium (arrow) from epicardium. The proximity of this lucency to the cardiac border suggests a normal pericardium. Abnormal separation of this fat from the adjacent cardiac border would suggest pericardial thickening or effusion. (*From* Ellis, K., and King, D. L.: Pericarditis and pericardial effusions. Radiologic and echocardiographic diagnosis. Radiol. Clin. North Am. *11*:393–413, 1973.)

structures, however, as judged by the movement of epicardial fat or coronary calcifications within a larger, nearly immobile, outer margin of the heart silhouette clearly suggests a large pericardial effusion.

Angiocardiography

Venous and selective right atrial angiocardiography remains an excellent, if somewhat cumbersome, method for the demonstration of pericardial effusions.[80] A separation of the midmargin of the opacified right atrium from the adjacent lung margin of more than 4.5 mm is abnormal. When this distance is over 10 mm (see Fig. 25–8B), especially when the thickness varies conspicuously with heart cycles, a significant pathologic condition is virtually always present. With cardiac tamponade, the atrial margins are actually compressed by the effusion (see Fig. 25–9C). Excessive thickening of the apparent heart wall at other margins or external to the opacified coronary arteries may also indicate pericardial fluid or thickening. Pleural effusion, mediastinal fat, and other pleural or mediastinal thickening must be considered in the differential diagnosis. Loculated pericardial effusions may be difficult to diagnose by any method.

Radionuclide techniques for imaging the blood pool, myocardium, lung, and liver in various combinations are useful in the diagnosis of large pericardial effusions. The increasing resolution and availability of these techniques promise much for the future. Right atrial angiocardiography using gas (for example, intravenous carbon dioxide) was a very popular and helpful diagnostic study prior to the wide availability of echocardiography. Although cardiac catheterization with angiocardiography (often combined with pericardiocentesis and the introduction of gas into the pericardium) remains essential to the complete diagnostic work-up of many cases of pericardial disease, M-mode and two-dimensional echocardiography have become the primary studies for the initial diagnosis of pericardial effusion.

Echocardiography in Pericardial Effusion

Echocardiography is the simplest and most sensitive means of visualizing and diagnosing the presence of a pericardial effusion.[12, 26, 30, 38, 73, 89] The fluid is seen as echo-free spaces anterior and posterior to the heart. The usual M-mode technique allows inspection of the pericardium surrounding the left ventricle in the region of the posterior papillary muscle (Fig. 25–13A and B). Anteriorly, the right or left ventricular wall is examined near its junction with the septum. The use of two-dimensional echocardiography increases the ease, speed, and reliability of the examination and is now the preferred method (Fig. 25–13E).

Effusions as small as 75 ml may be detected by echocardiography. Larger effusions loculated in regions inaccessible to the sound beam may go undiagnosed, however. In the absence of loculation, small effusions usually first appear adjacent to the posterior left ventricular wall. Occasionally, a left pleural effusion layering between the heart and the lung may simulate this finding. As the pericardial fluid increases in volume it also becomes detectable anterior to the heart. Its presence here indicates a moderate- or large-sized effusion. It is rare to detect fluid anterior to the heart and not posterior as well. The false positive diagnosis of an isolated anterior effusion is usually caused by the presence of large amounts of anterior mediastinal or epicardial fat.

PERICARDITIS

Acute Pericarditis

Roentgenographic manifestations of acute pericarditis are limited and may not be evident. Most typical is increasing cardiomegaly resulting from pericardial effusion. A sympathetic pleural effusion is not uncommon. When pneumonitis is present, it is usually an additional response to the primary underlying disease. Spontaneous pneumopericardium is very rare; when present it is usually caused by perforation of a peptic ulcer[40] or contiguous local abscess into the pericardium, but it can also be the result of trauma or gas dissection with high-pressure mechanical ventilation.

Acute pericarditis may be either a local inflammatory process or a manifestation of systemic disease. Since nearly all cases involve the epimyocardium, the condition might be regarded as myopericarditis. Acute idiopathic (or recurrent) pericarditis is most often of viral origin.

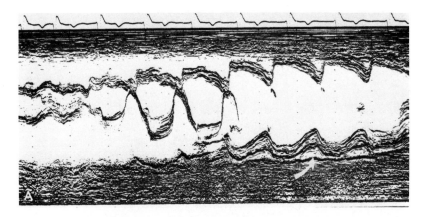

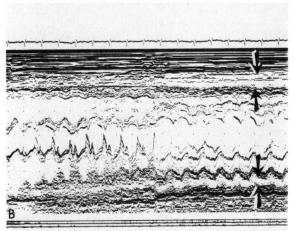

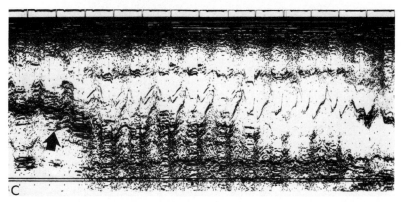

Figure 25–13. Echocardiography and pericardial effusion, calcification and thickening. *A,* A 56-year-old male with severe mitral regurgitation. Echocardiogram shows dilatation of the left atrium and the left ventricle, exaggerated motion of the mitral valve and ventricular walls, and a small effusion posterior to the left ventricular free wall (arrow). *B,* A sweep of the ultrasound beam from the aortic root (left) to the level of the chordae (right) shows an echo-free space (arrows) of a large pericardial effusion anterior to the right ventricle wall and posterior to the left ventricular free wall in this 23-year-old male with class IIIA Hodgkin's disease. *C,* A 57-year-old male with calcification of the apical pericardium. A sweep from the apex (left) to the mitral valve (right) shows an abrupt change in the character of the echoes posterior to the left ventricular free wall. At the apex, calcification produces strong echoes with shadowing behind (arrow). To the right, a more normal appearance is visible. The calcified wall shows diminished motion.

Illustration continued on the following page

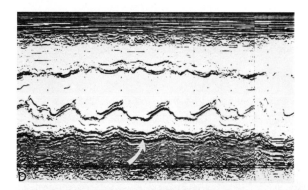

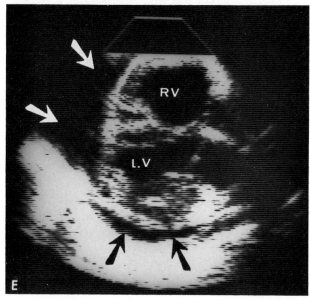

Figure 25-13 *Continued.* *D,* Chordal dimension recording showing an area thought to represent a thickened pericardium (arrow) in this 30-year-old male with a history of pericarditis and current constrictive pericarditis. Echocardiography cannot reliably measure pericardial thickness. *E,* Two-dimensional echogram showing echo-free pericardial effusion laterally (white arrows) and posterior (black arrows) to the left ventricle (LV). RV= right ventricle.

PURULENT PERICARDITIS. Purulent bacterial pericarditis is commonly the consequence of contiguous spread of infection from the lung, pleura, or mediastinum, or of infective endocarditis, but also it can arise from systemic bacteremia and as a postoperative complication.[51, 70] Formerly, the most common causal agent was the pneumococci of an accompanying pneumonia, but today *Staphylococcus aureus,* Gram-negative bacteria, and fungi (especially Candida and Aspergillus species) are more common in many centers. Virtually every organism has been reported to cause acute pericarditis. Amebic pericarditis (like amebic lung abscess) is not rare in some tropical regions.[45] Rarely, septic pericarditis[72] may complicate myocardial infarction or blunt trauma to the chest. Purulent pericarditis is frequently lethal and often not diagnosed before necropsy. Treatment with both appropriate antibiotics and surgical drainage is usually necessary for survival.

OTHER TYPES OF ACUTE PERICARDITIS. The sympathetic pericarditis that occurs in about 7 per cent of patients with cases of myocardial infarction[85] and some patients with cases of blunt chest trauma is the consequence of injury to the underlying myocardium. Some of these patients in subsequent weeks experience Dressler's syndrome, an equivalent of the postpericardiotomy syndrome (see further on). Acute bloody pericardial effusions may be seen during chronic anticoagulant therapy as well as secondary to various blood dyscrasias, Gaucher's disease, or rupture of a dissecting or other aneurysm.

Subacute and Chronic Pericarditis

PERICARDITIS DUE TO TUBERCULOSIS AND HISTOPLASMOSIS. Tuberculous pericarditis is becoming relatively rare[77]; it is usually subacute or chronic in its clinical presentation and is ten times more common in blacks. A chronic effusion, with progressive thickening of both the visceral and the parietal pericardium, is typical. With early intensive sustained chemotherapy the result is usually good. When treatment is begun later in the course of the disease, early pericardiectomy should probably also be considered. Pericarditis due to *Histoplasma capsulatum* has been well documented; typically, it affects young adults, is accompanied by local pneumonitis or hilar adenopathy or both, and spontaneously regresses without late constriction.[66] Pericardial calcification and pericardial constriction have been reported, however.

UREMIC PERICARDITIS AND EFFUSION. Pericarditis, acute and chronic with effusion, is increasingly seen because of the prolonged survival of uremic patients on chronic dialysis and those with renal transplants.[34] Tamponade as well as constriction is not rare. In cases of progressive effusion, surgical internal drainage or pericardiectomy may be required.

RADITION-INDUCED PERICARDITIS WITH EFFUSION. Postradiotherapy pericarditis with significant effusion is being increasingly observed following high-dose radiotherapy of the heart for lymphoma, breast or esophageal carcinoma, and other mediastinal tumors.[55] Like the pleura, the pericardium reacts to high-dose radiation first by a delayed but acute inflammatory reaction, followed by effusion and eventually by fibrous thickening. The effusions are delayed and may not become evident for as long as a year or more following treatment (90 per cent in the first year). Most of these effusions appear to begin with an episode of acute pericarditis. The resulting cardiac enlargement may be eccentric, the greater enlargement being on the side not sclerosed by the radiotherapy. Pericardiocentesis may be lifesaving, and at least a partial pericardiectomy is required eventually in many cases.[60] It must be remembered, however, that all layers of the heart may be damaged by irradiation.

CHRONIC PERICARDIAL EFFUSIONS. Chronic pericardial effusions, often large but with minimal symptoms, may be secondary to rheumatoid disease, lupus erythematosus, scleroderma, rheumatic heart disease, chronic heart failure, hypothyroidism, some chronic anemias, and idiopathic causes. In some cases, the pericardial effusion has been responsible for years of massive cardiomegaly[22] and is large enough to cause inversion of the diaphragm with severe episodic dyspnea (Fig. 25–14).

Constrictive Pericarditis

Of the chronic restrictive heart diseases, constrictive pericarditis is the most important to diagnose, since it is potentially curable by pericardiectomy. Constrictive pericarditis causes cardiac dysfunction primarily by limiting diastolic expansion of the ventricles, but sometimes also by locally obstructing flow across the atrioventricular valves[18] or the right ventricular outflow tract,[8] or in the vena cavae.

The origin of most cases is uncertain, since examination of the resected pericardium usually reveals only nonspecific scar tissue.[16, 82] Some cases are caused by tuberculosis, whereas other cases follow pericarditis due to viral,[11] bacterial, or fungal infection, rheumatoid disease, lupus erythematosus, drug idiosyncrasy,[83] radiation therapy,[42, 81] chronic uremia,[91] or trauma (including on rare occasions open heart surgery itself). Pericardial constriction due to a rare inherited syndrome — mulibrey nanism—has even been reported in children; it may be relieved by pericardiectomy.[86]

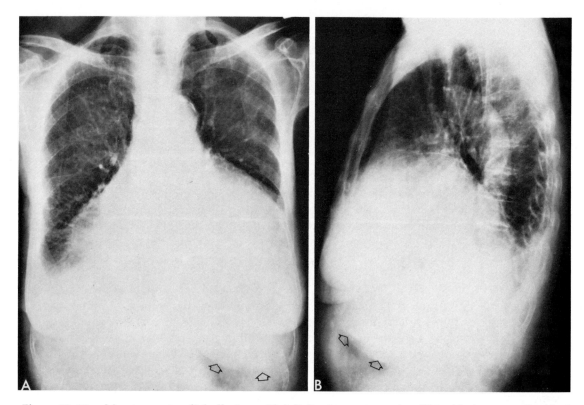

Figure 25–14. Massive pericardial effusion with left diaphragm inversion. This elderly woman had had a chronic pericardial effusion, probably secondary to congestive heart failure. The effusion became so large that the left diaphragm was inverted, causing the patient to experience extreme shortness of breath (arrows). *A,* Frontal view. *B,* Lateral view.

CHEST ROENTGENOGRAPHIC FINDINGS IN CONSTRICTIVE PERICARDITIS

CALCIFICATION OF THE PERICARDIUM (Fig. 25–15, see Fig. 25–13C). This finding implies significant chronic pericarditis, but not necessarily hemodynamic constriction. It is first recognized on plain chest films but is most sensitively detected by fluoroscopy or computerized tomography. The pericardial calcification tends to be more marked in the dependent regions and in the atrioventricular grooves. Distribution of the shell-like calcification over more than one cardiac chamber or region helps distinguish it from calcification in ventricular aneurysms, coronary arteries, and hydatid cyst, and from pleural calcification. Pericardial calcification is reported in 10 to 70 per cent of patients with pericardial constriction.

NORMAL OR SMALL HEART SIZE. A normal-sized or small heart in the presence of generally elevated venous pressures strongly implying cardiac failure suggests restrictive cardiac disease and, especially, constrictive pericarditis.[26] The great majority of patients have a normal- or small-sized heart; but if the heart is large, a combination of chronic pericardial effusion and constricting pericardial thickening is likely to be present (effusive-restrictive pericarditis) (Fig. 25–16)[43]. Many patients also have definite, though mild, disproportionate prominence of the left atrium and changes in the lung suggesting some elevation of pulmonary venous pressure. Conspicuous ascites is often the presenting clinical feature, and commonly an erroneous diagnosis of primary liver cirrhosis is made.

FLAT OR STRAIGHT HEART BORDER. A persistent flattened or straight heart border, especially at the margin of the right atrium in the presence of high systemic venous

Figure 25–15. Pericardial calcification. Frontal (*A*) and lateral (*B*) views of a young man with severe constrictive pericarditis. Nearly all of the extensive calcification was successfully removed by a subsequent pericardiectomy. Note the straight lower right heart border despite the marked elevation of right atrial pressure (mean 20 mm Hg).

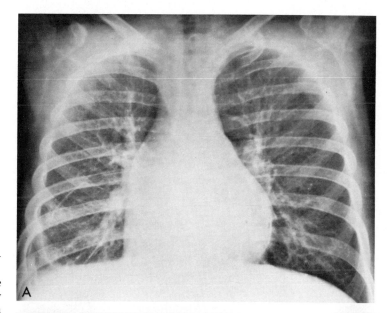
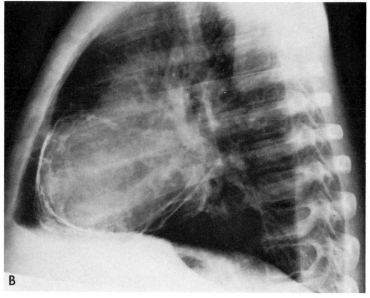

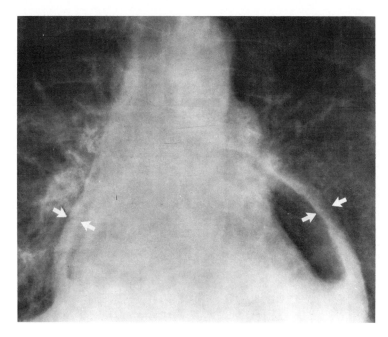

Figure 25–16. Tuberculous effusion with a thick pericardium. After pericardiocentesis, the introduction of some air into the pericardium shows a relatively small heart and a thickened pericardium (arrows). A similar thickening of the visceral pericardium caused severe constrictive pericarditis (effusive-constrictive pericarditis).[43] (*From* Ellis, K., and King, D. L.: Pericarditis and pericardial effusions. Radiologic and echocardiographic diagnosis. Radiol. Clin. North Am. *11*:393–413, 1973.)

pressure, strongly suggests the presence of constrictive pericarditis (Fig. 25–17). This feature implies stiffness of the wall of the heart, since the normally compliant pericardium and atrial diastolic wall tend to bulge more prominently when the atrial pressure is high. Some degree of flattening of the right atrial border is seen in over 50 per cent of patients with constrictive pericarditis.

CHRONIC RIGHT PLEURAL THICKENING. This finding, due to either fluid or chronic pleural thickening, is present in about one-third of the cases and, in conjunction with other signs, is helpful in suggesting the diagnosis (Fig. 25–17B).

FLUOROSCOPY. Fluoroscopy may help uncover the presence and extent of pericardial calcification. The cardiac border pulsation tends to be diminished in constrictive pericarditis, although pulsation may be very prominent in some regions. A diastolic snap[15] may be recognized, that is, sudden end to early diastolic expansion of a ventricle (see Angiocardiography in Constrictive Pericarditis).

ECHOCARDIOGRAPHY IN CONSTRICTIVE PERICARDITIS (Fig. 25–13D). Echocardiography is of little use in the specific diagnosis of constrictive pericarditis, although it may detect an associated pericardial effusion.[30, 67] Although thickening of the pericardium may, in some instances, be suggested from the echocardiogram, it is a subtle finding easily overinterpreted and easily overlooked. Echocardiography may sometimes demonstrate an abrupt cessation of ventricular expansion in diastasis producing a "flat" M-mode echocardiogram of septal and posterior wall motion. Other findings include paradoxical septal motion caused by the hemodynamic changes of constrictive pericarditis. The echocardiogram should be utilized to exclude other diagnostic possibilities.

ANGIOCARDIOGRAPHY IN CONSTRICTIVE PERICARDITIS. Besides helping to rule out other causes of cardiac failure, conventional angiocardiography usually demonstrates important diagnostic features: a flattened diastolic right atrial border and an increase in right-atrial-to-lung-wall thickness (the normal maximal thickness is 4.5 mm) (Fig. 25–17D).[44] Normal wall thickness does not absolutely exclude pericardial constriction, however.

Other findings consistent with but not specific for constrictive pericarditis include: decreased or normal diastolic size of the ventricles, an enlarged and often poorly

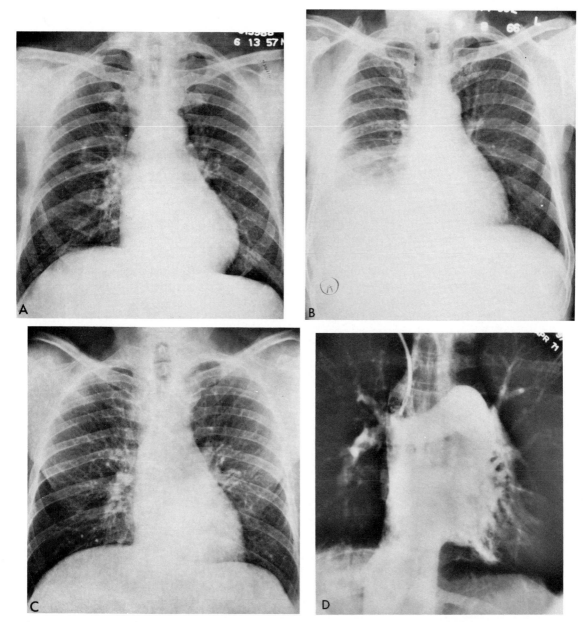

Figure 25–17. Typical frontal chest films in constrictive pericarditis. *A,* A 56-year-old man with a straight right heart border despite severely elevated right atrial pressure. *B,* A 42-year-old man with a normal-sized heart and chronic right-sided effusion and thickening of the pleura. *C,* A normal-sized heart and a relatively straight right heart border in a 45-year-old man with a case of severe constrictive pericarditis. *D,* Frontal angiocardiogram of the patient in *C* following an injection into the superior vena cava showing again the flat, somewhat thickened (8 mm) right atrial border.

contracting atrium,[68] caval dilatation, slow transit of contrast material through the lungs, a flat or inverting atrial septum,[24] evidence of upper lobe venous dilatation, and occasionally, local chamber deformities due to local constriction.[17] Poor systolic emptying of the left atrium is a common feature of patients with significant pericardial constriction.[68]

Cineangiocardiography demonstrates the cardiac chambers very well and often shows a diastolic snap[15] at the end of the rapid ventricular filling phase, which implies a sudden decrease in compliance (ventricular distensibility). Cine coronary arteriography may clearly reveal pericardial thickening between the epicardial coronary arteries and the adjacent lung[69] and relative immobility of the epicardial coronary arteries.

OTHER RADIOGRAPHIC FEATURES IN CONSTRICTIVE PERICARDITIS. In addition to ascites and peripheral edema, a few patients with constrictive pericarditis have a protein-losing enteropathy.[53] This may mimic intestinal lymphangiectasia both on biopsy and on the small bowel series, since enlarged mucosal folds are often seen. Lymphopenia secondary to loss of lymphocytes into the gut may cause anergy and a falsely negative tuberculin skin test.

The diagnosis of constrictive pericarditis, with its distinction from other restrictive cardiac diseases including restrictive cardiomyopathy, certain cases of coronary artery disease, and endomyocardial fibrosis,[9] may be extremely difficult.[35, 56, 74, 90] Normal contraction of the right ventricular infundibulum is characteristic of constrictive pericarditis, whereas contraction is poor in amyloid cardiomyopathy.[7] Systolic time interval,[48] and echocardiographic and volume expansion studies[5, 52] may be helpful in certain cases. The radiologic finding of a calcified or thickened pericardium or both is often critical to an accurate diagnosis. Computerized tomography may be useful for these determinations. Rarely, pericardial neoplasm may masquerade as constrictive pericarditis.

Following successful pericardiectomy for constrictive pericarditis, the heart is often permanently larger than it was preoperatively. Since success depends upon the completeness of the pericardial removal, most or all of the pericardial calcification is excised. Measurable atrophy of myocardial fibers has been demonstrated in long-standing constrictive pericarditis.[20] This factor may be responsible for the prolonged convalescence and substantial cardial dilatation seen postoperatively in a few patients.

POSTOPERATIVE PERICARDIUM

Most pericardial surgery today is incidental to cardiac exposure during operations on the heart valves, cardiac walls or septa, great vessels, and coronary arteries. Other indications for surgery include the treatment of constrictive pericarditis; tamponade or uncontrolled disease due to inflammatory processes; tumor; trauma; and finally, certain neoplasms of the lung, pleura, or mediastinum.

Serial postoperative chest roentgenograms are essential. In the early postoperative period, portable bedside x-ray equipment is required. Numerous special factors affect these x-ray examinations, including the patient's clinical status, position, and ability to respond; the cooperation of physicians and nurses; and chest drainage tubes, vascular catheters, ventilatory apparatus and tubing, chest wall swelling and emphysema, cardiac pacemaker wires and monitoring devices, and surgical dressings. Suboptimal film density, nonstandard film geometry, patient motion, and artifacts are common. Because of these variables, many apparent alterations are of no significance, but an attempt should be made to understand them. Gross or unexpected changes, such as pneumothorax, atelectasis, and large effusions, are more important. An optimal yield of useful information requires clear, complete, accurate knowledge of the clinical situation and the previous chest roentgenograms, and an understanding of the possible complications to be encountered.

Following convalescence from pericardial surgery, interpretation of the chest roentgenograms requires accurate knowledge of the operative findings and the exact surgical procedure. Correct interpretation is also dependent upon appreciation of the natural history of the underlying cardiac disease as well as of the expected late consequences of the cardiac surgery. Close cooperation and communication between the surgeon and the radiologist are critical for optimal patient care.

The roentgenographic manifestations of the most important complications of pericardial surgery are outlined as follows.[25]

Acute

POSTOPERATIVE HEMORRHAGE FROM THE PERICARDIUM. Excessive postoperative bleeding is the most common primary complication.[39] Blood loss is monitored both by continuous attention to the clinical state, including the fluid and blood requirements for maintenance of satisfactory arterial and venous pressures, cardiac output, hematocrit and blood volume, and by estimation of the cumulative losses of fluid and blood. Portable chest roentgenograms showing accumulations of pleural fluid or increasing size of the cardiomediastinal silhouette may afford crucial supporting evidence of excessive bleeding (Fig. 25–18).

When excessive bleeding continues, re-exploration of the chest is often necessary and may be lifesaving. This complication typically occurs within the first 48 hours after surgery. Excessive postoperative bleeding is more often encountered after prolonged operations, especially in cases in which numerous arterial collateral vessels were present and long suture lines involve high-pressure pulmonary arteries or the aorta. Postoperative massive chylopericardium is rare.[46]

POSTOPERATIVE PERICARDIAL HEMORRHAGE WITH TAMPONADE. Cardiac tamponade due to compression of the heart by accumulations of bloody fluid and clot in the pericardial space follows open heart surgery in 2 to 6 per cent of cases (see Figure 25–18).[28, 68] Since cardiac tamponade can rapidly cause death and may be confused with other low-output states, prompt correct diagnosis and treatment are crucial.

Despite wide fenestration and tube drainage of the pericardium, tamponade commonly presents within a few hours after operation (in most cases by 48 hours). Such patients usually have had excessive blood loss by tube drainage and rising central venous pressure together with progressive hypotension, tachycardia, acidoses, and diminishing urinary output. "Low-output syndrome" resulting from myocardial failure is the major alternative diagnosis. Roentgenographically, there is sometimes an impressive increase in cardiomediastinal size. In about half the cases, however, no striking change can be recognized on the portable chest films, since tamponade develops in a poorly compliant mediastinum. Immediate reoperation is required for the removal of blood and clot and the sustained relief of tamponade.

The much less common episodes of tamponade that occur late (after the first seven days) in the postoperative period are mainly the result of anticoagulant therapy.[27, 57] Late pericardial tamponade may also be associated with the postpericardiotomy syndrome or with perforation of the myocardium by a transvenous catheter.[3] The pericardial hemorrhage occurs slowly enough in some cases to allow progressive cardiac enlargement to be documented on chest roentgenograms. If tamponade develops

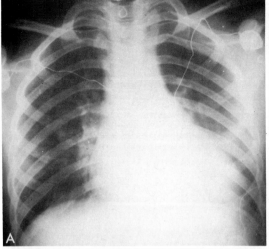

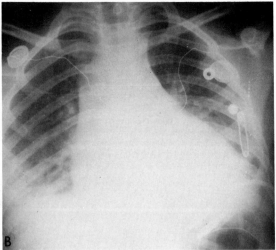

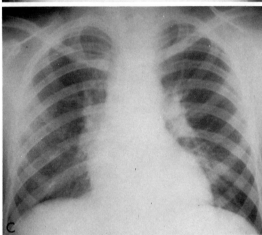

Figure 25–18. Postoperative pericardial bleeding and tamponade. *A,* Portable chest roentgenogram of this 13-year-old boy is unremarkable ten hours after surgical repair by median sternotomy of the ventricular septal defect with prolapse of the right coronary leaflet and aortic regurgitation of recent onset. An excessive — 1300 ml — of blood had drained from a mediastinal drainage tube. *B,* On the second postoperative day the mediastinum is much wider, raising the question of pericardial effusion. The patient was irritable and febrile, and complained of upper abdominal pain. Cardiac tamponade precipitated an arrest, and exploration of the mediastinum permitted the evacuation of much blood and large clots. *C,* One month later the heart is normal in size. (*From* Ellis, K., Malm, J. R., Bowman, F. O., Jr., and King, D. L.: Roentgenographic findings after pericardial surgery. Radiol. Clin. North Am. *9:*327–341, 1971.)

within a relatively stiff pericardium, the serial roentgenographic changes are not very impressive. If it develops suddenly, no chest film is likely to be obtained.

Tamponade is probably the most likely diagnosis when convalescing postoperative patients on anticoagulants and not in chronic heart failure experience sudden hypotension and an increase in venous pressure in the absence of pulmonary edema. Pulmonary embolism is the major alternative diagnosis. Echocardiography may be extremely valuable in these cases.

POSTOPERATIVE CARDIAC HERNIATION. Acute herniation of the heart through a pericardial defect with secondary cardiac strangulation is a rare catastrophic complication of the early postoperative period (Fig. 25–19). More than 40 cases have been reported, virtually all following thoracotomies in which the pericardium was opened in order to complete the resection of a thoracic tumor.[1, 21, 64] Most often a pneumonectomy had been performed.

The first signs are hypotension with distended neck veins and cyanosis — often suggesting superior vena caval obstruction. Tachypnea, chest pain, and ischemic electrocardiographic changes are frequently present, followed by shock and cardiac arrest. The chest roentgenogram shows a striking shift of the heart into the postopera-

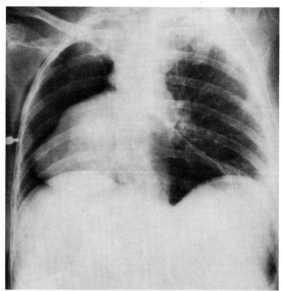

Figure 25–19. Postoperative cardiac herniation. Portable chest film taken immediately after a right pneumonectomy reveals herniation of the heart into the air-filled right chest. The air-containing "empty" pericardial cavity is evident left of the spine. In the supine position there was volvulus with caval obstruction. The herniation was reduced by prompt reoperation. (*From* Arndt, R. D., Frank, C. G., Schmitz, A. L., and Haveson, S. B.: Cardiac herniation with volvulus after pneumonectomy. Am. J. Roentgenol. *130*:155–156, 1978.)

tive chest (see Fig. 25–19). Air is seen in place of the heart in the residual pericardial sac, and sharp notches may be noted between the edges of the herniated heart and the adjacent mediastinum. An accurate early diagnosis is critical, since corrective surgery is usually curative.

Various postoperative maneuvers, such as placing a chest tube on suction, moving the patient, turning the patient onto the operated side, and extubation, have apparently precipitated herniation. Cardiac strangulation also occurs with congenital pericardial defects or post-traumatic rupture of the pericardium.

POSTOPERATIVE INFECTION OF THE PERICARDIUM. Infections of the pericardium are surprisingly infrequent (occurring in less than 1 per cent of cases) after heart surgery. Superficial mediastinal wound infections are more common, however.[71] Perioperative antibiotic coverage generally delays signs of infection until a week or more after operation. Increasing fever, irritability, electrocardiographic changes, often a little drainage from the mediastinal wound (in cases of median sternotomy), or wound disruption may herald such infection. In some cases, serial roentgenograms show a widening mediastinum as the first evidence of the pericardial infection. Infection is more likely when a vertical cleft is visible roentgenographically, indicating incomplete bony apposition at the sternotomy site.

Once wound infection is recognized, exploration to provide adequate drainage is usually necessary. Even infecting organisms of relatively low virulence are frequently difficult to eradicate. Pericardial infection is serious because of two catastrophic complications, either of which may cause sudden death: pericardial tamponade or lethal hemorrhage due to disruption of cardiac or great vessel suture lines (Fig. 25–20).

POSTPERICARDIOTOMY SYNDROME. This peculiar syndrome is seen in 10 to 40 per cent of patients undergoing pericardial surgery.[29, 50] It occurs after the first week and up to six months or more (but most commonly between the second and fourth weeks) after pericardiotomy. The patient develops fever or chest pain, or both, often pericardial or pleural in type. Some pleural or pericardial effusion is common, and friction rubs are heard in more than half the patients. The white blood count, erythrocyte sedimentation rate, and C-reactive protein level are usually elevated, and the electrocardiogram may reveal the nonspecific changes of pericarditis. Cultures are negative, but antiheart antibodies correlate closely with the clinical syndrome.[29] Differential diagno-

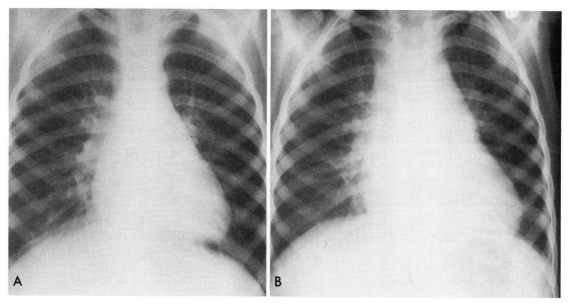

Figure 25–20. Postoperative pericardial infection with secondary aortotomy disruption. *A,* Unremarkable chest film taken six days after the repair of an ostium secundum atrial septal defect with a large left-to-right shunt. The ascending aorta had been cannulated for cardiac bypass. The postoperative course had been smooth, but subsequently increasing fever and irritability occurred. *B,* One week later the mediastinum has progressively widened despite massive antibiotic therapy. Purulent drainage (*Staphylococcus aureus*) from the median sternotomy wound was followed by cardiac arrest secondary to tamponade. Mediastinal exploration controlled bleeding from the aortotomy incision, and the pericardium was drained. No further bleeding occurred until one week later, when exsanguination followed sudden aortotomy wound disruption—the most dreaded consequence of postoperative pericardial wound infection. (*From* Ellis, K., Malm, J. R., Bowman, F. O., Jr., and King, D. L.: Roentgenographic findings after pericardial surgery. Radiol. Clin. North Am. *9:*327–341, 1971.)

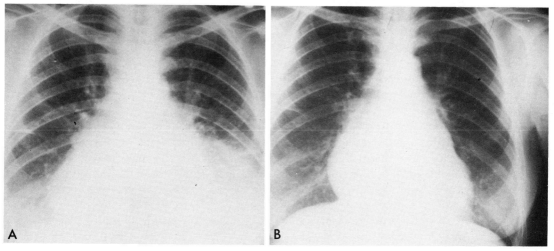

Figure 25–21. Postpericardiotomy syndrome. *A,* Chest roentgenogram of a 44-year-old woman taken because of acute onset of chest pain and fever eight weeks following a mitral commissurotomy. Marked cardiomegaly and a predominate left pleural effusion are seen. The earlier postoperative course had been uneventful, and the clinical result had seemed to be excellent. *B,* Six days later roentgenographic and clinical improvement had promptly followed acetylsalicylate therapy. (*From* Ellis, K., Malm, J. R., Bowman, F. O., Jr., and King, D. L.: Roentgenographic findings after pericardial surgery. Radiol. Clin. North Am. *9:*327–341, 1971.)

sis includes postoperative incisional pain; infection of the wound, including the pericardium; pulmonary embolus; myocardial infarction; aortic dissection; infective endocarditis; and pneumonia.

These clinical episodes are of variable duration. Most last about a week, but recurrent attacks during the next few months are not uncommon. Salicylates, rest, and if necessary, steroids relieve the symptoms. The precise origin of the postpericardio-tomy syndrome is unknown, although degenerating cellular material, including blood, in the pericardial cavity; viral infection; reactivated rheumatic process; trauma; and hypersensitivity with autoantibodies coincident with specific viral infections have been implicated. The pericardial injury that initiates the syndrome need not be heart surgery but may be the result of closed chest trauma, stab wounds, and diagnostic needle punctures.

Roentgenographic features consistent with pericardial effusion, pleural effusions, or basilar pulmonary infiltrates are typical. When these findings occur in an appropriate postoperative clinical setting, particularly in the absence of frank clinical heart failure or pneumonia, they are highly suggestive of the postpericardiotomy syndrome (Fig. 25–21). The diagnosis is supported by a response to aspirin or adrenal steroids, and a benign outcome in nearly all cases. Cardiac tamponade is a recognized, but relatively rare, complication of the syndrome.

Late or Chronic Postoperative Pericardial Complications

A variety of late complications of pericardial surgery are of interest.

1. Cardiac deformities or abnormal positions resulting from chronic herniation through pericardial defects (see Fig. 25–1E) may cause unusual mobility of the heart and its separation from the diaphragm (Fig. 25–22), and air in the pericardium in the presence of pneumothorax (Fig. 25–23).

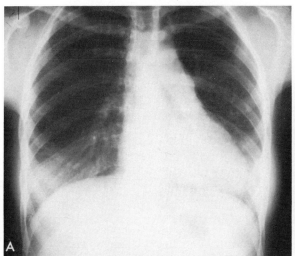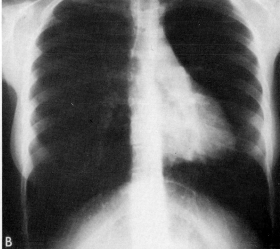

Figure 25–22. Postoperative left pericardial defect. *A*, Frontal chest roentgenogram of a 15-year-old girl in maximal expiration following repair of an anomalous pulmonary venous connection from the left upper lobe to the left innominate vein and an associated atrial septal defect. *B*, In this frontal chest roentgenogram taken in maximal inspiration the heart is widely separated from the left diaphragm be-cause of a surgically created defect in the pericardium. The patient is asymptomatic. (*From* Ellis, K., Malm, J. R., Bowman, F. O., Jr., and King, D. L.: Roentgenographic findings after pericardial surgery. Radiol. Clin. North Am. *9*:327–341, 1971.)

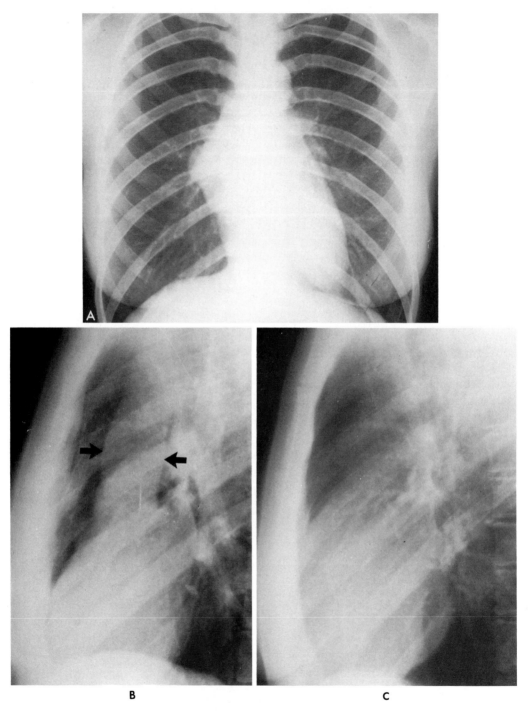

Figure 25–23. Pericardial emphysema secondary to a spontaneous right pneumothorax and a postoperative pleurapericardial defect. *A,* Preoperative chest roentgenogram of a 29-year-old woman showing mediastinal thymoma. During its resection a small 2 × 3-cm right-sided pericardial defect was created. *B,* Lateral chest roentgenogram taken five years later, during an episode of recurrent right-sided spontaneous pneumothorax, shows that air has entered the pericardial cavity, as evidenced by air contrast around the aortic root (arrows). *C,* After clearing of the pneumothorax the intrapericardial ascending aorta was no longer visible. When the leaking apical lung blebs were excised, the previously created pleuropericardial defect was again seen. (*From* Ellis, K., Malm, J. R., Bowman, F. O., Jr., and King, D. L.: Roentgenographic findings after pericardial surgery. Radiol. Clin. North Am. 9:327–341, 1971.)

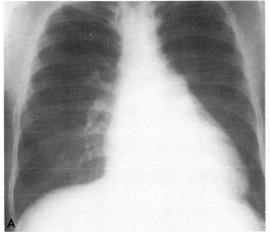

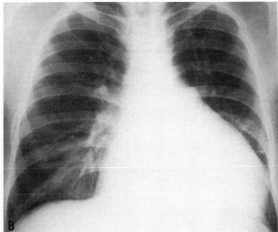

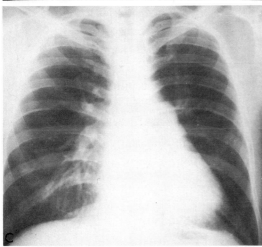

Figure 25–24. Postpericardiotomy syndrome with subsequent constrictive pericarditis. *A,* Chest roentgenogram of a 28-year-old man five weeks following the correction of a large congenital shunt from the left ventricle to the right atrium with excellent immediate postoperative results. *B,* Two weeks later increasing cardiomegaly resulting from pericardial effusion accompanies a clinically severe episode of the postpericardiotomy syndrome. *C,* One year later the heart is normal in size as the clinical picture of constrictive pericarditis develops. Pericardiectomy was performed with successful removal of the constricting fibrous pericardium and excellent clinical results. (*From* Ellis, K., Malm, J. R., Bowman, F. O., Jr., and King, D. L.: Roentgenographic findings after pericardial surgery. Radiol. Clin. North Am. *9:*327–341, 1971.)

2. Late presentation of pericardial infections.

3. Late presentation of postpericardiotomy syndrome.

4. Pericardial constriction requiring pericardiectomy has occasionally been reported following cardiac surgery (Fig. 25–24), including coronary artery bypass operations.[4, 10, 47] A number of these patients experienced the postpericardiotomy syndrome following the original operation.

5. Coronary artery bypass graft occlusion has been reported to occur in a high percentage of patients following only symptomatic treatment of postpericardiotomy syndrome. The incidence of graft occlusion was much lower after treatment of the postpericardiotomy syndrome with vigorous steroid therapy.[87]

References

1. Arndt, R. D., Frank, C. G., Schmitz, A. L., et al.: Cardiac herniation with volvulus after pneumonectomy. Am. J. Roentgenol. *130:*155–156, 1978.
2. Bartle, S. H., and Herman, H. J.: Acute mitral regurgitation in man: hemodynamic evidence and observations indicating an early role for the pericardium. Circulation *36:*839–851, 1967.
3. Bassan, M. M., and Merin, G.: Pericardial tamponade due to perforation with a permanent endocardial pacing catheter. J. Thorac. Cardiovasc. Surg. *74:*51–54, 1977.

4. Brown, D. F., and Older, T.: Pericardial constriction as a late complication of coronary bypass surgery. J. Thorac. Cardiovasc. Surg. 74:61–64, 1977.

5. Bush, C. A., Stang, J. M., Wooley, C. F., et al.: Occult constrictive pericardial disease. Diagnosis by rapid volume expansion and correction by pericardiectomy. Circulation 56:924–930, 1977.

6. Carty, J. D., Deverall, P. B., and Losowsky, M. S.: Pericardial defect presenting as acute pericarditis. Br. Heart J. 37:98–100, 1975.

7. Chang, L. W. M., and Grollman, J. H., Jr.: Angiocardiographic differentiation of constrictive pericarditis and restrictive cardiomyopathy due to amyloidosis. Am. J. Roentgenol. 130:451–453, 1978.

8. Chesler, E., Mitha, A. S., Matisoun, R. E., et al.: Subpulmonic stenosis as a result of noncalcific constrictive pericarditis. Chest 69:425–427, 1976.

9. Clark, G. M., Valentine, E., and Blount, S. G.: Endocardial fibrosis simulating constrictive pericarditis. N. Engl. J. Med. 254:349–355, 1956.

10. Cliff, W. J., Grobety, J., and Ryan, G. B.: Post operative pericardial adhesions. J. Thorac. Cardiovasc. Surg. 65:744–750, 1973.

11. Cooper, D. K. C., and Sturridge, M. F.: Constrictive epicarditis following Coxsackie virus infection. Thorax 31:472–474, 1976.

12. Cosio, F. G., Martinez, J. P., Serrano, C. M., et al.: Abnormal septal motion in cardiac tamponade with pulsus paradoxus. Chest 71:787–789, 1977.

13. Crittenden, I. H., Adams, F. H., and Mulder, D. G.: A syndrome featuring defects of the heart, sternum, diaphragm and anterior abdominal wall. Circulation 20:396–404, 1959.

14. Deenadayalu, R. P., Tuuri, D., Dewall, R. A., et al.: Intrapericardial teratoma and bronchiogenic cyst. J. Thorac. Cardiovasc. Surg. 67:945–952, 1974.

15. Desilets, D. T., Grollman, J. H., Jr., and MacAlpin, R. N.: Ciné angiocardiographic demonstration of diastolic snap in constrictive pericarditis. Radiology 86:1056–1063, 1966.

16. Deterling, R. A., Jr., and Humphreys, G. H., II: Factors in the etiology of constrictive pericarditis. Circulation 12:30–43, 1955.

17. Deutch, V., Miller, H., Yahini, J. H., et al.: Angiocardiography in constrictive pericarditis. Chest 65:379–387, 1974.

18. Dillon, J. C.: Tricuspid stenosis secondary to pericardial disease. Editorial. Chest 71:690–691, 1977.

19. Dimich, J., Grossman, H., Bowman, F. O., Jr., et al.: Congenital absence of left pericardium. Am. J. Dis. Child. 110:309–314, 1965.

20. Dines, D. E., Edwards, J. E., and Burchell, H. B.: Myocardial atrophy in constrictive pericarditis. Proc. Staff Meet. Mayo Clin. 33:93–99, 1958.

21. Dippel, W. F., and Ehrenhaft, J. L.: Herniation of the heart after pneumonectomy. J. Thorac. Cardiovasc. Surg. 65:207–209, 1973.

22. Dressler, W., Levin, E. J., and Axelrod, M.: Huge pericardial effusion of 15 years duration. J.A.M.A. 195:188–190, 1966.

23. Ellis, K., Leeds, N. E., and Himmelstein, A.: Congenital deficiencies in the parietal pericardium. Am. J. Roentgenol. 82:125–137, 1959.

24. Ellis, K., Kanter, I. E., and King, D. L., et al.: The atrial septal sign. Am. J. Roentgenol. 109:37–50, 1970.

25. Ellis, K., Malm, J. R., Bowman, F. O., Jr., et al.: Roentgenographic findings after pericardial surgery. Radiol. Clin. North Am. 9:327–341, 1971.

26. Ellis, K., and King, D. L.: Pericarditis and pericardial effusions. Radiologic and echocardiographic diagnosis. Radiol. Clin. North Am. 11:393–413, 1973.

27. Ellison, L. H., and Kirsh, M. M.: Delayed mediastinal tamponade after open heart surgery. Chest 65:64–66, 1974.

28. Engelman, R. M., Spencer, F. C., Reed, G. E., et al.: Cardiac tamponade following open heart surgery. Circulation 41–42(Suppl. II):II165–II171, 1970.

29. Engle, M. A., McCabe, J. C., Ebert, P. A., et al.: The postpericardiotomy syndrome and antiheart antibodies. Circulation 49:401–406, 1974.

30. Feigenbaum, H.: Echocardiography. Ed. 2. Philadelphia, Lea & Febiger, 1976, pp. 419–446.

31. Feigin, D. S., Fenoglio, J. J., McAllister, H. A., et al.: Pericardial cysts. A radiologic-pathologic correlation and review. Radiology 125:15–20, 1977.

32. Felner, J. M., Fleming, W. H., and Franch, R. H.: Echocardiographic identification of a pericardial cyst. Chest 68:386–387, 1975.

33. Figley, M. M., and Bagshaw, M. A.: Angiocardiographic aspects of constrictive pericarditis. Radiology 69:46–53, 1957.

34. Fox, H. E., Yee, J. M., Weaver, J. C., Jr., et al.: Pericardial drainage operations in the management of uremic pericardial effusions. J. Thorac. Cardiovasc. Surg. 73:504–508, 1977.

35. Gaasch, W. H., Peterson, K. L., and Shabetai, R.: Left ventricular function in chronic constrictive pericarditis. Am. J. Cardiol. 34:107–110, 1974.

36. Gibson, J. Y.: A large intrapericardial cyst presenting as a cardiac abnormality. Radiology 119:49–50, 1976.

37. Glancy, D. L., and Roberts, W. C.: The heart in malignant melanoma. Am. J. Cardiol. 21:555–571, 1968.

38. Goldberg, B. B., and Pollack, H. M.: Ultrasonically guided pericardiocentesis. Am. J. Cardiol. 31:490–493, 1973.

39. Gomez, M. M. R., and McGoon, D. C.: Bleeding patterns after open heart surgery. J. Thorac. Cardiovasc. Surg. 60:87–97, 1970.

40. Gossage, A. A. R., Robertson, P. W., and Stephenson, S. F.: Spontaneous pneumopericardium. Thorax 31:460–465, 1976.
41. Green, B., Zornoza, J., and Ricks, J. P.: Eccentric pericardial effusion after radiation therapy of left breast carcinoma. Am. J. Roentgenol. 128:27–30, 1977.
42. Greenwood, R. D., Rosenthal, A., Cassady, R., et al.: Constrictive pericarditis in childhood due to mediastinal irradiation. Circulation 50:1033–1039, 1974.
43. Hancock, E. W.: Subacute effusive-constrictive pericarditis. Circulation 43:183–192, 1971.
44. Holt, J. P.: The normal pericardium. Am. J. Cardiol. 26:455–465, 1970.
45. Ibarra-Perez, C., Green, L., Cavillo-Juarez, M., et al.: Diagnosis and treatment of rupture of amebic abscess of the liver into the pericardium. J. Thorac. Cardiovasc. Surg. 64:11–17, 1977.
46. Kansu, E., Fraimow, W., and Smullens, S. N.: Isolated massive chylopericardium. Chest 71:408–410, 1977.
47. Kendall, M. E., Rhodes, G. R., and Wolfe, W.: Cardiac constriction following aorta-to-coronary bypass surgery. J. Thorac. Cardiovasc. Surg. 64:142–153, 1972.
48. Khullar, S., and Lewis, R. P.: Usefulness of systolic time intervals in differential diagnosis of constrictive pericarditis and restrictive myocardiopathy. Br. Heart J. 38:43–46, 1976.
49. King, J. F., Crosby, I., Pugh, D., et al.: Rupture of pericardial cyst. Chest 60:611–612, 1971.
50. Kirsh, M. M., McIntosh, K., Kahn, D. R., et al.: Postpericardiotomy syndromes. Ann. Thorac. Surg. 9:158–179, 1970.
51. Klacsmann, P. G., Buckley, B. H., and Hutchins, G. M.: The changed spectrum of purulent pericarditis. An 86 year autopsy experience in 200 cases. Am. J. Med. 63:686–673, 1977.
52. Kliman, J. W., Bush, C. A., Wooley, C. F., et al.: The changing spectrum of pericardiectomy for chronic pericarditis: occult constrictive pericarditis. J. Thorac. Cardiovasc. Surg. 74:668–673, 1977.
53. Kumpe, D. A., Jaffe, R. B., Waldman, T. A., et al.: Constrictive pericarditis and protein losing enteropathy. An imitator of intestinal lymphangiectasia. Am. J. Roentgenol. 124:365–373, 1975.
54. Leagus, C. J., Gregorski, R. F., Crittenden, J. J., et al.: Giant intrapericardial bronchiogenic cyst. J. Thorac. Cardiovasc. Surg. 52:581–587, 1966.
55. Martin, R. G., Ruckdeschel, J. C., Chang, P., et al.: Radiation-related pericarditis. Am. J. Cardiol. 35:216–222, 1975.
56. Meaney, E., Shabetai, R., Bhargava, V., et al.: Cardiac amyloidosis, constrictive pericarditis and restrictive cardiomyopathy. Am. J. Cardiol. 38:547–556, 1976.
57. Merrill, W., Donahoo, J. S., Brawley, R. K., et al.: Late cardiac tamponade: a potentially lethal complication of open-heart surgery. J. Thorac. Cardiovasc. Surg. 72:929–932, 1976.
58. Miller, A. J., Pick, R., and Johnson, P. J.: The production of acute pericardial effusion. Am. J. Cardiol. 28:463–466, 1971.
59. Moene, R. J., Dekker, A., and vander Harten, H. J.: Congenital right-sided pericardial defect with herniation of part of the lung into the pericardial cavity. Am. J. Cardiol. 31:519–522, 1973.
60. Morton, D. L., Glancy, L., Joseph, W. L., et al.: Management of patients with radiation-induced pericarditis with effusion: a note on the development of aortic regurgitation in two of them. Chest 64:291–297, 1973.
61. Moulton, A. L., Jaretzki, A., Bowman, F. O., Jr., et al.: Massive lipoma of the heart. N. Y. State J. Med. 76:1820–1825, 1976.
62. Nasser, W. K., Helmen, C., Tavel, M. E., et al.: Congenital absence of the left pericardium. Circulation 41:469–478, 1970.
63. Nelson, R. M., Jensen, C. B., and Scott, W. M., III: Pericardial tamponade following open heart surgery. J. Thorac. Cardiovasc. Surg. 58:510–514, 1969.
64. Nogrady, M. B., and Nemee, J.: Partial congenital pericardial defect in childhood. Report of four cases. J. Can. Assoc. Radiol 21:116–119, 1970.
65. Peterson, D. T., Zatz, L. M., and Popp, R. L.: Pericardial cyst ten years after acute pericarditis. Chest 67:719–721, 1972.
66. Picardi, J. L., Kauffman, C. A., Schwarz, J., et al.: Pericarditis caused by Histoplasma capsulatum. Am. J. Cardiol. 37:82–86, 1976.
67. Pool, P. E., Seagreen, S. C., Abbasi, A. S., et al.: Echocardiographic manifestations of constrictive pericarditis. Chest 68:684–688, 1975.
68. Preger, L., Dayem, M. K. A., Goodwin, J. F., et al.: Pericarditis and pericardial effusion. Lancet 2:701–706, 1965.
69. Ramsey, H. W., Sbar, S., Elliott, L. P., et al.: The differential diagnosis of restrictive myocardiopathy and chronic constrictive pericarditis without calcification. Am. J. Cardiol. 25:635–637, 1970.
70. Rubin, R. H., and Moellering, R. C., Jr.: Clinical microbiologic and therapeutic aspects of purulent pericarditis. Am. J. Med. 59:68–78, 1975.
71. Sanfelippo, P. M., and Danielson, G. K.: Complications associated with median sternotomy. J. Thorac. Cardiovasc. Surg. 63:419–423, 1972.
72. Schatz, J. W., Wiener, L., Gallagher, H. S., et al.: Salmonella pericarditis: an unusual complication of myocardial infarction. Chest 64:267–269, 1973.
73. Settle, H. P., Adolph, R. J., Fowler, N. O., et al.: Echocardiographic study of cardiac tamponade. Circulation 56:951–959, 1977.
74. Shabetai, R., Fowler, N. O., and Guntheroth, W. G.: The hemodynamics of cardiac tamponade and constrictive pericarditis. Am. J. Cardiol. 26:480–489, 1970.

75. Shin, M. S., Tyndall, E. C., and Ronderos, A.: Pedunculated pericardial coelomic cyst. Chest 63:123–124, 1973.
76. Siegel, R. E.: Galen on surgery of the pericardium. Am. J. Cardiol. 26:524–527, 1970.
77. Somers, K., DeBuse, P. J., Patel, A. K., et al.: Childhood tuberculous pericarditis. Chest 60:2–28, 1971.
78. Spodick, D. H.: Medical history of the pericardium. Am. J. Cardiol. 26:447–454, 1970.
79. Spooner, E. W., Kuhns, L. R., and Stein, A. M.: Diagnosis of pericardial effusion in children: a new radiographic sign. Am. J. Roentgenol. 128:23–25, 1977.
80. Steinberg, I., von Gall, H., and Finby, N.: Roentgen diagnosis of pericardial effusions: new angiocardiographic observations. Am. J. Roentgenol. 79:321–332, 1958.
81. Stewart, J. R., Cohn, K. E., Fajardo, L. F., et al.: Radiation induced heart disease. Radiology 89:302–310, 1967.
82. Strauss, A. W., Santa-Maria, M., and Goldring, D.: Constrictive pericarditis in children. Am. J. Dis. Child. 129:822–826, 1975.
83. Sunder, S. K., and Shah, A.: Constrictive pericarditis in procainamide-induced lupus erythematosus syndrome. Am. J. Cardiol. 36:960–962, 1975.
84. Takita, H., and Mijares, W. S.: Herniation of the heart following intrapericardial pneumonectomy. J. Thorac. Cardiovasc. Surg. 59:443–446, 1970.
85. Toole, J. C., and Silverman, M. E.: Pericarditis of acute myocardial infarction. Chest 67:647–653, 1975.
86. Tuuteri, L., Perheentupa, J., and Rapola, J.: The cardiopathy of mulibrey nanism. Chest 65:628–631, 1974.
87. Urschel, H. C., Jr., Rassuk, M. A., and Gardner, M.: Coronary artery bypass occlusion secondary to postcardiotomy syndrome. Ann. Thorac. Surg. 22:528–531, 1976.
88. Van de Hauwaert, L. G.: Cardiac tumors in infancy and childhood. Br. Heart J. 33:125–132, 1971.
89. Vignola, P. A., Pohost, G. M., Curfman, G. D., et al.: Correlation of echocardiographic and clinical findings in patients with pericardial effusion. Am. J. Cardiol. 37:701, 1976.
90. Vogel, J. H. K., Horgan, J. A., and Strahl, C. L.: Left ventricular dysfunction in chronic constrictive pericarditis. Chest 59:484–492, 1971.
91. Wolfe, S. A., Bailey, G. F., and Collins, J. J., Jr.: Constrictive pericarditis following uremic effusion. J. Thorac. Cardiovasc. Surg. 63:540–544, 1972.
92. Wychulis, A. R., Connolly, D. C., and McGoon, D. C.: Pericardial cysts, tumors and fat necrosis. J. Thorac. Cardiovasc. Surg. 62:294–300, 1971.
93. Yeoh, C. B., Harris, P. D., Leff, E., et al.: Intrapericardial teratoma. N. Y. State J. Med. 76(5):708–710, 1976.

26

THE HEART

Part I
Cardiac Catheterization

DIANA F. GUTHANER, M.D.
LEWIS WEXLER, M.D.

INTRODUCTION

Forsmann's courageous act of introducing a rubber catheter into his own vein and passing it into the heart[31] heralded an era of remarkable observations of cardiac physiology and the development of cardiac angiography. Blood samples for oxygen saturation and hemodynamic measurements obtained through the cardiac catheter provide direct information about intracardiac shunts, valvular lesions, and cardiac function. In order to visualize the interior of cardiac chambers and dynamic blood flow within the heart and blood vessels, it is necessary to introduce nontoxic radiopaque materials into the blood stream without greatly altering normal function. The flowing blood, now rendered radiopaque, can be observed at fluoroscopy and recorded on x-ray film as a series of static events or in a cine format. Advances in all aspects of x-ray technology, pharmacology of radiographic contrast materials, and techniques of catheterization have enabled the present sophisticated clinical investigation known as cardiac angiography to develop.

Less than 50 years ago, Egas Moniz, a Portuguese pioneer in the field, performed the first intravascular injection of a relatively noxious radiopaque material (sodium iodide) in a living patient. The potential of this technique was further explored shortly thereafter with the performance of the first abdominal aortogram. Rousthöi, in 1933, succeeded in opacifying the cardiac chambers, aorta, and coronary arteries of a rabbit, using a catheter introduced into the ascending aorta from the carotid artery.[78] Interest lay dormant for some years; however, in 1947 Chávez pioneered the technique of selective angiocardiography by describing direct intracardiac injections.[17] Using a technique first developed in dogs and rabbits, Radner introduced a long needle through a sternal cannula and punctured the ascending aorta directly, injecting 20 to 30 ml of Thorotrast (thorium dioxide).[72] The radiographs he obtained showed the aortic root, but the film quality was poor.

Forsmann's operative technique for the introduction of a catheter into the central circulation was modified by Seldinger in 1953[83] to permit rapid placement of a catheter into the aorta by the simple and safe method of percutaneous puncture of a vessel. The catheter, with its preselected curve, could be directed under fluoroscopic guidance into any desired branch of the aorta or cardiac chamber. The development of rapid film changers and pressure injectors made it possible to deliver sufficient contrast volumes in a brief time while simultaneously obtaining several radiographs of the short-lived vascular events. Further refinements and developments occurred, including modification of the catheters to facilitate rapid large-volume injections. Initially, angiographers used open-ended catheters; later, closed-end catheters with multiple side holes were employed. More elaborate catheter designs with a variety of different-shaped terminal loops were introduced. In the mid-1950's, triiodobenzoic compounds, Urografin in Germany and Hypaque in the United States, were developed and found to have both minimal toxicity and satisfactory radiodensity.

In 1959, Sones poineered a method for "selective" coronary arteriography, a technique that could be performed safely and consistently.[89] Ricketts and Abrams in 1962, published the results of their attempts to adapt the percutaneous transfemoral approach to selective coronary catheterization.[75] They designed specially shaped catheters from materials familiar to cardiovascular radiologists that could be introduced percutaneously by Seldinger's method. Judkins made further improvements in this approach by modifying both catheter shape and material.[50, 51] He introduced a wire braid into the wall of the catheter which increased its torque response and facilitated more precise control of the position of the tip. The catheter tips were designed to be "coronary seeking." Amplatz,[5] Bourassa,[12] and Schoonmaker[82] have devised modifications in the catheter shapes which are also in use for selective percutaneous coronary catheterization.

TECHNIQUE

The angiographic aspects of cardiac catheterization and routine angiographic techniques, requirements, and complications will be discussed in this section. It is our belief that the angiographic technique should not be learned from a book. No description is an adequate explanation of the maneuvers required to catheterize a difficult vessel. The angiographer must learn the "feel" of a proper catheter placement, and this comes only after long hours of supervised experience.

A primary goal of the cardiac catheterization laboratory and its personnel is to ensure satisfactory, safe, and efficient patient handling with maximal patient comfort. To this end, the patient is prepared on the day prior to the procedure with complete but informal explanations of what to expect. Blood chemistry, with particular attention to renal function, is determined, and a baseline electrocardiogram is obtained. The patient is maintained on fluid prior to the procedure and premedicated with diazepam or a barbiturate. The order of the procedure is flexible, being tailored to individual requirements.

The routine in our laboratory commences with obtaining physiologic data and cardiac output, using either the Fick principle, a measurement of oxygen consumption and the arteriovenous oxygen difference, or an indicator dilution technique. Computer data processing is being used in many laboratories to establish various physiologic parameters. For localization and quantification of a central shunt, oxygen saturation of blood samples from the right heart chambers, the pulmonary artery, and a systemic artery is obtained. Inert radioactive gas techniques are more sensitive for the identification of small shunts. Electrocardiographic and continuous pressure monitoring at the catheter tip is utilized throughout the procedure. A pigtail catheter with multiple side holes is then manipulated across the aortic valve, usually by looping the catheter against the sinus of Valsalva. The optimal position for the catheter tip in a left ventriculogram is lying free within the body of the left ventricular chamber near the apex in the absence of ventricular extrasystoles. Occasionally, the catheter must be placed in the outflow tract in front of the mitral valve in order to minimize catheter-induced extrasystoles.

Although accurate measurements of left ventricular volume require biplane filming,[18, 24] quantitative ventriculography can be obtained from a single-plane cineangiographic study.[40] The change in ventricular volume can be calculated throughout the cardiac cycle and the ejection fraction derived from the end-systolic and end-diastolic images. The perimeter of the opacified left ventricle can be digitized by the use of a light pen and computer to perform calculations and produce an analog print-out. However, observation of the ventriculogram also provides an approximate estimation of ventricular function and segmental wall motion in addition to information concerning the presence of mitral regurgitation or a left-to-right shunt. To evaluate the septal and lateral walls in profile, a left anterior oblique projection is required; the left ventricular outflow tract is elongated by angling the tube in a craniocaudal direction.

For coronary arteriography, our experience has been entirely with the Judkins technique; the reader is referred to Gensini's text[36] for a detailed discussion of the Sones technique. With the use of the Judkins preshaped catheters, insertion into the right and left coronary arteries is readily accomplished. The left catheter seeks the left coronary orifice, while the right catheter is easily manipulated anteriorly into the right coronary ostium. The projection of the cardiac chambers or the coronary system into any desired obliquity is achieved with a fixed x-ray system by rotating the patient in a cradle mounted on a free-floating table top[97] or by rotating the x-ray system around the patient with newer "C" or "U" arm systems that accommodate complex projectional angles.[28]

Catheterization

APPROACH. Because methods of catheter entry for cardiac catheterization vary with the age of the patient, the vascular system to be investigated, and the existing disease, a single standard approach is precluded. In neonates during the first week of life, umbilical vessels usually permit access to the vascular system. For older infants, the preferred and most facile method of vessel entry is a modification of the percutaneous technique developed by Seldinger,[83] but if this is not possible, a direct cut-down on the vessel, either the artery or vein in the arm or the saphenous vein in the groin, can be performed.

The approach to the venous system, right heart, or pulmonary vasculature is via a peripheral vein, usually the femoral, median cubital, or internal jugular vein. The femoral artery is the preferred percutaneous access route to the arterial system or left heart. In the presence of iliofemoral occlusive disease, a percutaneous transaxillary approach is the method of choice for those experienced in the technique. An approach from the right allows ready access to the ascending aorta, and from the left the descending aorta is easily entered. The preshaped Judkins[50, 51] and Amplatz[98] catheters may be used without modification for coronary catheterization from the left axilla.[71] The alternative approach to the left heart and coronary vessels is via brachial arteriotomy.

Either percutaneous or cut-down techniques can be used safely, but the operator should choose one approach and gain expertise in it over a long period in a supervised training program.

CATHETERS. Considerable improvements have been made in the development of catheters and their application to the study of the vascular system over the past 50 years. Several preshaped catheters are manufactured from extruded polyethylene or polyurethane or from woven nylon or Dacron with a radiopaque coating. Ideally, a catheter system includes a relatively flexible tip to minimize inflicted trauma together with a more rigid basic design to allow manipulation. Incorporation of a wire mesh within the wall of the catheter improves torque control, so that a desired deflection of the tip is obtained by small twists of the catheter at its entry site.

Disposable, single-use catheters are available in a variety of shapes, number and position of side holes, and diameters (designated by a given French size). For example, catheters used for right heart catheterization and the Sones catheters are fabricated from woven Dacron and have side holes. Preshaped catheters, such as the Judkins, Amplatz, and pigtail catheters, are made of polyurethane or polyethylene with added torque control. The Judkins primary curve catheter for left coronary catheterization is available in several sizes, depending on the distance from the anchoring point on the right anterolateral aortic wall to a point below the coronary ostium. Patients with normal-sized aortas invariably accommodate a 4-cm curve. Older patients or those with hypertension and an ectatic or dilated aorta require larger curves of 5 or 6 cm.

CATHETER POSITIONS. Familiarity with typical and atypical catheter courses and positions may be of assistance during a hemodynamic study and in the evaluation of cinecardiograms.[93]

1. The course of a catheter positioned in the pulmonary artery via the right heart may be simulated by a catheter in the left superior vena cava draining into the coronary sinus (Fig. 26–1) or one in the left atrial appendage via a defect in the atrial septum. In

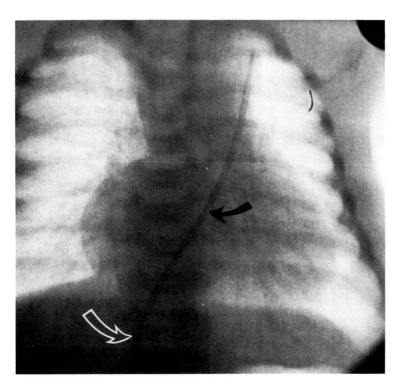

Figure 26–1. Frontal projection demonstrating a venous catheter passing from the inferior vena cava (open arrow) into a left superior vena cava via the coronary sinus (arrow). The position of the catheter across the heart is similar to the passage of a catheter through the right heart chambers into the pulmonary artery.

the lateral projection, the normal anterior course, across the tricuspid valve into the right ventricle anteriorly to enter the pulmonary artery, must be distinguished from a posterior position in the coronary sinus. In addition, the catheter position may be confirmed by a combination of pressure measurements, oximetry, or contrast injections.

2.   A catheter that enters the right heart via an azygos continuation of the inferior vena cava ascends along the right side of the spine posterior to the heart to enter the superior vena cava and then descends into the right atrium. In the lateral view it mimics a catheter passed retrograde in the aorta to the left ventricle. A similar appearance on the left side of the spine occurs in the presence of hemiazygos continuation of the inferior vena cava. In this case the catheter enters the coronary sinus behind the left atrial appendage in order to reach the right atrium (Fig. 26–2).

3.   A catheter that crosses the atrial septum and mitral valve to enter the left ventricle (Fig. 26–3) has a similar appearance in a frontal projection to a catheter that has crossed the septum and entered a left lower pulmonary vein. If on further advancement the catheter projects beyond the cardiac margin, it is likely to be in a pulmonary vein.

4.   Pulmonary veins may be entered directly from the superior vena cava in cases of anomalous drainage of the right upper pulmonary vein (Fig. 26–4). More frequently, a catheter will cross the atrial septum either through an atrial septal defect or through a patent foramen ovale and enter the right upper pulmonary vein from the left atrium. Because the atrial septum runs obliquely in the frontal projection, it appears as if the catheter has passed directly from the right atrium into the pulmonary vein; consequently, an erroneous diagnosis of anomalous pulmonary venous drainage may be made. If the catheter takes this course, an injection of contrast material with the patient positioned in the craniocaudal left anterior oblique view will demonstrate the relationship of the right upper pulmonary vein and the atrial septum.

5.   A venous catheter across a ventricular septal defect may be passed into the ascending aorta, which in its normal position lies medial and posterior to the pulmonary artery (Fig. 26–5). The descending aorta may be reached from the pulmonary

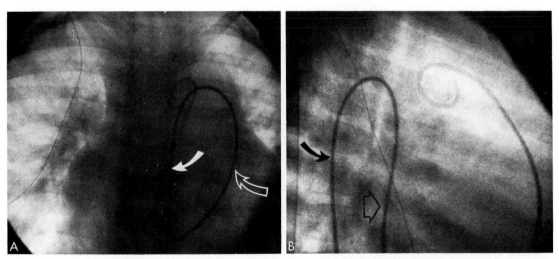

Figure 26–2.   Frontal (*A*) and lateral (*B*) projections of a child with polysplenia and complex congenital heart disease. The catheter, which was introduced into the venous system, traverses a hemiazygos continuation of the inferior vena cava (arrow) to the left of the spine to reach the coronary sinus (open arrow) and a common atrial chamber. The tip of the catheter has been advanced anteriorly into the pulmonary artery.

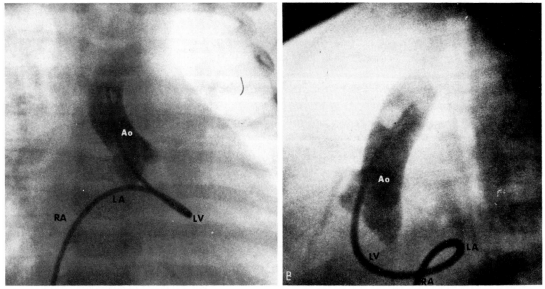

Figure 26–3. Frontal (*A*) and lateral (*B*) projections demonstrating a balloon-tipped catheter that has been passed from the inferior vena cava through the right atrium (RA), across the atrial septum, the left atrium (LA) and mitral valve into the left ventricle (LV), and finally into the ascending aorta (Ao) for an aortogram.

artery via a patent ductus arteriosus. This is a characteristic catheter course, confirmed by advancing the catheter well below the diaphragm (Fig. 26–6).

Angiographic Equipment

Cineangiographic equipment today includes a powerful three-phase, constant-potential x-ray generator capable of at least 1000 ma at 100 to 150 kv with short exposure

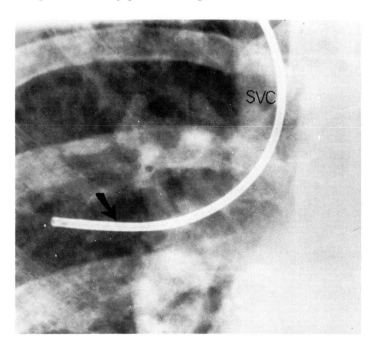

Figure 26–4. Atrial septal defect with partial anomalous pulmonary venous return. The catheter from the right basilic vein has been passed into the superior vena cava (SVC) and into an anomalous right upper lobe pulmonary vein (arrow) which drains into the superior vena cava. The patient also had a sinus venosus atrial septal defect.

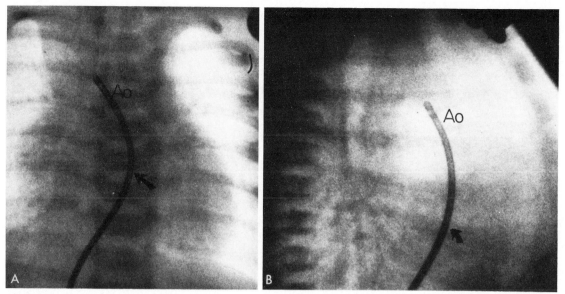

Figure 26–5. Frontal (*A*) and lateral (*B*) projections showing a venous catheter traversing the right heart chambers and crossing the ventricular septum via a ventricular septal defect (arrow), with the tip finally positioned in the aorta (Ao).

times of 1 to 10 milliseconds.[49] The use of a pulsing unit enables synchronization of radiation output with the open phase of the camera shutter. A high-speed, rotating anode x-ray tube with high heat capacity and focal spot size of between 0.3 to 0.6 mm is required. The image intensifiers introduced in 1971 utilize a cesium iodide input phosphor capable of very high resolution. By electronically varying the viewing field,

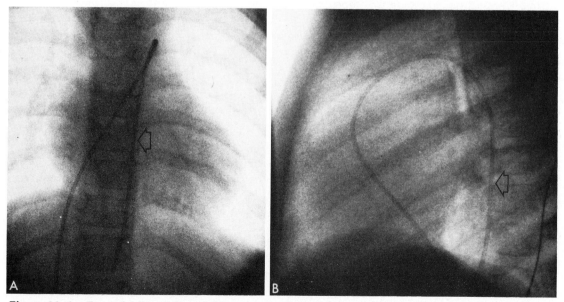

Figure 26–6. Frontal (*A*) and lateral (*B*) projections demonstrating the characteristic course described by the catheter from the right heart into the main pulmonary artery and across a patent ductus arteriosus into the descending aorta (open arrow).

one may obtain either large areas or magnified modes. Fluoroscopic images can be visualized constantly by use of a video system with instant replay on closed-circuit television with a minimum resolution of 50 line pairs per inch. For the study of dynamic cardiac events, our equipment includes a 35-mm cine camera capable of 30 to 60 frames per second. Cameras capable of higher speeds may be of value for the study of congenital heart disease. Spot film devices of 100 or 105 mm with film rates of 6 to 12 seconds can be used with the image intensifier. Serialographic films can also be obtained in a larger format, 14 inches by 14 inches, with high resolution at up to six films per second. A variety of tables with adjustable heights and "floating" table top motion can be fitted with rotating "cradles" for obtaining oblique views. Alternatively, the x-ray tube and image intensifier can be mounted on opposite ends of a "C" or "U" arm, which rotates around the patient to obtain oblique and complex angled views.

Ordinarily, single-plane capability is sufficient for the study of heart disease in adults. However, a multipurpose catheterization laboratory for the study of adult and congenital heart disease requires biplane imaging capability and instant video replay. This is because most complex congenital cardiac anomalies require at least two projections to visualize structures and their interrelationships. Since there are strict limitations to the volume of contrast medium that can be given to an infant, biplane cine filming is highly desirable for the study of congenital heart disease. Axial cineangiography, in addition to affording oblique rotational views, facilitates optimal visualization of specific cardiac chambers[10, 27, 28] and coronary circulation[3, 8, 60] by aligning the x-ray beam with the axis of the cardiac structure being studied.

Radiation workers are allowed a maximal dose of 5 rem per year under the National Center for Radiological Health (NCRH) guidelines, which are based on a presumed "acceptable risk" level with an added safety factor. By careful attention to the principles of radiation safety, exposure levels can be kept below 10 per cent of the maximal permissable dose (500 mrem per year). Particular attention should be paid to the lens of the eye and the thyroid gland of the operator; these parts have been shown to have the greatest exposure.[79] Important principles for exposure reduction include: (1) strict collimation of the x-ray beam to the viewing field; (2) minimal exposure times; (3) use of the inverse square rule; that is, personnel should remain as distant as possible from the x-ray source, particularly during cine or serial filming, and (4) use of adequate radiation shielding; that is, lead aprons should be worn by the operator, and lead-rubber and lead-glass shields should be interposed between the operator and the sources of primary and secondary radiation.

CONTRAST MEDIA

The available vascular contrast agents have varying proportions of sodium and N-methylglucamine (meglumine) salts attached to an anion — a triiodinated benzoic acid, either diatrizoate or iothalamate. In choosing a contrast agent for a particular study, one must consider the viscosity, the ratio of sodium (Na) and meglumine ion, the total iodine content, and whether calcium (Ca) and magnesium (Mg) ions are added to counteract calcium chelating agents.[29] Agents containing a higher or a very low proportion of sodium salts produce increased repolarization abnormalities and myocardial irritability leading to ventricular fibrillation.[4, 37, 101] Whether this is due to the protective effect of the large meglumine molecule or to the direct toxic effect of sodium has not been determined. The higher the proportion of meglumine, the higher the viscosity—a disadvantage when the high flow rates are required.

For the majority of angiocardiographic procedures, a diatrizoate preparation of intermediate viscosity with a large proportion of meglumine and a small percentage of sodium, e.g., a Na-methylglucamine ratio of 1:6.6 and a sodium content of 190 mmol per liter (Renografin 76 per cent, Hypaque 76 per cent), is advocated.[66, 87, 88] Metrizoate with a similar Na-meglumine ratio but with the addition of calcium and magnesium ions lowers toxicity and may prove superior to currently available agents.[15] Contrast agents containing less iodine, such as Renografin 60 per cent and Hypaque 50 per cent, are recommended for small infants, in whom contrast density is less important and toxicity of the more concentrated contrast agents must be considered.

Significant hemodynamic changes lasting several minutes result from a large intravascular injection of high-osmolarity contrast medium.[14, 34, 55, 68, 80] Peripheral vasodilatation and increased blood flow produce a subjective "flushing" sensation and a fall in diastolic pressure. The increased osmolarity causes blood volume expansion several minutes after the injection. This results in an elevation of the left ventricular filling pressure, while depression of myocardial function due to contrast toxicity results in a further fall in systolic pressure.[38, 61] Transient elevation of pulmonary vascular resistance occurs with pulmonary angiography.[9]

Selective coronary angiography produces the following transient changes, which last from 5 to 30 seconds:[21, 29, 45] sinus bradycardia or even asystole due either to direct[46] or to reflex suppression of the sinoatrial or atrioventricular node; electrocardiographic changes consisting of prolongation of PR, QRS, and QT intervals; axis shift; flattening and inversion of T waves; ST segment elevation or depression; a concomitant transient hypotension; and, rarely, ventricular fibrillation. During selective right coronary injections the electrocardiographic pattern[20, 65] produced is identical to that of inferior wall ischemia, while with a left coronary injection the transient electrocardiographic changes resemble those of anterior wall ischemia. These alterations may be related to transient ionic imbalance caused by the sodium ion, since electrocardiographic changes are minimized when sodium is balanced with other ions, such as calcium and magnesium.[94] Metrizamide, the new nonionic contrast agent currently undergoing trials, produces fewer incidences of ventricular fibrillation and electrocardiographic disturbances and has less effect on myocardial function.[47, 81]

In the absence of dehydration, reported data suggest that angiography utilizing up to 4 to 5 ml of contrast medium per kg of body weight can be performed satisfactorily and without significantly increased risk.[26] In infants a more dilute contrast agent, 60 per cent rather than 75 to 76 per cent, is preferable, and the total dose should be limited to 3 to 4 ml per kg.[32]

COMPLICATIONS

Cardiac angiographic procedures performed by experienced operators are relatively safe and have low morbidity and mortality. Even so, they carry a risk that is acceptable only when such investigation is warranted by the clinical status of the patient and the indications for the study. The incidence of serious complications for coronary arteriography, for example, has been reported to be 1.5 per cent, with a mortality rate of 0.1 per cent ranging from 0.09 per cent to 8 per cent (an unacceptable figure).[1, 77] However, the complication rate for catheterization in infants with severe complex congenital heart disease is significantly higher, being estimated at 2.9 per cent, with a mortality rate of 0.26 per cent, although postcatheterization death in the severely ill infant is common.[54, 90] Complications may be conveniently grouped into those associated with catheter introduction and manipulation in the vascular system; those associated with catheter manipulation in the heart; those related to coronary arteriography; and those due to the contrast medium injected. It is mandatory for a catheterization laboratory to be fully equipped to manage all cardiovascular emergencies with ventilatory assist devices, drugs, and a direct-current defibrillator.

Vascular Complications

INFECTION. Infection at the cut-down or puncture site that necessitates antibiotic therapy occurs rarely and seldom progresses to endocarditis. Patients with congenital heart lesions are placed on a prophylactic antibiotic regime.

CATHETER KNOTTING. Catheter knotting occurs occasionally and requires considerable manipulation of the catheter and guide wire for correction.[57] Separation of a portion of the catheter or sheath and removal of such a foreign body from the vascular system can be readily achieved by using a variety of devices such as baskets and claws.[2, 25]

THROMBOEMBOLISM. Thromboembolic complications account for the majority of problems encountered.[30] Thrombotic material may form on the surface of catheters.[48, 64] During a catheter exchange, this material is stripped off onto the guide wire at the entrance site (demonstrated by "pull-out" angiography)[85] and is then carried proximally with the introduction of the next catheter over the guide wire. To lower the incidence of local arterial thrombus and peripheral or cerebral emboli, meticulous attention to technique is required to minimize catheterization time. Certain plastics (polyurethane) are less thrombogenic than others (polyethylene).[11] Systemic heparinization (at a dose of 45 mg per kg) and addition of heparin to flush solutions combat the formation of adherent platelet thrombi.[95] The increased risk of hemorrhage is minor, and the heparin effect may be readily reversed by the administration of protamine sulfate at the conclusion of the procedure. Visceral or peripheral atheroemboli[62, 76] occur with dislodgment of atheromatous material from the aortic wall in the presence of advanced atherosclerosis or an aneurysm. This condition is marked by characteristic

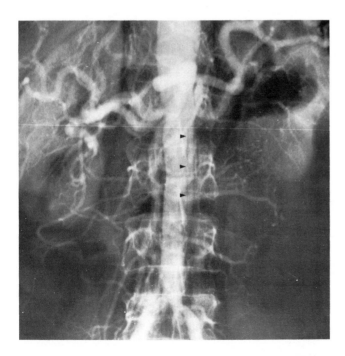

Figure 26–7. Abdominal aortogram in a frontal projection performed following apparent subintimal passage of the catheter. An intimal flap (arrowheads) is seen in the infrarenal aorta. There was associated pain but no further sequelae.

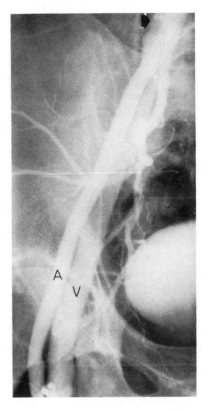

Figure 26–8. A femoral artery (A) to femoral vein (V) fistula is demonstrated several months following cardiac catheterization, at which time catheters were introduced into both vessels percutaneously. Early filling of the iliac vein and inferior vena cava is seen following contrast injection into the aorta.

skin discoloration (livedo reticularis) due to dissemination of cholesterol microemboli,[73, 74] retinal embolization, colicky abdominal pain and diarrhea, or peripheral ischemic manifestations. Atheroembolic disease of the kidneys severe enough to produce renal failure has been documented.[53]

VASCULAR INJURY. Iatrogenic dissection of a peripheral vessel or even the aorta[19] (Fig. 26–7) may occur, often without significant clinical sequelae, although the danger of aortic branch compromise, peripheral ischemia, and extension of the dissection must be kept in mind. An arteriovenous fistula is an occasional complication (Fig. 26–8), occurring more frequently with catheterization of both artery and vein on the same side.

BLOOD LOSS. Blood loss is a problem only in infants with small circulating blood volume, and blood replacement is required.

Cardiac Complications

ARRHYTHMIA. Transient arrhythmias occur commonly during intracardiac catheter manipulation. When the right ventricular or left ventricular outflow tracts are irritated, ventricular extrasystoles and, occasionally, sustained ventricular fibrillation may ensue. Right bundle branch block may result from trauma to the right side of the ventricular septum. Therefore, patients with pre-existing left bundle branch block should have prophylactic placement of a cardiac pacemaker prior to right heart catheterization or pulmonary arteriography. Other rhythm disturbances, such as atrial fibrillation or flutter, complete heart block, and supraventricular and ventricular tachycardias, occur less commonly and are usually transient, reverting spontaneously to

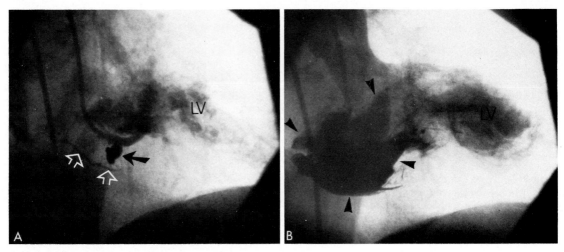

Figure 26–9. Early (A) and late (B) frames taken from a left ventriculogram (LV) in a right anterior oblique projection. A, There has been transmural extravasation of contrast (arrow) and early filling of thebesian veins (open arrows). B, In a later frame, the contrast has perforated into the pericardial cavity (arrowheads).

normal sinus rhythm following withdrawal of the catheter. If they persist, standard therapy for the specific arrhythmia should be instituted. Bradycardia associated with a vasovagal reaction responds promptly to the early administration of atropine. Some advocate routine premedication with atropine, and others premedicate only patients with aortic stenosis in whom a vasovagal episode may be more hazardous and reversal more difficult.

PERFORATION. Perforation of a cardiac chamber has become uncommon with the use of softer catheter material, balloon-tipped catheters, and pigtail catheters. The abnormal passage of the catheter outside the cardiac silhouette is indicative of perforation. Atrial perforation occurs most commonly and may be difficult to recognize because of the low pressure in both atrium and pericardial space. If contrast medium is injected into the pericardial sac, the hyperosmolarity of the agent promotes accumulation of fluid in the pericardial sac, with resultant danger of cardiac tamponade.[69] Intramyocardial extravasation of contrast (myocardial staining) (Fig. 26–9), if severe, may be associated with transient ischemic ST-T wave changes and arrhythmias. This risk exists when the injection is made into a small hypertrophied cardiac chamber through a straight catheter with an end hole.

HYPOXIA. Hypoxic episodes may be precipitated in a child with tetralogy of Fallot during passage of the catheter into the pulmonary artery, which further compromises the already stenotic outflow tract.

Complications Related to Coronary Arteriography

Although coronary arteriography is a low-risk procedure,[16, 77] the complications specifically related to it are dependent primarily on the experience and skill of the operator.[22, 39] The femoral route is more easily mastered and has a complication rate comparable to that of the brachial arteriotomy approach, which requires expert surgical technique to avoid loss or weakening of the radial pulse due to brachial artery occlusion.[63] Both techniques are associated with an increased mortality risk in the

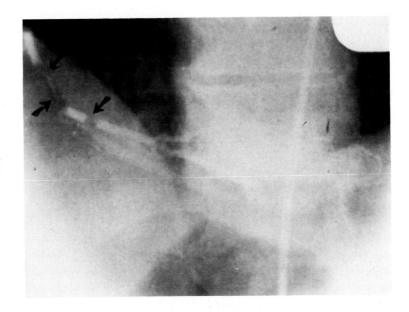

Figure 26–10. Detail of a right coronary arteriogram demonstrating several air emboli (arrows). The patient sustained an inferior myocardial infarction.

presence of left main coronary artery disease,[13, 23] unstable angina, congestive heart failure, and multiple ventricular extrasystoles.

EMBOLISM. The introduction of an air bubble or thrombus material into the coronary artery (Fig. 26–10) leads to myocardial ischemia and often infarction.[41, 92] Meticulous attention is necessary to avoid this complication; a closed system between the catheter, the manifold with contrast reservoir, and the injecting syringe should be used. After flushing with heparinized saline solution, the catheter is filled with contrast in the descending aorta, so that all subsequent manipulations into the coronary artery are performed with a closed system. Systemic heparinization also appears to decrease the risk of coronary embolus.[52]

VASCULAR INJURY. Iatrogenic dissection of the coronary artery (Fig. 26–11) occurs sporadically[42, 86] and can usually be recognized immediately by pressure damping and at fluoroscopy with small test injections of contrast in the false channel. A large subintimal hematoma usually compromises coronary flow, precipitating a myocardial infarction or, less frequently, resolving with minor sequelae.

SPASM. Spasm may occur locally at the catheter tip (Fig. 26–12). It is more frequent in the proximal segment of the right coronary artery but may occur in a segment remote from the ostium or in a segment with a fixed stenosis.[35] If catheter spasm is suspected it is important to perform several opacifications following nitroglycerin administration. Catheter-induced spasm[33] is not usually accompanied by chest pain or electrocardiographic changes and is not provoked by ergonovine maleate,[44] as occurs in patients with Prinzmetal's variant angina.

INJECTION OF CONTRAST INTO AN OCCLUDED VASCULAR SYSTEM. The catheter tip may occlude a small or narrowed coronary artery (narrowed either by a fixed lesion or by spasm) or an aortocoronary graft. If contrast medium is injected into the occluded coronary system, prolonged opacification of the arteries results. A dense, irregular myocardiogram or myocardial blush is produced by prolonged capillary filling as well as by early opacification of the coronary veins, particularly the small thebesian veins, which under normal conditions are not visualized. When a wedged injection is made, the catheter should be promptly removed from the vessel to allow blood flow, because if

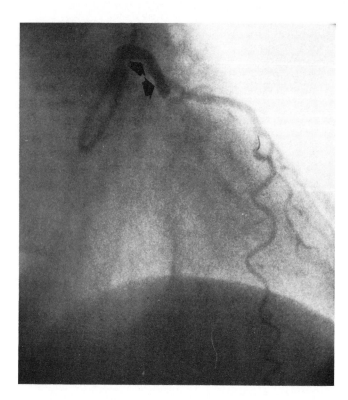

Figure 26–11. Left coronary arteriogram in a right anterior oblique projection. A subintimal dissection involves the left main coronary and proximal circumflex arteries (arrows). The circumflex coronary artery is occluded proximally. Six weeks later at coronary arteriography, the circumflex coronary artery was mildly narrowed by external compression from the clotted subintimal dissection, with good flow distally.

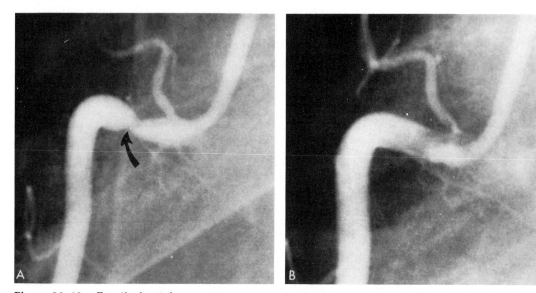

Figure 26–12. Detail of a right coronary arteriogram demonstrating spasm (arrow) at the tip of the catheter (*A*), which resolves (*B*) following administration of nitroglycerin.

the contrast remains in the occluded system for a prolonged time, irreversible damage to the myocardium may result.

Complications Related to Contrast Medium

Patterns of adverse reactions[59, 99] related to the intravascular use of iodine-containing radiographic contrast medium[7, 84] can be divided into (a) minor reactions, such as nausea, vomiting, and limited urticaria, and (b) major reactions, such as edema of the face or glottis, bronchospasm, collapse, or cardiac arrest. The incidence of nonfatal contrast reactions is 2.33 to 5 per cent, a fatal reaction occurs once in 10,000 cases.[6, 100] No consistently reliable and safe *in vivo* test has been developed to predict adverse reactions, but activation of the complement immune system has been implicated.[58] Patients with a previous history of allergic reaction during such studies are considered to be at increased risk. A recent uncontrolled study advocated a high-dose steroid regime both prior to and after the study and noted the protective role of steroids for patients with previous contrast reactions.[102]

Pulmonary edema may develop during or after angiography in patients with left ventricular failure or valvular heart disease. It is precipitated by the hypervolemia resulting from the osmotic effect of contrast and necessitates routine aggressive therapy, including intravenous diuretics, morphine, and oxygen.

Acute oliguric renal failure[43, 56, 70, 91, 96] is a recognized, albeit rare, complication of angiography and is seen particularly in the dehydrated, diabetic patient.[67] This nephrotoxicity has been attributed to a direct effect on the tubular epithelium, an acute uric acid nephropathy, precipitation of mucoprotein producing an obstructive uropathy in the presence of volume depletion, or decreased renal blood flow due to sludging of deformed erythrocytes.

References

1. Adams, D. F., Fraser, D. B., and Abrams, H. L.: The complications of coronary arteriography. Circulation 48:609–618, 1973.
2. Aldridge, H. E., and Lee, J.: Transvascular removal of catheter fragments from the great vessels and heart. Can. Med. Assoc. J. 117:1300, 1977.
3. Aldridge, H. E., McLoughlin, M. J., and Taylor, K. W.: Improved diagnosis in coronary cine arteriography with routine use of 110° oblique views and cranial and caudad angulations. Comparison with standard transverse oblique views in 100 patients. Am. J. Cardiol. 36:468–473, 1975.
4. Almen, T.: Effects of metrizamide and other contrast media on the isolated rabbit heart. Acta Radiol. (Suppl.) 335:216, 1973.
5. Amplatz, K., Formanek, G., Stanger, P., et al.: Mechanics of selective coronary artery catheterization via femoral approach. Radiology 89:1040–1047, 1967.
6. Ansell, G.: Adverse reactions to contrast agents. Scope of problem. Invest. Radiol. 5:374–391, 1970.
7. Ansell, G.: A national survey of radiological complications: interim report. Clin. Radiol. 19:175–191, 1968.
8. Arani, D. T., Bunnell, I. L., and Greene, D. G.: Lordotic right posterior oblique projection of the left coronary artery. A special view for special anatomy. Circulation 52:504–508, 1975.
9. Austen, W. G., Wilcox, B. R., and Bender, H. W.: Experimental studies of the cardiovascular responses secondary to the injection of angiographic agents. J. Thorac. Cardiovasc. Surg. 47:356–366, 1964.
10. Bargeron, L. M., Jr., Elliott, L. P., Soto, B., et al.: Axial cineangiography in congenital heart disease. I. Concept, technical and anatomic considerations. Circulation 56:1075–1083, 1977.
11. Bourassa, M. G., Cantin, M., Sandborn, E. B., et al.: Scanning electron microscopy of surface irregularities and thrombogenesis of polyurethane and polyethylene coronary catheters. Circulation 53:992–996, 1976.
12. Bourassa, M. G., Lesperance, J., and Campeau, L.: Selective coronary arteriography by the percutaneous femoral artery approach. Am. J. Roentgenol. 107:377–383, 1969.

13. Bourassa, M. G., and Noble, J.: Complication rate of coronary arteriography. A review of 5250 cases studied by a percutaneous femoral technique. Circulation 53:106–114, 1976.
14. Brown, R., Rahimtoola, S. H., Davis, G. D., et al.: The effect of angiocardiographic contrast medium on circulatory dynamics in man. Cardiac output during angiocardiography. Circulation 31:234–240, 1965.
15. Carter, A. M., and Olin, T.: Toxicity of roentgen contrast media at selective injection into the coronary artery in the rabbit. Invest. Radiol. 10:73–78, 1975.
16. Chahine, R. A., Raizner, A. E., and Miller, R. R.: The lesson from the complications of coronary arteriography. Chest 75:5, 1979.
17. Chavez, I., Dorbecker, N., and Celis, A.: Direct intracardiac angiography: its diagnostic value. Am. Heart J. 33:560–593, 1947.
18. Cohn, P. F., Gorun, R., Adams, D. F., et al.: Comparison of biplane and single plane left ventriculograms in patients with coronary artery disease. Am. J. Cardiol. 33:1–6, 1974.
19. Cooley, D. A., Wukasch, D. C., and Hallman, G. L.: Acute dissecting ascending aortic aneurysm resulting from coronary arteriography; successful surgical treatment. Chest 61:317–319, 1972.
20. Corliss, R. J., McKenna, D. H., Sialer, S., et al.: Hemodynamic responses of selective coronary arteriography in dogs. Angiology 18:734–740, 1967.
21. Coskey, R. L., and Magidson, O.: Electrocardiographic response to selective coronary arteriography. Br. Heart J. 29:512–519, 1967.
22. Davis, K., Kennedy, W. J., Kemp, H. G., Jr., et al.: Complications of coronary arteriography from the collaborative study of coronary artery surgery (CASS). Circulation 59:1105, 1979.
23. DeMots, H., Bonchek, L. I., Rösch, J., et al.: Left main coronary artery disease: risks of angiography, importance of coexisting disease of other coronary arteries and effects of revascularizaton. Am. J. Cardiol. 36:136–141, 1975.
24. Dodge, H. T., Sandler, H., Baxley, W., et al.: Usefulness and limitations of radiographic methods for determining left ventricular volume. Am. J. Cardiol. 18:10–24, 1966.
25. Dotter, C. T., Rösch, J., and Bilbao, M. K.: Transluminal extraction of catheter and guide fragments from the heart and great vessels: 29 collected cases. Am. J. Roentgenol. 111:467–472, 1971.
26. Doust, B. D., and Redman, H. C.: The myth of 1 ml/kg in angiography. A study to determine the relationship of contrast medium dosage to complications. Radiology 104:557–560, 1972.
27. Elliott, L. P., Bargeron, L. M., Jr., Bream, P. R., et al.: Axial cineangiography in congenital heart disease. II. Specific lesions. Circulation 56:1048–1093, 1977.
28. Fellows, K. E., Keane, J. F., and Freed, M. D.: Angled views in cineangiocardiography of congenital heart disease. Radiology 56:485–490, 1977.
29. Fischer, H. W., and Thomson, K. R.: Contrast media in coronary arteriography: a review. Invest. Radiol. 13:450, 1978.
30. Formanek, G., Frech, R. S., and Amplatz, K.: Arterial thrombus formation during clinical percutaneous catheterization. Circulation 41:833–839, 1970.
31. Forsmann, W.: Die Sondierung des rechten Herzens. Klin. Wochenschr. 8:2085, 1929.
32. Fox, K. M., Patel, R. G., Bonvicini, M., et al.: Safe amounts of contrast medium for angiocardiography in neonates and infants. Eur. J. Cardiol. 5:373–380, 1977.
33. Friedman, A. C., Spindola-Franco, H., and Nivatpumin, T.: Coronary spasm: Prinzmetal's variant angina vs. catheter-induced spasm; refractory spasm vs. fixed stenosis. Am. J. Roentgenol. 132:897, 1979.
34. Friesinger, G. C., Schaffer, J., Criley, J. M., et al.: Hemodynamic consequences of the injection of radiopaque material. Circulation 31:730–740, 1965.
35. Gensini, G. G., diGiorgi, S., Murad-Netto, S., et al.: Arteriographic demonstration of coronary artery spasm and its release after the use of a vasodilator in a case of angina pectoris in the experimental animal. Angiology 13:550–553, 1962.
36. Gensini, G. G.: Coronary Arteriography. Mt. Kisco, New York, Futura Publishing Co., 1975.
37. Gensini, G. G., and diGiorgi, S.: Myocardial toxicity of contrast agents used in angiography. Radiology 82:24–34, 1964.
38. Gootman, N., Rudolph, A. M., and Buckley, N. M.: Effects of angiographic contrast media on cardiac function. Am. J. Cardiol. 25:59–65, 1970.
39. Green, G. S., McKinnon, C. M., Rösch, J., et al.: Complicatons of selective percutaneous transfemoral coronary arteriography and their prevention. A review of 445 consecutive examinations. Circulation 45:552–557, 1972.
40. Greene, D. G., Carlisle, R., Grant, C., et al.: Estimation of left ventricular volume by one-plane cineangiography. Circualation 35:61–69, 1967.
41. Guss, S. B., Zir, L. M., Garrison, H. B., et al.: Coronary occlusion during coronary angiography. Circulation 52:1063–1068, 1975.
42. Haas, J. M., Peterson, C. R., and Jones, R. C.: Subintimal dissection of the coronary arteries: a complication of selective coronary arteriography and the transfemoral percutaneous approach. Circulation 38:678, 1968.
43. Heneghan, M.: Contrast-induced acute renal failure. Editorial. Am. J. Roentgenol. 131:1113, 1978.
44. Heupler, F. A., Jr., Proudfit, W. L., Razavi, M., et al.: Ergonovine maleate provocative test for coronary arterial spasm. Am. J. Cardiol. 41:631–640, 1978.
45. Higgins, C. B.: Effects of contrast media on the conducting system of the heart. Mechanism of action and identification of the toxic component. Radiology 124:599–606, 1977.

46. Higgins, C. B., and Feld, G. K.: Direct chronotropic and dromotropic actions of contrast media: ineffectiveness of atropine in the prevention of bradyarrhythmias and conduction disturbances. Radiology 121:205–209, 1976.
47. Higgins, C. B., and Schmidt, W.: Direct and reflex myocardial effects of intracoronary administered contrast materials in the anesthetized and conscious dog: comparison of standard and newer contrast materials. Invest. Radiol. 13:205, 1978.
48. Jacobsson, B., and Schlossman, D.: Angiographic investigation of formation of thrombi on vascular catheters. Radiology 93:355–359, 1969.
49. Judkins, M. P., Abrams, H. L., Bristow, J. D., et al.: Optimal resources for examination of the chest and cardiovascular system. Report of the Inter-Society Commission for Heart Disease Resources. Circulation 53:A-1, 1976.
50. Judkins, M. P.: Selective coronary arteriography. I. A percutaneous transfemoral technic. Radiology 89:815–824, 1967.
51. Judkins, M. P.: Percutaneous transfemoral selective coronary arteriography. Radiol. Clin. North Am. 6:467–492, 1968.
52. Judkins, M. P., and Gander, M. P.: Prevention of complications of coronary arteriography. Circulation 49:599–602, 1974.
53. Kassirer, J. P.: Atheroembolic renal disease. N. Engl. J. Med. 280:812–818, 1969.
54. Krovetz, L. J., Shanklin, D. R., and Schiebler, G. L.: Serious and fatal complications of catheterization and angiocardiography in infants and children. Am. Heart J. 76:39–47, 1968.
55. Krovetz, L. J., Mitchell, B. M., and Neumaster, T.: Hemodynamic effects of rapidly injected hypertonic solutions into the heart and great vessels. Am. Heart J. 74:453–462, 1967.
56. Krumlovsky, F. A., Simon, N., Santhanam, S., et al.: Acute renal failure. Association with administration of radiographic contrast material. J.A.M.A. 239:125–127, 1978.
57. Kuebler, W., Kirkham, B. C., and Read, R.: Removal of figure-8 knot in femoral-cerebral "headhunter I. V." catheter during angiography. South. Med. J. 68:650–651, 1975.
58. Lang, J. H., Lasser, E. C., and Kolb, W. P.: Activation of serum complement by contrast media. Invest. Radiol. 11:303–308, 1976.
59. Lasser, E. C.: Basic mechanisms of contrast media reactions: theoretical and experimental considerations. Radiology 91:63–65, 1968.
60. Lesperance, J., Saltiel, J., Petitclerc, R., et al.: Angulated views in the sagittal plane for improved accuracy of cinecoronary angiography. Am. J. Roentgenol. 121:565–574, 1974.
61. Lipton, M. J., Higgins, C. B., Wiley, A. A., et al.: The effect of contrast media on the isolated perfused canine heart. Invest. Radiol. 13:519, 1978.
62. Lonni, Y. G. W., Matsumoto, K. K., and Lecky, J. W.: Postaortographic cholesterol (atheromatous) embolization. Radiology 93:63–65, 1969.
63. Machleder, H. I., Sweeney, J. P., and Barker, W. F.: Pulseless arm after brachial artery catheterization. Lancet 19:407–409, 1972.
64. Nejad, M. S., Klaper, M. A., Steggerda, F. R., et al.: Clotting on the outer surfaces of vascular catheters. Radiology 91:248–250, 1968.
65. Ovitt, T., Rizk, G., Frech, R. S., et al.: Electrocardiographic changes in selective coronary arteriography: the importance of ions. Radiology 104:705–708, 1972.
66. Paulin, S., and Adams, D. F.: Increased ventricular fibrillation during coronary arteriography with a new contrast medium preparation. Radiology 101:45–50, 1971.
67. Pillay, V. K. G., Robbins, P. C., Schwartz, F. D., et al.: Acute renal failure following intravenous urography in patients with long-standing diabetes mellitus and azotemia. Radiology 95:633–636, 1970.
68. Popio, K. A., Ross, A. M., Oravec, J. M., et al.: Identification and description of separate mechanisms for two components of renografin cardiotoxicity. Circulation 58:520–528, 1978.
69. Popper, R. W., Schumacher, D., and Quinn, C. H.: Cardiac tamponade due to hypertonic contrast medium in the pericardial sac following cineangiography. Clinical observation and experimental study. Circulation 35:933, 1967.
70. Port, F. K., Wagoner, R. D., and Fulton, R. E.: Acute renal failure after angiography. Mayo Clin. Proc. 121:544–550, 1974.
71. Price, J. E., Jr., and Rösch, J.: Selective coronary arteriography by percutaneous left transaxillry approach using preshaped torque control catheters. Circulation 48:1321–1323, 1973.
72. Radner, S.: An attempt at the roentgenologic visualization of coronary blood vessels in man. Acta Radiol. 26:497, 1945.
73. Ramirez, G., O'Neill, W. M., Jr., Lambert, R., et al.: Cholesterol embolization. A complication of angiography. Arch. Intern. Med. 138:1430–1432, 1978.
74. Retan, J. W., and Miller, R. E.: Microembolic complications of atherosclerosis. Literature review and report of a patient. Arch. Intern. Med. 118:534–545, 1966.
75. Ricketts, H. J., and Abrams, H. L.: Percutaneous selective coronary cinearteriography. J.A.M.A. 181:620–624, 1962.
76. Roscher, A. A., and Endlich, H. L.: Atheroembolization. A complication of vascular surgery and/or diagnostic angiography. Int. Surg. 56:82–94, 1971.
77. Ross, R. S., and Gorlin, R.: Cooperative study on cardiac catheterization. Coronary arteriography. Circulation 37(III):67–73, 1968.
78. Rousthöi, P.: Über Angiokardiographie: vorlaufige Mitteilung. Acta Radiol. 14:419, 1933.

79. Rueter, F. G.: Physician and patient exposure during cardiac catheterization. Circulation 58:134–139, 1978.
80. Sako, Y.: Hemodynamic changes during arteriography. J.A.M.A. 183:253–256, 1963.
81. Salvesen, S., Nilsen, P. L., and Holtermann, H.: Effects of calcium and magnesium ions on the systemic and local toxicities of the N-methylglucamine (meglumine) salt of metrizoic acid (Isopaque). Acta Radiol. (Suppl.) 270:180, 1967.
82. Schoonmaker, F. W., and King, S. B.: Coronary arteriography by the single catheter percutaneous femoral technique. Experience in 6,800 cases. Circulation 50:735–740, 1974.
83. Seldinger, S. I.: Catheter replacement of the needle in percutaneous arteriography. A new technique. Acta Radiol. 39:368–376, 1953.
84. Shehadi, W. H.: Adverse reactions to intravascularly administered contrast media. A comprehensive study based on a prospective survey. Am. J. Roentgenol. 124:145–152, 1975.
85. Siegelman, S. S., Caplan, L. H., and Annes, G. P.: Complications of catheter angiography: study with oscillometry and "pullout" angiograms. Radiology 91:251–253, 1968.
86. Silverman, J. F., Gnekow, W., and Pfeifer, J. F.: Iatrogenic dissection of the right coronary artery. Radiology 110:712–714, 1974.
87. Simon, A. L., Shabetai, R., Lang, J. H., et al.: The mechanism of production of ventricular fibrillation in coronary angiography. Am. J. Roentgenol. 114:810–816, 1972.
88. Snyder, C. F., Formanek, A., Frech, R. S., et al.: The role of sodium in promoting ventricular arrhythmia during selective coronary arteriography. Am. J. Roentgenol. 113:567–571, 1971.
89. Sones, F. M., Jr., and Shirey, E. K.: Cine coronary arteriography. Mod. Concepts Cardiovasc. Dis. 31:735–738, 1962.
90. Stanger, P., Heymann, M. A., Tarnoff, H., et al.: Complications of cardiac catheterization of neonates, infants, and children. A three-year study. Circulation 50:595–608, 1974.
91. Swartz, R. D., Rubin, J. E., Leeming, B. W., et al.: Renal failure following major angiography. Am. J. Med. 65:31–37, 1978.
92. Takaro, T., Pifarre, R., Wuerflein, R. D., et al.: Acute coronary occlusion following coronary arteriography. Mechanisms and surgical relief. Surgery 72:1018–1029, 1972.
93. Taketa, R. M., Sahn, D. J., Simon, A. L., et al.: Catheter positions in congenital cardiac malformations. Circulation 51:749–757, 1975.
94. Tragardh, B., and Lynch, P. R.: ECG changes and arrhythmias induced by ionic and nonionic contrast media during coronary arteriography in dogs. Invest. Radiol. 13:233, 1978.
95. Walker, W. J., Mundall, S. L., Broderick, H. G., et al.: Systemic heparinization for femoral percutaneous coronary arteriography. N. Engl. J. Med. 288:826–828, 1973.
96. Weinrauch, L. A., Robertson, W. S., and D'Elia, J. A.: Contrast media-induced acute renal failure. Use of creatinine clearance to determine risk in elderly diabetic patients. J.A.M.A. 239:2018–2019, 1978.
97. Wexler, L.: Simplified serial coronary arteriography. Am. J. Roentgenol. 111:780–781, 1971.
98. White, R. I., Jr., Frech, R. S., and Amplatz, K.: An improved technique for right coronary artery catheterization. Am. J. Roentgenol. 113:562–566, 1971.
99. Wiedeman, M. P.: Vascular and intravascular responses to various contrast media. Angiology 14:107–109, 1963.
100. Witten, D. M., Hirsch, F. D., and Hartman, G. W.: Acute reactions to urographic contrast medium. Am. J. Roentgenol. 119:832–840, 1973.
101. Wolf, G. L., Kraft, L., and Kilzer, K.: Contrast agents lower ventricular fibrillation threshold. Radiology 129:215, 1978.
102. Zweiman, B., and Hildreth, E. A.: An approach to the performance of contrast studies in contrast material-reactive persons. Ann. Intern. Med. 83:159, 1975.

Part II
Congenital Heart Disease

INA L. TONKIN, M.D.
PETER R. BREAM, M.D.
LARRY P. ELLIOTT, M.D.

With advancing surgical techniques, survival rates are increasing for patients with all types of congenital heart lesions. Another major factor in this lowered mortality rate is improved postoperative care. It is important that all physicians dealing with the postoperative care of patients with congenital heart disease (CHD) be aware of the normal, as well as the abnormal, postoperative roentgenologic findings. In this section, we review the preoperative chest film appearances of the congenital lesions under discussion. The major emphasis is on those chest film appearances unique to each lesion.

SHUNT LESIONS

Preoperative Radiographic Diagnosis

The posteroanterior and lateral chest films, or ideally, four views of the chest with barium, are excellent tools for the preoperative diagnosis of congenital heart disease. However, a left-to-right shunt cannot be suggested unless the pulmonary vascularity is sufficiently prominent. Of the four major left-to-right shunts, the patent ductus arteriosus (PDA) is the only one with a definitive plain film appearance.

Ventricular Septal Defects

A ventricular septal defect (VSD) is the most common left-to-right shunt lesion that presents in infancy. It is often complicated by coarctation of the aorta or by a patent ductus arteriosus.

The small ventricular septal defect shows normal vascularity and heart size. Only the moderate- or large-sized ventricular septal defect exhibits shunt vascularity. In the infant with a large ventricular septal defect, there is often associated left ventricular failure. This appears on the chest film as ill-defined vascularity (perivascular edema) and air-space edema.[7] The body of the left atrium is often enlarged, strongly suggesting that the atrial septum is intact in the presence of a shunt. There are no definitive radiographic signs.

ANGIOGRAPHIC DATA FOR SURGICAL MANAGEMENT. Surgical management is not optimal unless the precise site and number of ventricular septal defects are known. For this reason, the definitive diagnosis is made by ciné left ventriculography utilizing axial views.[1, 5]

POSTOPERATIVE RADIOGRAPHIC FINDINGS. The normal postoperative appearance of totally corrected left-to-right shunts indicates a close correlation between the chest roentgenograms and the hemodynamic findings after surgery.[17] In the immediate postoperative period, the vascularity remains prominent. In the vast majority of cases, the pulmonary vascularity ultimately returns to normal (Fig. 26–13). This usually indicates a low pulmonary vascular resistance, normal pulmonary arterial pressure, or a residual shunt of small volume. A reduction in heart size almost invariably follows. A shuntlike pulmonary vasculature with some degree of left atrial enlargement may persist after the repair of a ventricular septal defect for as long as two years, however, in spite of normal postoperative catheterization findings. Finally, the complications of median sternotomy (see Part IV) may also occur with the repair of any septal defect.

The common complications unique to a ventricular septal defect repair are (1) a recurrent shunt; (2) cardiomegaly secondary to arterioventricular bundle damage; (3) damage to the tricuspid valve, resulting in tricuspid valve incompetence and reflected radiologically as right atrial enlargement; (4) complications associated with the banding of the pulmonary artery; and (5) subaortic obstruction created by a misplaced patch (especially in patients with a severe degree of overriding of the aortic valve).[3]

A recurrent shunt, with incomplete closure of a ventricular septal defect secondary

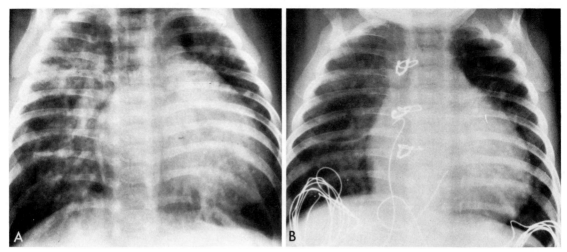

Figure 26–13. Shunt lesions (ventricular septal defects). *A,* Preoperative chest film shows cardiomegaly and shunt vascularity with perivascular edema in a one-month-old infant with a large ventricular septal defect. *B,* Significant regression of the heart size and pulmonary vascularity is evident on the seventh postoperative day.

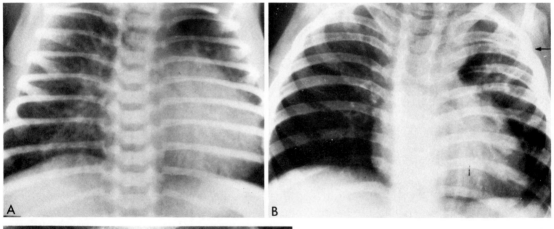

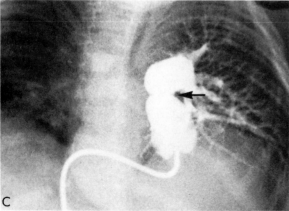

Figure 26–14. Pulmonary artery banding. *A,* A neonate with a large ventricular septal defect. There is profuse shunt vascularity and generalized cardiomegaly. *B,* Signs of a left thoracotomy (arrow). Note the decreased pulmonary vascularity of the right lung on the follow-up chest radiograph taken at 14 months of age. *C,* The anteroposterior pulmonary arteriogram with cranial angulation shows a tight distal pulmonary artery band (arrow). There is complete occlusion of the right pulmonary artery and partial restriction of the left pulmonary artery flow.

to patch disruption, has been reported in as high as 10 per cent of cases.[3] The postoperative chest film may show residual shunt vascularity and pulmonary venous hypertension (PVH) if left ventricular failure coexists.

Cardiomegaly secondary to arterioventricular bundle damage and complete heart block may be apparent. Patients with this complication may require a temporary ventricular pacing wire or a permanent pacing in the future.

Right atrial enlargement secondary to damage to the tricuspid valve and insufficiency may occur after the repair of a ventricular septal defect. Generally, the right atrial approach is preferred, especially in patients with increased pulmonary vascular resistance.[3] The tricuspid valve should be carefully retracted without incision of the tricuspid valve leaflets, to avoid valvular damage and postoperative tricuspid valve insufficiency. Also, in placing the patch over the ventricular septum, one must take care to avoid suturing the tricuspid valve leaflets.

The effects of banding of the pulmonary artery in different congenital anomalies, including ventricular septal defects, have been clinically evaluated and correlated with the roentgenographic findings.[10] Although in most institutions total repair is preferred to the banding of the pulmonary artery, the latter is still employed by some groups in the management of severe heart failure from a ventricular septal defect in infants.

Postoperative problems stemming from banding are related, in part, to the degree of stenosis it creates. The pulmonary vascularity remains increased, and cardiac failure may occur if the band is inadequate. If the band is too tight, a profound decrease in pulmonary vasculature, with progressive cyanosis resulting from right-to-left shunting at the ventricular level, may be expected. Also, dilatation of the pulmonary artery distal to the band may be seen, with aneurysmal dilatation of the left pulmonary artery. Rarely, the pulmonary arterial band migrates, occluding a pulmonary artery (Fig. 26–14) or damaging the pulmonary valve leaflets.

Subaortic obstruction created by faulty placement of a prosthetic patch is manifested as left ventricular enlargement and, eventually, left ventricular failure.

Patent Ductus Arteriosus

A patent ductus arteriosus is often seen in the premature infant owing to the child's low pulmonary vascular resistance and a lesser degree of hypertrophy of the media of the pulmonary arteries in comparison with that of the term infant. Also, delayed closure of the ductus arteriosus is seen in normal preterm infants as well as in infants with pulmonary disorders, such as hyaline membrane disease, bronchopulmonary dysplasia, and meconium aspiration. Therefore, premature infants with a patent ductus arteriosus or a ventricular septal defect may acquire congestive heart failure in the first week of life, with a large, high-pressure, high-flow left-to-right shunt.

The chest film shows shunt vascularity and left atrial enlargement. Cardiomegaly may be present, especially if congestive heart failure develops. The "ductus bump" seen on the chest film is diagnostic and is seen in approximately 50 per cent of cases of patent ductus arteriosus.[7]

POSTOPERATIVE RADIOGRAPHIC FINDINGS. In the neonate, one often sees marked improvement in the appearance of the pulmonary vascularity and cardiomegaly immediately after ductus ligation (Fig. 26–15). All of the findings associated with a left thoracotomy may be seen in the postoperative patient, however.

A pseudoaneurysm with calcification may occur at the site of the ductus ligation. Also, a recurrent left-to-right shunt may be seen, with occasional recanalization of the

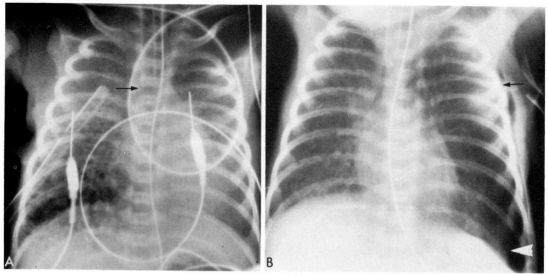

Figure 26–15. Preterm infant with patent ductus arteriosus. *A,* Preoperative chest film in a 1500 gm preterm infant showing changes of hyaline membrane disease with pulmonary interstitial emphysema of the right lower lobe. There is mild cardiomegaly and generalized interstitial pulmonary edema secondary to a patent ductus arteriosus. Note the low placement of the endotracheal tube (arrow). *B,* Following ligation the immediate postoperative chest radiograph shows signs of a left thoracotomy (arrow). There is a left pneumothorax (arrowhead) but marked improvement in the pulmonary edema and cardiomegaly.

ductus. Finally, a chylothorax may occur postoperatively if there is interruption of the thoracic duct (see Fig. 26–18).

Atrial Septal Defect

The atrial septal defect (ASD) rarely presents in infancy, but it is the most common shunt lesion found in the older child. In adults, more than nine of ten patients who present with shunt vascularity have an atrial septal defect. There is also a fourfold increase in the incidence of atrial septal defects in females.[7]

The preoperative chest film of a moderate or large atrial septal defect shows shunt vascularity with a prominent pulmonary trunk. The left atrium is usually normal. There may be left atrial enlargement, however, with severe mitral incompetence secondary to a ballooning mitral valve, which has an increased incidence in association with atrial septal defect. There is almost invariably some right-sided heart enlargement. The left ventricle and aorta are either normal or relatively small. In adults, cardiomegaly often develops secondary to tricuspid valve incompetence, atrial fibrillation, or right ventricular failure.

An anomaly recurring in 90 per cent of the cases of sinus venosa atrial septal defect is partial anomalous pulmonary venous connection of the right upper lobe pulmonary veins to the superior vena cava or right atrium. One can occasionally see the anomalous vein on the posteroanterior chest film (Fig. 26–16).

Another form of partial anomalous pulmonary venous connection is the scimitar syndrome, or hypogenetic right lung syndrome, in which the right pulmonary veins empty into the inferior vena cava. The posteroanterior chest film shows hypoplasia of the right lung and thorax, dextroposition of the heart, hypoplasia or absence of the right pulmonary artery, the anomalous right pulmonary vein in the shape of a scimitar, and

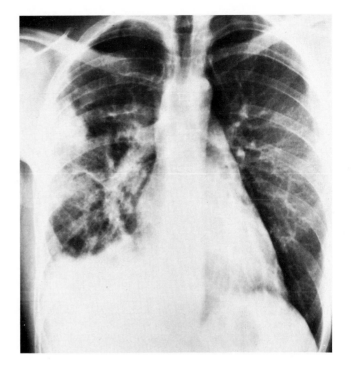

Figure 26–16. Atrial septal defect repair with pulmonary embolism. Postoperative chest film in a 28-year-old male with repair of an atrial septal defect and partial anomalous pulmonary venous connection. Radiographic signs of pulmonary embolism include the presence of a right pleural effusion and pleural-based densities secondary to pulmonary infarction.[7]

an anomalous subdiaphragmatic systemic arterial supply to the lower lobe of the right lung from the aorta or one of its major branches. Approximately 50 per cent of the cases have an associated atrial septal defect. A ventricular septal defect, tetralogy of Fallot, coarctation of the aorta, and absence of the right pulmonary artery have all been reported as associated findings.[7]

ANGIOGRAPHIC DATA FOR SURGICAL MANAGEMENT. An injection into the right upper lobe pulmonary vein, using axial cineangiography, accurately shows the size and the location or type of the atrial septal defect by placing the length of the atrial septum in profile.[1, 5] Anomalous pulmonary veins may also be diagnosed by this method. In patients with the scimitar syndrome, the diagnosis is confirmed by direct injection into the anomalous right pulmonary vein or by observing the venous phase of the right pulmonary arterial injection.

POSTOPERATIVE RADIOGRAPHIC FINDINGS. The repair of an atrial septal defect generally has extremely low rates of complication and mortality. Prosthetic patches are often used in defects greater than 25 mm in diameter, however, and recurrent shunt secondary to patch disruption has been reported.[9] A systolic murmur may be evident postoperatively secondary to mitral insufficiency, since there is an increased incidence of prolapsing mitral valve. Also, pulmonary thromboembolism may occur in older patients with atrial fibrillation after atrial septal defect repair.

The occurrence of cyanosis after the repair of an atrial septal defect should strongly suggest (1) the possibility of the diversion of the vena cava into the left atrium or (2) the communication of a left superior vena cava with the left atrium that was not recognized preoperatively. The diversion of the vena cava into the left atrium may occur with a large secundum atrial septal defect or with anomalous pulmonary veins, a factor that may make surgical repair and patching of these lesions difficult.[9]

The postoperative chest appearance of patients with the scimitar syndrome (Fig. 26–17) is similar to the preoperative appearance. The anomalous vein remains visible, as a tunnel is created through the atrial septal defect to the left atrium. Thrombosis or

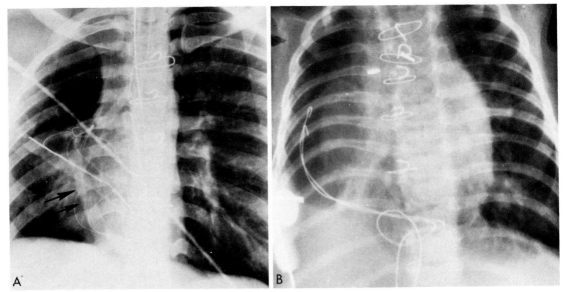

Figure 26–17. Postoperative chest in scimitar syndrome. *A,* The postoperative chest in this 26-year-old female clearly shows the anomalous right pulmonary vein (arrows). The vein has been tunneled with a graft through the atrial septal defect to the left atrium. *B,* The anomalous pulmonary vein is not easily seen in this four-month-old with a hypoplastic right pulmonary artery, hypoplastic right lung, and dextroposition of the heart.

stenosis of the re-established right lower pulmonary veins presents as a right-sided alveolar edema.

Persistent Common Atrioventricular Canal

The partial type (ostium primum atrial septal defect associated with a cleft anterior mitral valve leaflet) of persistent common atrioventricular canal (PCAVC) usually mimics the radiologic appearance of an atrial septal defect as long as the mitral valve is competent. The intermediate and complete forms show profound shunt vascularity and considerable cardiomegaly. The left atrium may be enlarged, depending on the amount of atrioventricular valve incompetence. The persistent common atrioventricular canal is the most common lesion with a large shunt and 3 to 4+ cardiomegaly. There is also a 30 to 40 per cent incidence of Down's syndrome in patients with the complete form of persistent common atrioventricular canal.[7]

The electrocardiogram is specific in that it shows left axis deviation (LAD) in 98 per cent of cases. In the partial type, the left axis deviation is mild to moderate; it is severe in the complete forms.

ANGIOGRAPHIC DATA FOR SURGICAL MANAGEMENT. The diagnosis is confirmed at cardiac catheterization with a left ventriculogram, using axial cineangiography.[1, 5] The location and number of ventricular septal defects can be accurately identified, since the entire length of the septum is seen. Also, the atrioventricular valve anatomy is well visualized, so that one can distinguish a formed, yet cleft, mitral valve from the common atrioventricular valve. Finally, the length of the atrial septum is visualized to show the size of the ostium primum atrial septal defect.

POSTOPERATIVE RADIOGRAPHIC FINDINGS. The repair of a partial atrioventricular canal may produce problems similar to those encountered with atrial septal defect repairs. With complete atrioventricular canal repair, however, one may see pulmonary venous hypertension and left atrial enlargement secondary to the suturing of the cleft mitral valve, which results in mitral stenosis, recurrent mitral insufficiency, and left ventricular outflow tract obstruction. Disruption of the atrial or ventricular patches may also occur. Finally, one may see persistent cardiomegaly secondary to atrioventricular bundle damage and complete heart block, which is the most frequent complication of total correction.

VALVULAR OBSTRUCTIVE LESIONS

Pulmonary Valvular Stenosis

Obstruction of the right ventricular outflow with an intact ventricular septum may result from infundibular stenosis, pulmonary valvular stenosis, or peripheral pulmonary artery stenosis. The radiographic finding in cases of moderate-to-severe pulmonary valvular stenosis is normal pulmonary vascularity, with a prominent pulmonary trunk secondary to post-stenotic dilatation. The key roentgen finding is unilateral dilatation of the proximal left pulmonary artery. The heart size is usually normal, but right ventricular prominence may be evident.

ANGIOGRAPHIC DATA FOR SURGICAL MANAGEMENT. The diagnosis is confirmed by biplane right ventriculography. The stenotic pulmonary valve may have the typical appearance of a truncated cone or may be dysplastic with thickened nonmobile pulmonary leaflets. Adequate anatomic visualization of the stenotic valve and its function, as well as pressure gradient data, is essential for the determination of the type of surgical repair.

POSTOPERATIVE RADIOGRAPHIC FINDINGS. Pulmonary regurgitation may be common after pulmonary valvotomy, but the regurgitant flow is apparently well tolerated. With moderate-to-severe pulmonary insufficiency, right heart enlargement occurs. These postoperative findings are best confirmed by pulmonary angiography.[11] A prosthetic pulmonary valve or valved external conduit may be required in those rare patients with a calcified or absent pulmonary valve.

Congenital Aortic Stenosis

The four types of obstruction that occur between the left ventricle and aorta are supravalvular, valvular, subvalvular of the discrete or fibromuscular type, and hypertrophic obstructive cardiomyopathic (asymmetric septal hypertrophy and so forth).

Infants may present with critical aortic stenosis with fibrosis of the myocardium, necrosis of the papillary muscles, and fibroelastosis. The neonatal radiographic findings are nonspecific; they include pulmonary venous hypertention, large left atrium, and cardiomegaly, with no evidence of a prominent ascending aorta.

In the older child with aortic stenosis, the radiographic findings are usually normal pulmonary vascularity and a normal-sized left ventricle. Pulmonary venous hypertension and left ventricular enlargement secondary to left ventricular failure are uncommon complications in this age group. Since these patients are too young to have valve calcification, poststenotic dilatation of the ascending aorta is the premier sign. It is present in the majority of patients, even those with mild degrees of valvular stenosis. The aortic valve is usually bicuspid or deformed and usually calcifies after the age of 30.

ANGIOGRAPHIC DATA FOR SURGICAL MANAGEMENT. As in the case of pulmonary valve stenosis, adequate anatomic demonstration of the stenotic valve by biplane cineangiography as well as by pressure measurements, helps to determine whether the surgical approach should be valvotomy or prosthetic valve replacement.

POSTOPERATIVE RADIOGRAPHIC FINDINGS. The normal postoperative radiographic findings include typical features of a median sternotomy, with prominence of the ascending aorta in the older postoperative patient.

Aortic valvular insufficiency after valvotomy may not cause any abnormal chest film findings. Aortic regurgitation rarely presents a problem in the early postoperative period, and small infants appear to tolerate mild insufficiency better than stenosis. In an adult patient with a normal-sized left ventricle, however, preoperative progressive left ventricular enlargement in the face of normal vascularity suggests postoperative aortic valve insufficiency. If the patient shows pulmonary venous hypertension and left ventricular enlargement as well, one should suspect severe aortic insufficiency, which may be associated with the additional complication of bacterial endocarditis.[12]

Re-stenosis may occur but is found less frequently than aortic regurgitation. Aortic valvular calcification may have a slightly increased incidence in those who have had a valvotomy and is found approximately ten years postvalvotomy.[12]

AORTIC ARCH ANOMALIES

Coarctation of Aorta

Coarctation of the aorta (CoA) in *infancy* is often associated with a left-to-right shunt resulting from a ventricular septal defect or patent ductus arteriosus. The chest radiograph shows shunt vascularity, often with superimposed pulmonary venous hypertension, which is usually caused by left ventricular failure and generalized cardiomegaly.

In the older child or adult with coarctation of the aorta, the chest film is almost always diagnostic. The pulmonary vascularity shows either normal vascularity or pulmonary venous hypertension secondary to left ventricular failure. The *sine qua non* is a disfigured transverse aortic arch, which has various configurations. Except for the presence of rib notching (which is seen most commonly in patients older than five years), increased density in the lower rib margins, and an altered aortic knob, the ascending aorta and cardiac configurations are identical to those of aortic stenosis and systemic hypertension.

ANGIOGRAPHIC DATA FOR SURGICAL MANAGEMENT. The diagnosis of coarctation is confirmed by biplane thoracic root aortography. The location and involvement of the brachiocephalic vessels are important, as well as the presence of an abnormal aortic valve, which is seen in 70 per cent of patients with coarctation of the aorta.

POSTOPERATIVE RADIOGRAPHIC FINDINGS. A hemothorax may occasionally result from the disruption of the anastomosis and hemorrhage from injured vessels. Chylothorax may also occur (Fig. 26–18). Postoperative hypertension, abdominal pain with mesenteric vasculitis, and paraplegia have also been reported.[11] Radiographic signs of congestive heart failure are seen in postoperative patients who have additional lesions, such as ventricular septal defects.

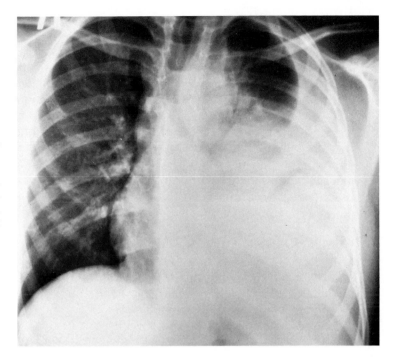

Figure 26–18. Repair of coarctation of the aorta with pleural effusion. On the fourth postoperative day, a large left pleural effusion developed. Although a hemothorax secondary to an anastomotic leak was considered likely, on reentry a chylothorax was evacuated.

Re-coarctation of the aorta occurs frequently in infants, who require early surgical intervention. In addition, calcification of the homograft may occur several years after surgery.

Vascular Rings

The most common vascular rings are (1) a double aortic arch and (2) a right arch with an aberrant left subclavian artery and left ductus or ligamentum arteriosus. Either may cause symptoms of stridor and dysphagia in infants. The lateral chest film of an infant with a double aortic arch may show an anterior indentation on the trachea and hyperaeration. The anteroposterior film of the esophagogram in cases of double aortic arch shows a high rightward aortic impression and a lower leftward impression, since 80 per cent of patients have a higher and larger right arch component. The lateral esophagogram shows a large posterior impression on the barium-filled esophagus. The right aortic arch with an aberrant left subclavian artery shows signs of a right arch and posterior left oblique impression on the barium-filled esophagus. There is no left-sided indentation on the esophagogram.

ANGIOGRAPHIC DATA FOR SURGICAL MANAGEMENT. The diagnosis of both types of vascular ring may be confirmed by thoracic root aortography. Axial angiography best demonstrates the type of vascular ring.[21] Intracardiac anomalies are rarely associated.

POSTOPERATIVE RADIOGRAPHIC FINDINGS. The signs of a left thoracotomy are seen in most patients following the repair of a double aortic arch or a right arch with an aberrant left subclavian artery or left ductus arteriosus. A right thoracotomy approach may be used in 20 per cent of the cases of double aortic arch in which the right arch component is smaller. The postoperative patient may have recurrent respiratory problems with hyperaeration and recurrent stridor. Also, failure to ligate the left ductus or ligamentum arteriosus may result in recurrent symptoms and incomplete disruption of the vascular ring.

Interrupted Aortic Arch

The radiographic appearance of an interrupted aortic arch in infants is nonspecific; the findings include a widened mediastinum and shunt vascularity secondary to ventricular septal defects, which are frequently associated with interrupted aortic arch. In the older child, one may note a prominent pulmonary trunk (secondary to the reversing ductus) filling the descending aorta and an absent aortic knob. The diagnosis and type of interruption are confirmed by ventriculography and aortography.

POSTOPERATIVE RADIOGRAPHIC FINDINGS. This lesion is frequently associated with intracardiac anomalies and has a high medical and surgical mortality rate. In neonates left thoracotomy complications are seen, as well as respiratory complications that require long-term ventilation (Fig. 26–19).

COMPLEX CYANOTIC HEART DISEASE

The complex cyanotic heart lesions include (1) cardiac anomalies with deficient pulmonary blood flow and (2) cardiac anomalies with excessive pulmonary flow.

Cardiac Anomalies with Deficient Pulmonary Blood Flow

A palliative systemic-to-pulmonary artery shunt to increase pulmonary flow is necessary for the management of all cases of severe pulmonary valve stenosis or atresia, regardless of the position of the pulmonary trunk, the number of ventricles, the ventriculoarterial connections, or the presence of left or right atrioventricular valve

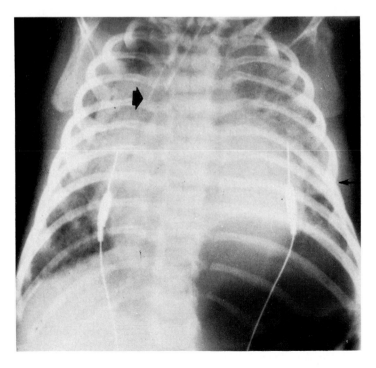

Figure 26–19. Repair of an interrupted aortic arch. The postoperative chest film of a one-month-old infant shows a left thoracotomy (small arrow), low endotracheal tube (arrowhead), and gastric distention. Note cardiomegaly and pulmonary edema secondary to an associated ventricular septal defect and left ventricular failure. The patient has chronic cystic lung changes secondary to bronchopulmonary dysplasia and oxygen toxicity.

atresia. A common example is tetralogy of Fallot in patients with an anatomy unfavorable for total repair owing to the presence of marked hypoplasia of the right ventricular outflow tract and the pulmonary annulus and arteries. Other examples include severe pulmonary stenosis or atresia with an intact ventricular septum, a single ventricle, and complete transposition of the great arteries with a ventricular septal defect and pulmonary stenosis or atresia.[8]

Palliation with a Glenn anastomosis may also be indicated — in preparation for a later Fontan procedure — in cases of tricuspid atresia and of a single ventricle of the double-inlet left ventricular type. The various types of systemic-to-pulmonary artery shunts are listed in Table 26–1 (p. 1802).

POSTOPERATIVE RADIOGRAPHIC FINDINGS OF PALLIATIVE SHUNTS. The normal postoperative findings of subclavian artery–to–pulmonary artery anastomosis (Blalock-Taussig shunt) include the signs of a thoracotomy, usually on the side opposite the aortic arch. Unilateral rib notching may be seen years later, because the dilated intercostal arteries act as collateral channels around the obliterated subclavian artery (Fig. 26–20). An adequate communication shows a bilateral increase in vascularity of the shunt type. Also, variable degrees of left atrial enlargement and cardiomegaly secondary to left ventricular enlargement are seen two weeks to six months after the performance of the shunt procedure.[4]

The normal postoperative findings of the ascending aorta–to–right pulmonary artery (Waterston-Cooley) operation are signs of a right thoracotomy with an increase in pulmonary vascularity confined to the right side (Fig. 26–21). Cardiomegaly with left atrial enlargement (LAE) occurs postoperatively when the shunt is of sufficient magnitude (Fig. 26–21).

The descending thoracic aorta–to–left pulmonary artery anastomosis (Potts-Smith-Gibson operation) is not used as frequently at present because of the difficulty of taking this anastomosis down at the time of total repair. It may be used in small neonates,

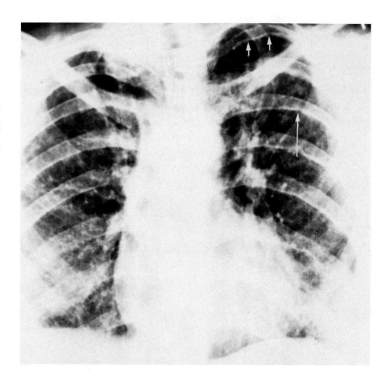

Figure 26–20. Blalock-Taussig shunt. Unilateral rib notching (arrows) and increased density of the lower rib margins in the left second through sixth ribs is the result of intercostal artery collaterals that developed after obliteration of the left subclavian artery. The radiographic findings of tetralogy of Fallot with pulmonary atresia are evident, with reticulated pulmonary vascularity, an inapparent pulmonary artery segment, and a prominent ascending aorta.

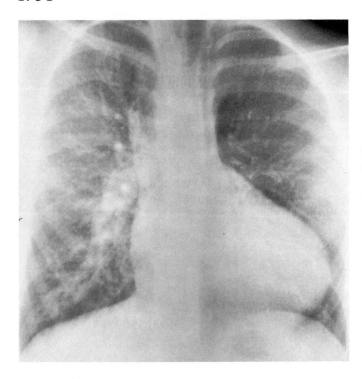

Figure 26–21. Waterston-Cooley shunt. The postoperative features of the ascending aorta–to–right pulmonary artery are demonstrated, with subtle signs of a right thoracotomy and an increase in pulmonary vascularity confined to the right lung.

however, and if performed correctly it provides relatively equal flow to both lungs.[8] A greater degree of cardiomegaly is seen after this procedure when the anastomosis is too large (5 mm or greater).[4]

POSTOPERATIVE COMPLICATIONS. The postoperative complications of a palliative shunt are (1) lack of function and (2) excessive shunting.

With an immediate nonfunctioning Blalock-Taussig shunt, there is no increase in the pulmonary vascularity of either lung. With Waterston's shunt the vascularity remains diminished on the side of the shunt.

In patients with an adequately patent Blalock-Taussig shunt that progressively narrows, there is a bilateral decrease in vascularity; in those patients with an originally patent, progressively narrowing Waterston shunt, there is a unilateral decrease in vascularity on the side of the shunt. Clinically, the shunt murmur may be absent, and there may be increased cyanosis. The presence of shunt obstruction is suggested by dynamic scintillation scanning and confirmed by angiocardiography.

The shunt may be patent but too wide, carrying excessive flow to the lungs. Excessive shunting commonly occurs with the Waterston-Cooley and Potts-Smith-Gibson anastomoses and is less common with the Blalock-Taussig type. It is manifested on plain films by an excessive increase in the pulmonary vasculature in one or both lungs (Fig. 26–22). Signs of congestive heart failure may be present, as well as pulmonary venous hypertension, pleural effusions, and left ventricular enlargement (Fig. 26–23). Pulmonary vascular obstructive disease may develop, accompanied by signs of pulmonary hypertension, that is, enlargement of the pulmonary trunk and central pulmonary arteries on serial chest films.[16]

Also, patients with palliative shunts, but with patent right-to-left shunts, may acquire systemic vascular thrombosis and brain abscesses from septic emboli. Furthermore, a chyloma with resultant chylothorax may occur after palliative shunt procedures or after total correction, with take-down of the shunt. A chylothorax usually occurs in

Figure 26–22. Potts-Smith-Gibson operation with excessive shunting. Signs of a left thoracotomy (arrow) are present in this patient with a single ventricle and pulmonary stenosis who had recently had Potts-Smith-Gibson anastomosis (descending thoracic aorta–to–left pulmonary artery). There is the combination of excessive shunting and pulmonary venous hypertension (PVH) reflected as ill-defined basal vessels and interstitial edema. The pulmonary venous hypertension is secondary to left ventricular failure.

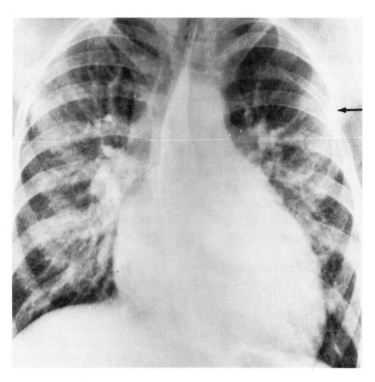

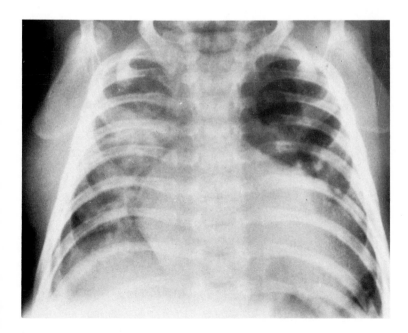

Figure 26–23. Excessive systemic pulmonary shunting. The posteroanterior chest film of this two-month-old child with complete transposition of the great arteries shows pulmonary edema in the right lung following Blalock-Taussig and Blalock-Hanlen procedures. Reentry and tightening of the right Blalock-Taussig shunt was necessary in this case.

the intermediate postoperative period and tends to be a large, unilateral, recurrent chylous effusion. This entity is discussed in Part IV of this chapter.

SYSTEMIC VENOUS SHUNTS

The superior vena cava–to–right pulmonary artery shunt (Glenn's anastomosis) is primarily used for patients with tricuspid atresia accompanied by severe pulmonary stenosis or atresia. The normal postoperative findings include signs of a right thoracotomy, early increased pulmonary vascular flow if the pulmonary vascular resistance is low, and prominence of the superior vena cava (SVC). Later, however, the pulmonary vascularity shows decreased perfusion in the upper and middle lobes and normal to slightly increased markings in the lower lobes.[4]

The complications of this procedure are secondary to increased pressure in the superior vena cava, which depends on the resistance of the right pulmonary arterial bed. Therefore, two main problems may arise from this superior vena caval hypertension: (1) chylothorax and (2) superior vena caval syndrome. As previously mentioned, chylothorax can result from the operative procedure, interrupting lymphatic channels as well as forming increased pressure in the superior vena cava.

Some degree of mild superior vena caval hypertension postoperatively may be well tolerated if the pulmonary vascular resistance is low. In the presence of significantly increased vascular resistance, however, there may be an immediate severe superior vena caval syndrome, resulting in the physiologic obstruction of flow through the shunt and death. This problem is seen most frequently in infants younger than six months of age.[4] The "late" form of superior vena caval syndrome (three years after the superior vena caval–right pulmonary artery anastomosis) may cause clinical signs of increasing cyanosis; a rising hematocrit; and severe headaches, with edema and dilated venous channels of the upper trunk, head, and neck. With obstruction of the superior vena cava, flow to the right lung is compromised first. Over a period of time, systemic collateral arteries from the aorta and major branches supply this area. As a result, the right upper lobe acquires a reticulated, disorganized appearance. The right lower lobe arteries maintain their normal tubular, organized appearance.

Angiocardiography is necessary to rule out an anatomic or mechanical cause for this syndrome, such as stricture or thrombosis of the anastomotic site or the presence of a persistent left superior vena cava or other significant venous collaterals. The occurrence of this late syndrome may also be due to decreasing flow in the left lung because of the development with age of increasing pulmonary stenosis. The late superior vena caval syndrome is reversible, and total correction of the cardiac lesions is recommended.[2]

OPEN CORRECTIVE PROCEDURES

Tetralogy of Fallot

PREOPERATIVE RADIOGRAPHIC DIAGNOSIS. The tetralogy of Fallot is the most common cyanotic congenital heart lesion. The chest radiograph is highly suggestive. The fundamental sign on a chest film is decreased pulmonary vascularity. The anatomic signs are an inapparent pulmonary artery and a normal-sized heart with an upturned cardiac apex secondary to right ventricular hypertrophy. There is an increased incidence of bony anomalies in patients with tetralogy of Fallot. Also, a right aortic arch is present in 25 to 30 per cent of the cases.[7] The diagnosis is confirmed by axial cine right ventriculography and aortography.[1, 5]

ANGIOGRAPHIC DATA FOR SURGICAL MANAGEMENT. Axial cineangiography demonstrates the entire pulmonary artery from the supravalvular area to and beyond its bifurcation. It is important to rule out stenoses of the origin of the left and right pulmonary arteries and to assess the pulmonary artery size, so that outflow tract patches may be extended over the proximal pulmonary artery stenosis. Axial cineangiography also easily demonstrates the size and position of and the number of defects in the entire ventricular septum.[5] Multiple ventricular septal defects occur in 10 to 15 per cent of cases of tetralogy of Fallot. The determination of the status of the atrioventricular valves by axial cineangiography helps rule out the possibility of associated persistent common atrioventricular canal or atrioventricular canal–type ventricular septal defects. Finally, axial cineangiography shows the origin and distribution of the coronary arteries. It is especially important to rule out the presence of an anomalous anterior anterior descending coronary artery's arising from the right cornary artery and coursing within the myocardium of the right ventricle.

POSTOPERATIVE RADIOGRAPHIC FINDINGS. The normal postoperative appearance often shows evidence of a palliative thoracotomy and a median sternotomy performed for total repair of tetralogy of Fallot. The usual postoperative radiographic findings include cardiomegaly, pulmonary edema, and pleural effusions; these symptoms often improve, giving way to residual cardiomegaly and a normal appearance by the seventh postoperative day. Residual cardiomegaly with normal or increased pulmonary vascularity is a usual finding, and the pulmonary trunk may become more prominent in serial films (Fig. 26–24).[16]

IMMEDIATE POSTOPERATIVE COMPLICATIONS. In the immediate postoperative period, excessive bleeding may occur secondary to collateral circulation or coagulation abnormalities (Fig. 26–25). This complication is manifested by a widened mediastinum, pleural effusions, or cardiomegaly due to hemopericardium. Another cause of bleeding and, possibly, arrhythmia leading to sudden death, is a right ventriculotomy resulting in ligation of an unrecognized coronary artery anomaly, that is, left anterior descending from the right coronary artery or from a single coronary artery. Cardiomegaly may also be secondary to complete heart block, the heart generally reverting to a more normal

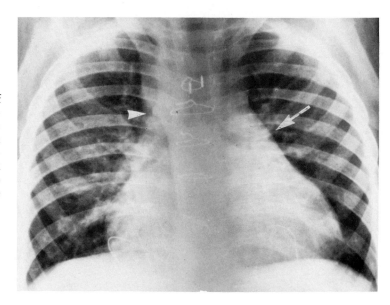

Figure 26–24. Total repair of tetralogy of Fallot. The usual postoperative findings include normal pulmonary vascularity with residual cardiomegaly and prominence of the pulmonary trunk (arrowhead). This patient also has a right aortic arch (large arrow).

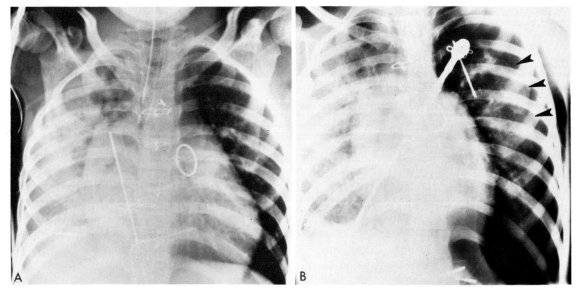

Figure 26–25. Postoperative radiographic complications of tetralogy of Fallot. *A,* Immediate postoperative chest film of an eight-year-old with severe pulmonary stenosis requiring a valved external conduit. There is unilateral alveolar right lung opacity suggestive of edema or pulmonary hemorrhage. Note the low placement of the endotracheal tube and the tip of the nasogastric tube in the midesophagus. *B,* Two days later the patient developed a large left tension pneumothorax (arrows) and subsequently died. At postmortem examination, unilateral pulmonary hemorrhage was found, with disruption of the patch extending to the right pulmonary artery.

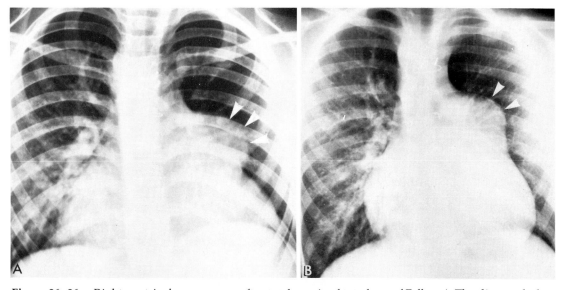

Figure 26–26. Right ventricular aneurysm after total repair of tetralogy of Fallot. *A,* The discrete bulge (arrowheads) in the upper left heart border represents an aneurysm of the right ventricle in a five-year-old boy who had had total correction of tetralogy of Fallot at the age of three years. *B,* Six months later the right ventricular aneurysm has calcified (arrowheads).

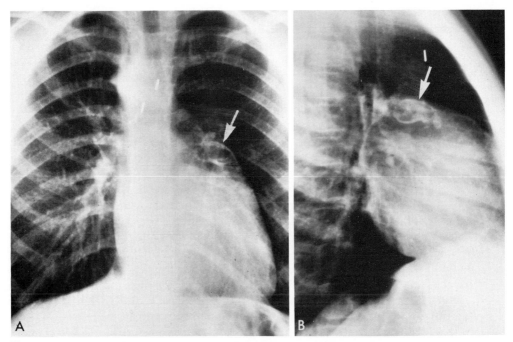

Figure 26–27. Calcification of outflow patch following total repair of tetralogy of Fallot. *A,* The frontal chest radiograph of a seven-year-old girl who had total repair of tetralogy of Fallot with patch reconstruction of the right ventricular outflow tract at one year of age. Note the linear calcification of the prosthetic patch on the anteroposterior (arrows) and lateral (*B*) projections, with some obstruction to flow demonstrated by decreased left pulmonary vascularity.

rhythm in a few weeks. Signs of right heart failure are seen with enlargement of the superior vena cava, azygous vein, and right heart in patients with significant postoperative pulmonary insufficiency.

LATE POSTOPERATIVE COMPLICATIONS. After the first six postoperative months, progressive cardiomegaly indicates a significant hemodynamic problem, such as a reopened or an unrecognized muscular ventricular septal defect, significant residual outflow tract obstruction, unrecognized or inadequate repair of stenosis at the bifurcation of the pulmonary trunk, outflow tract aneurysm, severe pulmonary insufficiency, atrioventricular dissociation, complete heart block, postsurgical coronary artery abnormalities, or a combination of these.[14] These hemodynamic complications may be confirmed at cardiac catheterization (and by angiocardiography).

An aneurysm of the right ventricle may be seen on the frontal chest film as a localized bulge beneath the pulmonary trunk (Fig. 26–26). This is usually secondary to infundibulectomy and ventriculotomy but may result from patch reconstruction of the outflow tract. These findings are confirmed by angiocardiography, but it is difficult to differentiate between true and false postoperative outflow tract aneurysms.[14] Linear calcification of the prosthetic patch of the outflow tract or ventricular septum can be seen on long-term follow-up (Fig. 26–27).

Pulmonary Atresia with Ventricular Septal Defect

PREOPERATIVE RADIOGRAPHIC FINDINGS. Patients with pulmonary atresia and a ventricular septal defect (most commonly tetralogy of Fallot with pulmonary atresia or pseudotruncus) often have a disorganized, reticulated pulmonary vascular pattern resulting from tortuous systemic collaterals supplying the lungs. The cardiac configuration is similar to that of tetralogy of Fallot. A major difference is that the heart is usually large and the apex more upturned. The aorta is prominent, since this is the only artery arising from the heart. A right aortic arch is found in 50 per cent of the cases.[7]

ANGIOGRAPHIC DATA FOR SURGICAL MANAGEMENT. Basically, the angiographic information required is the same as that for tetralogy of Fallot, except with regard to the detection of true and confluent pulmonary arteries. Aortography in the conventional anteroposterior and lateral views may show systemic collaterals and the true pulmonary arteries. With these conventional views, however, the pulmonary arteries may be superimposed in the labyrinth of systemic collaterals; they can be separated by changing the patient to an upright sitting position or angling the x-ray image intensifier toward the feet. The true confluent pulmonary arteries show a characteristic V-shaped configuration, the so-called sea gull sign.[5]

It is important to determine all sources of pulmonary blood flow, including systemic collaterals or patent surgical systemic-to-pulmonary anastomoses.[15] When the true pulmonary arteries cannot be seen by video tape replay at the time of catheterization, it is necessary to perform a wedged pulmonary vein injection on the side in question. With proper anesthesia and angiographic technique, this procedure is safe; it is essential to the visualization of the true pulmonary arteries.

POSTOPERATIVE RADIOGRAPHIC FINDINGS. These patients often require an initial palliative shunt to allow the confluent pulmonary arteries to increase in size. A valved external conduit (Rastelli's procedure), connecting the right ventricle to the pulmonary trunk or pulmonary arteries is often required. When valvular pulmonary atresia, a main pulmonary artery segment, and normally related great arteries are present, an outflow tract patch may be used in place of a valved external conduit.[18] Patch grafting of the proximal pulmonary arteries is required in cases of proximal pulmonary artery stenosis. The postoperative roentgenographic and angiocardiographic findings are similar to those after tetralogy of Fallot correction.

Severe Pulmonary Stenosis with Intact Ventricular Septum

PREOPERATIVE RADIOGRAPHIC DIAGNOSIS. These patients are cyanotic at birth owing to right-to-left atrial level shunts. The major x-ray findings include (1) decreased pulmonary vascularity, (2) an inapparent aorta, and (3) moderate-to-severe cardiomegaly secondary to right atrial enlargement resulting from massive tricuspid valve incompetence.

ANGIOGRAPHIC DATA FOR SURGICAL MANAGEMENT. It is important to demonstrate the size of the right ventricle, the degree of pulmonary valve obstruction, and the status of the pulmonary blood flow that is often visualized via a patent ductus arteriosus. These angiographic data can be obtained by good right ventriculograms and conventional anteroposterior and lateral cineangiocardiograms.

POSTOPERATIVE RADIOGRAPHIC FINDINGS. The surgical procedure performed to correct this condition depends on the size and the function of the right ventricle. If the ventricle is too small to receive and discharge a full complement of systemic venous return, a shunt procedure should be undertaken to increase the size of the pulmonary arteries. Occasionally, a pulmonary valvotomy or valved external conduit procedure can be performed at a later date.

If the right ventricle is sufficiently large, a pulmonary valvotomy (Brock's procedure) with closure of the atrial septal defect can be performed. Pulmonary vascularity is usually decreased for two months postoperatively. A murmur of pulmonary insufficiency is audible postoperatively in about 25 per cent of the patients, but the insufficiency may be demonstrated angiocardiographically and has little physiologic consequence.[8]

Tricuspid Atresia — Fontan's Operation

PREOPERATIVE RADIOGRAPHIC DIAGNOSIS.   Tricuspid atresia, or right atrioventricular valvular atresia, can mimic all forms of cyanotic heart disease, regardless of the type of vascularity.

Basically, with atresia of the right atrioventricular valve, there is a functional single left ventricle and a small right ventricle. With normally related great arteries, there is usually decreased vascularity owing to obstruction of the pulmonary blood flow. The vascularity may be increased by a large ventricular septal defect and the absence of pulmonary stenosis. In these cases of right atrioventricular valvular atresia in which the rudimentary right ventricle is on the left base of the heart (inverted position), there is often a discrete bulge along the left heart border. The most reliable diagnostic aid is the electrocardiogram, which nearly always shows left axial deviation.

ANGIOGRAPHIC DATA FOR SURGICAL MANAGEMENT.   The status of the pulmonary blood flow is the most important angiographic information obtained prior to surgery. If Glenn's anastomosis is present, the superior vena cava and left innominate vein should be injected to demonstrate the right pulmonary flow and any venous collaterals that may need ligation at the time of Fontan's procedure. In addition, an aortogram should be performed to visualize any systemic pulmonary collaterals. Information concerning the functional status of the right atrium, as well as the degree of pulmonary resistance, is necessary before the performance of Fontan's procedure.

POSTOPERATIVE RADIOGRAPHIC FINDINGS.   The usual radiographic findings after shunt operations, that is, the Glenn anastomosis and the Potts-Smith-Gibson procedure, have been previously described. Fontan's procedure, in which a conduit is placed from the hypertrophied right atrium or right ventricular outflow tract to the pulmonary artery, requires an adequate right atrium and normal vascular resistance with closure of the atrial septal defect. The usual radiographic findings after the performance of Fontan's procedure include mild pulmonary edema and cardiomegaly through the intermediate postoperative period. Occasionally, signs of systemic venous congestion are present as well as hepatomegaly, ascites, and edema.[8] Long-term evaluation may show calcification of the conduit.

Ebstein's Anomaly of Tricuspid Valve

PREOPERATIVE RADIOGRAPHIC DIAGNOSIS.   In infants with Ebstein's anomaly, the radiographic findings include decreased vascularity and cardiomegaly caused primarily by a large right heart; the anomaly has an appearance indistinguishable from that of pulmonary atresia with an intact ventricular septum. In the older child or the adult with massive cardiomegaly, right atrial enlargement, and decreased vascularity, Ebstein's anomaly is the most likely diagnosis, based on longevity statistics.

ANGIOGRAPHIC DATA FOR SURGICAL MANAGEMENT.   The preoperative assessment of the size and contractility of the atrialized chamber relative to those of the distal right ventricular chamber is important for surgical selection and can be accomplished with right ventriculography using biplane cineangiography. In those patients in whom

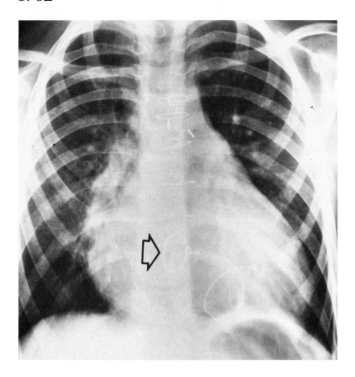

Figure 26–28. Tricuspid valve replacement in Ebstein's anomaly. A heterograft porcine valve replacement (arrow) performed on this patient shows satisfactory results with some residual cardiomegaly.

prosthetic valve replacement is indicated, it is important that the atrialized chamber show adequate volume variation.[13] The visualization of both right ventricular chambers can be achieved by adequate injections followed by cineangiography.

POSTOPERATIVE RADIOGRAPHIC FINDINGS. The treatment of Ebstein's anomaly may include plication of the tricuspid valve by direct suture and artifical valve replacement (Fig. 26–28).[13] The usual postoperative radiographic findings are residual cardiomegaly and gradual improvement in the pulmonary vascularity. The latter may not be apparent for several weeks. The complications of prosthetic valves persist, which include the complications of anticoagulation, possible pulmonary embolism, and infection.[8]

Excessive Pulmonary Blood Flow

There are two types of palliative procedures for this group of cyanotic patients with shunt vascularity or admixture lesions: the creation of an atrial septal defect and pulmonary artery banding.

CREATION OF ATRIAL SEPTAL DEFECT. A balloon atrial septostomy, or Rashkind's procedure, is life-saving for the newborn infant younger than two weeks with complete transposition of the great arteries. A surgical atrial septectomy, or Blalock-Hanlen procedure, which is rarely used, can be performed via a right thoracotomy. These palliative procedures are also performed for patients with total anomalous pulmonary venous connection. In most institutions, however, early open total correction of both complete transposition of the great arteries and total anomalous pulmonary venous connection is preferred to an intermediate Blalock-Hanlen procedure.

POSTOPERATIVE RADIOGRAPHIC FINDINGS. The previously described complications associated with a right thoracotomy, such as phrenic nerve paralysis, can be seen after the performance of the Blalock-Hanlen procedure. Occasionally, pulmonary overcir-

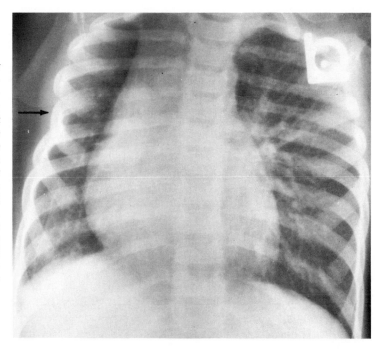

Figure 26–29. Right pulmonary vein occlusion following Blalock-Hanlen procedure. An atrial septectomy (Blalock-Hanlen) procedure was performed on this patient with complete transposition in the first week of life. At one year of age the posteroanterior chest film shows signs of a right thoracotomy (arrow) with decreased vascularity on the right and increased *left* pulmonary vascular markings. Note also the volume loss of the right lung with rotation of the heart to the right, which has developed secondary to decreased right pulmonary flow caused by pulmonary vein obstruction.

culation can result, with associated palliative shunts, causing pulmonary edema possibly requiring surgical re-entry and repair (Fig. 26–22). A rare complication is occlusion of the right pulmonary veins at the time of atrial septectomy. The postoperative chest film then shows decreased pulmonary blood flow to the right lung, with increased flow in the left pulmonary artery (Fig. 26–29).

PULMONARY ARTERY BANDING. The other palliative operation for cyanotic infants with increased pulmonary flow is pulmonary artery banding.[10] This technique can be utilized in infants with excessive pulmonary flow and uncontrollable cardiac failure in an effort to gain a better balance of systemic pulmonary flow. It is also employed (although infrequently) in an attempt to protect the pulmonary bed, in some infants with early evidence of elevated pulmonary vascular resistance. Candidates for pulmonary artery banding include those with any of the transposition complexes in association with a large ventricular septal defect, those with a single ventricle without pulmonary stenosis, and those with persistent truncus arteriosus. The postoperative radiographic complications are discussed in the section on ventricular septal defects (see p. 1743 and Fig. 26–14). In most situations, early total repair of cyanotic heart lesions is favored over surgical palliation and subsequent open total correction.

Complete Transposition of Great Arteries

PREOPERATIVE RADIOGRAPHIC DIAGNOSIS. The classic indication of complete transposition of the great arteries is cyanosis in a full-term male infant with no other congenital anomalies. The chest x-ray shows shunt vascularity with a narrow anterior mediastinum, the absence of a discrete pulmonary artery segment[19] and right atrial or right heart enlargement.

ANGIOGRAPHIC DATA FOR SURGICAL MANAGEMENT. The left ventriculogram using axial cineangiography gives the most information for surgical repair.[1, 5, 20] The precise location, size, and number of ventricular septal defects are easily demonstrated.

In addition, through the complete visualization of the left ventricular outflow tract and movement of the mitral valve, the type and degree of left ventricular outflow tract obstruction is demonstrated.[20] Pulmonary valve stenosis as well as branch stenosis of the pulmonary arteries is also nicely demonstrated. A right ventriculogram using axial cineangiography shows the location of the ventricular septal defect as well as anomalies of the aortic arch such as a patent ductus arteriosus or coarctation of the aorta.

POSTOPERATIVE RADIOGRAPHIC FINDINGS. The usual complications of a median sternotomy, such as a mediastinal hematoma, can be seen after the performance of this procedure. Pulmonary vascularity may be reticulated in the immediate postoperative period, but it returns to normal in six months, with mild residual cardiomegaly (Fig. 26–30).

Early complications following this procedure consist of damage to the conduction system, superior vena caval obstruction, pulmonary venous obstruction, inadequate size of the new right or left atrium, shriveling of the patch, leaks about the patch, and tricuspid insufficiency.[8]

Superior vena caval obstruction is indicated radiographically by prominence of the superior vena cava or azygous vein along the right upper heart border (Fig. 26–31A). The diagnosis is confirmed angiocardiographically by the injection of the superior vena cava and the demonstration of the obstruction with filling of the venous collaterals, that is, the azygous system, the ascending lumbar veins, and the inferior vena cava to the newly created venous atrium (Fig. 26–31B and C). Enlargement of the new pulmonary venous atrium with a piece of pericardium has prevented pulmonary venous obstruction.[8]

A common complication in the acute or intermediate stage after the performance of Mustard's procedure is the development of a chyloma (Fig. 26–65A). It appears radiographically as a mediastinal mass, with disappears as a unilateral chylothorax

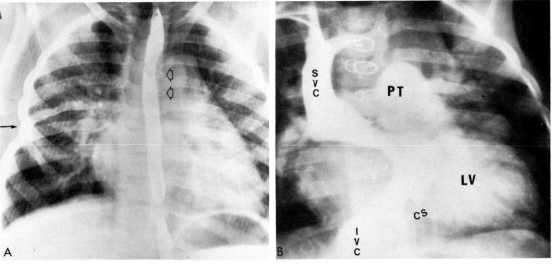

Figure 26–30. Postoperative Mustard operation in complete transposition. *A,* The postoperative chest film shows evidence of a right thoracotomy (arrow) following an atrial septectomy and median sternotomy for total correction. The sternal wires (open arrows) are often difficult to see when they overlie the spine. The pulmonary vascularity remains increased with residual cardiomegaly. *B,* The superior venacavagram (SVC) shows no evidence of stenosis at the junction of the pericardial baffle. The inferior vena cava (IVC) and coronary sinus (CS) opacify in a retrograde manner. There is normal flow of blood into the left ventricle (LV) and pulmonary trunk (PT).

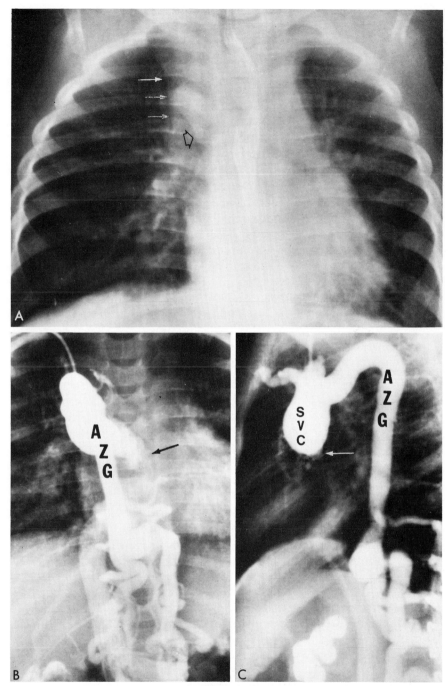

Figure 26–31. Postoperative Mustard operation with superior vena caval obstruction. *A,* Taken after a Mustard procedure in infancy, this posteroanterior chest film shows an abnormally prominent superior vena cava (arrows) and azygous vein (open arrow), indicating significant stenosis between the superior vena cava and the pericardial baffle. Note that pulmonary vascularity is within normal limits. Superior venacavagram in anteroposterior (*B*) and lateral (*C*) projections. The dilated superior vena cava (SVC) and azygous (AZG) vein are superimposed. In *B* and *C*, arrows indicate the site of obstruction at the superior vena caval–pericardial baffle anastomosis. The lateral view (*C*) unfolds the superimposed structures. The azygous vein acts as a collateral channel filling the hemiazygous system, ascending lumbar veins, and inferior vena cava to opacify the new "venous atrium."

develops. Occasionally, a chylothorax does not resolve with repeated thoracentesis, and re-entry and repair of the chylous leak is necessary.

Senning's procedure, now being used for total correction more frequently in some institutions, results less often in postoperative superior vena caval obstruction than Mustard's procedure. Pulmonary venous hypertension secondary to the obstruction of pulmonary veins may occur, however.

A long-standing complication is chronic fibrosis of the right ventricle. This is manifested as pulmonary venous hypertension and right ventricular enlargement. The left ventricle may also be affected. The fibrosis may stem from the cardioplegic solutions used at operative repair or from other sources that are not clear-cut.

With either Mustard's or Senning's procedure, a valved external conduit, or Rastelli's procedure, may occasionally be required to correct complete transposition of the great arteries with severe obstruction to pulmonary flow. A valved external conduit can also be used to correct other malformations of the transposition complexes, or conotruncal positional anomalies with a double-outlet right or left ventricle, with or without ventricular inversion. In order for open repair of these lesions to be performed, the ventricular septal defect must be located in such a way relative to the great arteries that the former may be closed and the blood flow routed in the correct physiologic direction using both Mustard's or Senning's procedure and Rastelli's procedure.

The complications of the valved external conduit procedure that can be demonstrated radiographically are obstruction resulting from kinking or clotting, residual cardiomegaly, and signs of right heart failure. Occasionally, long-term follow-up reveals calcification of the conduit, which may even erode into the sternum (Fig. 26–32).

Persistent Truncus Arteriosus

PREOPERATIVE RADIOGRAPHIC DIAGNOSIS. Anatomically, persistent truncus arteriosus is a large arterial vessel at the base of the heart from which the aortic arch, pulmonary trunk, and coronary arteries originate. Roentgenologically, it may mimic any of the other admixture lesions. Occasionally with a type-I persistent truncus arteriosus, one may see a straight upper left heart border or significantly elevated left pulmonary artery owing to anatomic origin from the single arterial trunk. The only significant roentgen finding is a right aortic arch, which occurs in approximately 35 per cent of patients with persistent truncus arteriosus. In addition, 50 per cent of these patients have extracardiac anomalies, especially those who have a left aortic arch.[7]

ANGIOGRAPHIC DATA FOR SURGICAL MANAGEMENT. Surgical planning requires preoperative determination of the relation of the truncus to the right or left ventricle, the origin of the pulmonary arteries, the presence of truncal valve stenosis or insufficiency, and the anatomy of the coronary arteries. These conditions as well as the size of the ventricular septal defect can be demonstrated by adequate right and left ventriculograms and truncal injections using biplane axial cineangiography.[1, 5]

POSTOPERATIVE RADIOGRAPHIC FINDINGS. The complications of pulmonary artery banding have been previously described. The most common type of persistent truncus arteriosus, type I, in which the pulmonary arteries emerge from the left basal aspect of the trunk in a normal position, has the best anatomy for Rastelli's procedure. This involves the closing of the ventricular septal defect and the placement of a graft with a valve to create an outflow from the right ventricle to the pulmonary arteries.

The postoperative complications shown radiographically include acute right heart failure secondary to obstruction with kinking of the conduit or even secondary to obstruction due to the pressure of the homograft and its valve against the sternum.

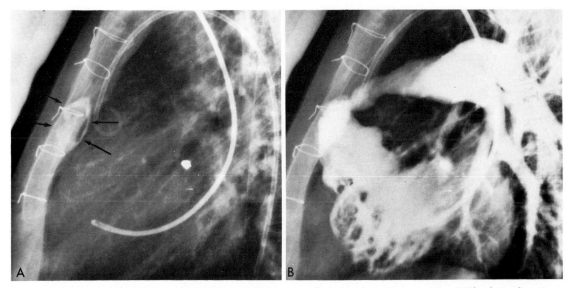

Figure 26–32. Calcification of prosthetic patch in complete transposition repair. *A,* The lateral projection of this 24-year-old female shows a calcified prosthetic patch (arrows) following repair of complete transposition (with the additional anomalies, pulmonary valve stenosis, and a ventricular septal defect) at an early age. Note that the conduit has eroded anteriorly into the sternum. *B,* The lateral right ventriculogram shows the anterior location of this patch, which is stenotic. This patient underwent a successful repair with a Hancock heterograft valved external conduit.

With a residual ventricular septal defect secondary to patch disruption, the roentgenographic findings include increased shunt vascularity and pulmonary edema associated with congestive heart failure.

Single Ventricle

PREOPERATIVE RADIOGRAPHIC DIAGNOSIS. The radiographic appearance depends on the type of single ventricle (SV). The vascularity is usually increased, as in the case of a large shunt or admixture lesion. When the single ventricle is on the left and the rudimentary right ventricle is along the left heart border, a discrete bulge is present. When the aorta arises from the inverted right ventricle, transposition of the great arteries usually exists, and the ascending aorta may form a convex bulge along the upper left heart border.

ANGIOGRAPHIC DATA FOR SURGICAL REPAIR. In order for surgical correction with a prosthetic septum to be performed, the determination of the status of the atrioventricular valves and their papillary muscle attachments is crucial. Axial cineangiography accomplishes this and easily demonstrates the position and anatomy of the outlet chamber, the trabecular pattern of the single ventricle, the type of pulmonary valve or subvalvular stenosis, and the coronary artery anatomy as well.[6, 15] The anterior descending coronary artery may arise from the right coronary artery in a large number of cases.[15]

POSTOPERATIVE RADIOGRAPHIC FINDINGS. A prosthetic septum can be constructed in patients with two atrioventricular valves and separate attachment of the papillary muscles. Since the cardiac conduction system is anomalous, the radiographic finding of cardiomegaly secondary to conduction system injury is frequent. With prosthetic septum disruption, the radiographic signs of cardiomegaly, pulmonary edema, and congestive heart failure are seen. Since no growth of the prosthetic septum can be anticipated, total correction is advised in children after the age of five.[8] However, despite its complications, banding of the pulmonary artery may be used as an early palliative procedure to reduce excessive pulmonary blood flow.

References

1. Bargeron, L. M., Jr., Elliott, L. P., Soto, B., et al.: Axial cineangiography in congenital heart disease. Section I. Concept, technical and anatomic considerations. Circulation 56:1075–1083, 1977.
2. Boruchow, I. B., Bartley, T. D., Elliott, L. P., et al.: Use of superior vena cava–right pulmonary artery anastomosis in congenital heart disease with decreased pulmonary blood flow. Circulation 44:777–784, 1969.
3. Cartmill, T. B., DuShane, J. W., McGoon, D. C., et al.: Results of repair of ventricular septal defect. J. Thorac. Cardiovasc. Surg. 52:486–499, 1966.
4. Curry, G. C., Victoria, B. E., Diacoff, G. R., et al.: Radiologic changes following repair and palliation of right-to-left admixture shunts. Radiol. Clin. North Am. 9:177–191, 1971.
5. Elliott, L. P., Bargeron, L. M., Jr., Bream, P. R., et al.: Axial cineangiography in congenital heart disease. Section II. Specific lesions. Circulation 56:1084–1093, 1977.
6. Elliott, L. P., Bream, P. R., and Gessner, I. H.: Single and common ventricle. In Moss, A. J., Adams, F. H., and Emmanouilides, G. C., (eds.): Heart Disease in Infants, Children and Adolescents. Baltimore, Williams & Wilkins Company, 1977, pp. 381–393.
7. Elliott, L. P., and Schiebler, G. L.: The X-ray Diagnosis of Congenital Heart Disease in Infants, Children and Adults. Pathologic, Hemodynamic and Clinical Correlations as Related to the Chest Film. Springfield, Illinois, Charles C Thomas, Publisher, 1979, pp. 115–401.
8. Engle, M. A.: Cyanotic congenital heart disease. Am. J. Cardiol. 37:283–308, 1976.
9. Goor, D. A., and Lillehei, C. W.: Congenital Malformations of the Heart. New York, Grune & Stratton, Inc., 1975, pp. 103–111.
10. Gyepes, M. T., Abrams, H. L., and Shumway, N. E.: Radiologic aspects of operable heart disease. VIII. The effects of pulmonary artery banding. Radiology 88:466–472, 1967.
11. Hipona, F. A., Paredes, S., and Lerona, P. T.: Roentgenologic analysis of common postoperative problems in congenital heart disease. Radiol. Clin. North Am. 9:229–251, 1971.
12. Jack, W. D., and Kelly, D. T.: Long-term follow-up of valvulotomy for congenital aortic stenosis. Am. J. Cardiol. 38:231–234, 1976.
13. Jugdutt, B. I., Brooks, C. H., Stern, L. P., et al.: Surgical treatment of Ebstein's anomaly. J. Thorac. Cardiovasc. Surg. 73:114–119, 1977.
14. Knight, L., Joransen, J., Marin-Garcia, J., et al.: Roentgenographic and angiocardiographic changes after total correction of tetralogy of Fallot. Am. J. Roentgenol. 123:691–702, 1975.
15. McCartney, F. J., Partridge, J. B., Scott, O., et al.: Common or single ventricle: an angiocardiographic and hemodynamic study of 42 patients. Circulation 53:543–554, 1976.
16. Marr, K., Giargiana, F. A., Jr., and White, R. I., Jr.: The radiographic diagnosis of pulmonary hypertension following Blalock-Taussig shunts in patients with tetralogy of Fallot. Am. J. Roentgenol. 122:125–32, 1974.
17. Silbiger, M. L., Stewart, S., Morrow, A. G., et al.: Correlation of chest roentgenograms and hemodynamic findings following surgical repair of ventricular septal defects. Radiology 90:90–93, 1968.
18. Soto, B., Pacifico, A. D., Luna, R. F., et al.: A radiographic study of congenital pulmonary atresia with ventricular septal defect. Am. J. Roentgenol. 129:1027–1037, 1977.
19. Tonkin, I. L., Kelley, M. J., Bream, P. R., et al.: The frontal chest film as a method of suspecting transposition complexes. Circulation 53:1016–1025, 1976.
20. Tonkin, I. L., Sansa, M., Elliott, L. P., et al.: Recognition of developing left ventricular outflow tract obstruction in complete transposition of the great arteries. Radiology 134:53–59, 1980.
21. Tonkin, I. L., Elliott, L. P., and Bargeon, L. M., Jr.: Concomitant axial cineangiography and barium esophagography in the evaluation of vascular rings. Radiology, in press.

Part III

Acquired Valvular Heart Disease

PETER R. BREAM, M.D.

INA L. TONKIN, M.D.

LARRY P. ELLIOTT, M.D.

ACQUIRED DISORDERS OF THE AORTIC VALVE

Aortic Stenosis

Isolated aortic valvular stenosis is almost invariably secondary to a congenital bicuspid valve defect. The bicuspid valve is not inherently stenotic but becomes so with increasing age. This acquired stenosis is secondary to valve calcification, which restricts the valve opening. The chest film findings are usually benign and include normal vascularity and normal heart size (Fig. 26–33). Pulmonary venous hypertension and an enlarged left ventricle occur late in the disease process, suggesting failure of the left ventricle; they are associated with a higher surgical mortality rate. The only specific x-ray sign for aortic stenosis is calcification of the aortic valve. Moderate-to-severe amounts of calcium in the aortic valve are best seen in the center of the cardiac density on a lateral chest film (Fig. 26–33B). Fluoroscopy, however, is needed for the detection of the mildly calcified aortic valve. Prominence of the ascending aorta secondary to poststenotic dilatation on the posteroanterior chest film is a helpful sign, but it is nonspecific and may be absent in cases of significant aortic stenosis.

Other causes of isolated aortic valvular stenosis are rare. Isolated rheumatic aortic valvular stenosis is unusual and almost always coexists with rheumatic mitral valvular

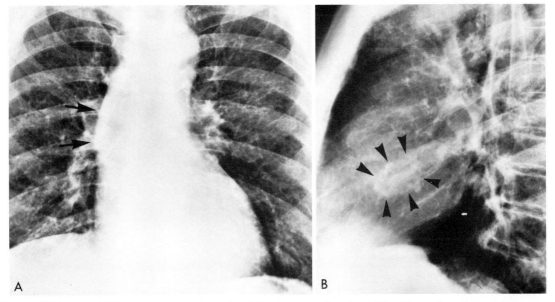

A   B

Figure 26–33. Calcific aortic valve stenosis. *A,* Posteroanterior chest film. The pulmonary vascularity and heart size are normal. The ascending aorta (arrows) is mildly prominent. *B,* Lateral chest film. The most important and specific finding is dense calcification (arrowheads) of the aortic valve.

disease. The x-ray characteristics of rheumatic aortic valvular stenosis are usually overshadowed by those of the mitral valve. The only specific finding is calcification of the aortic valve. Calcification of the aortic valve in cases of significant rheumatic aortic valvular stenosis is less frequent, however, and less extensive than that seen in cases of bicuspid valvular stenosis. Therefore, aortic valvular stenosis may be indicated by the chest x-ray of a patient with obvious rheumatic mitral valvular disease if there is a prominent ascending aorta with a normal descending aorta or if calcium is detected in the aortic valve.

Idiopathic hypertrophic subaortic stenosis (IHSS) is a dynamic type of acquired subaortic stenosis caused by the apposition of the hypertrophied superior septal wall and the free edge of the anterior leaflet of the mitral valve. The preoperative x-ray findings are nonspecific. This entity is indicated when there is a marked convexity of the left ventricular heart border together with an inapparent or normal-sized ascending aorta.

Aortic Valvular Insufficiency

Aortic valvular insufficiency has multiple origins but has a characteristic roentgenographic appearance. The chest film shows normal pulmonary vascularity and an enlarged left ventricle, with varying degrees of prominence of the ascending and the descending thoracic aorta (Fig. 26–34). The left ventricle may decompensate late in the course of disease, at which time the chest film shows pulmonary venous hypertension.

Aortic valvular insufficiency may be due to a primary disease of the aortic valve or

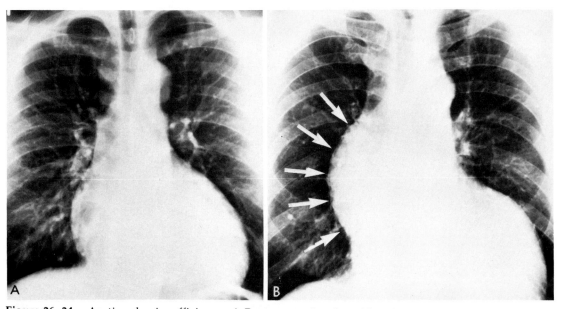

Figure 26–34. Aortic valve insufficiency. *A*, Posteroanterior chest film of a 19-year-old with rheumatic aortic valve insufficiency. The pulmonary vascularity is normal and the left ventricle is moderately enlarged. There is mild prominence of the ascending and descending aorta. *B*, Posteroanterior chest film of a 50-year-old with cystic medial necrosis. The x-ray findings (normal vascularity and large left ventricle) are similar except for the marked prominence of the ascending aorta (arrows). These findings indicate aortic insufficiency secondary to an abnormal ascending aorta.

to a disease of the ascending aorta with secondary involvement of the aortic valve annulus. Primary disease processes that cause aortic valvular insufficiency include congenital bicuspid aortic valve, with or without bacterial endocarditis; rheumatic heart disease; trauma; and congenital fenestration (Fig. 26–34A). Disease processes involving the ascending aorta that cause aortic valvular insufficiency include cystic medial necrosis (with or without Marfan's syndrome), dissection of the ascending aorta, and syphilitic or atherosclerotic aneurysm of the ascending aorta (Fig. 26–34B).

ACQUIRED MITRAL AND TRICUSPID VALVULAR DISEASE

Rheumatic fever is the most common cause of acquired mitral and tricuspid valvular disease. The radiographic findings of rheumatic heart disease are characteristic, in that pulmonary venous hypertension of varying degree and a triangular or "mitral-shaped" heart (Fig. 26–35) are usual. The mitral-shaped heart is produced by the enlargement of the left atrial appendage and the pulmonary trunk.

Mitral Valvular Stenosis

Mitral valvular stenosis is almost invariably secondary to rheumatic heart disease. Congenital mitral stenosis is rare, and other acquired diseases of the mitral valve cause

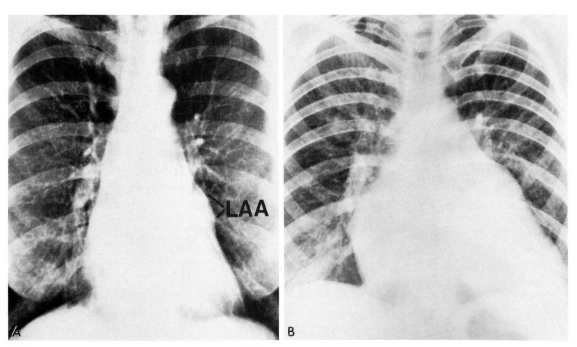

Figure 26–35. Rheumatic mitral valve disease. *A*, Posteroanterior chest film of a patient with mitral stenosis. There is moderate pulmonary venous hypertension and a normal-sized heart with a mitral configuration. The left atrial appendage (LAA) is large, and there is a mild increase in the size of the body of the left atrium. *B*, Posteroanterior chest film of a patient with mitral insufficiency. There is moderate pulmonary venous hypertension and an enlarged mitral-shaped heart. The body of the left atrium and the left ventricle are enlarged.

mitral valvular insufficiency. In cases of mitral stenosis the chest film usually shows moderate-to-severe pulmonary venous hypertension and a normal-sized, mitral-shaped heart (Fig. 26–35A). The left ventricle is normal to small in size, the body of the left atrium is mildly to moderately enlarged, and there is almost invariably a prominent pulmonary trunk and right atrium and ventricle. Calcium is occasionally detectable in the mitral valve. There may be calcium in the wall of the left atrium in severe, long-standing cases of mitral stenosis or in a thrombosed left atrial appendage. This is especially true in patients with atrial fibrillation.

Mitral Valvular Insufficiency

In contrast to mitral stenosis, the causes of mitral valvular insufficiency (MVI) are varied. The most common cause of significant mitral valvular insufficiency is rheumatic heart disease. Other causes include mitral valvular prolapse, bacterial endocarditis, and papillary muscle dysfunction or rupture.

Chest films of those patients with rheumatic mitral valvular insufficiency show mild-to-moderate pulmonary venous hypertension and enlargement, with a "mitral configuration" of the heart (Fig. 26–35B). The left atrium is moderately to severely enlarged, and the left ventricle is moderately enlarged. The pulmonary trunk is not prominent, and the "right heart" is normal in size.

Mitral valvular prolapse is a common clinical syndrome of diverse origins. Mitral valvular insufficiency is rarely associated; when present, it is usually mild. The chest film is usually normal, but thoracic bony anomalies may be detected.[2] Occasionally, associated mitral valvular insufficiency is severe enough to necessitate valve replacement. In these cases, the chest film findings may mimic those of rheumatic mitral valvular disease.

Tricuspid Valvular Disease

Acquired tricuspid valvular disease almost always coexists with severe rheumatic mitral valvular disease. Tricuspid stenosis is secondary to rheumatic valvulitis of the tricuspid valve and is a rare entity, usually coexisting with rheumatic mitral valvular stenosis. Tricuspid regurgitation, on the other hand, usually results from right heart dilatation. The latter has various causes, the most frequent being rheumatic mitral valvular disease. Other causes of acquired tricuspid valvular regurgitation include trauma, bacterial endocarditis, and carcinoid. Radiographically, tricuspid stenosis or insufficiency is suggested when there are signs of elevated systemic venous pressure or right heart enlargement (Fig. 26–36). Elevated systemic venous pressures are indicated on the upright posteroanterior chest film by prominence of the azygous vein or the superior vena cava.

POSTOPERATIVE FINDINGS

The surgical procedure for the treatment of most cases of acquired valvular heart disease is valve replacement. For this reason, it is convenient to group together the postoperative findings of all the acquired valvular diseases, since the complications are similar. The evaluation of the chest film of the patient who has undergone valve replacement should include the identification of the number and sites of previous

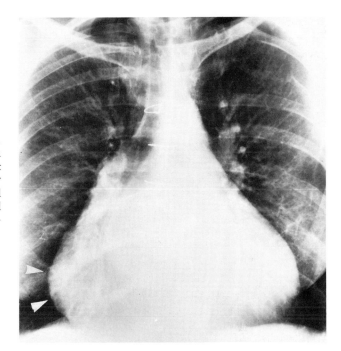

Figure 26–36. Tricuspid valve disease. Posteroanterior chest film in a patient with rheumatic heart disease status following left thoracotomy for mitral commissurotomy and median sternotomy for aortic and mitral valve replacement. The marked right atrial enlargement (arrowheads) indicates significant tricuspid valve insufficiency.

surgical procedures, the determination of the position and type of valve replacement, and a search for evidence of valve complications and new or coexistent disease.

Valve replacement is now always performed via a median sternotomy, regardless of the valve being replaced. The finding of evidence of other surgery (that is, right or left lateral thoracotomy) is important in that it gives a clue to the disease process. For instance, a patient with a left lateral thoracotomy and a median sternotomy for aortic valve replacement more than likely had coarctation of the aorta repaired via a left thoracotomy and replacement of a stenotic, bicuspid aortic valve via a median sternotomy. A right or left lateral thoracotomy in a patient with median sternotomy and mitral valve replacement usually indicates a previous commissurotomy for rheumatic mitral stenosis prior to the valve replacement.

The identification of the position and the type of valve replacement is important in directing the search for potential complications. The diseased valve may be replaced with a human aortic valve (homograft), porcine aortic valve (heterograft), or a prosthetic valve. There are two basic types of prosthetic valves: caged ball and tilting disc. The homograft valve has no metallic supporting structures and therefore cannot be detected radiographically unless it becomes calcified. The supporting apparatus for the porcine valve is metallic and therefore radiopaque. The caged-ball and tilting-disc prosthetic valves are radiopaque to varying degrees and can be identified by their radiographic appearance.[4]

The position of the valves can be routinely identified on the posteroanterior chest film. When there is any doubt, a lateral chest film is diagnostic (Fig. 26–37). The postoperative evaluation of valve position and motion is important, since postoperative complications are frequently related to valve dysfunction. Cardiac chamber size is more easily determined, since the prosthetic valve serves as an internal marker and the cardiac border as an external marker.

Different combinations of prosthetic valves are employed for the correction of different disease processes. Aortic-mitral valve replacement is the most common and is usually performed to correct rheumatic valve disease. Other valve replacement combi-

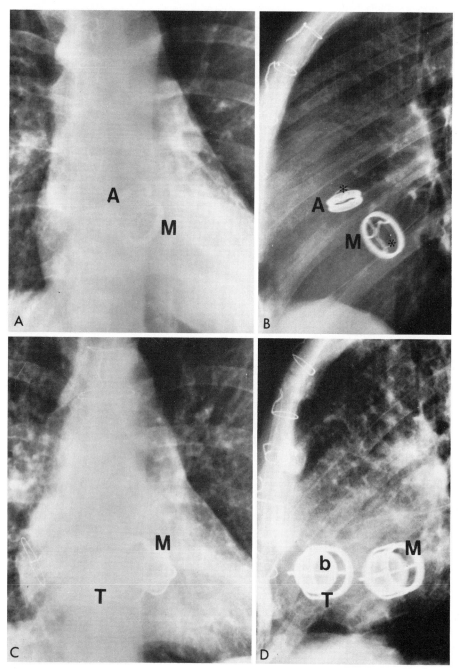

Figure 26–37. Prosthetic valves. Posteroanterior (*A*) lateral (*B*) chest films following aortic (A) and mitral (M) valve replacement with tilting-disc valves. Note that the identification of the type and position of prosthetic valve is easier on the lateral chest film. The thin metal markers (*) identify the position of the tilting disc. Posteroanterior (*C*) and lateral (*D*) chest films following mitral (M) and tricuspid (T) valve replacement with ball and cage valves. The ball (b) may be radiopaque.

nations used to correct rheumatic valve disease are mitral-tricuspid and mitral-aortic-tricuspid. If a pulmonary valve prosthesis is also seen, then combined congenital and acquired disease should be suspected.

The radiologist is in a front-line position for the detection of serious postoperative valve complications. The presence of complications should be suspected when significant pulmonary venous hypertension occurs in the postoperative period. A sudden increase in the degree of pulmonary venous hypertension on postoperative films suggests postoperative valve dysfunction. Cinefluoroscopy of the suspected valve should be part of the radiologic evaluation.

Common postoperative valve replacement complications include the calcification of homograft and heterograft valves, ball variance or ball shrinkage in caged-ball valves, thrombosis of disc-type valves, prosthesis detachment, hemolysis, and infection.

The radiologist should be familiar with the complications that cause specific x-ray findings. One is thrombosis of a tilting-disc valve prosthesis in the mitral or aortic

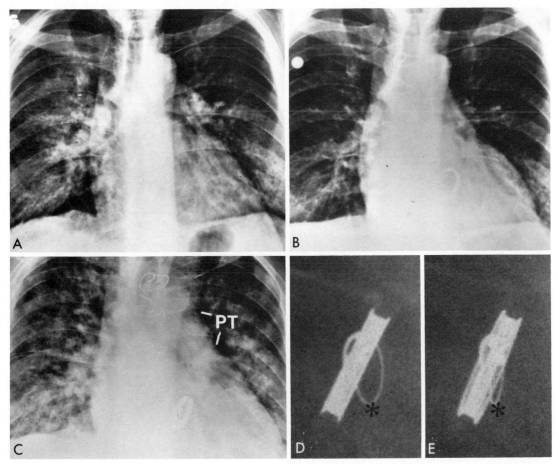

Figure 26–38. Thrombosis of the tilting disc valve. *A,* Preoperative posteroanterior chest film demonstrates findings typical of rheumatic mitral valve disease. *B,* Posteroanterior chest film following mitral valve replacement with a tilting disc prosthesis shows marked improvement. *C,* Posteroanterior chest film one week after cessation of anticoagulant therapy. The findings of severe pulmonary venous hypertension and enlargement of the pulmonary trunk (PT) suggest obstruction at or proximal to the mitral valve. *D* and *E,* Cinefluoroscopy of the mitral valve in the right anterior oblique position shows limited excursion of the disc (*) during diastole (D) and incomplete closure of the disc in systole (E). These findings indicate thrombosis of the valve prosthesis.

position. This can be recognized on plain films and more specifically with fluoroscopy through the evaluation of the radiopaque ring used to identify the position and movement of the disc (Fig. 26–38).[1] It should open fully (45 to 60 degrees) and have no restriction of movement. The disc should close completely and lie in the same plane as the radiopaque supporting ring.[1] The timing of the chest film x-ray exposure in relation to valve movement is such that the valve is usually fully open or fully closed on the chest film. *If the valve appears partially open, thrombosis should be suspected and fluoroscopy of the valve performed.*

Another valve complication that may be suggested on plain films and confirmed with fluoroscopy is prosthesis detachment. This occurs when some of the sutures or tissues holding the valve in place loosen. In such cases, a portion of the valve ring

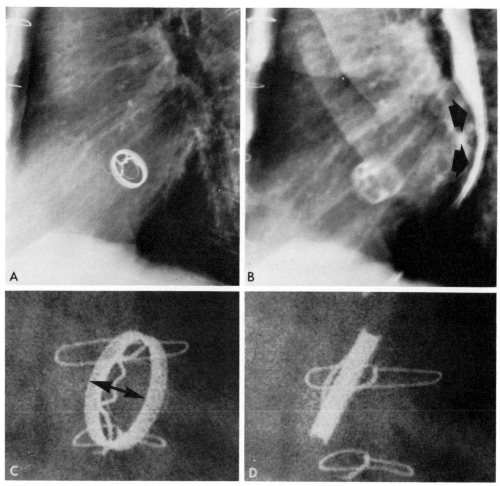

Figure 26–39. Loose mitral valve prosthesis (MVP). *A,* Lateral chest film following mitral valve replacement. The normal appearance of the metallic base ring serves as a radiographic baseline. *B,* Lateral chest film in the same patient following clinical deterioration and the appearance of a new murmur. The posterior deviation of the barium-filled esophagus (arrows) indicates left atrial enlargement. The base ring of the mitral valve prosthesis is blurred. These findings suggest a loose or partially detached MVP, especially with the normal appearance of the prosthesis on an earlier examination. *C* and *D,* Right anterior oblique cinefluroscopy of the mitral vlave prosthesis demonstrated excessive tilting of the base ring (arrows) from diastole (C) to systole (D). These cinefluoroscopic findings are diagnostic of a partially detached valve prosthesis, which is usually associated with severe paravalvular mitral insufficiency.

usually shows excessive movement, indicated on plain films by blurring of the prosthetic valve (Fig. 26–39), and there is associated paravalvular regurgitation. Fluoroscopy should be used to evaluate all suspicious valves. The "tilting" or "rocking" of the metallic support ring more than 12 degrees in the case of the mitral valve and more than 6 degrees in the case of the aortic valve is considered excessive motion.[5]

Even if there are no specific plain film findings of prosthetic valve dysfunction (that is, of a detached or thrombosed prosthesis), postoperative cardiac dysfunction may be indicated radiographically by a change in the pulmonary vascular pattern or an increase in heart or individual chamber size. In such situations, fluoroscopy is recommended for the evaluation of possible prosthetic valve dysfunction.

Surgery for idiopathic hypertrophic subaortic stenosis or fixed subaortic stenosis is aimed at relieving the subaortic gradient. This can usually be accomplished by myomectomy with or without mitral valve replacement. If obstruction remains, then a valved external conduit from the left ventricular apex to the distal thoracic or upper abdominal aorta may be performed to bypass the subaortic obstruction (Fig. 26–40). The aortic valve is intrinsically normal and does not need to be replaced.

Cystic medial necrosis and other aneurysms of the ascending aorta associated with aortic valve insufficiency usually require the replacement of both the aortic valve and the ascending aorta.[3] This may be accomplished by a composite prosthetic valve–graft. Complications following surgery are related not to the surgical procedure but to the progression of disease and include dissection and aneurysmal formation distal to the site of surgery (Fig. 26–41).

Mitral commissurotomy is an effective operation for the relief of noncalcified mitral stenosis. It may be performed from a right or left lateral thoracotomy or from a median

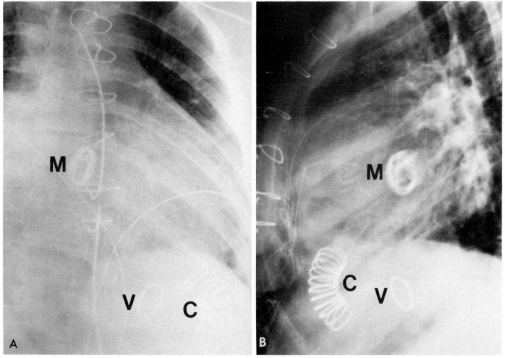

Figure 26–40. Left ventricular apex-to-aorta valved external conduit. Anteroposterior (*A*) and lateral (*B*) postoperative chest films. Myomectomy and mitral valve (M) replacement failed to relieve subaortic left ventricular outflow tract obstruction. The metallic spiral (C) represents a portion of the conduit, and the metallic ring (V) represents the site of the heterograft valve.

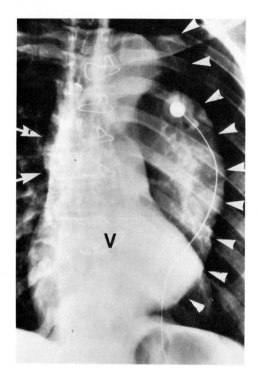

Figure 26–41. Surgery for cystic medial necrosis. Posteroanterior chest film following aortic valve and ascending aorta replacement for aneurysm of the ascending aorta and aortic valve insufficiency. The metallic ring (V) represents the base ring of a heterograft valve. The replaced ascending aorta (arrows) is now normal in appearance. The significant finding is marked prominence of the aortic arch and descending aorta (arrowheads). This represents an extension of the disease process distal to the ascending aorta graft.

sternotomy. Chest film findings after mitral commissurotomy include evidence of a previous thoracotomy, isolated prominence of the pulmonary trunk, and pulmonary venous hypertension. The left atrial appendage is usually absent owing to surgical removal (Fig. 26–42). Infrequently, however, it is still apparent on the film; in this case, the presence of a thoracotomy and a mitral-configuration cardiovascular silhouette indi-

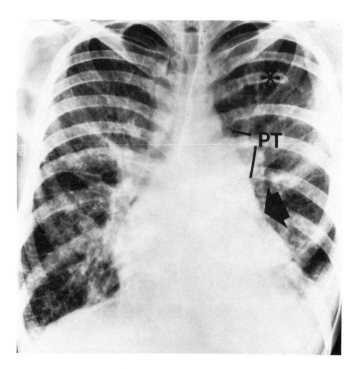

Figure 26–42. Mitral commissurotomy. Posteroanterior chest film shows signs of previous left thoracotomy (*), severe interstitial edema, prominence of the pulmonary trunk (PT), and inapparent left atrial appendage (arrow). These radiographic findings are secondary to restenosis of the mitral valve following commissurotomy via a left thoracotomy.

cates that a mitral valve commissurotomy was performed. In following a patient after mitral commissurotomy, one should carefully evaluate the degree of pulmonary venous hypertension, since restenosis of the valve after several years is common. The enlargement of the left atrium and left ventricle following mitral commissurotomy usually indicates significant mitral regurgitation. To follow progressive enlargement of the body of the left atrium, posteroanterior and lateral views with barium in the esophagus are suggested (see Fig. 26–39B).

Mitral annuloplasty, or valvuloplasty, may be used for repair in some cases of pure mitral regurgitation. The procedure is performed via a median sternotomy, and no radiopaque material is used. Its main advantages over prosthetic valve replacement are that anticoagulation is not needed and the potential complications of a valve prosthesis are avoided. Postoperative complications of valvuloplasty include recurrent mitral regurgitation.

SUMMARY

The postoperative chest film of the patient with acquired valvular heart disease can be used to monitor the patient's status. Knowledge of the location of surgery and the position and type of valve replacement allows more efficiency in the search for specific complications. Most significant complications cause pulmonary venous hypertension, a sudden increase in pre-existing hypertension, or a change in heart or individual chamber size. The fluoroscopic evaluation of the prosthetic valve suspected of malfunction is frequently diagnostic.

References

1. Bjork, V. O., Henze, A., and Hindmarsh, T.: Radiopaque marker in the tilting disc of the Bjork-Shiley heart valve. J. Thorac. Cardiovasc. Surg. 73:563–569, 1977.
2. Bon Tempo, C. P., Ronan, J. A. de Leon, A. C., et al.: Radiographic appearance of the thorax in systolic click–late systolic murmur syndrome. Am. J. Cardiol. 36:27–36, 1975.
3. Kouchoukos, N. T., Karp, R. B., and Lell, W. A.: Replacement of the ascending aorta and aortic valve with a composite graft: results in 25 patients. Ann. Thorac. Surg. 24(2):140–148, 1977.
4. Mehlman, D. J., and Resnekov, L.: A guide to the radiographic identification of prosthetic heart valves. Circulation 57:613–623, 1978.
5. White, A. F., Dinsmore, R. E., and Buckley, M. J.: Cineradiographic evaluation of prosthetic cardiac valves. Circulation 48:882–889, 1973.

Part IV
Postoperative Findings Common to Acquired and Congenital Heart Disease

PETER R. BREAM, M.D.
LARRY P. ELLIOTT, M.D.
ARTHUR S. SOUZA, Jr., M.D.
INA L. TONKIN, M.D.

The chest film is an indispensable aid in the management of the postoperative cardiac patient. Proper interpretation of these films involves three major principles:

1. The postoperative chest film is a *dynamic* affair, with rapid changes occurring within the first 72 hours.

2. The findings must be considered as being highly *relative*. What is normal in a 36-hour postoperative open-heart patient is grossly abnormal in a patient walking in from the street to the emergency room with chest pain.

3. There are certain abnormal findings whose origins and significance become apparent because they occur in a specific *time sequence*. In other words, the widening of the mediastinum at 24 hours may indicate bleeding, whereas the same finding at 5 days suggests a chyloma, the harbinger of a chylothorax.

We have divided the postoperative period into three stages: (1) the acute (0 to 72 hours), (2) the intermediate stage (3 to 14 days), and (3) the late stage (more than 2 weeks).

In order for the postoperative chest to be interpreted with any accuracy, the appropriate films must be available for comparison. The preoperative film should be compared with the initial postoperative film. In the first postoperative week, all films should be viewed in sequence. This is best accomplished if the films are hung on a multiple-panel viewer. In this way the entire sequence of postoperative films is continuously available for viewing. Discharge films (10 to 14 days postoperative) must be compared with preoperative films.

THE ACUTE POSTOPERATIVE PERIOD

The cardiac patient undergoes constant monitoring for the first 48 to 72 postoperative hours. During this period, several portable supine anteroposterior chest films are taken. The interpretation of this group of films involves the analysis of five specific areas: (1) assist devices, (2) skeletal structures and soft tissues, (3) cardiac and mediastinal structures, (4) pulmonary system, and (5) abdomen.

Assist Devices

The first step in the analysis of the chest film of the postoperative cardiac patient is a check for the proper positioning of the numerous assist and monitoring devices (Fig. 26–43). The tip of the endotracheal tube should be 2 to 5 cm above the level of the carina in the adult patient and 1 to 3 cm above the carina in the pediatric patient. There

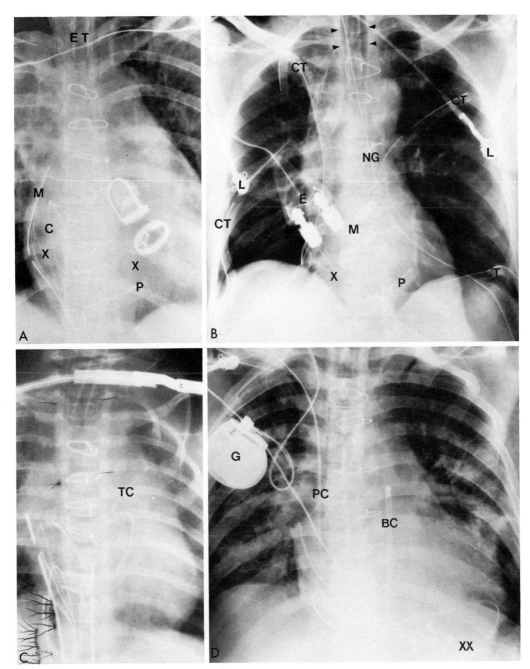

Figure 26–43. Acute postoperative anteroposterior chest films. *A,* Median sternotomy for aortic and mitral valve replacement. The endotracheal (ET) tube is well above the carina. The mediastinal (M) and pericardial (P) drains are properly positioned. Radiopaque transthoracic venous pressure catheter (C) and temporary atrial and ventricular pacing wires (X) are also present. *B,* Median sternotomy for aortic valve replacement. Endotracheal tube with cuff inflated (arrowheads) is properly positioned. M and P drains and pacing wires are present. Right and left chest tubes (CT) are also present. Electrical junction box (E) and EKG leads (L) are superimposed over the chest. The nasogastric (NG) tube is pulled to the left in the mid chest by a tortuous aorta. *C,* Median sternotomy for repair of tetralogy of Fallot. In addition to the usual assist devices, a radiopaque thermodilution catheter (TC) is properly positioned into the pulmonary artery. It enters the chest via the sternotomy, having been placed through the right ventriculotomy. *D,* Median sternotomy with the usual assist devices. Other such devices include the intra-aortic balloon assist catheter (BC), the permanent transvenous pacing catheter (PC) and generator (G), and the permanent epicardial pacing wires (XX).

may or may not be a radiopaque marker at the tip (Fig. 26–43A). The inflated cuff should be below the vocal cords (Fig. 26–43B). The endotracheal tube is usually removed 24 to 72 hours after surgery.

The use of mediastinal drains is customary after median sternotomy. There are usually two or three mediastinal drains, one of which is bent and positioned between the heart and the diaphragm to drain the inferior pericardial space (Fig. 26–43A and B). The one or more additional drains are straighter and drain the anterior mediastinum and pericardial space (Fig. 26–43A to D). The mediastinal drains are removed following the removal of other intracardiac assist devices, such as the right and left atrial pressure lines. This allows the monitoring of any potential bleeding. Intrathoracic drains and assist devices usually exit from the patient in the lower sternal area.

The nasogastric tube, when present, is usually in midline, although it may be deviated to the right by an enlarged left atrium or pulled to the left by a tortuous aorta (Fig. 26–43B). At the superior mediastinal level, deviation of the tube to the right may be the result of persistent bleeding or a large hematoma. The tip of the tube should reach well into the stomach.

Chest tubes are not usually inserted following median sternotomy but may be used if the pleural space was entered during surgery (Fig. 26–43B). After right or left thoracotomy a chest tube is always present on the ipsilateral side.

Temporary epicardial pacemaker wires are placed at the time of surgery and are brought out of the chest via a separate stab wound below the sternotomy. They remain in place until the intermediate postoperative period, when they are removed prior to the patient's discharge from the hospital. On the chest film they are seen as thin wires overlying the atrial and ventricular portions of the heart (Fig. 26–43A to C) Permanent epicardial pacemaker leads can also be placed at the time of operation and appear as "corkscrews" 1 cm long overlying the right ventricle. They are attached to thicker wires that run a variable course in the subcutaneous tissues (Fig. 26–43D).

Venous catheters are common in postoperative chests. The site of entrance and the location of the tip should be identified.

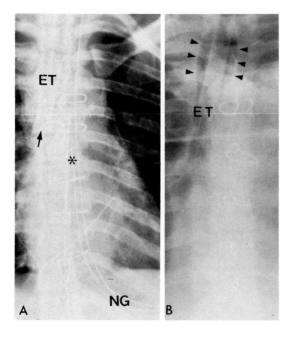

Figure 26–44. Abnormal endotracheal (ET) tube. A, Radiopaque marker (arrow) at tip of the endotracheal tube indicates abnormal placement into the right main stem bronchus. Also note that the nasogastric (NG) tube reaches the stomach, but its tip (*) is at the level of the midesophagus. B, The endotracheal tube is properly positioned, but its cuff (arrowheads) is overinflated.

Other monitor and assist devices encountered less commonly on the acute postoperative chest film include intra-aortic balloon assist devices, thermodilution catheters, and intracardiac pressure monitoring catheters.

An intra-aortic balloon assist device is a large catheter introduced surgically via the femoral artery and positioned into the proximal descending thoracic aorta. The balloon extends for 30 or 40 cm along the catheter and terminates at its tip. The tip of the catheter should be positioned between the level of the left bronchus inferiorly and the level of the aortic arch superiorly (Fig. 26–43D).

Thermodilution catheters are used to measure cardiac output in the immediate postoperative period. They may enter the vascular system peripherally or may be placed through the right ventricular wall at the time of operation (Fig. 26–43C). The type used, and hence its radiographic appearance, varies from one institution to another.

Intracardiac hemodynamic pressure monitoring devices placed through the right atrial appendage and the body of the left atrium are commonly present, but their visibility varies according to their degree of radiopacity (Fig. 26–43A). They are pulled out several hours before the removal of the mediastinal drainage tubes.

When an unusual placement or location of any assist device is discovered, the patient's physician must be notified immediately so that corrective action can be taken before a serious complication develops. The most common postoperative complication encountered in assist devices is malposition of the endotracheal tube (Fig. 26–44). If it is too low, unequal aeration of the lungs occurs, and significant atelectasis results if proper positioning is not achieved early. If it is too high, the inflated cuff may damage the vocal cords. Overinflation of the cuff (Fig. 26–44B) for long periods of time may cause tracheal necrosis.

Mediastinal and pleural tube malplacement is uncommon. The most common type

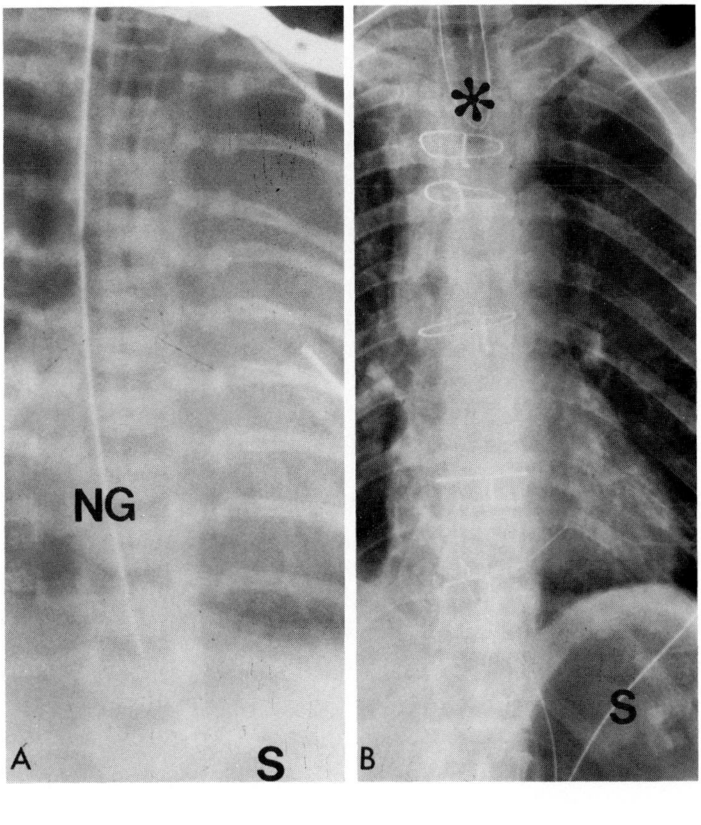

Figure 26–45. Abnormal nasogastric (NG) tube. A, The nasogastric tube fails to reach into stomach (S). B, The nasogastric tube is coiled in upper esophagus (*) of this patient with a dilated stomach.

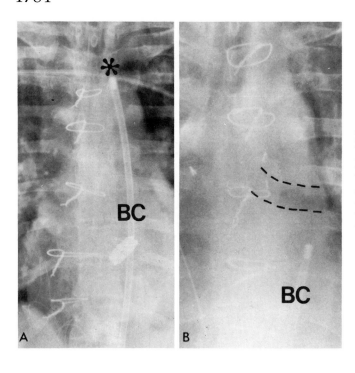

Figure 26–46. Abnormal intra-aortic balloon assist catheter (BC). *A,* The balloon assist catheter is too high, and its tip (*) is obstructing the left subclavian artery. *B,* The balloon assist catheter is too low, as its tip is below the left main bronchus (-----). In this position the balloon is less effective.

occurs when a side hole of the tube is outside the space to be drained. If the break in the radiopaque linear marker in the tube, which marks the most distal side hole in the tube, is identified outside the chest, a side hole of the tube is also outside and the function of the tube is lost.

The nasogastric tube is in an abnormal position when the tip fails to reach into the stomach (Figs. 26–44*A* and 26–45). The most common cause is insufficient advancement of the tube (Fig. 26–45*A*). An unusual problem, but one that is easily recognizable on the radiograph, is coiling of the tube within the stomach or esophagus (Figs. 26–44*A* and 26–45*B*).

The intra-aortic balloon assist catheter is abnormally positioned when the tip of the catheter is above the level of the aortic arch or below the level of the left bronchus, as seen on the anteroposterior film (Fig. 26–46). The high position may obstruct the origin of the left subclavian or the left common carotid artery. Since any intravascular catheter forms a clot with the potential for subsequent embolism, it is imperative that the catheter tip be kept well below the great arteries arising from the aortic arch.

Skeletal Structures and Soft Tissues

The usual radiographic skeletal and soft tissue findings in the postoperative chest are dependent upon the site of surgery (that is, the right or left thorax or the midline of the sternum).

In cases of right and left thoracotomy there is normally an asymmetric soft tissue density resulting from the unilateral soft tissue edema and dressings at the site of operation (Fig. 26–47). There is usually localized pleural thickening at the exact site of surgery or at the site of chest tube insertion. Bony changes may be present in the acute postoperative period but are almost always detectable in the late postoperative period.

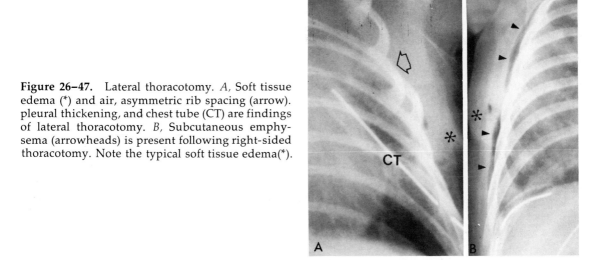

Figure 26–47. Lateral thoracotomy. *A,* Soft tissue edema (*) and air, asymmetric rib spacing (arrow). pleural thickening, and chest tube (CT) are findings of lateral thoracotomy. *B,* Subcutaneous emphysema (arrowheads) is present following right-sided thoracotomy. Note the typical soft tissue edema(*).

The appearance of soft tissue and bony changes involving a median sternotomy is readily appreciated. Sternal wires (see Fig. 26–43) are present, except in infants, in whom nonradiopaque sutures are sometimes used.

Abnormal findings encountered in the soft tissue structures in the acute postoperative period are infrequent. In the case of a right or a left thoracotomy, rib fractures near the site of thoracotomy may occur. Subcutaneous emphysema (Fig. 26–47B) is perhaps the most common complication and at times may be extensive. Localized pleural or soft tissue hematomas of considerable size occur rarely and must be differentiated from pulmonary parenchymal opacities.

Abnormal skeletal findings encountered in patients after the performance of a median sternotomy include fracture of the first or second rib (Fig. 26–48), sternal dehiscence, and evidence of surgical re-entry. Fracture of the first or second rib, or of both, is thought to occur at the time sternal spreaders are applied.[2] Sternal dehiscence is uncommon in the acute postoperative period but more common in the intermediate (3 to 14 days) and late (more than 14 days) periods. Re-entry of the chest is seen radiographically as a change from one film to another in all or some of the sternal wires. The most common reason for re-entry in the acute period is continued postoperative bleed-

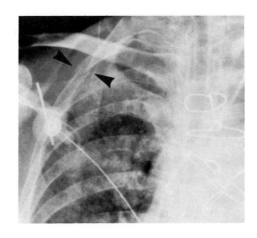

Figure 26–48. Rib fracture from sternotomy. There is a fracture of the right second rib (arrowheads) secondary to median sternotomy.

ing, which is reflected clinically in excessive amounts of mediastinal or chest tube drainage. Excessive bleeding is usually not radiographically evident until the chest tubes are removed, after which blood collects in the pericardium, mediastinum, or pleural spaces, which usually results in detectable radiographic changes.

Cardiac and Mediastinal Structures

Following cardiac surgery, there is usually widening of the cardiac-mediastinal structures. The normal amount of widening is further enhanced by the inherent magnification in portable anteroposterior films. It is important to compare multiple serial postoperative films, since small changes from one film to the next are difficult to appreciate. When several serially performed films are viewed at one time, significant changes from the first to the last film may become apparent. This is especially true in the case of mediastinal widening. Other expected postoperative findings that are often seen are small amounts of pneumomediastinum and pneumopericardium (Fig. 26–49).

Abnormal cardiac and mediastinal postoperative findings include extensive pneumo- or hemopericardium, extensive pneumo- or hemomediastinum, cardiac tamponade, and a chyloma.

Hemopericardium during the first 24 to 48 postoperative hours is a common complication. The stage of its development is indicated by the amount of blood drained from the mediastinal-pericardial tubes. Cardiac tamponade secondary to hemopericardium is possible even with drains and with pericardial-pleural communication, since blood clots may occlude the communications. Enlargement of the cardiac-mediastinal silhouette may or may not accompany the clinical signs of cardiac tamponade. The appearance of a left apical opacity in the acute period may represent blood leaking from the mediastinum into the extrapleural soft tissue and is an indirect sign of hemopericardium or hemomediastinum (Fig. 26–50).[8]

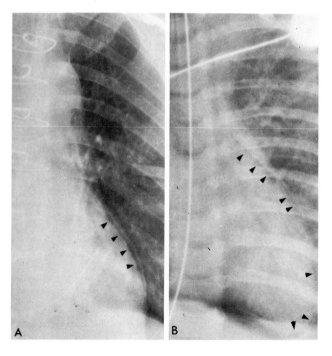

Figure 26–49. Pneumopericardium. Median sternotomy (A) and right thoracotomy (B). A small pneumopericardium (arrowheads) is an incidental finding in the acute postoperative period following cardiac surgery.

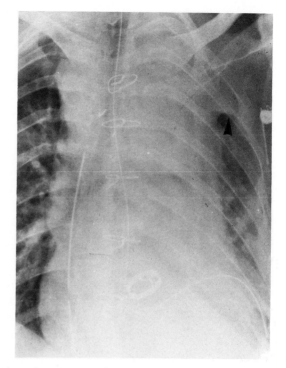

Figure 26–50. Mediastinal hematoma. There is a widened mediastinal and pericardial silhouette, representing excessive bleeding in the acute post-operative period following aortic valve replacement. The left apical opacity (arrowhead) is a finding of mediastinal bleeding with communication into the extrapleural space.

A chyloma is a localized mediastinal collection of chyle or lymph and is the forerunner of a chylothorax. A chyloma may be apparent in the acute postoperative period, whereas a chylothorax is usually not apparent until well into the intermediate period.[6] This complication is discussed in a later section (see The Intermediate Period, pp. 1795–1796; Fig. 26–65).

Pulmonary System

The lungs and pleural space are usually normal on the first chest film taken in the acute postoperative period. It is the rule rather than the exception, however, that varying degrees of left lower lobe atelectasis and left pleural effusion develop later in the acute postoperative period (Fig. 26–51). The exact reason for this is unknown. Possible reasons include (1) a lower level of surfactant in the left lower lobe, (2) the physical compression of the left lower lobe by the heart when the patient is in the supine position, and (3) mucous plugs not removed by endotracheal tube suction owing to the bronchial anatomy (that is, the right bronchus being easier to enter than the left). The radiologic findings include disappearance of the left hemidiaphragm (the silhouette sign) and increased opacity in the retrocardiac area. There may be air bronchograms in the left lower lobe. The increased opacity in the left lower lobe can be easily detected when this area is compared with the retrocardiac density to the right of the spine. They should normally have equal gray densities, but the postoperative problem in the left lower lobe causes a "white-out" in the left retrocardiac area.

Any pulmonary opacity other than the left lower lobe white-out should be considered to be abnormal. Pulmonary edema is usually diffuse but may occasionally be localized to one lobe or segment. Its rapid appearance or disappearance should help to distinguish it from other pathologic processes. Pneumonia is extremely unlikely to be the cause of a pulmonary opacity in the acute postoperative period.

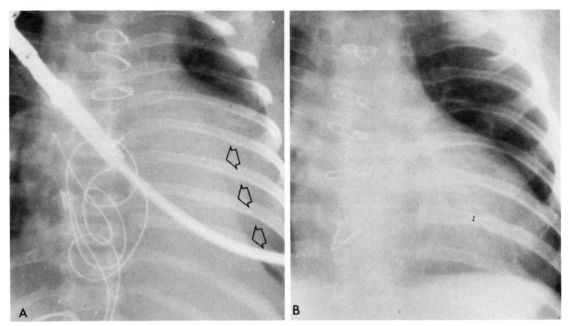

Figure 26–51. Left lower lobe atelectasis. *A,* Anteroposterior chest film 36 hours postoperatively with retrocardiac opacity (arrows) representing left lower lobe atelectasis. *B,* The same patient seven days postoperatively, showing complete clearing of left lower lobe atelectasis.

A diffuse lung opacity that at times mimics unilateral pulmonary edema is the posteriorly layered pleural effusion (Fig. 26–52). This is the normal distribution for pleural fluid in the supine patient. The distinguishing features are a small lateral or apical collection of pleural fluid (Fig. 26–52B), a left-sided location, and the appearance of normal vessels despite a diffuse opacity (Fig. 26–52). If doubt remains, a lateral decubitus or cross-table lateral film is definitive.

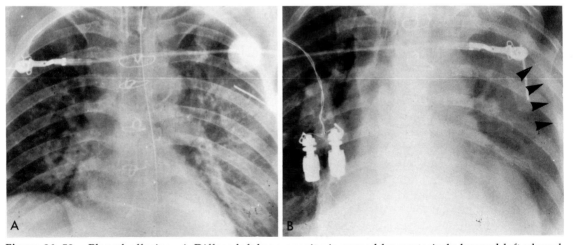

Figure 26–52. Pleural effusion. *A,* Diffuse left lung opacity is caused by posteriorly layered left pleural effusion. A characteristic finding differentiating this from a parenchymal opacity (pneumonia, edema, and so forth) is the normal appearance of the left lung vessels. *B,* Diffuse left lung and left pleural opacity (arrowheads) caused by large left pleural effusion.

Pulmonary contusion following lateral thoracotomy is unusual, but it is a possibility when a localized pulmonary opacity is present in the immediate postoperative period in a patient with an ipsilateral thoracotomy (Fig. 26–53). Operative pulmonary contusions are seen most often in the outer two thirds of the midlung zone. The opacity usually begins to resolve in the first several postoperative days.

Postoperative parenchymal atelectasis occurs infrequently outside the left lower lobe. It is demonstrated radiographically by a localized uniform opacity and reduced lung volume. On anteroposterior supine chest films, reduced volume is difficult to detect since common signs (elevated hemidiaphragm, shifted mediastinum, approximation of the ribs, compensatory overinflation, and so forth) are usually absent. A shift in the position or the orientation of the horizontal fissure is easily detected, however, and aids in the recognition of right-sided volume loss (Fig. 26–54).

Linear plates of focal atelectasis are not uncommon and are usually seen in the lower lung fields. These are thought to be related to the decreased respiratory excursions and pain-related suppression of cough. The linear densities can appear or disappear within hours or days.

Pneumothorax is a precarious condition in the patient who already has postoperative pulmonary dysfunction (Fig. 26–55). A careful search along the outer margins of the lung should be made on all films in order to detect the pneumothorax as early as possible (Fig. 26–55A). If a small pneumothorax is detected, its development may be followed by serial radiographic examinations. However, the postoperative intensive care personnel should be contacted in order to watch and prepare for any sudden increase in the size of the pneumothorax.

Occasionally, a vertical fissure line is mistaken for the lung margin of a small pneumothorax.[3] However, careful examination will reveal lung markings lateral to this line. The vertical fissure line is a thin radiopaque line paralleling the lateral thoracic wall in the lower portion of the chest (Fig. 26–56). It extends in a vertical direction from the lateral portion of the diaphragmatic dome and terminates at the level of the hilum.

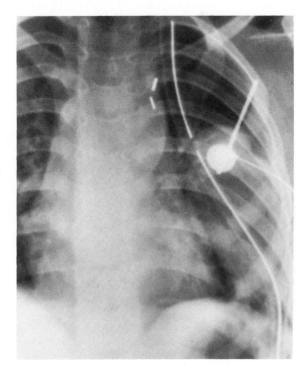

Figure 26–53. Pulmonary contusion. There is a localized peripheral left lower lung pulmonary opacity following ipsilateral thoracotomy.

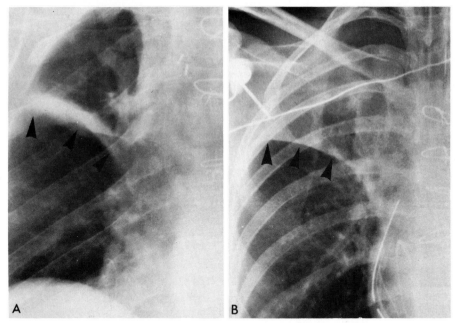

Figure 26–54. Right upper lobe atelectasis. Segmental (*A*) and diffuse (*B*) right upper lobe volume loss is detected by upward deviation of the horizontal fissure (arrowheads).

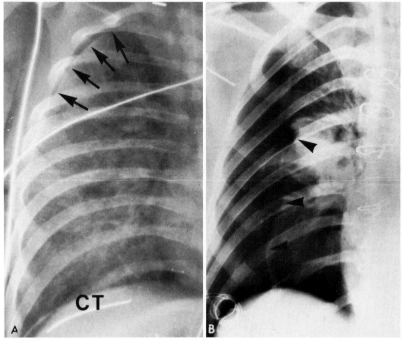

Figure 26–55. Pneumothorax. *A,* Postoperative right thoracotomy. There is a localized right apical pneumothorax (arrows) in the presence of a low right chest tube (CT). *B,* Postoperative median sternotomy with large right-sided pneumothorax (arrowheads).

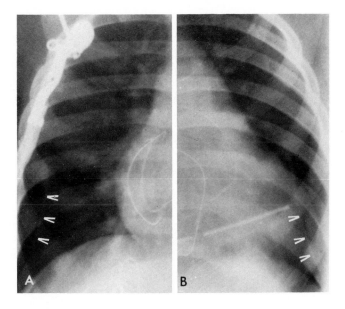

Figure 26–56. Vertical fissure line. Right-sided (*A*) and left-sided (*B*). A thin vertical line (arrowheads) parallels the lateral chest wall on the postoperative anteroposterior chest in two young patients. This line represents the lower portion of the major fissure seen end-on and should not be mistaken for the visceral pleura of a pneumothorax.

It is thought to represent the lower portion of the major fissure seen on end owing to an alteration in the position of the middle and lower lobes. It is seen more frequently on the right side (Fig. 26–56*A*) than on the left (Fig. 26–56*B*) and in infants and young children. It is most often seen in patients with cardiomegaly and congestive heart failure.[3]

Abdomen

The upper abdomen is usually readily seen on the postoperative chest film. Gastric distention is easily detected (see Fig. 26–45*B*). Pneumoperitoneum is more difficult to recognize in the supine chest film and small amounts of intraperitoneal air often go unnoticed (Fig. 26–57). Free intraperitoneal air in patients undergoing median sternot-

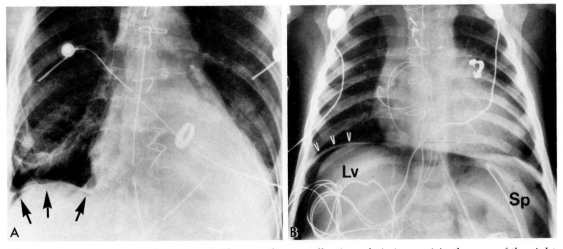

Figure 26–57. Pneumoperitoneum. *A,* The curvilinear collection of air (arrows) in the area of the right hemidiaphragm represents a small pneumoperitoneum. *B,* A massive pneumoperitoneum outlines liver (Lv), spleen (Sp), and diaphragm (arrowheads).

omy may be the result of the extension of the sternotomy incision into the abdomen. In the presence of pneumomediastinum, air may dissect from the mediastinum into the abdomen, usually retroperitoneally.

Postoperative ileus is not uncommon but is usually transient. A significantly progressive ileus should alert the radiologist to the possible development of ischemic nonobstructive enterocolitis, a reversible complication of shock or low cardiac output.

THE INTERMEDIATE PERIOD

The approach to chest films taken 3 to 14 days postoperatively is similar to that used in the acute period (0 to 48 hours), although the types of abnormalities and complications are different. The patient is no longer in the intensive care unit, he is ambulatory, and he is usually able to have upright posteroanterior and lateral chest films taken. The patient free of complications usually has only one or two sets of chest films made during this period.

Assist Devices

Assist and monitoring devices have usually been removed by this time. In fact, these devices usually remain in use only when the postoperative course is abnormal. The only assist devices normally present during this period are the temporary epicardial pacing wires (Fig. 26–58), and they are usually removed on the day before the patient's discharge from the hospital.

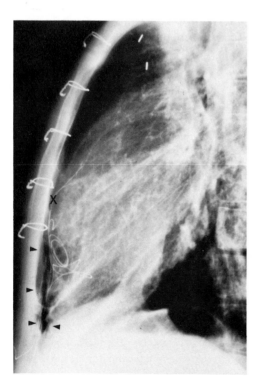

Figure 26–58. Normal seven-day postoperative chest. A small amount of lower retrosternal air (arrowheads) and thin radiopaque temporary pacing wires (X) are seen on the lateral chest film.

Skeletal Structures and Soft Tissues

Right and left lateral thoracotomies normally show predictable radiographic changes in the intermediate postoperative period. These include soft tissue edema, localized pleural thickening, and sometimes minor rib changes. The findings of a large soft tissue mass (hematoma) or air in the soft tissue (subcutaneous emphysema) are common minor complications (Fig. 26–59). A rib fracture near or at the site of the thoracotomy is a complication that may not be detected radiographically until the intermediate period, owing to the superior resolution of nonportable films.

The vast majority of patients undergoing median sternotomy have no complications related to the site of the incision. Occasionally, dehiscence of the wound occurs, however. Radiographically, this appears as broken sternal wires, and a widening "midsternal stripe" (Fig. 26–60).[5] Dehiscence tends to occur in patients undergoing prolonged mechanical ventilation or in those with a wound infection.

Cardiac and Mediastinal Structures

During the intermediate period there should be a return to the normal or preoperative state from the cardiac-mediastinal widening seen during the acute period. It is imperative that preoperative films be reviewed for comparison with films made during the intermediate period or before the patient's discharge. Slight increases in

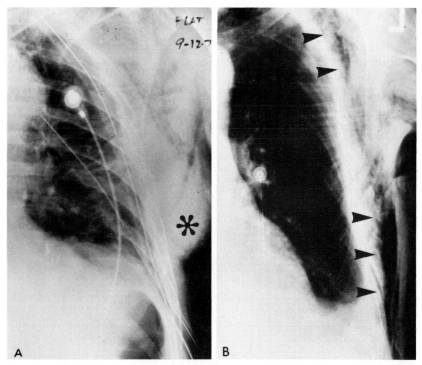

Figure 26–59. Abnormal findings of lateral thoracotomy on the intermediate postoperative chest film. A large soft tissue hematoma (A,*) and large amount of subcutaneous emphysema (B, arrowheads) complicate lateral thoracotomy in two different patients.

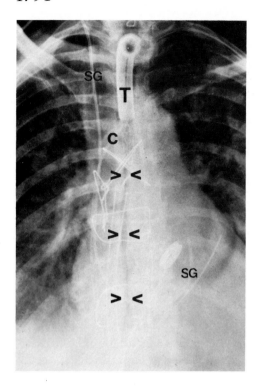

Figure 26–60. Sternal dehiscence. Radiographic signs of sternal dehiscence include the widened midsternal stripe (arrowheads) and additional sternal wires and mediastinal drains. Other assist devices include a tracheostomy tube (T), a Swan-Ganz catheter (SG), and a venous catheter (C).

mediastinal width or cardiac silhouette size are not uncommon or important, but any *significant* increase in the heart size or the width of the mediastinum is abnormal (Fig. 26–61). Possible causes of these conditions include hemopericardium, mediastinal hematoma, mediastinitis, cardiac tamponade, heart failure, and chyloma. Mediastinal hematoma is usually benign and tends to resolve with time. Mediastinitis should be

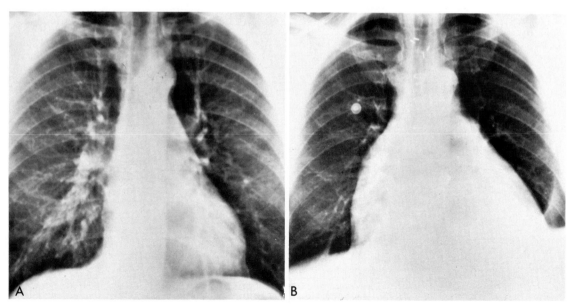

Figure 26–61. Hemopericardium. *A,* The preoperative chest film is normal. *B,* Seven days following aortic valve replacement there are bilateral pleural effusions and marked widening of the pericardial-cardiac silhouette.

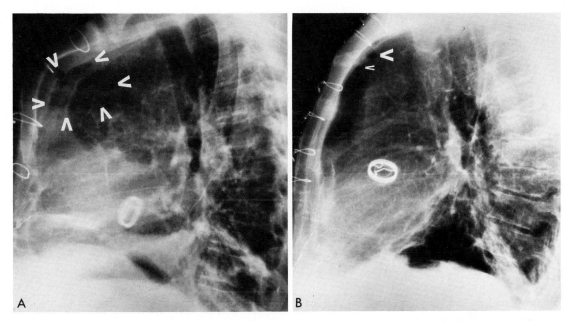

Figure 26–62. Mediastinitis. Superior retrosternal air bubbles (arrowheads) on the lateral chest films of two different patients following mitral (*A*) and aortic (*B*) valve replacement are an early radiographic sign of mediastinitis.

suspected when localized air bubbles or air-fluid levels are seen in the retrosternal area on the lateral film, with or without mediastinal widening (Fig. 26–62). Hemopericardium with cardiac tamponade is usually suggested by clinical deterioration and is seen radiographically as widening of the cardiomediastinal structures. *It is a true surgical emergency.*

A chyloma, as mentioned in the discussion of the acute postoperative period, is the forerunner of a chylothorax. It appears radiographically as a localized superior mediastinal mass that develops during the acute or intermediate period (Fig. 26–65). It resolves when the ipsilateral chylothorax develops. Rarely, chylopericardium may cause cardiac tamponade.

Pulmonary System

In the intermediate postoperative period, radiographic pulmonary abnormalities usually include some degree of opacity in the left lower lung. The opacity is the result of varying degrees of left lower lobe atelectasis or left pleural effusion. By the time of the patient's discharge the x-ray may show a small, residual opacity in the left lower lobe and left or bilateral small pleural effusions (Fig. 26–63). These abnormalities are the usual findings and should be regarded as such.

Significant postoperative abnormalities are usually apparent radiographically. The most common postoperative pulmonary problems are atelectasis and effusion. When small and localized to the left lower lobe, they are considered to be usual findings. When localized to the right lung or when large, they are considered significant postoperative abnormalities (Fig. 26–64). Pulmonary edema is typically generalized, but it may be localized and mimic pneumonia. Pneumonia and pulmonary infarction are unusual radiographic findings in the postoperative chest, however. Any right-sided

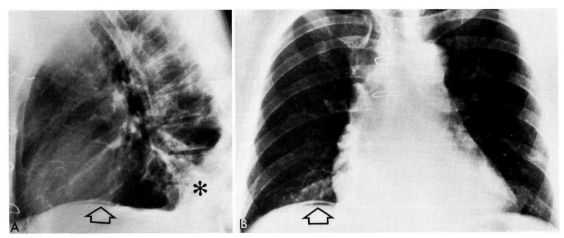

Figure 26–63. Usual findings on the intermediate postoperative chest film. Small bilateral pleural effusions and mild left lower lobe volume loss (*), both of which are better detected on the lateral (*A*) than on the posteroanterior (*B*) chest film, are the usual seven-day postoperative findings. Note the small pneumoperitoneum (arrow).

pulmonary abnormality is significant, and the usual radiographic criteria for diagnosis should be used.

The presence of chylothorax should be suspected when an effusion develops during the later part of the intermediate period, particularly when there was a preceding chyloma (Fig. 26–65). A chylothorax is most likely to occur in children following operations on or around the aortic isthmus, that is, a systemic-pulmonary artery shunt (initial procedure or removal at subsequent repair), coarctation repair, and the ligation of patent ductus arteriosus.[6] Rarely, chylothorax may develop following median sternotomy for intrapericardial surgery and is thought to originate from the anterior mediastinum in the region of the thymic tissue.[7] Chylothorax is usually large, unilateral (left- or right-sided) and recurrent even months after apparent resolution.

Phrenic nerve paralysis is usually first recognized when the patient is no longer on the respirator. It may be suspected in the acute period, but the findings are more specific in the intermediate period, in which films are made in the erect position. The primary sign is an elevated diaphragm. This complication may have to be distinguished from a subpulmonary effusion. If paralysis is suspected, inspiration and expiration films or fluoroscopy can be used to document the abnormality. Phrenic nerve paralysis is more common on the left side and may occur following cardiac operations from a lateral thoracotomy or a median sternotomy (Fig. 26–66 and 26–67).

Postoperative pneumothorax may first be detected in the intermediate period owing to the increased sensitivity of the upright chest film in detecting small amounts of pneumothorax. An expiratory film accentuates a questionable pneumothorax. A small apical pneumothorax in a clinically stable patient usually resorbs and can be followed radiographically.

Abdomen

Abnormal abdominal findings in the chest that may be detected in the intermediate postoperative period include splenomegaly secondary to the postperfusion syndrome,[1] hepatomegaly secondary to right heart failure, persistent ileus, and pneumoperitoneum. Pneumoperitoneum may first become evident in the upright films

Figure 26–64. Pleural effusions in the intermediate postoperative period. *A,* Posteroanterior chest film seven days postoperatively shows moderate bilateral pleural effusions (*). *B,* Posteroanterior and left lateral decubitus (*C*) chest film in another patient with left-sided subpulmonary pleural effusion. The subpleural effusion can be suspected from the posteroanterior chest (*A*) by the increased distance between the stomach (S) and the "apparent" left hemidiaphragm (arrow). Left lateral decubitus film (*C*) demonstrates a large left pleural effusion (arrowheads) freely layered in the dependent portion of the left chest.

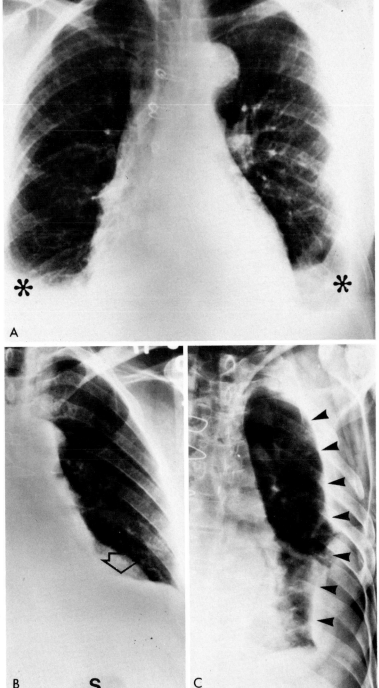

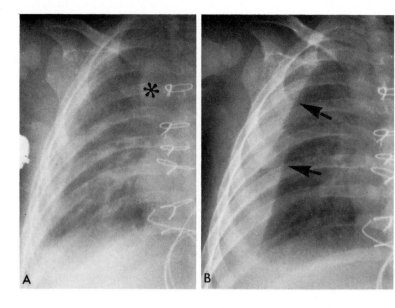

Figure 26–65. Chylothorax. *A,* A two-day postoperative chest film following repair of tetralogy of Fallot and ligation of a patent ductus arteriosus showing right paratracheal mass (*) representing a chyloma. *B,* A seven-day postoperative chest film demonstrating an increasing right pleural effusion (arrows) representing a chylothorax and resolution of the chyloma.

made during this period, since small or moderate amounts of pneumoperitoneum are difficult to detect in films taken with the patient in the supine position, which is required in the acute postoperative period (Fig. 26–67). The most common cause of pneumoperitoneum is inadvertent entrance of air into the peritoneal cavity at the time of median sternotomy. In our experience, the second most common cause of pneumoperitoneum is pneumomediastinum. This occurs most frequently in the postoperative patient requiring prolonged assisted ventilation. The pneumomediastinum itself may be small and clinically inapparent. If it is determined that neither of these conditions caused pneumoperitoneum then rupture of a hollow viscus should be suspected.

THE LATE POSTOPERATIVE PERIOD

Assist Devices

During the late postoperative period the patient usually has no assist or monitor devices. An exception is a patient requiring permanent pacemaker wires (see Fig. 26–43D). A patient who needs continued monitoring and assist devices more than two weeks after surgery usually has significant postoperative cardiac or pulmonary dysfunction. The analysis of assist devices during this period is similar to that in the acute postoperative period.

Skeletal Structures and Soft Tissues

The approach to the chest films of patients with known or suspected heart disease should always involve a systematic search of the soft tissues and bony structures for evidence of previous surgery. The radiographic indications of previous right or left lateral thoracotomy include asymmetry of the soft tissues, asymmetry of the ribs, and localized pleural thickening (Fig. 26–68). Previous median sternotomy is almost always demonstrated by the presence of radiopaque sternal wires, except when the surgery was performed in infancy, when nonradiopaque sutures may have been used.

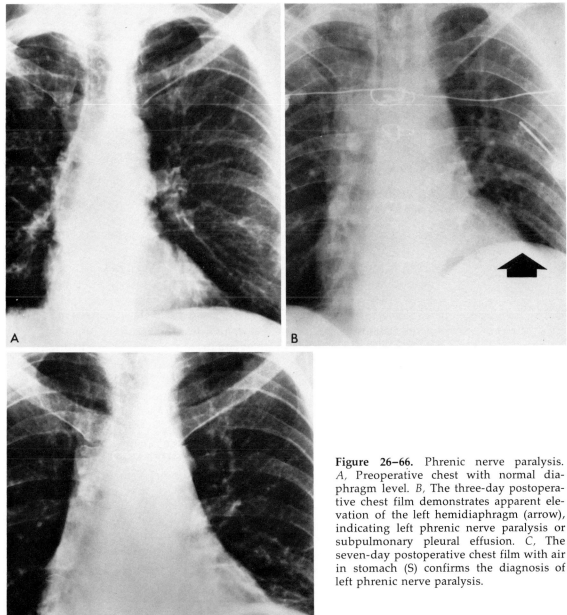

Figure 26–66. Phrenic nerve paralysis. *A,* Preoperative chest with normal diaphragm level. *B,* The three-day postoperative chest film demonstrates apparent elevation of the left hemidiaphragm (arrow), indicating left phrenic nerve paralysis or subpulmonary pleural effusion. *C,* The seven-day postoperative chest film with air in stomach (S) confirms the diagnosis of left phrenic nerve paralysis.

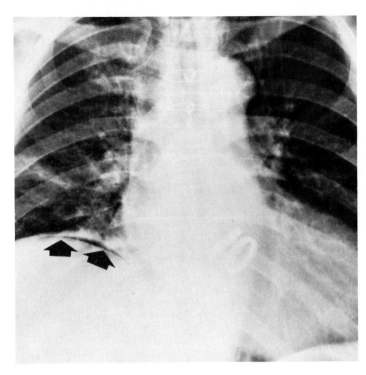

Figure 26–67. Right phrenic nerve paralysis and pneumoperitoneum. Elevation of the right hemidiaphragm was present on the erect chest film seven days following mitral and aortic valve replacement. The pneumoperitoneum (arrows) was small and resolved spontaneously.

Once previous surgery is detected, the type of operation, and thereby the type of cardiac abnormality, can usually be determined if one knows the common operations performed from a right or left thoracotomy or a median sternotomy. A partial listing is given in Table 26–1.

Combinations (a right or left thoracotomy and a median sternotomy) usually indicate that correction (median sternotomy) of cyanotic congenital heart disease (Fig. 26–68D) and a previous palliative procedure (right or left thoracotomy) were performed.

Postoperative osteomyelitis or wound dehiscence in the late postoperative period is rare. Broken sternal wires in an otherwise normal chest are usually not significant but should be noted, since they may be a source of localized postoperative chest pain (Fig. 26–69).

Cardiac and Mediastinal Structures and Pulmonary System

During the late postoperative period cardiac and mediastinal size and contour should return to normal, and the physiologic condition of the pulmonary vasculature (shunt, pulmonary venous hypertension) to normal or nearly normal. The repaired atrial septal defect and patent ductus arteriosus show prominent vascularity for several months. Once the patient's baseline postoperative x-ray appearance is established, any increase in the size or change in the contour of the heart, or change in the pulmonary vascular pattern (for example, from normality to pulmonary edema) must be considered in light of the previous surgery (Fig. 26–70). Specific complications are discussed in Parts II and III of this chapter.

Recurrent or late hemopericardium with cardiac tamponade may occur as late as two to four weeks postoperatively and is a true surgical emergency. The clinical signs may be varied. Widening of the cardiomediastinal structures may or may not be

Text continued on page 1804

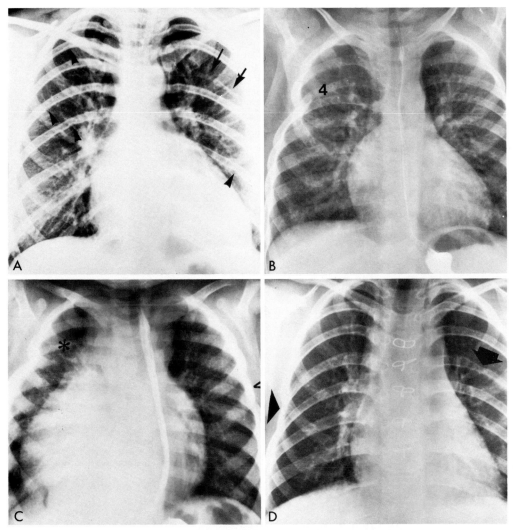

Figure 26–68. Previous surgery. *A,* Regeneration of the left fifth rib (arrows) and bilateral rib notching (arrowheads) indicate repair of coarctation of the aorta. The persistent rib notching does not necessarily indicate inadequate repair of the coarctation. *B,* Asymmetry of the rib cage with irregularities of the right fourth rib (4) indicates a previous right-sided thoracotomy. This patient has tricuspid atresia and a previous superior vena cava–right pulmonary artery (Glenn) anastomosis. *C,* Right fourth posterior rib (*) is small and irregular and indicates a previous right-sided thoracotomy (Glenn shunt). The left fifth rib is flattened laterally (arrowhead) and represents a subtle radiographic finding of previous right-sided thoracotomy (Blalock-Taussig shunt). This patient has a cardiac malposition and complex cyanotic congenital heart disease with severe obstruction to pulmonary flow. *D,* Postoperative left (arrow) and right (arrowhead) thoracotomies for palliative systemic-to–pulmonary artery shunts and median sternotomy for complete repair in patient with tetralogy of Fallot.

TABLE 26–1. OPERATIONS PERFORMED FROM RIGHT AND LEFT THORACOTOMIES AND MEDIAN STERNOTOMY

Right Thoracotomy	Left Thoracotomy	Median Sternotomy
Systemic-to-pulmonary artery shunts	Systemic-to-pulmonary artery shunts	Septal defect repair
Right subclavian artery to RPA (Blalock-Taussig) (Fig. 26–68D)	Left subclavian artery to LPA (Blalock-Taussig) (Fig. 26–68C and D)	Semilunar valve Valvotomy Replacement
Ao to RPA (Waterston)	PDA ligation	AV valve
SVC to RPA (Glenn) (Fig. 26–68B and C)	Coarctation repair (Fig. 26–68A)	Valvotomy or valvoplasty Replacement
Atrial septostomy (Blalock-Hanlon)	Pulmonary artery banding	Repair complex heart disease
ASD closure	Mitral valve commissurotomy (closed)	Tetralogy (Fig. 26–68D)
Mitral valve surgery (uncommon) Commissurotomy Replacement	Descending aortic aneurysm repair	Transposition (Mustard or Senning repair)
		Ascending aortic aneurysm repair
		Coronary artery bypass grafting (CABG)

Abbreviations:
Ao = aorta
ASD = atrial septal defect
AV = atrioventricular
LPA = left pulmonary artery

PDA = patent ductus arteriosus
RPA = right pulmonary artery
SVC = superior vena cava

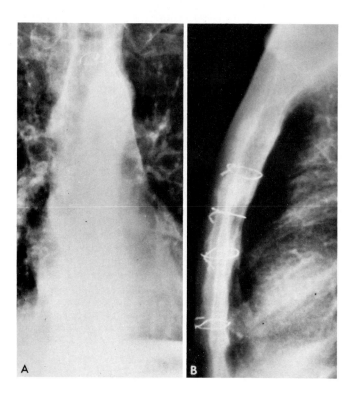

Figure 26–69. Broken sternal wires. Posteroanterior (*A*) and lateral (*B*) late postoperative chest film, with broken top (*A*) and bottom (*B*) sternal wires.

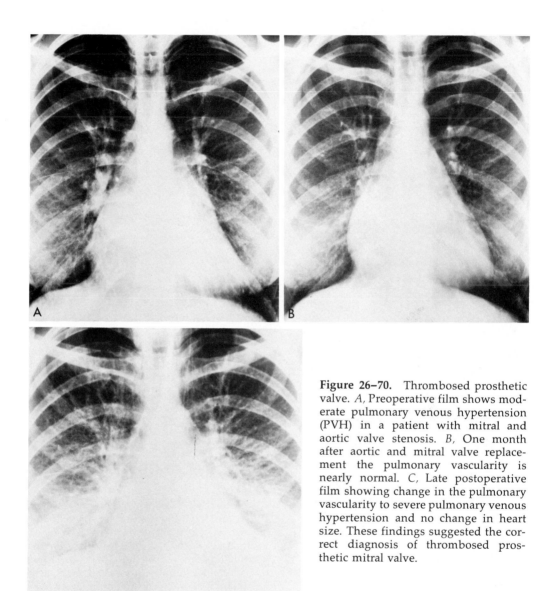

Figure 26–70. Thrombosed prosthetic valve. *A,* Preoperative film shows moderate pulmonary venous hypertension (PVH) in a patient with mitral and aortic valve stenosis. *B,* One month after aortic and mitral valve replacement the pulmonary vascularity is nearly normal. *C,* Late postoperative film showing change in the pulmonary vascularity to severe pulmonary venous hypertension and no change in heart size. These findings suggested the correct diagnosis of thrombosed prosthetic mitral valve.

present. A more specific radiographic finding is a change in the size or the configuration of the cardiac silhouette, detected by the comparison of serial films. Additional radiographic findings include nearly normal pulmonary vascularity and enlargement of the azygous vein and of the superior vena cava secondary to elevated right-heart filling pressure.

The postpericardiotomy syndrome consists clinically of fever, pericarditis, and pleurisy; it develops two to four weeks after surgery.[4] The radiologic manifestations include pericardial effusion and pleural effusions, usually on the left side (Fig. 26–71).

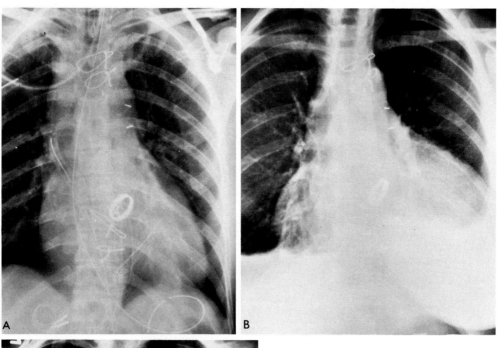

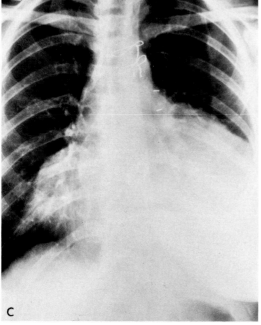

Figure 26–71. Postpericardiotomy syndrome. One-day (*A*), seven day (*B*), and fifteen-day (*C*) postoperative films in a patient with aortic valve replacement demonstrate enlarging heart size and bilateral pleural effusions (left greater than right) with normal pulmonary vascularity. These findings are nonspecific but should suggest the postpericardiotomy syndrome with enlarging pericardial effusion.

Occasionally, pulmonary infiltrates may be present. The diagnosis of the syndrome is made clinically and may be supported by the radiographic findings. These radiographic findings may mimic those seen in cases of hemopericardium and cardiac tamponade, however.

References

1. Austen, W. G., and Hutter, A. M.: Acquired mitral and tricuspid disease. *In* Sabiston, D.C. (ed.): Davis-Christopher Textbook of Surgery. Ed. 2. Philadelphia, W. B. Saunders Company, 1977, p. 2371.
2. Curtis, J. A., Libshitz., H. I., and Dalinka, M. K.: Fracture of the first rib as a complication of midline sternotomy. Radiology *115*:63–65, 1975.
3. Davis, L. A.: The vertical fissure line. Am. J. Roentgenol. *84*:451–453, 1960.
4. Ebert, P. A.: The pericardium. *In* Sabiston, D.C. (ed.): Davis-Christopher Textbook of Surgery. Ed. 2. Philadelphia, W. B. Saunders Company, 1977, p. 2174.
5. Escovitz, E. S., Okulski, T. A., and Lepayowker, M. S.: The midsternal stripe: a sign of dehiscence following median sternotomy. Radiology *121*:521–524, 1976.
6. Higgins, C. B., and Reinke, R. T.: Postoperative chylothorax in children with congenital heart disease. Radiology *119*:409–413, 1976.
7. Joyce, L. D., Lindsay, W. G., and Nicoloff, D. M.: Chylothorax after median sternotomy for intrapericardial cardiac surgery. J. Thorac. Cardiovasc. Surg. *71*:476–480, 1976.
8. Simeone, J. F., Minagi, H., and Putman, C. E.: Traumatic disruption of thoracic aorta: significance of the left apical extrapleural cap. Radiology *17*:265–268, 1975.

Part V
The Coronary Circulation

DIANA F. GUTHANER, M.D.
IVO OBREZ, M.D., Sc.D.
LEWIS WEXLER, M.D.

The aims of this chapter are to present coronary anatomy as visualized by coronary angiography[1, 8, 31] and to simplify the interpretation of coronary arteriograms by showing how the two-dimensional static radiographic image can be converted into a three-dimensional dynamic reality. This usually requires considerable effort, preferably aided by the use of a three-dimensional model of the heart. Common variations of the basic anatomic patterns of coronary arterial supply are described. These normal variations must be understood for proper interpretation prior to determination of therapy.

The pathophysiologic consequences of an obstruction in a given anatomic site are predictable, although not uniform, and should be looked for in a systematic way. The variety of roentgenographic changes seen on coronary arteriography include irregularity of contour; filling defects and stenoses, either eccentric or concentric; occlusion; dilatation; elongation and tortuosity; and aneurysm formation. These appearances represent pathologic processes of atherosclerosis; e.g., intimal plaque, hemorrhage beneath a plaque, increased thickness of intima and wall, superimposed thrombus, and weakening of muscular and elastic layers of media, respectively. As these changes are presented in two dimensions, one must imagine the cross-sectional anatomy they represent. Examples of nonatheromatous lesions of the coronary arteries encountered in adults are also illustrated, as they may produce symptoms identical to those of atherosclerotic disease. Congenital coronary anomalies that manifest themselves in adult life as myocardial ischemia or that may require modifications of angiographic techniques are also described.

NORMAL ANATOMY AND COMMON VARIATIONS

The spatial concept of the perpendicular relationship of the interventricular septum (IVS) and atrioventricular sulcus (AVS)[19, 44] is a helpful simplification in understanding coronary anatomy in three dimensions. The AVS separating the atria posteriorly and above from the ventricles is seen *en face* in the left anterior oblique projection and can be represented as an open circle. With rotation of the heart into a right anterior oblique projection, the circle closes until it is seen in profile. The IVS, lying perpendicular to the AVS, may similarly be considered as a segment of an open ellipse in the right anterior oblique projection but is seen in profile in the left anterior oblique projection in which the right ventricle lies to the right and the left ventricle to the left. The major coronary arteries lie in these two grooves. The right coronary artery (RCA) courses in the right aspect of the AVS, giving off the posterior descending coronary artery (PDA) at the crux, which then lies in the posterior IVS. The crux is the intersection of the AVS and IVS posteriorly. The left coronary artery (LCA) lies in the left AVS, giving off the left anterior descending coronary artery (LAD), which runs in the anterior IVS and continues in the left AVS as the left circumflex coronary artery (LCx). It is now not difficult to develop the anatomic picture by projecting the major coronary arteries on the AVS and IVS as seen in the oblique projections.

Branches from the RCA or LCx in the AVS can course posteriorly over the atria or anteriorly over the ventricles. Such ventricular branches are known as *marginal* arteries. Those arising from the RCA supplying the right ventricle are called acute marginal branches, while those from the LCx are known as obtuse marginal branches. The posterolateral, or diaphragmatic, surface of the left ventricle is supplied by terminal branches of the RCA, LCx, or both (see further on).

Branches from the arteries in the IVS, the anterior or posterior interventricular arteries, may penetrate the IVS from above or below to supply the septal wall. Epicardial branches of the anterior descending arteries run obliquely over the left ventricle to supply primarily the anterior wall and are known as *oblique,* or *diagonal,* branches. Quite often the first diagonal or first marginal branch is large, supplying a major portion of the anterior wall. If this artery arises near the junction of the LAD and LCx, it is known as the *ramus intermedius* or *intermediate* artery.

A reciprocity exists between adjacent vessels such that in some hearts the diagonal branches are large and the marginal branches small, while the reverse is true for other hearts. It is important for the angiographer to remember that every portion of viable functioning muscle must have a blood supply. Each region of the left ventricular wall should be scrutinized and its vascular supply identified before the examination can be considered complete.

Coronary Preponderance or "Dominance"

Although a multitude of variations occur in the distribution of the major coronary arteries, a reciprocity exists to maintain a uniform myocardial blood flow. This reciprocity involves not only the branches of the left coronary system but also the distribution of the terminal branches of the RCA and the LCx. In attempting to classify these variations in right and left coronary distribution, Banchi[9] defined as "dominant" the coronary artery providing the blood supply to the crux cordis and adjacent areas of the posterior left ventricular wall and IVS. Schlesinger[83] classified the coronary dominance on the basis of origin of the PDA. In essence, all the early definitions of coronary dominance were based on which coronary artery crossed the crux cordis; that is, it was the RCA in right dominance, the LCx in left dominance, and in balanced circulation both the RCA and the LCx reached the crux. Unfortunately, these classifications defining the local arterial distribution at the crux area were later erroneously extended to define the blood supply to the posterior portion of the left ventricle. By this definition, the RCA is dominant in the majority of the human hearts. If, on the other hand, one takes as the criterion of coronary dominance the amount of myocardium supplied by the right or left coronary artery, the LCA is dominant in a majority of hearts: It supplies the anterior and lateral left ventricular wall, most of the septum, and major portions of the left atrium.[48]

Comparative measurements of the diameter of right and left coronary arteries in postmortem perfusion studies as well as in angiograms confirm the concept that the LCA predominates in providing the blood supply in the majority of human hearts, even when the crux area and adjacent portions of the posterior ventricular wall and IVS are supplied by the RCA.[77] Consequently, the term "coronary preponderance" or "dominance" should be used only to define a specific topographic variant of arterial distribution at the crux area.

In the normal coronary system, the variations in coronary arterial distribution do not influence the cardiac blood supply. In diseased coronary arteries, however, the distribution of the right or left coronary artery may be of paramount importance in deciding whether coronary bypass surgery is indicated. Consequently, the definition of coronary dominance can be used to specify a vessel with sufficient run-off to be bypassed in the presence of a significant stenosis. "Right dominance" refers to the situation in which the RCA supplies the PDA and at least several branches to the posterior left ventricular wall. "Left dominance" implies that the LCx supplies the whole of the posterior left ventricular wall and the atrioventricular node artery (AVN) and terminates in the PDA. In this instance the RCA would be nonbypassable because of inadequate run-off even when significantly stenosed. A "balanced circulation" is one in which both the RCA and the LCx supply significant portions of the posterior circulation. Usually the RCA gives off the PDA and perhaps one or two small branches to the posterior wall, while the LCx supplies the major portion of the posterolateral segment. In this case, both RCA and LCx have sufficient flow to maintain patency of a bypass graft.

Coronary Sinuses (Aortic Sinuses of Valsalva)

The aortic valve ring at the base of the heart supports three cusps — the right located to the right anteriorly, the left located to the left and slightly posteriorly, and the noncoronary cusp, located posteriorly and to the right. The inclination of the valve ring brings the left aortic cusp to the highest location and the noncoronary cusp to the lowest position. The coronary ostia are usually situated in the upper portion of their respective sinuses of Valsalva.

Right Coronary Artery (RCA)

The proximal segment is directed toward the right and anteriorly and then curves almost at right angles downward to follow the right AVS. The RCA courses around the

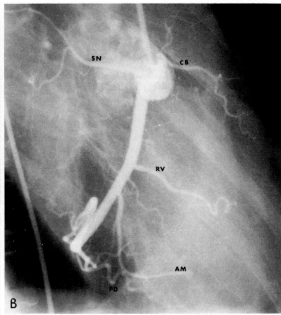

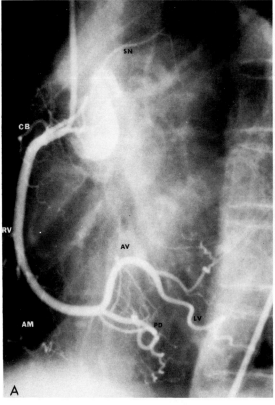

Figure 26–72. Right coronary arteriogram in left anterior oblique (*A*) and right anterior oblique (*B*) projections demonstrating a right dominant coronary system. CB = conus branch; SN = sinus node artery; RV = right ventricular branch; AM = acute marginal branch; PD = posterior descending artery; AV = atrioventricular node artery; LV = posterior left ventricular branch.

right ventricle, best displayed in a left anterior oblique projection (Fig. 26–72). At the acute margin of the heart, marked by an acute marginal branch, it passes posteriorly in the right AVS toward the posterior IVS (crux cordis), where it usually terminates.

The RCA gives rise to the PDA at the crux, the AVN, and branches to the left atrium and ventricle in almost 90 per cent of cases (so-called right dominant circulation) (Fig. 26–72). In the remaining cases, the RCA terminates with a branch to the acute margin (left dominant circulation). Paulin[77] reported that the PDA arose from the LCx in 16 per cent of the coronary arteriograms he reviewed (Fig. 26–73). A small percentage of cases exhibit two PDA's, one arising from the RCA and one from the LCx (balanced circulation). An association of left dominance of the coronary arteries and bicuspid aortic valve has recently been described.[42, 45] Occasionally, a minor variation occurs when the main RCA divides before it reaches the acute margin into a right ventricular branch and a parallel branch that courses along the AVS to give rise to the PDA posteriorly (Fig. 26–74).

PROXIMAL RCA. This segment, by definition, includes the RCA from the coronary ostium to the first major right ventricular branch and gives rise to the conus branch, the sinoatrial node artery (SN), and Kugel's artery. Occasionally the first major septal perforator arises from the proximal RCA (Fig. 26–75).

CONUS BRANCH. Schlesinger et al.[84] described and named this vessel as the third coronary artery and found a separate origin from the aorta in 51 per cent of examined hearts (Fig. 26–76). This incidence was confirmed by James in his studies of coronary artery casts.[47] Paulin was able to identify the pulmonary conus artery in angiograms in 173 cases; in 76 of them the artery arose separately from the aorta or from the right coronary ostium and in 97 cases as one of the first branches of the RCA.[77] He defined the

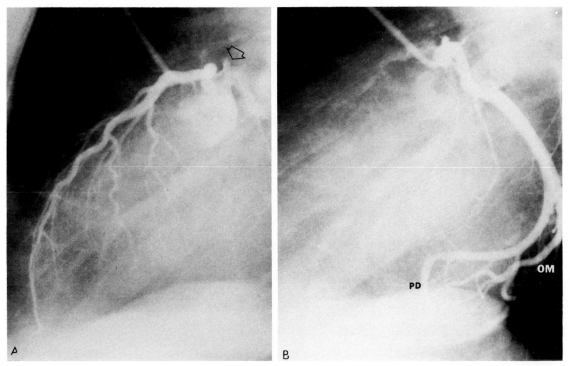

Figure 26–73. Left coronary arteriogram in a lateral projection demonstrates separate LAD and LCx origins. *A,* Selective LAD injection with the LCx origin (arrow) seen with reflux of the contrast. *B,* Selective LCx injection demonstrating a dominant left coronary system. PD = posterior descending artery; OM = obtuse marginal branch.

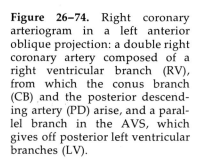

Figure 26–74. Right coronary arteriogram in a left anterior oblique projection: a double right coronary artery composed of a right ventricular branch (RV), from which the conus branch (CB) and the posterior descending artery (PD) arise, and a parallel branch in the AVS, which gives off posterior left ventricular branches (LV).

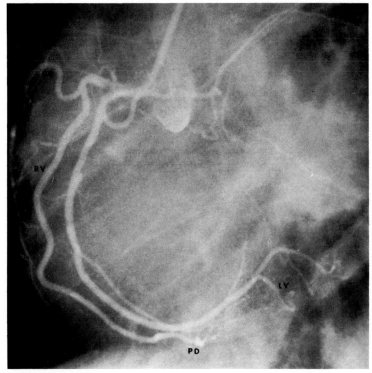

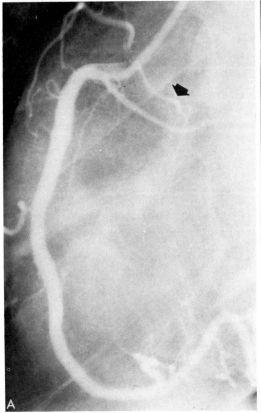

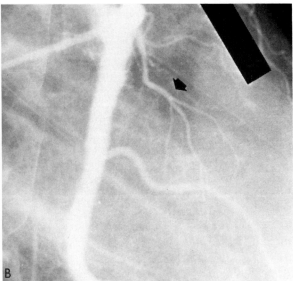

Figure 26–75. Right coronary arteriogram in a left anterior oblique projection (*A*) and detail from a right anterior oblique projection (*B*). The first major septal perforator arises from the proximal RCA (arrow).

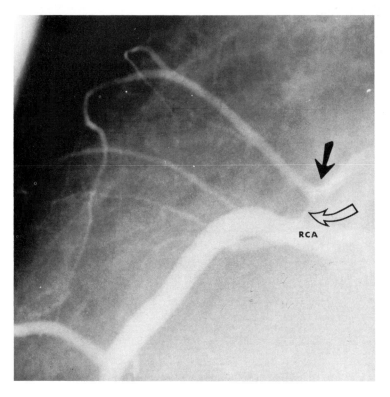

Figure 26–76. Detail from a right coronary arteriogram in the lateral projection: The conus artery arises from a separate ostium (closed arrow). The open arrow indicates the edge of the right aortic sinus. RCA = right coronary artery ostium.

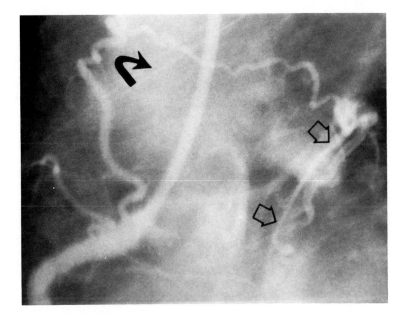

Figure 26–77. Detail of a selective right coronary arteriogram in the left anterior oblique projection: The conus branch fills the proximal LAD (open arrows) of an occluded LAD system via Vieussens' collateral pathway (closed arrow).

variability in caliber, length, and distribution of the vessel. Often, two or more branches run to the pulmonary conus area or one branch gives off several smaller vessels. On the basis of these findings, he classified the various types of right pulmonary conus artery. However, because of the angiographic techniques he used (aortic root injection), he was able to identify the pulmonary conus branches originating from the LAD in only a few cases. The importance of the pulmonary conus artery as a potential collateral pathway between the right and left coronary systems (proximal RCA and LAD) was recognized by Vieussens:[93] the "Vieussens collateral ring" was identified in coronary angiograms by Paulin (Fig. 26–77).[78]

In our experience, using selective coronary arteriography, the right and left pulmonary conus arteries can be identified in most cases unless they originate separately from the aorta. A reciprocity exists between the right and left conus arteries; usually the right conus artery dominates, but occasionally the left conus artery has a larger distribution. A single conus artery without side branches is not seen often. Usually, two or more branches run parallel to the conus area, or several smaller branches arise from a single trunk. If the pulmonary conus artery originates from the aorta at the right coronary ostium, it can be visualized by reflux of contrast medium during injection into the RCA. In fact, the catheter tip may pass directly into the orifice of the conus artery and occlude it. In an extreme variation, the conus artery may originate together with a large right anterior ventricular branch separately from the aorta. In a left anterior oblique projection, the conus branch can be seen doubling on itself from a rightward and cephalad course to a caudad and leftward direction. In a right anterior oblique projection, its course can be followed anteriorly to the right ventricular outflow tract to supply the infundibulum.

Sᴉɴᴜs Nᴏᴅᴇ Aʀᴛᴇʀʏ (SN)   The SN artery was first described by Keith and Flack in 1904.[51] The presence of an artery to the sinus node is constant; however, its origin, course, and distribution of branches may vary considerably. James,[47, 48] using an injection and corrosion technique in heart specimens, found that the SN artery originated from the RCA (usually from its proximal segment) in 54 per cent of cases and from the LCx in 42 per cent; in 2 per cent, both the RCA and the LCx supplied a branch to the sinus node. Other authors have found the SN artery to originate from the RCA in 60 to 65 per cent of cases.

The angiographic anatomy of the SN artery was described by Paulin.[77] In his material, the SN artery arose in 46 per cent from the RCA and in 36 per cent from the LCx. On angiograms, he identified the different levels of origin of the SN artery, the most common site being the proximal segments of the RCA and LCx. He also described some anatomic variations in the course of the SN artery and its terminal branches around the superior vena cava (SVC) as well as the proximal origin of the SN artery. The distribution of the site of origin of the SN artery was also studied in detail by DiGuglielmo and Guttadauro.[20, 21]

It is possible to visualize the sinoatrial trunk in the majority of cases: It passes posteriorly toward the junction of the SVC with the right atrium (RA), supplying two or more superior atrial branches to the right and left atria and terminating in the SN artery proper (see Fig. 26–79). As it encircles the SVC, it has a characteristic arch or parabolic course before it reaches the sinoatrial node. In right anterior oblique projection the conus branch coursing anteriorly is easily separated from the SN artery coursing posteriorly from the AVS (see Fig. 26–72).

Atrial branches coursing in the posterior interatrial septum represent an important potential collateral route between the right and left coronary circulation via the LCx.

KUGEL'S ARTERY. Kugel[55] originally described an atrial artery arising from the LCx and penetrating the atrial septum between the atrioventricular valves. It has three anatomic variations: Most commonly, the artery originates from the proximal portion of the LCx, running in the plane of the atrioventricular rings along the anterior atrial wall, penetrating the interatrial septum close to its connection with the IVS, and terminating posteriorly at the crux, where it anastomoses with branches of the AVN artery. The second variation is an anastomosis between the proximal RCA and LCx, both limbs connecting with terminal branches of the AVN artery. In the rare third variation, small branches in a reticular pattern connect the proximal RCA and LCx with the arterial system at the crux.

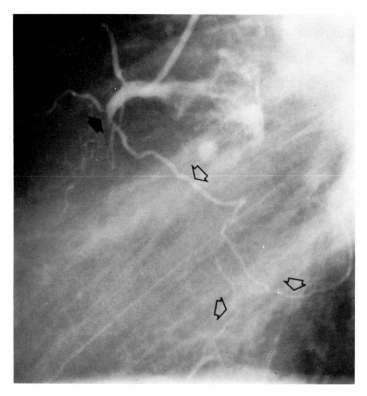

Figure 26–78. An occluded proximal RCA (closed arrow), with reconstitution of the distal vessel via Kugel's collateral pathway (open arrows) seen in the lateral projection.

Subsequent angiographic studies by Paulin[77] have demonstrated a similar inter-atrial branch that arises from the proximal RCA, passes under the right sinus of Valsalva, penetrates the atrial septum, and terminates in an anastomosis with the AVN artery in the ventricular septum. Sometimes this right Kugel's artery originates from the SN artery. Kugel's artery may provide partial blood supply to the AVN, but most importantly it represents a potential collateral pathway between the proximal and distal segments of the RCA (Fig. 26–78). Using postmortem specimens of the heart, Soto and colleagues[91] defined the angiographic anatomy of Kugel's artery more precisely. Although angiographically it is most frequently seen as a branch of the RCA, it can also be seen to arise from the LCx, as originally described by Kugel.

MID-RCA

RIGHT ATRIAL BRANCHES. These comprise varying number of branches passing backward over the right atrium. These branches have been roughly divided into superior, middle, and inferior groups, depending on their site of origin from the RCA.

RIGHT VENTRICULAR BRANCHES (RV). On a right anterior oblique projection, these branches are seen to pass anteriorly over the right ventricle, supplying muscular branches. In a left anterior oblique view, these ventricular branches are foreshortened. As they rise out of the AVS over the ventricular muscle they appear to course laterally and to the right in a loop from their origin at the RCA.

ACUTE MARGINAL BRANCH (AM). This is a large reasonably constant RV branch that courses along the acute margin of the right ventricle, supplying the anterior and diaphragmatic aspects.

DISTAL RCA. This segment extends from the acute margin to the origin of the PDA. Only small branches supplying the posterior ventricular wall arise from the distal RCA. At the crux, where the IVS meets the AVS posteriorly, the distal RCA forms a characteristic inverted U-curve as it passes beneath the posterior interventricular vein and terminates in the following branches.[47, 48]

ATRIOVENTRICULAR NODE ARTERY (AVN). The AVN artery originates, by definition, from the "dominant" coronary artery at the crux cordis. Keith and Flack[51] postulated that in the embryo the artery develops at the epicardial surface. Later, with invagination of the ventricular septum, the atrioventricular node pulls it deep into the myocardium. This process is an alternative explanation for the formation of the characteristic U turn of the posterior descending artery at the crux. In fact, Haas[35] has described two arteries: one providing the blood supply to the parts of the membranous septum, the atrioventricular node, and the bundle of His; and the second supplying borderline segments of the membranous and muscular septum and portions of the bundle branches. In injection and corrosive heart preparations, James[47, 48] has precisely described the topography of the artery and coined the term "atrioventricular node artery," because this vessel regularly supplies significant portions of the atrioventricular node. On the basis of these descriptions, Paulin[77] has identified the AVN artery in coronary arteriograms and has described the angiographic characteristics of the artery as follows: a constant origin from the "dominant" coronary artery at or near the crux; a straight course between the atria toward the noncoronary aortic cusp; a length of one third to three fourths the distance between the RCA and the aortic valve; a diameter of 1 to 1.5 mm; and a perpendicular course of its terminal branch toward the base of the heart (see Fig. 26–79).

We have been able to identify a few anatomic variations of the AV artery in arteriograms. In the most common variation, the AV artery terminated with two or three perpendicular branches. In another variation, two parallel arteries originated

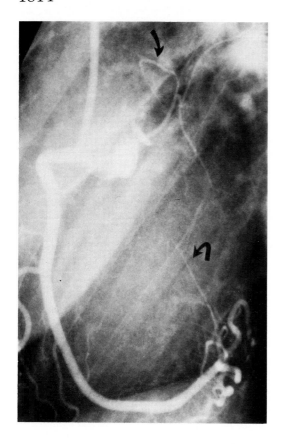

Figure 26–79. Lateral projection of a right coronary arteriogram: The SN branch of the RCA is seen in its characteristic course around the superior vena cava (arrow) and the vertical tail of the AV node artery (curved arrow).

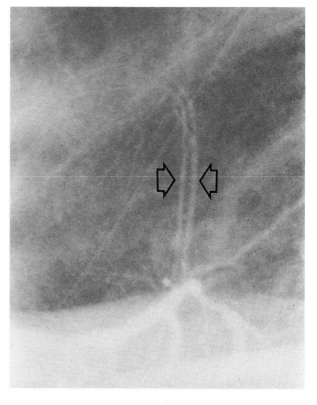

Figure 26–80. Detail of the crux region of a right coronary arteriogram demonstrating double AV node arteries (arrows).

from the "dominant" artery at the crux (Fig. 26–80). Both arteries showed angiographic characteristics of the AV artery. Possibly, this variation of the AV artery represents a simple duplication or an extreme form of the variation described by Haas.[35] Both arteries may contribute blood to the conduction system. It is important to be familiar with this variation, for if either or both arteries become occluded, conduction disturbances may result even though the angiographic findings are apparently normal. In cases of "left dominant" coronary artery, the AV artery originates from the LCx. Its angiographic characteristics are essentially the same as those described. In coronary artery disease, the AV artery may become an important intercoronary collateral route.

POSTERIOR DESCENDING ARTERY (PD). This vessel usually arises proximal to the crux and courses in the posterior IVS toward the apex. Septal branches pass at right angles to penetrate and supply the posterior septum. In a left anterior oblique projection, the PD is foreshortened as it is directed anteriorly. In a right anterior oblique view, it is seen as elongated and superimposed along the acute margin of the heart (see Fig. 26–72). The distal RCA bifurcation is displayed in a shallow left anterior oblique projection with cephalad angulation of the tube. A steep right anterior oblique (greater than 60 degree) projection also demonstrates the origin of the PD. Occasionally, two vessels run parallel along the posterior IVS. In the majority of cases, the PD does not reach the apex, which is then supplied by a recurrent LAD. Anatomic variations of the PD (23 per cent in one series)[58] include a double PD, early origin, and partial supply from acute marginal or posterior ventricular branches.

POSTEROLATERAL LEFT VENTRICULAR BRANCHES (LV). The continuation of the RCA courses in the posterior left AVS to give rise to epicardial branches supplying the posterolateral aspect of the left ventricle.

LEFT ATRIAL BRANCHES (LA). The most distal branches in the posterior left AVS are directed toward the left atrium. These branches may be quite large and completely supply the left atrium and may even give rise to the SN artery.

Left Coronary Artery (LCA)

The LCA supplies blood to most of the left ventricular myocardium. It is directed to the left from the left sinus of Valsalva.

LEFT MAIN CORONARY ARTERY (LMCA). The LMCA is of variable length and optimally is seen elongated in a left anterior oblique projection with craniocaudal angulation of the x-ray beam and in an anteroposterior or very slight right anterior oblique projection. Occasionally, the segment is absent, and the left anterior descending and circumflex coronary arteries arise from separate ostia (see Fig. 26–73). The left coronary artery bifurcates into circumflex branches that continue posteriorly in the left AVS, whereas the LAD courses anteriorly in the IVS, descending toward the apex.

LEFT ANTERIOR DESCENDING CORONARY ARTERY (LAD). The LAD is the direct continuation of the LMCA, coursing to the left and anterior to the main pulmonary artery and then descending toward the apex. From the apex it ascends in the posterior IVS for a varying distance to anastomose with distal branches of the right or left PD. Multiple projections are required to optimally visualize each segment of the LAD — the craniocaudal left anterior oblique or slight right anterior oblique for the proximal horizontal portion and the right anterior oblique or lateral for the mid- and distal LAD. With increasing obliquities of a right anterior oblique projection, the LAD approaches the left cardiac border. On a frontal and shallow right anterior oblique projection, the LAD forms a 90 degree angle as it enters the IVS at the point of origin of a major diagonal branch, which courses along the left heart border in these projections.

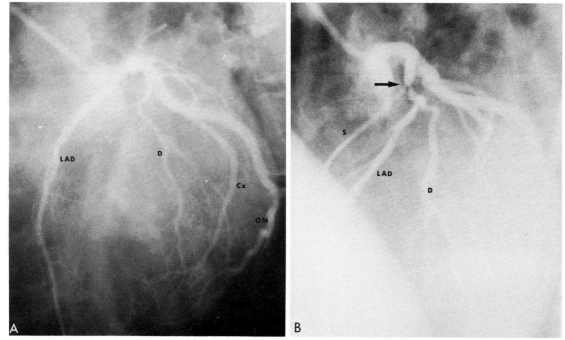

Figure 26–81. Left coronary arteriogram seen in a routine left anterior oblique projection (*A*). In the cranial-caudad left anterior oblique projection (*B*), the LMCA and proximal LAD are elongated, revealing a significant stenosis of the proximal LAD and origin of the first septal (arrow). LAD = left anterior descending artery; D = diagonal; S = septal; Cx = left circumflex artery; OM = obtuse marginal branch. (*From* Eldh, P., and Silverman, J. F.: Methods of studying the proximal left anterior descending coronary artery. Radiology *113*:738–740, 1974. Reproduced by permission.)

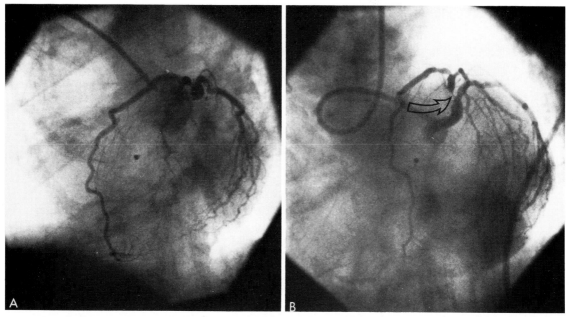

Figure 26–82. Left coronary arteriogram in a routine left anterior oblique projection (*A*) and a left anterior oblique view with caudal-cranial angulation of the x-ray tube ("spider view") (*B*), exposing a tight stenosis (arrow) in a high looping proximal LAD.

In a left anterior oblique projection the LAD courses almost vertically in the IVS. These projections demonstrate the mid- and distal vessel, but the proximal LAD and the region of the LMCA bifurcation are elongated and visualized to best advantage in a steep left anterior oblique projection (about 60 degrees), with a craniocaudal angulation of the tube at approximately 30 degrees (Fig. 26–81). A cephalad loop of the LMCA and proximal LAD is seen to advantage with a caudocranial angulation in a left anterior oblique projection (Fig. 26–82). The lateral projection is useful because it provides maximal separation of the LAD and circumflex coronary arteries and allows optimal visualization of the proximal and mid-LAD. Diagonal branches can be separated from the mid-LAD by angling the tube in a right anterior oblique projection. The LAD and the septal branches lying in the IVS move inward toward the base of the heart, aiding in their differentiation from diagonal and epicardial branches, which display an initial rotary outward motion in systole. Occasionally, the LAD exists as two short parallel branches with a paucity of apical branches.

Proximal LAD

The proximal LAD is the short segment from the origin to the first major septal branch. Rarely, the first major septal artery may arise from the LMCA or LCx near the bifurcation. James[47] also described an anatomic variation in which a major septal branch arose from the RCA and coursed behind the pulmonary artery to the IVS.

First Diagonal Branch.   This courses over the anterolateral aspect of the left ventricle between the IVS and the obtuse margins supplying the free wall.

Mid-LAD

The mid-LAD extends to the 90 degree angle formed by the LAD as it enters the IVS, which usually coincides with the origin of the second diagonal branch.

First Septal Branch.   This is usually the largest septal branch, coursing vertically in the anterior aspect of the septum. It is seen at right angles to the LAD in a right anterior oblique projection and parallel to the LAD in a left anterior oblique projection. A septal perforator occasionally arises from the proximal RCA.

Right Ventricular Branch (RV).   This branch either proceeds toward the infundibulum of the right ventricle, forming the anastomotic pathway of Vieussens with proximal occlusions of the LAD, or anastomoses with RV branches of the RCA to form a collateral pathway over the right ventricular surface.

Septal Branches.   These branches supply the major portion of the interventricular septum. In cases of "left dominant" coronary systems, the LAD and left PD may entirely supply the IVS. The identification of septal arteries in angiograms is usually not difficult. They branch off the LAD and PD almost perpendicularly and show a straight course in the septum with little change during systole. These branches anastomose in the IVS and are important collateral pathways between the LAD and PD.

Second Diagonal and Additional Diagonal Branches.   These branches are distributed to the anterolateral aspect of the left ventricle to the apex.

Apical or Terminal LAD

This is the portion of the LAD distal to the origin of the second diagonal branch, which extends to the apex, sometimes encircling it, and runs for a variable distance in the posterior IVS. The terminal apical branches are distributed to the anterolateral (recurrent lateral apical) and diaphragmatic (recurrent posterior) aspects of the apex.

Left Circumflex Coronary Artery (LCx).   The LCx exhibits considerable variation in its course and extent. It arises from the LMCA at a sharp angle, coursing anteriorly to enter the left AVS. It then proceeds posteriorly to terminate in the obtuse marginal branch in about 84 per cent of cases, and only in the remaining 16 per cent does it reach the crux of the heart to give rise to the left PDA.[77] Because of its close relationship to the AVS, the LCx exhibits an amplitude of motion, reflecting the atrial kick in diastole and a second excursion of movement in ventricular systole.

In a right anterior oblique projection, the LCx is directed caudally in the left AVS with the obtuse marginal (OM) branches coursing over the lateral surface of the left ventricle. In a left anterior oblique projection, it is directed first laterally and then posteriorly, projecting through the inferior third of the cardiac shadow as it runs in the posterior AVS toward the crux. With increasing steepness of a left anterior oblique projection to a lateral projection, the LCx is increasingly separated from the LAD. The proximal LCx is well visualized in a left or right anterior oblique projection with caudocranial angulation.

PROXIMAL LCx

The proximal LCx is a short segment from its origin in the LCA to the first major OM branch, often best displayed with caudocranial angulation of the tube in a right anterior oblique projection.

SINUS NODE ARTERY (SN).   This arises proximally from the LCx in about 50 per cent of cases and describes a sinuous course along the posterosuperior walls of the atria to reach the SVC–right atrial junction.

ATRIAL CIRCUMFLEX BRANCH.   Frequently this slender branch arises close to the origin of the LCx and courses on the atrial aspect of the AVS parallel to the LCx, giving rise to branches coursing posteriorly to supply the atrial walls.

OBTUSE MARGINAL BRANCHES (OM).   These comprise several, often large, branches in the region of the obtuse margin of the heart, which run across the lateral wall of the left ventricle toward the apex. They are best visualized in a right anterior oblique view. The most proximal OM branch may arise as a trifurcation from the LMCA and is then named an intermedius branch (Fig. 26–83).

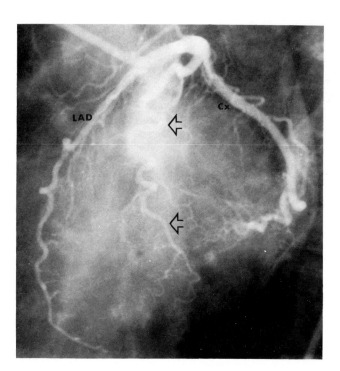

Figure 26–83.   Left coronary arteriogram in a left anterior oblique projection: An intermedius branch (open arrows) arises as a trifurcation from the LMCA. LAD = left anterior descending coronary artery; Cx = left circumflex coronary artery.

LEFT KUGEL'S ARTERY.   This branch penetrates the atrial septum, courses between the tricuspid and mitral valves to the posterior portion of the interventricular septum, and terminates near the AVN artery. Angiographically, it is less frequently seen than the right Kugel's artery.

DISTAL LCx

The distal portion is the continuation of the LCx in the posterior left AVS distal to the OM branches. The LCx may terminate in the OM branches, may continue beyond the OM branches toward the crux of the heart, or may continue from the crux as the left PDA in a "left dominant" circulation.

POSTEROLATERAL LEFT VENTRICULAR BRANCHES (PL).   Depending on the relative preponderance of the LCx, these branches supply a variable portion of the left ventricle. They are usually terminal branches of the LCx and are distributed to the posterolateral surface of the left ventricle. In a left anterior oblique projection, they tend to run diagonally from the obtuse margin toward the septum. Terminal branches of a dominant RCA run in the opposite diagonal direction from right to left. This difference is often useful to distinguish normal left posterolateral branches from posterolateral branches of an occluded RCA, which fill from collaterals during the LCA injection.

Coronary Venous System

The coronary sinus drains most of the blood from the heart. Two basic venous systems exist, but numerous anatomic variations occur.

The left ventricle is drained by several epicardial veins that tend to accompany the epicardial arteries.[19] They enter a large vein in the left AVS, the coronary sinus (CS), which empties into the right atrium. The great cardiac or anterior interventricular vein courses with the LAD from the apex to the base of the heart near the origin of the LCx artery, where it empties into the CS. A second major tributary of the CS is the middle cardiac or posterior interventricular vein, which runs with the PDA along the inferior cardiac surface from the apex to the base of the heart, where it enters the CS just before it enters the right atrium. Left diagonal and obtuse marginal veins drain the posterolateral wall of the left ventricle. The right ventricle is drained by the small cardiac or acute marginal vein, which courses along the acute margin of the heart and from the right AVS enters the CS inferiorly or the right atrium at a separate site. A network of veins — the anterior cardiac veins — encircle the right ventricular infundibulum to empty into the right atrium at the junction of the SVC and the right atrium. The oblique vein of Marshall or the left atrial vein, the vestige of the left superior cardinal vein, courses obliquely over the posterior surface of the left atrium and drains into the great cardiac vein. The CS, with the thebesian valve at its ostium, empties into the right atrium between the inferior vena cava and the tricuspid valve.

Thebesian veins[73] are tiny channels draining directly from the myocardium into the atrial and ventricular chambers.

Occasionally, an anomalous left superior vena cava, the remnant of the left anterior and common cardinal vein, empties directly into an enlarged coronary sinus as it passes behind the left atrial appendage (Fig. 26–84).

CORONARY COLLATERAL CIRCULATION

The concept of coronary arteries being "end arteries" is no longer held.[82]

An extensive network of intracoronary and intercoronary anastomoses can be

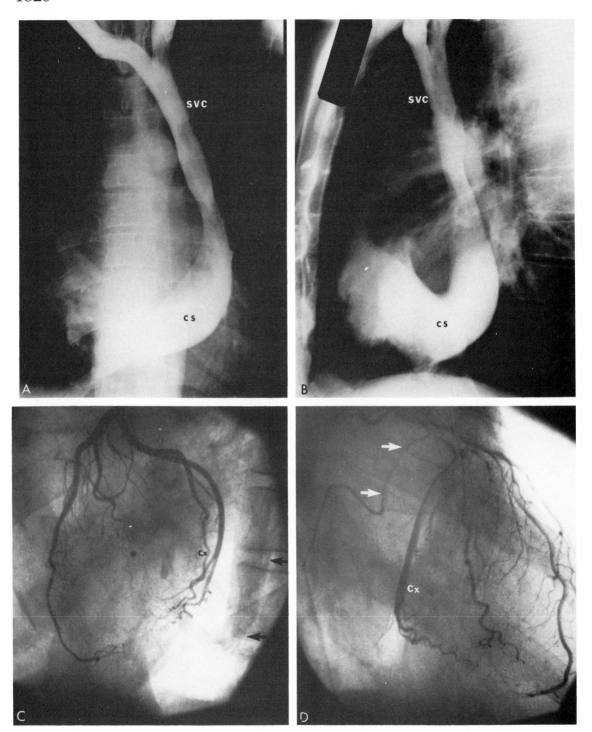

Figure 26–84. *A* and *B,* Superior venacavagram demonstrating a left superior vena cava (SVC) emptying into a large coronary sinus (CS), which is seen draining into the right heart in a frontal (*A*) and lateral (*B*) projection. *C,* Left coronary arteriogram in a left anterior oblique projection: The large coronary sinus occupies the space between the left circumflex artery (Cx) and the edge of the heart border (arrows). *D,* In the right anterior oblique projection the CS lies between the atrial circumflex branch (arrows) on the atrial aspect of the atrioventricular groove and the left circumflex artery.

demonstrated by infusion and corrosion studies even in normal hearts.[28, 49, 80] However-
er, these channels function only if a need arises.[97] A disparity therefore exists between
the anatomic presence of collateral channels and their functional patency.[57] One of the
principal stimuli for the functioning of these potential anastomoses is the development
of collateral circulation, as in response to a pressure gradient across a stenosis. With
resting flow, a pressure gradient exists across a stenosis when the stenosis exceeds 90
per cent. With higher flow demands, a less severe stenosis will cause a pressure
gradient. The extent and degree of myocardial ischemia is dependent on both the rate of
progression of a coronary obstructive lesion and the rate of development of functioning
collateral channels to ameliorate the decreased blood flow.[39]

The radiographic anatomy of the coronary collateral circulation has been studied by
Paulin,[78] Gensini and daCosta,[32] Jochem et al.,[50] and Sheldon.[88]

A. *Collateral circulation to LAD*

1. Intracoronary collaterals
   (a) Bridging collaterals from proximal to distal septal branches of LAD
   (b) Bridging collaterals from proximal diagonal to distal diagonal branches of
       LAD
2. Intercoronary collaterals from LCx
   (a) Proximal OM to proximal diagonal branches
   (b) Distal OM to distal LAD over the apex
   (c) Dominant LCx and AVN artery to LAD septal branches
3. Intercoronary Collaterals from RCA
   (a) Right PDA to LAD septal branches
   (b) Right ventricular branches to LAD
   (c) Right PDA or right acute marginal to LAD over the apex
   (d) RCA to LAD via conus branches of Vieussens' anastomotic ring

B. *Collateral circulation to LCx*

1. Intracoronary collaterals
   (a) Bridging collaterals from proximal to distal LCx
   (b) Proximal OM to distal OM branches
   (c) Left atrial Cx to distal LCx
   (d) Kugel's artery from proximal to distal Cx
2. Intercoronary collaterals from LAD
   (a) Diagonal to OM branches
   (b) LAD to distal OM over the apex
3. Intercoronary collaterals from RCA
   (a) Distal RCA to OM branches
   (b) Distal RCA or AVN artery to inferior atrial branches of LCx
   (c) Proximal RCA and right SN artery around atria to distal LCx
   (d) Proximal RCA to AVN artery via Kugel's artery and distal LCx in left dom-
       inant circulation

C. *Collateral circulation to RCA*

1. Intracoronary collaterals
   (a) Bridging collaterals from proximal to distal RCA (Fig. 26–85)
   (b) Proximal to distal acute marginal branches
   (c) Conus to lower acute marginal branches
   (d) Proximal RCA to distal RCA via Kugel's artery
   (e) Atrial branches, including SN artery, from proximal to distal RCA

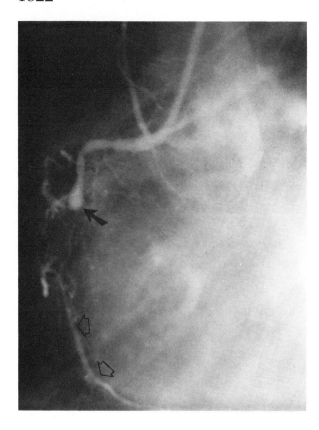

Figure 26–85. Right coronary arteriogram in a left anterior oblique projection: Occluded proximal RCA (closed arrow) is seen with reconstitution of the mid- and distal RCA (open arrows) via bridging intracoronary collaterals.

Figure 26–86. Left coronary arteriogram in a lateral projection: Septal intercoronary collaterals (arrow) from the LAD fill the PDA (open arrows) distal to an RCA occlusion.

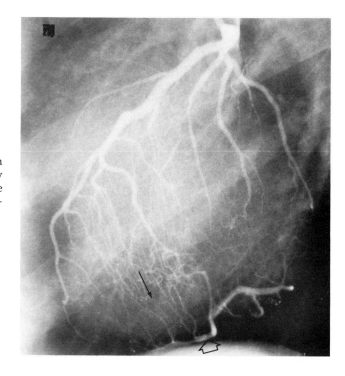

2. Intercoronary collaterals from LAD
   (a) Diagonal to right ventricular branches of RCA
   (b) LAD septal branches to PDA (Fig. 26–86)
   (c) LAD to right PDA over apex
   (d) LAD to proximal RCA via conus branches of Vieussens' ring
3. Intercoronary collaterals from LCx
   (a) Distal OM to posterolateral branches of RCA
   (b) Left atrial Cx to distal RCA or AVN artery
   (c) Proximal LCx to distal RCA via Kugel's artery

Other extracoronary channels, such as bronchial and mediastinal vessels, also contribute to collateral circulation. Two important collateral pathways were described by Kugel and Vieussens. In the presence of severe obstructive stenosis of the RCA or LCx, Kugel's artery[55] represents an important potential collateral pathway, which may connect the proximal portions of the LCx and RCA with the AVN artery and the posterior coronary arterial system (see Fig. 26–79). The importance of pulmonary conus arteries as a potential collateral pathway was recognized pathologically by Vieussens[93] and subsequently identified in coronary angiograms by Paulin.[77] The direction of blood flow through Vieussens' collateral ring over the pulmonary conus is usually from the right to the occluded LAD (see Fig. 26–77). However, cases in which Vieussens' ring developed in the presence of an occluded or severely stenotic proximal RCA have been reported.

Collateral channels have been shown to develop only with progression of obstructive lesions to greater than 75 per cent of the luminal diameter.[37] In general, it is believed that coronary collaterals will develop if luminal narrowing occurs slowly and increased coronary blood flow is stimulated, by exercise, for example. The recruitment of collateral anastomoses is available for improved resting flow and during periods of increased flow demands. In these instances, the preformed collaterals may be protective of myocardial damage in the presence of subsequent total occlusion of a previous stenosis. This concept may explain the paradox of single-vessel stenosis or occlusion leading to a large ventricular aneurysm, whereas severe three-vessel occlusion with numerous collaterals may occur with normal function of the myocardium. However, coronary collaterals cannot be relied on to protect against myocardial ischemia, at least as determined by treadmill exercise testing.[70]

CONGENITAL CORONARY ARTERY ANOMALIES

Anomalous Aortic Origin of Coronary Arteries

A variety of minor anomalies of the origin of the coronary arteries have been recognized, several of which have already been mentioned.[3, 13, 24, 74]

The conus branch may have a separate aortic origin, and the LAD and LCx may arise separately from the left sinus of Valsalva. Anomalous origin, however, implies that a coronary artery arises from an unusual portion of the aorta, e.g., the LCx from the right sinus of Valsalva. An unrecognized coronary anomaly may lead to errors in interpretation of coronary angiograms.[64] The danger of inadvertently injuring an anomalous coronary artery during valve replacement or excluding it from perfusion during open heart surgery has demanded the preoperative identification of such anomalies.[52] There have been isolated reports of sudden death associated with a major coronary artery coursing between the aorta and the main pulmonary artery.[11, 12, 16, 60] These anomalous vessels may be more likely to develop atheroma than normal vessels[89] because of their acute angle of origin[65] or because of the trauma resulting from their course between the great arteries. If one bears in mind that the entire regional myocardial blood supply to the left ventricle must be accounted for at coronary arteriography, it is unlikely that coronary anomalies will be overlooked.

ANOMALOUS LCx. The most common anomaly, that of the LCx originating from the proximal RCA or the right sinus of Valsalva (a reported frequency of 0.45 per cent,[15] was first described in 1933 by Antopol and Kugel[5] and in 1948 by White and Edwards.[94] In the majority of cases the LCx arises from the right sinus of Valsalva or the proximal RCA and follows a characteristic course posterior to the aorta.[76] A clue to the presence of this anomaly is a long nonbranched LMCA prior to continuation of the vessel in the IVS (Fig. 26–87).

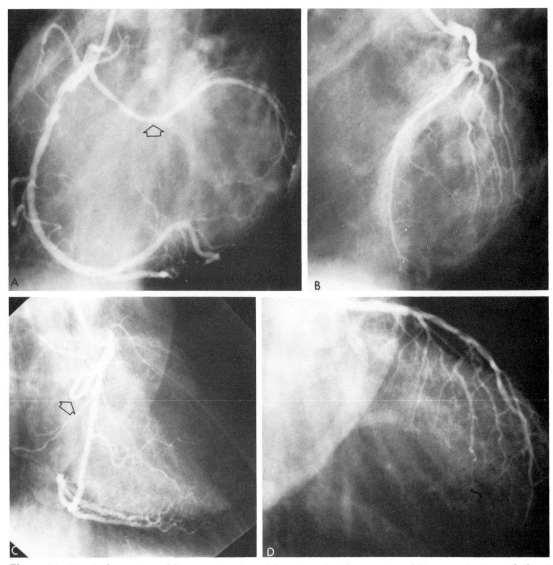

Figure 26–87. Left anterior oblique projections (above) and right anterior oblique projections (below) of right coronary arteriogram (*A* and *C*) and left coronary arteriogram (*B* and *D*): An anomalous circumflex (arrow) arises from the proximal RCA passing behind the aorta. The characteristic nonbranching segment of the LMCA is seen best in *B*.

Other less common anomalies include origin of both coronary arteries from the left sinus of Valsalva, the RCA coursing between the aorta and the pulmonary artery; origin of both coronary arteries from the right sinus of Valsalva, with the LMCA located either anterior or posterior to the aorta and then continuing between the aorta and pulmonary artery; origin of the LAD from the right sinus of Valsalva; and origin of the first septal perforator from the right sinus of Valsalva or the proximal RCA.

SINGLE CORONARY ARTERY (SCA). Single coronary artery is a rare congenital anomaly with an estimated incidence of 0.04 per cent.[33, 87] Approximately 40 per cent of

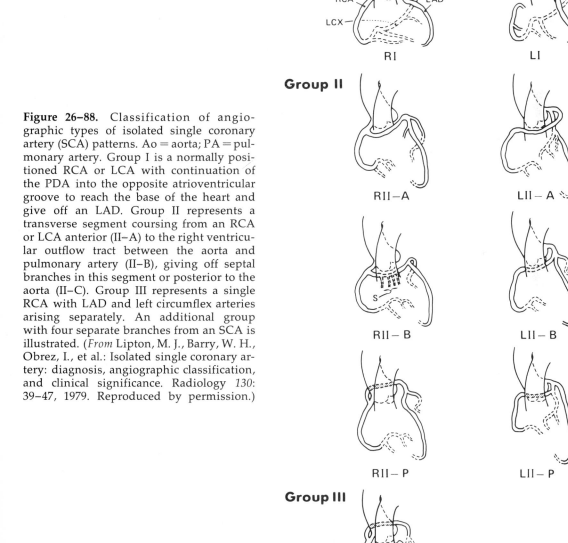

Figure 26–88. Classification of angiographic types of isolated single coronary artery (SCA) patterns. Ao = aorta; PA = pulmonary artery. Group I is a normally positioned RCA or LCA with continuation of the PDA into the opposite atrioventricular groove to reach the base of the heart and give off an LAD. Group II represents a transverse segment coursing from an RCA or LCA anterior (II–A) to the right ventricular outflow tract between the aorta and pulmonary artery (II–B), giving off septal branches in this segment or posterior to the aorta (II–C). Group III represents a single RCA with LAD and left circumflex arteries arising separately. An additional group with four separate branches from an SCA is illustrated. (*From* Lipton, M. J., Barry, W. H., Obrez, I., et al.: Isolated single coronary artery: diagnosis, angiographic classification, and clinical significance. Radiology *130:* 39–47, 1979. Reproduced by permission.)

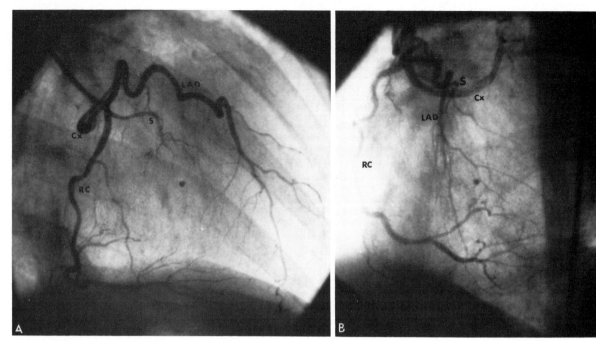

Figure 26–89. Right anterior oblique (*A*) and left anterior oblique (*B*) projections of a single right coronary artery (RC) that supplies an LAD, passing anterior to the pulmonary artery, a retroaortic circumflex (Cx), and a septal branch (S).

cases of SCA are associated with congenital cardiac anomalies. An angiographic classification has recently been proposed (Fig. 26–88).[62] We have seen an additional type in which the septal artery arose as a separate branch from the trifurcation of the SCA (Fig. 26–89). In effect, the SCA arose from the right sinus, divided into the RCA running in the right AVS, with the LCx coursing posterior to the aorta to the left AVS, the septal branch running between the aorta and the pulmonary artery, and the LAD passing anterior to the aorta to the IVS.

Anomalous Coronary Artery Arising from the Pulmonary Artery

Bland[14] first reported the detailed clinical and pathologic description of this anomaly, which in contrast to the previously described anomalies is hemodynamically significant.[59]

The LCA originates from the main pulmonary artery in 90 per cent of cases; the remainder include the more benign anomalous origin of the RCA from the pulmonary artery (Fig. 26–90).[56] The origin of the LAD as an accessory artery from the pulmonary artery has also been reported. Rarely, both RCA and LCA arise anomalously, a situation incompatible with survival. The majority of patients with anomalous LAD from the pulmonary artery (75 per cent) present as infants and children and die from myocardial ischemia and infarction. In 25 per cent of cases, they survive to adulthood, when they present with angina or mitral regurgitation.[46, 59] These patients are liable to sudden death because of inadequate myocardial blood supply from the LCA, which is perfused at low pressure and low oxygen tension. The presence of a coronary artery steal mechanism, secondary to the arteriovenous shunt created by blood passing from the RCA to the LCA via collaterals and retrograde into the pulmonary artery, was first described by Baue.[10] The greater the extent of collateralization and resulting shunt, the better the prognosis.

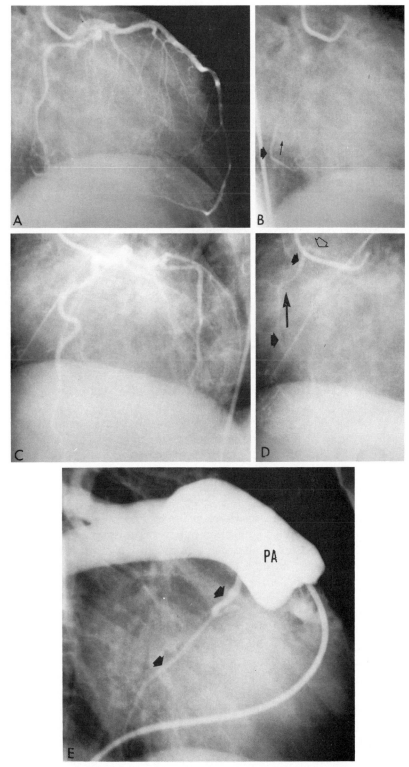

Figure 26–90. Early (*A* and *C*) and late (*B* and *D*) phases of a left coronary arteriogram in right anterior oblique (*A* and *B*) and left anterior oblique (*C* and *D*) projections: The RCA fills (arrows) in a retrograde direction to empty into the pulmonary artery (open arrow, *D*). Pulmonary artery injection (*E*) demonstrates the anomalous RCA (arrows) filling in an antegrade direction from the pulmonary artery (PA).

Supravalvular aortography or selective right coronary arteriography demonstrates a large, tortuous RCA, with the LCA filling via intercoronary collaterals retrograde into the pulmonary artery. Angiography is the most reliable method of demonstrating the small left-to-right shunt, with confirmation made only occasionally by a slightly elevated oxygen saturation in the pulmonary artery.

In the past, the surgical technique most frequently performed for anomalous LCA was ligation of the LCA at its origin from the pulmonary artery.[18, 36] The LCA was still supplied through the low-pressure collateral bed from the RCA, and there was a danger of recurrence with incomplete ligation in the presence of several openings into the pulmonary artery. The current surgical approach is the improvement of myocardial revascularization by use of an aortocoronary saphenous vein graft together with closure of the orifice in the pulmonary artery.[54]

Anomalous Coronary Arteries in Congenital Heart Disease

Coronary arterial patterns may be specific to certain congenital cardiac lesions and may even be useful in differentiating lesions, e.g., transposition complexes.[23] It is necessary to delineate the coronary anatomy preoperatively, so that major coronary branches are avoided during ventricular surgery. In both D-transposition and L-transposition, the noncoronary sinus, normally posterior, becomes the anterior right aortic sinus. In corrected or L-transposition with ventricular inversion, the coronary anatomy is inverted, matching the ventricles. The anatomic LCA originates from the right posterior sinus and gives rise to the LAD and a circumflex branch running in the right AVS. The right Judkins catheter will usually successfully catheterize this right-sided coronary artery, which supplies the systemic ventricle. The anatomic RCA arises from the left posterior aortic sinus and gives rise to the artery running in the left AVS. Angiographically, it looks like a mirror image of an RCA.

In D-transposition of the great vessels, a variety of coronary artery patterns have been described, but the most common is the origin of the RCA from the posterior right aortic sinus, to give rise to the LCx coursing posterior to the pulmonary artery. Their origins may be single or double. The LAD then arises from the left posterior aortic sinus, or the LCA arises from the left and the RCA from the right posterior sinus. Other variations include a single coronary artery arising from the posterior coronary sinus or the left sinus or the LCx arising from the LCA or from the posterior sinus.[23, 86] Coronary artery patterns may be useful as a guide to atrioventricular discordance, in that the course of the LAD delineates the position of the IVS.[34]

In the majority of cases of double-outlet right ventricle, the coronary artery is normally situated with the noncoronary sinus posterior.[23, 92] There have been occasional reports of coronary artery anomalies in double-outlet right ventricle. The coronary artery pattern in common ventricles corresponds to that most commonly seen with either dextro- or levo-looped ventricles.

In tetralogy of Fallot, an anomalous coronary artery distribution occurs in 4 to 9 per cent of patients.[26, 38, 53, 69] The origin of the LAD from the RCA or from a separate ostium in the right aortic sinus is the most frequent coronary anomaly associated with tetralogy of Fallot, or dextroposed aorta.[95] The LAD then courses over the anterior surface of the right ventricular outflow tract to reach the anterior IVS.[63] Secondary to right ventricular hypertrophy, the conus branch of the RCA is a large branch crossing anterior to the right ventricle. The preoperative recognition of the anomalous LAD or large conus branch is important to avoid inadvertent damage to them during right ventriculotomy.[29] The second most common coronary anomaly is an SCA originating from either the left or the right sinus. The LAD is again at risk when the LCA arises from the RCA and passes anteriorly over the right ventricle or when the RCA arising from the left sinus passes in front of the right ventricle.

Coronary Artery Fistulas

Coronary arteriovenous fistulas connect the major coronary artery (arising from the RCA in just over 50 per cent of cases, from the LCA in just under 50 per cent and from both in up to 10 per cent)[7, 96] directly with a cardiac chamber or vessel (Fig. 26–91).[68] In over 90 per cent of cases, the fistula empties into right-sided structures (right ventricle, right atrium, pulmonary artery, SVC, or CS), resulting in a small left-to-right shunt. The remaining fistulas drain into the left atrium or ventricle.[6]

In most cases a precordial continuous murmur prompts catheterization and angiography, often in asymptomatic patients.[59] However, older patients tend to develop symptoms secondary to atrial fibrillation and resulting cardiac failure, to subacute bacterial endocarditis, to myocardial ischemia secondary to a coronary steal phenomenon, or to rupture of the fistula or an associated aneurysm. Selective coronary arteriography demonstrates the fistulous origin from the proximal coronary artery, the enlarged, tortuous anastomotic channel(s) or plexus of vessels; its drainage into the recipient chamber or vessel; and the diminutive distal vessel attributed to the "steal" of coronary blood flow by the fistula.[71, 90]

Lesions with similar physical findings, such as patent ductus arteriosus, aortic–right ventricular fistula, aortopulmonary window, and a ventricular septal defect with aortic insufficiency, must be excluded.[71] Early prophylactic interruption of the fistula has been advocated because of the later development of symptoms and the increased postoperative complications in older patients.[61]

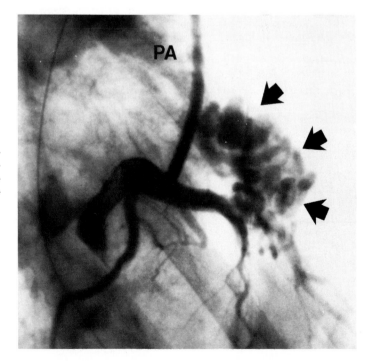

Figure 26–91. Left coronary arteriogram in a right anterior oblique projection demonstrating a fistulous communication (arrows) with the pulmonary artery (PA).

NONATHEROMATOUS OBSTRUCTIVE LESIONS

Myocardial Bridges

Occasionally, the large epicardial branches of the LCA, especially the LAD, leave the epicardial surface and turn for a variable distance a few millimeters within the myocardium. This intramyocardial segment is "bridged" by myocardial bands; it can be transiently compressed during systole, producing a "milking" effect, while flow remains normal during diastole (Fig. 26–92).[4, 30, 79] Although it is generally believed that the intramural segments of the coronary artery are protected against atheromatous development,[72, 79] this concept has not been confirmed in studies by Edwards et al.[22]

Myocardial bridging seen on coronary arteriography has long been considered of no clinical significance. However, symptomatic bridging[25, 72] of the coronary artery confirmed by electrocardiographic evidence of myocardial ischemia has been reported recently as well as lactate production during pacing, requiring surgical intervention, periarterial muscle resection, and bypass graft placement.

Coronary Artery Spasm

Coronary artery spasm has recently been implicated not only as the etiologic factor in Prinzmetal's variant angina but in some cases as the cause of myocardial infarction and typical angina.[43, 66, 67] The intermittent narrowing of a coronary artery, whether focal, involving multiple segments, or progressing to total occlusion, may occur spontaneously or following pharmacologic provocation and is reversible with vasodilators, such as nitroglycerin and the alpha-adrenergic blocker phentolamine.

In comparison with a fixed lesion, the hallmark of a spastic lesion is the dynamic range of the vessel caliber. Such coronary artery spasm causes significant myocardial ischemia and is associated with the clinical picture seen in patients with Prinzmetal's angina; chest pain occurs at rest with concomitant electrocardiographic changes, usually ST elevation, although T-wave inversion and ST depression have also been described. In this syndrome, spasm may be superimposed on severe proximal fixed lesions or may occur in the presence of minor narrowing or apparently normal coronary arteries.[41] The pathophysiology, however, has not been elucidated.[81]

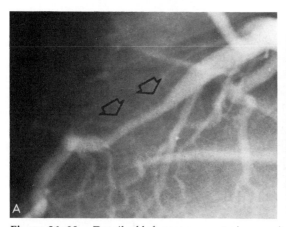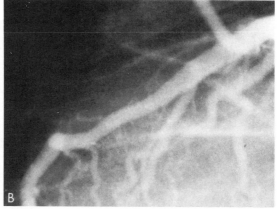

Figure 26–92. Detail of left coronary arteriogram in the lateral projection during systole (*A*) and diastole (*B*). A narrowing due to the intramyocardial course of the LAD, a "muscle bridge" (arrows), is seen on the systolic frame.

The use of ergonovine maleate as a provocative test for coronary artery spasm has been shown to be highly sensitive in patients with variant angina.[17, 40, 85] However, spasm demonstrated at the time of angiography must be differentiated from fixed stenoses and also from the more commonly encountered catheter-induced spasm.[27] The latter type occurs as an isolated lesion around the catheter tip, most frequently when the RCA is catheterized, and may extend distally or involve a segment remote from the catheter tip. Catheter-induced spasm is characterized by its reversibility following catheter removal or vasodilator therapy, the lack of pharmacologic reproducibility, and the absence of associated symptoms or electrocardiographic changes.

References

1. Abrams, H. L., and Adams, D. F.: Coronary arteriography. *In* Abrams, H. L. (ed.): Angiography. Vol. 1. Ed. 2. Boston, Little, Brown & Company, 1971, p. 401.
2. Adams, D. F., Abrams, H. L., and Ruttley, M.: The roentgen pathology of coronary artery disease. Semin. Roentgenol.7:319, 1972.
3. Alexander, R. W., and Griffith, G. C.: Anomalies of the coronary arteries and their clinical significance. Circulation *14*:800–805, 1956.
4. Amplatz, K., and Anderson, R.: Angiographic appearance of myocardial bridging of the coronary artery. Invest. Radiol. *3*:213–215, 1968.
5. Antopol, W., and Kugel, M. A.: Anomalous origin of the left circumflex coronary artery. Am. Heart J. *8*:802, 1933.
6. Arani, D. T., Greene, D. G., and Klocke, F. J.: Coronary artery fistulas emptying into left heart chambers. Am. Heart J. *96*:438, 1978.
7. Babb, J. D., and Field, J. M.: Double coronary arteriovenous fistula. Chest *72*:656–658, 1977.
8. Baltaxe, H. A., Amplatz, K., and Levin, D. C.: Coronary Angiography. Springfield, Illinois, Charles C Thomas, Publisher, 1963.
9. Banchi, A.: Morfologia delle arteriae coronariae cordis. Arch. Ital. Anat. Embriol. *3*:87, 1904.
10. Baue, A. E., Baum, S. Blakemore, W. S., et al.: A later stage of anomalous coronary circulation with origin of the left coronary artery from the pulmonary artery: coronary artery steal. Circulation *36*:878–885, 1967.
11. Benson, P. A.: Anomalous aortic origin of coronary artery with sudden death: case report and review. Am. Heart J. *79*:254–257, 1970
12. Benson, P. A., and Lack, A. R.: Anomalous aortic origin of left coronary artery: report of two cases. Arch. Pathol. *86*:214–216, 1968.
13. Blake, H. A., Manion, W. C., Mattingly, T. W., et al.: Coronary artery anomalies. Circulation *30*:927–940, 1964.
14. Bland, E. F., White, P. D., and Garland, J.: Congenital anomalies of coronary arteries: report of an unusual case associated with cardiac hypertrophy. Am. Heart J. *8*:787, 1933.
15. Chaitman, B. R., Lesperance, J., Saltiel, J., et al.: Clinical, angiographic and hemodynamic findings in patients with anomalous origin of the coronary arteries. Circulation *53*:122–131, 1976.
16. Cheitlin, M. D., Decastro, C. M., and McAllister, H. A.: Sudden death as a complication of anomalous left coronary origin from the anterior sinus of Valsalva: a not-so-minor congenital anomaly. Circulation *50*:780–787, 1974.
17. Cipriano, P. R., Guthaner, D. F., Orlick, A. E., et al.: The effects of ergonovine maleate on coronary arterial size. Circulation *59*:82, 1979.
18. Cooley, D. A., Hallman, G. L., and Bloodwell, R. D.: Definitive surgical treatment of anomalous origin of left coronary artery from pulmonary artery: indications and results. J. Thorac. Cardiovasc. Surg. *52*:798–808, 1966.
19. Daves, M. L.: Cardiac roentgenology: the loop and circle approach. Radiology *95*:157–160, 1970.
20. Diguglielmo, L., and Guttadauro, M.: A roentgenologic study of the coronary arteries in the living. Acta Radiol. (Suppl.) *97*:1–82, 1952.
21. Diguglielmo, L., and Guttadauro, M.: Anatomic variations in the coronary arteries: an arteriographic study in living subjects. Acta Radiol. *41*:393–416, 1954.
22. Edwards, J. C., Burnsides, C., Swarm, R. L., et al.: Arteriosclerosis in the intramural and extramural portions of coronary arteries in the human heart. Circulation *13*:235–241, 1956.
23. Elliott, L. P., Amplatz, K., and Edwards, J. E.: Coronary arterial patterns in transposition complexes: anatomic and angiocardiographic studies. Am. J. Cardiol. *17*:362–378, 1966.
24. Engel, H. J., Torres, C., and Page, H. L., Jr.: Major variations in anatomical origin of the coronary arteries: angiographic observations in 4,250 patients without associated congenital heart disease. Cathet. Cardiovasc. Diagn. *1*:157–169, 1975.

25. Faruqui, A. M. A., Maloy, W. C., Felner, J. M., et al.: Symptomatic myocardial bridging of coronary artery. Am. J. Cardiol. 41:1305–1310, 1978.

26. Fellows, K. E., Freed, M. D., Keane, J. F., et al.: Results of routine preoperative coronary angiography in tetralogy of Fallot. Circulation 51:561–566, 1975.

27. Friedman, A. C., Spindola-Franco, H., and Nivatpumin, T.: Coronary spasm: Prinzmetal's variant angina vs. catheter-induced spasm: refractory spasm vs. fixed stenosis. Am. J. Roentgenol. 132:897, 1979.

28. Fulton, W. F. M.: Arteriography, microanatomy and pathogenesis of obliterative coronary artery disease. In Fulton, W. F. M. (ed.): Coronary Arteries. Springfield, Illinois, Charles C Thomas, 1965.

29. Gadboys, H. L., Slonim, R., and Litwak, R. S.: The treacherous anomalous coronary artery. Am. J. Cardiol. 8:854–858, 1961.

30. Geiringer, E.: The mural coronary. Am. Heart J. 41:359–368, 1951.

31. Gensini, G. G.: Coronary Arteriography. Mt. Kisco, New York, Futura Publishing Company, 1975.

32. Gensini, G. G., and Bruto DaCosta, B. C.: The coronary collateral circulation in living man. Am. J. Cardiol. 24:393–400, 1969.

33. Gonzalez-Angulo, A., Reyes, H. A., and Wallace, S. A.: Anomalies of the origin of coronary arteries: special reference to single coronary artery. Angiology 17:96–103, 1966.

34. Guthaner, D., Higgins, C. B., Silverman, J. F., et al.: An unusual form of the transposition complex–uncorrected levo-transposition with horizontal ventricular septum: report of 2 cases. Circulation 53:190–195, 1976.

35. Haas, G.: Über die Gefässversorgung des Reizleitungs Systems des Herzens. Anatomischer Hefte 43:629, 1911.

36. Hallman, G. L., Cooley, D. A., and Singer, D. B.: Congenital anomalies of the coronary arteries: anatomy, pathology, and surgical treatment. Surgery 59:133–144, 1966.

37. Harris, C. N., Kaplan, M. A., Parker, D. P., et al.: Anatomic and functional correlates of intercoronary collateral vessels. Am. J. Cardiol. 30:611–614, 1972.

38. Hawe, A., Rastelli, G. C., Ritter, D. G., et al.: Management of right ventricular outflow tract in severe tetralogy of Fallot. J. Thorac. Cardiovasc. Surg. 60:131–143, 1970.

39. Hecht, S. H., Aroesty, J. M., Morkin, E., et al.: Role of the coronary collateral circulation in the preservation of left ventricular function. Radiology 14:305, 1975.

40. Heupler, F. A., Jr., Proudfit, W. L., Razavi, M., et al.: Ergonovine maleate provocative test for coronary arterial spasm. Am. J. Cardiol. 41:631–640, 1978.

41. Higgins, C. B., Wexler, L., Silverman, J. F., et al.: Clinical and arteriographic features of Prinzmetal's variant angina: documentation of etiologic factors. Am. J. Cardiol. 37:831–839, 1976.

42. Higgins, C. B., and Wexler, L.: Reversal of dominance of the coronary arterial system in isolated aortic stenosis and bicuspid aortic valve. Circulation 52:292–296, 1975.

43. Hillis, L. D., and Braunwald, E.: Coronary artery spasm. N. Engl. J. Med. 299:695–702, 1978.

44. Hood, J. H.: Anatomy of the coronary arteries. Semin. Roentgenol. 8:3–17, 1973.

45. Hutchins, G. M., Nazarian, I. H., and Bulkley, B. H.: Association of left dominant coronary arterial system with congenital bicuspid aortic valve. Am. J. Cardiol. 42:57–59, 1978.

46. Ihekwaba, F. N., Davidson, K. G., Ogilvie, B., et al.: Anomalous origin of the left coronary artery from the pulmonary artery with coronary artery steal in adults. Thorax 31:337–345, 1976.

47. James, T. N.: Anatomy of the Coronary Arteries. New York, Harper & Row, 1961.

48. James, T. N.: Anatomy of the coronary arteries in health and disease. Circulation 32:1020–1033, 1965.

49. James, T. N.: The delivery and distribution of coronary collateral circulation. Chest 58:183–203, 1970.

50. Jochem, W., Soto, B., Karp, R. B., et al.: Radiographic anatomy of the coronary collateral circulation. Am. J. Roentgenol. 116:50–61, 1972.

51. Keith, A., and Flack, M.: The form and nature of the muscular contractions between the primary division of the vertebrate heart. J. Anat. 41:172, 1907.

52. Kimbiris, D., Iskandrian, A. S., Segal, B. L., et al.: Anomalous aortic origin of coronary arteries. Circulation 58:606, 1978.

53. Kirklin, J. W., Ellis, F. H., Jr., McGoon, D. C., et al.: Surgical treatment for tetralogy of Fallot by open intracardiac repair. J. Thorac. Cardiovasc. Surg. 37:22–51, 1959.

54. Koops, B., Kerber, R. E., Wexler, L., et al.: Congenital coronary artery anomalies: experience at Stanford University Hospital (1963–1971). J.A.M.A. 226:1425–1429, 1973.

55. Kugel, M. A.: Anatomical studies on the coronary arteries and their branches. I. Arteria anastomotica auricularis magna. Am. Heart J. 3:260, 1927–1928.

56. Lerberg, D. B., Ogden, J. A., Zuberbuhler, J. R., et al.: Anomalous origin of the right coronary artery from the pulmonary artery. Ann. Thorac. Surg. 27:87, 1979.

57. Levin, D. C.: Pathways and functional significance of the coronary collateral circulation. Circulation 50:831–837, 1974.

58. Levin, D. C., and Baltaxe, H. A.: Angiographic demonstration of important anatomic variations of the posterior descending coronary artery. Am. J. Roentgenol. 116:41–49, 1972.

59. Levin, D. C., Fellows, K. E., and Abrams, H. L.: Hemodynamically significant primary anomalies of the coronary arteries: angiographic aspects. Circulation 58:25–34, 1978.

60. Liberthson, R. R., Dinsmore, R. E., and Fallon, J. T.: Aberrant coronary artery origin from the aorta: report of 18 patients, review of literature and delineation of natural history and management. Circulation 59:748, 1979.

61. Liberthson, R. R., Sagar, K., Berkoben, J. P., et al.: Congenital coronary arteriovenous fistula: report of 13 patients, review of the literature and delineation of management. Circulation 59:849, 1979.

62. Lipton, M. J., Barry, W. H., Obrez, I., et al.: Isolated single coronary artery: diagnosis, angiographic classification, and clinical significance. Radiology 130:39, 1979.

63. Longenecker, C. G., Reemtsma, K., and Creech, O., Jr.: Anomalous coronary artery distribution associated with tetralogy of Fallot: a hazard in open cardiac repair. J. Thorac. Cardiovasc. Surg. 42:258–262, 1961.

64. Longenecker, C. G., Reemtsma, K., and Creech, O., Jr.: Surgical implications of single coronary artery: a review and two case reports. Am. Heart J. 61:382–386, 1961.

65. Manninen, V., Rissanen, V. T., and Halonen, P. I.: Coronary ostium outside the aortic sinus. A factor in the etiology of ischemic heart disease. Adv. Cardiol. 4:94–98, 1970.

66. Maseri, A., L'Abbate, A., Baroldi, G., et al.: Coronary vasospasm as a possible cause of myocardial infarction: a conclusion derived from the study of "preinfarction" angina. N. Engl. J. Med. 299:1271, 1978.

67. Maseri, A., Severi, S., deNes, M., et al.: "Variant angina": one aspect of a continuous spectrum of vasospastic myocardial ischemia. Pathogenetic mechanisms, estimated incidence and clinical and coronary arteriographic findings in 138 patients. Am. J. Cardiol. 42:1019, 1978.

68. McNamara, J. J., and Gross, R. E.: Congenital coronary artery fistula. Surgery 65:59–69, 1969.

69. Meng, G. C. L., Eckner, F. A. D., and Lev, M.: Coronary artery distribution in tetralogy of Fallot. Arch. Surg. 90:363, 1965.

70. Most, A. S., Kemp, H. G., and Gorlin, R.: Postexercise electrocardiography in patients with arteriographically documented coronary artery disease. Ann. Intern. Med. 71:1043–1049, 1969.

71. Neufeld, H. M., Lester, R. G., Adams, P., Jr., et al.: Congenital communication of a coronary artery with a cardiac chamber or the pulmonary trunk (coronary artery fistula). Circulation 24:171–179, 1961.

72. Noble, J., Bourassa, M. G., Petitclerc, R., et al.: Myocardial bridging and milking effect of the left anterior descending coronary artery: normal variant or obstruction? Am. J. Cardiol. 37:993–999, 1976.

73. Nordenström, B.: The thebesian circulation in coronary angiography. Angiology 16:616–621, 1965.

74. Ogden, J. A.: Congenital anomalies of the coronary arteries. Am. J. Cardiol. 25:474–479, 1970.

75. Ogden, J. A., and Stansel, H. C., Jr.: Coronary arterial fistulas terminating in the coronary venous system. J. Thorac. Cardiovasc. Surg. 63:172–182, 1972.

76. Pape, H. L., Jr., Engel, H. J., Campbell, W. B., et al.: Anomalous origin of the left circumflex coronary artery: recognition, angiographic demonstration and clinical significance. Circulation 50:768, 1974.

77. Paulin, S.: Coronary angiography: a technical anatomic and clinical study. Acta Radiol. (Suppl.): 233:5, 1964.

78. Paulin, S.: Interarterial coronary anastomoses in relation to arterial obstruction demonstrated in coronary arteriography. Invest. Radiol. 2:147–159, 1967.

79. Polacek, P.: Relation of myocardial bridges and loops on the coronary arteries to coronary occlusions. Am. Heart J. 61:44, 1961.

80. Reiner, L., Molnar, J., Jimenez, F. A., et al.: Interarterial coronary anastomoses in neonates. Arch. Pathol. 71:103–112, 1961.

81. Ricci, D. R., Orlick, A. E., Cipriano, P. R., et al.: Altered adrenergic activity in coronary arterial spasm: insight into mechanism based on study of coronary hemodynamics and the electrocardiogram. Am. J. Cardiol. 43:1073, 1979.

82. Schlesinger, M. J.: An injection plus dissection study of coronary artery occlusions and anastomoses. Am. Heart J. 15:528–568, 1938.

83. Schlesinger, M. J.: Relation of anatomic pattern to pathologic conditions of the coronary arteries. Arch. Pathol. 30:403–415, 1940.

84. Schlesinger, M. J., Zoll, P. M., and Wessler, S.: The conus artery: a third coronary artery. Am. Heart J. 38:823–836, 1949.

85. Schroeder, J. S., Bolen, J. L., Quint, R. A., et al.: Provocation of coronary spasm with ergonovine maleate. New test with results in 57 patients undergoing coronary arteriography. Am. J. Cardiol. 40:487–491, 1977.

86. Shaher, R. M., and Puddu, G. C.: Coronary arterial anatomy in complete transposition of the great vessels. Am. J. Cardiol. 17:355–361, 1966.

87. Sharbaugh, A. H., and White, R. S.: Single coronary artery: analysis of the anatomic variation, clinical importance and report of five cases. J.A.M.A. 230:243–246, 1974.

88. Sheldon, W. C.: On the significance of coronary collaterals. Am. J. Cardiol. 24:303–304, 1969.

89. Silverman, K. J., Bulkley, B. H., and Hutchins, G. M.: Anomalous left circumflex coronary artery: "normal" variant of uncertain clinical and pathologic significance. Am. J. Cardiol. 41:1311–1314, 1978.

90. Silverman, J. F., Obrez, I., and Kriss, J. P.: Coronary artery fistula: diagnosis and evaluation by selective contrast and radioisotope coronary arteriography. Assoc. Can. Radiol. 25:310–315, 1974.

91. Soto, B., Russell, R. O., Jr., and Moraski, R. E.: Radiographic Anatomy of the Coronary Arteries, an Atlas. Mt. Kisco, New York, Futura Publishing Company, 1976.

92. Udoff, E. J., Roland, J. M., and White, R. I., Jr.: Coronary artery anomaly in double outlet right ventricle. Am. J. Roentgenol. 131:710, 1978.

93. Vieussens, R.: Nouvelles découvertes sur le coeur. Paris, 1706.

94. White, N. K., and Edwards, J. E.: Anomalies of the coronary arteries: report of four cases. Arch. Pathol. 45:766–771, 1948.

95. White, R. I., Jr., Frech, R. S., Castaneda, A., et al.: The nature and significance of anomalous coronary arteries in tetralogy of Fallot. Am. J. Roentgenol. 114:350–354, 1972.

96. Yenel, F.: Coronary arteriovenous communication: report of a case and review of the literature. N. Engl. J. Med. *265*:577–580, 1961.
97. Zoll, P. M., Wessler, S., and Schlesinger, M. J.: Interarterial coronary anastomoses in the human heart, with particular reference to anemia and relative cardiac anoxia. Circulation 4:797, 1951.

Part VI
Bypass Graft Angiography

DIANA F. GUTHANER, M.D.
LEWIS WEXLER, M.D.

INTRODUCTION

Over the past 40 years a variety of surgical approaches have been introduced to revascularize the myocardium for the treatment of coronary athero-occlusive disease. Early attempts to augment myocardial blood flow were indirect, including myocardial poudrage to stimulate collateral flow. In the late 1940's, Vineberg suggested tunneling the internal mammary artery into the left ventricular myocardium to establish connections with the coronary vessels. Direct myocardial revascularization was accomplished in 1957 with coronary artery endarterectomy. In May 1967 aortocoronary saphenous vein bypass grafts were first performed by Favaloro at the Cleveland Clinic. Immediate myocardial revascularization is achieved by interposition of a reversed segment of saphenous vein between the aorta and the coronary artery distal to the obstruction. This technique has enjoyed increasing acceptance, but its long-term results and final place in the therapeutic spectrum of coronary artery disease remain unresolved. The beneficial effect of complete myocardial revascularization for relief of anginal symptoms has been established,[4] with excellent correlation of patency of bypass grafts and symptomatic relief.[1, 14, 20, 23, 40] Reports of late symptomatic deterioration, as coronary artery disease inexorably progresses, are now appearing, however.[11, 12, 45, 52] Although selected subgroups of patients appear to derive improved life expectancy,[4, 9, 32, 33, 50, 51] more prolonged follow-up and late angiographic studies are warranted to evaluate survival following surgery and to compare longevity with that obtained using medical therapy.

LEFT VENTRICULAR FUNCTION

Postoperative angiographic evaluation includes left ventriculography in a 30 degree right anterior oblique projection. Improved left ventricular function depends both on the patency of the bypass graft subserving the abnormally contracting segment of the left ventricle and on the viability of the perfused ventricular segment. The latter may remain ischemic with potential reversibility of the contraction abnormality. If irreversible myocardial replacement by fibrous tissue has already occurred, however, improvement is unlikely. Sublingual nitroglycerin, isoproterenol, and postextrasystolic potentiation have been proposed in attempts to predict the benefit of bypass surgery by differentiating reversible from irreversible contraction disorders.[6, 24] Left ventriculography, therefore, enables one to evaluate areas of abnormal segmental wall motion contraction patterns.[39] The presence of a normally contracting segment indicates adequate myocardial perfusion either from the native coronary artery system or via a patent bypass graft supplying the segment.

Currently, fairly accurate estimates of focal ischemia can also be obtained from myocardial perfusion radionuclide studies with intravenous thallium-20 (see Volume I, pp. 33–34). This technique is helpful in the selection of patients for coronary arteriography and for the evaluation of graft patency in some patients without recourse to arteriography.

GRAFT PATENCY

Major factors determining early graft patency include (1) caliber of recipient vessel (greater than 90 per cent patency with coronary diameter of greater than 1.5 mm)[26]; (2) distal coronary blood flow measured intraoperatively using electromagnetic flow meters (90 per cent patency rate with flows greater than 40 ml per minute)[19, 26]; (3) presence of athero-obstructive disease distal to graft insertion; (4) area of myocardium perfused (correlation between graft patency and area of perfusion)[34]; (5) location of coronary artery and its surgical accessibility (80 to 85 per cent left anterior descending graft patency, 75 to 85 per cent right graft patency, and only 40 to 73 per cent patency rate of circumflex and posterior grafts)[1]; (6) quality of the autologous vein; for example,

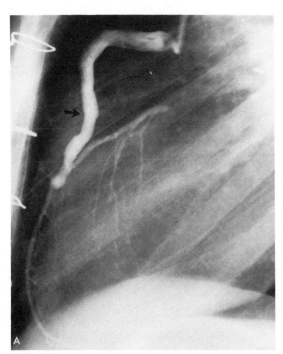 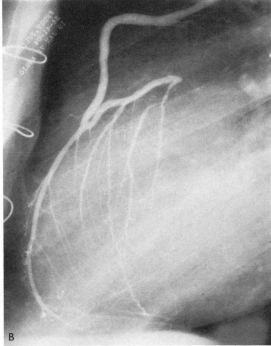

Figure 26–93.   Selective graft angiogram in the lateral projection (*A*) demonstrates a patent LAD graft (arrow) in the early postoperative period. One years postoperatively (*B*), selective graft angiography demonstrates diffuse reduction in caliber of the functioning vein graft, an angiographic appearance of intimal hyperplasia. (*From* Guthaner, D. F., and Wexler, L.: Radiologic evaluation of patients with coronary bypass. *In* Moseley, R. D., Jr. et al. (eds.): Current Problems in Diagnostic Radiology. Chicago, Year Book Medical Publishers, Inc., 1976. Reproduced by permission.)

technically faulty grafts (too long, angulated veins, veins subjected to trauma), or Y-grafts[17]; (7) technically inadequate distal anastomoses; and (8) bypass graft surgery combined with distal endarterectomy that is associated with substantially decreased graft patency rate.[54]

The literature is replete with reports of aortocoronary graft patency rates of 70 to 85 per cent, six to twelve months postoperatively.[1, 23, 43, 47, 49] Early graft closures can, therefore, be attributed predominantly to technical factors. In fact, a graft patent at early follow-up appears to have an excellent likelihood of being patent at late follow-up, with a reported annual attrition rate of about 1.8 per cent.[25, 35] Progressive intimal fibrous proliferation occurs in all grafts, however, and is probably related to arterialization of the vein graft after one to two months *in situ*.[8, 27, 29, 55] Histologically, there is circumferential fibrous myointimal thickening, proliferation of smooth muscle cells, and subsequent medial fibrosis. These appearances manifest angiographically as a smooth or irregular, diffuse or localized reduction of graft diameter (Fig. 26–93). It was initially feared that progressive intimal hyperplasia would affect the late patency rate. Long-term follow-up studies, however, suggest that intimal hyperplasia does not appear to be a significant factor in the long-term patency of vein grafts.[10, 18, 31, 35, 36]

GRAFT ANGIOGRAPHY

Technique[22]

Pari passu with progress in coronary artery surgery, there have been developments in techniques of selective coronary angiography. This modality, introduced by Sones and Shirey in 1958,[48] was first modified to a percutaneous transfemoral approach by Ricketts and Abrams in 1962.[44] Judkins[28] introduced catheters made of polyurethane incorporating a wire braid that allowed improved torque control and preshaped their terminal loops to facilitate engagement of either the right or the left coronary ostium. For selective graft angiography, we prefer a modified right coronary catheter with a shorter curve (3 cm) and a smooth downward-directed terminal portion, or a hook shape with a horizontal terminal segment, similar to the Amplatz right coronary catheter.[3] Any catheter may be modified to suit a particular aorta. In the presence of aortofemoral athero-occlusive disease, the percutaneous transaxillary approach is feasible for those experienced in the technique. Many centers prefer the brachial approach of Sones, using the standard Sones coronary catheter.

In some institutions, the aortic graft ostia are marked by a metallic clip or ring to facilitate locating the graft orifice during selective catheterization. However, caution is necessary, as markers may move in relation to the graft and then become misleading rather than helpful.

If selective catheterization of vein grafts is unsuccessful, aortography may be indicated. However, aortography is not the optimal method for graft visualization. Grafts arise proximally from the anterior surface of the aorta. As contrast medium layers posteriorly in a supine patient, the anterior grafts may not reliably be filled. In searching for left-sided grafts that arise to the left and higher from the ascending aorta, a shallow right anterior oblique projection (RAO) is advocated, a left anterior oblique projection (LAO) is recommended for right-sided grafts arising to the right. If the graft is occluded, a small stump at the graft orifice may be seen in profile in the appropriate projection either on aortography or on selective catheterization (Fig. 26–94). These outpouchings are readily visualized with the use of selective catheters that tend to engage the orifice of the occluded vessel.

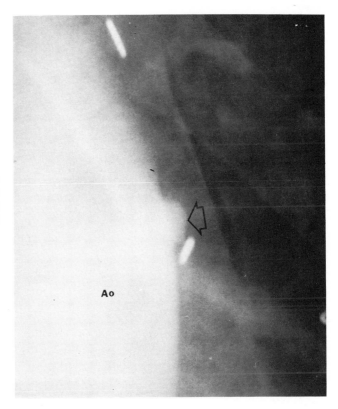

Figure 26–94. Detail of a supravalvular aortogram demonstrating deformity due to proximal occlusion of the graft (arrow). The lower metallic clip marks the aortic ostium of the graft. Ao = ascending aorta.

Ao

Graft Anatomy (Fig. 26–95)

The graft to the right coronary artery usually arises anteriorly and to the right from the aorta, just above the right coronary sinus. It may occasionally be placed more posteriorly. It courses inferiorly parallel to the right atrioventricular groove to reach the distal right coronary artery (Fig. 26–96). Grafts to the left coronary vessels arise higher and to the left from the anterior aspect of the aorta. The graft to the left anterior descending coronary artery is usually placed lowest, while diagonal and obtuse marginal grafts are inserted higher on the aorta. They pursue a leftward, horizontal course as they arch over the main pulmonary artery segment to reach the interventricular septum and anterolateral left ventricular wall (Fig. 26–97). Here the graft is anastomosed distal to the stenosis, to the mid–left anterior descending coronary artery, and occasionally more distally. In some instances, grafts to the circumflex or obtuse marginal branches arise posteriorly and descend in the transverse sinus behind the pulmonary artery, where they overlie the left atrium. The grafts are selectively opacified in turn, and cineangiograms are performed in at least two orthogonal projections.[5]

Graft Anastomoses

PROXIMAL. The aortic ostia of the vein graft, when widely patent, appear funnel-shaped. They may arise perpendicular to the aorta or at a more acute angle. In a small series of patients evaluated five to eight years after coronary artery bypass surgery, proximal anastomotic stenoses occurred in about 20 per cent.[21] The majority of the proximal stenoses occurred in about 20 per cent.[21] The majority of the proximal stenoses remained stable (see Fig. 26–97). Late graft occlusion was difficult to predict from the appearance of the graft or the anastomosis.

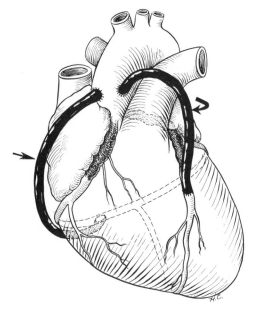

Figure 26–95. Diagrammatic representation of saphenous vein aortocoronary bypass grafts. The graft to the right coronary artery (straight arrow) courses inferiorly to anastomose posteriorly with the distal right coronary artery. The graft to the left anterior descending coronary artery (curved arrow) arches anteriorly over the main pulmonary artery to reach the mid- or distal left anterior descending artery. (*From* Guthaner, D. F., and Wexler, L.: Radiologic evaluation of patients with coronary bypass. *In* Moseley, R. D., Jr. et al. (eds.): Current Problems in Diagnostic Radiology. Chicago, Year Book Medical Publishers, Inc., 1976. Reproduced by permission.)

DISTAL. The majority of stenoses involve the distal anastomosis, either the graft itself or the coronary artery in the region of the anastomotic site. Again, we found it impossible to predict which grafts, whether tightly stenotic or not, would progress to occlusion (Fig. 26–98). A common technical problem results from mobilizing the left anterior descending coronary artery for the distal anastomosis. If retraction of the graft occurs, tenting of the left anterior descending coronary artery results, often with distortion and associated mild stenosis that tends to remain stable. Pseudoaneurysms occur at the distal anastomosis, probably as a result of leakage at a suture site (Fig. 26–99). Thrombus may partially occlude the aneurysm and even encroach on the graft lumen to compromise graft blood flow. Some of these aneurysms may be completely occluded by thrombus and hence no longer be evident on subsequent angiography.

Figure 26–96. Selective right coronary graft injection in the lateral projection demonstrating a functioning graft with intimal hyperplasia in its midportion (arrow). The distal right coronary fills well, but there is poor retrograde filling of the mid–right coronary artery (arrowheads).

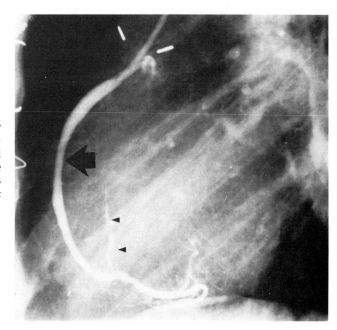

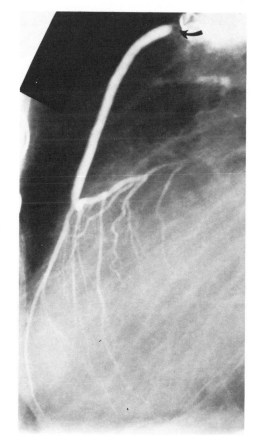

Figure 26–97. Selective left anterior descending graft injection in the lateral projection one year after surgery. There is antegrade filling of the distal left anterior descending and retrograde filling of the proximal left anterior descending, diagonal, and septal branches. The stenosis of the proximal anastomosis (arrow) remained unchanged in appearance on a repeat angiogram 75 months after bypass graft surgery.

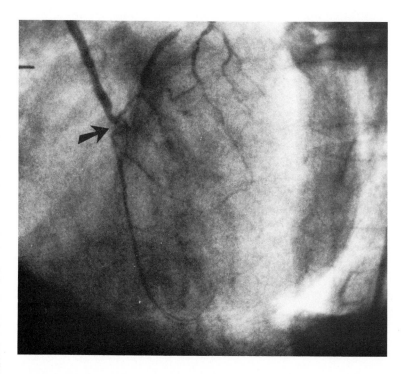

Figure 26–98. Selective left anterior descending graft angiogram in a left anterior oblique projection. There are stenoses in the graft at the distal anastomosis and the left anterior descending coronary artery, both proximal and distal to the anastomosis (arrow), which persisted at late follow-up.

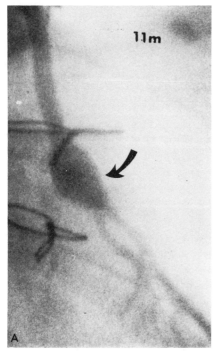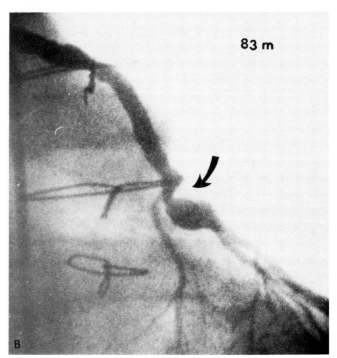

Figure 26–99. Selective left coronary graft injections in a right anterior oblique projection in the early postoperative period (*A*) and 83 months postoperatively (*B*). There is an aneurysm (arrow) involving the distal anastomosis, which at late follow-up is partially obliterated by thrombus with compromise of the lumen. (*From* Guthaner, D. F., Robert, E. W., Alderman, E. L., et al.: Long-term serial angiographic studies after coronary artery bypass surgery. Circulation *60*:250–259, 1979. Reproduced by permission.)

Because of their propensity to thrombose the side branch, Y-grafts are no longer performed routinely. "Snake" or skip grafts are currently popular, utilizing side-to-side anastomoses to one or more branches with a final distal end-to-side anastomosis.

Graft Body

There is often considerable disparity in the size of the vein grafts compared with the native coronary artery. Over a period of about one year, there is ordinarily a decrease in graft caliber owing to intimal hyperplasia, so that the graft more closely approximates the size of the native coronary artery (see Fig. 26–93). Angiographic features of intimal hyperplasia include a diffuse, smooth narrowing, although sometimes a shagginess may occur and findings may be limited to a short segment. Long-term follow-up studies show that there may be continued progressive intimal hyperplasia in a graft but that this does not inevitably lead to occlusion.[18] On high-quality films, the normal venous valves may be visualized in the graft as linear radiolucent lines, which may become the site of excess intimal hyperplasia.

Functional Considerations

From a selective graft injection, good antegrade filling of the distal recipient coronary artery and its branches occurs. A poorly functioning or occluded graft is reflected by poor or no filling of the distal coronary artery. Retrograde filling of the native coronary artery proximal to the graft anastomosis may occur if this segment is patent. A bidirectional flow pattern in this proximal segment of the native bypassed coronary artery has been attributed to antegrade diastolic flow in the coronary artery (nonopacified blood) and retrograde systolic filling via the graft (opacified blood) and is considered important in assessing graft function and proximal coronary artery patency.[37]

INTRINSIC CORONARY CIRCULATION

For a routine postoperative follow-up study, selective native coronary arteriography is also performed.

Bypassed Coronary Vessels

The coronary artery proximal to the graft anastomosis, if patent, is visualized either by retrograde filling from the graft injection or from the selective native coronary injection. It may be difficult, however to ascertain whether the native circulation is patent or occluded at the site of previous narrowing. Nonvisualization of the coronary

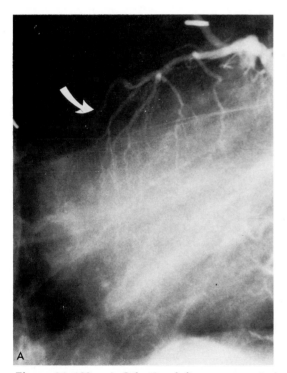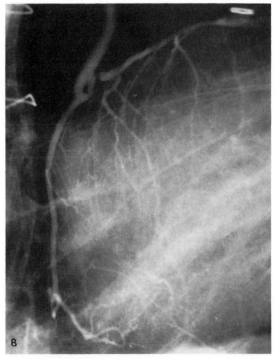

Figure 26–100. *A,* Selective left coronary arteriogram in the lateral projection shows absent opacification or pseudo-occlusion (arrow) of the distal left anterior descending coronary artery. *B,* Selective left anterior descending graft injection in the lateral projection demonstrates a patent graft, which fills both the distal and the proximal left anterior descending coronary artery. (*From* Guthaner, D. F., and Wexler, L.: Radiologic evaluation of patients with coronary bypass. *In* Moseley, R. D., Jr. et al. (eds.): Current Problems in Diagnostic Radiology. Chicago, Year Book Medical Publishers, Inc., 1976. Reproduced by permission.)

vessel distally may be due to good inflow of nonpacified blood from the patent graft. This "pseudo-occlusion" phenomenon gives the impression of an occluded native coronary artery (Fig. 26–100).[46] These findings may be misleading when progression of proximal coronary artery disease is being considered. The presence of a bidirectional flow pattern on selective graft angiography confirms the patency of the coronary artery proximally.[37] Accelerated progression of proximal coronary artery stenosis to occlusion has been established.[2, 7] Presumably there is decreased flow through the bypassed

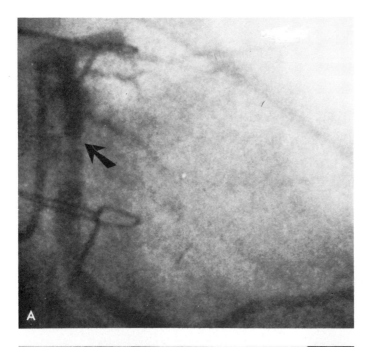

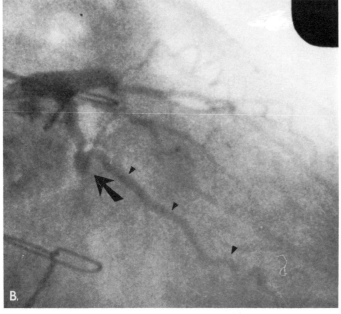

Figure 26–101. Selective native coronary arteriogram in the right anterior oblique projection demonstrates occlusion of the proximal left anterior descending coronary artery. *A,* On the initial postoperative study, the circumflex branch has a significant stenosis (arrow), which was not bypassed. *B,* At follow-up 71 months following surgery, the distal circumflex coronary artery is occluded (arrow). The second obtuse marginal branch (arrowheads) has hypertrophied to supply collaterals to the lateral wall of the left ventricle.

segment in the presence of a patent graft, which predisposes to thrombosis. The incidence of progression of disease in the coronary artery distal to the graft anastomosis has been more controversial, however. Earlier reports suggested increased progression of distal stenoses attributable to turbulence created by graft inflow.[17, 41] These findings have not been supported either by our study or by those of other investigators.[21]

Nonbypassed Coronary Vessels

Recrudescence of symptoms and late symptomatic deterioration have been attributed to progression of disease in the nongrafted arteries. Bypass grafting is therefore a palliative procedure, which in no way deters the progress of coronary atherosclerosis but merely directs myocardial blood flow where there has already been compromise. The progression of athero-occlusive disease and its location remain unpredictable (Fig. 26–101).

Collateral Pathways

The changing patterns of collateral flow reflect graft function and severity of coronary artery athero-occlusive disease.[42] An excellent correlation exists between graft patency and regression of previously demonstrable intercoronary collateral channels.[13] In the presence of an occluded graft, the collateral pathways persist.[53] Reversal of flow through pre-existing collateral channels may occur, or new collateral channels may develop when a nonbypassed stenotic coronary artery becomes dependent on flow from a patent graft (Fig. 26–102).

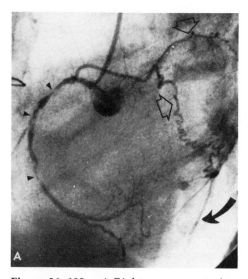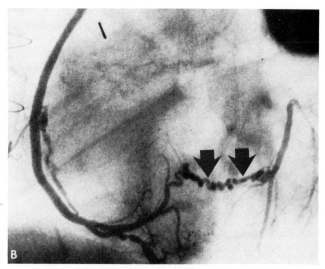

Figure 26–102. *A,* Right coronary arteriogram in the left anterior oblique projection demonstrates significant stenoses of the proximal and mid–right coronary artery (arrowheads), which were not successfully bypassed at the first surgery. Atrial collaterals encircling the left atrium (open arrows) re-form the distal left circumflex artery and left posterolateral branches (arrow). *B,* Following repeat surgery and right coronary graft insertion, collaterals to supply the left circumflex system now arise in the atrioventricular groove from the distal right coronary artery (arrows).

INTERNAL MAMMARY–CORONARY ARTERY GRAFTS

Satisfactory myocardial revascularization has also been accomplished using the internal mammary artery with direct anastomosis to a coronary artery.[15, 16, 38] The intraoperative blood flows achieved are not as high as those obtained from saphenous vein grafts,[31] but the reported patency rate tends to be higher (95 per cent), contributing to the reported improved overall survival. Although this is the preferred technique in many centers reporting excellent results, to the best of our knowledge there is currently no good comparative long-term angiographic evaluation of both techniques. Selective internal mammary artery injections may be performed via the percutaneous femoral route, using a catheter similar to a modified right Judkins coronary catheter with a longer, more acutely angled tip.[30]

THALLIUM-201 MYOCARDIAL SCAN

Thallium-201 radionuclide myocardial scans are becoming a valuable adjunct or complement to coronary arteriography, both before and after bypass surgery. Introduced in 1975, thallium-201 was found to distribute itself in the myocardium proportionate to the coronary blood flow. Imaging can be done at rest or during exercise.

Exercise imaging can supplement cardiac catheterization studies; it gives valuable information concerning the viability of the myocardium and aids in assessment of the functional role of collaterals. The scan results can be important in deciding whether a bypass graft would be physiologically effective. After bypass surgery, an exercise scan can provide direct proof of the efficacy of the graft. The scan can also help in the selection of patients for repeat coronary angiography and possible revascularization surgery, when symptoms develop months or years after bypass surgery.

References

1. Alderman, E.L., Matlof, H.J., Wexler, L., et al.: Results of direct coronary artery surgery for the treatment of angina pectoris. N. Engl. J. Med. *288*:535–539, 1973.
2. Aldridge, H.E., and Trimble, A.S.: Progression of proximal coronary artery lesions to total occlusion after aortocoronary saphenous vein bypass grafting. J. Thorac. Cardiovasc. Surg. *62*:7–11, 1971.
3. Amplatz, K., Formanek, G., Stanger, P., et al.: Mechanics of selective coronary artery catheterization via femoral approach. Radiology *89*:1040–1047, 1967.
4. Anderson, R.P., Rahimtoola, S.H., Bonchek, L.I., et al.: The prognosis of patients with coronary artery disease after coronary bypass operations. Circulation *50*:274–282, 1974.
5. Baltaxe, H.A., and Levin, D.C.: Angiographic demonstration of complications related to the saphenous aortocoronary bypass. Am. J. Roentgenol. *119*:484–492, 1973.
6. Banka, V.S., Bodenheimer, M.M., Shah, R., et al.: Intervention ventriculography. Comparative value of nitroglycerin, post-extrasystolic potentiation and nitroglycerin plus post-extrasystolic potentiation. Circulation *53*:632–637, 1976.
7. Bourassa, M.G., Goulet, C., and Lesperance, J.: Progression of coronary arterial disease after aortocoronary bypass grafts. Circulation *48* (Suppl. III):127–131, 1973.
8. Brody, W.R., Angell, W.W., and Kosek, J.C.: Histologic fate of the venous coronary artery bypass in dogs. Am. J. Pathol. *66*:111–130, 1972.
9. Cameron, A., Kemp, H.G., Shimomura, S., et al.: Aortocoronary bypass surgery — a 7 year follow-up. Circulation *60*:1, 1979.
10. Campeau, L., Lesperance, J., Corbara, F., et al.: Aortocoronary saphenous vein bypass graft changes 5 to 7 years after surgery. Cardiovasc. Surg. (Suppl. to Circulation) *58*:1, 1978.
11. Campeau, L., Lesperance, J., Hermann, J., et al.: Loss of the improvement of angina between 1 and 7 years after aortocoronary bypass surgery. Correlations with changes in vein grafts and in coronary arteries. Circulation *60*:1, 1979.

12. Carey, J.S., and Cukingnan, R.A.: Subjective multivariable analysis by computer for evaluation of coronary artery bypass. Arch. Surg. 3:769–772, 1976.
13. Glassman, E., Spencer, F.C., Krauss, K.R., et al.: Changes in underlying coronary circulation secondary to bypass grafting. Circulation 50 (Suppl. II):80–83, 1974.
14. Gott, V.L.: Outlook of patients after coronary artery revascularization. Am. J. Cardiol. 33:431–437, 1974.
15. Green, G.E., Spencer, F.C., Tice, D.A., et al.: Arterial and venous microsurgical bypass grafts for coronary artery disease. J. Thorac. Cardiovasc. Surg. 60:491–503, 1970.
16. Green, G.E.: Internal mammary artery-to-coronary artery anastomosis. Three year experience with 165 patients. Ann. Thorac. Surg. 14:260–271, 1972.
17. Griffith, L.S.C., Achuff, S.C., Conti, C.R., et al.: Changes in intrinsic coronary circulation and segmental ventricular motion after saphenous-vein coronary bypass graft surgery. N. Engl. J. Med. 288:589–595, 1973.
18. Grondin, C.M., Lesperance, J., Bourassa, M.G., et al.: Serial angiographic evaluation in 60 consecutive patients with aortocoronary artery vein grafts 2 weeks, 1 year, and 3 years after operation. J. Thorac. Cardiovasc. Surg. 67:1–6, 1974.
19. Grondin, C.M., Lepage, G., Castonguay, Y.R., et al.: Aortocoronary bypass graft. Initial blood flow through the graft and early postoperative patency. Circulation 44:815–819, 1971.
20. Guiney, T.E., Rubenstein, J.J., Sanders, C.A., et al.: Functional evaluation of coronary bypass surgery by exercise testing and oxygen consumption. Circulation 48 (Suppl. III):141–145, 1973.
21. Guthaner, D.F., Robert, E.W., Alderman, E.L., et al.: Long-term serial angiographic studies after coronary artery bypass surgery. Circulation 60:250–259, 1979.
22. Guthaner, D.F., and Wexler, L.: The radiologic evaluation of patients with coronary bypass. In Mosely, R.D., Jr. et al. (eds.): Current Problems in Diagnostic Radiology. Chicago, Year Book Medical Publishers, Inc., 1976.
23. Hartman, C.W., Kong, Y., Margolis, J.R., et al.: Aortocoronary bypass surgery: correlation of angiographic, symptomatic and functional improvement at 1 year. Am. J. Cardiol. 37:352–357, 1976.
24. Helfant, R.H., Pine, R., Meister, S.G., et al.: Nitroglycerin to unmask reversible asynergy: correlation with postcoronary bypass ventriculography. Circulation 50:108–113, 1974.
24a. Iskandrian, A.S., Wasserman, L., and Segal, B.L.: Thallium-201 myocardial scintigraphy. Arch. Intern. Med., 140:320–327, 1980.
25. Itscoitz, S.B., Redwood, D.R., Brauer, L.E., et al.: Long-term durability of patient saphenous vein aortocoronary bypass grafts (Abstract). Am. J. Cardiol. 33:146, 1974.
26. Johnson, W.D.: Surgical techniques of myocardial revascularization: an overview. Bull. N.Y. Acad. Med. 48:1146–1156, 1972.
27. Jones, M., Conkle, D.M., Ferrans, V.J., et al.: Lesions observed in arterial autogenous vein grafts. Light and electron microscopic evaluation. Circulation 48 (Suppl. III):198–221, 1973.
28. Judkins, M.P.: Selective coronary arteriography. I. A percutaneous transfemoral technique. Radiology 89:815–824, 1967.
29. Kern, W.H., Dermer, G.B., and Lindesmith, G.C.: The intimal proliferation in aortic-coronary saphenous vein grafts. Light and electron microscopic studies. Am. Heart J. 84:771, 1972.
30. Kittredge, R.D., and Kemp, H.G.: Left internal mammary artery-coronary artery bypass anatomy. Am. J. Roentgenol. 128:395–401, 1977.
31. Lawrie, G.M., Lie, J.T., Morris, G.C., et al.: Vein graft patency and intimal proliferation after aortocoronary bypass: Early and long-term angiopathologic correlations. Am. J. Cardiol. 38:856–862, 1976.
32. Lawrie, G.M., Morris, G.C., Chapman, D.W., et al.: Patterns of patency of 596 vein grafts up to seven years after aortocoronary bypass. J. Thorac. Cardiovasc. Surg. 73:443–448, 1977.
33. Lawrie, G.M., Morris, G.C., Howell, J.F., et al.: Improved survival after 5 years in 1,144 patients after coronary bypass surgery. Am. J. Cardiol. 42:709, 1978.
34. Lesperance, J., Bourassa, M.G., Biron, P., et al.: Aorta to coronary artery saphenous vein grafts, preoperative angiographic criteria for successful surgery. Am. J. Cardiol. 30:459–465, 1972.
35. Lesperance, J., Bourassa, M.G., Saltiel, J., et al.: Late changes in aortocoronary vein grafts: angiographic features. Am. J. Roentgenol. 116:74–81, 1972.
36. Lesperance, J., Bourassa, M.G., Saltiel, J., et al.: Angiographic changes in aortocoronary vein grafts: lack of progression beyond the first year. Circulation 48:633–643, 1973.
37. Levin, D.C., Baltaxe, H.A., and Carlson, R.G.: Angiographic demonstration of bidirectional coronary artery blood flow following aortocoronary bypass vein grafts. Am. J. Roentgenol. 113:554–561, 1971.
38. Loop, F.D., Irarrazaval, M.J., Bredee, J.J., et al.: Internal mammary artery graft for ischemic heart disease. Effect of revascularization on clinical status and survival. Am. J. Cardiol. 39:516–522, 1977.
39. Martin, E.C., Wixson, D., and Baltaxe, H.A.: Regional ejection fractions in patients with patent and thrombosed grafts after coronary artery vein bypass surgery. Invest. Radiol. 12:205–209, 1977.
40. Matlof, H.J., Alderman, E.L., Wexler, L., et al.: What is the relationship between the response of angina to coronary surgery and anatomical success? Circulation 48 (Suppl. III):168–172, 1973.
41. Maurer, B.J., Oberman, A., Holt, J.H., et al.: Changes in grafted and nongrafted coronary arteries following saphenous vein bypass grafting. Circulation 50:293–300, 1974.
42. McLaughlin, P.R., Berman, N.D., Morton, B.C., et al.: Saphenous vein bypass grafting. Changes in native circulation and collaterals. Circulation 52 (Suppl. I):66–71, 1975.

43. Morris, G.C., Reul, G.J., Howell, J.F., et al.: Follow-up results of distal coronary artery bypass for ischemic heart disease. Am. J. Cardiol. *29*:180–185, 1972.
44. Ricketts, H.J., and Abrams, H.L.: Percutaneous selective coronary cine arteriography. J.A.M.A. *181*:620–624, 1962.
45. Robert, E.W., Guthaner, D.F., Wexler, L., et al.: Six-year clinical and angiographic follow-up of patients with previously documented complete revascularization. Circulation *58* (Suppl. I):194, 1978.
46. Ross, A.M., Hammond, G.L., Cohen, L.S., et al.: Angiographic evaluation of saphenous vein bypass grafts: Artifactual "occlusion" caused by dual sources of flow. Am. J. Cardiol. *39*:384–389, 1977.
47. Sheldon, W.C., Rincon, G., Effler, D.B., et al.: Vein graft surgery for coronary artery disease, survival and angiographic results in 1000 patients. Circulation *48* (Suppl. III):184–189, 1973.
48. Sones, F.M., Jr., and Shirey, E.K.: Cine coronary arteriography. Mod. Concepts Cardiovasc. Dis. *31*:735–738, 1962.
49. Steele, P., Battock, D., Pappas, G., et al.: Correlation of platelet survival time with occlusion of saphenous vein aortocoronary bypass grafts. Circulation *53*:685–687, 1976.
50. Stiles, Q.R., Lindesmith, G.G., Tucker, B.L., et al.: Long-term follow-up of patients with coronary artery bypass grafts. Circulation *54* (Suppl. III):32–34, 1976.
51. Talano, J.V., Scanlon, P.J., Meadows, W.R., et al.: Influence of surgery on survival in 145 patients with left main coronary artery disease. Circulation *52* (Suppl. I):105–111, 1975.
52. Tecklenberg, P.L., Alderman, E.L., Miller, D.C., et al.: Changes in survival and symptom relief in a longitudinal study of patients after bypass surgery. Circulation *52* (Suppl. I):98–104, 1975.
53. Uflacker, R., and Enge, I.: The behaviour of collateral circulation after coronary artery bypass surgery. Cardiovasc. Radiol. *1*:225, 1978.
54. Urschel, H.C., Razzuk, M.A., Wood, R.E., et al.: Factors influencing patency of aortocoronary saphenous vein grafts. Surgery *72*:1048–1063, 1972.
55. Vlodaver, Z., and Edwards, J.E.: Pathologic changes in aortic coronary arterial saphenous vein grafts. Circulation *44*:719–728, 1971.

Part VII
Ventricular Aneurysm

DIANA F. GUTHANER, M.D.
LEWIS WEXLER, M.D.

CLINICAL PICTURE

The frequency of left ventricular aneurysms following myocardial infarction is reported to be 3 to 20 per cent with a five-year mortality rate of 88 per cent.[18, 22, 50] Left ventricular aneurysms often manifest clinically with refractory congestive heart failure, ventricular tachyarrhythmias, and systemic emboli. Left ventricular end-diastolic volume and left ventricular end-diastolic pressures are frequently elevated, resulting in a low resting cardiac output[22] and pulmonary congestion.[33] The degree of left ventricular dysfunction depends on the extent of aneurysmal involvement of the left ventricle, the quality of left ventricular function, and the contractility of the remainder of the left ventricular myocardium.[22, 52] These factors, as reflected in the measured ejection fraction and the cardiac index (cardiac output per square meter of body surface area), and, in addition, the presence of mitral regurgitation, significantly influence the surgical risk of the patient.[8] The overall long-term survival rate following surgery has improved substantially to 60 per cent at five years, with the majority of the patients reaching a functional class I or II.[8] Aneurysmectomy is often combined with myocardial revascularization in the presence of multivessel coronary artery disease, in an attempt to improve both the longevity and the functional status of the patient.[54] Therefore, left ventricular function assessed by left ventriculography and routine hemodynamic indices prior to surgery is a significant determinant of the postoperative prognosis.[1, 35, 40, 42, 53, 54]

TYPES OF LEFT VENTRICULAR ANEURYSMS

True Aneurysm

With the advent of contrast left ventriculography in the early 1960's, left ventricular contraction abnormalities have been more readily demonstrated.[22] The angiographic definition of a left ventricular aneurysm is a dyskinetic or paradoxical systolic expansion of the noncontractile left ventricular segment that protrudes beyond the end-diastolic outline of the left ventricle. This definition is at variance with the pathologic definition, which instead indicates the underlying fibrosis secondary to

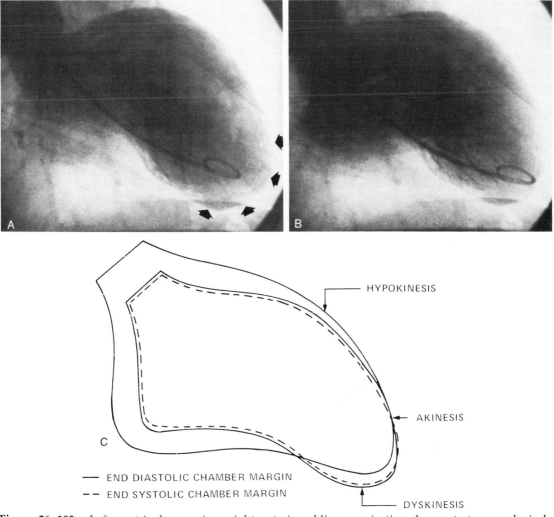

Figure 26–103. Left ventriculogram in a right anterior oblique projection demonstrates paradoxical systolic expansion of a left ventricular aneurysm (arrows) on a systolic frame (*A*) and a diastolic frame (*B*). Diagrammatic representation of the left ventricular contour in end-diastole and end-systole (*C*).

myocardial infarction and the lack of residual contractile ability.[57] An abnormally contracting segment may contain a variable amount of viable myocardium, however. Dyskinetic or paradoxical motion may be observed clinically when myocardium has only been rendered ischemic and transmural infarction has not occurred.[4, 57] But, in the presence of dense fibrous scar tissue or thrombosis, left ventricular segmental compliance may be decreased, interfering with the classic picture of paradoxical segmental systolic expansion.

Aneurysm is derived from the Greek word meaning "to dilate." A left ventricular aneurysm refers to the abnormal dilatation of a diseased segment of the left ventricular wall, often with replacement by full-thickness scar tissue.

The most common form of a left ventricular aneurysm is a true aneurysm that usually results from transmural myocardial infarction (Fig. 26–103). The wall of a true aneurysm contains all the components of the original wall, now largely replaced by scar tissue or fibrosis.

Pseudoaneurysm

A pseudoaneurysm of the left ventricle, in contrast with a true aneurysm, is a communication from the ventricular chamber to the pericardial sac, where it is limited by pericardium and fibrous adhesions.[17, 20] Pseudoaneurysms, therefore, imply rupture of the myocardial wall. Although the pathogenesis of both true and false aneurysms may be myocardial necrosis following myocardial infarction, pseudoaneurysm may also be caused by trauma with penetration of the myocardium by a foreign body or rupture following myocardial contusion.

The diameter of a pseudoaneurysm sac is larger than its narrow mouth. In response to the left ventricular pressure, the aneurysmal sac may progressively enlarge.[46] The frequency of spontaneous and fatal rupture is significant.[59] It is impossible to differentiate true from false aneurysms on clinical grounds, including the use of electrocardiography. However, ventriculography does allow differentiation by demonstrating the narrow orifice of the pseudoaneurysm (Fig. 26–104).[46, 61] Because of the relative danger

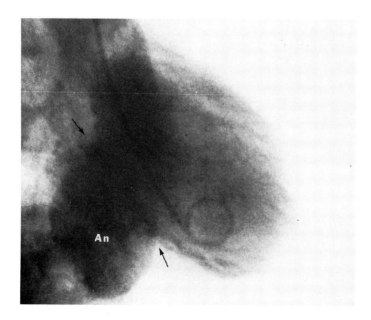

Figure 26–104. Left ventriculogram in a right anterior oblique projection demonstrating a pseudoaneurysm (An) following myocardial infarction involving the posterobasal and septal segments of the left ventricle. Arrows demonstrate the neck of the aneurysm.

of rupture of a pseudoaneurysm, aggressive surgical intervention is both warranted and effective and accurate diagnosis is therefore essential.[21] Echocardiography may also enable differentiation by demonstrating a large echo-free space lying posterior or anterior to the ventricular cavity, the communicating orifice being visualized as a discontinuity of the respective left ventricular wall.[39, 41, 47]

Mycotic Aneurysm

The formation of abscesses in the myocardial wall may complicate subacute bacterial endocarditis, especially if *Staphylococcus aureus* is the causative organism.[48] These abscess cavities may lead to perforation and saccular aneurysm or to pseudoaneurysm formation (Fig. 26–105). A mycotic aneurysm of the left ventricle most commonly involves the membranous septum or mitral-aortic intervalvular area.

Traumatic Contusion

Traumatic contusion of the heart and subsequent fibrous replacement may result from severe blunt trauma and lead to true aneurysm formation.[2, 5] In contrast, a penetrating injury may be complicated by development of a pseudoaneurysm with an accompanying change in the cardiac contour on chest radiography, fluoroscopy, and angiography.

Congenital Left Ventricular Diverticulum

Congenital ventricular diverticula occur rarely as isolated lesions in certain African natives, such as South African Bantu tribes, and in Negroes,[11, 12] or occur in association with other cardiac anomalies or midline defects in the pericardium, diaphragm, and

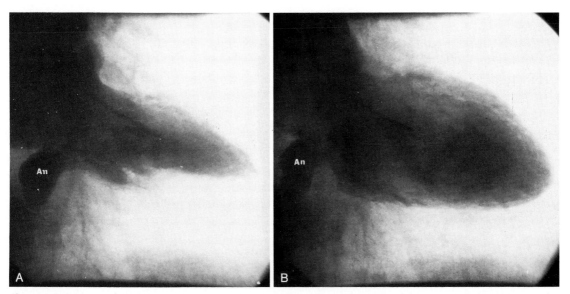

Figure 26–105. Left ventriculogram in a right anterior oblique projection in systole (*A*) and diastole (*B*), showing a pseudoaneurysm (An) in a subvalvular location secondary to infective endocarditis.

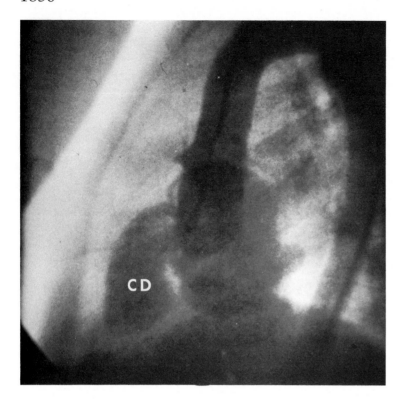

Figure 26–106. Left ventriculogram in a lateral projection showing a large congenital diverticulum (CD) extending anteriorly into the interventricular septum.

anterior abdominal wall (Fig. 26–106).[9, 19] These congenital ventricular diverticula arise most frequently in the subvalvular area in intimate relationship to the mitral or aortic valves or, more rarely, at the left ventricular apex. Angiography reveals paradoxical systolic expansion of the diverticulum. In the muscular type of congenital left ventricular diverticulum, normal trabeculae and contractility reflect the possible origin of the diverticulum as an accessory outpouching from the primitive ventricle.[58] A normal trabecular pattern is not, however, invariably present. A second form of congenital aneurysm, the fibrous type, is described. This is characterized by an absence of trabeculae in the wall of the aneurysm, which appears as a smooth, thin-walled sac. The aneurysm forms at the site of a congenital weakness in the left ventricular wall. The congenital diverticula only rarely display systemic embolic events, probably owing to the relatively small mouth of the diverticulum or aneurysm.

A great variety of other etiologies of left ventricular aneurysms have been reported in the early literature and include rheumatic carditis,[43] syphilitic carditis,[3] tuberculosis often associated with a calcified aneurysm,[13] and interstitial myocarditis.[13]

DIAGNOSTIC MODALITIES

Noninvasive Techniques

The frontal chest radiograph usually demonstrates generalized cardiac enlargement but may reveal a classic localized bulge or irregularity of the left ventricular cardiac contour. Occasionally, calcification occurs in the necrotic myocardium or mural thrombus (Fig. 26–107). Left ventricular aneurysm may also be seen on the lateral chest film as an increased density superimposed on the cardiac shadow in the retrosternal

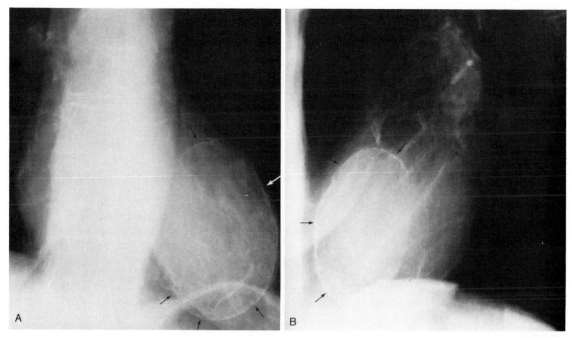

Figure 26–107. Frontal (*A*) and lateral (*B*) chest radiographs of a patient with a left ventricular aneurysm outlined by calcification (arrows).

position.[31] Cardiac fluoroscopy was first recommended in 1939 for the evaluation of abnormal left ventricular wall motion. The infarcted and thinned myocardium demonstrates either decreased systolic pulsations or paradoxical systolic motion.[34] An anterior aneurysm is most readily recognized fluoroscopically.[6, 10, 49] Other noninvasive techniques, including cinefluoroscopy and variations of kymography, were introduced soon after as screening tests.[14, 51] In one series, about 75 per cent of patients with abnormal left ventricular contraction were identified by electrocardiographic and pathologic correlation.[36, 37] The outer contour of the heart shadow, including the surrounding pericardial fat, however, is a silhouette that does not accurately reflect the true magnitude of endocardial systolic motion.[32, 55] In fact, left ventricular aneurysms may readily be overlooked, both on a routine chest radiograph and with cinefluorography.

Present noninvasive diagnostic techniques include echocardiography and radionuclide left ventriculography. Evaluation of regional left ventricular wall motion following intravenous injection of radioactive tracers by first-pass (Fig. 26–108) or gated cardiac blood pool scanning[7, 62] correlates well with results of left ventricular volumes, ejection fractions, and segmental left ventricular wall motion obtained at left ventriculography. Segmental asynergy may be detected on routine M-mode echocardiography. Newer techniques of two-dimensional cross-sectional imaging, however, allow improved visualization of left ventricular wall motion and delineation of junctional areas between normally contracting wall segments and dyskinetic or akinetic segments (Fig. 26–109). Apicobasal views (the right anterior oblique equivalent and the four-chambered view) allow reliable detection and characterization of left ventricular aneurysms, including apical aneurysms.[60] The application of gating techniques to computed tomography (CT) allows the determination of left ventricular wall motion. A left ventricular aneurysm can be detected on a routine CT scan through the cardiac structure at ventricular level by the lobulated anterolateral contour of the heart.[26]

Text continued on page 1854

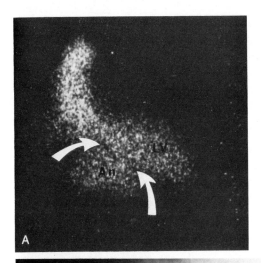

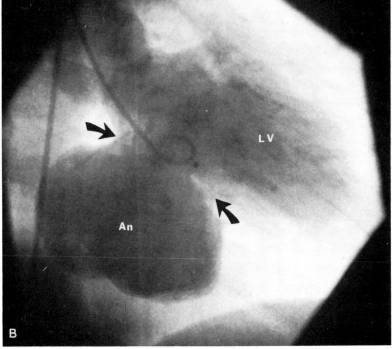

Figure 26–108. First-pass nuclear angiocardiogram (*A*) and left ventriculogram in a right anterior oblique projection (*B*) demonstrating a false aneurysm (An) arising from the inferior aspect of the left ventricle (LV). Arrows indicate the narrow neck of the aneurysm.

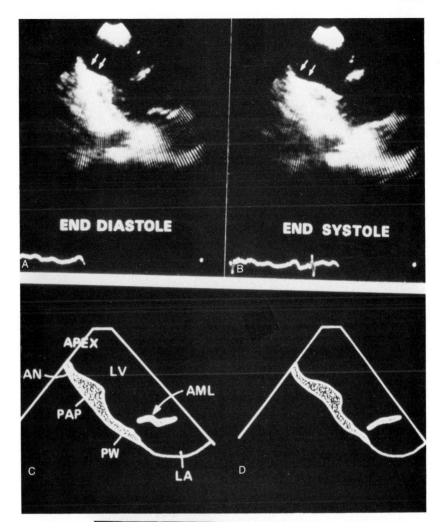

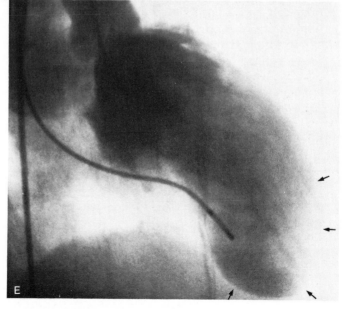

Figure 26–109. Long-axis cross-sectional echogram of the left ventricular apex demonstrates the left ventricular aneurysm (arrows) in end-diastole (*A*) and paradoxical expansion at end-systole (arrows) (*B*) with corresponding explanatory diagrams (*C* and *D*). The apex of the left ventricle (LV) is on the left. Left ventriculogram in the same patient in a right anterior oblique projection (*E*) confirms an aneurysm involving the anterolateral and apical aspects of the enlarged left ventricle (arrows). AN = aneurysm; PAP = papillary muscle; PW = posterior left ventricular wall; AML = anterior mitral valve leaflet; LA = left atrium. (Parts *A* to *D* courtesy of Robert Fowles, M.D.)

Cine Left Ventriculography

Contrast left ventriculography reflects endocardial systolic contraction but does not always demonstrate evidence of previous myocardial infarction because the fibrosis may be patchy. Segments that are seen to contract abnormally correspond to the anatomic site of myocardial infarction, however.

Replacement of systolic contraction by paradoxical regional expansion of the left ventricular wall determines the presence of a left ventricular aneurysm.[25] In addition, ventriculography contributes information regarding the location, size, and shape of the aneurysm as well as the presence of mural or intracavity thrombus and contractility of the remainder of the left ventricle. Conventionally, the left ventriculogram is performed in a 30 degree right anterior oblique projection. This projection allows assessment of apical, anterolateral, and inferior left ventricular wall aneurysms (see Fig. 26–103). The left anterior oblique projection with cranial angulation is required to assess septal motion and the left ventricular posterolateral wall.

Aneurysms involve the anterior and apical segments of the left ventricle more frequently. Although inferior and posterior myocardial infarctions occur commonly, the development of a left ventricular aneurysm involving the posterior left ventricular wall is rare. Athero-occlusive vascular disease usually diffusely involves the major coronary arteries. One explanation of the predilection of aneurysm formation for the anterolateral and apical segments is that the blood supply of this area comes solely from the left anterior descending coronary artery. In contrast, both the circumflex and the right coronary arteries contribute to the myocardial perfusion of the posterior and inferior surfaces. Similarly, the left ventricular septum with its dual blood supply from left anterior descending and right coronary arteries is rarely involved by aneurysm formation. It therefore follows that the left anterior descending coronary artery and often a major diagonal branch will be severely diseased in the presence of an apical or anterolateral aneurysm and that both right and circumflex coronary arteries are severely affected if an inferior aneurysm is seen.[28] Perhaps the diaphragm serves as a support to counteract the development of inferior aneurysms. Severe and diffuse occlusive coronary artery disease may lead to an ischemic cardiomyopathy with global hypokinesis of the left ventricle. Assessment of localized contraction abnormalities of the left ventricle can be made at ventriculography, enabling improved prognostication and determination of surgical therapy, such as planned aneurysmal resection.

Not all patients develop ventricular aneurysms following myocardial infarction.[15] Those patients with mild coronary artery disease and minimal prior stimulus for the development of intercoronary collaterals or those who have sustained major infarction are more susceptible to the development of a large infarcted segment.[18, 22] If, however, coronary arteriography reveals extensive coronary athero-occlusive disease, revascularization of the remainder of the jeopardized myocardium may be indicated at the time of aneurysmectomy. In the region of the aneurysm, the coronary arteries may appear as sparse fine branches, widely separated as they skirt the aneurysm, with areas of avascularity between.

INTRACAVITY THROMBUS

The occurrence of thrombus on the endocardial surface of a ventricular aneurysm is common and is often clinically manifest by peripheral systemic emboli.[15, 22] A pseudoaneurysm with its narrow neck has a lower incidence of systemic emboli, although a thrombus itself may lie freely within the sac. The diagnosis of a mural

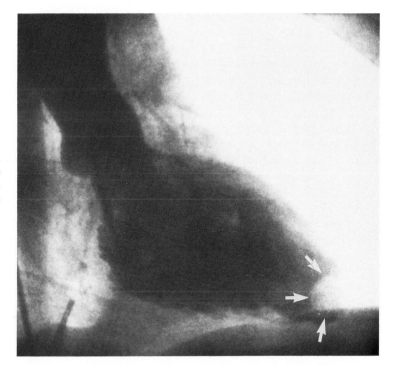

Figure 26–110. Left ventriculogram in a right anterior oblique projection demonstrating a circular filling defect (arrows) due to thrombus in an apical aneurysm.

thrombus on contrast ventriculography is based on the demonstration of a filling defect persisting throughout the cardiac cycle (Fig. 26–110).[27] The filling defect is most commonly located at the apex of the left ventricle and in a true aneurysm is often organized and adherent to the myocardial wall. A mural thrombus may be indicated only by a smooth wall with loss of normal apical left ventricular contour (Fig. 26–111).

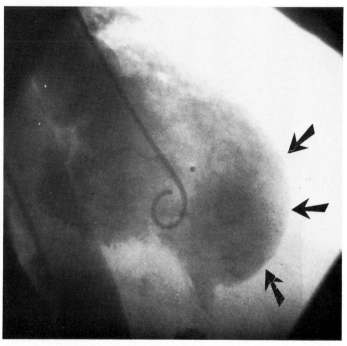

Figure 26–111. Left ventriculogram in a right anterior oblique projection demonstrating an anterolateral-apical left ventricular aneurysm. The contour is smooth (arrows) owing to a layered mural thrombus.

The accuracy of angiographic demonstration of left ventricular thrombi is poorly defined in the literature but is probably low. In pathologic series the incidence of left ventricular aneurysm thrombi is high.[50] In a series of patients evaluated for angina, however, the frequency of mural thrombi was 4.8 per cent.[27] Left ventricular thrombi have been shown to occur commonly with left ventricular aneurysm secondary to an acute myocardial infarction, classically located on the endocardial surface adjacent to the infarcted myocardium. They may become adherent to the wall and develop a pseudointima. Most commonly, they occur at the apex but may extend to the anterior free wall or septum.

M-mode echocardiographic features include multiple fine echoes within the left ventricular cavity.[30] Because of technical factors, however, this modality is not always reliable. Two-dimensional wide-angle echocardiography using apical (apex four-chamber or apex frontal view) and subxiphoid transducer positions allows improved visualization of the left ventricular apex and has been useful in the detection of left ventricular masses.[16, 28, 44] Although the acoustic impedance of a ventricular thrombus is similar to that of endocardium, dense echoes occur with a more organized thrombus and allow the distinction between thrombus and myocardial wall to be easily recognized (see Fig. 26–109). During coronary arteriography, an abnormal vascular blush with direct flow of contrast material into the left ventricular chamber may be demonstrated. This abnormal vascularity appears similar to tumor blush and is due to neovascularity extending from the myocardium into the left ventricular mural thrombus.[24, 56]

References

1. Aranda, J. M., Befeler, B., Thurer, R., et al.: Long-term clinical and hemodynamic studies after ventricular aneurysmectomy and aorto-coronary bypass. J. Thorac. Cardiovasc. Surg. 73:772, 1977.
2. Arenberg H.: Traumatic heart disease: a clinical study of 250 cases of non-penetrating chest injuries and their relation to cardiac disability. Ann. Intern. Med. 19:326, 1943.
3. Aronstein, C. G., and Neuman, L.: Syphilitic aneurysm of the heart: case report with review of the literature. Am. J. Clin. Pathol. 11:128, 1941.
4. Banka, V.S., and Helfant, R. H.: Temporal sequence of dynamic contractile characteristics in ischemic and nonischemic myocardium after acute coronary ligation. Am. J. Cardiol. 34:158, 1974.
5. Berkoff, H. A., Rowe, G. G., Crummy, A. B., et al.: Asymptomatic left ventricular aneurysm. A sequela of blunt chest trauma. Circulation 55:545, 1977.
6. Bjork, L.: Roentgen diagnosis of left ventricular aneurysm. Am. J. Roentgenol. 97:338, 1966.
7. Borer, J. S., Jacobstein, J. G., Bacharach, S. L., et al.: Detection of left ventricular aneurysm and evaluation of effects of surgical repair: The role of radionuclide cineangiography. Am. J. Cardiol. 45:1103, 1980.
8. Burton, N. A., Stinson, E. B., Oyer, P. E., et al.: Left ventricular aneurysm. Preoperative risk factors and long-term postoperative results. J. Thorac. Cardiovasc. Surg. 77:65, 1979.
9. Cantrell, J. R., Haller, J. A., and Ravitch, M. M.: A syndrome of congenital defects involving the abdominal wall, sternum, diaphragm, pericardium and heart. Surg. Gynecol. Obstet. 107:602, 1958.
10. Cheng, T. O.: Incidence of ventricular aneurysm in coronary artery disease. An angiographic appraisal. Am. J. Med. 50:340, 1971.
11. Chesler, E., Tucker, R. B. K., and Barlow, J. B.: Subvalvular and apical left ventricular aneurysms in the Bantu as a source of systemic emboli. Circulation 35:1156, 1967.
12. Chesler, E., Joffe, N., Schamroth, L., et al.: Annular subvalvular left ventricular aneurysms in the South African Bantu. Circulation 32:43, 1965.
13. Clearkin, K. P., and Bunje, H.: Rare cardiac aneurysm in a young adult. Thorax 10:42, 1954.
14. Dack, S.: The ventricular pulsations in myocardial infarction: a fluoroscopic and kymography study. Dis. Chest 27:282, 1955.
15. Davis, R. W., and Ebert, P. A.: Ventricular aneurysm: A clinical-pathologic correlation. Am. J. Cardiol. 29:1, 1972.
16. DeMaria, A. N., Bommer, W., Neumann, A., et al.: Left ventricular thrombi identified by cross-sectional echocardiography. Ann. Intern. Med. 90:14, 1979.
17. Diethrich, E. B., Koopot, R., and Kinard, S. A.: Pseudoaneurysm of atrioventricular groove. A late complication of mitral valve replacement. J. Thorac. Cardiovasc. Surg. 74:47, 1977.
18. Dubnow, M. H., Burchell, H. B., and Titus, J. L.: Post infarction ventricular aneurysm: a clinicomorphologic and electrocardiographic study of 80 cases. Am. Heart J. 70:753, 1965.

19. Edgett, J. W., Jr., Nelson, W. P., Hall, R. J., et al.: Diverticulum of the heart: part of the syndrome of congenital cardiac and midline thoracic and abdominal defects. Am. J. Cardiol. 24:580, 1969.

20. Fallah-Nejad, M., Abelson, D. M., and Blakemore, W. S.: Left ventricular pseudoaneurysm. A rare complication of open-heart surgery with unusual Doppler manifestations. Chest 61:90, 1972.

21. Favaloro, R. G., Effler, D. B., Groves, L. K., et al.: Ventricular aneurysm — clinical experience. Ann. Thorac. Surg. 6:227, 1968.

22. Gorlin, R., Klein, M. D., and Sullivan, J. M.: Prospective correlative study of ventricular aneurysm. Mechanistic concept and clinical recognition. Am. J. Med. 42:512, 1967.

23. Graber, J. D., Oakley, C. M., Pickering, B. N., et al.: Ventricular aneurysm: an appraisal of diagnosis and surgical treatment. Br. Heart J. 34:830, 1972.

24. Grollman, J. H., Jr., Hoffman, R. B., Price, J. E., Jr., et al.: Abnormal vascularity in left ventricular mural thrombus demonstrated by selective coronary arteriography. Radiology 113:591, 1974.

25. Grondin, P., Kretz, J. G., Bical, O., et al.: Natural history of saccular aneurysms of the left ventricle. J. Thorac. Cardiovasc. Surg. 77:57, 1979.

26. Guthaner, D. F., Wexler, L., and Harell, G.: CT demonstration of cardiac structures. Am. J. Roentgenol. 133:75, 1979.

27. Hamby, R. T., Wisoff, B. G., Davison, E. T., et al.: Coronary artery disease and left ventricular mural thrombi: clinical, hemodynamic and angiocardiographic aspects. Chest 66:488, 1974.

28. Helfant, R. H., Kemp, H. G., and Gorlin, R.: Coronary atherosclerosis, coronary collaterals and their relation to cardiac function. Ann. Intern. Med. 73:189, 1970.

29. Herman, M. V., and Gorlin, R.: Implications of left ventricular asynergy. Am. J. Cardiol. 23:538, 1969.

30. Horgan, J. H., O'Mshiel, F., and Goodman, A. C.: Demonstration of left ventricular thrombus by conventional echocardiography. J. Clin. Ultrasound 4:287, 1976.

31. Kittredge, R. D., Gamboa, B., and Kemp, H. G.: Radiographic visualization of left ventricular aneurysms on lateral chest film. Am. J. Roentgenol. 126:1140, 1976.

32. Kittredge, R. D., and Cameron, A.: Abnormalities of left ventricular wall motion and aneurysm formation. Am. J. Roentgenol. 116:110, 1972.

33. Klein, M. D., Herman, M. V., and Gorlin, R.: A hemodynamic study of left ventricular aneurysm. Circulation 35:614, 1967.

34. Kurtzman, R. S., and Lofstrom, J. E.: Detection and evaluation of myocardial infarction by image amplification and cinefluorography. Radiology 81:57, 1963.

35. Lee, D. C. S., Johnson, R. A., Boucher, C. A., et al.: Angiographic predictors of survival following left ventricular aneurysmectomy. Circulation 56:12, 1977.

36. Master, A. M., Gubner, R., Dack, S., et al.: Form of ventricular contraction in cardiac infarction: fluoroscopic studies. Proc. Soc. Exp. Biol. Med. 41:89, 1939.

37. Master, A. M., Gubner, R., Dack, S., et al.: The diagnosis of coronary occlusion and myocardial infarction by fluoroscopic examination. Am. Heart J. 20:475, 1940.

38. Meltzer, R. S., Guthaner, D. F., Rakowski, H., et al.: Diagnosis of left ventricular thrombi by two-dimensional echocardiography. Br. Heart J. 42:261, 1979.

39. Mills, P. G., Rose, J. D., Brodie, B. R., et al.: Echophonocardiographic diagnosis of left ventricular pseudoaneurysms. Chest 72:365, 1977.

40. Moran, J. M., Scanlon, P. J., Nemickas, R., et al.: Surgical treatment of postinfarction ventricular aneurysm. Ann. Thorac. Surg. 21:107, 1976.

41. Morcerf, F. P., Duarte, E. P., Salcedo, E. E., et al.: Echocardiographic findings in false aneurysm of left ventricle. Cleve. Clin. Q. 43:71, 1976.

42. Mullen, D. C., Posey, L., Gabriel, R., et al.: Prognostic considerations in the management of left ventricular aneurysms. Ann. Thorac. Surg. 23:455, 1977.

43. Parkinson, J., Bedford, D. E., and Thomson, W. A. R.: Cardiac aneurysm. Q. J. Med. 31:455, 1938.

44. Ports, T. A., Cogan, J., Schiller, N. B. et al.: Echocardiography of left ventricular masses. Circulation 58:528, 1978.

45. Recchia, F., Orzan, F., Krajcer, Z., et al.: Determinants of perioperative mortality and morbidity with left ventricular aneurysmectomy. Experience in 96 patients. Circulation 56(III):59, 1977.

46. Roberts, W. C., and Morrow, A. G.: Pseudoaneurysm of the left ventricle: an unusual sequel of myocardial infarction and rupture of the heart. Am. J. Med. 43:639, 1967.

47. Roelandt, J., Van den Brand, M., Vletter, W. B., et al.: Echocardiographic diagnosis of pseudoaneurysm of the left ventricle. Circulation 52:466, 1975.

48. Saksena, F. B., Kramer, N. E., Towne, W. D., et al.: Infective aneurysm of the left ventricle: angiographic and echocardiographic features. Am. Heart J. 96:384, 1978.

49. Schattenberg, T. T., Guiliani, E. R., Campion, B. C., et al.: Post-infarction ventricular aneurysm. Mayo Clin. Proc. 45:13, 1970.

50. Schlichter, J., Hellerstein, H. K., and Katz, L. N.: Aneurysm of the heart: Correlative study of 102 proved cases. Medicine 33:43, 1954.

51. Schwedel, J. B., Samet, P., and Mednick, H.: Electrokymographic studies of abnormal left ventricular pulsations. Am. Heart J. 40:410, 1950.

52. Sharma, S. D., Ballantyne, F., and Goldstein, S.: The relationship of ventricular asynergy in coronary artery disease to ventricular premature beats. Chest 66:385, 1974.

53. Shaw, R. C., Connors, J. P., Hieb, B. R., et al.: Postoperative investigation of left ventricular aneurysm resection. Circulation 56(II):7, 1977.

54. Smulyan, H., Eich, R. H., Johnson, L. W., et al.: An evaluation of the results of left ventricular

aneurysmectomy: use of a simplified method for analysis of the left ventriculogram. Am. Heart J. 96:596, 1978.

55. Sos, T. A., Sniderman, K. W., Levin, D. C., et al.: Cinefluoroscopy in evaluating left ventricular contractility and aneurysms. Radiology 133:31, 1979.

56. Soulen, R. L., Grollman, J. H., Paglia, D., et al.: Coronary neovascularity and fistula formation. A sign of mural thrombus. Circulation 56:663, 1977.

57. Tennant, R., and Wiggers, C. J.: The effect of coronary occlusion on myocardial contraction. Am. J. Physiol. 112:351, 1935.

58. Treistman, B., Cooley, D. A., Lufschanowski, R., et al.: Diverticulum or aneurysm of left ventricle. Am. J. Cardiol. 32:119, 1973.

59. VanTassel, R. A., and Edwards, J. E.: Rupture of heart complicating myocardial infarction: analysis of 40 cases including nine examples of left ventricular false aneurysm. Chest 61:104, 1972.

60. Weyman, A. E., Peskoe, S. M., Williams, E. S., et al.: Detection of left ventricular aneurysms by cross-sectional echocardiography. Circulation 54:936, 1976.

61. Yakierevitch, V., Vidne, B., Melamed, R., et al.: False aneurysm of the left ventricle. J. Thorac. Cardiovasc. Surg. 76:556, 1978.

62. Zaret, B. L., Strauss, H. W., Hurley, P. J., et al.: A noninvasive scintiphotographic method for detecting regional ventricular dysfunction in man. N. Engl. J. Med. 284:1165, 1971.

Part VIII
Cardiac Neoplasms

PAUL R. CIPRIANO, M.D.
RANDOLPH P. MARTIN, M.D.
LEWIS WEXLER, M.D.

INTRODUCTION

Neoplastic heart diseases are uncommon and can be simply categorized. The majority of cardiac neoplasms are metastatic. Most primary tumors of the heart have benign histology. Primary tumors of the heart that have malignant histology are rare, but they usually occur in children and young adults. Occasionally, extracardiac tumors produce pharmacologically active substances, which circulate systemically and have marked effects on cardiac structure and function. Metastases and primary cardiac neoplasms are frequently advanced by the time they produce cardiac symptoms and are detected. Many cardiac tumors have been successfully treated, however, since the advent of recently developed noninvasive methods of cardiac imaging that provide spatial orientation of cardiac structures throughout the cardiac cycle. Two-dimensional echocardiography and computed transmission tomography may allow early detection, localization, and accurate quantification of even small cardiac tumors. Newer methods of cardiac imaging promise to be important in developing methods of detecting and successfully treating neoplastic diseases of the heart. Current advances in cardiac surgical techniques permit the successful resection of many cardiac tumors, while cardiac transplantation may be required for patients having more advanced disease.

METASTATIC NEOPLASMS

Incidence

Metastases occur 16 to 40 times more frequently than primary neoplasms of the heart in autopsy studies.[11, 19, 29] Tumors may metastasize hematogenously by lymphatics and by direct extension to involve pericardium, myocardium, and cardiac chambers. Either grossly visible or microscopic metastases involve the heart in 3 to 21 per cent of patients who die of extracardiac neoplasms.[1, 3, 9, 15] Symptoms are usually related to the location of cardiac metastases, but the extent of metastatic involvement does not appear to correlate well with clinical manifestations of heart disease.[3, 25] In less than one third of patients with cardiac metastases are cardiac symptoms or signs detected clinically, nor do they contribute to death. There is nearly always widespread involvement of other organ systems in the presence of metastases to the heart.[3, 12, 25]

A few primary neoplasms account for most cardiac metastases. Bronchogenic carcinoma and breast carcinoma are the most common tumors to metastasize to the heart, with metastases occurring in more than 30 per cent of patients having disseminated disease.[3] Other primary neoplasms that occur less commonly than carcinoma of the lung and breast metastasize to the heart more frequently. Notably, there is evidence of metastases to the heart and pericardium in an estimated 40 to 60 per cent of patients having malignant melanoma.[3, 10] Infiltration of the heart occurs in 37 to 44 per cent of patients with leukemia,[3, 20] in approximately 60 per cent of patients with lymphocytic leukemia, and in 40 per cent of patients with myelogenous leukemia. Twenty-four per cent of patients with lymphoma have cardiac infiltration with tumor. This occurs in approximately 25 to 40 per cent of patients with reticulum cell sarcoma, 10 to 40 per cent of patients with lymphosarcoma, and 5 to 30 per cent of patients with Hodgkin's disease.[3, 5, 21] Rhabdomyosarcoma, a disease that occurs primarily in childhood, metastasizes to the heart in approximately one third of patients.[18] Other cardiac metastases originate from a variety of tumors that involve the heart much less frequently than the aforementioned lesions.

Pericardial Metastases (See also Chapter 25)

The pericardium is a frequent site of metastatic disease.[1, 3, 5, 25] Pericardial fluid, in the presence or absence of cardiac tamponade, may be the first sign of cardiac involvement with neoplasm. As pericardial metastases become more advanced, there may be associated invasion of the myocardium and encasement of the heart with tumor.[8, 25] Pericardial metastases have been reported to be either the primary cause of death or a contributing factor in less than one third of patients with pericardial involvement.[15, 25] Atrial or ventricular arrhythmias, electrocardiographic abnormalities, and congestive heart failure due to cardiac constriction may all be nonspecific signs of pericardial metastases. Malignant pericardial fluid may be suggested by chest roentgenograms that demonstrate a uniformly enlarged cardiac silhouette.[2, 15, 23] Less commonly, metastatic masses will be observed in the cardiac silhouette. A widened pericardial space and straightening of the lateral border of the right atrial chamber may be demonstrated by right angiocardiography in the presence of sufficient malignant pericardial fluid. Echocardiography, however, is currently the recommended method for detecting and quantitating even small amounts of pericardial fluid.[14]

Neoplastic involvement of the pericardium is demonstrated by the cytology of pericardial fluid and by histologic examination of pericardial tissue that is obtained by biopsy at the time of pericardiocentesis. Pneumopericardium, produced by introducing air into the pericardial space following pericardiocentesis, may be helpful in demonstrating the extent and distribution of pericardial thickening and masses due to metastases.[2, 4] Although the prognosis for most patients who have metastatic pericardial disease is poor, the adverse hemodynamic effects of this condition may be relieved by pericardiocentesis or pericardiectomy.[25] Some pericardial metastases, notably those due to leukemia or lymphoma, may be successfully palliated with chemotherapy and radiation therapy.[2, 8, 20]

Myocardial Metastases

Metastases are found in the myocardium less commonly than in the pericardium.[1] Metastatic myocardial disease is detected clinically and is associated with serious cardiac dysfunction much less frequently than pericardial metastases. Myocardial metastases may produce arrhythmias and, if located in the conduction system, heart block.[8, 15] There is usually insufficient replacement of myocardial mass by metastases to produce congestive heart failure.[8]

Endocardial Metastases

Endocardial metastases are less common than either pericardial or myocardial metastases, and they seldom produce signs or symptoms of heart disease.[15] Endocardial metastases, however, may have marked hemodynamic effects. Neoplasms may seed the endocardium of the right heart by return of systemic blood to the heart.[5] Although endocardial metastases are initially silent, they are a source of pulmonary or systemic emboli, and as they enlarge they may obstruct blood flow and produce symptoms of right heart failure. Intracavitary metastases can usually be clearly demonstrated by angiography (Fig. 26–112B) and two-dimensional echocardiography (Fig. 26–113). These methods of imaging the heart allow the location and size of tumors to be accurately determined if surgical treatment is being considered. The most common intracavitary metastatic tumors to the heart are renal cell carcinoma and Wilms' tumor, which can grow into the renal vein and then extend into the inferior vena cava to the right atrium. They may obstruct venous return or block the tricuspid valve. Intracavitary metastases can be successfully palliated by surgical removal.

Extracardiac Cardioactive Tumors

Occasionally, extracardiac tumors, notably malignant carcinoid and pheochromocytoma, release pharmacologically active substances that affect the heart as they circulate systemically. When carcinoid tumor metastasizes to the liver, sufficient amounts of serotonin (5-hydroxytryptamine) maybe released to produce endocardial thickening, primarily of the chambers and valves of the right side of the heart.[8, 11] This results in decreased mobility and retraction of the leaflets of the tricuspid valve and pulmonic valve, which may produce tricuspid valvular stenosis, with or without regurgitation and pulmonic valvular stenosis. The pharmacologic effect of serotonin is reduced as blood passes through the pulmonary circulation; therefore, there is usually no endocardial thickening of the chambers of the left side of the heart.[8, 11] Clinical signs and symptoms of carcinoid heart disease are usually due to right heart failure with tricuspid regurgitation and, less frequently, pulmonic stenosis. Enlargement of the right ventricle or right atrium or both may be evident on chest roentgenograms (Fig. 26–114A). Tricuspid regurgitation may be detected noninvasively by two-dimensional echocardiography.[16] Tricuspid stenosis and regurgitation, right ventricular function, and pulmonic valvular stenosis in this disorder may be quantitated by cardiac catheterization and cardioangiography (Fig. 26–114B). Although the prognosis of patients

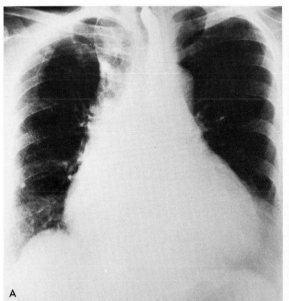

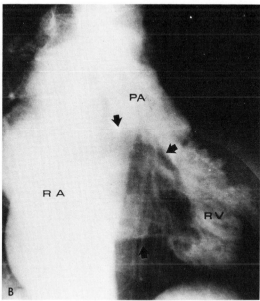

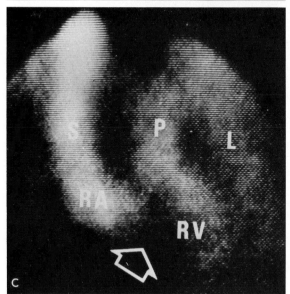

Figure 26–112. Metastasis to right ventricle. *A,* Chest roentgenogram of a 67-year-old woman with a recurrent carcinoma of the recto-sigmoid colon that metastasized to the right ventricle. Cardiac contour is moderately enlarged and globular owing to pericardial fluid. *B,* Frontal view of a right angiocardiogram. The large metastatic tumor (arrows) causes a filling defect in the right ventricle. *C,* Frontal view of a radioisotopic angiocardiogram performed after injection of an intravenous bolus of 99m-Tc pertechnetate. The defect in the right ventricle (arrow) is caused by the metastatic tumor. Megavoltage radiation therapy did not reduce the size of this tumor. Postmortem examination showed that the metastatic tumor occupied 85% of the right ventricular cavity and involved the endocardium, myocardium, and pericardium. L = lung; P and PA = pulmonary artery; RA = right atrium; RV = right ventricle; S = superior vena cava. (*From* Steiner, R. M., Bull, M. I., Kumpel, R., et al.: The diagnosis of intracardiac metastases of colon carcinoma by radioisotopic and roentgenographic studies. Am. J. Cardiol. *26*:300, 1970. Reproduced by permission.)

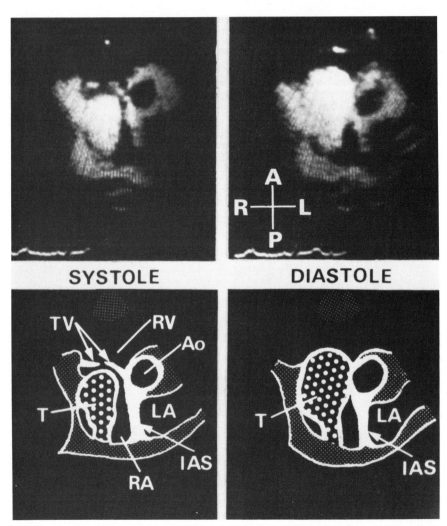

Figure 26–113. Metastasis to right atrium; echocardiogram. Two-dimensional echocardiogram and explanatory diagram in the short-axis view during ventricular systole and diastole in a 54-year-old woman with a renal cell carcinoma extending from the inferior vena cava into the right atrium. The tumor appears as a large mass of echoes filling the right atrium, attached to the posterior wall of the right atrium, and prolapsed into the orifice of the tricuspid valve during ventricular diastole. The left kidney containing a hypernephroma, which extended into the inferior vena cava and right atrium, was successfully removed by surgery. A = anterior; Ao = aorta; IAS = inter-atrial septum; L = left; LA = left atrium; P = posterior; R = right; RA = right atrium; RV = right ventricle; T = tumor, TV = tricuspid valve.

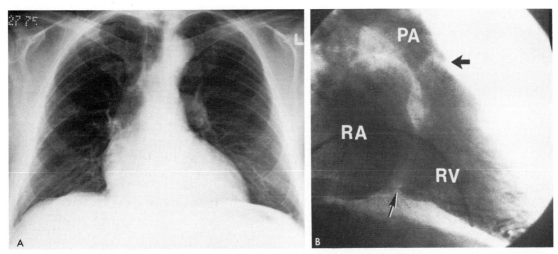

Figure 26–114. Carcinoid syndrome; tricuspid and pulmonic valve involvement. *A,* Chest roentgeno-gram of a 55-year-old man with tricuspid valvular stenosis and regurgitation and pulmonic valvular stenosis due to malignant carcinoid syndrome. There is cardiomegaly and an enlarged right atrial silhouette. *B,* A right ventricular angiogram in the right anterior oblique view shows marked tricuspid regurgitation (black and white arrow) with filling of an enlarged right atrium. The leaflets of the pul-monic valve are thickened (black arrow), as is seen with valvular pulmonic stenosis. PA = pulmonary artery; RA = right atrium; RV = right ventricle.

with carcinoid heart disease is poor, we have observed improved cardiac hemodynamics in this condition following replacement of the tricuspid valve with a prosthesis.

Pheochromocytomas are chromaffin cell tumors of the sympathoadrenal system, which produce the catecholamines epinephrine and norepinephrine. Focal myocardial damage has been produced by large amounts of circulating catecholamines.[27] The tu-mors may be isolated, or they may be associated with neurocutaneous syndromes, Sip-ple's syndrome, and other conditions.

BENIGN NEOPLASMS

Although primary neoplasms of the heart are much less common than metastases, 80 per cent of primary cardiac tumors have benign histology[11] and many can be surgically removed if found early. Unfortunately, histologically benign cardiac tumors may produce serious complications due to systemic emboli before they are detected. These tumors may also enlarge and result in death, which frequently occurs in infants and children.[6] Myxomas and rhabdomyomas constitute the majority of all benign cardiac neoplasms. Fibroelastic papillomas of various sizes occur relatively commonly on the ventricular surface of semilunar valves or the atrial surfaces of atrioventricular valves (Fig. 26–115).[13]

Myxomas

Myxomas are endocardial tumors that originate from multipotential mesenchymal cells.[7] These tumors usually occur in adults, and they constitute approximately one half

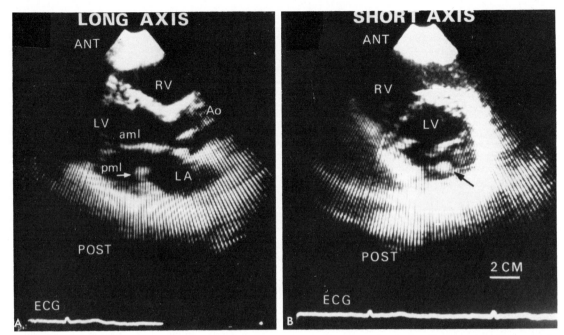

Figure 26–115. Papillary fibroma of mitral valve. Two-dimensional echocardiogram in (*A*) long axis and (*B*) short axis views in a 35-year-old man with systemic emboli that induced a right cerebral hemisphere infarct and a myocardial infarct. Cerebral angiograms showed multiple emboli in the distribution of the right and left middle cerebral arteries. Coronary arteriograms, the levophase of a pulmonary angiogram, and a left ventriculogram were normal. The posterior leaflet of the mitral valve was thickened on the two-dimensional echocardiogram (arrows). A 0.6 by 1.0 by 0.6 cm mulberry-shaped papillary fibroma of the posterior mitral valve leaflet with superficial thrombi was successfully removed by surgery. Ao = aorta; aml = anterior mitral valve leaflet; ANT = anterior; LV = left ventricle; pml = posterior mitral valve leaflet; POST = posterior; LA = left atrium; RV = right ventricle.

of all benign cardiac neoplasms.[11, 15, 19] Three fourths of myxomas are located in the left atrium.[11] They frequently project into the left atrial cavity from their attachment on the interatrial septum. Myxomas occur, in decreasing order of frequency, in the right atrium, right ventricle, left ventricle, or more than one chamber. They may obstruct blood flow, and a murmur of mitral stenosis due to left atrial myxoma may be detected intermittently. Often, there is a systemic reaction with elevation of the erythrocyte sedimentation rate, and frequently there are abnormalities of serum protein, demonstrated by electrophoresis, which return to normal after the tumor is removed.[8] Plain chest roentgenograms may demonstrate pulmonary venous or pulmonary arterial hypertension or both.[4] Approximately 10 per cent of myxomas contain calcium, which can occasionally be seen on chest roentgenograms or by fluoroscopy. These tumors are best demonstrated by angiocardiography (Fig. 26–116) and by two-dimensional echocardiography (Fig. 26–117). An atrial branch of the left coronary artery may terminate in a left atrial myxoma, and a collection of radiographic contrast within the tumor has been demonstrated during coronary angiography (Fig. 26–118).[17] Myxomas of the left atrium may result in serious complications or death owing to obstruction of the mitral valve orifice or systemic embolization of the tumor. Microscopic examination of material removed at arterial embolectomy may demonstrate the tumor. Surgical removal of myxomas is usually successful, although these tumors may metastasize to sites more distal in the systemic circulation, and they may recur following surgical removal.

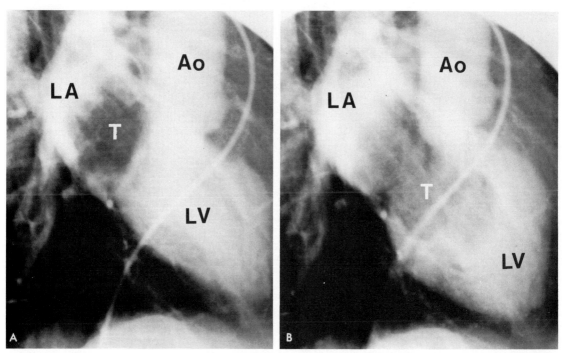

Figure 26–116. Left atrial myxoma. *A,* Levophase of a pulmonary angiogram in the lateral view during ventricular systole in an adult patient, which shows a large filling defect in the left atrium due to a myxoma. *B,* During ventricular diastole the tumor is demonstrated to prolapse through the mitral valve into the left ventricle. The myxoma was successfully removed by surgery. Ao = aorta; LA = left atrium; LV = left ventricle; T = tumor. (Courtesy of Thomas A. Sos, M.D., New York.)

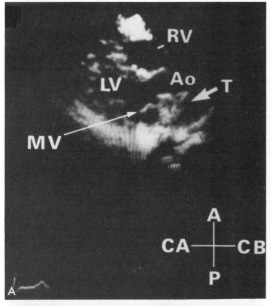

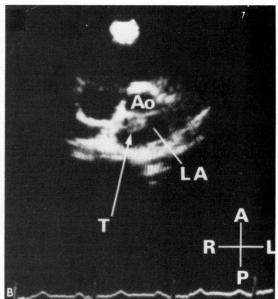

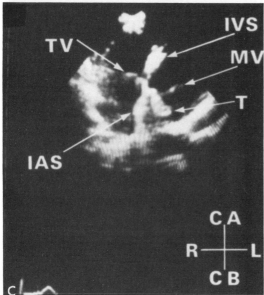

Figure 26–117. Left atrial myxoma; echocardiogram. Two-dimensional echocardiograms in the long-axis view (*A* and *C*) and the short-axis view (*B*) in a 29-year-old woman with nonspecific constitutional symptoms and evidence of a systemic embolus. A mobile left atrial mass is seen attached to the interatrial septum. Cardiac cineangiography was not performed. A 3 by 3 by 2 cm pedunculated myxoma, which was attached to the left side of the interatrial septum, was removed surgically. A = anterior; Ao = aorta; CA = cardiac apex; CB = cardiac base; IAS = interatrial septum; IVS = interventricular septum; L = left; LA = left atrium; LV = left ventricle; MV = mitral valve; P = posterior; RV = right ventricle; T = tumor; TV = tricuspid valve.

Rhabdomyomas

Rhabdomyomas are the second most common primary heart tumor, accounting for approximately 20 per cent of benign cardiac neoplasms.[11] The nearly exclusive incidence of these tumors in infants and children, their multifocality, and their microscopic appearance suggest that rhabdomyoma is a hamartoma (Fig. 26–119) or a malformation rather than a true cardiac neoplasm.[6] These tumors are usually multiple, and frequently they become large intracavitary cardiac masses. Physical findings and electrocardiographic changes are not specific for this tumor. However, once an intracavitary mass has been demonstrated in an infant or young child, it is much more likely to be a rhabdomyoma than a myxoma.[6] Rhabdomyomas occur in males twice as frequently as

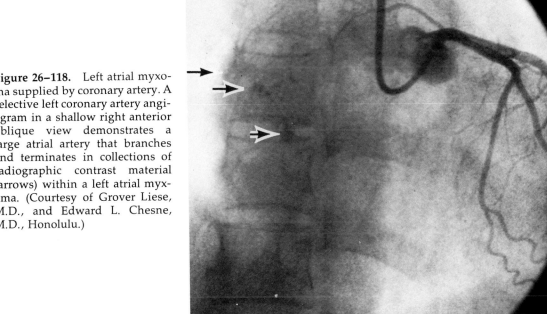

Figure 26–118. Left atrial myxoma supplied by coronary artery. A selective left coronary artery angiogram in a shallow right anterior oblique view demonstrates a large atrial artery that branches and terminates in collections of radiographic contrast material (arrows) within a left atrial myxoma. (Courtesy of Grover Liese, M.D., and Edward L. Chesne, M.D., Honolulu.)

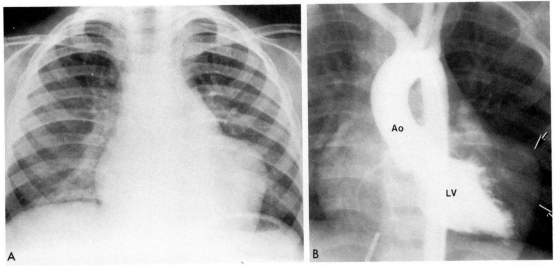

Figure 26–119. Hamartoma of left ventricle. *A,* Chest roentgenogram of a child with ventricular tachycardia due to a hamartoma of the left ventricle. A marked convexity of the left ventricular cardiac silhouette is present. *B,* A left ventricular angiogram in the frontal view shows a mass in the free wall of the left ventricle (arrows) representing the tumor. The tumor was successfully removed by surgery. Ao = aorta; LV = left ventricle. (Courtesy of Thomas A. Sos, M.D., New York.)

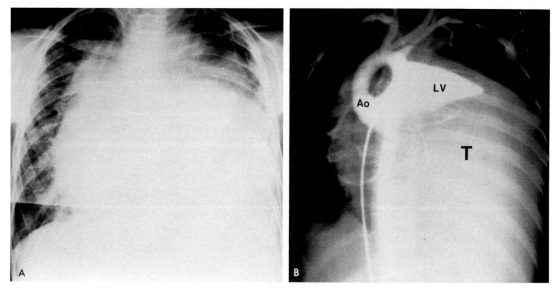

Figure 26–120. Fibrosarcoma of left ventricle. *A,* Chest roentgenogram of a seven-year-old boy who had rapidly enlarging globular cardiac silhouette. In addition to the large cardiac silhouette there is evidence of pulmonary venous congestion and increased interstitial lines, as is seen in left ventricular failure. *B,* A left ventricular angiogram, using a venous catheter passed across the interatrial septum, shows that the relatively small left ventricular chamber is markedly elevated and that most of the cardiac silhouette is occupied by the tumor. The left coronary artery overlies the tumor. The patient died following an operation to remove this malignant fibrosarcoma, which appeared to originate in the left ventricle. Ao = aorta; LV = left ventricle; T = tumor. (Courtesy of Phillip Caves, M.D.)

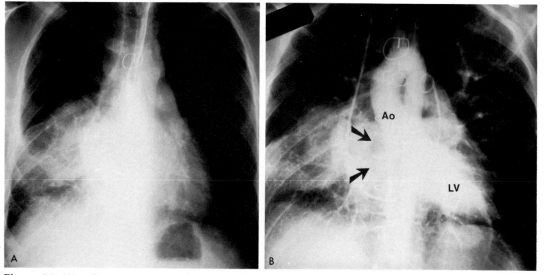

Figure 26–121. Recurrent mesenchymoma of atrial septum; plain film and angiogram. *A,* Chest roentgenogram of an 18-year-old boy with local recurrence of a malignant mesenchymoma that originated from the interatrial septum and extended into the left atrium. The multiple metallic clips are related to previous resection of the left atrial tumor. There is faint calcification of the tumor, which was better seen by fluoroscopy. The tumor invaded the middle and lower lobes of the right lung and compressed the intermediate bronchus. There are interstitial lines in the right lower lobe owing to obstruction of lymphatics and pulmonary veins. *B,* Frontal view of the levophase of a pulmonary angiogram shows a large filling defect (arrows) due to recurrent tumor in the left atrium. The patient died following an operation to resect the recurrent tumor. Ao = aorta; LV = left ventricle.

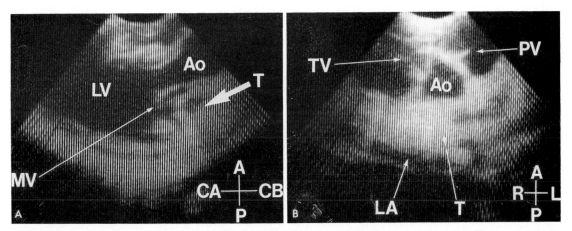

Figure 26–122.   Recurrent mesenchymoma; echocardiogram. Two-dimensional echocardiograms in (*A*) long-axis view and (*B*) short-axis view of the patient in Figure 26–121. The recurrent tumor appears as a large mass of echoes filling the left atrium. A = anterior; Ao = aorta; CA = cardiac apex; CB = cardiac base; L = left; LA = left atrium; LV = left ventricle; MV = mitral valve; P = posterior; PV = pulmonic valve; T = tumor; TV = tricuspid valve.

in females, and 30 to 50 per cent of these tumors are associated with tuberous sclerosis.[6, 11] Approximately 20 per cent of these tumors contain microscopic calcium, as do other benign cardiac neoplasms.[4] In fact, myocardial calcification in a child is very likely to be a neoplasm. Although the tumors are frequently multiple and death due to rhabdomyoma is common below the age of one year, many patients with rhabdomyoma appear to be good candidates for surgical resection of all or part of the tumor.[6]

MALIGNANT NEOPLASMS

Malignant primary cardiac tumors are rare, but they usually occur in children and young adults. No predisposing factors are known. These tumors consist primarily of various types of sarcomas,[1, 11, 28] particularly hemangiosarcoma, rhabdomyosarcoma, and mesenchymomas. These neoplasms may originate within any cardiac chamber, and they may involve cardiac valves.[4] Ventricular arrhythmias, obstruction to cardiac blood flow, and valvular dysfunction may occur. These tumors usually produce an enlarging cardiac silhouette on chest roentgenograms (Fig. 26–120*A*). Their size and location can best be demonstrated by angiocardiography (Figs. 26–120*B* and 26–121*B*) and by two-dimensional echocardiography (Fig. 26–122). The large majority of malignant primary pericardial tumors are mesotheliomas.[4] Although the prognosis for patients with primary cardiac neoplasms is poor, surgery or radiation therapy has been successful in some cases.[22, 26]

References

1. Abrams, H. L., Spiro, R., and Goldstein, N.: Metastases in carcinoma. Analysis of 1000 autopsied cases. Cancer 3:74–85, 1950.
2. Abrams, H. L., Adams, D. F., and Grant, H. A.: The radiology of tumors of the heart. Radiol. Clin. North Am. 9:299–326, 1971.
3. Bisel, H. F., Wroblewski, F., and LaDue, B.: Incidence and clinical manifestations of cardiac metastases. J.A.M.A. 153:712–715, 1953.

4. Davis, G. D., Kincaid, O. W., and Hallermann, F. J.: Roentgen aspects of cardiac tumors. Semin. Roentgenol. *4*:384, 1969.
5. DeLoach, J. F., and Haynes, J. W.: Secondary tumors of heart and pericardium. Review of the subject and report of one hundred thirty-seven cases. Arch. Intern. Med. *91*:224–249, 1953.
6. Fenoglio, J. J., McAllister, H. A., and Ferrans, V. J.: Cardiac rhabdomyoma: a clinicopathologic and electron microscopic study. Am. J. Cardiol. *38*:241–251, 1976.
7. Ferrans, J. J., and Roberts, W. C.: Structural features of cardiac myxomas: histology, histochemistry, and electron microscopy. Hum. Pathol. *4*:111–146, 1973.
8. Freiman, A. H.: Cardiovascular disturbances associated with cancer. Med. Clin. North Am. *50*:733–746, 1966.
9. Gassman, H. S., Meadows, R., Jr., and Baker, C. A.: Metastatic tumors of the heart. Am. J. Med. *19*:357–365, 1955.
10. Glancy, D. L., and Roberts, W. C.: The heart in malignant melanoma. Am. J. Cardiol. *21*:555–571, 1968.
11. Griffiths, G. C.: Primary tumours of the heart. Clin. Radiol. *13*:183–194, 1962.
12. Hanbury, W. J.: Secondary tumors of the heart. Br. J. Cancer *14*:23–27, 1960.
13. Heath, D.: Pathology of cardiac tumors. Am. J. Cardiol. *21*:315–327, 1968.
14. Horowitz, M. S., Schultz, C. S., Stinson, E. B., et al.: Sensitivity and specificity of echocardiographic diagnosis of pericardial effusion. Circulation *50*:239–247, 1974.
15. Hurst, J. W., and Cooper, H. R.: Neoplastic disease of the heart. Am. Heart J. *50*:782–802, 1955.
16. Lieppe, W., Behar, V. S., Scallion, R., et al.: Detection of TR with 2-dimensional echocardiography and peripheral vein injections. Circulation *57*:128–132, 1978.
17. Marshall, W. H., Steiner, R. M., and Wexler, L.: "Tumor vascularity" in left atrial myxoma demonstrated by selective coronary angiography. Radiology *93*:815–816, 1969.
18. Pratt, C. B., Dugger, D. L., Johnson, W. W., et al.: Metastatic involvement of the heart in childhood rhabdomyosarcoma. Cancer *31*:1492–1497, 1973.
19. Prichard, R. W.: Tumors of the heart: review of the subject and report of one hundred and fifty cases. Arch. Pathol. *51*:98–128, 1951.
20. Roberts, W. C., Bodey, G. P., and Wertlake, P. T.: The heart in acute leukemia. Am. J. Cardiol. *21*:388–412, 1968.
21. Roberts, W. C., Glancy, D. L., and DeVita, U. T., Jr.: Heart in malignant lymphoma (Hodgkin's disease, lymphosarcoma, reticulum cell sarcoma and mycosis fungoides). A study of 196 autopsy cases. Am. J. Cardiol. *22*:85–107, 1968.
22. Sagerman, R. H., Hurley, E., and Bagshaw, M.: Successful sterilization of a primary cardiac sarcoma by supervoltage radiation therapy. Am. J. Roentgenol. *92*:942–946, 1964.
23. Steiner, R. E.: Radiologic aspects of cardiac tumors. Am. J. Cardiol. *21*:344–356, 1968.
24. Steiner, R. M., Bull, M. I., Kumpel, F., et al.: The diagnosis of intracardiac metastasis of colon carcinoma by radioisotopic and roentgenographic studies. Am. J. Cardiol. *26*:300–304, 1970.
25. Thurber, D. L., Edwards, J. E., and Achor, R. W.: Secondary malignant tumors of the percardium. Circulation *26*:228–241, 1962.
26. Van der Hauwaert, L. G.: Cardiac tumours in infancy and childhood. Br. Heart J. *33*:125–132, 1971.
27. Van Vliet, P. D., Burchell, H. B., and Titus, J. L.: Focal myocarditis associated with pheochromocytoma. N. Engl. J. Med. *274*:1102–1108, 1966.
28. Whorton, C. M.: Primary malignant tumors of the heart. Cancer *2*:245–260, 1949.
29. Wood, P.: Diseases of the Heart and Circulation. London, Eyre and Spottiswood, 1956.

PART IX
Cardiac Pacemakers

IRVING EHRLICH, B.S., M.D.

HISTORY

Although Zoll, in 1952, was the first person to accomplish sustained external control of cardiac rate in a living human,[79] electrical stimulation of muscle tissue dates back to Galvani's experiments with frogs' legs.[12] In 1809, Burns advocated the use of electrical discharge in the treatment of cardiac arrest,[7] and in 1819 Aldini, perhaps somewhat morbidly, attempted to apply this dictum when he tried to activate the arrested hearts of decapitated criminals by means of electrical stimulation.[1] Again in 1887, McWilliam demonstrated that electrical shocks could be used to sustain the heartbeat in animals after vagally induced cardiac standstill.[38] In 1912, Erlanger devised a method of sinoatrial stimulation by means of a bipolar platinum electrode, which was introduced directly through the chest wall,[14] and in 1932, Hyman first used the term "artificial pacemaker" in reference to an external electrical pulse generator connected to percutaneous needle electrodes inserted into the right atrium.[25] Sweet, in 1947, showed that electrical stimulation could be accomplished in the arrested heart by sinoatrial node stimulation in two patients who acquired asystole during thoracotomy.[67] Then, in 1952, Zoll demonstrated the feasibility of transthoracic cardiac stimulation.[79] His method required high voltages and was very painful but proved lifesaving and served as the impetus for further research into the application of electrical stimulation of the heart.

After Zoll, development of a true cardiac pacemaker proceeded rapidly. Lillehei, in 1957, first affixed electrodes directly to the cardiac ventricle during open heart surgery as a means of treating iatrogenic heart block.[73] His generator was externally located. The following year, however, Senning used an internally powered unit that was recharged from outside the body.[61] Then, in 1960, Chardack introduced the first truly autonomous pacemaker, with a mercury cell battery system.[9]

Up until 1959, aside from the early external electrodes, all pacing was accomplished through electrodes implanted directly into the myocardium. In 1959, Furman and Schwedel introduced transvenous endocardial pacing with an electrode inserted through the jugular vein.[17] This method significantly reduced the mortality and morbidity associated with the open thoracotomy previously required.

From the early 1960's until the present, advances in pulse generators, energy sources, and electrodes have produced more reliable and longer-lived pacing systems.

INDICATIONS

Originally, cardiac pacing was used primarily in the treatment of the conduction defects producing the Stokes-Adams syndrome. With refinement of the various techniques of cardiac pacing, however, the range of indications has broadened considerably. In general, the choice of temporary or permanent, myocardial or transvenous pacing depends on the expected duration of the defect as well as the clinical condition of the patient. Currently, four main clinical categories are indications for pacing.[36]

The Stokes-Adams Syndrome

These patients have a high-grade or complete heart block with atrioventricular dissociation resulting in idioventricular rhythms or asystole and concomitant cerebral ischemia resulting in loss of consciousness. The block may be the result of coronary artery disease, rheumatic heart disease, diphtheria, syphilis, cardiomyopathy, collagen disease, sarcoidosis, amyloidosis, metastatic disease, or congenital defects, or it may be surgically induced. Most cases, however, are the result of idiopathic fibrosis and degeneration of the conducting system. The mortality rate of untreated patients with Stokes-Adams syndrome has been estimated at 50 per cent within one year after onset.[28]

Patients with congenital heart block are usually asymptomatic, especially if there are no other cardiac defects.[20] The incidence of syncope being in the range of 10 per cent, there is a predisposition to sudden death, however.

Bradycardias

These include sinus bradycardia, sinoatrial node block or standstill, the "sick sinus syndrome," and any other condition resulting in cardiac decompensation with congestive failure, such as atrial flutter or fibrillation with a slow ventricular response.

Acute Myocardial Infarction

Most commonly, these patients require only temporary pacing. Their conduction defects — first degree, second degree, or complete block — are usually the result of transient edema around the atrioventricular node secondary to ischemia of the adjacent myocardium. This type of block is found in diaphragmatic infarctions and is usually slowly progressive, but almost never permanent; it usually reverts to normal during the first week.[66] On the other hand, anterior wall infarctions produce heart block as the result of destruction and necrosis of the conducting fibers of the right bundle and of part of the left. The block is sudden in onset, usually permanent, and long-term survival is poor even with pacing.

Overdrive

The object in this case is to increase the cardiac rate in order to subdue life-threatening ectopic mechanisms. The pacemaker may be used alone or in combination with drugs. It may also be used in the treatment of drug-induced dangerous rhythms, such as those produced by digitalis, quinidine, and procainamide.[78]

IDENTIFICATION

There are three main categories of pacing systems.[20] The first, and best known, is the implantable pulse generator with either endocardial or myocardial electrodes, which is used for long-term permanent pacing. The second type is the temporary pacer, which is external; a battery-powered pulse generator is connected to exteriorized electrodes of either the transvenous endocardial or the transthoracic myocardial variety. The third type is the console battery or AC-powered unit, which is known more commonly as a cardioverter or defibrillator. These units are mainly used with cutaneous electrodes; however, they may at times function with endocardial or myocardial electrodes as alternatives to the strap on battery-powered pulse generators of the second category for temporary pacing.

The fully implanted pulse generators come in a variety of circuit configurations, including asynchronous, atrial synchronous, ventricular synchronous, and ventricular inhibited types. No one type of mechanism is best; under certain circumstances, however, one type may be preferred to another. For example, an atrial synchronous pacer may give better results in a patient with a healthy myocardium, allowing for physiologic increase in cardiac output with effective atrial contraction (Fig. 26–123), whereas in a patient with complete heart block and no effective atrial mechanism, the

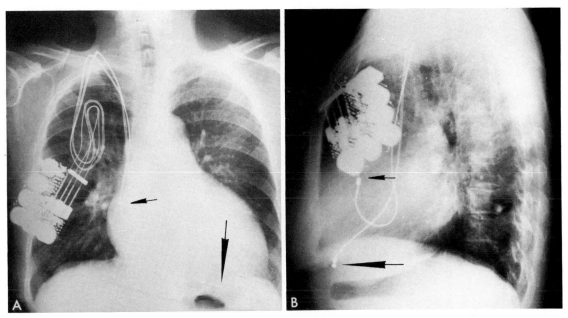

Figure 26–123. *A* and *B,* Atrio-ventricular synchronous transvenous pacemaker. Two bipolar lead systems are present, one in the right atrial appendage (small arrow) and the second at the apex of the right ventricle (large arrow). (Courtesy of D. Morse, M.D., and R. Steiner, M.D.)

asynchronous type with its inherent simplicity and greater reliability is preferable. The ventricular inhibited variety is used in patients with intermittent block and a fairly rapid spontaneous rate (80 to 90), whereas the ventricular synchronous type is useful in patients who have only occasional spontaneous activity.[21]

Two types of endocardial electrode configurations are currently in use — unipolar and bipolar. They differ in their inherent sensitivity to both intracardiac and extracardiac impulses. The unipolar electrode can be differentiated from the bipolar radiographically by the single radiopaque button on its end; the bipolar catheter has both the end button and an opaque collar several millimeters proximal. The unipolar electrode is more sensitive to impulses arising in the heart, but it also is more sensitive to external interference and is about ten times more likely to supply false signals to the pulse generator than is the bipolar lead.[36] This difference can be important when the unipolar electrode is used in conjunction with the popular "demand" or noncompetitive pulse generators of the ventricular synchronous or inhibited type.

Unipolar pulse generators have a single electrode connection, whereas bipolar units have two. It is not unusual to see a unipolar generator used with bipolar electrodes, however (Fig. 26–124). Also, care must be exercised in the evaluation of possible disconnection of one side of a bipolar lead, since in cases of fracture or some other cause of failure a bipolar generator may be connected to only one side of a bipolar electrode catheter, the circuit being completed by utilization of an indifferent lead close to the generator.[62] In this case, the negative or cathodal lead is intracardiac.

At times, several lead systems can be seen in one patient. This results when one fails but is left in place to avoid tearing of the endocardium or tricuspid valve in cases of adhesion of the electrode catheter to these structures, and a different catheter is inserted transvenously or myocardial leads are implanted.

Several charts of the physical and radiographic appearance of pulse generators have been published.[44, 71, 72] Most of these have become outdated, however, owing to the

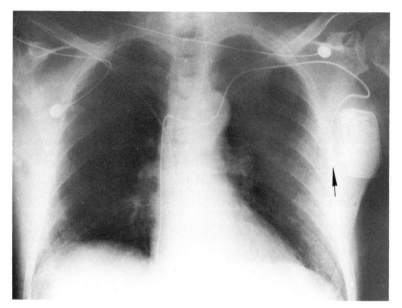

Figure 26–124. Bipolar transvenous electrode catheter connected to a unipolar pulse generator. Such configurations are not uncommon, so that care must be exercised in distinguishing them from cases of lead disconnection; the distinguishing factor is the presence of only one electrode boot connector on a unipolar pulse generator. Note the unused lead of the catheter (arrow).

proliferation of the various pulse generator varieties (Fig. 26–125). Some manufacturers now include a radiopaque coding identification schema in their pulse generators to allow the radiologist to determine which type is implanted in a patient.[62]

NORMAL POSITIONING

In the early days of cardiac pacing, myocardial electrodes were the most common method of permanent pacing. The pulse generator was usually implanted in the subcutaneous tissues of the left upper abdomen. The metallic leads were then tunneled subcutaneously up to the level of the cardiac apex, penetrated the intercostal space, and were sewn into the myocardium at a relatively avascular location. It was important to leave enough slack in the lead to accommodate body movements, respiratory motion, and cardiac contraction.[24] Myocardial implantation is still used occasionally, especially if the endocardial surface is too sensitive to an intracardiac electrode, causing ectopic activity not controllable by drug therapy.[33] It may also be preferred in children in order to leave enough slack to compensate for subsequent growth, which might displace an endocardial lead.[36] Sutureless epicardial electrodes have been introduced that can be inserted through a subxiphoid incision and screwed into either the left or the right ventricular wall without the need for an open thoracotomy (Fig. 26–126).[40] Temporary epicardial atrial or ventricular wires are commonly used to control cardiac rhythm after open heart surgery. These leads are subsequently removed.

The transvenous endocardial electrode approach is more commonly used today (Figs. 26–127 and 26–128). In 1965, Chardack recommended that the catheter "lie on the inferior wall of the right ventricle wedged into place and pointing towards the apex of the right ventricle."[10] This description has been reiterated recently by others.[50] Escher stated that the percutaneous transvenous electrode may be passed either to the right atrium or ventricle through the right or left subclavian vein either by the infra- or supraclavicular route. The right or left femoral, brachial, and external and internal jugular veins may also be used,[15] although the longer intravenous routes allow more motion of the lead system, predisposing to displacement from proper position. These longer routes are mostly used for temporary pacing (Figs. 26–129 and 26–130).

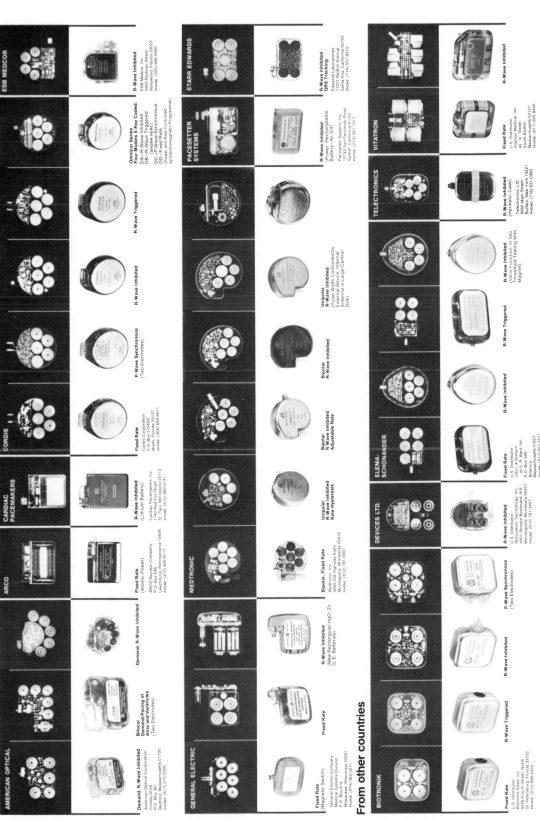

Figure 26–125. Identification chart for various pacemakers. Such charts become outdated rapidly as new and improved units become available. (Reproduced with the permission of Eastman Kodak Company and D. Morse, M.D.)

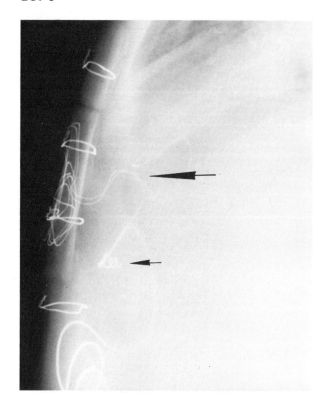

Figure 26–126. Myocardial screw-type electrode (small arrow). Such electrodes can be inserted via a simple subxiphoid incision, without an open thoracotomy. Thus, the rates of operative mortality and morbidity usually associated with the installation of myocardial leads are reduced. Note the temporary pacing wires inserted at surgery in a patient with a congenital cardiac defect (large arrow). These are removed by simply pulling them out at the incision site.

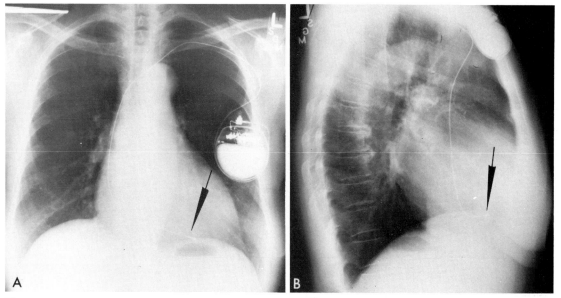

Figure 26–127. *A* and *B*, The normal placement of a unipolar pacer-electrode system. The pulse generator is in a subcutaneous pocket in the left anterior chest wall. The electrode catheter has a smooth course in the subcutaneous tissue, until it enters the venous system. Its course is via the left subclavian vein, superior vena cava, and right atrium, and into the right ventricle. Note the anterior location of the electrode tip on the lateral projection (arrow).

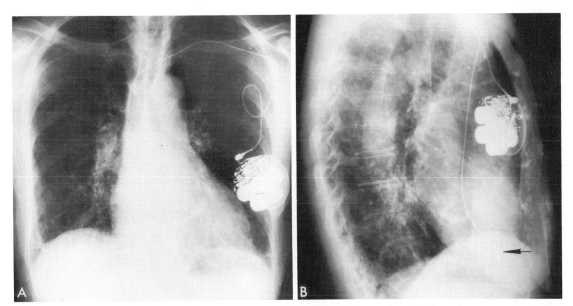

Figure 26–128. *A* and *B,* Normal placement. Note the strain-relieving loop in the subcutaneous portion of the electrode's course. Also, note the slight downward angulation of the tip of the electrode on the lateral view as it extends beneath the trabeculae carneae of the right ventricle (arrow).

For permanent insertions, the left cephalic vein approach has been suggested, being more stable than others.[39] Entrance into the venous system is just inferior to the clavicle near the junction of the cephalic and axillary veins. This allows a more gradual curving of the catheter, thereby decreasing the amount of stress on the wires.[32] The pulse generator is then buried in the subcutaneous tissues of the chest wall or beneath the pectoralis major muscle.[24] The pacing pocket is drained routinely for 24 hours.[11] The use of routine antibiotics is disputed, however.[11, 23] The procedure is usually performed under local anesthesia and with fluoroscopic control. The catheter is wedged beneath the trabeculae carneae in the anterior portion of the right ventricle. Conklin suggested aiming for a pacing threshold of 0.6 ma or lower and a sensing threshold of 4 mv or higher.[11] Such levels are necessary, since the threshold for stimulation may increase by as much as a factor of 10 during the first few days, probably secondary to local tissue reaction.[36]

Although the insertion of the transvenous catheter is done with the aid of image-intensification fluoroscopy, it is important for the radiologist to carefully evaluate the position of the tip of the catheter as well as its course. Both frontal and lateral radiographs are necessary, since accidental coronary sinus location may appear perfectly normal on a frontal view, but the incorrect posterior location is seen only on the lateral view. Of course, it is important to be in close contact with the clinician, since the coronary sinus position may be used as an alternative site for permanent atrial pacing in a patient with adequate atrioventricular conduction.[46, 47]

If the catheter enters a persistent left superior vena cava, it will enter the right atrium via a persistent sinus venosum, and positioning of the electrode tip is not compromised (see Fig. 26–157).

The amount of slack within the ventricle is important, since too much allows for early displacement of the electrode. Although the patient may continue to pace with the catheter tip in an abnormal position, the threshold of stimulation is necessarily increased, causing premature failure.[37] This is especially true in cases of myocardial penetration or perforation.

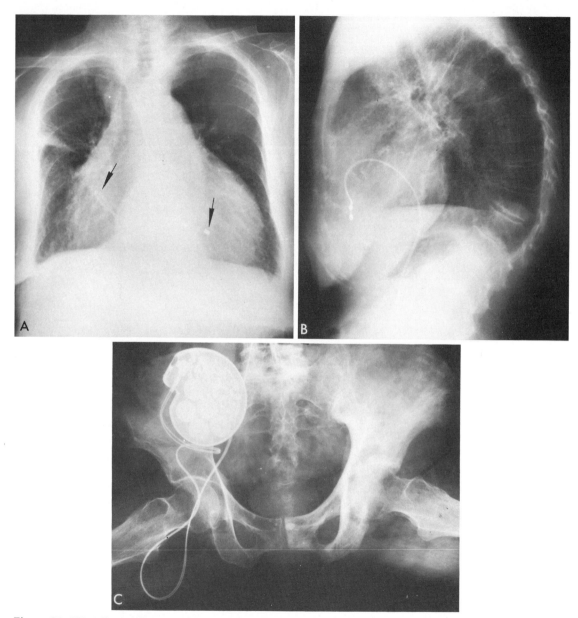

Figure 26–129. Femoral pacemaker insertion. Anteroposterior (*A*) and lateral (*B*) views of the chest show a bipolar electrode catheter entering the right atrium from the inferior vena cava (arrows). *C*, View of the pelvis demonstrates a bipolar pulse generator, with the electrode catheter inserted into the femoral vein. Such installations are more prone to lead displacement initially because of the long course of the catheter; they are mostly limited to temporary insertions.

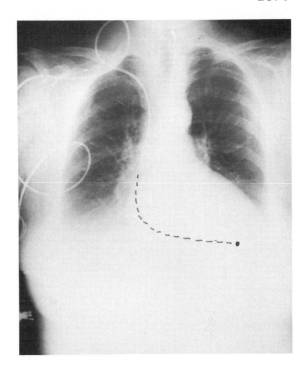

Figure 26–130. Temporary transvenous electrode catheter. The catheter is inserted into the right subclavian vein percutaneously. The procedure is usually done under fluoroscopic guidance. In an emergency, however, it can be performed blindly. Other sites of insertion include the jugular, brachial, and femoral veins.

Finally, Wright in 1973 suggested that a "pulse generator in the infraclavicular fossa may interfere with the swing of a golf club and thus remove one of the last remaining pleasures for the elderly."[75]

ENERGY SOURCES

Originally, large external pulse generators were used for temporary pacing. Power for these devices was easily obtained. With the miniaturization of the circuitry, however, new, small power sources were sought. The early, fully implantable pulse generators needed a small, relatively long-lasting energy source. Various types were tried, including radiofrequency or electromagnetically coupled implants, rechargeable nickel-cadmium cells, and other sources using body chemistry or mechanical motion. These sources were limited for one reason or another, and it was not until the zinc-mercuric oxide cell was employed that a reliable totally implantable pulse generator could be made. These cylindric cells are combined in 4 to 6 cell batteries with an output of approximately 8 volts and a current output that is stable for 80 to 90 per cent of its life. The terminal phase of the voltage decay takes place relatively rapidly over several weeks and is accompanied by a change in the pacer rate.[36] Recently, the lithium iodide cell has been utilized. Together with the P^{238} oxide generators it promises even longer service than the old mercury cells (Figs. 26–131 to 26–134).

COMPLICATIONS

Patients with cardiac pacemakers are managed mainly by cardiologists and thoracic surgeons. The complications associated with pacemakers have become less frequent as the technology has improved. Pacemaker clinics now employ sophisticated electronic

Text continued on page 1882

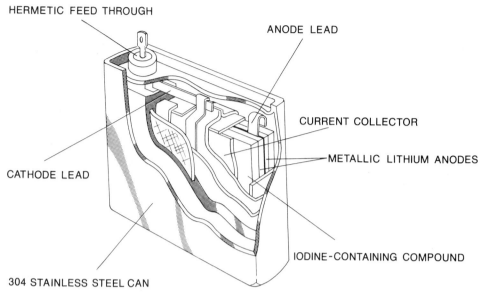

HERMETIC FEED THROUGH

ANODE LEAD

CURRENT COLLECTOR

METALLIC LITHIUM ANODES

CATHODE LEAD

IODINE-CONTAINING COMPOUND

304 STAINLESS STEEL CAN

Figure 26–131. Diagram of a lithium-iodide battery. Such batteries offer longer life-times in comparison with the older mercury cells. They are made in a variety of sizes and shapes, so that it is easy to distinguish them from their cylindric mercury predecessors. (Courtesy of D. Morse, M.D. and R. Steiner, M.D.)

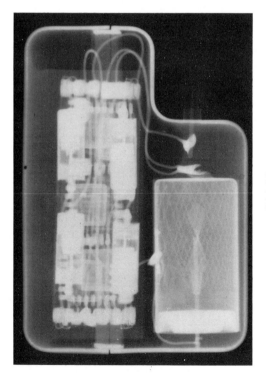

Figure 26–132. Radiograph of an Arco lithium battery-powered pulse generator. (Courtesy of D. Morse, M.D., and R. Steiner, M.D.)

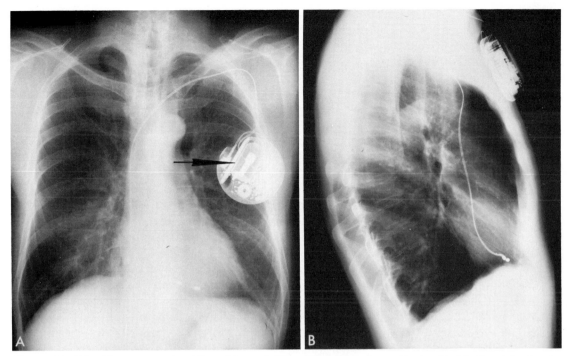

Figure 26–133. Posteroanterior (*A*) and lateral (*B*) radiographs of a patient with Medtronic's atomic-powered pulse generator. Note the radioactive isotope container in place of a chemical battery pack (arrow). Such generators offer a greater life expectancy than mercury cells, allowing a longer interval between generator changes.

Figure 26–134. Lateral radiograph of a patient with a Cordis atomic-powered pulse generator using a unipolar myocardial electrode. Note the half dumbbell–shaped radioactive isotope containing the power cell (arrow). The circular open-ended wire structure is an old myocardial electrode that was cut during the surgery for the replacement of a previous pulse generator.

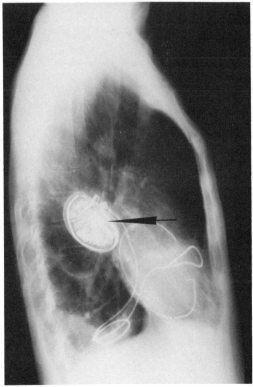

equipment in the detection of complications, such as increasing threshold, exit block, and perforations, as well as in the prediction of impending battery exhaustion. The radiologist can often be helpful in detecting some of these complications, however, and in certain instances may be the key person for ascertaining a particular complication.

Inadequate Positioning and Lead Displacement

Youmans et al. stated that electrode displacement occurred in three of four cases as an early complication of endocardial units in 1967.[76] This was attributed to improper stabilization and excessive intracardiac lead length. In a series of 1376 pacemaker placements, 698 of which were of the transvenous type, they reported 78 cases of electrode displacement. Forty-six of these occurred within two weeks of the initial placement; one case occurred four and one half years after surgery.[23] Sites of displacement include the right atrium, outflow tract of the right ventricle, pulmonary artery, and superior and inferior vena cava (Figs. 26–135 and 26–136). Posterior positioning in the coronary sinus is sometimes desirable but is usually an error in initial placement.[62] Ragaza and Shapiro reported two cases of malposition in the coronary sinus and posterior cardiac vein with adequate pacing function.[57] The EKG pattern was that of right bundle branch block — as opposed to the expected left bundle branch block — and thus indicative of malplacement. Meyer and Miller also reported five cases of coronary sinus placement with intermittent failure to pace appearing 6 hours to 2 weeks postinsertion (Fig. 26–137),[43] whereas Spitzberg et al. had a case in which the electrode

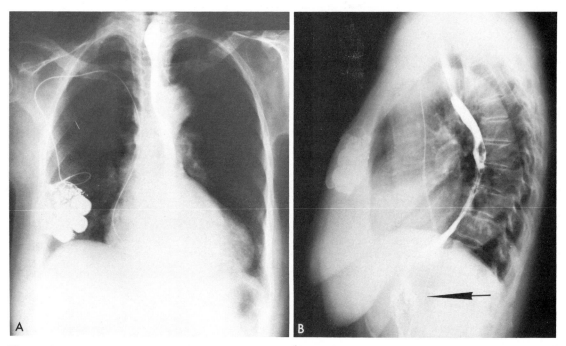

Figure 26–135. Displacement of the electrode into the inferior vena cava. Posteroanterior (*A*) and lateral (*B*) radiographs of a patient who presented with failure to pace and hiccups. The unipolar electrode catheter is clearly seen to extend below the diaphragm in the inferior vena cava on the lateral view (arrow). Such displacements are the result of inadequate initial positioning of the electrode tip, too much slack in the course of the catheter, or poor fixation by fibrous tissue at the endocardial surface. (Courtesy of G. Popky, M.D.)

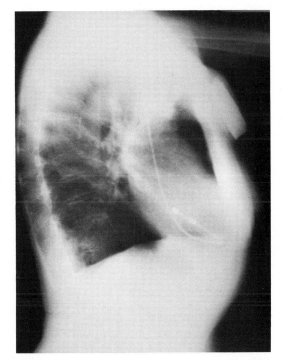

Figure 26–136. The bipolar electrode catheter is coiled in the right ventricle. This may result in failure to pace or intermittent pacing. In most cases, even if there is adequate function, battery life is substantially reduced. (Courtesy of M. M. McHenry, M.D.)

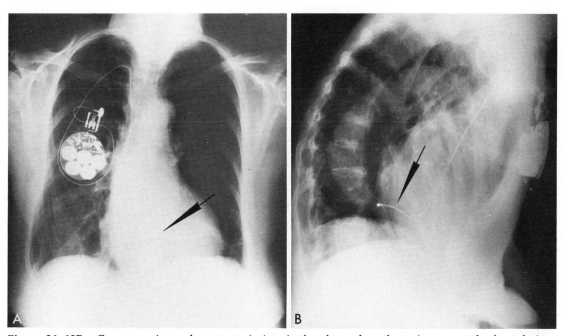

Figure 26–137. Coronary sinus placement. *A,* A unipolar electrode catheter is seen on the frontal view crossing the midline and pointing toward the apex of the right ventricle, a "normal" appearance (arrow). *B,* On the lateral view, however, the tip of the catheter is posteriorly located in the coronary sinus (arrow). (*From* Meyer, J. A., and Millar, K.: Malplacement of pacemaker catheters in the coronary sinus. Recognition and clinical significance. J. Thorac. Cardiovasc. Surg. *57:*511–518, 1969.)

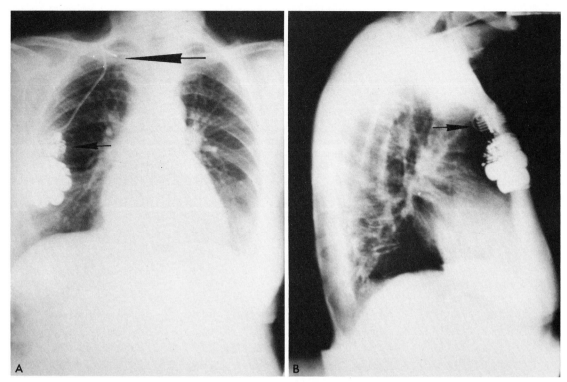

Figure 26–138. *A* and *B,* Twiddler's syndrome — the iatrogenic displacement of an electrode catheter caused by the patient's manipulation of the pulse generator in its subcutaneous pocket. Note the coiling of the catheter around the connector boot (small arrow) and the tip of the electrode at the level of the clavicle (large arrow), resulting in failure to pace. (*From* Bayliss, C. E., Beanlands, D. S., and Baird, R. J.: The pacemaker twiddler's syndrome. Can. Med. Assoc. J. *99*:371–373, 1968.)

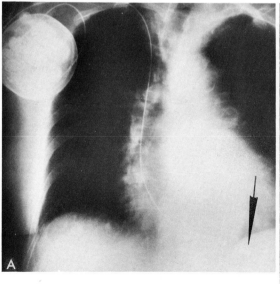

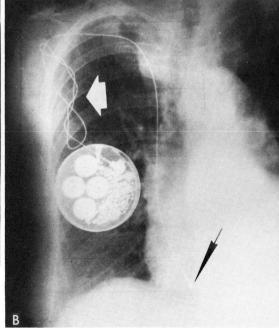

Figure 26–139. Twiddler's syndrome—an example of patient manipulation of the pulse generator. *A,* Electrode catheter is in good position (arrow). *B,* Three months later, the electrode has been withdrawn to a more proximal location within the right ventricle (large arrow), with twisting of the more proximal portion (arrowhead).

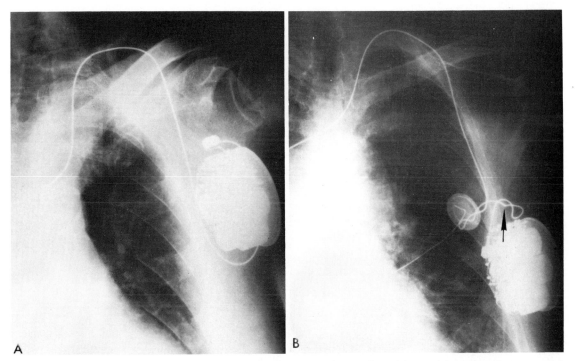

Figure 26–140. Twiddler's syndrome. *A,* Pulse generator in good position, with a smooth contour of the electrode catheter. *B,* The generator is rotated, and the electrode is twisted. Such manipulation may result in lead breaks (note the sharp angulation [arrow]) as well as in the intermittent or complete failure of pacing. These consequences can be avoided by the adequate fixation of both the pulse generator and the proximal electrode catheter. (*From* Meyer, J. A., Fruehan, C. T., and Delmonico, J. E., Jr.: The pacemaker twiddler's syndrome, a further note. J. Thorac. Cardiovasc. Surg. *67*:903–907, 1974.)

was in the middle cardiac vein with good pacing for 18 months.[63] Imparato and Kim noted that soft, small catheters (2 mm) displaced 25 per cent of the time, whereas larger ones (greater than 3.2 mm) displaced only 10 per cent of the time.

Position changes may be patient-induced, as was first reported by Bayliss et al. in 1968 and termed the twiddler's syndrome (Fig. 26–138). The surgeon must secure both the pulse generator and the electrode catheter to prevent manipulation by the patient and to allow tissue fixation by endocardial fibrosis. Withdrawal of the electrode in cases of twiddler's syndrome not only can cause failure to pace but also may cause phrenic nerve stimulation produced by the electrode in the superior vena cava or brachial plexus stimulation through the jugular vein location (Figs. 26–139 and 26–140).[3]

Perforation (Figs. 26–141 to 26–143)

Perforation of the right ventricular myocardium by transvenous endocardial electrodes can be an early or late complication. It has been reported by many authors and in most cases is a relatively benign complication.[8, 12, 16, 41, 48] The perforation may be partial (penetration) or complete and may present as intermittent or complete failure to pace,[42] phrenic nerve stimulation,[12, 42] or epigastric muscle stimulation[3] or may be asymptomatic, with only EKG changes suggesting the diagnosis. Radiographically, perforation is suggested on serial x-rays by a change in the position of the catheter tip in relation to the cardiac silhouette. Frank perforations are easy to recognize, but the subtle ones test the radiologist's diagnostic ability. Ormond et al. suggested the use of

Text continued on page 1888

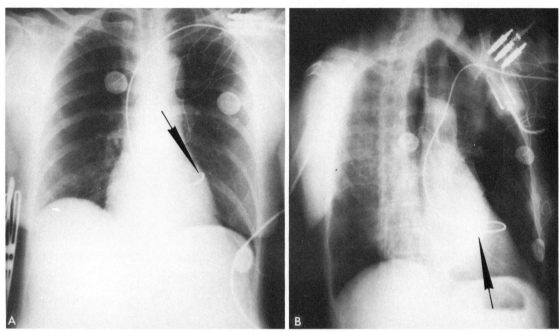

Figure 26–141. *A* and *B,* Perforation of the right ventricle. The temporary electrode catheter has perforated the right ventricular wall and is seen wrapping itself around the heart within the pericardial sac (arrows). Such perforation is more common with the stiffer types of catheters, as well as during insertions done without the benefit of fluoroscopy. (*From* Meyer, J. A., and Millar, K.: Perforation of the right ventricle by electrode catheters. Ann. Surg. *168*:1048–1060, 1968.)

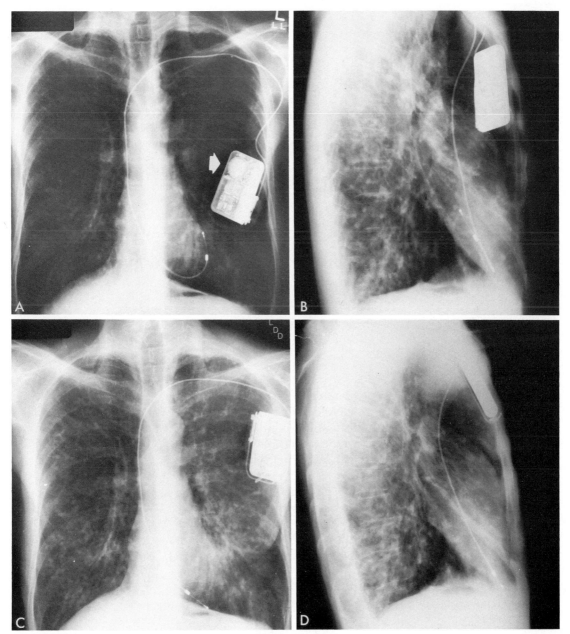

Figure 26–142. Perforation of the right ventricle. *A* and *B,* Note abnormal position of the electrode catheter, indicating perforation with the distal portion within the pericardial sac. The pulse generator is powered by rechargeable nickel-cadmium batteries (arrow). *C* and *D,* The perforation was corrected by the withdrawal of the transvenous electrode near the pulse generator until the tip was within the lumen of the right ventricle. Such treatment usually causes little or no pericardial hemorrhage when the electrode has a small diameter.

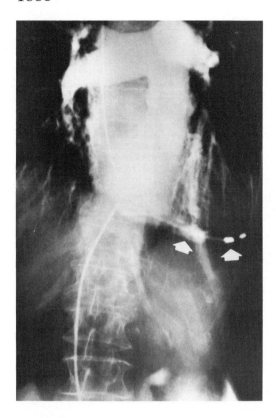

Figure 26–143. Perforation of the right ventricle. This right ventricular angiogram demonstrates the extension of the electrode catheter beyond the confines of the opacified ventricular lumen (arrows). (*From* Kennedy, P. A., Shipley, R. E., Prozan, G. B., et al.: Three years' experience with long-term endocardiac pacing. Am. J. Surg. *116*:164–169, 1968.)

fluoroscopically guided spot films to evaluate possible penetration or perforation.[50] They stated that if the tip of the endocardial electrode is within 3 mm of the epicardial fat pad that normally covers the anterior and inferior walls of the heart, penetration has occurred, and if the tip is within the fat pad, complete perforation has taken place (Fig. 26–144). They reported that one third of their patients had some degree of penetration. Others have reported the incidence of perforation to range from 4 to 20 per cent in temporary pacers and from 5 to 7 per cent in permanent placements, with an overall incidence of 29 per cent penetration or perforation over a 36-month follow-up period.[2, 4, 19, 48, 60]

The repositioning of electrodes, initial placement with the guide wire in place, and use of small-sized tips have been related to an increased incidence of perforation.[26, 36]

Although extracardiac perforations are relatively benign, serious complications, such as tamponade, have been reported in up to 10 per cent of cases.[24] The size of the electrode catheter has also been linked to possible tamponade. Although they generally have a lower incidence of perforation, catheters larger than 3.8 mm had a 100 per cent incidence of tamponade in one series.[26] In most cases, treatment of perforation is merely the withdrawal of the catheter until the tip of the electrode is within the lumen of the right ventricle.[8] Withdrawal may be difficult in some cases because of fibrous tissue formation adherent to the catheter.[13] Even in these cases, however, withdrawal may be possible by a method of graded skin traction on the catheter over a period of several days (Fig. 26–145).[27]

Perforation of the intracardiac septum may also occur and may be diagnosed by a change in the EKG pattern or position of the catheter on x-ray.[64]

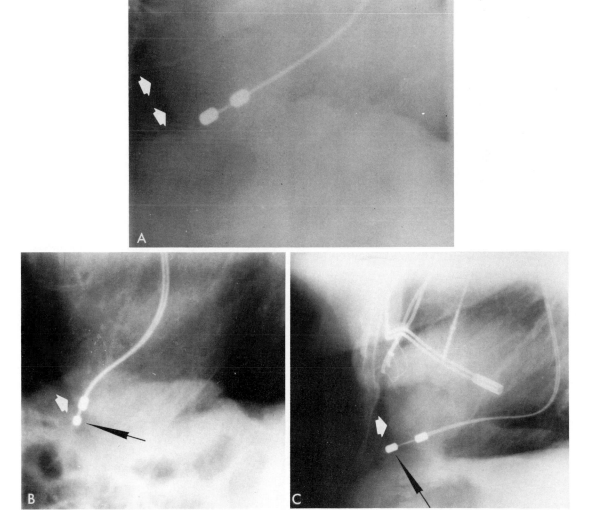

Figure 26–144. *A,* Normal positioning. The tip is well behind the anterior border (arrows) of the right ventricle. *B* and *C,* Perforation of the tip of the electrode in two patients (black arrows). The electrode tips (black arrows) are beyond the confines of the ventricle (white arrows). (Courtesy of M. Rubenfire, M.D.)

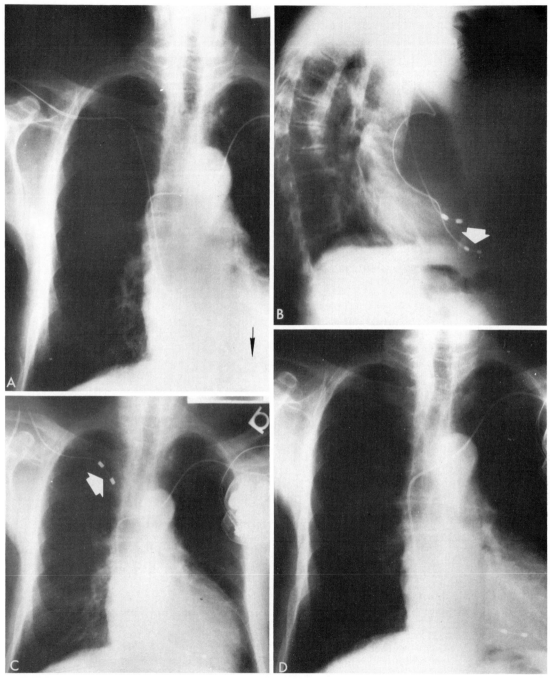

Figure 26–145. Withdrawal of the electrode catheter by graded skin traction. Posteroanterior (*A*) and lateral (*B*) radiographs demonstrating two bipolar transvenous electrode catheters. The one entering from the left side is in good position at the apex of the right ventricle (arrow). The second is higher and resulted in intermittent pacing. Attempts at withdrawal of the malpositioned catheter at surgery were thwarted because of the presence of endocardial fibrous adhesions. *C,* Following nine days of traction on the electrode catheter, its tip is seen in the subclavian vein (arrow). *D,* The catheter was then easily removed. (Courtesy of A. M. Imparato, M.D.)

Electrode Fractures (Figs. 26–146 to 26–150)

Although electrode fractures have become less common owing to the development of new alloys, they are still a significant cause of pacing failure of both the myocardial and the transvenous methods.[33] As battery life is extended, they will probably become even more significant. In a study of pacemaker wires in 1973, 80 per cent were of the helical coil type made of Elgiloy (a mixture of cobalt, chromium, iron, and nickel, with small amounts of molybdenum and manganese,[37] platinum-iridium, or stainless steel. The remainder were braided stainless steel wires, which had the highest incidence of fractures (28 per cent). The platinum-iridium alloy had a 15 per cent incidence; Elgiloy, 4.1 per cent, and the coiled stainless steel, 2.7 per cent. The frequency of fracture did not increase with the age of the electrode. Epicardial lead systems had an overall incidence of 19 per cent, whereas transvenous, endocardial electrodes were shown to break in only 3.9 per cent of cases. Electrode breaks were less common when the pulse generator was implanted in the chest than when it was in the abdomen, probably because of the increased support capability afforded by the ribs.[53]

The most common sites of fracture are at points of stress, such as the vicinity of the pulse generator,[23, 24] the place where the epicardial leads penetrate the intercostal space,[24, 62] the point of insertion of the epicardial terminals into the myocardium,[24, 62] and creases in the skin.[24] The point of entry into the venous system and the level of the clavicle are also common sites in transvenous systems.[23, 29]

Whereas most fractures cause failure to pace, partial fractures may give intermittent pacing.[36, 51] These may be position-related.[33] With demand pacers, sensing failure may be the only sign of fracture, owing to the increase in electrical resistance at the site of the fracture.[49] A pinched lead caused by a tight suture may resemble a true fracture radiographically.[62]

Fractures may be diagnosed electrocardiographically or radiographically. Some fractures can be seen on routine chest films, but in many cases, fluoroscopy and cineradiography may be necessary for adequate visualization.[33, 37]

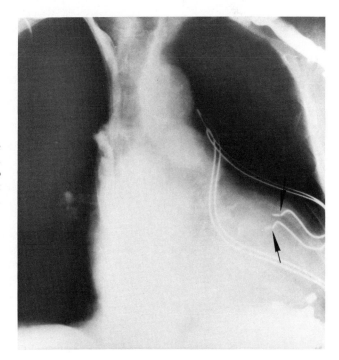

Figure 26–146. Myocardial lead breaks. Note the site of wire fractures at the entrance of electrode into the myocardium (arrows). This is a common site of fracture owing to the constant flexion produced by cardiac contraction. (*From* Rembert, F. M., and Cooley, R. N.: Implantable cardiac pacemakers: radiologic appearance. Texas Med. *63*:72–78, 1967.)

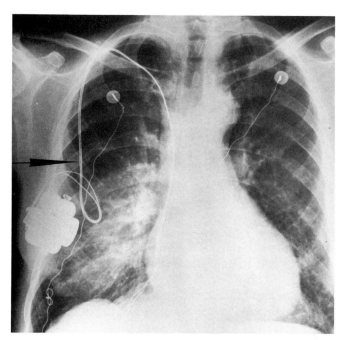

Figure 26–147. Lead break. Note the radiolucent line through one conductor of the bipolar catheter (arrow). Such fractures are less common now because of the improved alloys used in electrode construction. (Courtesy of D. Morse, M.D., and R. Steiner, M.D.)

Figure 26–148. Lead break. Fracture of electrode catheter at the site of its entry into venous system (arrow). Sharp angulations of the wires are suspicious for breaks, which at times may be demonstrable only by fluoroscopy or cineradiography. (*From* Kennedy, P. A., Shipley, R. E., Prozan, G. B., et al.: Three years' experience with long-term endocardiac pacing. Am. J. Surg. *116*:164–169, 1968.)

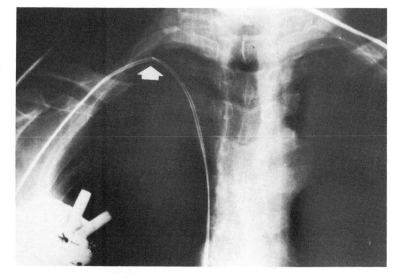

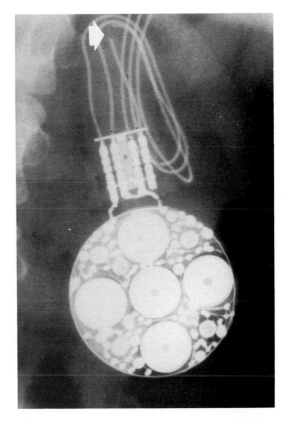

Figure 26–149. Lead break. Fracture of one conductor near the pulse generator (arrow). (*From* McHenry, M. M., and Grayson, C. E.: Roentgenographic diagnosis of pacemaker failure. Am. J. Roentgenol. *109*:94–100, 1970.)

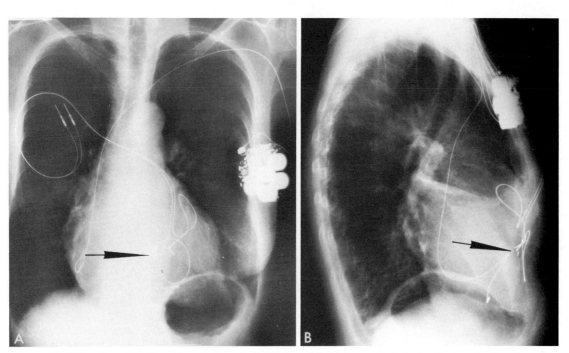

Figure 26–150. *A* and *B,* Lead break. The end of one of the myocardial electrodes has broken (arrow), necessitating replacement with a transvenous system.

Mercury Cell Exhaustion

Until recently, the mercury cell battery was the predominant type of energy source for totally implantable pacemakers. Four to six zinc–mercuric oxide cells are connected in a series to form a battery with an average output of 5.6 to 8.4 volts.[33] This configuration maintains a stable current output for 80 to 90 per cent of the battery's life, with rapid decay occurring during the final weeks or days before total depletion.

The primary cell consists of a radiopaque central zinc anode "ring" with a hollow radiolucent core. Around the anode is a thin radiolucent ring containing the electrolyte (sodium hydroxide). The outer opaque third ring consists of the mercuric oxide depolarizer. A metallic case contains all of this material. In new batteries, the three concentric rings are of approximately similar width (Fig. 26–151A). As the battery is used, mercuric oxide is converted to metallic mercury,[37] and the lucent rings become irregular and smaller. The zinc anode also degenerates, and the central lucent core becomes smaller and irregular, eventually filling in with liquid mercury (Fig. 26–151B). To obtain an undistorted *en face* view of the pacemaker, the patient is rotated until such a view is seen fluoroscopically and then recorded on a spot film. Rembert and Cooley in 1967 stated that at 30 per cent exhaustion the inner lucent ring was obscured, and both rings were filled in at 50 per cent depletion.[58] Collapse of the hollow zinc anode occurred at the end of the battery's life. This method has relatively low reliability in predicting the exact charge state of the battery and its depletion characteristics over a period of time because of the difficulty in obtaining serial films in the same position. It can help identify markedly depleted batteries in asymptomatic patients.[69] Electrocardiographic determination is much more accurate in predicting charge, since most modern pacemakers exhibit a detectable decrease in rate as the battery becomes depleted. There

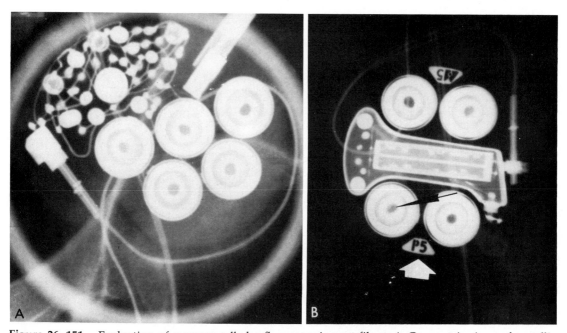

Figure 26–151. Evaluation of mercury cells by fluoroscopic spot films. *A,* Concentric rings of metallic and radiolucent densities, with smooth, sharp margins, indicating that these cells are relatively new. *B,* Irregularities of the margins, thinning of the concentric rings, and some filling in of the hollow anode core indicate some degree of depletion of these cells (arrow). The exact state of the charge cannot be determined by this method, however. Also note the identification code of the pulse generator (large arrow).

have been instances of "runaway rate" pacemakers, but circuitry changes have done much to eliminate this reaction to battery depletion.

Mercury batteries have a life expectancy that does not exceed 3 years, the average for the asynchronous type being approximately 23 to 25 months. Demand-type pacemakers have a shorter life expectancy owing to the greater complexity of their circuitry.[36]

The newer lithium-based batteries and atomically powered pacemakers are believed to have an inherently longer life span than the older mercury cells. This has been estimated to be in the range of five to ten years.[52] No radiographically based method has been found for their evaluation at the present time.

Thrombosis and Pulmonary Embolism

Although relatively uncommon, thrombosis of the right atrium and ventricle have been reported by several authors.[30, 35, 56, 59, 76] Youmans reported a case of thrombus formation on an electrode catheter in the superior vena cava demonstrated angiographically without evidence of pulmonary embolus.[76] Goldberg reported a case of fatal pulmonary embolus following the development of right ventricular thrombus.[22] Death from right atrial and ventricular thrombosis with associated pulmonary embolus was reported by Kennedy et al.[32] Two cases of air embolus demonstrated under fluoroscopy during the insertion of a permanent pacemaker via the jugular vein have also been reported.[77] Thrombosis in an arm vein has been found to be a relatively common occurrence with temporary pacemakers. The frequency and severity of the clotting, as demonstrated by venography, are greater with the cephalic than with the basilic vein approach.[74] Venous thrombosis has also been found to be common with permanent pacers, although it is not usually associated with arm or facial edema (Fig. 26–152).[65]

Wound Infections and Other Complications

Air around a newly inserted pulse generator is a relatively common finding on chest radiographs, since some air is normally introduced into the pocket at surgery (Figs. 26–153 and 26–154). Progressive accumulation of gas or fluid may indicate infection, however.[62] Bayliss et al. reported a tendency for fluid to accumulate in the pacemaker pocket without clinical evidence of infection.[3] Campo et al. reported 10 cases of infection, in 460 insertions.[8] Treatment consisted of removal of the pacemaker, together with administration of systemic antibiotics. A case of septic pulmonary emboli as a result of pacemaker pocket infection was reported in 1972.[70] Although such infections are usually limited to the generator pocket itself, the entire unit, including the electrode, should be removed. Insertion of a new permanent pacer should be delayed until the infection has been controlled.

Extrusion of the pulse generator has been reported[18, 33] and is related to reoperation for pulse generator replacement or electrode repositioning.[53] Its occurrence is also related to local pressure effects and the amount of subcutaneous tissue overlying the pacemaker.

Phrenic Nerve Stimulation

Although hiccupping and diaphragmatic stimulation have been related to perforation of an endocardial electrode, they may occur without perforation.[5, 45] Phrenic nerve

Text continued on page 1898

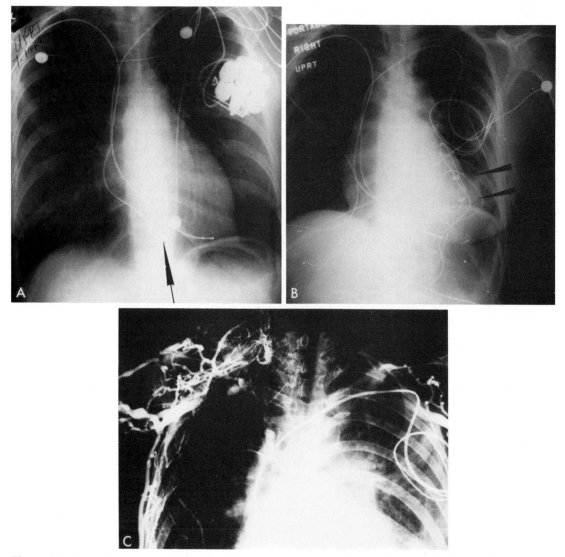

Figure 26–152. Venous occlusion following pacemaker insertion. *A,* Permanent bipolar transvenous pacemaker, its intracardiac lead in poor position (arrow). Premature failure resulted, requiring the placement of a temporary pacemaker via the right brachial route. *B,* Bipolar epicardial leads have been inserted. The old pulse generator has been removed, but the electrode catheter is still in place. The temporary electrode is still seen. Note the localized reaction at the site of epicardial lead placement (arrows). *C,* Bilateral arm venogram was performed because of painful edema of the right arm. There is occlusion of the right brachiocephalic vessels, with the development of collaterals secondary to the presence of the temporary electrode catheter. Note the occlusion of the left side, which was asymptomatic.

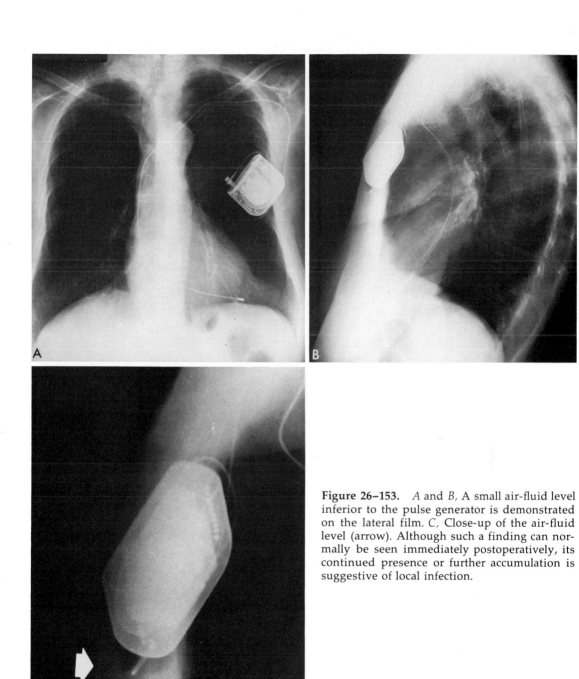

Figure 26–153. *A* and *B,* A small air-fluid level inferior to the pulse generator is demonstrated on the lateral film. *C,* Close-up of the air-fluid level (arrow). Although such a finding can normally be seen immediately postoperatively, its continued presence or further accumulation is suggestive of local infection.

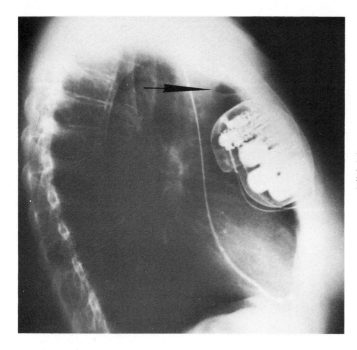

Figure 26-154. Air-fluid level in the pacemaker pocket (arrow). (Courtesy of D. Morse, M.D., and R. Steiner, M.D.)

stimulation is also a complication of epicardial lead placement and can be prevented by insulating the electrode from the adjacent nerve at the time of insertion.[16, 54] Fluoroscopy may be helpful in making the diagnosis.

Postcardiotomy Syndrome

Although this syndrome is usually seen after cardiac surgery, myocardial infarction, and blunt or penetrating trauma to the chest, Kaye et al. reported a case in which they noted an increase in heart size on chest x-ray, fever, malaise, pedal edema, pericardial rub, and pleural effusion with pleuritic chest pain beginning two weeks after pacemaker implantation and lasting for approximately three months (Fig. 26–155).[31] The diagnosis of pericardial effusion was made using carbon dioxide instilled into the pericardial sac. The pacer wire was in a good position and functioned well. The authors believe the findings to be consistent with the postcardiotomy syndrome because the effusion developed six weeks prior to the fever, a fact that virtually rules out viral pericarditis.

Others have reported asymptomatic pericardial friction rubs developing following pacemaker insertion.[45]

Other Complications

Pneumothorax caused by perforation of a vein during insertion of a temporary pacemaker via the subclavian or jugular route, although rare (0.7 per cent), has been reported.[8, 15] Extravascular, intrapleural electrode passage is a rare occurrence.[15] Localized myocardial hematoma at the site of an epicardial electrode insertion has been demonstrated radiographically in one case.[24] This should not be confused with an occasionally visualized prominence at the site of electrode insertion resulting from the

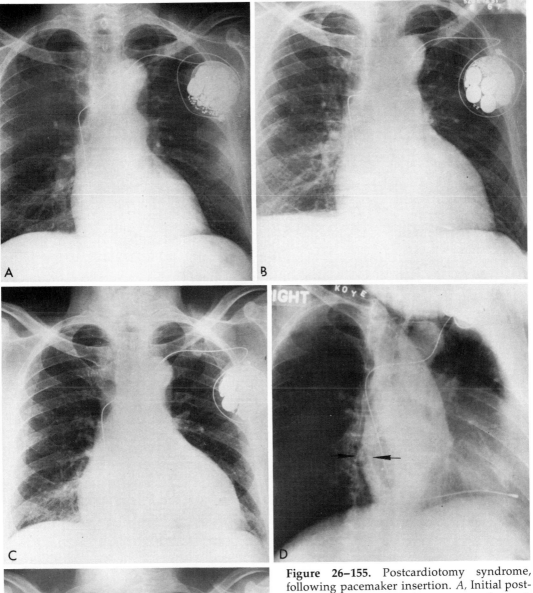

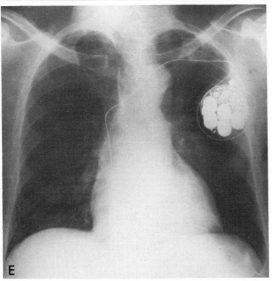

Figure 26–155. Postcardiotomy syndrome, following pacemaker insertion. *A,* Initial postoperative radiograph demonstrates the unipolar pacemaker and electrode catheter to be a good position. The heart is normal-sized. *B,* Follow-up examination three weeks later shows the cardiac silhouette to be slightly larger, with a small right pleural effusion. *C,* Approximately eight weeks postoperatively, the cardiac silhouette is even larger. *D,* Left lateral decubitus radiograph taken after the intravenous injection of carbon dioxide demonstrates the presence of a pericardial effusion (arrows). *E,* Repeat examination shows the return of the cardiac silhouette to normal size approximately three months postoperatively. No therapy was given during this time aside from the continued administration of 0.25 mg of digoxin each day. (*From* Kaye, D., Frankl, W., and Arditi, L. I.: Probable postcardiotomy syndrome following implantation of a transvenous pacemaker. Am. Heart J. 90:627–630, 1975.)

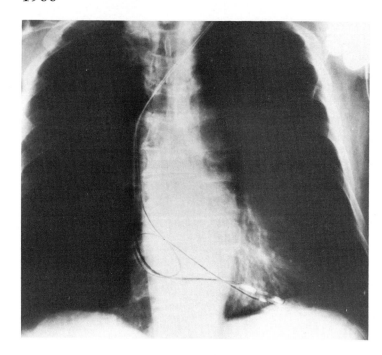

Figure 26–156. Looped catheters. Coiling of permanent and temporary transvenous catheters is demonstrated. Such complications are more frequent when the permanent catheter is inserted from the same side as the temporary catheter. (*From* Kennedy, P. A., Shipley, R. E., Prozan, G. B., et al.: Three years' experience with long-term endocardiac pacing. Am. J. Surg. *116*:164–169, 1968.)

Figure 26–157. Persistent left superior vena cava. The unipolar electrode catheter is seen within a persistent left superior vena cava (arrows). The catheter enters the right atrium via the sinus venosum and electrode positioning is not affected. (Courtesy of D. Morse, M.D., and R. Steiner, M.D.)

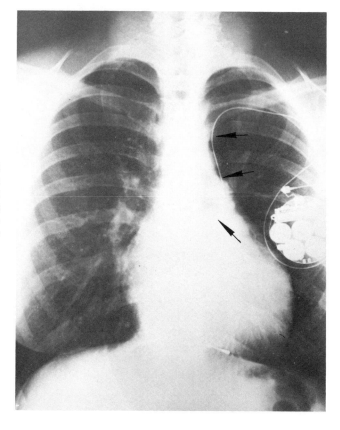

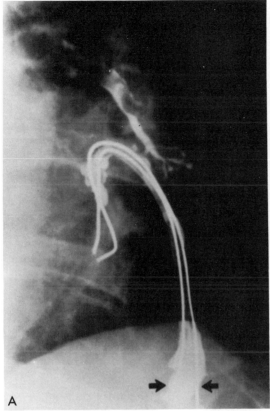

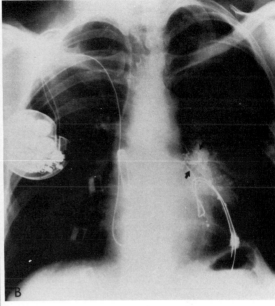

Figure 26–158. *A,* Fistulogram demonstrating the subcutaneous tract along the path of the epicardial leads, with fistulation into the lingular bronchus. *B,* Posteroanterior view demonstrating the lingular infiltrate and contrast material in the bronchial tree. Reproduced with permission from Tegtmeyer, C. J., Hunter, J. G. Jr., and Keats, T. E.: Bronchocutaneous fistula as a late complication of permanent epicardial pacing. Am. J. Radiol. *121:*614–616, 1974.

surgical mesh or sponge that is sometimes used for stabilization.[69] Knotting of electrodes has also been reported. This complication occurred during insertion of a permanent pacemaker electrode through the same vein in which a temporary electrode had been left in place (Fig. 26–156).[6, 55] Tricuspid insufficiency was reported in two of eight patients who had more than one endocardial electrode as a result of the physical presence of the catheters.[23] It thus seems prudent to remove electrodes that are not being used, if at all possible. A bronchocutaneous fistula developed in a patient with an epicardial pacemaker. The pulse generator had been removed because of infection, but the epicardial leads had been left in place. The infection then spread along the lead tracts, causing a lingular infiltrate with eventual development of the bronchial fistula (Fig. 26–158).[68] Finally, a pacemaker may cause a defect on a radionuclide lung scan simply by its absorption of the radiation emitted by the radiopharmaceutical in the lung beneath it. Multiple views are thus necessary for accurate evaluation (Fig. 26–159).[69]

SUMMARY

Cardiac pacemakers have progressed from experimental curiosities to universally accepted treatment modalities. They are effective and reliable. Their true complications are relatively uncommon and, for the most part, easily treated. Although pacemakers are primarily the responsibility of the cardiologist and thoracic surgeon, the radiologist may be helpful in diagnosing certain complications associated with these devices. Good posteroanterior and lateral radiographs are essential for evaluating the position

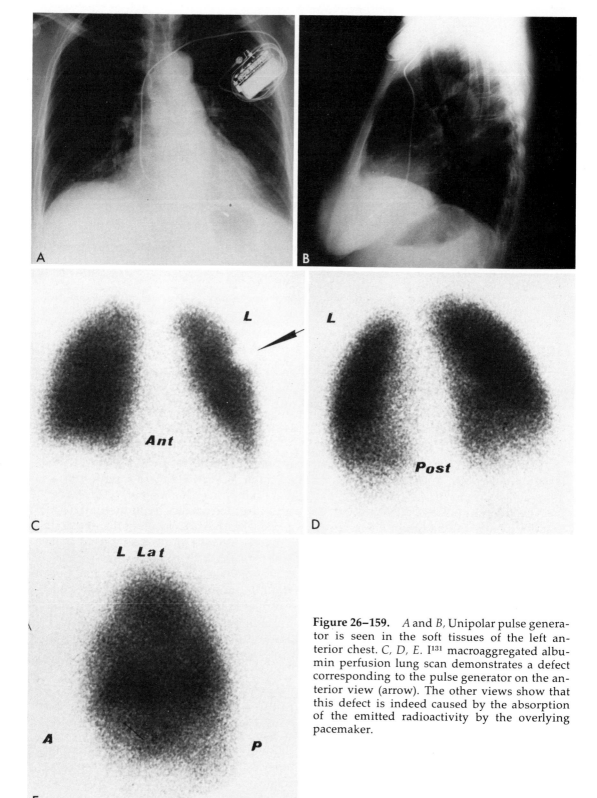

Figure 26–159. *A* and *B,* Unipolar pulse generator is seen in the soft tissues of the left anterior chest. *C, D, E.* I[131] macroaggregated albumin perfusion lung scan demonstrates a defect corresponding to the pulse generator on the anterior view (arrow). The other views show that this defect is indeed caused by the absorption of the emitted radioactivity by the overlying pacemaker.

and condition of catheter electrodes. Spot films can help diagnose possible perforation not obvious on regular films. They are also useful for evaluating the condition of the mercury cell batteries. Cineradiography can localize small electrode fractures; fluoroscopy is useful in determining displacement of electrodes through cardiac motion and phrenic nerve stimulation. Such methods are useful aids to primary physicians in the management of cardiac pacemaker patients.

References

1. Aldini, J.: General Views on the Application of Galvanism to Medical Purposes: Principally in Cases of Suspended Animation. London, J. Callow, 1819.
2. Barold, S., and Center, S.: Electrocardiographic diagnosis of perforation of the heart by pacing catheter electrode. Am. J. Cardiol. 24:274–278, 1969.
3. Bayliss, C. E., Beanlands, D. S., and Baird, R. J.: The pacemaker-twiddler's syndrome: a new complication of implantable transvenous pacemakers. Can. Med. Assoc. J. 99:371–373, 1968.
4. Bernstein, V., Rotem, C. E., Pertz, D. I., et al.: Permanent pacemakers: 8 year follow up study. Ann. Intern. Med. 74:361–369, 1971.
5. Birch, L. M., Berger, M., and Thomas, P. A.: Synchronous diaphragmatic contraction: a complication of transvenous cardiac pacing. Am. J. Cardiol. 21:88–90, 1968.
6. Boal, B. H., Keller, B. D., Ascheim, R. S., et al.: Complication on intracardiac electrical pacing — knotting together of temporary and permanent electrodes. N. Engl. J. Med. 280:650–651, 1969.
7. Burns, A.: Observations on Some of the Most Frequent and Important Diseases of the Heart. Edinburgh, Thomas Bryce and Company, 1809.
8. Campo, I. N., Garfield, G. J., Escher, D. J. W., et al.: Complications of pacing by pervenous subclavian semifloating electrodes including two extraluminal insertions. Am. J. Cardiol. 26:627, 1970.
9. Chardack, W. M., Gage, A. A., and Greatbatch, W.: A transistorized, self-contained implantable pacemaker for the long term correction of complete heart block. Surgery 48:643–654, 1960.
10. Chardack, W. M., Gage, A. A., Federico, A. J., et al.: Five years' clinical experience with an implantable pacemaker: an appraisal. Surgery 58:915–922, 1965.
11. Conklin, E. F., Giannelli, S., Jr., and Nealon, T. F., Jr.: Four hundred consecutive patients with permanent transvenous pacemakers. J. Thorac. Cardiovasc. Surg. 69:1–7, 1975.
12. Cosby, R. S., Penido, J. R. F., and Cotton, B. H.: Catheter perforation of the ventricle after intracardiac pacing. Geriatrics 22:182–186, 1967.
13. Danielson, G. K., Shabetai, R., and Bryant, L. R.: Failure of endocardial pacemaker due to late myocardial perforation. J. Thorac. Cardiovasc. Surg. 54:42–48, 1967.
14. Erlanger, J.: Sinus stimulation as a factor in the resuscitation of the heart. J. Exp. Med. 16:452–469, 1912.
15. Escher, D. J. W.: Types of pacemakers and their complications. Circulation 47:1119–1131, 1973.
16. Fabris, F., Morea, M., Vincenzi, M., et al.: Failures and complications observed in 34 patients treated with temporary and permanent electric cardiac stimulation. J. Cardiovasc. Surg. 8:110–113, 1967.
17. Furman, S., and Schwedel, J. B.: An intracardiac pacemaker for Stokes-Adams seizures. N. Engl. J. Med. 261:943–948, 1959.
18. Furman, S.: Complications of pacemaker therapy for heart block. Am. J. Cardiol. 17:439–440, 1966.
19. Furman, S., Escher, D. J. W., and Solomon, N.: Experiences with myocardial and transvenous implanted cardiac pacemakers. Am. J. Cardiol. 23:66–72, 1969.
20. Furman, S., and Escher, D. J. W.: Principles and Techniques of Cardiac Pacing. New York, Harper & Row, 1970.
21. Furman, S., Escher, D. J. W., and Parker, B.: The failure of triggered pacemakers. Am. Heart J. 82:28–38, 1971.
22. Goldberg, E.: Complications of pacemaker therapy for heart block. Am. J. Cardiol. 17:439, 1966.
23. Grögler, F. M., Frank, G., Greven, G., et al.: Complications of permanent transvenous cardiac pacing. J. Thorac. Cardiovasc. Surg. 69:895–904, 1975.
24. Hall, W. M., and Rosenbaum, H. D.: The radiology of cardiac pacemakers. Radiol. Clin. North Am. 9:343–353, 1971.
25. Hyman, A. S.: Resuscitation of the stopped heart by intracardial therapy. Experimental use of an artificial pacemaker. Arch. Intern. Med. 50:283–305, 1932.
26. Imparato, A. M., and Kim, G. E.: Electrode complications in patients with permanent cardiac pacemakers. Arch. Surg. 105:705–710, 1972.
27. Imparato, A. M., and Kim, G. E.: The trapped endocardial electrode: removal by prolonged graded skin traction. Ann. Thorac. Surg. 14:605–608, 1972.
28. Johansson, B. W.: Adams-Stokes syndrome: review and follow-up study of forty-two cases. Am. J. Cardiol. 8:76–93, 1961.

29. Kantrowitz, A., Rubenfire, M., and Wajszczuk, W.: Complications of permanent transvenous pacemaker therapy. *In* Thalen, H. J. T. (ed.): Cardiac Pacing: Proceedings of the Fourth International Symposium on Cardiac Pacing. The Netherlands, Van Gorcum & Company, 1973, pp. 244–252.

30. Kaulbach, M. G., and Krukonis, E. E.: Pacemaker electrode-induced thrombosis in the superior vena cava with pulmonary embolization. Am. J. Cardiol. 26:205–207, 1970.

31. Kaye, D., Frankl, W., and Arditi, L. I.: Probable postcardiotomy syndrome following implantation of a transvenous pacemaker: report of the first case. Am. Heart J. 90:627–630, 1975.

32. Kennedy, P. A., Shipley, R. E., Prozan, G. B., et al.: Three years' experience with long-term endocardiac pacing: complications: their care and prevention. Am. J. Surg, 116:164–169, 1968.

33. Kosowsky, B. D., and Barr, I.: Complications and malfunctions of electrical cardiac pacemakers. Prog. Cardiovasc. Dis. 14:501–514, 1972.

34. Lillehei, C. W., Cruz, A. B., Johnsrude, I., et al.: A new method of assessing the state of charge of implanted cardiac pacemaker batteries. Am. J. Cardiol. 16:717–721, 1965.

35. London, A. R., Runge, P. J., Balsam, R. F., et al.: Large right atrial thrombi surrounding permanent transvenous pacemakers. Circulation 40:661–664, 1969.

36. Lown, B., and Kosowsky, B. D.: Artificial cardiac pacemakers. N. Engl. J. Med. 283:907–916, 1970.

37. McHenry, M. M., and Grayson, C. E.: Roentgenographic diagnosis of pacemaker failure. Am. J. Radiol. 109:94–100, 1970.

38. McWilliam, J. A.: On electrical stimulation of the mammalian heart. *In* Hamilton, J. B. (ed.): Transactions of the International Medical Congress. Ninth Session. Vol. 3. Washington, D.C., 1887, pp. 253–255.

39. Mansour, K. A., Dorney, E. R., Tyras, D. H., et al.: Cardiac pacemakers: comparing epicardial and pervenous pacing. Geriatrics 3:151–155, 1973.

40. Mansour, K. A., Fleming, W. H., and Hatcher, C. H., Jr.: Initial experience with a sutureless screw-in electrode for cardiac pacing. Ann. Thorac. Surg. 16:127–132, 1973.

41. Meckstroth, C. V., Shoenfeld, C. D., and Wardwell, G. A.: Myocardial perforation from a permanent endocardial electrode. J. Thorac. Cardiovasc. Surg. 54:16–21, 1967.

42. Meyer, J. A., and Millar, K.: Perforation of the right ventricle by electrode catheters: a review and report of nine cases. Ann. Surg. 168:1048–1060, 1968.

43. Meyer, J. A., and Millar, K.: Malplacement of pacemaker catheters in the coronary sinus: recognition and clinical significance. J. Thorac. Cardiovasc. Surg. 57:511–518, 1969.

44. Morse, D., et al.: Guide to Identification of Pacemakers. Rochester, New York, Eastman Kodak Company, Radiography Markets Division, Chart M4-62A, 1974.

45. Morris, J. J., Jr., Whalen, R. E., McIntosh, H. D., et al.: Permanent ventricular pacemakers: comparison of transthoracic and transvenous implantation. Circulation 36:587–597, 1967.

46. Moss, A. J., Rivers, R. J., Jr., and Cooper, M.: Long term pervenous atrial pacing from the proximal portion of the coronary vein. J.A.M.A. 209:543–545, 1969.

47. Moss, A. J., Rivers, R. J., Jr., and Kramer, D. H.: Permanent pervenous pacing from the coronary vein: long term follow-up. Circulation 49:222–225, 1974.

48. Nathan, D. A., Center, S., Pina, R. E., et al.: Perforation during indwelling catheter pacing. Circulation 33:128–130, 1966.

49. Nevins, M. A., Landau, S., and Lyon, L. J.: Failure of demand pacemaker sensing due to electrode fracture. Chest 59:110–113, 1971.

50. Ormond, R. S., Rubenfire, M., Anbe, D. T., et al.: Radiographic demonstration of myocardial penetration by permanent endocardial pacemakers. Radiology 98:35–37, 1971.

51. Parsonnet, V., Gilbert, L., Zucker, I. R., et al.: Complications of the implanted pacemaker. J. Thorac. Cardiovasc. Surg. 45:801–812, 1963.

52. Parsonnet, V.: Power sources for implantable cardiac pacemakers. Chest 61:165–173, 1972.

53. Parsonnet, V., Gilbert, L., and Zucker, I. R.: The natural history of pacemaker wires. J. Thorac. Cardiovasc. Surg., 65:315–322, 1973.

54. Peleska, B., and Buda, J.: Stimulation of the phrenic nerve as a complication of implanted battery pacemaker: management without thoracotomy. J. Cardiovasc. Surg. 6:477–481, 1965.

55. Pomfret, D., Polansky, B. J., and Huvos, A.: Dangerous complication of temporary floating pacing electrodes. N. Engl. J. Med. 280:651–652, 1969.

56. Prozan, G. B., Shipley, R. E., Madding, G. F., et al.: Pulmonary thromboembolism in the presence of an endocardiac pacing catheter. J.A.M.A. 206:1564–1565, 1968.

57. Ragaza, E. P., and Shapiro, R.: Radiologic recognition of unusual sites of a transvenous catheter pacemaker. J. Can. Assoc. Radiol. 21:214–216, 1970.

58. Rembert, F. M., and Cooley, R. N.: Implantable cardiac pacemakers: radiologic appearance. Texas Med. 63:72–78, 1967.

59. Reynolds, J., Anslinger, D., Yore, R., et al.: Transvenous cardiac pacemaker, mural thrombosis, and pulmonary embolism. Am. Heart J. 78:688–691, 1969.

60. Rubenfire, M., Anbe, D. T., Drake, E. H., et al.: Clinical evaluation of myocardial perforation as a complication of permanent transvenous pacemakers. Chest 63:185–188, 1973.

61. Senning, A.: Prevention of post-hypercapneic ventricular fibrillation in dogs. J. Thorac. Cardiovasc. Surg. 38:630–642, 1959.

62. Sorkin, R. P., Schuurmann, B. J., and Simon, A. B.: Radiographic aspects of permanent cardiac pacemakers. Radiology 119:281–286, 1976.

63. Spitzberg, J. W., Milstoc, M., and Wertheim, A. R.: An unusual site of ventricular pacing occurring during the use of the transvenous catheter pacemaker. Am. Heart J. 77:529–533, 1969.

64. Stillman, M. T., and Richards, A. M.: Perforation of the interventricular septum by transvenous pacemaker catheter. Am. J. Cardiol. *24*:269–273, 1969.

65. Stoney, W. S., Addlestone, R. B., Alford, W. C., Jr., et al.: The incidence of venous thrombosis following long-term transvenous pacing. Ann. Thorac. Surg. 22:166–170, 1976.

66. Sutton, R., Chatterjee, K., and Leathan, A.: Heart block following acute myocardial infarction: treatment with demand and fixed-rate pacemakers. Lancet 2:645–648, 1948.

67. Sweet, W. H.: Stimulation of the sino-atrial node for cardiac arrest during operation. Bull. Am. Coll. Surg. *32*:234, 1947.

68. Tegtmeyer, C. J., Hunter, J. G., Jr., and Keats, T. E.: Bronchocutaneous fistula as a late complication of permanent-epicardial pacing. Am. J. Radiol. *121*:614–616, 1974.

69. Tegtmeyer, C. J.: Roentgenographic assessment of causes of cardiac pacemaker failure and complications. C.R.C. Crit. Rev. Diagn. Imaging 9:1–50, 1977.

70. Waisser, E., Kuo, C. S., and Kabins, S. A.: Septic pulmonary emboli arising from a permanent transvenous cardiac pacemaker. Chest *61*:503–505, 1972.

71. Walter, W. H., and Wenger, N. K.: Radiographic identification of commonly used implanted pacemakers. N. Engl. J. Med. *281*:1230–1231, 1969.

72. Walter, W. H.: Radiographic identification of commonly used pulse generators — 1970. J.A.M.A. *215*:1974–1975, 1971.

73. Weirich, W. L., Gott, V. L., and Lillehei, C. W.: The treatment of complete heart block by the combined use of a myocardial electrode and an artificial pacemaker. Surg. Forum *8*:360–363, 1957.

74. Wernitsch, W., van de Weyer, K. H., and Richter, G.: Thrombotic changes with temporary cubital pacemaker electrode. Fortschr. Roentgenstr. *110*:371–377, 1969.

75. Wright, K. E., and McIntosh, H. D.: Artificial pacemakers: indications and management. Circulation *47*:1108–1118, 1973.

76. Youmans, C. R., Jr., Derrick, J. R., and Wallace, J. M.: Considerations of complications of permanent transvenous pacemakers. Am. J. Surg. *114*:704–710, 1967.

77. Zeft, H. J., Harley, A., Whalen, R. E., et al.: Pulmonary air embolism during insertion of a permanent transvenous cardiac pacemaker. Circulation *36*:456–459, 1967.

78. Zelis, R., Mason, D. T., Spann, J. F., Jr., et al.: Effects of ventricular stimulation and potassium administration on digitalis induced arrhythmias. Am. J. Cardiol. *25*:428–433, 1970.

79. Zoll, P. M.: Resuscitation of the heart in ventricular standstill by external electric stimulation. N. Engl. J. Med. *247*:768, 1952.

Part X
Assisted Circulation

CARL E. RAVIN, M.D.

The continued high mortality associated with cardiogenic shock has prompted extensive efforts to develop mechanical support for the failing circulatory system. Numerous avenues have been explored, ranging from systems that augment compromised myocardial pumping ability to those that totally replace cardiac function with mechanical devices.

Currently, the most commonly employed assisted circulation devices are those designed to support the circulation for a finite period of time, during which the damaged heart can recover sufficient function to maintain adequate circulation on its own. Most often, such support is required following acute myocardial infarction or cardiac surgery. Support and improvement of myocardial function during the period following the acute insult allows sufficient time for natural healing and recovery of function to occur. Of such devices, the intra-aortic counterpulsation balloon has been the most widely used. The circulatory system can also be supported for finite periods by extracorporeal membrane oxygenators, which offer the additional advantage of oxygenating the blood in the setting of pulmonary failure. Development of mechanical hearts remains an experimental endeavor and has not yet gained wide acceptance as a clinical treatment modality.

INTRA-AORTIC COUNTERPULSATION BALLOON

Counterpulsation, provided by intra-aortic ballon assist, has been established both experimentally and clinically as an effective way of providing temporary assistance to the compromised myocardium.[4, 5, 10, 11, 22, 23] Because it is structurally simple, relatively safe, and therapeutically effective, this device has gained wide acceptance as a method of improving cardiac function in patients with low-output cardiac failure.

Theory of Operation

Several models of the intra-aortic counterpulsation balloon (IACB) are available, but the basic designs are similar.[9] All consist of a cylindric or fusiform inflatable bag, approximately 26 cm long, surrounding a catheter (Fig. 26–160). The balloon is inflated with 20 to 40 cc of gas (depending upon balloon size) during cardiac diastole and forcibly deflated during systole. Inflation-deflation timing is electrically determined by linkage to the electrocardiogram. The goals of counterpulsation include augmentation of coronary artery perfusion during diastole and reduction of impedance to ventricular ejection, and thus ventricular work, during systole. Most coronary blood flow to the left ventricular myocardium occurs during cardiac diastole, and the goal of intra-aortic counterpulsation is to elevate mean aortic root diastolic pressure, thereby improving coronary artery perfusion. This is achieved by inflating the balloon during cardiac diastole, thus obstructing the aortic lumen. The ability of the IACB to elevate mean aortic root diastolic pressure is dependent upon several variables, including the position of the balloon within the aorta, the volume of blood displaced by the balloon, the relationship of the balloon diameter to the aortic lumen diameter, and the duration of balloon inflation-deflation.[23] The most effective increases in mean aortic root diastolic pressures are achieved by placing the balloon as close as possible to the aortic valve. In a clinical setting, however, the risk of cerebral embolism from such positioning is so high that the balloon must be placed no closer to the valve than the origin to the left subclavian artery. Similarly, although 100 per cent occlusion of the aortic lumen is likely to produce the largest increment in mean aortic root pressure, this could potentially damage the aortic wall and red blood cells. Therefore, optimal occlusivity is generally set in the 90 to 95 per cent range.

Inflation-deflation timing is determined by electronic linking with the electrocar-

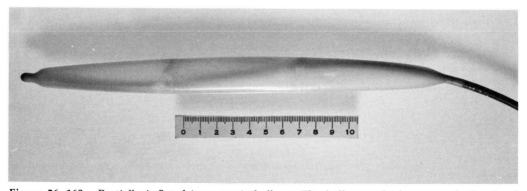

Figure 26–160. Partially inflated intra-aortic balloon. The balloon, which surrounds the distal portion of the catheter, is fusiform. (*From* Hyson, E. A., Ravin, C. E., Kelley, M. J., et al.: Intra-aortic counterpulsation balloon: radiographic considerations. Am. J. Roentgenol. *128*:915–918, 1977. Reproduced by permission.)

diogram. Ideally, the balloon should inflate at the end of ventricular ejection, coincident with closure of the aortic valve. Premature inflation obstructs ventricular ejection and is counterproductive. Deflation ideally occurs as the aortic valve opens. Forced deflation of the balloon by vacuum imparts a forward momentum to the blood remaining in the aortic root and thereby decreases impedance to ventricular ejection.

Both carbon dioxide and helium have been used as the driving gas for IACB's. Helium is advantageous in that its lower density and viscosity make for more rapid inflation-deflation capabilities, but it is potentially lethal if balloon rupture occurs.[6] Because of this, many systems employ carbon dioxide, which is rapidly absorbed into the blood in the event of balloon leakage or rupture. The response characteristics of such systems have not been severely limited by the increased viscosity of the carbon dioxide.

Intra-aortic counterpulsation, by increasing mean aortic root pressure during diastole, improves coronary artery perfusion. By imparting a forward momentum to the blood remaining in the aortic root at the time of ventricular ejection, it reduces impedance to ventricular ejection and thus reduces myocardial work. Consequently, myocardial oxygenation is improved while myocardial work and oxygen requirements are reduced, with resultant improvement in myocardial function.

Radiographic Features

The IACB is inserted through a Dacron graft placed end-to-side to the common femoral artery. The balloon is advanced in a retrograde fashion until its distal tip lies at the level of the aortic knob, as seen on a routine chest radiograph. This position assures that the balloon lies distal to the origin of the left subclavian artery, thereby reducing the potential risk of cerebral embolism. Correct positioning maximizes augmentation of coronary artery blood flow while minimizing the risk of cerebral embolus, occlusion of the left subclavian artery, or intermittent occlusion of the renal arteries by the balloon itself. During systole, when the balloon is deflated, the IACB is seen as a radiopaque catheter. During diastole, with the balloon inflated, a lucent area (corresponding to the gas-filled balloon) is seen paralleling the distal portion of the catheter (Fig. 26–161).[9, 21]

Occasionally, because of extensive atherosclerotic changes in the abdominal or thoracic aorta, placement of the balloon via the usual retrograde approach may not be possible. In these situations, the balloon may be placed in an antegrade fashion, through the aortic arch (Fig. 26–162).[17, 19] This approach requires a thoracotomy, however, for both the insertion and the removal of the balloon.

Potential Complications

The most common radiographically apparent complications associated with use of intra-aortic counterpulsation balloons result from incorrect positioning. A balloon that is positioned too high may enter the left subclavian artery (Fig. 26–163) or one of the cerebral vessels and, if such a position is not corrected, may result in arterial laceration, obstruction, or embolism.[15]

The inability to advance the balloon to the level of the aortic knob results in decreased effectiveness of counterpulsation and, if positioned too low, may result in the obstruction of major abdominal arteries, such as the celiac, superior mesenteric, or renal arteries.

Text continued on page 1910

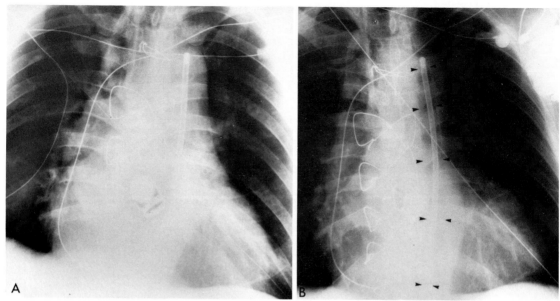

Figure 26–161. *A,* Chest film illustrating the appearance of an intra-aortic counterpulsation balloon during systole (note that the prosthetic aortic valve is in the open position). The balloon, when deflated during systole, is not visible radiographically. *B,* Chest film obtained during diastole (note that the prosthetic aortic valve is closed) illustrating the gas-filled balloon, which is projected as a radiolucent cylinder (arrowheads) paralleling the distal portion of the catheter. (*From* Hyson, E. A., Ravin, C. E., Kelley, M. J., et al.: Intra-aortic counterpulsation balloon: radiographic considerations. Am. J. Roentgenol. *128:*915–918, 1977. Reproduced by permission.)

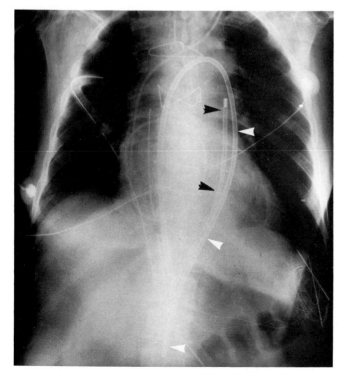

Figure 26–162. Postoperative chest film demonstrating two intra-aortic counterpulsation balloons. Preoperatively, it had only been possible to place a 20-cc balloon (black arrowheads) via the usual retrograde route because of significant atherosclerotic changes in the patient's aorta and femoral artery. This small balloon did not achieve maximal counterpulsation effects because of its decreased occlusivity. Therefore, at the time of thoracotomy, a second, larger, IACB (white arrowheads) was placed in an antegrade fashion through the aortic arch. It was subsequently possible to remove the smaller IACB and to sustain effective circulatory support using the larger IACB. This was subsequently removed via a repeat thoracotomy.

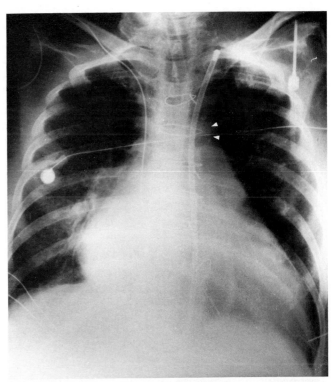

Figure 26–163. Incorrect positioning of IACB. Chest film demonstrating an IACB advanced above the level of the aortic arch (arrowheads) into the left subclavian artery. This position can result in damage to both the subclavian artery and the thoracic aorta. (*From* Ravin, C. E., Putnam, C. E., and McLoud, T. C.: Hazards of the intensive care unit. Am. J. Roentgenol. *126*:423–431, 1976. Reproduced by permission.)

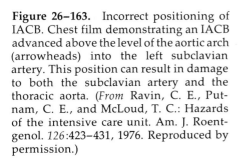

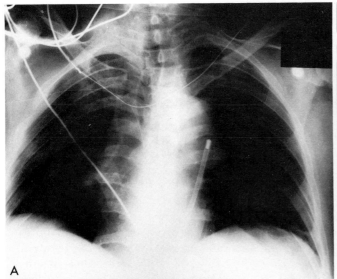

A

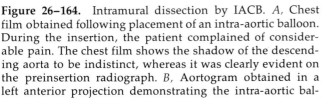

B

Figure 26–164. Intramural dissection by IACB. *A,* Chest film obtained following placement of an intra-aortic balloon. During the insertion, the patient complained of considerable pain. The chest film shows the shadow of the descending aorta to be indistinct, whereas it was clearly evident on the preinsertion radiograph. *B,* Aortogram obtained in a left anterior projection demonstrating the intra-aortic balloon to be outside the aortic lumen. The IACB was removed, and the patient sustained no adverse clinical effect from the inadvertent intramural position of the balloon at the time of insertion. (*From* Hyson, E. A., Ravin, C. E., Kelley, M. J., et al.: Intra-aortic counterpulsation balloon: radiographic considerations. Am. J. Roentgenol. *128*:915–918, 1977. Reproduced by permission.)

An additional risk associated with the use of this device is dissection of the aortic wall.[9, 16] This results from the inadvertent dissection of the catheter into the aortic wall during initial placement and is frequently associated with complaints of pain by the patient during insertion of the balloon. The loss of definition of the descending aorta on the chest radiograph after placement of the intra-aortic balloon may be an early clue to such intramural positioning (Fig. 26–164).

Other complications associated with the intra-aortic balloon are generally not apparent on routine radiographic examinations. These include wound infections at the site of balloon insertion, red cell hemolysis, platelet destruction, and arterial insufficiency in the catheterized limb.[1, 3, 16] Thromboembolism involving the aorta or the renal, celiac, or mesenteric arteries has been decreased by systemic heparinization and by the maintenance of the balloon in the pumping, rather than in the stationary, mode.[2]

EXTRACORPOREAL PUMPING WITH MEMBRANE OXYGENATION

Membrane oxygenators are a logical outgrowth of the membrane lungs used during cardiac surgery and of renal hemodialysis equipment. In large part, the development of membrane oxygenators depended upon technical improvements in the structure of the membranes themselves.[7] The development in 1966 of a silicone-polycarbonate copolymer was a major advance and has allowed the subsequent development of a functioning extracorporeal membrane oxygenator (ECMO). Such a device can now provide circulatory support and gas exchange adequate to meet the needs of a normothermic adult. Refinements in equipment have reduced the damage to the various blood components and allowed use of these devices for periods of days or weeks.

The major advantage of this system compared with the intra-aortic counterpulsation balloon is that it allows both gas exchange and circulatory support. It is far more costly than the IACB, however, and requires considerable technical support.

Theory of Operation

Three systems of circulatory bypass can be employed with the ECMO.[8] The venovenous route drains venous blood from the inferior vena cava just below the diaphragm and forwards it to the membrane oxygenator. Oxygenated blood is returned from the ECMO to the superior vena cava via the internal jugular vein. Use of this route provides the entire circulation (both systemic and pulmonary) with well-oxygenated blood. Because of the high flow rates necessary with this system, however, pressures in the pulmonary circuit are maintained at relatively high levels.

The venoarterial route obviates the problem of persistently high pressures in the pulmonary circuit, thus improving the potential for pulmonary recovery. Venous blood is withdrawn from the right atrium, and oxygenated blood is returned into the abdominal or descending thoracic aorta. The upper regions of the thoracic aorta serve as the site of mixing of the oxygenated blood returning from the ECMO, with the blood returning from the patient's lung and ejected by the left ventricle. Unfortunately, this can sometimes result in the carotid and coronary arteries receiving desaturated blood. This problem is corrected to some extent by advancing the cannula that is returning oxygenated blood as far as possible toward the aortic root. This bypass system markedly reduces flow through the pulmonary circuit and reduces pulmonary artery pressures to below normal levels. Such a reduction in pressure, however, may be undesirable for the healing of damaged pulmonary parenchyma.

Further improvements can be obtained by combining the two systems into a venovenous-venoarterial system. This adds a second arterial catheter placed into the right ventricle to the venoarterial system. Thus, oxygenated blood is returned to both the systemic and the pulmonary systems, and, by appropriate control of return to the right ventricle, pulmonary artery pressures may be maintained at more normal levels, theoretically facilitating healing of damaged lung tissue.

Radiographic Features

The radiographic features of ECMO systems are limited and consist only of identification of the radiopaque cannulas used to collect and return blood (Fig. 26–165). In order to determine whether the cannulas are correctly positioned, one must know which of the previously described systems (that is, the venovenous, venoarterial, and venovenous-venoarterial systems) is being utilized. The membrane oxygenator itself is extracorporeal and is thus not visualized on radiographs.

As this device is generally employed when there is significant pulmonary failure, with or without associated myocardial failure, the changes associated with the adult respiratory distress syndrome and its complications may be seen on the radiographs. (See Adult Respiratory Distress Syndrome, p. 20, Chapter 1.)

IMPLANTABLE ARTIFICIAL HEART

Attempts to develop a satisfactory mechanical heart have been ongoing for more than two decades. These devices are desirable in situations in which the heart is not

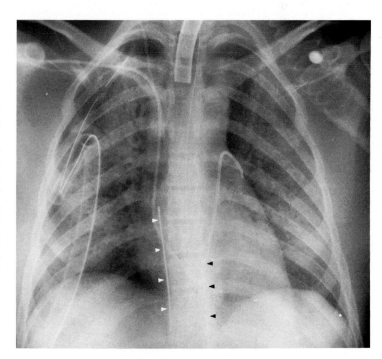

Figure 26–165. Anteroposterior supine chest radiograph of a patient with adult respiratory distress syndrome on an extracorporeal membrane oxygenator. The cannulas related to the use of this device are evident. The venous catheter (white arrowheads) is positioned in the right atrium, and the arterial catheter (black arrowheads) is in the distal thoracic aorta. (Courtesy of A. Morris, M.D., and J. Armstrong, M. D., Salt Lake City, Utah.)

expected to recover sufficient function to support life. Multiple attempts at development of such mechanical devices have been made, but several factors continue to limit their success. For a number of years, thrombus formation within the artificial heart was the significant limiting factor.[12, 14, 18] Recently, however, this problem has been significantly reduced by the capability to manufacture an extremely smooth polyurethane surface for the mechanical heart.[18] In addition, improvement in the design features related to blood flow through the device have aided in reducing or preventing thrombus formation. Pharmacologic advances modifying platelet adhesiveness have also reduced the risk of thrombus formation. At present, the major problem limiting artificial hearts has been mechanical failure resulting from tearing of the surfaces lining the chambers through which the blood is pumped at their points of maximal flexion.[18] Anticipated improvements in the polymers used in the construction of these devices may obviate this problem.

In addition to the full mechanical replacement of the heart, mechanical left ventricular assist devices have been developed. Such devices have been employed in situations in which balloon counterpulsation (IACB) is unable to effectively support the circulatory system. These units are placed either on the external chest wall or intra-abdominally and pump blood from the left ventricular apex to the aorta.[13, 20] Although such devices can maintain a maximal blood flow of 7 liters per minute for as long as 30 days, they are limited both by mechanical failures and by the risk of infections occurring where they penetrate the chest wall.

The radiographic features of these various total mechanical replacements or left ventricular assist devices vary owing to differences in design.

References

1. Berger, R. L., Saini, V. K., Ryan, T. J., et al.: Intra-aortic balloon assist for postcardiotomy cardiogenic shock. J. Thorac. Cardiovasc. Surg. 66:906–915, 1973.
2. Bernstein, E. R., and Murphy, A. E., Jr.: The importance of pulsation in preventing thrombosis from intra-aortic balloons. J. Thorac. Cardiovasc. Surg. 62:950–956, 1971.
3. Butner, A. N., Krakauer, J. S., Rosenbaum, A., et al.: Clinical trial of phase-shift balloon pumping in cardiogenic shock: results in 29 patients. Surg. Forum 20:199–200, 1969.
4. Curtis, J. J., Barnhorst, D. A., Pluth, J. R., et al.: Intra-aortic balloon assist. Initial Mayo Clinic experience and current concepts. Mayo Clin. Proc. 52:723–730, 1977.
5. Dunkman, W. B., Leinbach, R. C., Buckley, M. J., et al.: Clinical and hemodynamic results of intra-aortic balloon pumping and surgery for cardiogenic shock. Circulation 46:465–477, 1972.
6. Furman, S., Vijaynagar, R., Rosenbaum, R., et al.: Lethal sequelae of intra-aortic balloon rupture. Surgery 69:121–129, 1971.
7. Galletti, P. M.: Background and technical aspects of membrane oxygenation. In Bregman, D.: Mechanical Support of the Failing Heart and Lungs. New York, Appleton-Century-Crofts, 1977, pp. 129–142.
8. Hill, J. D.: Clinical experience with ECMO: future needs. In Bregman, D.: Mechanical Support of the Failing Heart and Lungs. New York, Appleton-Century-Crofts, 1977, pp. 165–182.
9. Hyson, E. A., Ravin, C. E., Kelley, M. J., et al.: Intra-aortic counterpulsation balloon: radiographic considerations. Am. J. Roentgenol. 128:915–918, 1977.
10. Kantrowitz, A., Tjonneland, S., Krakauer, J. S., et al.: Mechanical intra-aortic cardiac assistance in cardiogenic shock. Arch. Surg. 97:1000–1004, 1968.
11. Kantrowitz, A., Krakauer, J. S., Rosenbaum, A., et al.: Phase-shift balloon pumping in medically refractory cardiogenic shock. Arch. Surg. 99:739–743, 1969.
12. Kolff, W. J.: Removing limiting factors for total cardiac replacement. Transplant. Proc. 3(4):1449–1457, 1971.
13. Norman, J. C., Fuqua, J. M., Hibbs, C. W., et al.: An intracorporeal (abdominal) left ventricular assist device. Arch. Surg. 112:1442–1451, 1977.
14. Olsen, D. B., Unger, F., Oster, H., et al.: Thrombus generation within the artificial heart. J. Thorac. Cardiovasc. Surg. 70:248–255, 1975.
15. O'Rourke, M. F., and Shepherd, K. M.: Protection of the aortic arch and subclavian artery during intra-aortic balloon pumping. J. Thorac. Cardiovasc. Surg. 65:543–546, 1973.
16. Pace, P., Tilney, N., Couch, N., et al.: Peripheral arterial complications of intra-aortic balloon counterpulsation. Abstract. Circulation 54(Suppl. 2):13, 1976.

17. Pappas, G.: Intrathoracic intra-aortic balloon insertion for pulsatile cardiopulmonary bypass. Arch. Surg. *109*:842–843, 1974.
18. Pierce, W. S., Brighton, J. A., Donachy, J. H., et al.: The artificial heart. Progress and promise. Arch. Surg. *112*:1430–1438. 1977.
19. Printup, C. A., Dietrick, W. R., Getzen, J. H., et al.: Ascending aorta insertion of the dual-chambered intra-aortic balloon for counterpulsation during cardiac operations. Ann. Thorac. Surg. *20*:694–697, 1975.
20. Radvany, P., Pine, M., Weintraub, R., et al.: Mechanical circulatory support in postoperative cardiogenic shock. J. Thorac. Cardiovasc. Surg. *75*:97–103, 1978.
21. Ravin, C. E., Putman, C. E., and McLoud, T. C.: Hazards of the intensive care unit. Am. J. Roentgenol. *126*:423–431, 1976.
22. Scheidt, S., Wilner, G., Mueller, H., et al.: Intra-aortic balloon counterpulsation in cardiogenic shock. N. Engl. J. Med. *288*:979–984, 1973.
23. Weber, K. T., and Janicki, J. S.: Intra-aortic balloon counterpulsation. Ann. Thorac. Surg. *17*:602–636, 1974.

Part XI

Clinical Echocardiography

MORRIS N. KOTLER, M.D., F.R.C.P.

GARY S. MINTZ, M.D.

BERNARD L. SEGAL, M.D.

WAYNE R. PARRY

Echocardiography is widely accepted as a safe and essential diagnostic tool in the evaluation of patients with a variety of cardiac disorders. M-mode (single-dimension) echocardiography is the cornerstone of diagnostic pulse-reflected ultrasound. It provides accurate, reliable, and reproducible information at no known risk to the patient, and it is relatively inexpensive. It remains the technique of choice in obtaining quantitative measurements of heart size, wall thickness, and left ventricular function. This study can be performed on critically ill postoperative patients in the surgical intensive care unit. Serial studies, especially in the assessment of a pharmacologic agent, can be performed at regular intervals at the bedside. However, particular skill and expertise are essential to obtain high-quality and reproducible echocardiograms. The major disadvantage of M-mode echocardiography is that it yields a limited, "ice pick," one-dimensional view of the heart. The entire left ventricular cavity, apex of the left ventricle, right atrium, and three leaflets of the tricuspid valve cannot always be evaluated by this modality. In addition, intracardiac structures are displayed in an unfamiliar format that bears little resemblance to the cardiac anatomy. Spatial orientation of intracardiac structures cannot always be readily appreciated by M-mode techniques.

Two-dimensional echocardiography provides spatial orientation and allows lateral as well as axial distances between structures to be appreciated. The images obtained by the various two-dimensional systems resemble heart structures. The newer real-time, two-dimensional imaging devices are capable of extraordinarily rapid image formation times, offering the viewer a remarkable appreciation of the heart in motion. With the sophisticated phased-array systems or the newer mechanical arc scanners, 80- to 90-degree sector scans of the heart can be obtained. This allows complete visualization of the entire left ventricular cavity, cardiac apex, right ventricle, right and left atria, and interatrial septum as well as the tricuspid and pulmonary valves and the great vessels.

The disadvantages of two-dimensional echocardiographic systems include considerable cost, bulky nontransportable equipment, and limited resolution. As with M-mode echocardiography, suboptimal two-dimensional images may be obtained on obese, emphysematous patients, on patients with chest deformities, or on patients on a respirator.

A detailed knowledge of cardiac anatomy and physiology and the basic principles of ultrasound are essential in understanding both M-mode and two-dimensional echocardiography. An appreciation of the pitfalls and limitations of both techniques should temper the physician's interpretation. Overinterpretation and acceptance of poor-quality tracings or recordings may be even more hazardous than underinterpretation, especially in the critically ill postoperative patient.

PHYSICAL PRINCIPLES

M-mode echocardiography depends on sound waves of very high frequency that are generated by a piezoelectric crystal incorporated into a transducer that converts electrical to vibratory or sound wave energy. While ultrasound generally represents vibrations above 20,000 cycles per second (cycles per second = Hertz [Hz]; 1000 cycles per second = 1 megahertz [MHz]), the sound frequencies used in echocardiography range from 1 to 10 MHz. The piezoelectric crystal is used both as a signal transmitter and as a receiver and generates high-frequency vibrations, generally in the range of 2 to 5 MHz. Most instruments transmit sound for approximately 1 microsecond and receive sound for the remaining 999 microseconds. All transmitted sound from a single pulse travels through the thorax and returns before the next pulse, so that there is no interference between sequential pulses. The high-frequency sound waves are reflected best from the interface between tissues of different acoustic impedance (density). The subsequent returning sound energy is converted to an electrical impulse that can be displayed on a strip chart recording coupled with other parameters for timing of cardiac events, such as the elctrocardiogram or phonocardiogram.

Velocity of sound in soft tissues of the body is approximately 1546 meters per second. Velocity is equal to wavelength times frequency: the higher the frequency, the smaller the wavelength. For a typical 2.25 MHz transducer, the wavelength is approximately 0.7 mm. The wavelength determines the axial resolution, or ability to resolve two structures aligned parallel with the axis of the sound beam. Very short wavelength permits resolution of small distances. However, there is a reciprocal relationship between resolution and penetration of soft tissue. Thus, in pediatric cardiology, the use of high-frequency transducers of 5 MHz with short penetration provides high resolution. However, in adults lower frequency transducers are needed to produce enough energy to penetrate the chest, with a consequent loss in axial resolution. As a sound pulse travels through soft tissue it loses energy by reflection, by refraction, and by absorption. Thus, sound returning from distant structures in relation to the transducer has lower energy than that reflected from structures near the transducer. For this reason, a depth compensation circuit is used in most commercial instruments so that the intensity of echoes near the transducer is attenuated or reduced, while more distant echoes are relatively enhanced. Most commercial ultrasound systems employ focused transducers, which collimate the emitted sound beam and thus reduce the lateral spread.

There are esssentially three modes of displaying the processed echo data on the oscilloscope monitor. In the "A" mode, echoes are displayed as vertical spikes along the horizontal baseline. The amplitude, or height, corresponds to the relative intensity of the echo, while the depth of echo origin is indicated on the abscissa or X-axis. In the

"B" mode, brightness format, the echoes remain unchanged but are now displayed as dots rather than spikes. The more intense the echo, the greater the brightness of the dot. M-mode, which is commonly used in echocardiography, is achieved by sweeping a B-mode display across the oscilloscope at a uniform speed. For easy viewing the B-mode display is usually rotated 90 degrees in a clockwise direction and swept across the screen from left to right. In this presentation, the depth of an echo is shown along the vertical, or Y, axis, and time is represented on the horizontal, or X, axis. The intensity of an echo is still proportional to brightness, but the dots now appear as undulating lines. In effect, M-mode recording is a continuous plot of the depth of structures with respect to time.

One of the technical problems encountered is poor lateral resolution, or insufficient distinction of structures lying in close proximity to each other. Even with focused transducers an ultrasonic beam cannot be accurately focused over the entire depth range of the beam. The beam spreads out at a finite angle, causing some echoes to appear as if they arise from structures in the central beam, whereas in fact they are echoes recorded from structures off the main axis. These spurious echoes are displayed in a plane where there is no directly corresponding structure. A classic example of the lateral beam resolution problem occurs in patients with a mitral Starr-Edwards prosthesis.[74] Spurious echoes arising from the suture ring or even the ball may be recorded behind the aortic root within the left atrial cavity when the suture ring is actually attached to the mitral annulus.

Other potential problems may be related to technique and interpretation. These include the following:

1. Drop-out phenomenon, or the sudden disappearance of echoes that should be normally recorded from a specific anatomic structure within the ultrasound beam.

2. Reverberations or false echoes recorded twice as far from the transducer as the first interphase, since ultrasound waves can be reflected more than once before returning to the transducer. This may result in an erroneous impression of a structure recorded behind the heart.

3. Considerable interobserver and intraobserver variability can occur, especially when echocardiographic measurements are performed. In addition, the greater the distance from the chest wall of an intracardiac structure, the greater the error in measurement. In the measurement of left ventricular wall thickness, a difference of 2 to 3 mm may be of considerable significance. A recent attempt at standardization of all echocardiographic measurements has been undertaken.[77]

With regard to two-dimensional systems, the original multielement linear array system consisted of a transducer with 20 separate crystals in linear arrangement.[11] Each crystal was pulsed sequentially, and the image was displayed as a series of single-line reflections. The large transducer size, low-line density, and wide beam size resulted in overall poor resolution and discontinuity of images from the underlying ribs. A mechanical scanner was subsequently introduced, consisting of a single crystal transducer that was allowed to oscillate rapidly by means of an electronic motor through a 30° arc.[31] This system is relatively inexpensive and provides good-quality images. More recently, a wide-angle (80 to 90 degree) mechanical sector scan using multiple rotating crystals has been developed. The phased-array system represents a distinct advantage in two-dimensional echocardiography.[40] An 80 degree sector scan of the heart is obtained at a scan rate of 30 frames per second. The crystals (up to 32 piezoelectric crystals) are excited almost simultaneously but slightly out of phase, so that the crystal on one end of the transducer is excited slightly before the next one. By alternation of the sequence of crystal excitation the ultrasonic wave front is electronically steered in an 80 degree sector. Images are represented in real-time, and the sector images or frames at 30 per second are recorded on ½-inch video tapes. Generally, individual frames can be photographed by a Polaroid R camera attachment. Since each video tape frame consists of two interlacing fields and the stop frame mode consists of only a single field, there is half of the information, and therefore significant degradation of image quality can result. For this reason an idealized diagram accompanies most of the two-dimensional illustrations.

TECHNIQUE

With the patient in the supine or semirecumbent position and with the trunk elevated between 15 and 45 degrees, an M-mode transducer is applied to the chest wall

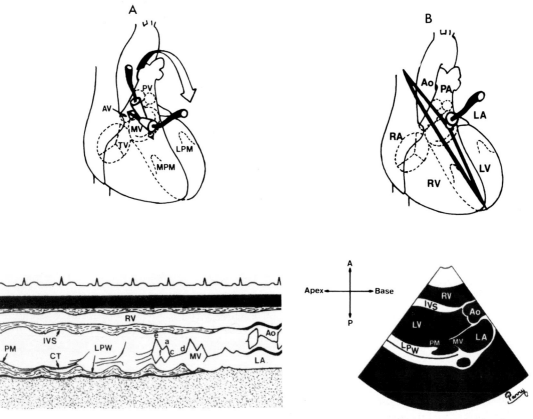

Figure 26–166. *A*, The M-mode transducer in the third interspace pointing toward the mitral valve as well as toward the aortic valve. An M-mode echocardiographic sweep from the aortic root to the left ventricular cavity is shown diagramatically below this. The electrocardiogram is demonstrated for timing events. Anteriorly, the right ventricular wall, cavity, and septum are demonstrated. Posteriorly, the left ventricular cavity and posterior wall structures are identified. Ao = aorta; LA = left atrium; MV = mitral valve; IVS = interventricular septum; CT = chordal structures; PM = papillary muscle; LPW = left ventricular posterior wall; MPM = medial papillary muscle; LPM = lateral papillary muscle. *B*, A two-dimensional transducer placed in the long axis of the left ventricle. Shown is an idealized diagram of an image frame of the long-axis plane of the left ventricle. Anteriorly and to the right is the aorta, and posteriorly is the left atrium. The right ventricular cavity is separated from the left ventricular cavity by the interventricular septum. The circular structure posterior to the atrioventricular junction is the descending aorta. PA = pulmonary artery; Ao = aorta; RA = right atrium; IVS = interventricular septum; PM = papillary muscle; RV = right ventricle; LV = left ventricle; LA = left atrium; AV = aortic valve; TV = tricuspid valve; PV = pulmonary valve.

in the third or fourth interspace, 1 to 5 cm lateral to the left sternal border. A water-soluble gel (Aquasonic) is used to ensure contact between the transducer and the skin. The transducer is directed slightly medially from a true anteroposterior direction to locate the mitral valve. The mitral valve is usually found at the depth of 5 to 8.5 cm from the chest wall. Maximum amplitude of mitral valve motion is obtained by directing the ultrasound beam to the tip of the mitral valve. Once the mitral valve has been identified, the septum and left ventricular posterior wall can also be recognized by angulating the transducer inferolaterally away from the tip of the mitral valve. As the transducer is rotated toward the apex, the posterior mitral leaflet merges into postero-chordal structures and papillary muscles (Fig. 26–166A). The two mitral leaflets (anterior and posterior) move in diastole in an M-shaped mirror image pattern. At the onset of systole, the leaflets merge at the C-point. During systole the two leaflets move slightly anteriorly to the D-point. With the onset of diastole, the leaflets open to the E-point. The early diastolic velocity of the leaflets, "E to F slope," is dependent upon the rate of filling of the left ventricle. If the transducer is rotated from the mitral valve position in a medial-cephalad direction, the aortic root can be identified.

The aortic root consists of two undulating intense echoes that move anteriorly during systole and posteriorly during diastole. Two aortic valve leaflets may be seen within the aortic root: They separate in systole, creating a boxlike appearance, and come together in diastole. Portions of the tricuspid valve may be identified during systole and diastole when the transducer is directed medially and toward the spine. When identified, the tricuspid valve is contiguous with the anterior aortic wall. The posterior aortic wall and anterior mitral valve are in continuity as are the anterior aortic wall and septum (Fig. 26–166A). During systole, the interventricular septum and left ventricular posterior wall thicken. The septum moves in a posterior direction, and the left ventricular posterior wall moves in an anterior direction; thus, there is reduction in the diameter of the left ventricle and shortening of the minor axis. The right ventricle is usually seen anterior to the septum, and the left atrium is posterior to the aortic root.

The long-axis view of the left ventricle, as obtained by two-dimensional echocardiography, is shown in Figure 26–166B. The transducer is positioned in the third or fourth interspace, and the ultrasound beam is directed in a plane parallel to a line joining the right shoulder to the left flank, thus producing an 80 degree arc. The image obtained represents a section through the long axis of the left ventricle. The image is oriented so that the aorta is displayed to the right, the cardiac apex to the left, the chest wall and right ventricle anteriorly, and the left ventricular posterior wall and left atrium posteriorly (Fig. 26–166B). In this view, practically the entire left ventricular cavity can be seen except for a small portion of the apex. The long axis of the left ventricle allows visualization of the aortic root and the aortic valve leaflets. The aortic valve leaflets appear as a thin line during diastole in the midline of the aortic root. With the onset of systole, the leaflets open abruptly and come to align themselves nearly parallel to the aortic wall. The long-axis view allows visualization of the anterior and posterior leaflets of the mitral valve as well as the chordal and papillary muscle attachments. Generally, the anterior leaflet appears larger than the posterior leaflet. With the onset of diastole, the anterior leaflet opens and approximates the left ventricular septal surface. The posterior leaflet moves in a posterior direction and has a much smaller excursion compared with the anterior leaflet. During systole the mitral leaflets coapt at a point inferior to the atrioventricular groove. The descending aorta is frequently seen as a circular structure posterior to the atrioventricular groove (Fig. 26–166B).[63]

The tricuspid valve, or portions of it, is visualized by M-mode techniques with a transducer in the third or fourth interspace but directed more medially toward the patient's spine. Unless the right ventricle is grossly enlarged, only the systolic and portions of the diastolic motion can be recorded (Fig. 26–167A). However, with two-dimensional echocardiography, a long-axis view of the right ventricular inflow tract can be readily obtained (Fig. 26–167B).[96] With the transducer in the same interspace (either third or fourth intercostal), and with inferomedial and slight clockwise rotation of the transducer, a long-axis view of the right ventricle and right atrium is obtained. The chest wall is anterior, the right atrium is on the right and posterior, and the right ventricular apex is anterior and to the left of the image (Fig. 26–167B). This view enables the right atrial cavity, the tricuspid anterior and posterior leaflets, and the right ventricular inflow portion of the right ventricle to be seen.[96] The position and motion of the tricuspid leaflets are very well demonstrated in this view. The anterior leaflet is a relatively larger and longer structure and has slightly increased excursion compared with the posterior tricuspid leaflet.

The pulmonary valve can be located by M-mode echocardiography.[109] The transducer is positioned in the second intercostal space, and the beam is angulated in a

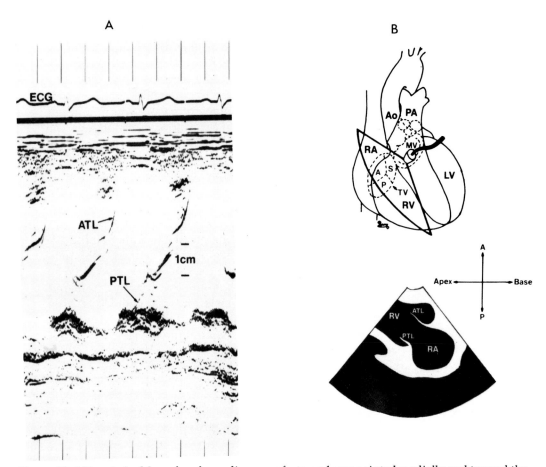

Figure 26–167. *A,* An M-mode echocardiogram of a transducer pointed medially and toward the spine showing portions of the tricuspid valve. ATL = anterior tricuspid leaflet; PTL = posterior tricuspid leaflet. *B,* Two-dimensional view of the right ventricular inflow tract with a transducer placed in the third intercostal space and rotated slightly clockwise. In the idealized diagram the right ventricle is anterior, the right atrium is posterior, and two leaflets of the tricuspid valve are clearly visualized. ATL = anterior leaflet; RV = right ventricle; PTL = posterior leaflet; RA = right atrium; Ao = aorta; PA = pulmonary artery; MV = mitral valve; TV = tricuspid valve; LV = left ventricle.

lateral and cephalad direction (Fig. 26–168A). The pulmonary artery is identified as a sonolucent space, 1 to 2 cm from the anterior chest wall, and is anterior to and left of the aorta. Generally, the posterior cusp of the pulmonary valve can be recognized in the majority of subjects. It opens during systole and has a fairly prominent *a* wave (Fig. 26–168A). The *a* wave represents the effect of atrial contraction on the pulmonic leaflet. Point "b" represents the position of the leaflet at the onset of ventricular ejection. Point "c" represents the maximal opening position of the posterior pulmonic leaflet. Points "d" to "e'" represent diastolic closure, and points "e'" to "f" represent the leaflet in the closed position during diastole.

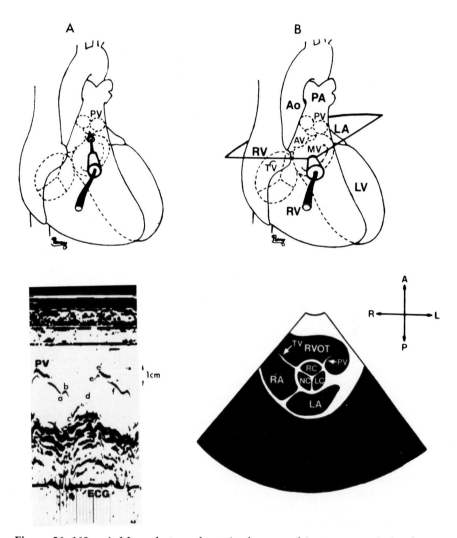

Figure 26–168. *A,* M-mode transducer in the second interspace pointing laterally toward the left shoulder. The pulmonary valve is superior, anterior, and lateral to the aortic valve. The recording of the posterior pulmonic leaflet is depicted below. Points a, b, c, d, e, e', and f are described in the text. *B,* Cross-sectional view at the level of the great vessels. The aorta appears as a circle with a trileaflet aortic valve. Anteriorly, the outflow tract of the right ventricle (RVOT) is sausage-shaped in appearance, and the pulmonic valve (PV) can be seen. The tricuspid valve is medial, and the interatrial septum separates the left and right atrium. LA = left atrium; RA = right atrium; RC = right coronary cusp; NC = noncoronary cusp; LC = left coronary cusp.

In order to record the pulmonic valve by two-dimensional techniques, the transducer is placed in the parasternal position in the third or fourth intercostal space, and the short-axis view of the heart is obtained by rotating the transducer so that the plane of the ultrasound beam is perpendicular to the plane of the long axis of the left ventricle (Fig. 26–168B).[96] The transducer is pointed cephalad, and the great arteries are sectioned transversely (Fig. 26–168B). The aorta appears as a circle with a trileaflet aortic valve, which during diastole has the appearance of the letter "Y" (Fig. 26–168B). The right ventricular outflow tract crosses anterior to the aorta and has a sausage-like appearance (Fig. 26–168B). The pulmonary valve is visualized anterior and to the right of the aorta. During systole the pulmonary valve leaflets open and approximate the anterior and posterior pulmonary artery walls. The anterior leaflet of the tricuspid valve can also be seen on the left of the image. Other structures recorded in this view include the left atrium, the interatrial septum, and the right atrium to the left of the image. From this position the transducer can be rotated slightly clockwise and tilted beyond the pulmonary valve, allowing the main pulmonary artery and its bifurcation to be visualized.

Additional cross-sectional views of the left ventricle can be obtained by two-dimensional techniques by inferior tilting of the transducer. At the level of the body of the left ventricle where the transducer beam transects the mitral valve, the anterior and posterior mitral leaflets are widely separated, creating a fish-mouth appearance during diastole (Fig. 26–169A and B). During systole the leaflets are in a closed position and appear in a single line. The circular left ventricular myocardium can be seen contracting during systole and relaxing during diastole. Anterior and to the left, the right ventricle can be seen. As the transducer beam is tilted further inferiorly, a cross section at the level of the papillary muscles is obtained (Fig. 26–169A and C). The left ventricular myocardium is represented as a circular structure. The wall thickness and motion during each phase of the cardiac cycle can readily be appreciated. The anterolateral and posteromedial papillary muscles project into the left ventricular cavity and are visualized approximately at 4 and 8 o'clock positions, respectively (Fig. 26–169C). Further transducer angulation in an inferior direction displays a cross-sectional view at the ventricular apex. The ventricular cavity is small and surrounded by thickened circular myocardium (Fig. 26–169A and D).

Two-dimensional echocardiography has enhanced the ability to record the entire left ventricular cavity and apex, and the apical four-chambered view has been particularly valuable in evaluation of patients with a variety of cardiac disorders.[91] In order to record the apical image, the patient is positioned in the left lateral decubitus position. The apical impulse is localized, and the transducer is placed at, or in the immediate vicinity of, the point of maximal impulse. Once the apex is located the transducer beam is directed toward the base (Fig. 26–170A and B). The beam plane is perpendicular to the ventricular and atrial septa and passes through the plane of the mitral and tricuspid valve orifices. All four chambers of the heart, including the ventricular and atrial septa and the crux of the heart, are displayed (Fig. 26–170A and B). The image orientation is such that the apex is at the top and the atria at the bottom. Insertion of the tricuspid valve leaflet is slightly inferior and apical in relation to the mitral valve. In addition, on occasion the pulmonary veins can be identified entering the left atrium. The apical two-chambered or right anterior oblique equivalent view of the left ventricle is obtained by placing the transducer at the point of maximal impulse and rotating it so that the beam is directed in a plane nearly parallel to the ventricular septum (Fig. 26–170A and C). In this view, the apex of the left ventricle is displayed at the top right of the image, the aorta is at the bottom left, and the left atrium is situated posteriorly. The anterolateral and inferior walls of the left ventricle as well as the cardiac apex, left atrium, right ventricle, and

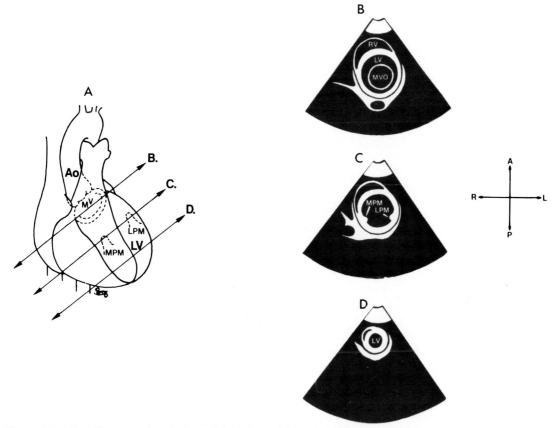

Figure 26–169. Cross-sectional view of the left ventricle. *A,* A diagrammatic view of the heart showing various cross-sectional planes taken from the level of the mitral valve toward the apex of the left ventricle. *B,* Cross-sectional view of the left ventricle at the level of the mitral valve. The right ventricle (RV) is anterior and to the left of the left ventricle (LV). The left ventricle appears as a circular structure. The mitral valve orifice (MVO) has a fish-mouth appearance during diastole. *C,* A cross-sectional view of the left ventricle at the level of the papillary muscles. The anterolateral papillary muscle (LPM) and the posteromedial papillary muscle (MPM) project in the left ventricular cavity at approximately the 4 and 8 o'clock positions. *D,* A cross-sectional view of the left ventricle at the apex of the left ventricle. The left ventricle is small and surrounded by thick circular muscle. R = right; A = anterior; L = left; P = posterior.

descending aorta are visualized. This view resembles a left ventricular angiogram obtained in the right anterior oblique plane and is particularly useful in detecting cardiac aneurysms and regional wall motion abnormalities.

The suprasternal notch position is obtained by positioning the transducer in the suprasternal notch with the beam angulated inferiorly and slightly posteriorly (Fig. 26–171*A* and *B*).[96] The ascending aorta is on the left and the descending aorta on the right. The origins of the brachiocephalic vessels, the right pulmonary artery, and the left atrium are visualized (Fig. 26–171*A*). This view allows visualization of a coarcted segment in patients with coarctation of the aorta and is extremely valuable for looking at the anatomic arrangement of the aortic arch and its branches.

The subcostal position has been very useful in patients with chronic obstructive lung disease and emphysema, when the usual precordial ultrasonic window may become obliterated because of hyperinflated lungs.[21] With two-dimensional techniques, it is particularly useful in evaluating infants and children with a variety of congenital cardiac disorders.[46] The subcostal examination is performed by placing the

Text continued on page 1924

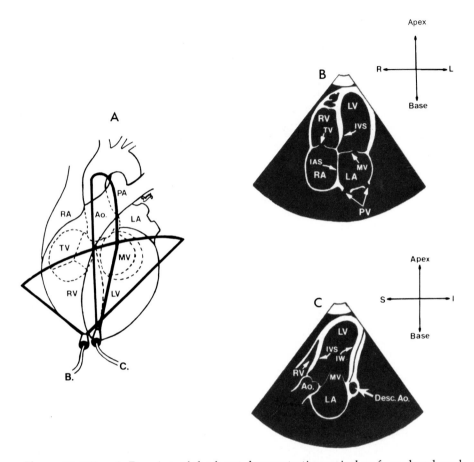

Figure 26–170. *A,* Drawing of the heart demonstrating apical or four-chambered view (position B), and the right anterior oblique view of the left ventricle (position C). The transducer is placed at the apex of the heart and angulated toward the base of the heart. *B,* Apical or four-chambered view of the heart. The interventricular septum (IVS) separates the right and left ventricles (RV and LV). The interatrial septum (IAS) separates the left and right atrium (RA and LA). The attachments of the tricuspid valve (TV, inferiorly situated) and mitral valve (MV) are seen. Pulmonary veins (PV) may be seen entering the left atrium. The apices of both ventricles are situated anteriorly, and the base of the heart is situated posteriorly. *C,* Right anterior oblique view of the left ventricle. The beam is parallel to the plane of the ventricular septum. The left ventricle and apex are anterior and to the right, and the aorta (Ao) is posterior and to the left. The inferior wall (IW) of the left ventricle is best seen in this view. R = right; L = left; S = superior; I = inferior; RA = right atrium; PA = pulmonary artery. (*From* Kotler, M. N., Mintz, G. S., Segal, B. L. et al.: Clinical uses of echocardiography. Am. J. Cardiol. 45:1061–1082, 1980. With permission.)

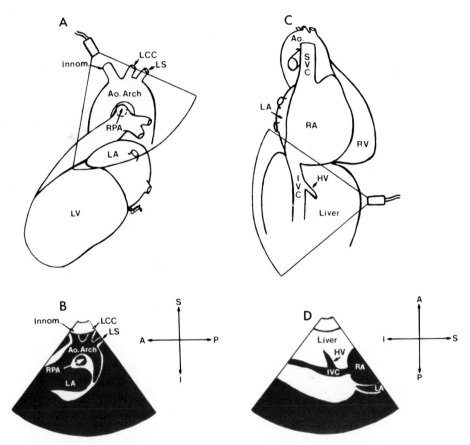

Figure 26–171. *A,* Drawing of the heart and great vessels with the transducer in the suprasternal notch position and directed inferiorly and slightly posteriorly. *B,* Diagrammatic representation of the sector scan. The ascending aorta (Ao) is on the left, the aortic arch is anterior, and the descending aorta is on the right. The origins of the brachiocephalic vessels can be seen, as can a cross section of the right pulmonary artery (RPA). Posteriorly, the left atrium can be seen. *C,* Drawing of the heart with the transducer in subxiphoid position and angulated toward the patient's spine. *D,* Diagrammatic representation of sector scan. Anteriorly, the liver and junction of the hepatic vein (HV) and the inferior vena cava (IVC) are seen. The junction of the inferior vena cava and right atrium (RA) is also demonstrated. The interatrial septum and left atrium (LA) may also be seen. Innom= innominate; LCC= left common carotid; LS = left subclavian artery; SVC = superior vena cava; S= superior; I= inferior; A = anterior; P = posterior. (*From* Kotler, M. N., Mintz, G. S., Segal, B. L., et al.: Clinical uses of echocardiography. Am. J. Cardiol. 45:1061–1082, 1980. With permission.)

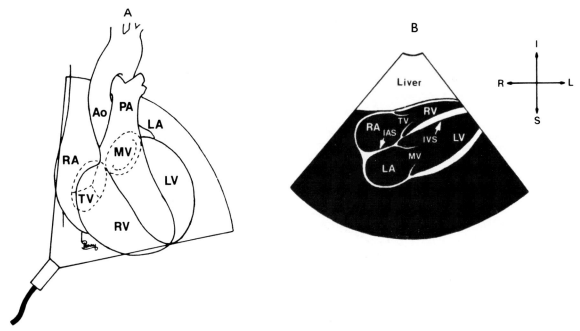

Figure 26–172. *A,* Subxiphoid view of a two-dimensional echocardiogram with the transducer placed in the subxiphoid position and angulated toward the base of the heart. *B,* Diagrammatic representation of sector scan. The right atrium and right ventricle are anteriorly situated, and the left atrium and left ventricle are posteriorly situated. The interatrial and interventricular septa and the tricuspid and mitral valves are also demonstrated. IAS = interatrial septum; IVS = interventricular septum; MV = mitral valve; TV = tricuspid valve; RV = right ventricle; LV = left ventricle; RA = right atrium; Ao = aorta; PA = pulmonary artery; LA = left atrium.

transducer in the midline or slightly to the patient's right, with the transducer pointed toward the spine. In this position the liver, hepatic veins, and inferior vena cava are identified (Fig. 26–171*C* and *D*). With slight tilting of the transducer, the junction of the hepatic veins into the inferior vena cava can also be identified (Fig. 26–171*C* and *D*).[96] The inferior vena cava to right atrium communication is also best assessed in this view. The transducer can also be placed along a coronal plane parallel to a line between the patient's shoulders, with a scan plane tilted about 45 degrees downward from the plane of the anterior chest wall.[96] This view allows visualization of both of the atrial cavities, the atrial septum, the ventricular septum, both of the ventricular cavities, and the atrioventricular valves (Fig. 26–172). Because both the interatrial septum and the membranous portion of the interventricular septum are somewhat perpendicular to the ultrasound beam and are usually completely imaged, there is very little echo drop-out. Therefore, this approach allows evaluation of the size and shape of both atria and ventricles as well as visualization of interatrial and ventricular septal defects.

POSTOPERATIVE ECHOCARDIOGRAPHIC CHANGES

Postoperative Patients and Ventricular Septal Motion

After coronary artery bypass surgery and valve replacement, septal motion is frequently abnormal in the immediate postoperative period. It is estimated that

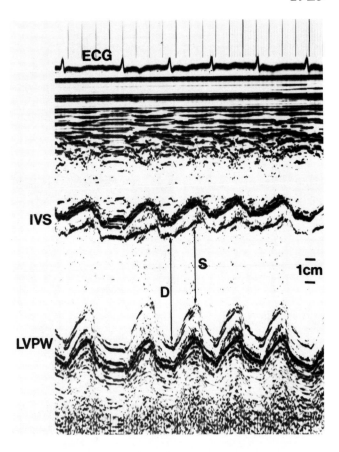

Figure 26–173. M-mode echocardiogram of a patient who had recently undergone aortic valve surgery, demonstrating the abnormal motion of the septum. The septum moves anteriorly during systole and fails to thicken normally. There is vigorous contraction of the posterior wall. D = diastolic dimension; S = systolic dimension; IVS = septum; LVPW = left ventricular posterior wall.

approximately 90 per cent of patients with aortic valve replacement and approximately 40 per cent of patients with mitral valve replacement demonstrate abnormal septal motion.[7] When such individuals are evaluated two months postoperatively, the abnormal septal motion disappears in those with mitral valve replacement and remains in approximately one third of those who have had aortic valve replacement (Fig. 26–173).[7] Early normalization of septal motion may suggest a paravalvular leak.[7] The reasons for abnormal septal motion are unclear but may be related to uneven myocardial perfusion and cooling during cardiopulmonary bypass. Abnormal septal motion is not a nonspecific finding after thoracotomy and may result from clinically inapparent septal ischemia during cardiopulmonary bypass.[102] A significant reduction in septal thickening was demonstrated postoperatively in those patients with abnormal motion, whereas no change in septal thickening was demonstrated in those with normal motion.[102] Abnormal intrathoracic cardiac motion as a result of right ventricular sternal adhesions may also account for the abnormal postoperative septal motion.[38] This theory is supported by the finding of an enlarged right ventricular cavity confirmed by echocardiography and gated blood pool nuclear scans.[102]

Pericardial Effusion

Both M-mode and two-dimensional echocardiography are the techniques of choice in the diagnosis of pericardial effusion. However, there are pitfalls and limitations in recognizing pericardial effusion, and proper gain setting and identification of the left

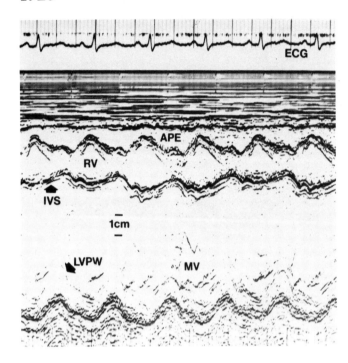

Figure 26–174. An M-mode echocardiogram on a patient with a loculated anterior pericardial effusion following open heart surgery. APE = anterior pericardial effusion; RV = right ventricle; IVS = interventricular septum; LVPW = left ventricular posterior wall; MV = mitral valve. *Note:* There is no posterior pericardial effusion.

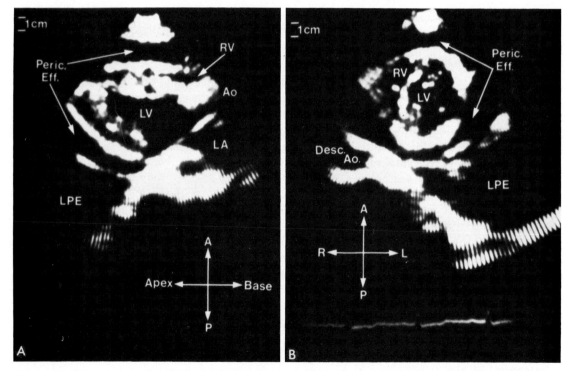

Figure 26–175. A two-dimensional echocardiogram (A) in the long-axis view and (B) in the cross-sectional view. The clear differentiation of a pericardial effusion from a left pleural effusion (LPE) is evident in both views. In addition, there is right ventricular compression owing to the large anterior pericardial effusion. Desc. Ao = descending aorta; RV = right ventricle; Ao = aorta; LA = left atrium; LV = left ventricle.

ventricular posterior wall structures are essential. Initially, fluid accumulates, usually posteriorly, and produces a posterior echo-free space. As the fluid increases, an anterior space develops. However, in the postoperative patient, on rare occasions an anterior loculated effusion may occur (Fig. 26–174). A false positive echo-free space posteriorly may be recorded when the transducer is angulated toward the mediastinum or toward the annulus. Mitral annular calcification may frequently be confused with the posterior wall, and the echo-free space posteriorly may be mistaken for pericardial effusion.[68] In most instances, fluid is not recorded behind the left atrium; however, in large effusions, fluid may be recorded behind the left atrium.[47]

Frequently, the distinction between pericardial and pleural effusions, particularly in a postoperative setting, is extremely difficult. We have found two-dimensional echocardiography helpful in differentiating the two conditions (Fig. 26–175). In addition, two-dimensional echocardiography may allow recognition of pericardial adhesions. This is important, because if adhesions are present in the apical area a subcostal pericardiocentesis may be inadvisable.

Cardiac tamponade remains a clinical diagnosis. It is most important to recognize this disorder in the immediate postoperative state. Echocardiography may be valuable in assessing whether fluid is producing mechanical compression. With marked fluid accumulation, a large echo-free space may be demonstrated posteriorly or even loculated anteriorly. Two-dimensional echocardiography may also demonstrate right ventricular compression,[82] which should be regarded as a dangerous sign postoperatively. Cardiac compression is localized at the apex of the right ventricle. However, vigorous systolic motion of the right ventricular outflow tract and right atrium can be noted. Other signs of cardiac tamponade include marked decrease in ventricular wall amplitude with acute tamponade, oscillations of the heart within the pericardial sac at one half the frequency of the heart rate, and reciprocal changes in size of the right and left ventricular chambers accompanied by alterations in mitral excursion and E-F slope with inspiration and expiration. Any of these findings may be present, but the sensitivity of each finding remains to be determined. Two-dimensional echocardiography may be more reliable than M-mode echocardiography in assessing the degree of pericardial fluid accumulation.[55]

Constrictive Pericarditis

In our experience, the echocardiogram is generally unreliable in constrictive pericarditis, although some helpful features have been reported.[83] These include a double band of narrowly separating intense echoes with parallel motion in the area of the pericardium. Abnormal motion of the septum has also been recorded. On occasion, very dense echoes recorded from pericardial calcification may be present. In addition, an abrupt change in left ventricular wall motion in diastole from rapid filling to a period of diastasis may be demonstrated.

Prosthetic Valves

The utility of echocardiography in the assessment of prosthetic valve function depends on a number of factors. First, familiarity with the basic types of prosthetic heart valves and their characteristics is essential. The motion of the disc Beall valve is considerably different from that of the eccentric monocuspid valve, such as the Bjork-Shiley. It should be noted that the Bjork-Shiley valve has a normal tilting motion, and depending on transducer beam angulation, the disc may appear below the aortic root, in the aortic root, or above the aortic root. Second, technique is of the utmost importance in the evaluation of mitral or aortic valve prostheses. The transducer should be placed at the cardiac apex and the beam angulated toward the annulus so that it is directed along the longitudinal axis of mitral valve opening motion. Aortic prosthetic valves are more difficult to evaluate. The transducer should be placed in the right supraclavicular or right second intercostal space. Third, there are many tilting discs that do not produce loud opening clicks; consequently, a simultaneous phonocardiogram to determine the A_2 mitral valve opening interval is essential. This interval, which usually measures about 0.08 to about 0.11 seconds, is shortened or lengthened, depending on the magnitude of left atrial pressure, obstruction to the valve orifice, and left ventricular dysfunction.[5] Fourth, the patient should be used as his or her own control, particularly in the follow-up examination. Shown in Figure 26–176A is a patient who had a normal mitral Bjork-Shiley valve inserted with an immediate postoperative recording. Six months later the patient presented with acute pulmonary edema. Echocardiography was unable to demonstrate valve opening and closing motion (Fig. 26–176B). The patient had extensive thrombus formation, and clot ingrowth, extending from the suture ring and left atrium, enveloped both the ventricular and the atrial side of the disc.

The M-mode characteristics of the newer bioprosthetic valves include recording of

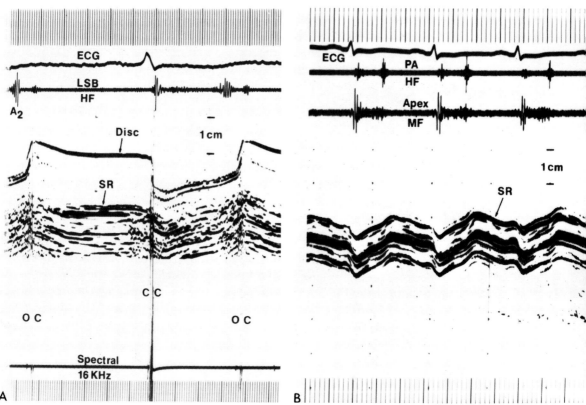

Figure 26–176. *A,* Simultaneous electrocardiogram, phonocardiogram, M-mode echocardiogram, and spectral analysis of a normal functioning mitral Bjork-Shiley valve. The opening and closing motion of the disc in conjunction with clearly recorded clicks is evident. *B,* Simultaneous electrocardiogram, phonocardiogram, M-mode echocardiogram, and spectral analysis of same patient. Individual leaflet motion is not apparent, and dense echoes are recorded from the suture ring (SR). The phonocardiogram demonstrates a holosystolic murmur compatible with mitral regurgitation.

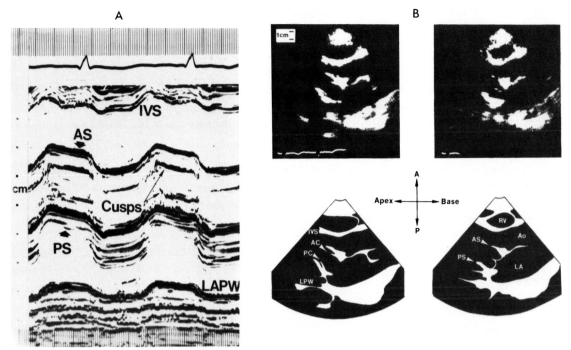

Figure 26–177. *A,* M-mode echocardiogram of a patient with a porcine mitral valve heterograft, showing the cusps clearly separated in diastole and merging during systole. The anterior stent (AS) and posterior stent (PS) are clearly visualized. LAPW = left atrial posterior wall. *B,* Two-dimensional echocardiogram in the same patient in the long-axis view. The stents point toward the apex. During diastole, both leaflets are seen to open (AC = anterior cusp, and PC = posterior cusp). During systole, both leaflets close.

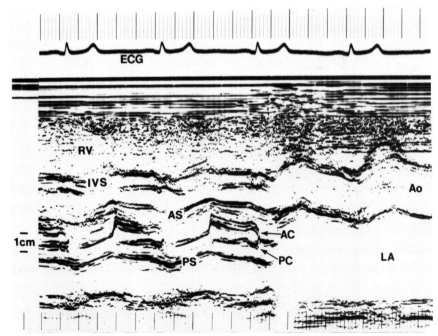

Figure 26–178. An M-mode echocardiogram on a patient with a porcine mitral valve heterograft, demonstrating early degenerative changes of both the anterior and the posterior cusps. The leaflets are thickened, and the mobility and excursion are decreased. AC = anterior cusp; PC = posterior cusp; AS = anterior stent; PS = posterior stent.

stents and individual cusps (Fig. 26–177A).[36] During systole the stents move anteriorly, and during diastole they move posteriorly. The leaflet opening motion of the mitral bioprosthetic valve occurs during diastole in a boxlike fashion, with the two leaflets merging with the onset of systole (Fig. 26–177A). The excursion of the heterograft aortic valve is similar to that of native aortic leaflets and is generally less than the excursion of the native mitral valves. Late dysfunction of bioprosthetic valves occurs as a result of disruption of leaflet tissue or calcification of the tissue leaflets, resulting in valvular insufficiency or stenosis. In addition, calcific degeneration of a bioprosthetic valve may occur, and dense echoes and limited motion may be recorded (Fig. 26–178). Two-dimensional echocardiography generally allows more accurate visualization of anterior and posterior stents as well as individual leaflet motion (see Fig. 26–177B). M-mode echocardiography has not always been able to define distinct leaflet motion, and in our experience, two-dimensional echocardiography can reveal individual leaflet motion more precisely. In addition, M-mode echocardiography may not always detect a vegetation of the tricuspid prosthetic valve, whereas two-dimensional echocardiography is more likely to demonstrate the valvular vegetation. Two-dimensional echocardiography can differentiate between valvular problems and left ventricular dysfunction.[80]

CLINICAL APPLICATIONS OF ECHOCARDIOGRAPHY

Contrast Echocardiography

Contrast echocardiography was introduced primarily for confirmation of ultrasonic cardiac anatomy.[30] Indocyanine green, saline infusion of blood, and injection of dextrose solution can produce a cloud of echoes. The exact cause of this echo production remains uncertain. A combination of factors, such as acoustic impedance differences, microbubbles in solution, turbulence, difference in temperature, and cavitation, appears to account for the echo-contrast effect.[88]

Recently, contrast echocardiography has been expanded with M-mode and two-dimensional echocardiography to include detection and localization of right-to-left and left-to-right intracardiac shunts. Since the contrast effect is lost on a single transit through the lungs, echoes do not normally appear on the left side of the heart following injection into a peripheral vein.[86] Most patients with an atrial septal defect have a predominantly left-to-right shunt; some may have an additional right-to-left shunt, as shown by the simultaneous appearance of echoes in the left atrium and ventricle. With peripheral vein injection of saline, tricuspid regurgitation can be readily appreciated by two-dimensional echocardiography even in the absence of clinical signs.[50] It appears to be superior to M-mode echocardiography, in which the findings are nonspecific for right ventricular volume overload and include an enlarged right ventricle and abnormal septal motion. The characteristic two-dimensional findings in tricuspid regurgitation include the appearance of contrast in the inferior vena cava (Fig. 26–179) and movement of contrast bubbles back and forth across the tricuspid valve. This technique is extremely useful and can be reliably used in the postoperative state in evaluating the residual degree of tricuspid regurgitation after corrective mitral valve surgery. By placement of the two-dimensional transducer in the epigastrium, high-quality images of the inferior vena cava and the right atrial junction may also be obtained. Vigorous pulsation of the inferior vena cava during systole may be confirmatory evidence of tricuspid regurgitation. The use of indwelling intracardiac catheters for contrast studies has proved successful in delineating residual intracardiac shunts in postoperative patients.[101] It

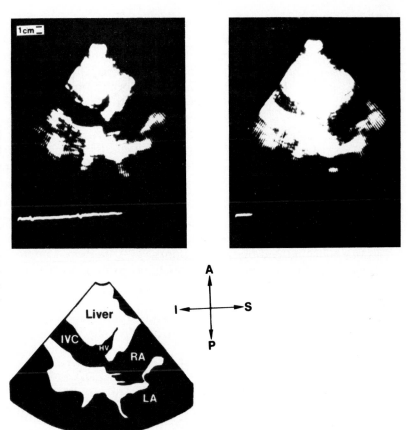

Figure 26–179. Subxiphoid view of a two-dimensional echocardiogram in a patient with tricuspid regurgitation. Left-hand panel shows a dilated inferior vena cava (IVC) entering the dilated right atrium (RA). Right-hand panel of the systolic frame following the peripheral injection of saline. Microcavitation and persistent cloud of echoes are demonstrated in the inferior vena cava and lower right atrium.

appears that contrast echocardiography may be more sensitive than the indicator-dilution technique. In patients with residual right-to-left shunts at the atrial level the left atrium and mitral orifice are opacified with echoes following contrast injection into a central venous catheter.[95] When right-to-left shunting occurs at the ventricular level, injection into the central venous line reveals an opacification of the left ventricle and aortic root without an opacification of the left atrium and mitral orifice.[95]

Left Ventricular Function

The left ventricular chamber is prolate ellipsoid in shape. Volume (V) of the ellipsoid is given by the formula

$$V = \frac{4}{3} \pi \, (L/2) \, (D_1/2)(D_2/2)$$

where L = long axis of the ventricle or distance from the aortic valve to the apex, and D_1 and D_2 = the short or minor axes that lie in perpendicular planes and bisect the major axis. The most accurate angiographic estimates of left ventricular volume are based upon this formula.[19] The minor axis dimensions are nearly identical in perpendicular views. In dilatation of the left ventricle, the ventricle becomes more spherical, with a resultant increase predominantly in the minor axis.

LEFT VENTRICULAR VOLUMES, STROKE VOLUME, AND EJECTION FRACTION. The calculation of left ventricular internal dimensions depends on the simultaneous recording of left ventricular septal echoes and left ventricular posterior endocardial echoes. The transducer is angulated caudally and laterally to a position just below the mitral valve leaflets to record left ventricular internal dimensions. (Fig. 26–180). The end-diastolic diameter (Dd) is the perpendicular distance between the echoes of the left side of the septum and the posterior endocardium at the time of onset of the QRS complex. The end-systolic diameter (Ds) is the shortest perpendicular distance between the echoes from the same structures and is usually measured at the time of peak movement of the posterior wall (Fig. 26–180).

Left ventricular volume can be calculated by various formulas.[25, 67, 69, 97] The first method relies on the assumption that the minor axis is the same in all planes and that in the normal ventricle the long axis is approximately twice the minor axis. Therefore, volume (V) of a prolapse ellipsoid $= \frac{\pi}{3} D^3 = 1.047 D^3$. Thus, volume may be estimated by cubing the echocardiographic minor axis.[67, 69] In larger ventricles, this method overestimates the volume. Separate regression equations have been derived to calculate end-systolic and end-diastolic volumes.[25, 97] The more commonly used formula is that derived by Teichholz et al.,[97] in which a correction for the change in ratio of L/D with increasing ventricular volume is taken into account. Volume $(V) = \left(\frac{7.0}{2.4 + D} \right) (D^3)$. The volumes obtained by this regression equation show good correlation with angiographic measurements even for dilated ventricles.[97] Stroke Volume (SV) = EDV − ESV. Ejection Fraction = SV/EDV.

The problems of measurement of left ventricular volumes by M-mode echocardiography have been emphasized.[52] Minor discrepancies between the ultrasonic beam and the minor axis can result in a 5 to 10 per cent error in minor axis measurements.[52] In addition, it cannot necessarily be assumed that the major to minor axis ratio is 2:1, especially in dilated or asynergic ventricles.[97]

Although M-mode echocardiography reliably estimates left ventricular function when the ventricular wall motion is uniform, it may be inaccurate in estimating left ventricular function in the presence of regional asynergy.[22, 97] When there is a localized wall abnormality that is not in the plane of the ultrasound beam, M-mode echocardiography tends to overestimate ejection fraction. If a localized wall abnormality is present in the septum or the left ventricular posterior wall, the ejection fraction may be underestimated by M-mode echocardiography. Recently, the mitral valve E-point to septal separation measurement has been introduced, which may be partially independent of regional variations in ventricular wall function.[57] On the basis of two studies,[48, 57] the E-point septal separation measurement provided a more accurate assessment of left ventricular function than M-mode determination of ejection fraction in patients with regional wall motion abnormalities.

Left ventricular ejection fraction as determined by two-dimensional echocardiography has been accurately correlated with ejection fraction by angiography.[9] In addition, differentiation between localized and diffuse left ventricular dysfunction can be accomplished with this technique.[15] Two-dimensional echocardiography may be more reliable than M-mode echocardiography for estimating left ventricular ejection fraction, especially in patients with coronary artery disease.[9] However, two-dimensional echocardiography may not always reliably detect and localize the endocardial surfaces because of oblique impingement of the ultrasound beam. Possibly for this reason, end-diastolic volumes are consistently underestimated and are probably unreliable when determined by two-dimensional techniques.

LEFT VENTRICULAR MASS. The thickness of the interventricular septum and the posterior wall of the left ventricle is measured from the echocardiogram of the ventricle in the area inferior to the tips of the mitral valve. The septal thickness is measured as the distance from the right to the left side of the septum, and posterior wall thickness is measured as the distance from the endocardium to the epicardial border of the posterior wall left ventricular mass.[99]

$$(LVM) = \text{Total ventricular volume} - \text{volume of left ventricular cavity} =$$
$$(Dd + 2 \text{ (wall thickness) })^3 - (Dd)^3.$$

This volume when multiplied by the specific gravity of muscle (1.05) gives left ventricular mass.

VELOCITY OF CIRCUMFERENTIAL FIBER SHORTENING. Measurement of "circumferential," or internal, chord shortening velocity is an excellent method for assessing left ventricular performance during ejection, since both the extent of shortening and the time factor (i.e., the rate of shortening) are considered.[56] It may reflect muscle function more directly than the more familiar ejection fraction.

$$\text{Velocity of circumferential} \quad Vcf = \frac{Dd - Ds}{Dd \times dt}$$
$$\text{fiber shortening}$$

where dt is the duration of minor axis shortening and is measured from the echocardiogram as the time from onset to peak posterior wall movement or, more accurately, as the ejection time measured from an externally recorded pulse tracing (see Fig. 26–180). VcF,

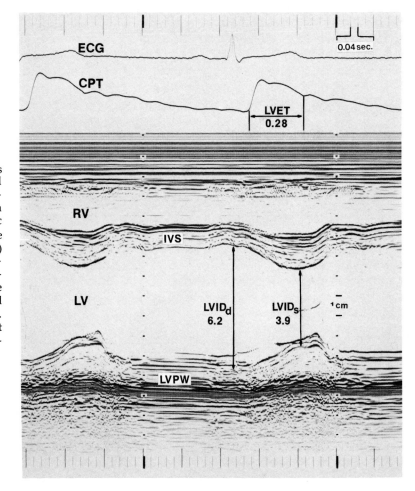

Figure 26–180. Simultaneous electrocardiogram, carotid pulse tracing (CPT), and M-mode echocardiogram of a normal patient. The diastolic dimension (LVID$_d$) and the systolic dimension (LVID$_s$) are clearly shown. In addition, the left ventricular ejection time is derived from the onset of the carotid pulse till the diacrotic notch (LVET). Vcf in this particular patient is calculated to be 1.32 circumferences per second.

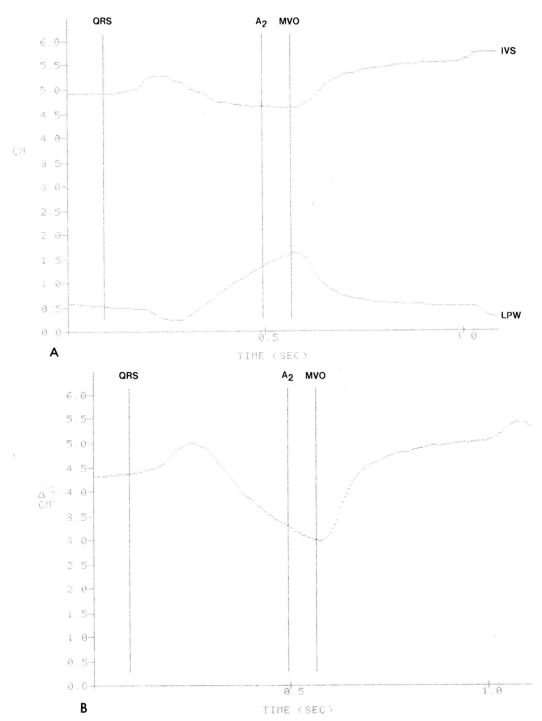

Figure 26–181. A digitized tracing of the left ventricular cavity dimension. *A,* Endocardial tracing of the interventricular septum and left ventricular posterior wall. *B,* Change in diameter of the left ventricular cavity over time (T).

Legend continued on the opposite page

as determined echocardiographically, has been shown to correlate well with the angiographically determined Vcf and is reproducible. The average value in normal subjects is 1.29 circumferences per second.[37] Because of abnormal septal motion. Vcf and ejection fraction cannot always be employed as a useful index of left ventricular function in the immediate postoperative period. The per cent of internal diameter shortening may be calculated as follows:[37]

$$\frac{\text{End-diastolic diameter} - \text{End-systolic diameter}}{\text{End-diastolic diameter}} \times 100$$

The lower limit of normal for this calculation is 28 per cent and correlates well with mean Vcf.

WALL THICKENING INDICES. Indices describing the extent and velocity of wall thickening are useful in assessing ventricular performance.[56] The extent of wall thickening or per cent of systolic thickening (% ΔT) may be calculated as follows:

$$\% \Delta T = \frac{Ts - Td}{Td} \times 100$$

where T is wall thickness; the per cent of systolic thickening of the interventricular septum or left ventricular posterior wall or both can thus be determined.

LEFT VENTRICULAR WALL MOTION. The wave form of the posterior wall resembles an inverted ventricular volume curve, whereas that of the septum is of smaller amplitude and is notched.[100] This lack of symmetry occurs as a result of two movements. The major motion is due to contraction and expansion of the ventricle. Superimposed on this is an anterior movement of the entire heart during systole and a

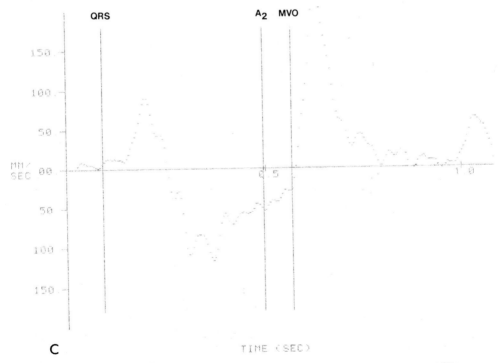

Figure 26–181 *Continued.* C, Rate of change in the diameter (the first derivative $\frac{dD}{dt}$). MVO = mitral valve opening.

posterior movement during diastole. Posterior wall velocity has been utilized as a measure of left ventricular function, but this measurement correlates poorly with angiographic ejection fraction or Vcf. The assessment of left ventricular functions from digitized echocardiograms appears to be a promising technique.[27] Ventricular endocardial echoes can be processed by a computer, permitting ventricular dimension and its rate of change to be calculated throughout the cardiac cycle (Fig. 26–181). Echocardiograms must be of optimal quality, and the recordings should be performed at a paper speed of 100 mm per second. By measuring the rate of change of dimension as well as recording the left ventricular dimension curve during diastole, Gibson et al.[27] were able to assess the effects of mitral valve surgery. Successful mitral commissurotomy is associated with an increase in peak filling rate and a return of filling pattern toward normal. Increased rates may result from surgically induced mitral regurgitation. Evaluation of mitral prostheses by this technique appears to be promising. Patterns of left ventricular wall movement during diastole may be abnormal in a variety of cardiac disorders, such as idiopathic hypertrophic subaortic stenosis and ischemic heart disease.

Echocardiography has been used to evaluate left ventricular function during open heart surgery.[93] However, the recording of suitable echocardiograms is not always technically feasible. Recently, transesophageal echocardiography has been utilized for the continuous monitoring of left ventricular dimensions during open heart surgery.[58] With this method, echocardiograms can be recorded at the same location throughout the entire procedure and sterilization of the probe is not required. The drop in cardiac output as determined by echocardiography appears to be secondary to decreased distensibility of the ventricular cavity as a result of mechanical constriction caused by closure of the pericardium and the chest wall.[59] Echocardiography has been utilized in assessing left ventricular performance after mitral valve replacement.[84] In patients with mitral regurgitation who have moderate left ventricular dilatation and a normal ejection fraction preoperatively, there is regression of myocardial hypertrophy and only minimal reduction of left ventricular per cent shortening after mitral valve replacement.[84] However, in patients with mitral regurgitation who exhibit grossly dilated left ventricles and a normal to low ejection fraction before surgery, left ventricular function may deteriorate and chamber dilatation and hypertrophy persist.[84]

Aortic Stenosis

Left ventricular outflow obstruction can be classified as being caused by valvular, subvalvular, or supravalvular aortic stenosis. In turn, each of these types can be subdivided according to etiologic, morphologic, and clinical characteristics. Valvular aortic stenosis may be due to an intrinsically stenotic congenital valve, either unicuspid, bicuspid, or tricuspid. A patient with a congenital bicuspid aortic valve can be asymptomatic for many years but can present during the fourth or fifth decade with severe aortic stenosis and heavy valve calcification. Discrete aortic stenosis on a normal trileaflet valve echo generally results from either rheumatic valve involvement or calcific disease of the elderly. In either event, when the valve becomes significantly narrowed and calcified the clinical and echocardiographic features may be indistinguishable from those of congenitally abnormal valvular stenosis and calcification. In calcific diseases of the elderly, dense echoes may be recorded within the aortic root during systole and diastole, and yet hemodynamic significant aortic stenosis may not be present.

BICUSPID AORTIC VALVE. M-mode echocardiography allows detection of a bicuspid valve in approximately 75 per cent of patients.[72] The characteristic M-mode finding is an eccentric position of the aortic leaflets in diastole (Fig. 26–182A). The leaflets

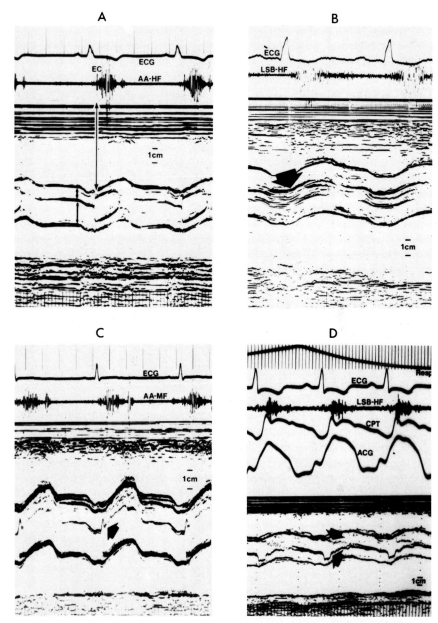

Figure 26–182. Composite M-mode series in bicuspid aortic valve (*A*), in aortic calcific stenosis (*B*), in discrete subaortic stenosis (*C*), and in idiopathic hypertrophic subaortic stenosis (*D*). *A,* A loud crescendo-decrescendo systolic murmur is recorded with an ejection click (EC) coinciding with maximal aortic valve opening. The aortic leaflet is in an eccentric position during diastole. *B,* A crescendo-decrescendo systolic murmur is recorded by phonocardiography. The aortic echocardiogram demonstrates increased echo densities during systole and diastole with inability to demonstrate individual leaflet motion. *C,* Crescendo-decrescendo murmur is recorded by phonocardiography. The aortic echocardiogram demonstrates normal aortic valve opening. In addition, there is early systolic closure with partial reopening, and coarse fluttering is present. The reclosure movement is demonstrated by a large arrow. *D,* Simultaneous electrocardiogram, phonocardiogram, and carotid pulse tracing apexcardiogram in a patient with typical IHSS. Midsystolic closure of both aortic valve cusps is present.

also may show multiple echoes during diastole, suggestive of redundant leaflet.[72] Furthermore, M-mode echocardiography may not demonstrate the actual valvular stenosis. The valves dome in systole, and unless the tip of the valve leaflet is intersected by the ultrasound beam the leaflets may be normally separated for much of their length. Two-dimensional echocardiography has demonstrated increased echodensity, abnormal leaflet motion, and abnormal systolic doming of the valve cusps in the parasternal long-axis view.[111] In diastole, the thickened aortic leaflets may be seen to bow backwards toward the cavity of the left ventricle. In the parasternal cross-sectional view, the bicuspid aortic valve can be visualized as two distinct cusps separated by a horizontal commissure. Occasionally, a median raphe of the anterior cusp may be present. In a recent study, two-dimensional echocardiography correctly identified a bicuspid valve in 95 per cent of patients.[26] The parasternal short-axis view was the most reliable in identifying the bicuspid valve.[26]

CALCIFIC AORTIC VALVULAR DISEASE. In acquired aortic valvular calcific stenosis, M-mode echocardiography has not been shown to be reliable in predicting the valve gradient by assessing the mobility and degree of thickening of the cusps. In addition, with heavy calcified valves, marked restriction of aortic valve motion is noted, and dense echoes may be recorded in systole and diastole (see Fig. 26–182B). When dense echoes are recorded in the aortic root during systole, or diastole, excessive calcification or fibrosis of the aortic valve is suggestive of, without necessarily implying, critical stenosis. The aortic valve orifice size can also be affected by cardiac output. With decreased cardiac output the amplitude of aortic valve motion is decreased.

Other indirect echocardiographic parameters may be useful in the assessment of patients with aortic stenosis. These include concentric hypertrophy of the left ventricle and decreased diastolic closures slope of the mitral valve. There have been several reports attesting to the value of M-mode echocardiography in interpreting the systolic left ventricular pressure and, indirectly, the severity of aortic stenosis, particularly in congenital aortic stenosis.[1, 3] With the use of regression equations, some investigators have demonstrated that pressure is proportional to posterior wall thickness divided by the left ventricular internal dimension and multiplied by a constant factor.[1, 3] The correlation appears to be more helpful in children than in adults.

SUBVALVULAR AORTIC STENOSIS. Discrete subvalvular aortic stenosis can be divided into three subtypes: (1) the discrete membranous types, (2) the fibromuscular collar, and (3) the fibromuscular tunnel. The membranous type is by far the most common. The M-mode echocardiographic features of subaortic stenosis due to the membranous type include early systolic closure of the aortic valve (see Fig. 26–182C), the presence of abnormal echoes within the left ventricular outflow tract, and the presence of left ventricular hypertrophy.[44] In the majority of instances, aortic regurgitation is present, and therefore diastolic fluttering of the mitral valve may also be observed. Aortic valve fluttering is generally observed, and the valve seldom reopens to a normal position. The left ventricular outflow tract is particularly narrowed, but caution is needed when measuring outflow tract, since it will vary depending on where the measurement is made and on transducer angulation.[44] The abnormality of early aortic valve closure is similar to that seen in hypertrophic subaortic stenosis (IHSS) but usually occurs earlier in systole. Partial closure in IHSS is usually more midsystolic (see Fig. 26–182D). Partial aortic valve closure can also occur on occasion in patients with isolated ventricular septal defect. Aortic valve echocardiographic abnormalities do not correlate with left ventricular aortic pressure gradients. It should be noted that the membrane is not consistently recorded by M-mode techniques because frequently the membrane is oriented parallel to the ultrasound beam. Two-dimensional echocardiography has been shown to be more reliable than M-mode in detecting discrete subvalvular membrane and in demonstrating the fibromuscular type of subaortic stenosis.[112] Discrete membrane may be seen as a distinct linear echo within the outflow tract. The membrane may, in addition, exhibit dynamic motion that can be readily recognized. Patients with a fibromuscular lesion show diffuse or shelflike narrowing of the outflow tract. Postoperatively, these lesions may completely disappear.

IDIOPATHIC HYPERTROPHIC SUBAORTIC STENOSIS OR HYPERTROPHIC OBSTRUCTIVE CARDIOMYOPATHY. The echocardiographic features of this disorder have been well described with an increased septal to posterior wall thickness ratio.[34] The septum is usually thicker than 1.5 cm, and the ratio of septal thickness to posterior wall

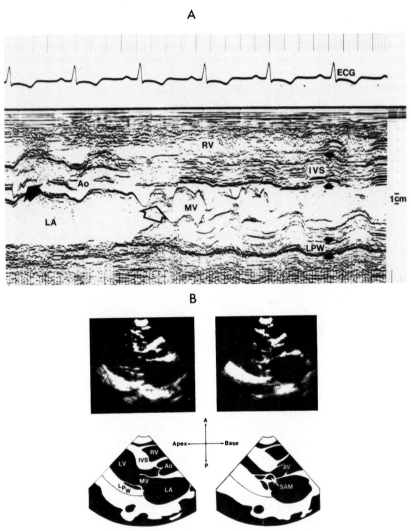

Figure 26–183. *A,* M-mode echocardiogram in a patient with IHSS. The large dark arrow (left) shows midsystolic closure of the aortic valve. The light arrow (middle) shows systolic anterior motion (SAM). The thickness of the interventricular septum is clearly seen between the two small dark arrows. The left ventricular posterior wall is normal in size compared with the septum. *B,* Two-dimensional echocardiogram in a patient with IHSS. Left-hand panel shows the thickened interventricular septum and normal mitral valve opening. Right-hand panel during systole demonstrates a thick septum in relation to the posterior wall. In addition, the tip of the mitral leaflet appears to be bent and drawn up into the left ventricular outflow tract (SAM motion).

thickness is usually above 1.5 to 1. Some investigators have regarded the ratio of 1.3 to 1 as suggestive of asymmetric septal hypertrophy. Other echocardiographic features include a hypodynamic septum with a hyperdynamic posterior wall, failure of the septum to thicken appreciably during systole (generally less than 20 per cent), and systolic anterior motion of the mitral valve (Fig. 26–183A).[68] Other features include a narrow left ventricular outflow tract, diastolic collision of the mitral valve and the septum, a decreased mitral valve E-F slope, and midsystolic closure of aortic valve leaflets.[68] However, these findings alone and in combination may be described in other conditions. Approximately 10 per cent of patients with left ventricular hypertrophy due to valvular aortic stenosis or hypertension have asymmetric septal hypertrophy as an isolated finding. Caution should be used in the measurement of the right side of the septum, as chordal structures within the right ventricular cavity can easily be mistaken for the right side of the septum.[41] In the absence of a typical systolic anterior motion (SAM) or murmur, the use of amyl nitrite or Valsalva's maneuver may be helpful in eliciting these findings.

Two-dimensional echocardiography provides very little additional diagnostic information compared with M-mode echocardiography in the assessment of idiopathic hypertrophic subaortic stenosis. In the parasternal long-axis view, two-dimensional echocardiography may localize the exact area of septal hypertrophy (Fig. 26–183B).[54] In the short-axis views, the mitral apparatus, including the papillary muscles, is usually anteriorly displaced.[54] Following septal myomectomy, two-dimensional echocardiography may be superior in delineating the extent of the myomectomy.[81] Two-dimensional echocardiography may also allow differentiation between the systolic anterior motion of the chordae tendineae and the systolic anterior motion of the mitral leaflets. However, it is not always possible to ascertain whether SAM occurs at the chordal end of the mitral leaflets or involves the entire mitral valve apparatus.[54]

Patients with fixed valvular, subvalvular, or supravalvular aortic stenosis may have coexistent dynamic subvalvular obstruction due to hypertrophic obstructive cardiomyopathy.[11] This distinction is not always made by cardiac catheterization. It is most important to distinguish the two coexistent lesions, since correcting the valvular aortic obstruction may enhance the dynamic subvalvular obstruction. M-mode echocardiographic recognition of idiopathic hypertrophic subaortic stenosis has been reported in combination with discrete subvalvular aortic stenosis, aortic valvular stenosis, and discrete supravalvular stenosis; this modality appears to be the technique of choice in the recognition of the coexistent disorder.

SUPRAVALVULAR AORTIC STENOSIS. Supravalvular aortic stenosis is an uncommon malformation, with heterogenous anatomic features and a high incidence of associated congenital heart defects. In patients with supravalvular aortic stenosis, a reduction in aortic dimension can be observed with a continuous M-mode sweep above the valve. Recently, two-dimensional echocardiography has been shown to be helpful in the differentiation of localized tubular hypoplasia from the discrete membranous form of supraventricular left ventricular outflow obstruction.[107]

Coarctation of the Aorta

Two-dimensional echocardiography, particularly when employing the suprasternal approach, is useful in visualization of the coarcted segment in a majority of patients (Fig. 26–184).[108] The aortic arch with all the branches proximal to the descending aorta can be visualized. The coarcted segment can be recognized as a localized area of narrowing, usually distal to the left subclavian artery figure.[108] Following resection, the normal aortic lumen is apparent.

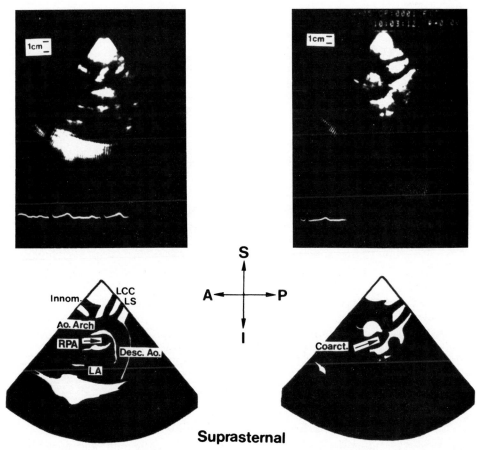

Suprasternal

Figure 26–184. A suprasternal view of the two-dimensional echocardiogram of the aortic arch in a normal subject (left-hand panel) and in a patient with coarctation (right-hand panel). In the normal subject, the aortic arch and its branches are visualized. The narrow segment is clearly visualized on the right-hand panel. Innom = right innominate artery; LCC = left common carotid artery; LS = left subclavian artery; Desc. Ao = descending aorta; Coarct = coarctation. (*From* Kotler, M. N., Mintz, G. S., Segal, B. L., et al.: Clinical uses of echocardiography. Am. J. Cardiol. *45*:1061–1082, 1980. With permission.)

Pulmonary Valve

The M-mode echocardiographic features of pulmonary valve stenosis may be useful in confirming the clinical diagnosis. The characteristic finding is a marked increase in the posterior deflection of the posterior pulmonic leaflet following atrial contraction.[109] The echocardiographic features may be explained by the decreased right ventricular compliance and the forceful right atrial contraction. This results in a high right ventricular end-diastolic pressure, which may exceed the pulmonary artery pressure and cause presystolic opening of the pulmonary valve (Fig. 26–185). M-mode echocardiography may be of limited value in the diagnosis of pulmonary stenosis because of difficulty in recording the pulmonary valve and because an exaggerated "A" wave is a nonspecific finding that can occur in a variety of disorders.[106] In addition, a normal echocardiogram may be recorded in patients with mild valvular pulmonary stenosis. Postoperatively, the pulmonary valve echocardiogram returns to normal, with less apparent increase in the depth of the "A" wave and inability to demonstrate

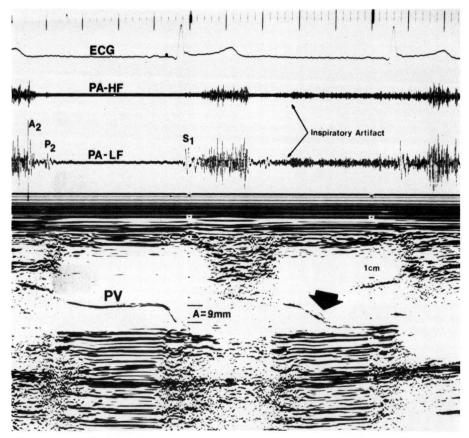

Figure 26–185. Simultaneous electrocardiogram, phonocardiogram, and M-mode echocardiogram in a patient with pulmonic stenosis. Note the large "a" wave of the pulmonary valve echocardiogram measuring 9 mm with presystolic opening during inspiration (dark arrow). The loud crescendo-decrescendo systolic murmur is recorded. PA = pulmonary area; HF = high frequency; LF = low frequency.

presystolic opening of the pulmonary valve. The two-dimensional echocardiographic features of valvular pulmonary stenosis are characterized by systolic doming of the pulmonary leaflet.[113] Normally, the pulmonary leaflets move rapidly apart during systole and remain parallel to the margin of the pulmonary artery. It appears that two-dimensional echocardiography may be more sensitive than M-mode in the diagnosis of valvular pulmonary stenosis[113] and may be useful in the evaluation of postoperative patients who have undergone pulmonary valve commissurotomy.

Mitral Stenosis

The echocardiographic features of mitral stenosis include reduced diastolic closure slope (E-F), thickened mitral leaflet, reduced "A" wave amplitude, and increased systolic closure slope (Fig. 26–186A). Following mitral valve commissurotomy the E-F slope improves, the "A" wave becomes more apparent, and the posterior leaflet motion may on occasion return to normal, although it usually still shows parallel motion to the anterior leaflet (Fig. 26–186B). The left atrium may demonstrate reduction in size following commissurotomy (Fig. 26–186C and D).

The major usefulness of echocardiography in evaluating patients with mitral stenosis has been to demonstrate a reduction in the early diastolic closure slope and the anterior mitral leaflet and anterior motion of the posterior leaflet. Recently, doubt has been cast on the specificity of these two observations.[13] The mitral E-F slope correlates poorly with the calculated mitral valve area.[13] Some investigators have shown that amplitude of closure of the mitral valve correlates better with the severity of mitral stenosis.[98] However, this measurement varies with heart rate and with the diastolic E-F slope.[98] Other investigators demonstrated that the rate of diastolic apposition of the anterior and posterior leaflets may correlate better with mitral valve area.[89] Further investigation into this measurement is needed.

Mitral valve orifice can be evaluated by cross-sectional echocardiography using a cross-sectional plane (Fig. 26–187). Several studies have correlated size of mitral valve

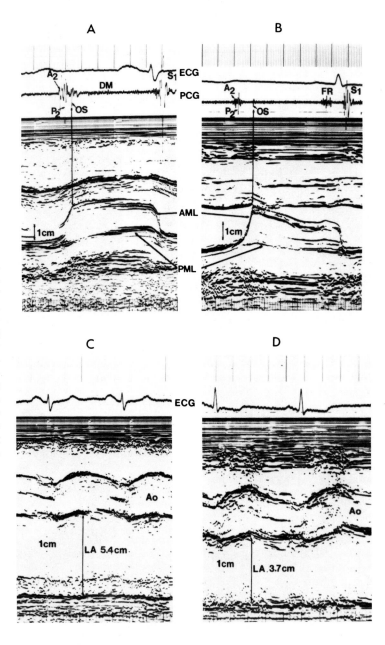

Figure 26–186. *A,* M-mode echocardiogram in a patient with mitral stenosis showing a parallel motion and thickening of both anterior and posterior leaflets (AML and PML). The phonocardiogram records an opening snap coinciding with E-point, and a diastolic murmur is recorded. *B,* Post-commissurotomy, the E-F slope is increased, and normal "A" wave is apparent. Parallel motion of both leaflets is still present. *C,* An enlarged left atrium, pre-commissurotomy. *D,* Reduction in left atrial size post-commissurotomy.

orifice obtained by cross-sectional echocardiography with mitral valve area and the size measured at the time of surgery or calculated from catheterization data.[35, 65, 105] However, there are limitations and pitfalls in evaluating mitral valve area by cross-sectional echocardiography. In some patients, an adequate examination cannot be obtained because of chest wall deformities and emphysema. In addition, the transducer must be aligned so as to locate the smallest valve area separating the atrium and the ventricle. Measurements must be made at the tips of the mitral leaflets. The mitral valve area determination may be inaccurate because of irregularity at the margin of the orifice or because of persistence of line thickness of the video imaging system. In addition, heavy calcification or dense fibrosis of the valve tips may result in spuriously small valve areas, especially if the gain attenuation is markedly increased. Severe calcification of the leaflet produces excessive echo reflection and may cause the leaflets to appear thicker and the mitral valve orifice to appear smaller than its actual size. Lateral-beam resolution problems and image drop-out, particularly in the region of commissures, may be contributing factors in errors in measurement.

In the parasternal longitudinal axis view, two-dimensional echocardiography demonstrates a classic obtuse angle bend of the anterior mitral leaflet during diastole. The tips of the leaflets are held together by thickened chordae, and the posterior leaflet moves minimally. In addition, in about 40 per cent of patients, the midportion of the

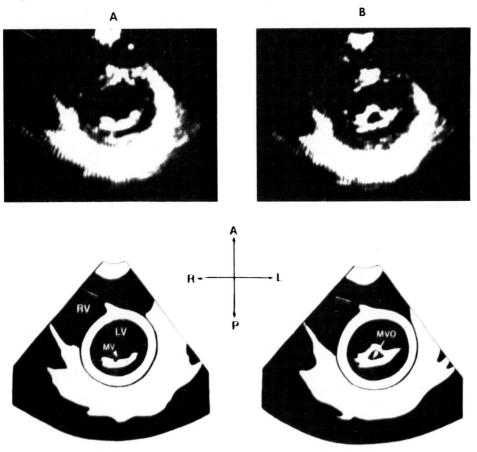

Figure 26–187. A cross-sectional view of a patient with mitral stenosis, during systole (*A*), and during diastole (*B*), showing decreased mitral valve orifice measuring 0.5 cm².

anterior leaflet can be seen to bulge above the level of the mitral ring and into the left atrium during systole.[65] This phenomenon should not be confused with mitral valve prolapse. Two-dimensional evaluation of the mitral valve area has been shown to be useful in following patients after commissurotomy, especially with regard to restenosis.[33]

Mitral Regurgitation

Mitral regurgitation may occur as a result of abnormal function of mitral annulus, mitral valve leaflets, chordae tendineae, papillary muscles, and left ventricular myocardium. In our institution the most common cause of mitral regurgitation is mitral valve prolapse; rheumatic mitral valve insufficiency is second in frequency.[61] Less common causes include ruptured chordae tendineae, papillary muscle dysfunction, mitral annular calcification, cleft mitral valve leaflet, idiopathic hypertrophic subaortic stenosis, and atrial myxoma.

MITRAL VALVE PROLAPSE. Diagnostic M-mode echocardiographic features of mitral valve prolapse include midsystolic buckling or abrupt posterior motion of the posterior mitral leaflet and frequently the anterior leaflet as well (Fig. 26–188A). Pansystolic hammock-like posterior motion of the mitral valve leaflet, with the greatest posterior displacement of the leaflets more than 3 mm from the "C" point, may also be demonstrated. Additional criteria include increased diastolic mitral valve excursion and multiple leaflet echoes recorded during systole. The incidence of mitral valve prolapse has been reported to range between 6 and 12 per cent; however, approximately 10 per cent of patients demonstrating the clinical syndrome may have a negative echocardiogram. Moreover, patterns of holosystolic posterior motion may be recorded in normal subjects, particularly with excessive inferior transducer angulation from a high acoustic window.

The diagnosis of mitral valve prolapse may be enhanced by two-dimensional technique.[29] Two-dimensional echocardiography may also demonstrate precise leaflet prolapse. Characteristic abnormalities are best seen in the parasternal longitudinal view but may also be demonstrated in the apical view. The abnormal leaflets are seen to arch superiorly above the mitral annular ring and into the left atrium. In addition, abnormal leaflet motion has been localized to the body of the leaflets with an intact coaptation point. Further echocardiographic findings include vigorous inferior systolic annular motion and anterior displacement of the coaptation point.

RHEUMATIC MITRAL REGURGITATION. The diagnosis of rheumatic mitral regurgitation cannot always be reliably made by echocardiography. Generally, the amplitude of the mitral valve is increased, and there is an increased E-F slope. The mitral leaflets may be thickened, and the posterior mitral leaflet may parallel the anterior leaflet (Fig. 26–188B). The two-dimensional features of rheumatic mitral regurgitation in the parasternal longitudinal axis view are very similar to those of mitral stenosis. However, in the parasternal cross-sectional view, the mitral valve area is generally larger than in pure stenosis. In addition, failure of closure of small areas of either the medial or the lateral aspect of the valve is associated with minimal regurgitation.[104] In patients with significant mitral regurgitation, failure of both sides of the valve leaflets to close in the center has been reported.[104] Two-dimensional echocardiography may be more precise than cardiac catheterization in determining the mitral valve area in patients with mixed mitral regurgitation and stenosis.

MITRAL ANNULAR CALCIFICATION. Mitral annular calcification can be recognized as a dense band of echoes between the posterior mitral leaflet and left ventricular posterior wall (Fig. 26–188C). Generally, the band of echoes starts at the atrioventricular groove and extends slightly into the body of the left ventricular cavity (Fig. 26–188C). Frequently, there is associated aortic valve sclerosis and aortic root thickening. Two-dimensional echocardiography allows the dense, crescent-shaped area of calcification to be seen in parasternal short-axis views between the posterior leaflet and the

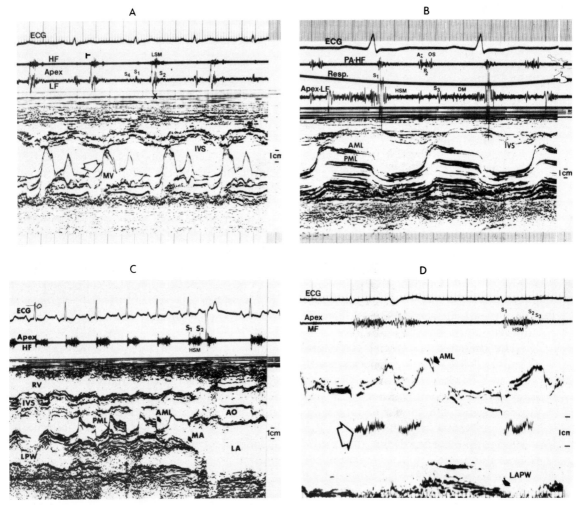

Figure 26–188. *A,* Simultaneous electrocardiogram, phonocardiogram, and M-mode echocardiogram in a patient with typical mitral valve prolapse. Note the systolic clicks (X), with late systolic murmur (LSM). The M-mode echocardiogram shows late systolic motion of the mitral valve leaflet (large arrow). *B,* Simultaneous electrocardiogram, phonocardiogram, and M-mode echocardiogram in a patient with mixed rheumatic mitral valve disease. A typical holosystolic murmur (HSM) in addition to the loud first sound, opening snap, third heart sound, and diastolic murmur is recorded. The mitral anterior and posterior leaflets (AML and PML) are thickened with reduced excursion, and the posterior mitral leaflet parallels the motion of the anterior leaflet. *C,* Simultaneous electrocardiogram, phonocardiogram, and M-mode echocardiogram in an 80-year-old patient with a calcified mitral annulus. A holosystolic murmur at the apex is recorded. A band of echoes extending from the atrioventricular junction at the body of the left ventricle is recorded. The band of echoes lies posterior to the posterior mitral leaflet and anterior to left ventricular posterior wall. The left atrium is enlarged. *D,* Simultaneous electrocardiogram, phonocardiogram, and M-mode echocardiogram in a patient with a flail posterior mitral leaflet. A holosystolic murmur (HSM) and S_3 are recorded. Chaotic systolic (large arrow) and diastolic fluttering of the posterior leaflet and abnormal motion of posterior leaflet during diastole are present.

left ventricular myocardium. A recent study has demonstrated that most calcific deposits occurring in elderly patients are in the submitral region and not in the true annulus.[16] Two-dimensional echocardiography appears to be more precise than M-mode echocardiography in accurately localizing the area of calcific deposit.

RUPTURED CHORDAE TENDINEAE. M-mode criteria of flail leaflet include systolic left atrial echoes, systolic mitral valve flutter, diastolic mitral valve flutter, and chaotic paradoxical diastolic leaflet motion (Fig. 26–188D). There is vigorous contraction of the septum and the posterior left ventricular wall. In addition, the left atrium may be minimally enlarged or normal-sized. The sensitivity of M-mode echocardiography in the diagnosis of flail anterior or posterior leaflet is generally about 60 per cent in our institution. However, the sensitivity of two-dimensional echocardiography has been reported to be as high as 90 per cent. The two-dimensional echocardiographic criteria include motion of the affected leaflet beyond the tip of the line of the mitral valve closure.[62] Two-dimensional echocardiography affords precise identification with regard to which leaflet is flail.

PAPILLARY MUSCLE DYSFUNCTION. Generally, the posteromedial papillary muscle is involved to a greater extent than the anterolateral in ischemic heart disease. Two-dimensional echocardiography can reliably discern diffuse or segmental wall motion abnormalities,[66] and on the parasternal short axis view, akinesis or hypokinesis of the affected papillary muscle may be detected (Fig. 26–189).

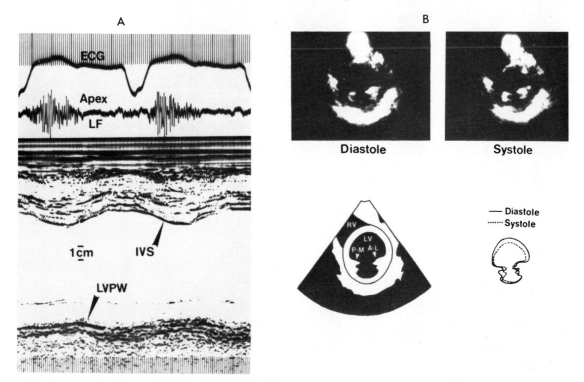

Figure 26–189. A, Simultaneous electrocardiogram, phonocardiogram, and M-mode echocardiogram in a patient with papillary muscle dysfunction. An enlarged left ventricle with marked hypokinesis of the left ventricular wall is demonstrated. A crescendo-decrescendo systolic murmur is recorded. B, A two-dimensional echocardiogram from a patient with significant papillary muscle dysfunction and infero-medial and lateral wall hypokinesis second to severe coronary disease. On cross section, both papillary muscles are dense and sclerotic, and there is virtually no movement of both papillary muscles. In addition, hypokinesis of the medial portion of the septum, inferior wall, and lateral wall is present. Movements of the left ventricular wall during systole (dotted lines) as compared with diastole (closed line) are demonstrated.

Cardiac Masses

Although there have been isolated reports[43, 92, 117] describing the usefulness of M-mode echocardiography in the diagnosis of cardiac tumors and left atrial and left ventricular thrombi, two-dimensional echocardiography appears to be superior in detecting intracardiac tumors and thrombi.[18, 70, 85] The apical view appears to be most useful in detecting left ventricular and left atrial thrombi. In two cases (Fig. 26–190), M-mode echocardiography could not detect the ventricular or the left atrial thrombus. The precise location of the mass, mobility, and point of attachment can be assessed by two-dimensional echocardiography. M-mode echocardiography allows identification of an atrial myxoma and can be helpful in the long-term postoperative evaluation of these patients (Fig. 26–191). However, the demonstration of a left atrial myxoma by M-mode techniques may not always be precise. Intracavitary echoes recorded within the left atrium may not always be due to myxoma but may be artifactual.[41] Two-dimensional echocardiography makes this distinction. Because myxomas may recur in the late postoperative period, echocardiography is an excellent technique for following such patients.

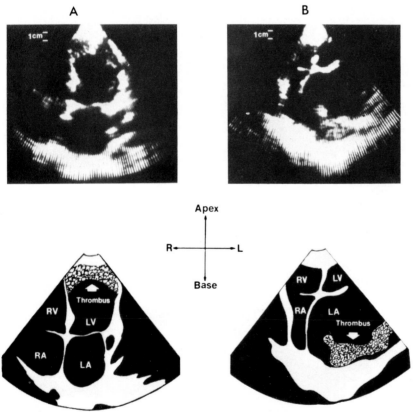

Figure 26–190. *A,* An apical view of a two-dimensional echocardiogram of the left ventricle. A large apical thrombus and an anteroapical aneurysm is visualized. *B,* An apical view of a two-dimensional echocardiogram in a patient with rheumatic mitral valve disease and enlarged left atrium. A large left atrial thrombus attached to the posterior left atrial wall is evident. The thrombus was not detected by M-mode echocardiography. The large left atrial thrombus was confirmed at surgery. (*From* Kotler, M. N., Mintz, G. S., Segal, B. L., et al.: Clinical uses of echocardiography. Am. J. Cardiol. 45:1061–1082, 1980. With permission.)

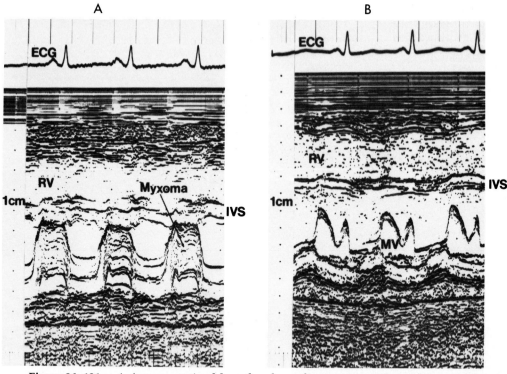

Figure 26–191. *A,* A preoperative M-mode echocardiogram in a patient with an atrial myxoma. A dense cloud of echoes is recorded behind the posterior mitral leaflet, separated from the mitral valve by a clear space. *B,* Same patient after resection of the myxoma. A normalized pattern of mitral valve movement is seen.

Ischemic Heart Disease

M-mode echocardiography may discern the indirect consequences of coronary artery disease, which include segmental areas of abnormal wall motion,[14] left ventricular dilatation, and myocardial scarring (Fig. 26–192).[73] Scarring is classically recognized as increased wall density, decreased motion, and reduced thickness usually measuring 7 mm or less. Unfortunately, M-mode echocardiography produces a limited "ice pick" view of the heart, and only large areas of asynergy may be detected. Two-dimensional echocardiographic scanning can yield more reliable information with regard to wall motion abnormalities[39] and ventricular aneurysms (Fig. 26–193).[114] Most patients with apical aneurysms demonstrate an abrupt bulge and a shelflike separation from the normal left ventricular myocardium. In addition, thrombi may be detected within the aneurysm.[18] Two-dimensional echocardiography can reliably identify a pseudoaneurysm[10] and differentiate a pseudoaneurysm from a true aneurysm. Following surgery and resection of a large aneurysm, reduction in heart size and disappearance of the bulge may be evident.

M-mode and two-dimensional echocardiography have been useful in differentiating cardiomyopathy from coronary artery disease. In cardiomyopathy, left ventricular dilatation and diffuse hypokinesis are present, in contrast to the segmental wall abnormality of coronary artery disease. In addition, echocardiography may be helpful in diagnosing other causes of chest pain syndrome, such as aortic stenosis, idiopathic hypertrophic subaortic stenosis, pericarditis, and mitral valve prolapse. Preliminary

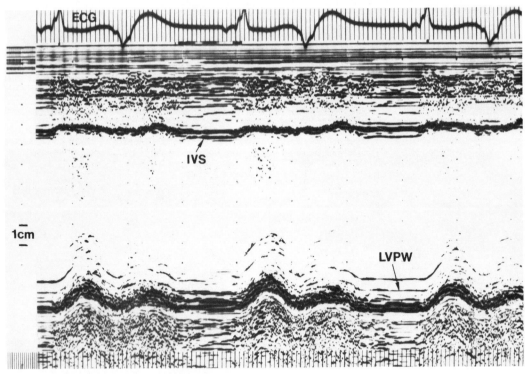

Figure 26–192. M-mode echocardiogram through the body of the left ventricle below the tips of the mitral leaflet. Septal scarring is evident by recording dense echoes of 6 mm. thickness as well as failure of the septum to thicken during systole. In addition, the left ventricle is grossly enlarged.

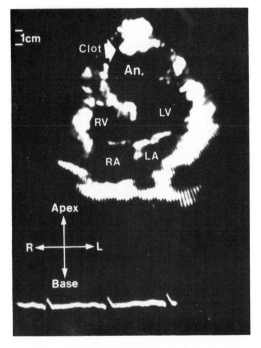

Figure 26–193. An apical view of a two-dimensional echocardiogram in a patient with a large anteroapical aneurysm secondary to left anterior descending coronary artery occlusion. In this systolic frame a large aneurysmal bulge is evident. In addition, dense echo-producing material in the apex is recorded, consistent with the presence of a clot. An = aneurysm. (*From* Kotler, M. N., Mintz, G. S., Segal, B. L., et al.: Clinical uses of echocardiography. Am. J. Cardiol. *45*:1061–1082, 1980. With permission.)

studies have now demonstrated that two-dimensional echocardiography may be useful in assessing regional cardiac dilatation[20] and prognosis after acute myocardial infarction[75] as well as in detecting left main coronary artery stenosis[110] and predicting the operability of patients with ventricular aneurysms.[2] Further studies are needed to confirm these initial exciting reports.

Endocarditis

M-mode echocardiography can detect vegetations in approximately one third of patients with proven diagnosed bacterial endocarditis.[103] Generally, the M-mode echocardiographic features include thickening of the valve and a shaggy appearance caused by the vegetation. It is estimated that M-mode technique detects only vegetations larger than 5 mm. In addition, M-mode echocardiography may visualize only limited areas of valvular and annular surfaces. Two-dimensional features of bacterial endocarditis and valvular vegetations have been reported.[28, 60] These lesions appear as rapidly oscillating masses that either are attached to or have replaced normal valve tissue. Masses can be localized in an individual leaflet, and the size and mobility of the lesions can be readily assessed. Although two-dimensional and M-mode echocardiography have comparable success in the detection of vegetations of the mitral and aortic valves, the former is more reliable in discerning complications of endocarditis, such as a flail leaflet, aortic root abscess, or ruptured sinus of Valsalva aneurysm.[60] Tricuspid valve vegetations may also be more readily identified by two-dimensional echocardiography.

Aortic Aneurysms

While the M-mode echocardiographic features of dissection of the ascending aorta have been described, frequent false positive results are obtained.[6] The entire ascending aorta cannot always be visualized by M-mode techniques, and for this reason two-dimensional echocardiography appears to be superior for the detection of aneurysms of the ascending aorta.[17] Two-dimensional echocardiographic features include excessive bulging and enlargement as well as demonstration of a spiral aortic tear separating the true lumen and the false lumen (Fig. 26–194).[17] The course of the descending thoracic aorta can be mapped using the parasternal long-axis and short-axis views.[63] In addition, the intimal flap separating a true from a false lumen has been reported in patients with type 3 dissection.

Congenital Heart Lesions

ATRIAL SEPTAL DEFECT. Although M-mode echocardiography is useful in detecting right ventricular volume overload (increased right ventricular dimension and abnormal septal motion), it is by no means specific for diagnosing atrial septal defects (Fig. 26–195A). This nonspecific finding of right ventricular volume overload is classically caused by atrial septal defects but can also be seen in patients with total or partial anomalous pulmonary venous return, pulmonary regurgitation, or tricuspid regurgitation. In addition, patients with a large left-to-right shunt may show early diastolic fluttering of the tricuspid valve. Postoperatively, the right ventricular cavity may be decreased in size and septal motion returned to normal (Fig. 26–195B). In secundum

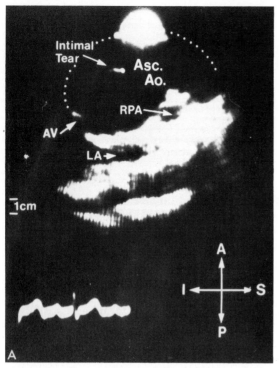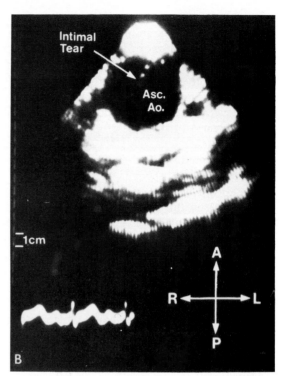

Figure 26–194. *A,* A long-axis view of the ascending aorta in a patient with a large aneurysm of the ascending aorta secondary to dissection. The dotted line represents the extent of the aneurysm, and the intimal tear is depicted by the white arrow. The transducer in this position was placed in the second right intercostal space, and therefore the right pulmonary artery (RPA) and left atrium are evident. The aortic valve below the aneurysm is seen. AV = aortic valve. *B,* A cross-sectional view of the same patient taken in the second right intercostal space showing the enlarged circular saccular aneurysm with the intimal tear (white arrow).

type atrial septal defect, there is normal anterior mitral leaflet attachment and continuity, with preservation of the posterior border of the aortic root. Mitral valve prolapse is commonly associated in patients with secundum defects. In some patients, total anomalous pulmonary venous drainage may be suspected from the presence of an echo-free space posterior to the left atrial wall or an abnormally small left atrial dimension. Patients with primum atrial septal defect have abnormal attachments of the mitral valve to the septum. The left ventricular outflow tract is narrowed, and there is prolonged diastolic apposition of the mitral valve against the septum.

In patients with atrial septal defects, two-dimensional echocardiography is particularly useful.[51, 115] In some patients with an ostium primum defect, the cleft mitral valve leaflet may be clearly visualized in the cross-sectional view.[51] The subcostal approach has been particularly useful in delineating the atrial septal defect. Use of contrast injection of indocyanine green dye has enhanced the diagnosis of atrial septal defect. In some patients, minimal amounts of contrast cross the defect from the right to the left atrium. In others, a contrast echo-free area can appear in the right atrium at the site of the atrial septal defect (Fig. 26–196). This negative contrast shadow occurs as a result of the blood flow from the left to right atrium washing out the effect of dye that was present in the right atrium. With the use of two-dimensional echocardiography and contrast techniques, residual shunts may be demonstrated in the postoperative period.

PATENT DUCTUS ARTERIOSUS. In infants with patent ductus arteriosus, the left atrium is enlarged and the ratio of left atrial diameter to aortic diameter (LA/Ao) is

A   B

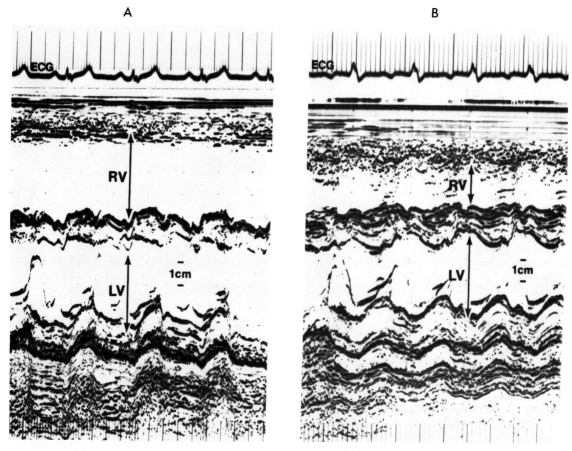

Figure 26–195. *A,* An M-mode echocardiogram in a patient with an ostium secundum atrial septal defect showing a large right ventricle and abnormal septal motion. *B,* A postoperative echocardiogram of the same patient two weeks following surgical closure of the interatrial septal defect. The right ventricle is considerably reduced in size, and normalization of septal motion has occurred. A small echo-free space behind the left ventricular posterior wall is compatible with a small pericardial effusion.

greater than 1:3.[90] Serial determinations of both the LA/Ao ratio and the estimate of circumferential fiber shortening can be used to assess the magnitude of the left-to-right shunt and the response to therapy.[90] Unfortunately, an elevated LA/Ao ratio is not specific for the diagnosis of patent ductus arteriosus. An abnormal ratio may be found in infants with congestive heart failure and a left-to-right shunt of other causes. Following ligation of the ductus arteriosus, the left atrial size returns to normal and the LA/Ao ratio falls below 1:3.[90] The patent ductus arteriosus has been visualized by two-dimensional echocardiography, which represents an important and exciting approach to the evaluation of patients with this disorder.[76]

VENTRICULAR SEPTAL DEFECT. Visualization of the usual isolated ventricular septal defect (VSD) by M-mode echocardiography is unrealiable. The standard M-mode echocardiogram of patients with an uncomplicated small ventricular septal defect is normal, whereas a ventricular septal defect of moderate size with a large left-to-right shunt may enlarge both ventricles and the left atrium. With M-mode echocardiography, septal "drop-out" may occur because the transducer beam may not be directed at right angles to the septum. When the interventricular septum appears to be absent echocardiographically, single ventricle,[24] complete atrioventricular canal, corrected transposi-

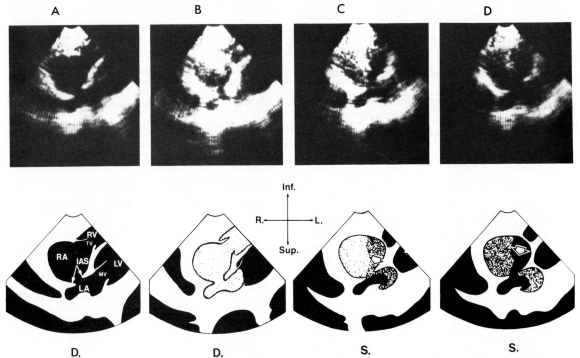

Figure 26–196. A subxiphoid two-dimensional echocardiogram in a patient with an atrial septal defect. *A,* An enlarged right atrium and an absent distal interatrial septum. *B,* Indocyanine green dye is injected and shows evidence of microcavitation, with echo densities filling the entire right and left atria. *C* and *D,* Wash-out effect of unopacified blood from the left atrium into the right atrium produces the so-called negative-contrast effect shown as the dark space (white arrow) in the idealized diagram.

tion of the great arteries,[23] and a straddling tricuspid valve[45] must be differentiated from a large ventricular septal defect.

The size of the left atrium has been found to be useful in distinguishing patients with ventricular septal defects and hemodynamically significant shunts from those with inconsequential shunts.[49, 78] M-mode echocardiographic visualization of aneurysms of the membranous septum causing obstruction of the ventricular septal defect has been reported.[79] Two-dimensional echocardiography has been reported to be useful in visualizing the size and location of an isolated ventricular septal defect.[87] In one study, the majority of isolated anterior ventricular septal defects could be visualized in the parasternal long-axis view or in intermediate views between the long-axis view of the left ventricle and the long-axis view of the right ventricle.[87] In the apical four-chambered view, posterior ventricular septal defects could be located.[87] In parasternal cross-sectional views, which included simultaneous visualization of the pulmonic valve and the mitral valve, the detection of subpulmonic ventricular septal defects could be accomplished.[87] In only 3 out of 25 patients was the ventricular septal defect unable to be visualized. Generally, when the ventricular septal defect is less than 5 mm or when the left-to-right shunt is less than 20 per cent, visualization is unlikely.[87]

COMPLETE ATRIOVENTRICULAR CANAL. Several definitive M-mode echocardiographic patterns can be identified as specific diagnostic features of complete atrioventricular canal.[116] These patterns vary with leaflet morphology and transducer position.[116] All three variations can be recorded in the same patient, depending on transducer position and angulation.[41]

In the most common pattern, separate mitral and tricuspid portions can be seen

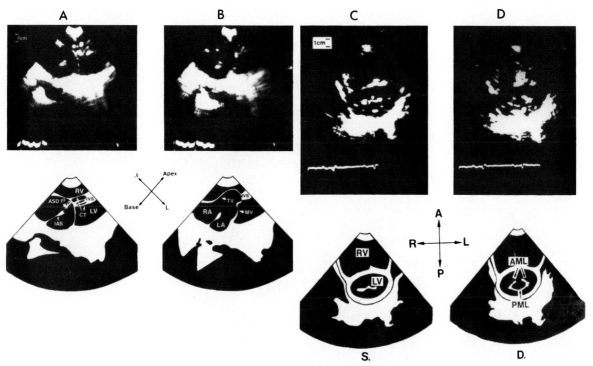

Figure 26–197. *A* and *B*, An apical view of a two-dimensional echocardiogram in a patient with a complete endocardial cushion defect (type 1A Rastelli). A common attached atrioventricular valve that is septally attached and appears to be divided during diastole is demonstrated. *C* and *D*, Systolic and diastolic frames in a patient with a partial endocardial cushion defect and cleft mitral valve. The cleft mitral valve ("drawbridge sign") during diastole is clearly evident (two large black arrows).

without an intervening septum.[116] In patients with a common undivided leaflet, a single atrioventricular valve can be seen to move from a posterior position within the left ventricular cavity to the anterior heart border across the interventricular septum.[116] In the third pattern, one leaflet opens anteriorly in diastole into the right ventricle and the other posteriorly into the left ventricle.[116] Two-dimensional echocardiography allows precise and accurate anatomic detail in patients with atrioventricular canal defects.[53] With the use of the apical view, differentiation between types A, B, and C of complete atrioventricular canal defects can be accomplished. The apical view also allows differentiation of divided and undivided and attached and free-floating common anterior valve leaflets (Fig. 26–197A).[32] In addition, a cleft in the anterior mitral leaflet can be demonstrated in the short-axis view (Fig. 26–197B).

TETRALOGY OF FALLOT. The echocardiographic spectrum in tetralogy of Fallot, truncus arteriosus, and pulmonary atresia with associated ventricular septal defect has been well described and includes:[12, 64, 94] (1) a large single systemic arterial trunk overriding the ventricular septum, (2) mitral semilunar continuity, (3) increased right ventricular dimension, and (4) normal septal motion but invariably increased septal thickness.

Figure 26–198A shows a preoperative echocardiogram in a patient with tetralogy of Fallot, and Figure 26–198B shows a postoperative patient with tetralogy of Fallot. In these patients, continuity of the anterior wall of the systemic arterial trunk and the ventricular septum was re-established by an identifiable prosthetic material. Displacement of the arterial trunk over the septum is still present in these patients postoperatively. Visualization of the pulmonary valve helps differentiate tetralogy of Fallot from truncus

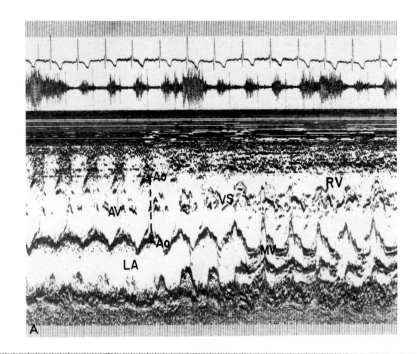

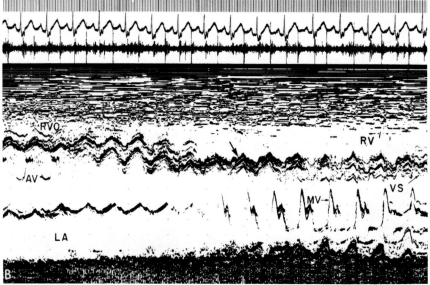

Figure 26–198. *A,* A four-year-old boy with tetralogy of Fallot. The M-mode echocardiogram scan is from the aortic valve to the base of the heart. The echocardiogram reveals a large aortic root (Ao) and aortic valve (AV) overriding the ventricular septum (VS). MV = mitral valve; RV = right ventricle. *B,* A 25-year-old woman after repair of tetralogy of Fallot. The echocardiographic scan from the aorta to the base of the heart reveals continuity of aortic root with the ventricular septum (VS). Note that the continuity is established by a septal patch, which appears as a dense intervening echo (arrow). Also note that the echocardiographic aortic ventricular septal override can still be appreciated. RVO = right ventricular outflow; LA = left atrium; AV = aortic valve; MV = mitral valve; RV = right ventricle. (*In* Kotler, M., and Segal, B. (Eds.): Clinical Echocardiography. *From* Seward, J. B., and Tajik, A. J.: Cyanotic congenital heart disease. Philadelphia, F. A. Davis Company, 1978. Reproduced by permission.)

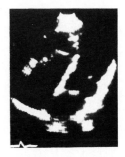

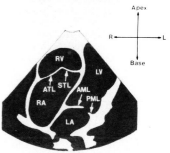

Figure 26–199. Four-chamber or apical view of two-dimensional echocardiogram in a patient with proven Ebstein's anomaly of the tricuspid valve. The inferior displacement of the tricuspid valve in relation to the mitral valve is visualized. The right ventricle is reduced in size; an enlarged right atrium or atrialized right ventricle is also demonstrated. ATL = anterior tricuspid valve leaflet; STL = septal tricuspid valve leaflet.

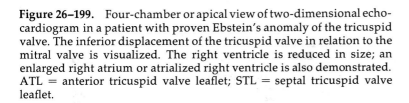

arteriosus and pulmonary atresia.[12] However, this is not always possible by M-mode echocardiography. Recently, two-dimentional echocardiography has been found useful in the pre- and postoperative patient with tetralogy of Fallot.[8] The pulmonary valve was recorded in 90 per cent of patients by two-dimensional echocardiography, whereas it was recorded in only 26 per cent by M-mode.[8] The ventricular septal defect was detected in 95 per cent of patients with tetralogy of Fallot by two-dimensional echocardiography but in only 76 per cent of patients by M-mode echocardiography.[8] Two-dimensional echocardiography reliably predicted the size of the right ventricular outflow tract both pre- and postoperatively.[8]

EBSTEIN'S ANOMALY OF THE TRICUSPID VALVE. The M-mode echocardiographic features of Ebstein's anomaly have been well described.[42, 53] They usually include delayed closure of the tricuspid valve, and a varying tricuspid valve (E-F slope). Additional features include a large atrialized portion of the right ventricle and abnormal septal motion. On occasion, M-mode echocardiography may be nondiagnostic in patients with Ebstein's anomaly, since precise tricuspid and mitral valve closure cannot always be observed simultaneously. Two-dimensional echocardiography using the apical view can detect inferior tricuspid displacement in relation to the mitral valve insertion (Fig. 26–199).[71] The marked inferior displacement of the tricuspid leaflet, with a small right ventricular cavity and a huge atrialized right ventricle, is characteristic of Ebstein's anomaly of the tricuspid valve (Fig. 26–199). In addition, associated tricuspid regurgitation and a right-to-left shunt can be detected by the use of contrast echocardiography. No systematic two-dimensional echocardiographic study has been performed on the postoperative evaluation of patients with Ebstein's anomaly of the tricuspid valve.

References

1. Aziz, K. U., VanGrondelle, A., and Paul, M. H.: Echocardiographic assessment of the relation between left ventricular wall and cavity dimensions and peak systolic pressure in children with aortic stenosis. Am. J. Cardiol. *40*:775–780, 1977.

2. Barrett, M., Charuzi, Y., Davidson, R., et al.: Assessment of left ventricular function in the presence of aneurysm by cross-sectional echocardiography. Circulation 58 (II): 189, 1978 (Abstract).

3. Bennet, D. H., Evans, D. W., and Raj, M. V. J.: Echocardiographic left ventricular dimensions in pressure and volume overload. Their use in assessing aortic stenosis. Br. Heart J. 37:971–977, 1975.

4. Bom, M., Lancee, C. T., vanZwieten, G., et al.: Multiscan echocardiography I. Technical description. Circulation 48:1066–1074, 1973.

5. Brodie, B. R., Grossman, W., and McClaurin, L.: Diagnosis of prosthetic mitral valve malfunction with combined echo-phonocardiography. Circulation 53:93–100, 1976.

6. Brown, O. R., Popp, R. L., and Kloster, F. E.: Echocardiographic criteria for aortic root dissection. Am. J. Cardiol. 36:17–20, 1975.

7. Burggraf, G. W., and Craige, E.: Echocardiographic studies of left ventricular wall motion and dimensions after valvular heart surgery. Am. J. Cardiol. 35:473–480, 1975.

8. Caldwell, R. L., Weyman, A. E., Hurwitz, R. A., et al.: Right ventricular outflow tract assessment by cross-sectional echocardiography in tetralogy of Fallot. Circulation 59:395–402, 1979.

9. Carr, K. W., Engler, R. L., Forsythe, J. R., et al.: Measurement of left ventricular ejection fraction by mechanical cross-sectional echocardiography. Circulation 59:1196–1206, 1979.

10. Catherwood, E., Mintz, G. S., Kotler, M. N., et al.: Pseudoaneurysm of the left ventricle complicated by Salmonella typhimurium infection: recognition by two-dimensional echocardiography. Am. J. Med. 68:782–786, 1980.

11. Chung, K. J., Alexson, C. G., Manning, J. A., et al.: Echocardiography in truncus arteriosus — the value of pulmonic valve detection. Circulation 48:281–286, 1973.

12. Chung, K. J., Gramiak, R., and Manning, J. A.: Echocardiographic diagnosis of hypertrophic obstructive cardiomyopathy coexisting with fixed left ventricular outflow obstruction in children. Circulation 48 (Suppl. IV):126, 1973 (Abstract).

13. Cope, G. D., Kisslo, J. A., Johnson, M. L., et al.: A reassessment of the echocardiogram in mitral stenosis. Circulation 52:664–670, 1975.

14. Corya, B. C., Rasmussen, S., Feigenbaum, H., et al.: Systolic thickening and thinning of the septum and posterior wall in patients with coronary artery disease, congestive cardiomyopathy and atrial septal defect. Circulation 55:109–114, 1977.

15. Davidson, R., Charuzi, Y., Davidson, S., et al.: Differentiation between localized and diffuse left ventricular dysfunction of two-dimensional echocardiography. Circulation 56 (Suppl. III):152, 1977 (Abstract).

16. D'Cruz, I., Panetia, F., Cohen, H., et al.: Submitral calcification or sclerosis in elderly patients: M-mode and two-dimensional echocardiography in mitral annulus calcification. Am. J. Cardiol. 44:31–38, 1979.

17. DeMaria, A. N., Bommer, W., Neumann, A., et al.: Identification and localization of aneurysms of the ascending aorta by cross-sectional echocardiography. Circulation 59:755–761, 1979.

18. DeMaria, A. N., Neumann, A., Bommer, W., et al.: Left ventricular thrombi identified by cross-sectional echocardiography. Ann. Intern. Med. 90:14–18, 1979.

19. Dodge, H. T., Sandler, H., Ballow, D. W.: Use of biplane angiography for the measurement of left ventricular volume in man. Am. Heart J. 60:762–776, 1960.

20. Eaton, L. W., Weiss, J. L., Bulkley, B. H., et al.: Regional cardiac dilatation after acute myocardial infarction. N. Engl. J. Med. 300:57–62, 1979.

21. Feigenbaum, H.: Echocardiography. Ed. 2. Philadelphia, Lea & Febiger, 1976, p. 79.

22. Feigenbaum, H., Corya, B. C., Dillon, J. C., et al.: Role of echocardiography in patients with coronary artery disease. Am. J. Cardiol. 37:775–786, 1976.

23. Felner, J. M.: Echocardiography: a cyanotic congenital heart lesion. In Kotler, M. N., and Segal, B. L., (eds.): Clinical Echocardiography. Philadelphia, F. A. Davis Company, 1978, pp. 251–267.

24. Felner, J. M., Brewer, D. B., and Franch, R. H.: Echocardiographic manifestations of single ventricle. Am. J. Cardiol. 38:80–84, 1976.

25. Fortuin, N. J., Hood, W. P., and Sherman, M. E.: Determination of left ventricular volumes by ultrasound. Circulation 44:575–584, 1971.

26. Fowles, R. E., Martin, R. P., Abrams, J. M., et al.: Two-dimensional echocardiographic features of bicuspid aortic valve. Chest 75:434–440, 1979.

27. Gibson, D. G., and Brown, D. J.: Continuous assessment of left ventricular shape in man. Br. Heart J. 37:904–910, 1975.

28. Gilbert, B. W., Haney, R. S., Crawford, F., et al.: Two-dimensional echocardiographic assessment of vegetative endocarditis. Circulation 55:346–353, 1977.

29. Gilbert, B. W., Schatz, R. A., vonRamm, O. T., et al.: Mitral valve prolapse. Two-dimensional echocardiographic and angiographic correlation. Circulation 54:716–723, 1976.

30. Gramiak, R., Shah, P. M., and Kramer, D. H.: Ultrasound cardiography: contrast studies in anatomy and function. Radiology 92:939–948, 1969.

31. Griffith, J. M., and Henry, W.: A sector scanner for real-time two-dimensional echocardiography. Circulation 49:1147–1152, 1974.

32. Hagler, D. J., Tajik, A. J., Seward, J. B., et al.: Real-time wide-angle sector echocardiography: atrioventricular canal defects. Circulation 59:140–150, 1979.

33. Heger, J. J., Wann, L. S., Weyman, A. E., et al.: Long-term changes in mitral valve area after successful commissurotomy. Circulation 59:443–448, 1979.

34. Henry, W. L., and Clark, C. E.: Asymmetric septal hypertrophy: echocardiographic identification of the pathognomonic anatomic abnormality of IHSS. Circulation *47*:225–233, 1973.
35. Henry, W. L., Griffith, J. M., Michaelis, L. L., et al.: Measurement of mitral orifice in patients with mitral valve disease by real-time two-dimensional echocardiography. Circulation *57*:827–831, 1975.
36. Horowitz, M. S., Tecklenberg, P. L., Goodman, D. J., et al.: Echocardiographic evaluation of the stent mounted aortic bioprosthetic valve in the mitral position. In vitro and in vivo studies. Circulation *54*:91–96, 1976.
37. Karliner, J. S.: Clinical reliability of determining left ventricular function by echocardiography. *In* Kotler, M. N., and Segal, B. L. (eds.): Clinical Echocardiography. Ed. 1. Philadelphia, F. A. Davis Company, 1978, p. 151.
38. Kerber, R., and Doty, D.: Abnormalities of interventricular septal motion following cardiac surgery. Cross-sectional echocardiographic studies. Am. J. Cardiol. *41*:372, 1978 (Abstract).
39. Kisslo, J. A., Robertson, D., Gilbert, B. W., et al.: A comparison of real-time, two-dimensional echocardiography and cineangiography in detecting left ventricular asynergy. Circulation *55*:134–141, 1977.
40. Kisslo, J., vonRamm, O. T., and Thurstone, F. L.: Cardiac imaging using a phased-array ultrasound II clinical techniques and application. Circulation *53*:262–267, 1976.
41. Kotler, M. N., Segal, B. L., Mintz, G. S., et al.: Pitfalls and limitations of M-mode echocardiography. Am. Heart J. *94*:227–249, 1977.
42. Kotler, M. N., and Tabatznik, B.: Recognition of Ebstein's anomaly by ultrasound technique. Circulation *44* (Suppl. 2):34, 1971 (Abstract).
43. Kramer, N. E., Rathod, R., Chawla, K. K., et al.: Echocardiographic diagnosis of left ventricular mural thrombi occurring in cardiomyopathy. Am. Heart J. *96*:381–383, 1978.
44. Krueger, S. K., French, J. W., Forker, A. D., et al.: Echocardiography in discrete subaortic stenosis. Circulation *59*:506–512, 1979.
45. LaCorte, M. A., Fellows, K. E., and Williams, R. G.: Overriding tricuspid valve: Echocardiographic and angiographic features. Am. J. Cardiol. *37*:911–919, 1976.
46. Lange, L. W., Sahn, D. J., Allen, H. D., et al.: Subxiphoid cross-sectional echocardiography in infants and children with congenital heart disease. Circulation *59*:513–524, 1979.
47. Lemire, F., Tajik, A. J., Guiliami, E. R., et al.: Further echocardiographic observations in pericardial effusion. Mayo Clin. Proc. *51*:13–18, 1976.
48. Lew, L. V., Henning, H., Schelbert, H., et al.: Assessment of mitral valve E-point septal separation as an index of left ventricular performance in patients with acute and previous myocardial infarction. Am. J. Cardiol. *41*:836–845, 1978.
49. Lewis, A. B., and Takahashi, M.: Echocardiographic assessment of left-to-right-shunt volume in children with ventricular septal defect. Circulation *54*:78–82, 1976.
50. Lieppe, W., Behar, V. S., Scallion, R., et al.: Detection of tricuspid regurgitation with two-dimensional echocardiography and peripheral vein injections. Circulation *57*:128–132, 1978.
51. Lieppe, W., Scallion, R., Behar, V. S., et al.: Two-dimensional echocardiographic findings in atrial septal defect. Circulation *56*:447–456, 1977.
52. Linhart, J. W., Mintz, G. S., Segal, B. L., et al.: Left ventricular volume measurements by echocardiography. Fact or fiction? Am. J. Cardiol. *36*:114–118, 1975.
53. Lündstrom, N. R.: Echocardiography in the diagnosis of Ebstein's anomaly of the tricuspid valve. Circulation *47*:597–605, 1973.
54. Martin, R. P., Rakowski, H., French, J., et al.: Idiopathic hypertrophic subaortic stenosis viewed by wide-angle, phased-array echocardiography. Circulation *59*:1206–1217, 1979.
55. Martin, R. P., Rakowski, H., French, J., et al.: Localization of pericardial effusion with wide angle phased-array echocardiography. Am. J. Cardiol. *42*:904–916, 1978.
56. Mason, S. J., and Fortuin, N. J.: The use of echocardiography for quantitative evaluation of left ventricular function. Prog. Cardiovasc. Dis. *21*:119–132, 1978.
57. Massie, B. M., Schiller, N. B., Ratshin, R. A., et al.: Mitral-septal separation: a new echocardiographic index of left ventricular function. Am. J. Cardiol. *39*:1008–1016, 1977.
58. Matsumoto, M., Oka, Y., Lin, Y. T., et al.: Transesophageal echocardiography for assessing ventricular function. N.Y. State J. Med. *79*:19–21, 1979.
59. Matsumoto, M., Oka, Y., Strom, J., et al.: The application of transesophageal echocardiography for continuous intraoperative monitoring of left ventricular performance. Am. J. Cardiol., in press.
60. Mintz, G. S., Kotler, M. N., Segal, B. L., et al.: A comparison of two-dimensional and M-mode echocardiography in the evaluation of patients with infective endocarditis. Am. J. Cardiol. *43*:738–744, 1979.
61. Mintz, G. S., Kotler, M. N., Segal, B. L., et al.: Two-dimensional echocardiographic evaluation of patients with mitral insufficiency. Am. J. Cardiol. *44*:670–678, 1979.
62. Mintz, G. S., Kotler, M. N., Segal, B. L., et al.: Two-dimensional echocardiographic recognition of ruptured chordae tendineae. Circulation *57*:244–250, 1978.
63. Mintz, G. S., Kotler, M. N., Segal, B. L., et al.: Two-dimensional echocardiographic recognition of the descending aorta. Am. J. Cardiol. *44*:232–238, 1979.
64. Morris, D. C., Felner, J. M., Schlant, R. C., et al.: Echocardiographic diagnosis of tetralogy of Fallot. Am. J. Cardiol. *36*:908–913, 1975.

65. Nichol, P. M., Gilbert, B. W., and Kisslo, J. A.: Two-dimensional echocardiographic assessment of mitral stenosis. Circulation 55:120–128, 1977.

66. Ogawa, S., Hubbard, F. E., Mardelli, T. J., et al.: Cross-sectional echocardiographic spectrum of papillary muscle dysfunction. Am. Heart J 97:312–321, 1979.

67. Pombo, J. F., Troy, B. L., and Russel, R. O., Jr.: Left ventricular volumes and ejection fraction by echocardiography. Circulation 43:480–490, 1971.

68. Popp, R. L.: Echocardiographic assessment of cardiac disease. Circulation 54:538–552, 1976.

69. Popp, R. L., and Harrison, D. C.: Ultrasonic cardiac echocardiography for determining stroke volume and valvular regurgitation. Circulation 41:493–502, 1970.

70. Ports, T. A., Cogan, J., Schiller, N. B., et al.: Echocardiography of left ventricular masses. Circulation 58:528–536, 1978.

71. Ports, T. A., Silverman, N. H., and Schiller, N. B.: Two-dimensional echocardiographic assessment of Ebstein's anomaly. Circulation 58:336–343, 1978.

72. Radford, D. J., Bloom, K. R., Izukawa, T., et al.: Echocardiographic assessment of bicuspid aortic valves. Circulation 53:80–85, 1976.

73. Rasmussen, S., Corya, B. C., Feigenbaum, H., et al.: Detection of myocardial scar tissue by M-mode echocardiography. Circulation 57:230–237, 1978.

74. Roelandt, J., Van Dorp, W. C., and Bom, M.: Resolution problems in echocardiography: a source of interpretation error. Am. J. Cardiol. 37:256–262, 1976.

75. Rogers, E. W., Weyman, A. E., Feigenbaum, H., et al.: Predicting survival after myocardial infarction by cross-sectional echocardiography. Circulation 58 (II):907, 1978.

76. Sahn, D. J., and Allen, H. D.: Real-time cross-sectional echocardiographic imaging and measurement of the patent ductus arteriosus in infants and children. Circulation 58:343–354, 1978.

77. Sahn, D. J., DeMaria, A., Kisslo, J., et al.: The committee of M-mode standardization of the American Society of Echocardiography: recommendations regarding quantitation in M-mode echocardiography: results of a survey of echocardiographic measurements. Circulation 58:1072–1083, 1978.

78. Sahn, D. J., Vaucher, Y., Williams, D. F., et al.: Echocardiographic detection of large left-to-right shunts and cardiomyopathies in infants and children. Am. J. Cardiol. 38:73–79, 1976.

79. Sapire, D. W., and Black, I. F. S.: Echocardiographic detection of aneurysms of the interventricular septum associated with ventricular septal defect. A method of noninvasive diagnosis and follow-up. Am. J. Cardiol. 36:797–801, 1978.

80. Schapira, J. N., Martin, R. P., Fowles, R. E., et al.: Two-dimensional echocardiographic assessment of patients with bioprosthetic valves. Am. J. Cardiol. 43:510–519, 1979.

81. Schapira, J. N., Stemple, D. R., Martin, R. P., et al.: Single and two-dimensional echocardiographic visualization of the effects of septal myomectomy in idiopathic hypertrophic subaortic stenosis. Circulation 58:850–860, 1978.

82. Schiller, N. B., and Botvinick, E. H.: Right ventricular compression as a sign of cardiac tamponade. An analysis of echocardiographic ventricular dimensions and their clinical implications. Circulation 56:774–779, 1977.

83. Schnittger, I., Bowden, R. E., Abrams, J., et al.: Echocardiography: pericardial thickening and constrictive pericarditis. Am. J. Cardiol. 42:388–395, 1978.

84. Schuler, G., Peterson, K. L., Johnson, A., et al.: Temporal response of left ventricular performance to mitral valve surgery. Circulation 59:1218–1231, 1979.

85. Seward, J. B., Gura, G. M., Hagler, D. J., et al.: Evaluation of M-mode echocardiography and wide-angle two-dimensional sector echocardiography in the diagnosis of cardiac masses. Circulation 58 (Suppl. II):234, 1978 (Abstract).

86. Seward, J. B., Tajik, A. J., Hagler, D. J., et al.: Peripheral venous contrast echocardiography. Am. J. Cardiol. 39:202–212, 1977.

87. Seward, J. B., Tajik, A. J., Hagler, D. J., et al.: Visualization of isolated ventricular septal defect with wide-angle two-dimensional sector echocardiography. Circulation 58 (Suppl. II):202, 1978 (Abstract).

88. Seward, J. B., Tajik, A. J., Spangler, J. G., et al.: Echocardiographic contrast studies: initial experience. Mayo Clin. Proc. 50:163–192, 1975.

89. Shiu, M. F.: Mitral valve closure index. Echocardiographic index of severity of mitral stenosis. Br. Heart J. 39:839–843, 1977.

90. Silverman, N. H., Lewis, A. B., Heymann, M. A., et al.: Echocardiographic assessment of ductus arteriosus shunts in premature infants. Circulation 50:821–825, 1974.

91. Silverman, N. H., and Schiller, N. B.: Apex echocardiography. A two-dimensional technique for evaluating congenital heart disease. Circulation 51:503–511, 1978.

92. Spangler, R. D., and Okin, J. T.: Echocardiographic demonstration of a left atrial thrombus. Chest 67:716–718, 1975.

93. Strom, J., Becker, R. M., Frishman, W., et al.: Effects of hypothermic hyperkalemic cardioplegic arrest on ventricular performance during cardiac surgery. N.Y. State J. Med. 78:2210–2212, 1978.

94. Tajik, A. J., Gau, G. T., Ritter, D. G., et al.: Echocardiogram in tetralogy of Fallot. Chest 64:107–108, 1973.

95. Tajik, A. J., and Seward, J. B.: Contrast echocardiography. In Kotler, M. N., and Segal, B. L., (eds.): Clinical Echocardiography, Ed. 1. Philadelphia, F. A. Davis Company, 1978, p. 317.

96. Tajik, A. J., Seward, J. B., Hagler, D. J., et al.: Two-dimensional real-time ultrasonic imaging of the heart and great vessels. Technique, image orientation, structure identification and validation. Mayo Clin. Proc. 53:271–303, 1978.

97. Teichholz, L. E., Kreulen, T., Herman, M. V., et al.: Problems in echocardiographic volume determinations: echocardiographic-angiographic correlations in the presence or absence of asynergy. Am. J. Cardiol. 37:7–11, 1976.

98. Toutouzas, P., Velimezis, A., Karayannis, E., et al.: End-diastolic amplitude of mitral valve echocardiogram in mitral stenosis. Br. Heart J. 39:73–79, 1977.

99. Troy, B. L., Pombo, J., and Rackley, C. E.: Measurement of left ventricular wall thickness and mass by echocardiography. Circulation 45:602–611, 1972.

100. Upton, M. T., and Gibson, D. G.: The study of ventricular function from digitized echocardiograms. Prog. Cardiovasc. Dis. 20:359–384, 1978.

101. Valdes-Cruz, L. M., Pieroni, D. R., Roland, J. M., et al.: Recognition of residual postoperative shunts by contrast echocardiography techniques. Circulation 55:148–152, 1977.

102. Vignola, P. A., Boucher, C. A., Curfman, G. D., et al.: Abnormal interventricular septal motion following cardiac surgery: clinical surgical echocardiographic and radionuclide correlates. Am. Heart J. 97:27–34, 1979.

103. Wann, L. S., Dillon, J. C., Weyman, A. E., et al.: Echocardiography in bacterial endocarditis. N. Engl. J. Med. 295:135–139, 1976.

104. Wann, L. S., Feigenbaum, H., Weyman, A. E., et al.: Cross-sectional echocardiographic detection of rheumatic mitral regurgitation. Am. J. Cardiol. 41:1258–1263, 1978.

105. Wann, L. S., Weyman, A. E., Feigenbaum, H., et al.: Determination of mitral valve area by cross-sectional echocardiography. Ann. Intern. Med. 88:337–341, 1978.

106. Weyman, A. E.: Pulmonary valve echo motion in clinical practice. Am. J. Med. 62:843–855, 1977.

107. Weyman, A. E., Caldwell, R. L., Hurwitz, R. A., et al.: Cross-sectional echocardiographic characterization of aortic obstruction. I. Supravalvular aortic stenosis and aortic hypoplasia. Circulation 57:491–497, 1978.

108. Weyman, A. E., Caldwell, R. L., Hurwitz, R. A., et al.: Cross-sectional echocardiographic detection of aortic obstruction. (II) Co-arctation of the aorta. Circulation 57:498–502, 1978.

109. Weyman, A. E., Dillon, J. C., Feigenbaum, H., et al.: Echocardiographic patterns of pulmonary valve motion in valvular pulmonary stenosis. Am. J. Cardiol. 34:644–651, 1974.

110. Weyman, A. E., Feigenbaum, H., Dillon, J. C., et al.: Non-invasive visualization of the left main coronary artery by cross-sectional echocardiography. Circulation 54:169–174, 1975.

111. Weyman, A. E., Feigenbaum, H., Hurwitz, R. A., et al.: Cross-sectional echocardiographic assessment of the severity of aortic stenosis in children. Circulation 55:773–778, 1977.

112. Weyman, A. E., Feigenbaum, H., and Hurwitz, R. A.: Cross-sectional echocardiography in evaluating patients with discrete subaortic stenosis. Am. J. Cardiol. 37:358–365, 1976.

113. Weyman, A. E., Hurwitz, R. A., Girod, D. A., et al.: Cross-sectional echocardiographic visualization of the stenotic pulmonary valve. Circulation 56:769–774, 1977.

114. Weyman, A. E., Peskoe, S. M., Williams, E. S., et al.: Detection of left ventricular aneurysms by cross-sectional echocardiography. Circulation 54:936–943, 1976.

115. Weyman, A. E., Wann, L. S., Caldwell, R. L., et al.: Negative contrast echocardiography: a new technique for detecting left-to-right shunts. Circulation 59:498–505, 1979.

116. Williams, R. G., and Rudd, M.: Echocardiographic features of endocardial cushion defects. Circulation 49:418–422, 1974.

117. Wolfe, S. B., Popp, R. L., and Feigenbaum, H.: Diagnosis of atrial tumors by ultrasound. Circulation 39:615–622, 1969.

27

ORGAN TRANSPLANTATION

Part I
Renal Allografts

AUDREY R. WILSON, M.D.

HISTORY AND CURRENT STATUS

Between 1963 and 1977, 25,108 kidney transplantations were reported to the Renal Transplant Registry by 301 institutions worldwide.[1] The terminal report, presented to the Sixth International Congress of the Transplantation Society in New York, summarized the accumulated experience of scientists and clinicians and was a record of accurate data about renal transplantation. The early 1960's saw the beginning of a new era in medicine — the widespread clinical application of renal transplantation for the treatment of chronic kidney failure. An exciting and exacting art was born and in an unprecedented way, the medical profession coordinated its efforts to improve the quality and prolong the life of patients who were afflicted by what had once been a uniformly fatal disease.

In the mid-1960's an unwarranted optimism prevailed. By the mid-1970's, it was apparent that the immunologic problems of rejection were poorly understood and that elaborate tissue-typing techniques did not significantly improve survival statistics. Some transplants succeeded while others were rejected, and the science remained an enigma. The surgical technique was quickly mastered, the complications were readily recognized and treated, and the art of juggling doses of prednisone and azathioprine was refined. Nevertheless, survival statistics have not improved since the late 1960's.

Since 1968, transplants from living related donors have had an 80 per cent one-year survival, whereas cadaveric donor transplants have had a 50 per cent one-year survival.[62] Increasing sophistication in histocompatibility typing and better understanding of immunosuppressive therapy with the introduction of antilymphocyte globulin have not significantly altered survival statistics.[38]

Figures based on 19,631 patients in whom follow-up data were available from the Transplant Registry reveal that 68.18 per cent were alive in 1977 and 45.3 per cent had functioning grafts, while 22.88 per cent had nonfunctioning or removed grafts and were maintained on dialysis. Another 31.58 per cent died; of these, 20.41 per cent had functioning grafts and 11.17 per cent died without graft function.[1] The distribution of diseases requiring transplantation had not changed in the 15 years during which the Transplant Registry collected data. Since then, many programs utilizing transplantation as the primary mode of therapy for juvenile diabetics with end-stage renal disease have been initiated. Glomerulonephritis accounted for 54.7 per cent of grafts; pyelonephritis, 12.3 per cent; nephrosclerosis, 5.6 per cent; polycystic disease, 5.5 per cent; unspecified conditions, 6.7 per cent; and other causes, 15.2 per cent in the Transplant Registry data.

Management of the transplant patient is based on the skilled management of rejection in its various stages and on the treatment of complications of immunosuppressive therapy and of end-stage renal disease. The technical skills required for transplantation were well developed at the turn of the century when Alexis Carrel published his technique for the anastomosis of arteries and veins.[6] His description of the histologic picture of extensive lymphocytic infiltration in the transplanted kidneys in animals is among the earliest observations of the rejection process. In 1914, he wrote: "The technical problems of organ grafting were solved but from a histologic standpoint no conclusion has thus far been reached because the interaction of the host and of the new organ are practically unknown."[8] That observation is still partly true today. Only with the advent of immunosuppressive therapy in the early 1960's did clinical organ grafting became a practical treatment for kidney failure.

The history of renal transplantation is divided into four periods:[18]

1. The earliest unsuccessful attempts.

2. Transplantation prior to immunosuppressive therapy, in which many heroic attempts were made, with a multitude of recorded failures but an occasional documented dramatic success, notably between monozygous twins.

3. The earliest attempts at immunosuppression with total-body radiation, in which results were almost uniformly fatal.

4. The burgeoning growth in the 1960's, after the discovery of the effectiveness of prednisone and azathioprine in suppressing rejection.

The first attempts at human transplantation were made with sheep, pig, goat, and subhuman primate donors. None of these attempts worked, and the recipients invariably died shortly after the insertion of the graft. The immunologic basis of rejection was not known until Medawar's classic studies with rodent skin grafts were published in 1944.[37] The first human-to-human kidney transplantation was reported by Voronoy, a Russian surgeon, in 1936.[69] The cadaver donor was B-positive blood type, while the recipient was O-positive. A small amount of urine was produced, but the patient died on the third postoperative day. The first clinical description of a renal transplantation in an intra-abdominal location was reported by Lawler in 1950.[29] One of the polycystic kidneys of a uremic patient was resected, and a transplant was anastomosed to the blood vessels and ureter. Clinical improvement was observed, and the transplanted kidney functioned briefly and excreted dye. The classic technique of placing the graft in the iliac fossa and anastomosing renal artery and vein to iliac vessels, still used today, was developed by Kuss and his colleagues in France. In 1951, eight attempts were reported from France in which the kidneys originated from living donors, but no clinical improvement in the recipients was observed.[18]

By 1953, Hume and his associates had performed eight transplants at Peter Bent Brigham Hospital by anastomosing renal blood vessels to the femoral artery and vein and placing the kidney subcutaneously in the thigh.[21] The eighth patient produced urine for six months; this was the first instance in which a transplant sustained life for any length of time. The first successful isograft from an identical twin was performed at the same institution in 1954, and lasting function was obtained.[40] Subsequent attempts to transplant free or cadaveric kidneys were undertaken in Boston, Los Angeles, Cleveland, and London with uniformly discouraging results. A total of 36 free or cadaveric transplants were reported without immunosuppressive therapy with only one encouraging result in which life was prolonged by six months.[18] It became clear that a way to suppress immune response must be found. Remarkable successes were achieved by Murray and coworkers with monozygous twins, however, seven successful cases being reported in 1958.[41] In the late 1950's, immunosuppression by total-body irradiation was attempted in 32 patients, but only four survived more than a year. This technique proved too hazardous and unpredictable in preventing rejection.

The great advance in renal transplantation in 1962 resulted from the discovery of azathioprine and 6-mercaptopurine and the introduction of corticosteroid therapy as an immunosuppressive agent.[42] The experimental basis for the use of steroids was laid in 1951 by Billingham, Krohn, and Medawar, but the clinical application to transplant rejection did not occur for another decade. Thiopurine compounds and 6-mercaptopurine and its imidazole derivative, azathioprine, were developed by Hitchings and Elion and reported in 1959. It is difficult to attribute the clinical application of azathioprine and steroids to a specific group.[58] In 1959, Calne successfully administered mercaptopurine to the recipient of human renal transplant.[20] Goodwin was one of the first to use corticosteroids.[17] The combination of azathioprine and prednisone soon became standard therapy as renal transplantation developed into a medical specialty. Successes were reported by Starzl,[62] Hume, Goodwin and Murray, and Calne.

Adjuvant surgical techniques, such as thymectomy, nephrectomy, and splenectomy, were advocated by some, then abandoned by many except in special circumstances. Thoracic duct cannulation and drainage has been attempted with inconclusive results. Terasaki and his group pioneered histocompatibility antigens, and the first application of histocompatibility testing to select the most suitable donor-recipient combination came in 1964.[64] Waksman and Woodruff[70] developed antilymphocyte globulin (ALG) in 1966; it was first used extensively by Starzl. The efficacy of ALG remains controversial. Early optimism regarding tissue typing and matching proved premature. Dramatic advances in organ preservation have also failed to improve survival statistics. Local radiation therapy to the graft is of questionable value as well.

Successful renal transplantation remains the province of the skilled surgeon and experienced nephrologist. The only contraindications to transplantation are uneradicable foci of infection and known malignancy. Although patients with diabetes mellitus,[59] particularly of juvenile onset, burned-out collagen vascular disease, and metabolic disorders are poor transplant candidates, they are worse candidates for maintenance dialysis.[43] Neither advanced age nor pre-existing systemic disease precludes the possibility of transplantation.[63]

A functioning transplant offers a better quality of life and a greater chance for rehabilitation than maintenance dialysis does. However, the mortality rate is higher during the first six months after transplantation, and the discomfort is greater. The short-term risk of transplantation is considerable, and the most common cause of death is sepsis. As the immunosuppressive drug dosage is tapered, the likelihood of serious infection diminishes, as do all the other complications of immunosuppressive therapy. If a functioning transplant is achieved, lipid metabolism may improve and blood pressure is likely to return to normal, thus reducing the risk of accelerated atherosclerosis common in dialysis patients. If a transplant patient survives with graft function into the second or third postoperative year, his life expectancy approaches that of the general population.

Allografts from HLA-identical siblings have a 90 per cent probability of sustaining life in the recipient five years after transplantation.[71] Transplants from parent to child or child to parent or between siblings sharing one haplotype have a 55 per cent success rate after five years.[71] Transplants from cadavers have a 36 per cent chance of functioning at five years.[71] The likelihood of a second transplant functioning at five years is similar to that of the first transplant. Because the five-year survival statistics are the same after the second transplant as after the first, a second attempt is worthwhile. Although graft survival has remained the same or diminished slightly for the past 15 years, recipient survival, particularly with cadaver kidneys, has improved. The complications of immunosuppressive therapy are more quickly recognized, and rejected kidneys are removed earlier.

Long-term dialysis has an overall annual mortality of 9 per cent, and compared with transplantation the initial phase is relatively problem-free.[7] Later on, however, abnormal lipid metabolism and hypertension result in accelerated atherosclerosis with increasing risk of myocardial infarction and cerebrovascular accident.[66] Hyperparathyroidism, neuropathy, and cerebral atrophy are additional risks of prolonged dialysis. Most patients, given the choice, will accept the risk of transplantation.

In the past two decades, transplantation as a cure for organ failure has become one of the most challenging and frustrating aspects of medicine, requiring unprecedented cooperation and coordination among the disciplines it crosses. Both society and the medical profession have been confronted with a new set of philosophic, political, and economic problems. Ethical and moral dilemmas have been created, and, more than ever, the value of the individual and the right to improved quality of life have been challenged and affirmed.

MEDICAL COMPLICATIONS

Infection

Sepsis is the major cause of death in renal transplant recipients, followed by atherosclerotic heart disease and cerebrovascular accidents. Sixty to 70 per cent of all transplant deaths are caused by infection and its sequelae. Although the urinary tract is most frequently invaded by bacteria, mortality is lowest (3 to 5 per cent) for infections at this site.[13] Pneumonia and septicemia are associated with the highest mortality. Bacterial agents are responsible for most fatalities, viral, fungal, and protozoal infections occurring relatively less frequently. Viral infections behave differently in immunosuppressed patients. The course of the disease is both prolonged and clinically altered. There may be an association between viral infection and graft rejection. The relationship between cytomegalovirus and rejection is particularly interesting. The role of hepatitis B virus infection in transplant patients has recently aroused interest. Of the fungal infections that proved fatal, *Candida*, *Cryptococcus*, *Aspergillus*, and *Nocardia* were the most frequent offenders. The lung and central nervous system were the most common sites of infection, followed by the gastrointestinal and genitourinary tracts and the skin.

Septicemia in transplant recipients is associated with a 36 per cent mortality.[36] Because these patients are receiving immunosuppressive therapy, the usual evidence for septicemia may not be present, and the diagnosis may be overlooked until a catastrophe such as septic shock occurs. Fever is readily mistaken for a symptom of acute rejection. Blood cultures should be obtained early and repeated often in the febrile transplant patient. The portal of entry may be lung, urinary tract, or wound site.

Pneumonia is difficult to recognize since it may appear radiographically like idiopathic post-transplant pulmonary congestion, postoperative atelectasis, fluid overload, or pulmonary embolism. Septicemic pneumonia is often fatal in patients who are vigorously immunosuppressed. Common bacterial infections are the usual cause but are much more severe and more frequently fatal because of immunosuppression. Early aggressive management is essential. When the urinary tract is the portal of entry, the organism is a gram-negative bacillus, most commonly *Escherichia coli.*

Cardiopulmonary complications seen on the chest x-ray include pulmonary edema or hemorrhage, pleural effusion, opportunistic infection, metastatic pulmonary calcification (rare), and mediastinal widening due to steroid-induced fat deposition (rare).[44] Infectious complications head the list in importance. Overwhelming infection is most likely to occur two to four weeks following transplantation, a period when the graft is most likely to be rejected and when corticosteroid and azathioprine doses are maximal. In the immediate postoperative period, an infiltrate may represent atelectasis, aspiration pneumonia, pulmonary edema, or pulmonary embolism.

The incidence of opportunistic infection correlates with the dosage of immunosuppressive drugs and prior or prolonged treatment with multiple antibiotics. Bacterial pneumonia may be more aggressive in transplant patients, but the distribution of organisms is no different from that in the average population. In the absence of antibiotic therapy, the organisms tend to be the same as those causing pneumonia in the nonimmunosuppressed patient. Unusual and opportunistic infections tend to occur in association with alterations of normal flora. Resistant and bizarre organisms flourish in the presence of prolonged antibiotic therapy. *Pneumocystis carinii* infection and fungal disease are particularly dangerous. Cavitation, when it occurs, is usually due to gram-negative organisms, such as *Klebsiella, Escherichia coli,* or *Pseudomonas,* although gram-positive cocci, fungi, and anaerobes may also cause cavitation. A pleural effusion associated with pneumonia should be considered empyema until proved otherwise.

Fungal infections encountered include *Aspergillus, Candida,* and *Cryptococcus. Histoplasma* and *Coccidioides* should be considered in endemic areas. This group of pathogens most commonly presents as cavitation, usually multiple. *Nocardia* infection and actinomycosis, though rare, may also present as cavitation within a mass or infiltrate.[44] Tuberculosis may be severe and fulminant in the immunosuppressed transplant patient. Typical symptoms are masked by steroids, and lung biopsy may be necessary to establish the diagnosis.

Noninfectious complications include cardiovascular problems, gastrointestinal complications, hyperparathyroidism, steroid-induced diabetes and bone disease, neurologic and ocular problems, and *de novo* neoplasia.

Cardiovascular Complications

Atherosclerotic heart disease is, after sepsis, the most common cause of death in transplant recipients. Hypertension, hyperlipidemia, hyperparathyroidism, steroid administration, myocarditis and pericarditis due to renal failure, and the metabolic problems of uremia are all contributing factors to increased atherosclerotic heart disease. Hyperlipidemia occurs in a high percentage (22 to 73 per cent) of transplant recipients.[11] The etiology is unclear but may be related to corticosteroid therapy or to increased plasma levels of insulin. Up to 4 per cent of transplant recipients die of cerebrovascular accidents (CVA).[11] Nephrosclerosis and polycystic disease predispose to CVA at an early age, suggesting that hypertension or congenital vascular malformations may be etiologic factors.

Hypertension is a frequent post-transplant problem and may be transient or permanent. A number of known factors play a role, but often the mechanism is obscure. Removal of the remnant kidneys may cure the hypertension. Since acute rejection frequently causes severe hypertension, treatment of the rejection may resolve the problem. Prednisone therapy, renal artery stenosis at the anastomotic site, and renal insufficiency due to chronic rejection are well-known causes. Early transient post-transplant hypertension may be associated with increased renin activity, suggesting ischemic damage to the grafted kidney. Persistent post-transplant hypertension varies from 36 per cent in recipients of living donor kidneys to 83 per cent in recipients of cadaveric kidneys.[11]

Since renal artery stenosis is a recognized complication of transplantation, arteriography is recommended in recipients whose hypertension persists or is uncontrollable. In a study of 100 consecutive transplant patients, routine arteriograms demonstrated stenosis in 25 per cent.[28] In hypertensive transplant recipients the probability of graft artery stenosis rose to 33 per cent, a finding confirmed by Bennett's series, in which 31 per cent of hypertensive graft recipients had renal artery stenosis.[5] Lacombe reported immediate resolution of hypertension following corrective surgery in all 14 patients operated on for graft artery stenosis in whom hypertension could not be controlled medically. The hypertension was generally not accompanied by elevated renal vein renin values, suggesting that this measurement was of no use in predicting surgical correctibility in transplant patients. Recurrence of stenosis was common and may have been due to excessive fibrosis, which is part of the rejection phenomenon. The recipient's own kidneys may be responsible for post-transplant hypertension. Again, renin levels are not a reliable index. If renal artery stenosis and chronic rejection have been excluded and hypertension is medically unmanageable, bilateral nephrectomy is indicated. Finally, glomerulonephritis may recur in the transplanted kidney, causing hypertension.

Gastrointestinal Complications

Gastrointestinal complications occur in approximately one third of transplant recipients.[22] Because these complications are frequently catastrophic, early diagnosis and treatment are essential. Such complications may occur anywhere along the gastrointestinal tract and include bleeding, peptic and stress ulcers, gastritis, pancreatitis, hepatitis, acute colitis, intestinal perforation, and intestinal obstruction.[45] Frequently, symptoms are masked by immunosuppressive therapy; therefore, a vigorous prophylactic and diagnostic approach is appropriate. Useful techniques include plain films, barium studies, ultrasound, angiography, and any other procedure that lends itself to the clinical problem.

Post-transplant reflux esophagitis may occur with or without a preoperative history of peptic esophagitis. The symptoms may be incapacitating. Esophagoscopy is the most reliable diagnostic tool. Monilial esophagitis is a common problem in debilitated individuals, and immunosuppression accelerates its course. The patient presents with painful swallowing; esophagoscopy reveals the characteristic plaques of moniliasis with associated mucosal changes. A barium esophagogram is diagnostic. Careful follow-up is suggested, since severe strictures may develop in spite of prompt therapy.

Massive gastrointestinal bleeding and perforated ulcer are frequent causes of death in transplant patients. Prophylactic ulcer surgery is indicated in selected cases. Aggressive management instituted immediately at the onset of symptoms is necessary. Steroid therapy masks the symptoms of perforation, delaying diagnosis.

The frequency of peptic ulcer disease in post-transplant patients is as high as 16 per cent.[67] In some institutions, an upper gastrointestinal series is part of the pretransplant work-up. If there is a prior history of ulcer disease, a prophylactic vagotomy and pyloroplasty or antrectomy may be justified.[31] In the immunosuppressed transplant recipient, wound healing and anastomotic breakdown present serious problems. Medical management of ulcer disease is also less likely to be effective in the immunosuppressed patient. When upper gastrointestinal hemorrhage occurs after transplantation, mortality is in the range of 60 per cent, so prophylactic ulcer surgery may be the treatment of choice.[12] There is a relatively higher incidence of gastric ulcers compared with duodenal ulcers in transplant patients; otherwise, the radiologic picture is the same. Since the ulcers may be superficial, endoscopy is a more useful diagnostic device than upper gastrointestinal series, although current double-contrast studies rival endoscopy in accuracy. If perforation is suspected, a water-soluble contrast agent should be used.

Peptic ulcer is the most probable cause of massive and often fatal gastrointestinal hemorrhage in transplant patients. Gastritis and superficial ulcerations in small and large bowel, particularly the cecum, are occasionally encountered. If bleeding is from the upper gastrointestinal tract, endoscopy is preferable. Emergency angiography may be useful both diagnostically and therapeutically, since it offers the possibility of pharmacologic control or catheter embolization. An upper gastrointestinal series is least useful and, in fact, may delay angiography because of the presence of residual barium.

If the clinical picture suggests lower gastrointestinal hemorrhage, angiography is unquestionably the procedure of choice. Barium is contraindicated if angiography is anticipated. In any event, a barium study of the colon is unlikely to reveal the bleeding site, and the presence of barium in the gut will eliminate the possibility of identifying the bleeding site with a water-soluble contrast agent in the vascular tree. Again, angiography offers the possibility of therapy as well as accurate localization. About two thirds of lower gastrointestinal bleeds can be controlled through the vascular catheter.

Renal transplant patients suffer an unusually high incidence of ileal and colonic perforation, which are frequently fatal. Perforation of the colon is often associated with diverticular disease. There is an increased incidence of diverticulitis with steroid therapy, possibly because of atrophy of intestinal lymphoid collections and consequent decreased resistance to bacterial invasion. Furthermore, when diverticulitis is present, a perforation is less likely to wall off if the patient is on steroid therapy. Consequently, generalized peritonitis and a fatal outcome are more frequent in the immunosuppressed transplant patient receiving steroids.

Ileal and colonic perforations due to fecal impactions have been attributed to nonabsorbable antacids, polystyrene sulfonate (Kayexalate) enemas, ischemia, and infectious colitis. Again, the symptoms of perforation are masked by steroid therapy, and almost all of these patients will die. Positive radiologic findings precede clinical evidence of perforation and peritonitis. Therefore, careful examination of plain films in multiple projections for free air or extraluminal air caused by abscess is essential. Water-soluble contrast enema is indicated immediately when unexplained abdominal pain is present. Since the ileum and colon perforate more readily than the stomach or duodenum, a water-soluble contrast enema should precede the upper gastrointestinal series when extraluminal air is present unless clinical evidence suggests otherwise.

Acute colitis has been reported in 0.9 to 3.8 per cent of post-transplant patients.[49] Intestinal perforation or obstruction may be a complication. Mortality is very high, particularly with perforation. Most cases are due to acute ischemic colitis, but pseudomembranous colitis, *Staphylococcus, Candida,* and cytomegalovirus infection are also reported etiologic factors. Barium enema shows thumbprinting, saw-tooth irregularity of the mucosa, pseudopolypoid filling defects, tubular narrowing of the colon, sacculations, and strictures.

Fecal impaction may cause mechanical obstruction resulting in bowel necrosis, especially in the right colon and ileum. This has been attributed to the use of nonabsorbable antacid gels such as aluminum hydroxide. Adynamic ileus occurs in the immediate postoperative period. Adhesions may cause mechanical obstruction.

Pancreatitis, with a mortality rate of 50 per cent, occurs in 2 to 6 per cent of all renal transplant patients. Hyperparathyroidism associated with chronic renal disease and steroid therapy is a causative factor. Cytomegalovirus has been found in the pancreas in post-transplantation patients with pancreatitis. Complications include hemorrhage from erosion into a major blood vessel, pseudocyst, and abscess. Symptoms are masked by steroid therapy. The radiographic findings are the same as in nontransplant patients.

Steroid-dependent diabetes is described in 3 per cent of living related donor kidney recipients and in 8 per cent of cadaver donor recipients (probably owing to higher steroid dosage).[55] Females, patients with a family history of diabetes, and those over 50 years old are more likely to be affected. Steroid-dependent diabetes is probably a manifestation of adult-onset diabetes.

Other Complications

Central nervous system complications include cerebrovascular accidents, infection, cancer, and central pontine myelinolysis. There is an increased incidence of both primary and secondary central nervous system tumors.

Transplant recipients are predisposed to thromboembolism because in the immediate postoperative period the coagulation abnormalities of chronic renal failure are rapidly corrected, resulting initially in the hypercoagulable state. Blood viscosity may be elevated, as are triglyceride, cholesterol, and fibrinogen levels. Steroids probably contribute to the pathogenesis of thromboembolism. The most common cause of death in the first 24 hours postoperatively is pulmonary embolism.

Pulmonary edema may occur during a rejection episode and is related to salt and water retention. It accounts for about one quarter of abnormal chest x-rays in transplant patients. Radiographic abnormalities on chest film include cardiomegaly, enlarged upper-zone vessels with hazy margins, bronchial wall edema, Kerley B lines, diminished lung volume, and pleural effusion. Other causes of pulmonary edema are uremia, metabolic acidosis, myocardial infarction, sepsis, pancreatitis, embolism, aspiration, and cerebral edema.[44] Pulmonary hemorrhage indistinguishable from pulmonary edema is rare but occurs as a result of azathioprine-induced thrombocytopenia. Pleural effusion in a transplant patient is most likely due to pulmonary edema or empyema but may be caused by uremic fibrinous pleuritis.

GRAFT COMPLICATIONS

Graft failure in the first two postoperative weeks is generally due to acute renal failure (ARF) or rejection. The most frequent cause of immediate post-transplant failure is acute renal failure. Thirty-two per cent of cadaver transplants undergo acute renal failure, whereas the incidence is only 11 per cent in grafts obtained from living related donors.[30] The occurrence of acute renal failure in cadaver kidneys is related to ischemia in the agonal period of hypotension. Grafts from living donors, which have multiple renal arteries, are more subject to acute renal failure. Iodinated contrast material should be administered judiciously and sparingly to transplant recipients, since if given rapidly in high doses in the dehydrated patient, it can cause acute renal graft failure.

A graft that never functions usually has acute renal failure, although, occasionally, hyperacute rejection may be the cause. While acute renal failure, usually presents with oliguria, both anuric and polyuric forms occur in post-transplant renal failure. If the recipient's own kidneys are present, they may be the source of urine output. Hyperacute rejection is usually noted at the operating table immediately after anastomosis of the blood vessels, when blood flow is established in the transplant. Immediate removal of the kidney is indicated. Occasionally, however, hyperacute rejection does not manifest until 12 to 48 hours after the transplant operation. It then becomes necessary to differentiate acute renal failure from hyperacute rejection. Patients with acute renal failure are usually asymptomatic and clinically stable, whereas patients with hyperacute rejection are sick. The ^{131}I-iodohippurate (Hippuran) renogram shows good graft uptake in acute renal failure, while poor isotope uptake suggests rejection but does not rule out acute renal failure. Repeat scans every 24 to 48 hours help differentiate acute renal failure from rejection. The prognosis for acute renal failure when properly managed is excellent. Surprisingly, neither patient nor graft survival statistics are made worse when acute renal failure occurs, provided that medical management of the temporary renal failure is appropriate.

Hyperacute rejection is usually obvious at the operating table as soon as the recipient's blood flows through the graft. Usually, the graft never functions and it is immediately removed before closing. Occasionally, there is initial urine output, but function ceases within 12 to 48 hours. Hyperacute rejection presents as rapidly progressive vascular thrombosis leading to complete cortical thrombosis and vasculonecrosis. The graft becomes flabby, mottled, and cyanotic as soon as the graft renal artery and vein are anastomosed to the patient's iliac vessels and blood flow is initiated. The immunologic basis for hyperacute rejection is preformed circulating antibodies against donor tissue, usually against donor HLA antigens. It is an exclusively humoral phenomenon. ABO blood incompatibility also results in hyperacute rejection, the pathologic basis being infarction due to vascular disruption. Occasionally, the sudden changes described are delayed by several hours, and the diagnosis can no longer be made by direct inspection of the graft. The renogram will show poor or absent uptake of isotope, and the arteriogram will show severe vasculitis, multiple infarctions, and cortical necrosis. Graft nephrectomy is inevitable since the changes are irreversible.

Acute rejection is generally manifested by fever, oliguria, hypertension, weight gain due to fluid retention, and graft pain and tenderness. Laboratory values indicate decrease in renal function, and proteinuria is seen. The diagnosis is usually obvious clinically, but occasionally biopsy is necessary to confirm the diagnosis or to exclude other causes of renal failure. Arteriography and venography are indicated when other complications, particularly vascular disorders, cannot be excluded. The ^{131}I-Hippuran scan shows poor or diminished uptake. The most frequent cause of graft failure and loss is acute rejection.

The immunologic basis for acute rejection is a mixed humerocellular reaction of antibody formation against donor tissue combined with a direct cellular infiltration. The pathologic findings include massive cellular infiltrate — predominantly round cells — in glomerular, interstitial, and perivascular areas of the kidney. Diffuse edema is seen, and frequently thrombosis of some small and medium-sized vessels is noted. The first acute rejection reaction typically occurs between 7 and 21 days following transplantation. Multiple episodes are the rule. The first rejection episode is usually the most clinically dramatic, subsequent rejection reactions tending to be progressively milder and more subtle.

Accelerated rejection occurs between four and seven days after transplantation and represents an anamnestic response to prior sensitization to donor antigens. Its clinical presentation is the same as in acute rejection except that it tends to be both clinically and pathologically more severe and violent. Acute rejection is altered and modified by immunosuppressive therapy.

When graft failure occurs in the immediate postoperative period, an arterial problem, although rare, must always be considered and excluded. This requires an arteriogram. Thrombosis of the transplant blood supply may be the result of rejection, ABO incompatibility, or a hypercoagulable state. Mechanical obstruction of the artery may occur from intimal damage caused by the perfusion catheter tip or by surgical manipulation. The graft may be rotated, twisted, or stretched. Extrinsic compression from a hematoma can cause occlusion of the graft artery. A leak at the arterial anastomotic site may be caused by infection or by a mechanical problem. Acute arterial complications may arise precipitously and immediately, or there may be a delay of several weeks. They may manifest as sudden oliguria or anuria, gross hematuria, evidence of retroperitoneal bleeding, and extragraft thromboembolic process.

The renogram will show poor or absent isotope uptake. The arteriogram will be diagnostic. If the problem of acute arterial occlusion is recognized and corrected promptly, graft function may occasionally be salvaged. Catastrophic hemorrhage from an infarcted necrotic graft or dehiscence of the arterial anastomosis may be prevented by immediate surgical intervention.

Graft artery stenosis, a more common arterial problem, usually develops slowly and becomes apparent several months after transplant surgery. However, if the stenosis is a part of the rejection phenomenon, it may be seen at three to four weeks.

Venous complications may be acute and precipitous or delayed and gradual in their development. They include thrombosis from rejection, mechanical problems, and hypovolemia or thromboembolic disease. Early acute thrombosis presents with pain and swelling of the graft and ipsilateral thigh and leg and usually is seen in the first two weeks. Hematuria is quickly followed by anuria.

The slow, insidious development of graft thrombosis later in the postoperative period is generally a part of the rejection process. Graft function deteriorates gradually, proteinuria increases, and systemic thromboembolic episodes occur. Thrombectomy or anticoagulation is unlikely to reverse the process and restore graft function. Other venous problems include embolism, ligation of an accessory graft vein, and anastomotic leak, which may be massive.

Acute recurrence of original disease occasionally accounts for graft failure. Focal glomerulosclerosis and rapidly progressive glomerulonephritis may recur early and should be considered when massive proteinuria is seen after transplantation. Diabetic nephropathy may also arise in the immediate post-transplant period. By and large, the pathologic findings of rejection and of recurrent disease tend to be similar and to obscure each other. It is therefore difficult to determine if recurrence of the original disease is present in a significant number of transplanted kidneys. Perhaps if the original disease clearly recurs early in the first transplant, a second graft should not be attempted since recurrence will be more likely.

Other early graft complications include renal tubular acidosis and acute hypercalcemia associated with graft failure. The latter is treated with emergency parathyroidectomy. Injudicious use of antacids may result in metabolic disorders. Calcium carbonate antacids may cause hypercalcemia. Phosphate-binding antacids may cause phosphate depletion syndrome, and magnesium-containing antacids may lead to hypermagnesemia.

Spontaneous graft rupture is a rare complication, usually occurring in the first postoperative week during or after a rejection episode. Emergency nephrectomy is usually necessary, but occasionally the rupture may be repaired and the graft salvaged. Late graft rupture at five months has been reported. Papillary necrosis, another rare complication, is generally associated with rejection but may be caused by infection.[24]

The most important late graft complication is chronic rejection. The clinical course is that of progressive, slow, inexorable deterioration in renal function. Hypertension and proteinuria are features of chronic rejection. The pathologic findings are interstitial fibrosis, small vessel intimal proliferation, and thrombosis. The end result of chronic rejection is loss of graft function. The recurrence of primary renal disease may be a late graft complication.

The development of glomerulonephritis in renal grafts from identical twins (presuming absence of histoincompatibility) first drew attention to the possibility of recurrence of original kidney disease in renal transplants. Glassock and associates reported the development of glomerular disease in 11 of 17 isografts transplanted into recipients whose original renal disease was glomerulonephritis. Similar recurrence of glomerulonephritis was subsequently found in renal allografts. The conclusion was based on the finding of identical morphologic lesions both in the allograft and in the recipient's original kidneys. The diagnosis of recurrence of disease in a graft is almost always based on the similarity or identity of the morphologic lesions observed in the graft and in the original kidneys. Based on this definition, the incidence of recurrence of glomerulonephritis in allografts ranges from 5 to 18 per cent. The higher incidence of recurrence of glomerulonephritis in isografts is attributed to absence of immunosuppressive therapy, without which allografts could not survive. Renal disease secondary to systemic disorders also may recur in the transplanted kidney.

Diabetic vascular lesions develop in normal kidneys transplanted into recipients with diabetes mellitus. Primary oxalosis consistently recurs in the transplanted kidney. Renal Fanconi syndrome, amyloidosis, and malignant nephrosclerosis may develop in a normal kidney transplanted into a recipient suffering from these diseases. Glomerulonephritis in renal allografts may also arise *de novo*.

DE NOVO NEOPLASMS

The incidence of *de novo* tumors in human allograft recipients is approximately 100 times greater than in the general population of the same age range.[19] Of particular interest is the disproportionately high incidence of lymphoma and its predilection for the central nervous system. If nonmelanoma skin cancers and carcinoma in situ of the cervix are excluded, 33 per cent of all tumors in renal transplant recipients are lymphomas, whereas in the general population only 3 to 4 per cent of tumors are lymphomas.[47] Of lymphomas in the transplant group, 62 per cent are reticulum cell sarcomas, while only 2 per cent are Hodgkin's disease. The latter is the most common lymphoma in the general population. Reticulum cell sarcoma is 350 times more likely to occur in a transplant recipient than in the average person.[48] There is a remarkably high incidence of central nervous system involvement in renal transplant patients who develop lymphoma. The likelihood of central nervous system involvement in the transplant group is 42 per cent, whereas in lymphoma of the general population, it is only 2 per cent. When lymphoma does invade the central nervous system in transplant patients, 87 per cent of the time it is confined to this site. Thus, it is evident that central nervous system symptoms in a transplant recipient require a careful tumor work-up.

The most common cancer among renal allograft recipients is cancer of skin and lower lip, constituting 40 per cent of the total, with an unusually high proportion of squamous cell carcinoma compared with basal cell carcinoma. Patients tend to be younger, and multiple tumors are more frequent. The incidence of prostate, colon, rectal, breast and lung cancer is lower, probably because transplant patients as a group are relatively young. There is an unexpectedly high incidence of Kaposi's sarcoma.

In patients with renal failure from neoplasm, a delay of at least one year is recommended before transplantation is considered because of the increased risk of recurrence in the transplant patient. The average time of appearance of *de novo* neoplasms is 34 months after transplantation. Lymphoma occurs earlier, at an average of 23 months.

RENAL OSTEODYSTROPHY (See also Chapter 31)

Secondary hyperparathyroidism with altered calcium metabolism is frequently associated with chronic renal disease.[11] Hyperparathyroidism and hypercalcemia may persist after successful renal transplantation. Parathormone levels may be elevated, but calcium levels may remain normal. Hypercalcemia is usually seen within the first postoperative month; it is mild and transient and disappears in 3 to 12 months. Late appearance does occur, however.

The mechanism of post-transplant hyperparathyroidism is similar to that of uremic secondary hyperparathyroidism.[51] Early hyperparathyroidism is related to phosphorus depletion, mobilization of calcium, and persistence of pretransplant hyperparathyroidism from slow involution. Persistent secondary hyperparathyroidism and hypercalcemia beyond six months are due to a variety of problems: (1) slow involution of parathyroid glands, (2) steroid therapy suppressing serum calcium and thus provoking parathormone production, (3) phosphate binding antacids causing hypophosphatemia and consequently hyperparathyroidism, (4) effects of vitamin D therapy, and (5) magnesium deficiency.

Factors predisposing to hyperparathyroidism include the state of phosphate depletion, the severity of pretransplant hyperparathyroidism, and the level of graft function. Persistent secondary hyperparathyroidism in the post-transplant period should result in hypercalcemia, hypophosphatemia, hyperphosphaturia, and increased parathormone levels. However, serum calcium elevation may be masked by poor graft function or suppressed by steroid therapy. The diagnosis of hyperparathyroidism may be made in almost all cases by bony changes seen on x-ray (see Chapter 31).[53] These include subperiosteal, intracortical, endosteal, subchondral, and trabecular bone resorption and brown tumors.

Subperiosteal bone resorption is seen along the radial aspect of the proximal and middle phalanges, particularly of the second and third digits, producing a characteristic lacy pattern that may progress to scalloped osseous erosion. Other locations are proximal medial tibia, humerus and femur, superior rib margins, terminal phalanges, and lamina dura of the teeth. Osteolysis is seen at tendon and ligament attachments on the calcaneus, ischium, trochanter, and distal clavicle.[53]

Intracortical bone resorption occurs as linear striations, usually in the second metacarpal, and accompanies subperiosteal bone resorption. Endosteal bone resorption appears as localized pockets or scallop defects along the inner margin of the cortex of the bones in the hands. Subchondral bone resorption with substitutive fibrosis is seen beneath the cartilaginous surfaces at the sacroiliac, acromioclavicular, sternoclavicular, and temporomandibular joints and symphysis pubis. Further manifestation of subchondral bone resorption includes erosive arthritis of peripheral joints.

Trabecular bone resorption is seen throughout the skeleton and produces a granular appearance. It is most obvious in the skull, where intradiploic resorption produces a salt-and-pepper pattern. Brown tumors, or osteoclastomas, appear as well-defined eccentric lesions which are frequently cortical in location; these lesions, however, are much more frequently encountered in primary hyperparathyroidism. Osteopenia — diminution in both quality and quantity of bone — is characteristic of renal osteodystrophy. Fewer trabeculae are visible, and there is biconcave deformity of vertebral bodies. Soft tissue and vascular calcification may be the result of secondary hyperparathyroidism. Subcutaneous and periarticular calcifications may regress after transplantation, but vascular calcifications usually do not. Renal osteodystrophy may be complicated by epiphysiolysis. The most common site for slipped epiphysis is the proximal femur, and the condition is usually bilateral. The typical patient is an adolescent male with long-standing uremia who has undergone dialysis or transplantation around the time of puberty.

Although aseptic necrosis is attributed to steroid therapy, it may be seen in patients with chronic renal disease on long-term hemodialysis who have severe secondary hyperthyroidism but who have never been on steroids. The usual site is the femoral head, but the distal femur, humeral head, condyles, talus, or cuboid and carpal bones may be affected. Spontaneous tendon rupture may result from hyperparathyroidism.

Because hyperparathyroidism is such a serious and insidious problem, pretransplant parathyroidectomy may be justified in selected cases.[31] Indications include medically uncontrollable and progressive hypercalcemia, bony complications such as pathologic fractures or aseptic necrosis, and deterioration of renal function due to hypercalcemia, nephrolithiasis, and nephrocalcinosis.

UROLOGIC COMPLICATIONS

Increasing experience with renal transplantation over the past 15 years has resulted in a decline in surgical complications with improved survival, although this has not been matched by a corresponding improvement in graft survival statistics. More is known about the use of immunosuppressive drugs, and patients are better prepared with dialysis. The surgeon is better equipped today by cumulative experience in deciding whether to sacrifice the graft in the interest of patient survival.

Urologic complications vary from as high as 25 per cent to as low as 3 per cent, depending on how recently the data were collected.[14] There has been significant improvement in morbidity and mortality statistics of urologic complications as technical ability in harvesting and reimplanting the donor ureter has improved. With meticulous attention to the preservation of the ureteral blood supply at the time of harvesting, most urologic complications can be avoided.

Urologic complications are associated with decrease in graft function. In the immediate postoperative period, when renal function diminishes, the differentiation between a mechanical problem that is potentially correctable by surgery and acute rejection or acute renal failure is crucial. Early recognition is essential since a urologic complication is often a surgical emergency. Untreated urinary tract fistula has a 50 per cent mortality, whereas immediate repair may reduce the mortality to 1 per cent.[9]

A mechanical urologic problem mistakenly attributed to rejection and treated unnecessarily with increased immunosuppressive therapy has its own significant morbidity. Careful use of all available diagnostic techniques is essential. When renal failure occurs, the possibility of a urologic complication should always be considered. Of the potential technical problems, urologic complications are far more likely than vascular complications. Urologic complications are due to extravasation, obstruction, or extraurinary collections.[4] Immediate complications include vesicocutaneous, ureterocutaneous, and calyceal-cutaneous fistulas with resulting extravasation.[9] Obstruction due to ureteral necrosis occurs in the immediate postoperative period. Immediate extraurinary collections include hematoma and abscess. Lymphocele, the most frequent complication, usually occurs late.[39] Less common late complications include urinary tract infection, vesicoureteral reflux, calculus formation, and papillary necrosis.

Early diagnosis of urologic complications with immediate surgical repair is necessary if the graft is to be salvaged.[56] Uncontrolled infection and sepsis or overwhelming rejection in association with a urologic complication, however, require graft removal in the interest of patient survival. The diagnosis of a urologic complication may prove difficult since acute renal failure, rejection, and mechanical problems all present as failing graft function. Furthermore, a urologic problem may be associated with rejection or acute renal failure. The surgical problem is easily overlooked while rejection is treated with steroids and antimetabolites, which only worsen the urologic complication.

Increasing reliance is being placed on sonography for detection of the suspected complications of hematoma, urinoma, abscess, lymphocele, and hydronephrosis.

Extravasation

Vesicocutaneous fistula almost always occurs along the bladder suture line. If a drain is left in place, persistent wound leakage is seen and intravenous indigo carmine or methylene blue dye stains the dressings. If there is no drain, vesicle fistula presents as extravasation along the anterolateral surface of the bladder where it has been opened for ureteroneocystostomy. The bladder extravasation is extraperitoneal and may extend along the anterior abdominal wall. The diagnosis may not be immediately obvious. Clinical evidence includes decreased urine output, lower abdominal tenderness, abdominal distention, and fever in the first two weeks postoperatively. A cystogram will confirm the diagnosis. A radionuclide study on the first and seventh postoperative days may be routinely obtained to reaffirm urinary tract continuity. Closure and excision of the fistula tract are almost always necessary.

Ureterocutaneous fistulas are a serious complication, since they generally indicate an interruption of ureteral blood supply during donor nephrectomy. The distal ureter normally has only marginal vascularity. The added insult of postoperative inflammatory response, plus a rejection episode involving the ureter along with the kidney and further compromising ureteral blood supply, may combine to create a ureteral fistula. Ureteral necrosis and fistula formation are more common in live donor graft recipients.[10] This is probably related to more extensive dissection of the hilar portion of the renal artery when the flank approach is used, as opposed to the anterior approach used in cadaver nephrectomy. Kidneys with multiple renal arteries are more liable to ureteral fistulas because of damage to ureteral blood supply during the increased dissection required as well as the inherently poor vascularity when more than one artery supplies a kidney. There is an increased incidence of fistula formation in diabetic patients.

The blood supply to the ureter may be affected by a severe rejection, resulting in ureteral necrosis, sloughing, and fistula formation. The combination of compromised ureteral blood supply during organ procurement and a mild rejection episode may be enough to cause vascular insufficiency and necrosis. Neglecting a ureteral fistula results in infection, sepsis, and death; immediate recognition and surgical repair are essential.[57] The reported incidence of ureteral fistulas is from 3 to 10 per cent,[46] though Salvatierra, Kountz, and Belzar report a rate of 0.5 per cent in 500 consecutive transplants.[56] The low complication rate is attributed to proper kidney removal with attention to ureteral blood supply and careful management of multiple renal arteries. Ureterocutaneous fistulas present with diminished urine output and failing graft function. The radionuclide scan will show an extravesical collection of urine before any other study is diagnostic. A cystogram is required to rule out vesical fistula. Intravenous pyelography best demonstrates ureteral extravasation, but if function is significantly impaired, retrograde or antegrade pyelography may be necessary. However, sonography can accurately depict confined extravasation (urinoma) but may not distinguish it from a hematoma.

Calyceal fistulas are rare but may occur if polar vessels are interrupted during nephrectomy or are occluded post-transplantation. Segmental ischemia, infarction, and calyceal fistula formation result, particularly if the occluded polar artery supplies more than 10 per cent of the renal mass. Extravasation from the proximal ureter, ureteropelvic junction, or calyces may occur with distal obstruction, especially after administration of diuretics. Calyceal fistula is a rare complication of transplant biopsy.

Diagnostic studies for detecting extravasation include the radionuclide scan, intravenous urography, cystography, and retrograde pyelography.

Obstruction

Ureteral obstruction may be due to distal ureteral necrosis at the ureteroneocystostomy site as a result of vascular insufficiency caused by a technical error, or it may occur because of rejection and subsequent fibrosis. Obstruction may be caused by kinking or compression of the ureter by the kidney, ureteral torsion, anastomotic stricture, blood clots, spermatic cord obstruction, retroperitoneal fibrosis, abscess, lymphocele, pyeloureteral kink, improper ureteral placement, fungus ball, and, last but not least, stones. Urinary obstruction is likely to be a late development, whereas extravasation and fistula formation are more frequent in the immediate postoperative period.

The radionuclide study supplies the first clue to obstruction in the failing graft, and urography confirms the diagnosis. If function is too poor to provide opacification of the collecting system, retrograde pyelography may be necessary. Sonography demonstrates the presence of hydronephrosis (see Fig. 3–36, p. 80, Vol. I) but does not localize the obstruction. Ureteral obstruction may occur years after renal transplantation. Predisposing factors are multiple surgical procedures, retroperitoneal fibrosis with adhesions, vascular insufficiency with intrinsic fibrosis, repeated rejection episodes, and urinary tract infection.

Extraurinary Collections

A mass displacing the kidney, bladder, or ureter in the immediate postoperative period is a urinoma, hematoma, or abscess. Immediate recognition of the mass and identification of its nature are essential. The usual signs of an inflammatory process may not accompany an abscess in the immunosuppressed patient. The presence of a urinoma, evidenced by extravasation from the collecting system, must be recognized if a urinary tract fistula is to be surgically repaired. Lymphocele,[50] the most common paratransplant fluid collection, is a late complication and is usually preceded by a rejection episode. The lymph originates either from the patient's interrupted lymphatics, which can be demonstrated by lymphangiography, or from lymphatic leakage in the transplanted kidney (shown by lymphocytic typing). The lymphocele presents with diminished renal function because the extraurinary collection has a mass effect, compressing the kidney or obstructing the ureter. Additional evidence for lymphocele is edema of the external genitalia and adjacent thigh or leg, thrombophlebitis due to iliac venous compression by the mass, and swelling over the graft site and suprapubic area.

If an extraurinary collection is suspected, a radionuclide study should be done.[65] If the mass picks up radionuclide activity, it is a urinoma. If it does not, it is an abscess, hematoma, or, in the late postoperative period, a lymphocele. Occasionally, a high-output lymphatic fistula may mimic a urinoma, presumably because of lymphatic diffusion of the isotope.

Needle aspiration and analysis of the contents of the fluid collection should be diagnostic. Lymph is similar to plasma, whereas urine contains creatinine, potassium, and urea nitrogen in higher concentrations. Sonic guidance may facilitate the aspiration. In addition, aspiration of a lymphocele may result in cure. Sonography is useful in determining the characteristics of the fluid collection.[26, 50] Urinoma, lymphocele,[34] and fresh hematoma all appear as a liquid-containing mass, but an organized hematoma is less transonic and an abscess initially has levels of echoes[2] (see Fig. 3–39 and text, p. 81, Vol. I).

Any mass may compress or occlude the renal vein, causing nephrotic syndrome. Ultrasonic Doppler flow studies of the venous system may be useful.

The treatment of lymphocele, the most common extraurinary collection, depends on its size and the degree of graft failure. Aspiration may be curative in some cases; some lymphoceles regress spontaneously, and others require surgical excision. Lymphoceles tend to recur; they may compress and obstruct the ureter and the pelvic veins. Repeated aspiration may cause infection, and marsupialization may be necessary.

Renal calculi may be secondary to hyperparathyroidism, antacid therapy, steroids, chronic infection, or renal tubular acidosis.[54] Infection is a serious associated problem because of the immunosuppressive therapy. Intravenous urography is indicated if a stone is suspected. Immediate removal of the stone and parathyroidectomy to control hyperparathyroidism are indicated.[32]

Infection

One of the most common sources of sepsis in the transplant patient is the urinary tract. Ascending urinary tract infection and pyelonephritis are usually associated with ureteral obstruction or fistula. Organisms include *Escherichia coli*, enterococci, and *Proteus*, but fungi and staphylococci are occasional offenders.

Vesicoureteral reflux occurs in one quarter of transplant recipients, probably as a result of surgical technique, and is generally of no clinical significance. Reflux up the native ureters is probably due to lack of normal peristalsis in the absence of urine production and flow.

Papillary necrosis is an exceedingly rare transplant complication. It is thought to be the result of rejection and periglomerular fibrosis with subsequent papillary ischemia and necrosis.[24]

TRANSPLANT ANGIOGRAPHY

Renal arteriography is the most accurate diagnostic tool for evaluating early transplant anuria, graft rejection, and hypertension.[3, 15] Graft rejection and acute renal failure, the most common causes of early postoperative transplant failure, can usually be differentiated on the arteriogram, particularly if selective injection and magnification techniques are used.[23] The renal arteriogram is the definitive technique for evaluating potentially correctable renal artery stenosis, frequently the cause of hypertension. Since angiography is an invasive technique, which is associated with discomfort and the potential for accelerating or provoking renal failure, it should be used judiciously. A review of the clinical indications is useful.

In the initial postoperative period, acute anuria is the primary indication for angiography in order to distinguish between vascular occlusion, acute rejection, and acute renal failure. Later on, gradual deterioration of graft function with rising blood urea nitrogen (BUN) and creatinine may be considered a relative indication. Uncontrolled hypertension either in the immediate postoperative period or later on requires angiographic evaluation because the graft may be salvaged and the hypertension surgically corrected if renal artery or anastomotic stenosis is found. A combination of deterioration of function and hypertension more than 40 days after transplant surgery is an indication for arteriography. The presence of a bruit with or without associated hypertension or deterioration of graft function requires angiographic evaluation.

In order to be diagnostically useful, particularly in differentiating between rejection and acute renal failure, a good-quality selective arteriogram in multiple projections with magnification should be obtained. The additional information obtained from selective injection directly into the internal iliac artery to which the transplant renal artery is anastomosed is worthwhile, and no additional risk is incurred when the study is done by an experienced angiographer. It is likely that the decreased amount of contrast material used with the selective technique makes for a safer procedure than the nonselective midstream injection into the aorta or common iliac artery. If multiple renal arteries are anastomosed to the common iliac or external iliac artery, however, a complete picture of the kidney can be obtained only with a common iliac injection. It is essential to know the nature of the anastomosis before undertaking arteriography. The most frequently used anastomosis is end-to-end transplanted renal artery to recipient internal iliac artery. This anastomosis lends itself readily to selective injection. In most cases, neither guide wire nor catheter needs to cross the suture line. The contralateral femoral artery is punctured using the Seldinger technique, a preshaped 5F or 6F polyethylene catheter is introduced over a guide wire, the aortic bifurcation is saddled, and the internal iliac artery to which the renal artery is attached is easily catheterized. Each injection requires no more than 10 ml. of Hypaque 75. The delivery rate and program of filming depend upon the flow rate through the kidney and the intrarenal vascular resistance. Usually all the necessary information can be obtained with two projections using no more than 20 ml. of contrast material. Contrast material should be used sparingly and judiciously, since the possibility exists of accelerating or provoking a rejection episode. In addition, high doses of contrast material injected into an already damaged kidney in a dehydrated patient may cause acute renal failure.

The causes of immediate postoperative anuria are most commonly acute rejection, acute renal failure (also known as acute tubular necrosis or acute vasomotor nephropathy), and renal artery thrombosis. These three are readily differentiated on the arteriogram. Rejection in the acute phase is primarily a vascular phenomenon, and the findings are demonstrated angiographically if good films are obtained. Acute humoral rejection causes capillary and arteriolar thrombosis at the cortical level (Fig. 27–1). With progression of the rejection process, larger and more proximal interlobar branches become occluded until complete and irreversible rejection results in thrombosis of segmental branches and ultimately of the renal artery itself (Fig. 27–2). Angiographic findings thus depend on the stage of acute rejection and whether or not there has been reversal with immunosuppressive therapy. In the early phase, when capillary and

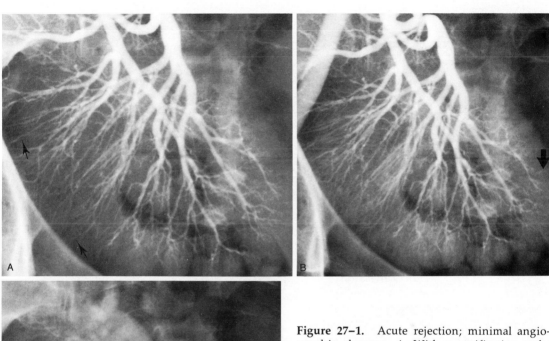

Figure 27–1. Acute rejection; minimal angiographic changes. *A,* With magnification technique, vasculitis is seen only in small vessels (arrows). There is minimal irregularity of distal interlobar branches. Straightening of interlobar vessels suggests moderate edema. *B,* At two seconds, arcuate and interlobular branches are seen, indicating cortical flow (arrow). *C,* A fairly good nephrogram is seen at four or five seconds, and the cortex is noted. Minor cortical defects suggest small infarcts (arrow) caused by small vessel occlusions. Venous drainage is noted. This kidney recovered well with increased dosage of azathioprine and prednisone.

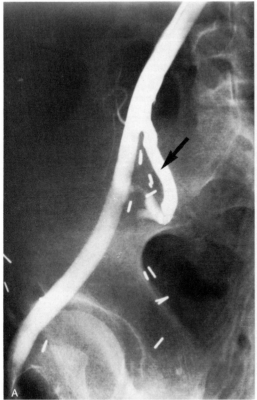

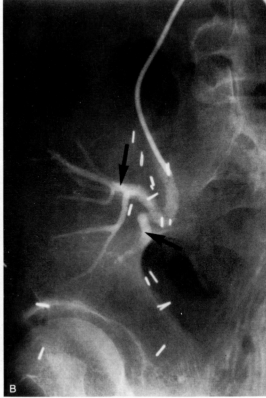

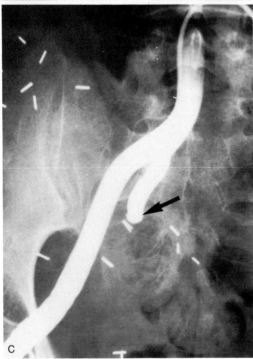

Figure 27–2. Advanced irreversible acute rejection: Angiogram. *A,* A selective injection is made into the hypogastric artery (arrow) to which the transplanted renal artery is anastomosed. There is marked increase in the intrarenal vascular resistance, with abundant reflux into the common iliac and external iliac arteries. *B,* Twenty seconds later, there is no nephrogram. The renal artery, dorsal, and ventral branches (arrows) and proximal interlobar branches still hold contrast material, and there is no flow. Although the major blood vessels are still patent, the kidney is completely infarcted and there is no hope of reversing the rejection process. Nephrectomy is unavoidable. *C,* Four days later, repeat arteriogram with injection into the common iliac artery demonstrates complete occlusion (arrow) of the renal artery attached to the hypogastric artery by end-to-end anastomosis. Renal artery occlusion secondary to rejection is demonstrated. An intact anastomosis was seen on the initial arteriogram.

arteriolar thrombosis occurs at the cortical level, the arteriogram shows a prolonged arterial clearance time, increased intrarenal vascular resistance, blanched cortex, and a featureless nephrogram. As rejection progresses and distal interlobar arteries are involved, occluded branches are seen. The interlobar arteries have an irregular, beaded appearance with areas of discrete or tubular narrowing, and vessels stretched and displaced by interstitial edema are seen. Arborization becomes progressively more disorganized. Depending on the level at which interlobar branches occlude and on the number occluded, the nephrogram will become irregular, patchy, and prolonged.

There is a correlation between the severity of angiographic changes and the degree of functional impairment (Figs. 27–3 and 27–4). To a certain extent, the arteriogram has prognostic value. The reversibility of the rejection process can be predicted by the extent of the angiographic changes. The greater the number of interlobar arteries occluded, the more proximal the occlusion, the more prolonged the arterial clearance time, and the poorer the nephrogram, the more severe is the rejection process and the less likelihood there is of reversibility (Fig. 27–5). Frequently, the angiographic appearance of the kidney provokes the decision for nephrectomy or persuades the clinician to continue a vigorous immunosuppressive regimen. Renal angiography is indicated when progressive graft deterioration has occurred and when confirmatory evidence of rejection is needed so that a timely transplant nephrectomy may be performed and immunosuppressive therapy discontinued. Text continued on page 1984

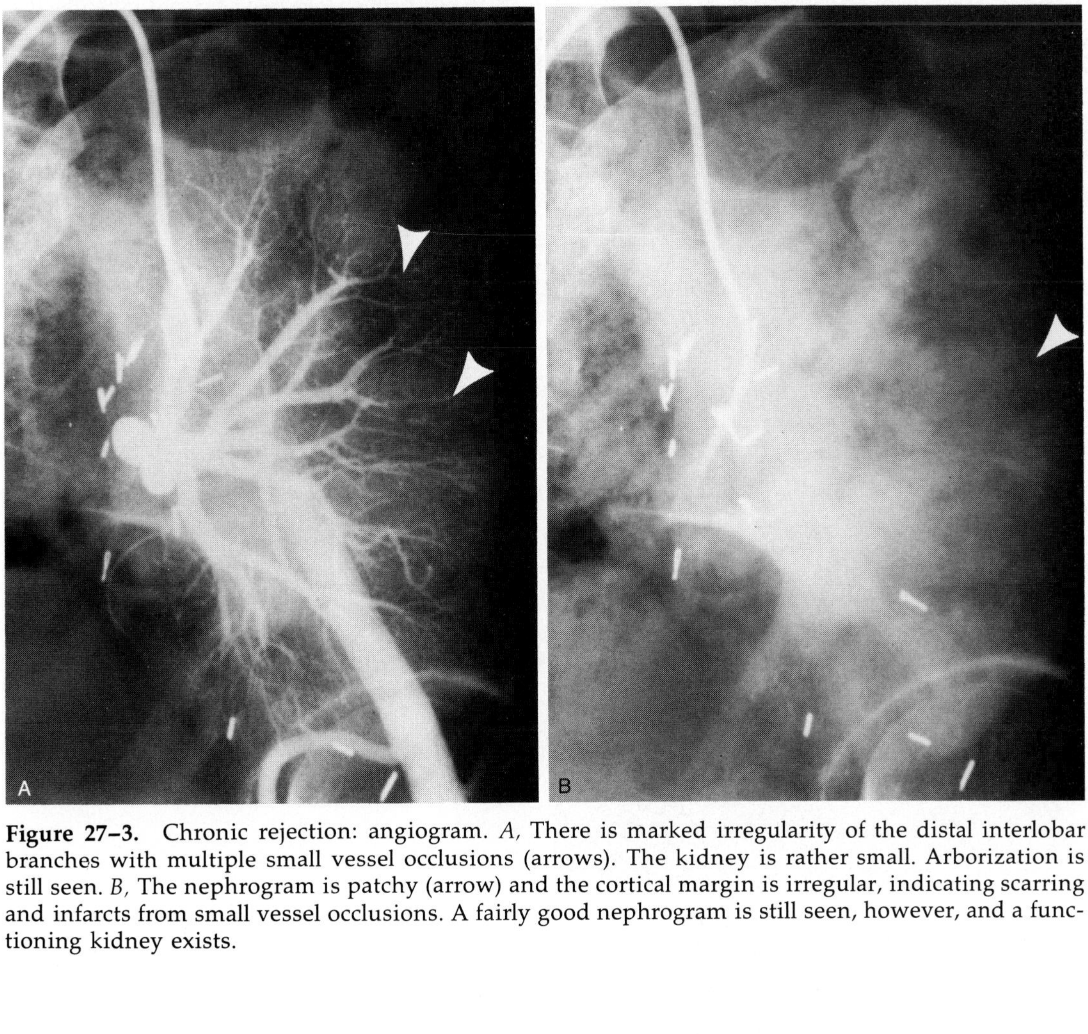

Figure 27–3. Chronic rejection: angiogram. *A,* There is marked irregularity of the distal interlobar branches with multiple small vessel occlusions (arrows). The kidney is rather small. Arborization is still seen. *B,* The nephrogram is patchy (arrow) and the cortical margin is irregular, indicating scarring and infarcts from small vessel occlusions. A fairly good nephrogram is still seen, however, and a functioning kidney exists.

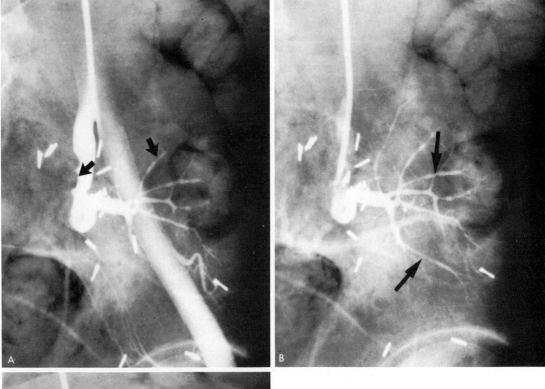

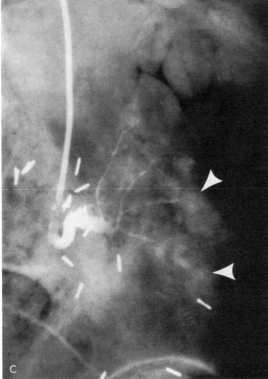

Figure 27–4. Chronic rejection: irreversible changes. *A,* The renal artery is irregular owing to perirenal fibrosis (left arrow). Proximal inter-lobar branches are markedly attenuated with an irregular, beaded appearance (right arrow). There is a marked increase in intrarenal vascular resistance with a large amount of reflux into the external iliac artery. *B,* Ten seconds later, the attenuated interlobar branches (arrows) still retain contrast material, indicating very poor blood flow to the destroyed cortex. Almost all of the distal interlobar branches are occluded, resulting in complete absence of arborization. *C,* At 20 seconds, a very poor quality nephro-gram with patchy irregularities (arrowheads) is seen. The kidney is almost completely destroyed by the chronic rejection process, and there is no possibility of salvage.

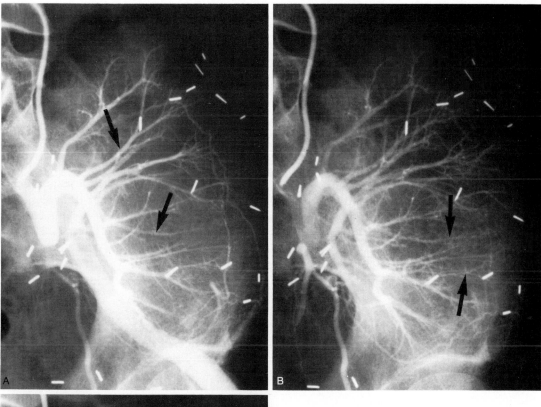

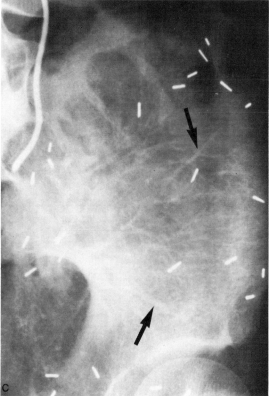

Figure 27–5. Subacute rejection: angiogram. *A,* At four weeks, selective injection into the hypogastric artery to which the transplanted renal artery is anastomosed end-to-end shows marked displacement and straightening of interlobar branches (arrows) secondary to edema. Arborization is poor, and only moderate reflux is present. *B,* Beading and irregularity (arrows) of the distal interlobar branches is seen, but the proximal branches remain intact. The extent of the cortical destruction is deceptive. *C,* An extremely poor nephrogram is seen. Veins (arrows) fill throughout the kidney, indicating arteriovenous shunting. There is no cortical blush. The rejection is irreversible.

Angiographic findings after acute humoral rejection are due to extensive occlusion of glomerular and intertubular capillaries and arterioles of the renal artery by platelet and fibrin thrombi. These develop secondary to humoral antibody attachment to cell surface histocompatibility antigens, which activates the complement system. If such a kidney is left in place for two to three weeks, extensive endothelial proliferation occurs in the larger arteries, producing serial stenoses readily identified on the arteriogram. The pathologic basis for the angiographic findings of rejection is the progressive obliteration of the microcirculation of the glomeruli.

Acute renal failure is the result of ischemic damage to the kidney. This may be an agonal event, or it may occur during perfusion and transportation of the cadaver kidney, or it may happen during the transplantation procedure. Acute renal failure is the most likely cause of anuria or oliguria when it occurs immediately following surgery, and spontaneous reversal occurs without treatment. Acute rejection is most likely when oliguria or renal function is delayed more than 48 hours after transplantation in a patient whose kidney initially functioned well and in whom there is no other demonstrable cause for decline in renal function. Other signs of rejection, such as fever, leukocytosis, hypertension, and swelling, are usually present.

In acute renal failure, the angiogram has many normal findings (Fig. 27–6). Vasculitis is absent. The appearance of the arborization is remarkably normal, except that the cortex is blanched owing to reduced cortical perfusion and the nephrogram is featureless because of absence of cortical blush. The interlobar arteries are smooth and regular. There is no beading, and no occlusions are seen. There is no excretion of contrast material in the collecting system. Flow is decreased, and there is some increased intrarenal vascular resistance as evidenced by reflux into the external iliac artery. Renal vein opacification is delayed.

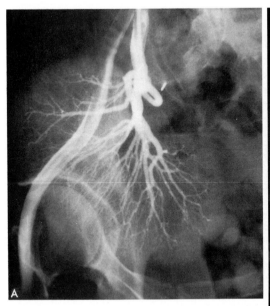
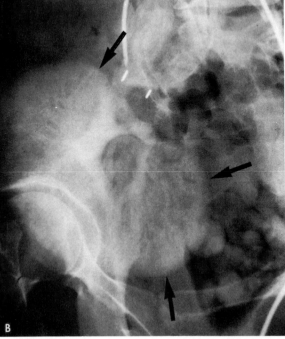

Figure 27–6. Acute renal failure. *A,* At three weeks, a normal-sized kidney with minimal edema and fairly good arborization is seen in spite of absence of urine output and a creatinine of 12. This represents acute renal failure rather than rejection. *B,* A good nephrogram with smooth cortical margin (arrows) is seen. The kidney has a rather poor corticomedullary junction, suggesting poor cortical flow.

Acute renal failure usually occurs only in kidneys transplanted from cadavers and is related to the agonal events in the cadaver of origin and to the method of harvest and preservation. Renal ischemia is thought to be the cause of acute renal failure. Acute renal failure generally subsides without treatment, and only watchful waiting is required. A rejection episode, on the other hand, requires increased immunosuppression, increasing the risk of infection and all the other problems resulting from high doses of corticosteroids and antimetabolites. The correct diagnosis is crucial, but the decision is difficult. The issue is further confused because an episode of rejection may precipitate acute renal failure or acute renal failure may precede rejection.

Ninety per cent of the cadaver kidneys undergo rejection in one form or another. During the first postoperative week, if the kidney never begins to function or after a short period of function begins to fail, the very difficult distinction between rejection and acute renal failure must be made. Acute renal failure presents as poor renal function or reduction in function in the first or second postoperative day. Fever and kidney tenderness — the symptoms of rejection — are usually absent.

Other than angiography, the diagnostic modalities available for differentiating between acute renal failure and rejection are intravenous pyelography, radionuclide studies, and sonography. Evaulation of the graft is divided into perfusion and functional components. Technetium pertechnetate flow studies may be used to evaluate vascular integrity. The normal perfusion time is five seconds. The visualization time of the kidney may be compared to that of the iliac artery and the radioactivity of the kidney to that of the adjacent tissue. Iodohippurate may be used to assess function of the graft. The kidney extraction time is 30 seconds. Maximum intensity is seen at between two and five minutes. Excretion in ureter and bladder occurs in 12 to 15 minutes, and at 30 minutes the kidney should have almost completely cleared the isotope, which is now in the bladder. Sonography may be used to evaluate increase in kidney size precisely. The echo pattern may delineate the kidney margin and localize abnormal fluid collections (see Transplant Kidney, p. 79, Chapter 3 and also Figures 3–35 to 3–40).

Neither radionuclide studies nor sonography differentiate between acute renal failure and rejection in the postoperative period. Increase in size occurs in both conditions. The technetium pertechnetate scan shows decreased opacification time and decreased clearance by the kidney. The iodohippurate scan shows decreased uptake, prolonged accumulation, and delayed excretion from the kidney in both cases. There is some evidence that cortical perfusion is greater in acute renal failure than during rejection, but this has not yet been confirmed. Retrospectively, improved renal function without increased immunosuppression suggests acute renal failure.

Vascular complications have been reported in as many as 30 per cent of patients after transplantation. The most common problem is renal artery stenosis, but arterial occlusion, either due to technical problems or as the ultimate end point of rejection, may occur. Anastomotic dehiscence, usually from infection and venous thrombosis, is a rare complication. Renal artery stenosis is associated with hypertension, deteriorating function, and, sometimes, a bruit. The anastomotic site, the hypogastric artery proximally, the renal artery distally, or intrarenal segmental branches may be stenotic, depending on the etiology of the problem. The rejection process itself may cause stensois by provoking an exuberant fibrous reaction either at the anastomotic site or distal to it. The stenosis may be discrete and bandlike or long and tubular, involving segmental branches. Stenoses at the anastomotic site may be technical, owing to a discrepancy in the size of the anatomosed vessels, the suture line, malrotation of the renal artery, or volvulus of the transplanted kidney. In the immediate postoperative period, stenosis may be caused by extrinsic compression at the anatomosis from edema or a hematoma.

Late in the history of the transplanted kidney, stenosis at the origin of the hypogastric artery may be caused by the formation of an atherosclerotic plaque. Stenosis proximal or distal to the suture line may result from the use of vascular clamps or from trauma and tears in the intima during perfusion.[16]

In his review of 306 renal transplants, Lacombe[28] found renal artery stenosis in 38 cases. In all cases, the diagnosis was made based on the arteriogram, the primary indication being refractory hypertension. This author advocates routine renal angiography of all transplant recipients periodically as a screening procedure, since the stenosis can in most cases be surgically repaired, curing the hypertension and preventing deterioration of function. He suggests that the incidence of renal artery stenosis in all transplant recipients is as high as 25 per cent and that normotensive patients with stenosis should have surgical repair to improve graft survival. The presence of renal artery stenosis may lead to subsequent deterioration of graft function with ultimate loss of the transplanted kidney.

There are sound arguments favoring an immunologic cause for renal artery stenosis. Similarities are found in the histologic changes in the stenosed renal arteries and the vascular lesions of renal allograft rejection. The two have in common subintimal fibrosis and intimal proliferation. In addition, there are some cases in which vascular lesions of allograft rejection with identical histologic appearances affect the whole arterial tree from main renal artery to renal capillaries. The first stage in the process seems to be the deposition of fibrin and platelets on the endothelium, leading to endothelial proliferation and intimal fibrosis. Thus, the development of renal artery stenosis may be attributed to the rejection process as well as to the trauma associated with kidney harvesting, preservation, and surgical anastomosis.

Although some instances of transplant renal artery stenosis are due to technical faults,[25] most are the result of acute angulation caused by dense periarterial fibrous tissue or by segmental subintimal fibrous thickening and cellular proliferation of the transplant renal artery. This is possibly a manifestation of the rejection phenomenon. Angulation stenosis results from a sharp angulation or kinking of the vessels at the end-to-end anastomosis of hypogastric to renal artery, resulting in dense adhesions that bind the renal artery posteriorly where it crosses the external iliac artery. Lysis of the adhesions may effect a cure.

Hypertension is found in 37 per cent of post-transplant patients. Etiologic factors include fluid overload associated with steroid therapy, acute rejection episodes, recurrence of primary renal disease in the transplanted kidney, production of excessive renin by the host kidney when bilateral nephrectomy is not done, or transplant renal artery stenosis. Hypertension from renal artery stenosis responds poorly to medical management.

Anuria immediately after transplantation may be due to acute humoral rejection, acute renal failure, renal artery thrombosis, urinary leakage, ureteral or urethral obstruction, or pressure from a lymphocele or a hematoma. A renal scintigram should precede the arteriogram because it will demonstrate ureteral leak. If absent or poor blood flow is demonstrated, then the diagnosis of acute rejection or renal artery thrombosis is confirmed or excluded by renal angiography. Functional deterioration of the graft, in which confirmatory evidence of rejection or renal artery stenosis is necessary in order to proceed with definitive surgery, is sufficient indication for an arteriogram. Hypertension and anuria also are persuasive reasons for arteriography. Vascular complications commonly present with marked decrease in graft function or with the appearance or exacerbation of hypertension. Angiography permits recognition of common causes of post-transplant dysfunction, including acute renal failure, rejection, ureteral obstruction, renal artery occlusion, and renal vein thrombosis. Although angiography is an invasive procedure, it enables diagnosis of all the common causes of post-transplant dysfunction. In contrast with isotope techniques, angiography differentiates arterial or venous obstruction from acute rejection. In most cases, it distinguishes acute renal failure from acute rejection. In addition, it is of prognostic value in predicting irreversibility when cortical necrosis is present.

The most important findings of histologically acute rejection are interstitial and perivascualr infiltrates of mononuclear cells and fibrinoid necrosis of small arteries, arterioles, and glomerular capillaries. This is associated with marked interstitial edema. Vascular changes may lead to renal ischemia, resulting in cortical necrosis, hemorrhages, and infarcts.

Angiographic changes reflect well the pathologic anatomic changes. The kidney is enlarged and edematous, vasculitis produces vessel stenosis or obliteration, arterial washout time is prolonged, poor cortical perfusion is evident from sparsely filled cortical vessels and ill-defined corticomedullary junction, and the nephrogram is poor. Concentration of contrast material in veins is usually so low that venous filling cannot be recognized. Simultaneous filling of arteries and veins may occur, however. This is a sign of redistribution of intrarenal blood flow, and it indicates severe cortical ischemia.

Abnormal findings of prognostic value on the arteriogram include:[23] (1) large vessel vasculitis, (2) prolonged arterial washout time, (3) poor filling of cortical vessels, (4) ill-defined corticomedullary junction, (5) poor nephrogram, and (6) arteriovenous shunting (see Fig. 5). Involvement of large vessels by irreversible vasculitis and arteriovenous shunting are indicative of severe cortical ischemia and are prognostically bad signs. A mild or focal rejection showing few vascular changes, normal arterial washout time, relatively good filling of cortical vessels, a good nephrogram, and appreciable venous filling without shunting usually indicates reversible rejection.

The newest method for treating transplant renal artery stenosis is percutaneous transluminal balloon dilatation.[27] This technique, which is applicable to transplanted kidneys as well as to native kidneys with renal artery stenosis, works admirably in controlling hypertension and preserving renal function.

References

1. Advisory Committee to the Renal Transplant Registry: The 13th Report of the Human Renal Transplant Registry. Transplant. Proc. 9:9–26, 1977.
2. Bartrum, R. J., Smith, E. H., D'Orsi, C. J., et al.: Evaluation of renal transplants with ultrasound. Radiology 118:405–410, 1976.
3. Beachley, M. C., Pierce, J. C., Boykin, J. V., et al.: The angiographic evaluation of human renal allotransplants. Arch. Surg. 111:134–142, 1976.
4. Becker, J. A., and Kutcher, R.: Urologic complications of renal transplantation. Semin. Roentgenol. 13(4):341–349, 1978.
5. Bennett, W. M., McDonald, W. J., Lawson, R. K., et al.: Post-transplant hypertension: studies of cortical blood flow and the renal pressor system. Kidney Int. 6:99–108, 1974.
6. Carrel, A.: La technique operatoire des anastomoses vasculaires et transplantation des visceres. Lyon Med. 98:859, 1902.
7. Cattran, D. C., Fenton, S. S., Wilson, D. R., et al.: Defective triglyceride removal in lipemia associated with peritoneal dialysis and hemodialysis. Ann. Intern. Med. 85:29–33, 1976.
8. Converse, J. D., and Casson, P. R.: The historical background of transplantation. In Rapaport, F. T., and Duasset, J. (eds.): Human Transplantation. New York, Grune & Stratton, 1968, p. 6.
9. Cook, G. T., Cant, J. D., Crassweller, P. O., et al.: Urinary fistulas ater renal transplantation. J. Urol. 118:20–21, 1977.
10. Corry, R. J., Thompson, J. S., Freeman, R. M., et al.: Critical comparison of renal transplant survival between recipients of live related donor and cadaver organs. Surg. Gynecol. Obstet. 146:519, 1978.
11. David, D. S., Sakai, S., Brennan, B. L., et al.: Hypercalcemia after renal transplantation. N. Engl. J. Med. 289:398, 1977.
12. Ehrlich, R. M., and Smith, R. B.: Surgical complications of renal transplantation. Urology 10:43–56, 1977.

13. Ehrlich, R. M. (ed.): Renal transplantation: Medical aspects. Part I. Urology 9 (Suppl. 6), 1977.
14. Ehrlich, R. M. (ed.): Renal transplantation: Surgical aspects. Part II. Urology 10(Suppl. 1), 1977.
15. Foley, W. D., Bookstein, J. J., Tweist, M., et al.: Arteriography of renal transplants. Radiology 116:271–277, 1975.
16. Goldman, M. H., Vineyard, G. C., Lakes, H., et al.: A twenty year survey of arterial complications of renal transplantation. Surg. Gynecol. Obstet. 141:758, 1975.
17. Goodwin, W. E., Kaufman, J. J., Mims, M. M., et al.: Human renal transplantation. I. Clinical experiences with 6 cases of renal homotransplantation. J. Urol. 89:13–24, 1963.
18. Groth, C. G.: Landmarks in clinical renal transplantation. Surg. Gynecol. Obstet. 134:323–328, 1972.
19. Hoover, R., and Fraumeni, J. F.: Risk of cancer in renal-transplant recipients. Lancet 2:55–57, 1973.
20. Hopewell, J., Calne, R. Y., and Beswick, I.: Three clinical cases of renal transplantation. Br. Med. J. 1:411–413, 1964.
21. Hume, D. M., Merrill, J. P., Miller, B. F., et al.: Experiences with renal homotransplantation in the human; report of nine cases. J. Clin. Invest. 34:327–382, 1955.
22. Julien, P. J., Goldberg, H. I., Margulis, A. R., et al.: Gastrointestinal complications following renal transplantation. Radiology 117:37, 1975.
23. Kaude, J. V., and Hawkins, I. F., Jr.: Angiography of renal transplant. Radiol. Clin. North Am. 14:295–308, 1976.
24. Kaude, J. V., Stone, M., Fuller, T. J., et al.: Papillary necrosis in kidney transplant patients. Radiology 120:69–74, 1976.
25. Kauffman, H. M., Sampson, D., Fox, P. S., et al.: Prevention of transplant renal artery stenosis. Surgery 81:161, 1977.
26. Koehler, P. R., Kanemoto, H. H., and Maxwell, J. G.: Ultrasonic "B" scanning in the diagnosis of complications in renal transplant patients. Radiology 119:661–664, 1976.
27. Kuhlmann, U., Vetter, W., Furrer, J., et al.: Renovascular hypertension: treatment by percutaneous transluminal dilatation. Ann. Intern. Med. 92:1–6, 1980.
28. Lacombe, M.: Arterial stenosis complicating renal transplantation in man: study of 38 cases. Ann. Surg. 181:283–288, 1975.
29. Lawler, R. H., West, J. W., McNulty, P. H., et al.: Homotransplantation of the kidney in the human. J.A.M.A. 144:844–845, 1950.
30. Lee, D. B. N., Prompt, C. A., Upham, A. T., et al.: Medical complications of renal transplantation. Urology 9 (Suppl. 6):7–30, 1977.
31. Lee, H. M., Madge, G. E., Gerardo, M. P., et al.: Surgical complications of renal transplant recipients. Surg. Clin. North Am. 58(2):285–304, 1978.
32. Leapman, S. B., Vidne, B. A., Butt, K. M., et al.: Nephrolithiasis and nephrocalcinosis after renal transplantation: a case report and review of the literature. J. Urol. 115:129–132, 1976.
33. Lindfors, O., Laasonen, L., Fyhrquist, F., et al.: Renal artery stenosis in hypertensive renal transplant recipients. J. Urol. 118:240–243, 1977.
34. Lipshultz, L. I., Wein, A. J., Arger, P. H., et al.: Post-transplantation lymphocyst: use of ultrasound as adjunct in diagnosis. Radiology 7:624, 1976.
35. Margules, R. M., Belzer, F. O., and Kountz, S. L.: Surgical correction of renovascular hypertension following allotransplantation. Arch. Surg. 106:13–16, 1973.
36. McHenry, M. C., Braun, W. E., Popowniak, K. L., et al.: Septicemia in renal transplant recipients. Urol. Clin. North Am. 3:647–666, 1976.
37. Medawar, P. B.: Immunity to homologous grafted skin. I. The suppression of cell division in grafts transplanted to immunized animals. Br. J. Exp. Pathol. 27:15–24, 1946.
38. Monaco, A. P., Campion, J. P., and Kapnick, S. J.: Clinical use of antilymphocyte globulin. Transplant. Proc. 9:1007–1018, 1977.
39. Mott, C., and Schreiber, M. H.: Lymphoceles following renal transplantation. Am. J. Roentgenol. 122:821–827, 1974.
40. Murray, J. E., Merrill, J. P., and Harrison, J. H.: Renal homotransplantation in identical twins. Surg. Forum 6:432, 1955.
41. Murray, J. E., Merrill, J. P., and Harrison, J. H.: Kidney transplantation between seven pairs of identical twins. Ann. Surg. 148:343, 1958.
42. Murray, J. E., Merrill, J. P., Dammin, G. J., et al.: Kidney transplantation in modified recipients. Ann. Surg. 156:337–355, 1962.
43. Najarian, J. S., Kjellstrand, C. M., and Simmons, R. L.: High risk patients in renal transplantation. Transplant. Proc. 9:107–111, 1977.
44. Nelson, J., Bragg, D. G., and Armstrong, J. D., Jr.: Cardiopulmonary complications of renal transplantation. Semin. Roentgenol. 13(4):311–318, 1978.
45. Owens, M. L., Wilson, S. E., Salzman, R., et al.: Gastrointestinal complications after renal transplantation. Arch. Surg. 111:467–471, 1976.
46. Palmer, J. M., and Chatterjee, S. N.: Urologic complications in renal transplantation. Surg. Clin. North Am. 58:305–319, 1978.
47. Penn, I.: Tumor incidence in human allograft recipients. Transplant. Proc. 11(1):1047–1051, 1979.
48. Penn, I.: Development of cancer as a complication of clinical transplantation. Transplant. Proc. 9:1121–1127, 1977.
49. Perloff, L. J., Chon, H., Petrella, E. J., et al.: Acute colitis in the renal allograft recipient. Am. J. Surg. 183:77–83, 1976.

50. Phillips, J. F., Neiman, H. L., and Brown, T. L.: Ultrasound diagnosis of post-transplant renal lymphocele. Am. J. Roentgenol. 126:1194–1196, 1976.
51. Pletka, P. G., Strom, T. B., Hampers, C. L., et al.: Secondary hyperthyroidism in human kidney transplant recipients. Nephron 17:371–381, 1976.
52. Prompt, C. A., Lee, D. B. N., Upham, A. T., et al.: Medical complications of renal transplantation. II. Noninfectious complications in recipients. Urology 9(Suppl. 6):32–48, 1977.
53. Resnick, D.: Abnormalities of bone and soft tissue following renal transplantation. Semin. Roentgenol. 13(4):329–336, 1978.
54. Rosenberg, J. C., Arnstein, A. R., Ing, T. S., et al.: Calculi complicating a renal transplant. Am. J. Surg. 129:326–330, 1975.
55. Ruiz, J. O., Simmons, R. L., Callender, C. O., et al.: Steroid diabetes in renal transplant recipients. Pathogenic factors and prognosis. Surgery 73:759–765, 1973.
56. Salvatierra, O., Jr., Olcott, C., IV, Ament, W. J., Jr., et al.: Urological complications of renal transplantation can be prevented or controlled. J. Urol. 117:421–424, 1977.
57. Schiff, M., Jr., McGuire, E. J., Weiss, R. M., et al.: Management of urinary fistulas after renal transplantation. J. Urol. 115:251–256, 1976.
58. Schwartz, R., and Dameshek, W.: Drug-induced immunological tolerance. Nature 183:1682–1683, 1959.
59. Simmons, R. L., Payne, W. D., Sutherland, D. E. R., et al.: Special problems in diabetic renal transplantation. Urol. Clin. North Am. 3:691–699, 1976.
60. Smellie, V. M., Vinik, M., and Hume, D. M.: Angiographic investigation of complicating human renal transplantation. Surg. Gynecol. Obstet. 5:963, 1969.
61. Smith, R. B., Cosimi, A. B., Lordon, R., et al.: Diagnosis and management of arterial stenosis causing hypertension after successful renal transplantation. J. Urol. 115:639–642, 1976.
62. Starzl, T. E., Marchioro, T. L., and Waddel, W. R.: The reversal of rejection in human renal homografts with subsequent development of homograft tolerance. Surg. Gynecol. Obstet. 117:385–395, 1963.
63. Stuart, F. P.: Selection, preparation and management of kidney transplant recipients. Med. Clin. North Am. 62(6):1381–1397, 1978.
64. Terasaki, P. I., Vredevoe, D. L., Mickey, M. R., et al.: Serotyping for homotransplantation. VI. Selection of kidney donors for thirty-two recipients. Ann. N.Y. Acad. Sci. 129:500–520, 1966.
65. Texter, J. H., and Haden, H.: Scintiphotography in the early diagnosis following renal transplantation. J. Urol. 116:547–549, 1976.
66. Thomas, F. T., and Lee, H. M.: Factors in the differential rate of arteriosclerosis between long surviving renal transplant recipients and dialysis patients. Ann. Surg. 184:342–351, 1976.
67. Thompson, W. M., Meyers, W., Seigler, H. F., et al.: Gastrointestinal complications of renal transplantation. Semin. Roentgenol. 13(4):319–328, 1978.
68. Vinde, B. A., Leapman, S. B., Butt, K. M., et al.: Vascular complications in human renal transplantations. Surgery 79:77, 1976.
69. Voronoy, U.: Sobre el bloqueo del aparato reticuloendotelial del hombre en algunas formas de intoxicacion por el sublimado y sobre la transplantacion del rinon cadaverico como metodo de tratamiento de la anuaria consecutiva a aquella into icacion. Siglo. Med. 97:296, 1936.
70. Waksman, B. H., Arbouys, S., and Arnason, B. G.: The use of specific "lymphocyte antisera" to inhibit hypersensitive reactions of the delayed type. J. Exp. Med. 114:997–1022, 1961.
71. Williams, G. M.: Status of renal transplantation today. Surg. Clin. North Am. 58(2):273–284, 1978.

Part II

Liver Homotransplantation

JOHN O. TAUBMAN, M.B., Ch.B., M.R.C.P.E., D.M.R.D., F.R.C.R.

WILLIAM C. KLINGENSMITH III, M.D.

INTRODUCTION

Since the first liver replacement with a homograft on March 1, 1963,[18] more than 176 liver transplants have been performed at the University of Colorado Medical Center. The introduction of newer surgical and imaging techniques in recent years has resulted in a significant reduction in lethal complications, particularly biliary obstruction.[22] Currently, emphasis is being placed upon the role of radionuclide studies, transhepatic cholangiography (THC), endoscopic retrograde cholangiopancreatography (ERCP), ultrasound, and computerized tomography (CT).

PREOPERATIVE EVALUATION OF DONORS

Brain Death

Unlike renal transplantation, liver homotransplantation is completely dependent on cadaver donors. The establishment of brain death is essential in obtaining donor livers that have not been damaged by prolonged agonal ischemia.[21] Radionuclide evaluation of cerebral perfusion in the anterior projection is a reliable method of confirming brain death.[14] The cardinal findings are the absence of the anterior and middle cerebral arteries during the arterial phase of the first circulation and, most importantly, the absence of activity in the superior sagittal sinus in the anterior equilibrium image (Fig. 27–7).

Aortography

When time permits, a single high abdominal aortic injection should be made to reveal any anomaly of hepatic arterial supply and to identify unsuspected vascular or hepatic disease. A second injection filmed in an oblique projection may be necessary,

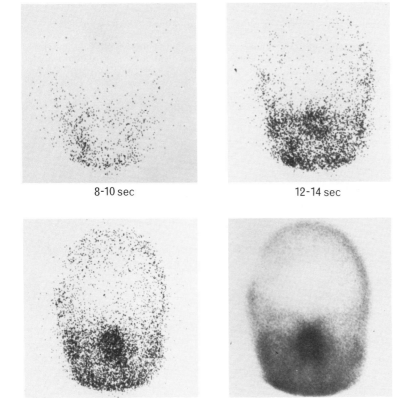

8-10 sec

12-14 sec

20-22 sec

1 min

Figure 27–7. Anterior cerebral perfusion study of a patient who had shot himself in the head. The two-second images at 8 to 10, 12 to 14, and 20 to 22 seconds after injection demonstrate flow in the external carotid system to the scalp without evidence of anterior or middle cerebral artery flow. The one-minute image shows no evidence of activity in the superior sagittal sinus. There is decreased scalp activity on the right side of the head in the region of the gunshot wound.

but selective studies should be avoided. Projections should include the renal arterial supply, in anticipation of renal transplantation. The recognition of anomalies of vascular supply prior to surgery reduces operative time. If there is a triple supply to the liver (as, for example, when the left gastric artery supplies the left lobe from an aortic origin, and the celiac and superior mesenteric arteries supply separate branches to the right lobe), a decision may be made preoperatively to abandon attempts at transplantation. When there is a double supply (for example, from the celiac and superior mesenteric arteries), vascular reconstruction may permit transplantation. No attempt is made to evaluate the portal venous system.

PREOPERATIVE EVALUATION OF RECIPIENTS

Extent of Liver Disease

Radionuclide studies play a prominent role in the preoperative evaluation of potential liver transplant recipients. To establish whether the patient's liver disease is terminal ^{99m}Tc sulfur colloid studies of phagocytic clearance by the hepatic Kupffer cells and ^{99m}Tc-N, α (2, 6-diethylacetanilide) iminodiacetic acid (^{99m}Tc diethyl IDA) studies of the hepatobiliary system are employed. In the ^{99m}Tc sulfur colloid study the findings of mottled liver activity, with relatively decreased clearance compared with that of the spleen, a small right hepatic lobe; a large spleen; relatively increased bone marrow clearance; and marked activity in the lungs indicate severe liver disease (Fig. 27–8).[9] In the

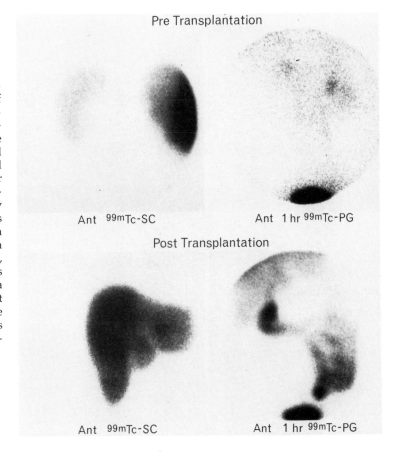

Pre Transplantation

Ant 99mTc-SC   Ant 1 hr 99mTc-PG

Post Transplantation

Ant 99mTc-SC   Ant 1 hr 99mTc-PG

Figure 27–8. Prior to liver transplantation, the anterior image of the ^{99m}Tc sulfur colloid (^{99m}Tc-SC) study demonstrates a shrunken liver with very little clearance of ^{99m}Tc-SC and an enlarged spleen with relatively increased activity. The anterior one-hour image from the ^{99m}Tc pyridoxylidegeneglutamate (^{99m}Tc-PG) study of the hepatobiliary system shows a large amount of renal excretion without identifiable activity in the liver. Post-transplantation, good clearance of ^{99m}Tc-SC is demonstrated in the liver (a splenectomy was performed at the time of transplantation). The one-hour ^{99m}Tc-PG study shows normal hepatic clearance and excretion of activity.

hepatobiliary study the findings of poor clearance of radiotracer, as judged by the liver-to-background ratio in early images, and markedly delayed or absent excretion of radiotracer into the intestine indicate severe liver disease (see Fig. 27–8). In patients being considered for transplantation because of primary hepatic malignancy, it is important to establish that the malignancy is not resectable. By demonstrating whether the malignancy spares one or more hepatic segments, ^{99m}Tc sulfur colloid studies are helpful in making this determination. If the malignancy is not resectable, it is important to exclude the diagnosis of asymptomatic bone metastases with a ^{99m}Tc phosphate bone study.

Biliary Tract Anatomy

The use of endoscopic retrograde cholangiopancreatography (ERCP) on the recipient identifies unsuspected disease or anomaly of the distal biliary tract.[21] The anatomy of the distal biliary tract in the recipient is of particular importance when a common duct–to–common duct anastomosis is performed.

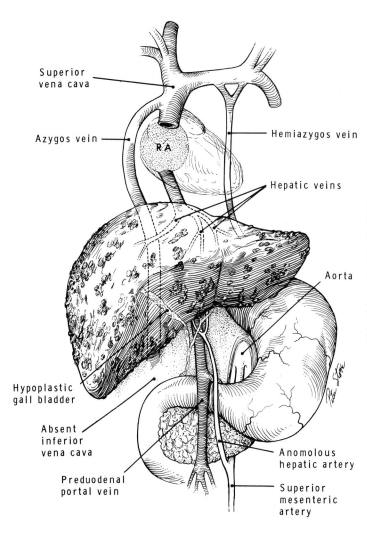

Figure 27–9. Diagram of the composite vascular malformation, consisting of absent inferior vena cava, preduodenal portal vein, and anomalous origin of the hepatic artery, encountered in three children with biliary atresia. (*From* Lilly, J. R., and Starzl, T. E.: Liver transplantation in children with biliary atresia and vascular anomalies. J. Pediatr. Surg. 9:707–714, 1974. Reproduced by permission.)

Inferior Venacavography

Patency of the inferior vena cava must be confirmed when the clinical situation indicates the possibility of the Budd-Chiari syndrome.[16] The prior recognition of the absence of the inferior vena cava combined with azygos continuation is important in infants and children who are to receive a liver transplant for biliary atresia. The association of extrahepatic biliary atresia with a composite vascular anomaly has been described.[13] These patients may have an absent inferior vena cava, azygos continuation, preduodenal portal vein, and anomalous origin of the hepatic artery (Fig. 27–9). In a large series of patients with biliary atresia, those patients with vascular anomalies also had visceral malformations.[12] Barium studies to detect gut malrotation, radionuclide studies to detect liver asymmetry or polysplenia, and inferior venacavography may identify children who have this composite anomaly, which may be lethal at surgery.

Through careful scrutiny one may detect the absence of the normal retrocardiac caval shadow on lateral chest films and an enlarged azygos vein on frontal chest films (Fig. 27–10).[23]

INTRAOPERATIVE EVALUATION OF RECIPIENT AND DONOR BILIARY TRACTS

Cholangiography

Operative cholangiography is not used routinely but may be important when a biliary tract anomaly is suspected upon exploration of the donor or recipient, perhaps to confirm preoperative ERCP findings. Low insertion of the cystic duct must be

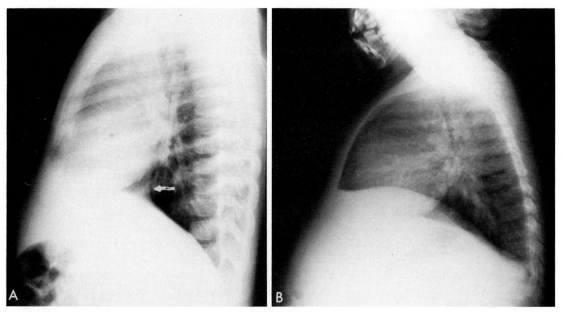

Figure 27–10. Lateral chest film showing the absence of the inferior vena cava. A, Retrocardiac density due to a normally located inferior vena cava (arrow). B, The retrocardiac space is "empty" owing to the absence of the inferior vena cava. (*From* Lilly, J. R., and Starzl, T. E.: Liver transplantation in children with biliary atresia and vascular anomalies. J. Pediatr. Surg. 9:707–714, 1974. Reproduced by permission.)

determined by direct inspection or cholangiography when drainage via the donor cystic duct and gallbladder, or via a common duct–to–common duct anastomosis, is planned. An anomalous double-barreled channel of cystic and common duct has led to complications in several patients.[21]

POSTOPERATIVE EVALUATION OF RECIPIENTS

Radionuclide Imaging and Normal Postoperative Appearance

We routinely evaluate our postoperative liver transplant patients with both ^{99m}Tc sulfur colloid and ^{99m}Tc diethyl IDA studies. The ^{99m}Tc sulfur colloid study provides better spatial resolution for the detection of focal intrahepatic lesions. The ^{99m}Tc diethyl IDA study evaluates hepatocyte clearance and biliary tract patency.

A normal postoperative ^{99m}Tc sulfur colloid study shows a homogeneous distribution of activity in the liver. The size of the transplanted liver is initially determined by the size of the donor. Splenectomy is often performed at the time of transplantation; when the spleen is not removed and is enlarged preoperatively, it may remain enlarged. Preoperative increased lung and bone marrow activity usually disappears or is significantly decreased following successful liver transplantation.

A normal postoperative ^{99m}Tc diethyl IDA study demonstrates a high liver-to-background activity ratio that peaks within five minutes, and an intestinal activity that peaks within ten minutes. Normal nondilated intrahepatic ducts are occasionally visualized.

Acute Hepatocyte Necrosis

Acute tubular necrosis is a frequent complication following renal transplantation. The frequency of acute hepatocyte necrosis secondary to prolonged warm ischemic time during liver transplantation is unknown. The typical findings in acute tubular necrosis are a marked decrease in renal clearance and relatively preserved perfusion. Hepatic flow studies are usually not performed, because only 6 mCi of ^{99m}Tc diethyl IDA or ^{99m}Tc sulfur colloid are used. In one of our patients, however, a ^{99m}Tc diethyl IDA study was done within 24 hours of a difficult transplantation that resulted in prolonged warm ischemia of the donor liver. Hepatocyte clearance was markedly decreased. Inspection of the transplanted liver through the fresh surgical wound at this time revealed a normally perfused pink liver, suggesting that this patient had acute hepatocyte necrosis.

Rejection

Although rejection is less common in liver transplant patients than in renal transplant patients, it is still a frequent complication.[20] Both phagocytic and hepatocytic function are affected by rejection, but ^{99m}Tc diethyl IDA hepatobiliary studies are more sensitive to the presence of rejection or a change in the degree of rejection. Figure 27–11 shows one patient who had moderate rejection (total bilirubin = 13.4 mg/dL) 17 days post-transplantation and 23 days later, after increased immunosuppressive therapy, showed improved liver function (total bilirubin = 5.0 mg/dL). The ^{99m}Tc diethyl IDA study shows significant improvement whereas the ^{99m}Tc sulfur colloid study is

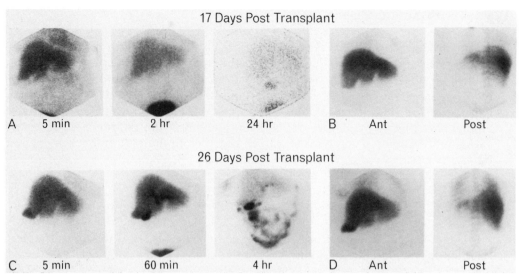

Figure 27–11. Rejection: radionuclide studies. Seventeen days following transplantation the patient was undergoing moderate rejection (total bilirubin = 13.4 mg/dL). The ^{99m}Tc-diethyl-IDA images (*A*) demonstrate poor clearance of radiotracer at 5 minutes, no intestinal activity at 2 hours, and only a small amount of intestinal activity at 24 hours. The ^{99m}Tc sulfur colloid images (*B*) show mild increased bone marrow activity. Twenty-six days post-transplantation, rejection had subsided (total bilirubin = 5.0 mg/dL). The ^{99m}Tc-diethyl-IDA images (*C*) demonstrate improved clearance at 5 minutes, initial extrahepatic activity at 60 minutes, and a large amount of small bowel activity at 4 hours. The ^{99m}Tc sulfur colloid images (*D*) show no change in bone marrow activity and a mild increase in lung activity.

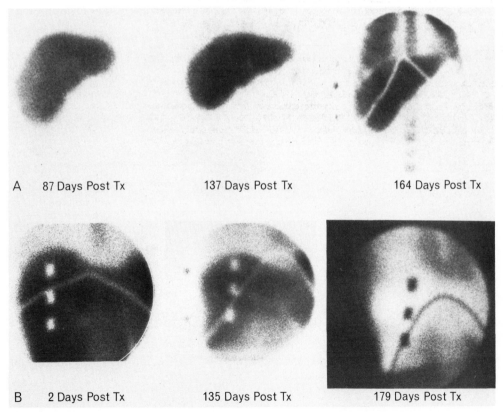

Figure 27–12. Rejection. Serial ^{99m}Tc sulfur colloid studies are shown in two liver transplant patients (*A* and *B*) who died of liver failure secondary to rejection nine and ten days, respectively, after the last images. There is markedly increased lung activity only in the last study before death.

1995

essentially unchanged (see Fig. 27–11). Although the ^{99m}Tc sulfur colloid studies often do not reflect change in the degree of rejection to the extent that the ^{99m}Tc diethyl IDA studies do, they sometimes signal the terminal stage of rejection by demonstrating a relatively large amount of ^{99m}Tc sulfur colloid in the lungs (Fig. 27–12).[6, 8, 9] Change in hepatocyte function secondary to rejection is most easily evaluated in serial ^{99m}Tc diethyl IDA studies by simple visual determination of the ratio of hepatic activity to background activity at some standardized time before the radiotracer has entered the biliary tract (for example, two to five minutes).

Hepatitis

Hepatitis and other diffuse diseases of hepatocytes are indistinguishable from rejection in ^{99m}Tc diethyl IDA and ^{99m}Tc sulfur colloid studies.

Vascular Complications

Angiography is necessary when arterial or venous occlusion is suspected.

Recurrent Tumors

In patients receiving liver transplants for hepatoma or cholangiocarcinoma, persistent tumor may invade the transplanted liver.[20, 24]

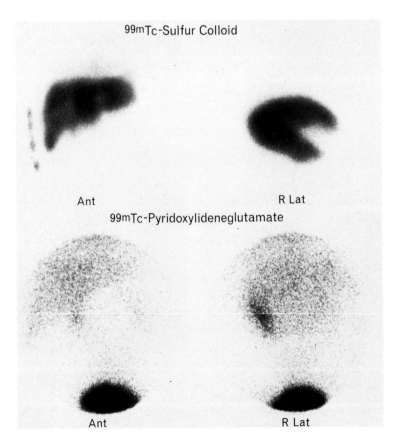

Figure 27–13. Hepatic abscess. Anterior and right lateral ^{99m}Tc sulfur colloid images clearly demonstrate a right hepatic lobe lesion, which proved to be an abscess. The hepatobiliary study images (^{99m}Tc pyridoxylideneglutamate) taken in the same projections do not delineate the focal lesion because of the poorer concentration of radiotracer.

Intra- and Extrahepatic Abscesses

Infection is the most common complication in liver transplant patients, occurring in 70 per cent of 93 patients at our institution.[17, 20] Gallium-67 citrate has been disappointing in identifying abscesses in both liver and renal transplant patients, in our experience. It is possible that the immunosuppressive regimen in these patients decreases gallium localization in the abscess and inhibits the host's defense against infection. Consequently, other radiopharmaceuticals and imaging modalities are relied upon for the delineation of abscess.

Intrahepatic abscesses are usually first visualized with ^{99m}Tc sulfur colloid. Better visualization of focal lesions is provided by ^{99m}Tc sulfur colloid images than by ^{99m}Tc diethyl IDA images because of the higher contrast obtained with ^{99m}Tc sulfur colloid (Fig. 27–13).[19] Intrahepatic abscesses may progress rapidly and contain bile secondary to the disruption of bile ducts (Fig. 27–14). Computed tomography (Fig. 27–14) and ultrasound are helpful in demonstrating both intra- and extrahepatic abscesses.

Figure 27–14. Hepatic abscess. *A,* ^{99m}Tc diethyl IDA images taken at 45 minutes and 24 hours demonstrate a round lesion in the left lobe of the liver, with a bile leak into the lesion. *B,* ^{99m}Tc sulfur colloid images taken 11 days apart show rapid development of a large left hepatic lobe lesion. *C,* Computed tomography demonstrates a large left hepatic lobe lesion containing gas. A left hepatic lobe abscess containing bile was found and drained at surgery.

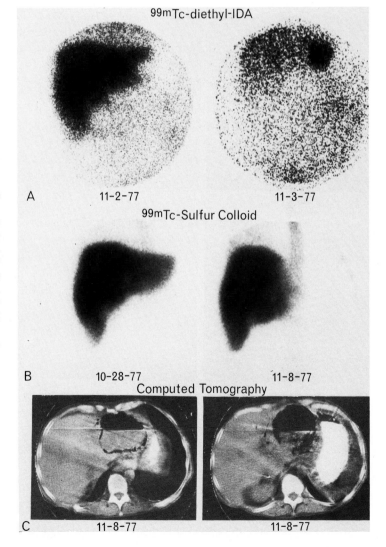

Fistulas

In a review of 93 liver transplant patients there were 8 examples of biliary fistulas.[22] Bile fistulas may be detected noninvasively with ^{99m}Tc diethyl IDA (Figs. 27–15 and 27–16). If precise anatomic detail is required, percutaneous transhepatic cholangiography or endoscopic retrograde cholangiopancreatography is performed.

Biliary Obstruction

Of the 93 patients described 24 had biliary obstruction.[22] Biliary obstruction is almost always secondary to cystic duct obstruction or a defective bile duct anastomosis.[22] Partial biliary obstruction may be diagnosed and differentiated from moderate hepatocellular disease or complete obstruction by hepatobiliary radiopharmaceuticals. In partial obstruction, serial images reveal dilated bile ducts, an abrupt termination of biliary tract dilatation, and delayed entrance of radiotracer into the small intestine (Fig. 27–17). The functional significance of the partial obstruction can be evaluated by determining the time at which activity in the liver parenchyma peaks or the time at which activity appears in the biliary ducts. In functionally significant partial obstruction, the time of peak liver activity and the time of bile duct activity are delayed (Fig. 27–17); in functionally insignificant partial obstruction, these times are normal. Complete obstruction cannot be reliably differentiated from severe hepatocellular disease with ^{99m}Tc diethyl IDA because the intestine is not visualized for 24 hours in either case.[3, 10, 11] However, hepatocyte clearance as determined by the liver-to-background activity ratio in initial images tends to be much better in the case of complete mechanical obstruction than in severe hepatocellular disease.

When the results of radionuclide imaging are inconclusive in distinguishing mechanical biliary tract obstruction from severe hepatocellular disease in a patient with clinical symptoms of jaundice, fever, and bacteremia, clarification of the cause must be made by early and, if necessary, repeated T-tube or transhepatic cholangiography or

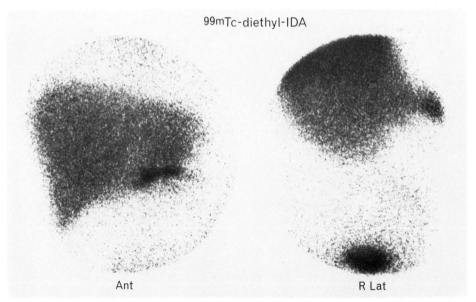

99mTc-diethyl-IDA

Ant   R Lat

Figure 27–15. Choledochocutaneous fistula. Anterior and right lateral ^{99m}Tc diethyl IDA images demonstrate excreted activity extending from the region of the porta hepatis to the left and anteriorly in a patient with a choledochocutaneous fistula.

Figure 27-16. Choledochoduo-denal fistula demonstrated by ERCP. Anastomosis was a choled-ochocholedochostomy (see Fig. 27-19D). *A* = dilated donor common duct; *B* = recipient common duct; *C* = duodenal bulb. The arrow indicates stricture at the site of anastomosis; the arrowhead indicates the fistula.

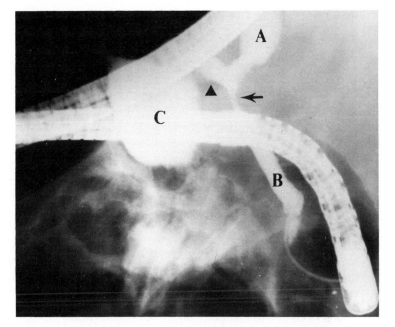

ERCP. Ultrasound or CT may show dilated ducts, but transhepatic cholangiography or ERCP is necessary to localize the site of obstruction (Fig. 27-18).

Cholangiographic Procedures

The choice of cholangiographic procedure is determined by the anastomotic technique used at surgery (Fig. 27-19). Currently, choledochocholedochostomy (Fig. 27-19D) is the procedure of choice for adult transplants under favorable anatomic conditions. Roux-en-y cholecystojejunostomy (Fig. 27-19B) may be used for children or adults with small ducts and has been used frequently as the initial procedure. Choledochojejunostomy (Fig. 27-19C) is an anastomosis used when the method shown in Figure

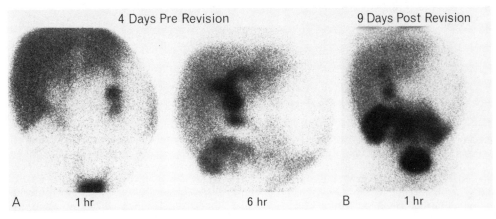

Figure 27-17. Revision of choledochojejunostomy. *A,* A hepatobiliary study with ^{99m}Tc pyridoxylideneglutamate four days prior to the revision of a choledochojejunostomy reveals no biliary activity at one hour (renal activity is present bilaterally) and dilated biliary ducts with a small amount of intestinal activity at six hours. *B,* Nine days after surgical revision, a repeat study demonstrates a normal amount of intestinal activity at one hour and no ductal dilatation.

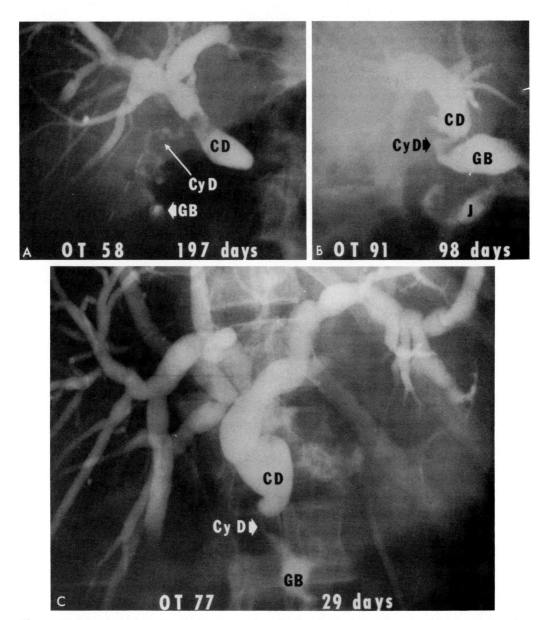

Figure 27–18. Transhepatic cholangiography. Cystic duct obstruction in three patients after cholecystoenterostomy. *A,* After this transhepatic cholangiogram, conversion was made to choledochoduodenostomy. At operation, the filling defect near the exit of the cystic duct consisted of chalklike sludge. *B* and *C,* After these cholangiograms, conversion was made to choledochojejunostomy. The patients recovered and remain well. CD = common bile duct; CyD = cystic duct; GB = gallbladder; J = Roux-en-Y limb of jejunum. (*From* Starzl, T. E., et al.: Orthotopic liver transplantation in 93 patients. Surg. Gynecol. Obstet. *142*:487–505, 1976. By permission of Surgery, Gynecology & Obstetrics.)

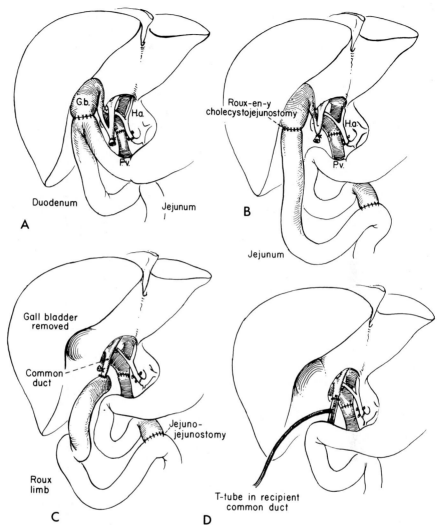

Figure 27–19. Cholangiographic procedures related to techniques of biliary duct reconstruction. *A,* Cholecystoduodenostomy. The methods shown in *B, C,* and *D* are now preferred to this. Transhepatic cholangiography or ERCP is used. *B,* Cholecystojejunostomy. This has been used frequently as the initial procedure, particularly for children or adults with small ducts. Transhepatic cholangiography is used. The Roux limb prohibits the use of ERCP. *C,* Choledochojejunostomy, after the removal of a gallbladder. This is used when cholecystojejunostomy fails or for reconstruction following biliary obstruction. Transhepatic cholangiography is used. The Roux limb prohibits the use of ERCP. *D,* Choledochocholedochostomy. The procedure of choice under favorable conditions for adults. T-tube cholangiography is convenient and simple. ERCP is employed after T-tube removal; transhepatic cholangiography is used if ERCP fails. G.b = gallbladder; H.a = hepatic artery; P.v = portal vein. (*From* Starzl, T. E., et al.: Orthotopic liver transplantation in 93 patients. Surg. Gynecol. Obstet. *142:*487–505, 1976. By permission of Surgery, Gynecology & Obstetrics.)

27–19 fails or for reconstruction following biliary obstruction. Cholecystoduodenostomy (Fig. 27–19A) is not now used but was the anastomosis most commonly used in the early series.

Appropriate procedures for cholangiography include transhepatic cholangiography or ERCP (Fig. 27–19A, B, and C); or T-tube cholangiography (see Fig. 27–19D) and ERCP after T-tube removal or transhepatic cholangiography if ERCP fails. Transhepatic cholangiography must be used when a Roux limb separates the jejunojejunostomy from the biliary anastomosis.

Of the 24 patients with biliary obstruction in the 93 consecutive transplants previously mentioned, 6 developed biliary cast formation sufficiently extensive to prevent surgical treatment.[20] In each of the six patients, obstruction of the large bile ducts was not clearly appreciated. The belief that mechanical obstruction is a cause for the cast syndrome has been questioned by the studies of Javitt et al. and Waldram et al.[7, 23]

Transhepatic cholangiography is done under fluoroscopy with the Chiba needle from the lateral approach.[1, 5, 15] In the presence of obstruction, dilated ducts may be noted, but significant obstruction may be present without obvious ductal dilatation when the liver is firm in texture or when the obstruction is early. If doubt exists, repeated cholangiography may be necessary to detect early progressive mechanical obstruction. At fluoroscopy, careful attention is paid to delayed flow through narrowed sites, such as the cystic duct.

When a cholecystojejunostomy has been performed, it is essential to pay scrupulous attention after the operation to the possibility of obstruction, repeated transhepatic cholangiographies and liver biopsies being performed when necessary. If obstruction develops, it is almost always at the level of the cystic duct, the narrow part of the drainage system (see Fig. 27–18). These patients often recover uneventfully after conversion from cholecystojejunostomy to choledochojejunostomy.[20, 22]

AUXILIARY LIVER TRANSPLANTS

Occasionally, auxiliary liver transplantation is performed. These transplants can be evaluated by ^{99m}Tc sulfur colloid and ^{99m}Tc diethyl IDA studies, using the same strategy as that used in orthotopic liver transplants.[4]

References

1. Ariyama, J., Shirakabe, H., Ohashi, K., et al.: Experience with percutaneous transhepatic cholangiography using the Japanese needle. Gastrointest. Radiol. 2:359–365, 1978.
2. Berdon, W. E., and Baker, D. H.: Plain film findings in azygos continuation of the inferior vena cava. Am. J. Roentgenol. 104:452–457, 1968.
3. Brown, D. W., and Starzl, T. E.: Radionuclides in the postoperative management of orthotopic human organ transplantation. Radiology 92:373–376, 1969.
4. Faris, T. D., Dickhaus, A. J., Marchioro, T. L., et al.: Radioisotope scanning in auxiliary liver transplantation. Surg. Gynecol. Obstet. 123:1261–1268, 1966.
5. Fraser, G. M., Cruikshank, J. G., Sumerling, M. D., et al.: Percutaneous transhepatic cholangiography with the Chiba needle. Clin. Radiol. 29:101–112, 1978.
6. Groth, C. G., Brown, D. W., Cleaveland, J. D., et al.: Radioisotope scanning in experimental and clinical orthotopic liver transplantation. Surg. Gynecol. Obstet. 127:808–816, 1968.
7. Javitt, N. B., Shiu, M. H., and Fortner, J. C.: Bile salt synthesis in transplanted human liver. Gastroenterology 60:405–408, 1971.
8. Klingensmith, W. C., and Ryerson, T. W.: Lung uptake of ^{99m}Tc sulfur colloid. J. Nucl. Med. 14:201–204, 1973.
9. Klingensmith, W. C., Yang, S. L., and Wagner, H. N.: Lung uptake of ^{99m}Tc sulfur colloid in liver and spleen imaging. J. Nucl. Med. 19:31–35, 1978.
10. Klingensmith, W. C., Koep, L. J., Fritzberg, A. R., et al.: Clinical comparison of ^{99m}Tc-diethyl-IDA, ^{99m}Tc-pyridoxylideneglutamate, and ^{131}I-rose bengal in liver transplant patients. Radiology 130:435–441, 1979.

11. Launois, B., Corman, J. L., Porter, K. A., et al.: Radioiodinated rose bengal kinetics in extrahepatic biliary obstruction and hepatic homograft rejection in dogs. Surg. Forum 23:338–339, 1972.
12. Lilly, J. R., and Chandra, R. S.: Surgical hazards of co-existing anomalies in biliary atresia. Surg. Gynecol. Obstet. 139:49–54, 1974.
13. Lilly, J. R., and Starzl, T. E.: Liver transplantation in children with biliary atresia and vascular anomalies. J. Pediatr. Surg. 9:707–714, 1974.
14. Mishkin, F.: Determination of cerebral death by radionuclide angiography. Radiology 115:135–137, 1975.
15. Okuda, K., et al.: Non-surgical percutaneous transhepatic cholangiography. Am. J. Dig. Dis. 19:21–36, 1974.
16. Putnam, C. W., Porter, K. A., Weil, R., et al.: Liver transplantation for Budd-Chiari syndrome. J.A.M.A. 236:1142–1143, 1976.
17. Schroter, G. P. J., Hoelscher, M., Putnam, C. W., et al.: Infections complicating orthotopic liver transplantation. Arch. Surg. 111:1337–1347, 1976.
18. Starzl, T. E., and Putnam, C. W.: Experience in Hepatic Transplantation. Philadelphia, W. B. Saunders Company, 1969.
19. Starzl, T. E., Van Houtte, J. J., Brown, D. W., et al.: Radiology and organ transplantation. Radiology 95:3–18, 1970.
20. Starzl, T. E., Porter, K. A., Putnam, C. W., et al.: Orthotopic liver transplantation in ninety-three patients. Surg. Gynecol. Obstet. 142:487–505, 1976.
21. Starzl, T. E., and Putnam, C. W.: Liver homotransplantation. In Sabiston, D. C. (ed.): Davis-Christopher Textbook of Surgery. Ed. 11. Philadelphia, W. B. Saunders Company, 1977, pp. 526–539.
22. Starzl, T. E., Putnam, C. W., Hansbrough, J. F., et al.: Biliary complications after liver transplantation: With special reference to the biliary cast syndrome and techniques of secondary duct repair. Surgery 81:212–221, 1977.
23. Waldram, R., Williams, R., and Calne, R. Y.: Bile composition and bile cast formation after transplantation of the liver in man. Transplantation 19:382–387, 1975.
24. Williams, R., Smith, M., Shilkin, K. B., et al.: Liver transplantation in man: the frequency of rejection, biliary tract complications, and recurrence of malignancy based on an analysis of 26 cases. Gastroenterology 64:1026–1048, 1973.

Part III

Cardiac Homotransplantation

JAMES F. SILVERMAN, M.D.
RONALD A. CASTELLINO, M.D.

The utilization of radiographic techniques to evaluate pulmonary and cardiac findings in patients following cardiac transplantation has markedly changed since the inception of this surgical procedure in 1968. Initially, it was felt that only frontal and lateral chest radiographs were needed to determine the presence of infection, rejection, contour changes, and other postoperative hemodynamically and nonhemodynamically induced abnormalities. Indeed, the chest radiograph remains the premier method for monitoring routine postoperative cardiac cases of all types, including transplants. In some areas, however, the plain chest radiograph as been found to be less useful than more complex methods of diagnosis, such as echocardiography, angiography, and pulmonary and myocardial biopsies. These topics are considered in the ensuing section. The discussion of the more routine postoperative complications, such as atelectasis and pneumothorax, as well as of findings related to intravenous and drainage tubes, is limited, since they are not peculiar to transplantation patients.

PREOPERATIVE FINDINGS

As of 1978, over 125 cardiac transplantations have been performed at Stanford University Hospital. All of these patients have had a thorough clinical, hemodynamic, and angiographic evaluation. All have had maximal trials of medical or surgical

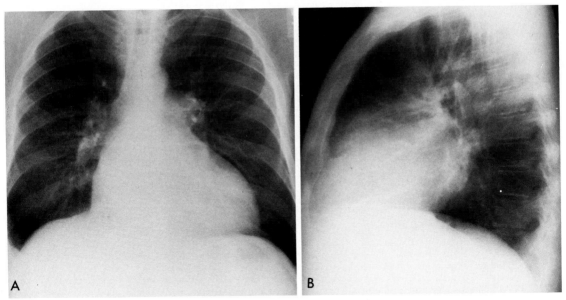

Figure 27–20. Posteroanterior (*A*) and lateral (*B*) chest films of a patient with end-stage coronary artery disease who was a transplant candidate. There is left ventricular and left atrial enlargement, a right pleural effusion, and mild pulmonary venous congestion.

management, or both, which were judged to be unsuccessful before the possibility of transplantation was considered. Approximately 75 per cent of patients who have undergone transplants have had coronary artery disease as their primary cardiac problem; most of the remainder have had cardiomyopathies. Thus, the common chest radiographic appearances seen in this group of patients include cardiomegaly, which is usually left-sided or biventricular; left atrial enlargement due to mitral regurgitation, which is almost always secondary to left ventricular dysfunction; and changes due to congestive heart failure with pulmonary venous congestion or frank pulmonary edema (Fig. 27–20).

The contraindications to cardiac transplantation are the following:

1. The presence of pulmonary inflammatory changes or pulmonary infarction due to the propensity of infection in the post-transplantation period.

2. The overage of the patient. Patients older than 55 years are poor risks owing to their concurrent peripheral and carotid vascular disease as well as to the metabolic problems, particularly osseous, that occur with steroid and immunosuppressive therapy.

3. Insulin-dependent diabetes mellitus, since insulin control is often unmanageable in patients on large steroid doses.

4. Pulmonary hypertension, since increases in pulmonary pressures are progressive and have led to death in several patients.

Apart from these objective contraindications, a subjective analysis is also utilized, since the follow-up care, including intensive drug and catheterization studies, are mentally demanding and require a reasonable degree of emotional stability in the recipient. This careful selection process for patients for cardiac transplantation has been reviewed in detail elsewhere.[5, 7]

POSTOPERATIVE FINDINGS

Radiographic management following transplantation is not dissimilar to that employed for patients undergoing more routine cardiac surgical procedures. Multiple

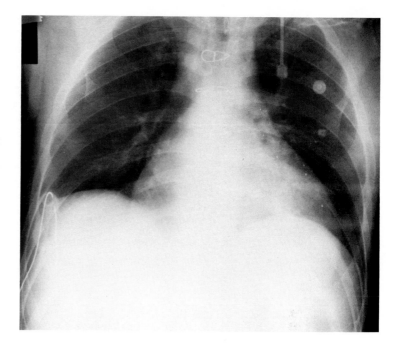

Figure 27–21. Portable chest radiograph three days post–cardiac transplantation. Note the left retrocardiac subsegmental atelectasis and the radiopaque markers overlying the left ventricular contours.

portable chest radiographs are taken daily to evaluate cardiac size, pulmonary interstitial and parenchymal changes, pneumothorax, tube positions during surgery, and tubes inserted and removed postoperatively. The immediate postoperative course in the cardiac transplant recipient is not particularly unusual, and the radiographic findings should not be interpreted differently from those in a patient who has had more routine cardiac surgery. Parenchymal segmental or subsegmental changes manifested by patchy consolidations, particularly in the retrocardiac areas in the first few days, are

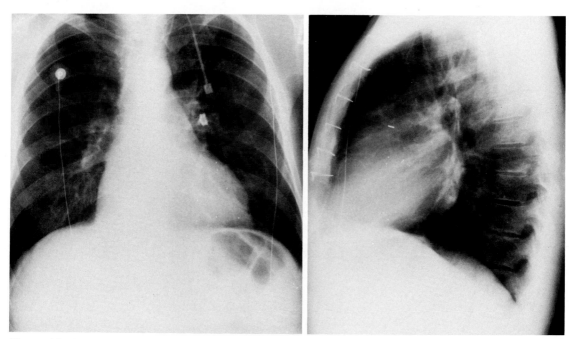

Figure 27–22. Posteroanterior and lateral chest radiograph ten days postsurgery. The cardiac size is returning to normal. The lungs are clear, with normal pulmonary vascular distribution. Again, note the radiopaque markers over the left ventricle.

common (Fig. 27–21). Small areas of atelectasis related to drainage tube position are usual. A small pneumothorax associated with tube removal is often seen, but this resolves in the usual manner. Such cardiopulmonary findings are commonplace and should not be considered unusual because of the nature of this surgical procedure.

A postoperative finding in the cardiac transplant group at the Stanford University Hospital is the presence of small radiopaque markers overlying the heart contour. These are myocardial screws placed as closely as possible to the endocardial surface of the left

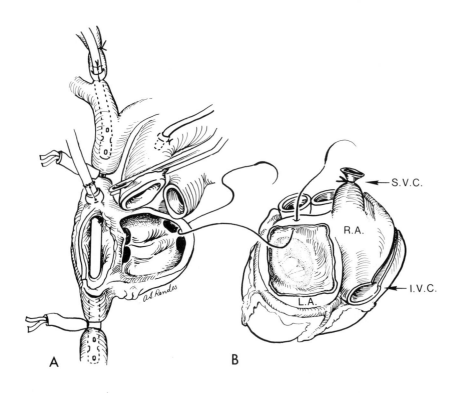

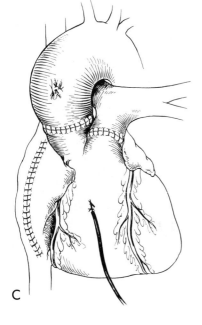

Figure 27–23. *A*, Recipient right and left atrial beds. The cannula is in the superior vena cava, the inferior vena cava, and the aorta. A clamp occludes the aortic root. *B*, The posterior aspect of the donor heart. Since the posterior wall of the donor right atrium, plus that of the recipient right atrium is often excessive, a redundant right atrial wall is produced. *C*, A frontal graphic of the completely sutured donor and recipient segments. Suture lines are seen in the right atrium, the aortic root, and the main pulmonary artery. (*From* Silverman, J. F., Griepp, R. B., and Wexler, L.: Radiographic changes in cardiac contour following cardiac transplantation. Radiology 3:303–306, 1974.)

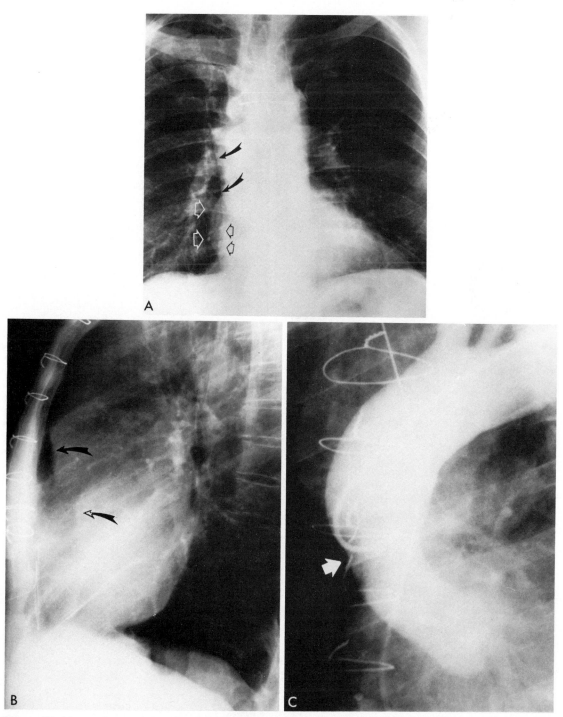

Figure 27–24. *A,* Posteroanterior chest radiograph with open white arrows pointing to the right atrial edge, and to the more medial second atrial edge (open black arrows), and solid arrows pointing to the prominent aortic shadow. *B,* Lateral chest radiograph. The lower arrow shows an extra-arterial shadow, and the upper arrow points to the broadened aortic contour. *C,* An ascending aortogram demonstrating the step-off (arrow) between the smaller donor and larger recipient ascending aortas.

ventricle at the time of surgery and utilized to evaluate noninvasively left ventricular function in the early and late postoperative periods (Figs. 27–21 and 27–22).

Within five to ten days, the cardiac size returns toward normal and the lungs become clear (Fig. 27–22). Continued improvement to a final cardiac size that is within normal limits is common. Once the postoperative changes are resolved, subsequent radiographic studies are obtained primarily for the evaluation or surveillance of opportunistic pulmonary infections.

Contour changes of the mediastinum are commonly noted following transplanta-

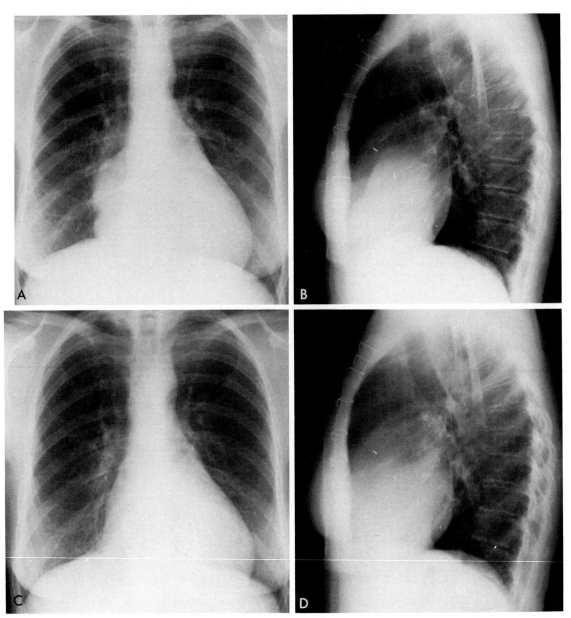

Figure 27–25. Posteroanterior (*A*) and lateral (*B*) radiographs revealing an unusual right heart contour after operation. Note the additional density overlying the cardiac shadow on the lateral view. *C* and *D*, The same patient several weeks later, showing spontaneous resolution of fluid collection adjacent to right atrium.

tion.[10] These changes are usually caused by the surgical technique related to the anastomosis between the donor and the recipient heart segments. The technique of closure must take into consideration the problems of suturing the normal-sized donor heart segment to the usually enlarged recipient segment. Because of the size differences, there is often mild distortion, producing contour abnormalities. Such changes are of no clinical significance but must be recognized as being related to the surgical anastomoses (Figs. 27–23 and 27–24). Unusual collections of fluid can also cause contour changes, but because of the time of their appearance and their spontaneous resolution, they are readily recognizable (Fig. 27–25A and B).

REJECTION

Acute Rejection

Early in our experience with these patients, we evaluated the ability of the chest radiograph to detect rejection of the transplanted heart. We found that other methods are clearly more sensitive than standard chest radiographs. Initially, the electrocardiographic change of R-wave diminution and the echocardiographic changes in posterior wall velocity were utilized. At present, endomyocardial biopsy is commonly employed together with the findings of electrocardiography or echocardiography. With these techniques, evidence of transplant rejection has been found at a much earlier time.

In cases of acute rejection there is pathologic evidence of edema surrounding the myocardial fibers, which appears to cause cardiac dysfunction. Although the obvious clinical manifestations of left ventricular failure may or may not be present, the electrocardiogram (EKG), the echocardiogram, and the myocardial biopsy are usually diagnostic. When the diagnosis of rejection is established, immunosuppressive therapy is increased; in this way, the process is usually reversed.

Radiographs taken during an episode of acute rejection may be unremarkable, or they may show signs of heart failure, consisting of increasing cardiomegaly and pulmonary congestive changes. These changes return to baseline following successful treatment of the rejection episode but progress if the rejection episode is not arrested by medication (Fig. 27–26).

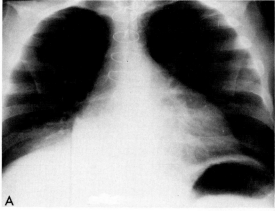
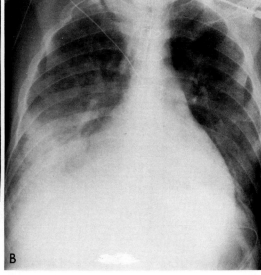

Figure 27–26. Rejection. *A* and *B*, Portable chest radiographs taken at one-day intervals of a patient who was asymptomatic. The patient developed fulminant pulmonary edema and eventually died.

The radiographs may be more useful in detecting rejection as the follow-up intervals become longer, since some patients become less critical of, or even deny, their symptoms. At times, such periodic radiographs may be the first evidence of congestive heart failure, leading to treatment and reversal of the rejection episode.

Chronic Rejection

These episodes are defined as the development of coronary artery disease, which is seen in the late postoperative period. Although they could theoretically be the result of any cause of failure of the homotransplanted heart, the late deaths stemming from a cardiac source have all been the result of progressive coronary artery disease with associated left ventricular failure. The coronary lesions are atheromatous and identical to those found in a nontransplanted heart (Fig. 27–27). Because of denervation, no pain is perceived by these patients, who may experience a decrease in myocardial blood flow.

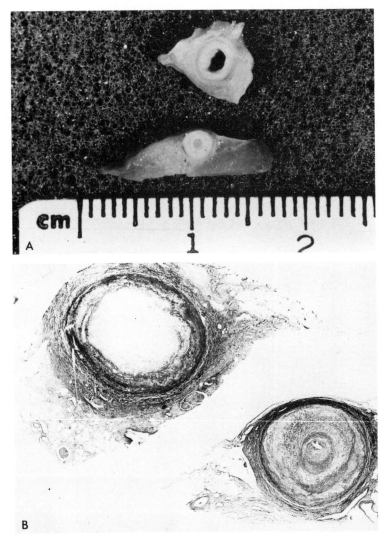

Figure 27–27. Gross (A) and microscopic (B) specimens of the distal left anterior descending coronary artery revealing partial and complete occlusions of the arterial lumen. (From Silverman, J. F., Lipton, M. J., Graham, A., et al.: Coronary arteriography in long-term human cardiac transplantation survivors. Circulation 50: 838–843, 1974.)

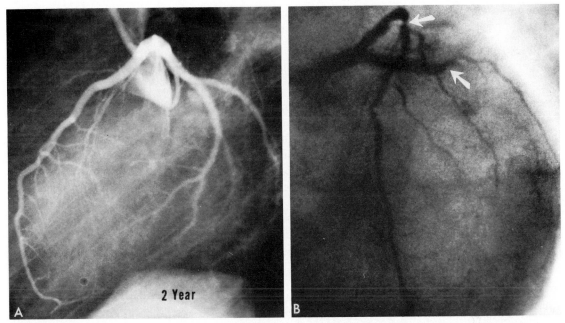

Figure 27–28. *A,* Left coronary artery injection (lateral projection) revealing normal vessels two years post-transplant. *B,* An abnormal left coronary artery injection showing advanced atheromatous disease (arrows). (*B* from Silverman, J. F., Lipton, M. J., Graham, A., et al.: Coronary arteriography in long-term human cardiac transplantation survivors. Circulation *50:*838–843, 1974.)

For this reason, coronary arteriography is routinely performed on a yearly basis to evaluate the coronary arteries in long-term survivors.[10]

As more patients survive longer, more coronary artery disease appears (Fig. 27–28). Yearly follow-up studies have shown progression of coronary artery disease in approximately 40 per cent of the long-term survivors. Some have acquired left ventricular dysfunction secondary to their progressive coronary artery disease.

OPPORTUNISTIC PULMONARY INFECTIONS

As in the case of patients who have received renal transplants, patients with cardiac transplants are at increased risk for acquiring infection. These infectious episodes may be caused by organisms that affect the normal population, as well as by opportunistic organisms that manifest increased pathogenicity in patients with immunologic compromise. Such infectious episodes are often rapidly progressive, leading to morbidity and mortality unless diagnosed early and treated vigorously. Furthermore, such infections may be present and progress rapidly while the infected patients are relatively asymptomatic, a fact that compounds the problems of early diagnosis.

The experience at Stanford University Hospital in the cardiac transplant program indicates, as expected, a high incidence of infectious episodes in this group of patients.[12] Furthermore, infections are the primary cause of death in 40 per cent of all three-month survivors. The lungs are the most frequent primary site of such infections, and pulmonary infections account for almost one half of all infectious episodes. Thus, the chest radiograph and ancillary techniques often play an important role in the initial identification of an infectious process, in the diagnostic work-up, and in the determination of the response to treatment.

Roentgenographic Aspects

The radiographic appearance of a pulmonary infection is nonspecific, and other possible diagnoses, such as pulmonary infarction, focal areas of pulmonary edema, and neoplasia, must be first excluded from consideration. Once it is established that an infection is the cause of a pulmonary lesion, then the specific causative organism or organisms must be determined. Each organism may be responsible for a variety of radiographic manifestations, and conversely, each radiographic manifestation can be produced by a variety of organisms. Thus, the chest radiograph cannot indicate which specific agent is responsible for a particular infectious episode.[2, 3]

In most instances, abnormalities noted in the lung fields within the first 30 days of cardiac transplantation are related to the immediate surgical procedure and consist of the usual postoperative complications, as detailed earlier. The development of a new parenchymal abnormality after this 30-day period must be viewed with concern and generally must be presumed to represent an infection until proved otherwise.[6] An exception is the development of infiltrates compatible with congestive failure in patients with other evidence of cardiac decompensation or cardiac rejection or both. This situation can be confusing, since the early radiographic manifestations of *Pneumocystis carinii*, for example, can mimic the early findings of pulmonary venous congestion (Fig. 27–29). Another exception is the development of a lesion caused by a neoplasm, since immunosuppressed transplant patients are at higher risk for the development of tumors, particularly the non-Hodgkin's lymphomas (Fig. 27–30).

The radiographic manifestations of pulmonary opportunistic infections are varied and nonspecific. Certain radiographic appearances are more frequently associated with specific organisms or groups of organisms, however, and thus may be helpful in guiding the diagnostic maneuvers for the determination of the etiologic agent.[2]

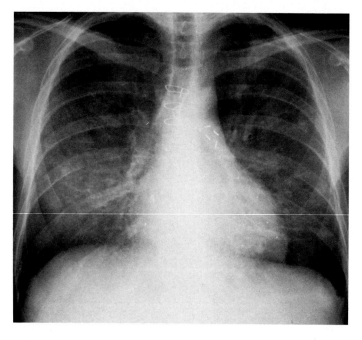

Figure 27–29. *Pneumocystis carinii.* This 35-year-old male who had received a cardiac transplant developed a diffuse bilateral pulmonary infiltrate, which was mostly interstitial in radiographic appearance. An extensive work-up was negative, and therefore a percutaneous needle aspiration was performed. Since the infiltrates were diffuse and fluoroscopic guidance was not required, the aspiration was performed at the bedside and revealed *Pneumocystis carinii* organisms on smear.

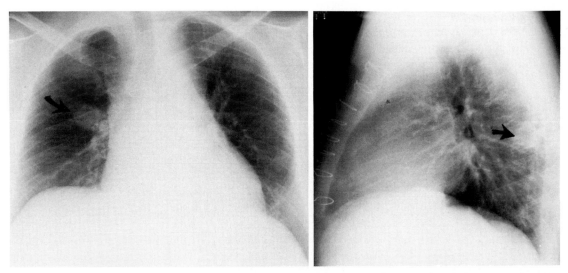

Figure 27–30. Malignant lymphoma. This 28-year-old male who had received a cardiac transplant developed an ovoid density in the superior segment of the right lower lobe. An extensive work-up failed to reveal the cause of this lesion, and the patient therefore underwent fluoroscopically guided percutaneous needle aspiration. Cultures from the aspirate were negative, but microscopic examination of the aspirated material raised the possibility of a malignant process. The aspirated material was not diagnostic, however, and the patient subsequently underwent a diagnostic thoracotomy with resection of the nodule, which proved to be a malignant lymphoma.

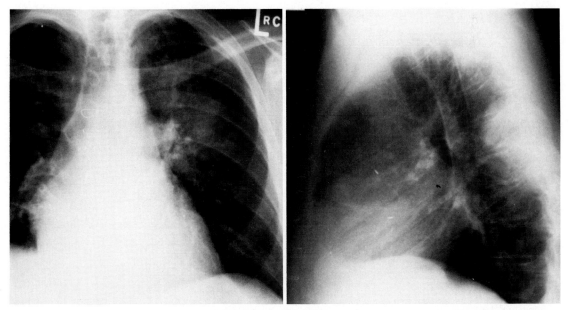

Figure 27–31. *Proprionibacterium acnes* infection. This 33-year-old male who had received a cardiac transplant developed a 5- by 6-cm infiltrate in the superior segment of the left lower lobe. Because an extensive work-up was negative, a percutaneous needle aspiration under fluoroscopic guidance was performed. This procedure yielded anaerobic *Proprionibacterium acnes* organisms.

Although a distinct radiographic appearance should not be accepted as being diagnostic for a specific organism, at times the clinical situation forces the institution of empirical therapy — based upon probable causative organisms as determined by the radiographic appearance — while the results of cultures and other diagnostic techniques are awaited.

LOBAR AND SEGMENTAL CONSOLIDATIONS. These are generally caused by bacterial infections, although it is not possible to distinguish between the various

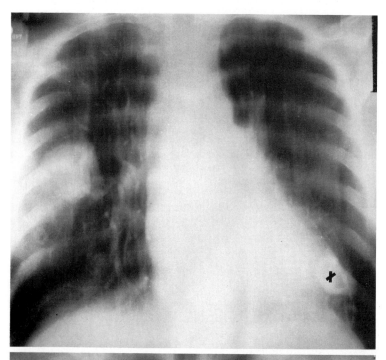

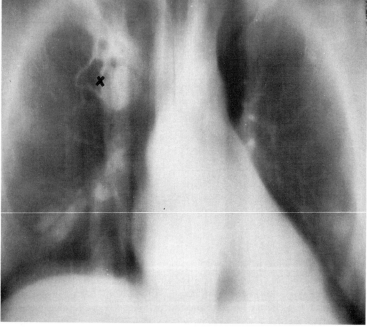

Figure 27–32. *Aspergillus* and *Nocardia* infection. This 45-year-old woman developed multiple pulmonary nodules (some with cavitation) 42 days post–cardiac transplantation. A percutaneous needle aspiration (X) yielded *Aspergillus* (tomogram on top) for which she was treated with amphotericin B, with gradual resolution of symptoms and most radiographic signs. Multiple cavitary lesions again appeared 558 days post transplantation, concomitant with clinical evidence of infection. This time *Nocardia* organisms were recovered on percutaneous needle aspiration (X) (tomogram on bottom). (*From* Blank, N., Castellino, R. A., and Shad, V.: Radiographic aspects of pulmonary infection in patients with altered immunity. Radiol. Clin. North Am. *11*:175–190, 1973.)

bacterial agents (Fig. 27–31). Necrotizing pneumonias are frequently accompanied by convex margins or bulging fissures and are often caused by gram-negative bacteria, particularly *Escherichia coli, Pseudomonas,* and *Klebsiella.* The rapid appearance of cavitation within such consolidation should raise the possibility of infection by anaerobic organisms; at times, fungi and gram-positive cocci produce similar findings, however.

MULTIPLE NODULAR LESIONS. Such lesions are typical of fungi, particularly *Aspergillus* and *Mucor,* and *Nocardia* (Fig. 27–32). The nodules often show rapid growth or cavitation or both. Likewise, solitary nodules or consolidations with or without cavitation may also be due to fungi. Other organisms, particularly anaerobic bacteria, are also frequently associated with cavitation.

DIFFUSE BILATERAL PARENCHYMAL INFILTRATES. These should suggest the possibility of infection by *Pneumocystis carinii, Toxoplasma,* viral pneumonia (especially cytomegalovirus), or mixed pathogens (see Fig. 27–29). *Pneumocystis carinii* pneumonia has received considerable attention in the literature and is usually bilaterally diffuse at the time of diagnosis. It can begin as a more focal infiltrate, however, although it is usually not diagnosed at this stage.

Percutaneous Needle Aspiration with Fluoroscopic Guidance

As noted previously, the radiographic appearance can be suggestive but certainly not diagnostic of a specific etiologic agent. However, the radiologic technique of fluoroscopically guided percutaneous pulmonary aspiration can frequently identify the causative organisms, thus guiding therapy.[1, 4] This technique is similar to that employed for the evaluation of undiagnosed pulmonary lesions suspected of being neoplasms. The procedure is performed in the Radiology Department under sterile conditions. Fluoroscopic guidance is used to ensure that the needle is placed within the lesion, to maximize the chances of obtaining diagnostic material. The study is performed with local anesthesia of the chest wall and pleura, and the aspiration is accomplished with an 18-gauge thin-walled spinal needle. The aspirated material is used for preparing slides, which must be appropriately stained, and for culture. The aspirated material is placed immediately into a sealed vial that contains media from which cultures can be obtained for anaerobic organisms as well as for aerobic bacteria and fungi.

Complications encountered include pneumothorax, which at times requires tube drainage, and transient hemoptysis. Contraindications include an uncontrolled bleeding diathesis, pulmonary arterial hypertension, severe underlying respiratory disease, extensive bullae or blebs in the needle path, and lack of patient cooperation.

To date, we have performed fluoroscopically guided percutaneous needle aspiration of pulmonary lesions in the examination of 83 presumed episodes of pulmonary infections in cardiac transplant recipients.[8] These patients were referred for this procedure only after an extensive work-up, including transtracheal aspirations, was negative or inconclusive. The overall diagnostic yield from this procedure was approximately 75 per cent. Not infrequently, two or more organisms were recovered in the same aspiration.

The advantages of this technique are its ability to recover material from the lesion in question directly and rapidly; the fact that it can be performed under local anesthesia; and its ability to be repeated at a later date, should the clinical need arise. Its major disadvantage is that only small amounts of tissue are sampled, so that the information gained may not be representative of the entire pathologic process. On

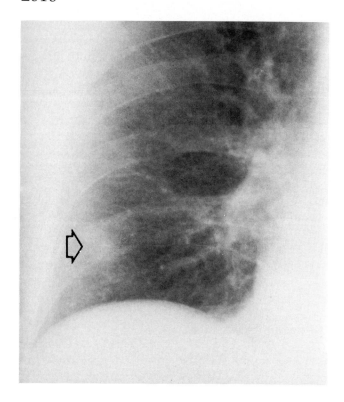

Figure 27–33. *Cryptococcus* infection. This 54-year-old man, who had received a cardiac transplant, developed a poorly defined nodular infiltrate in the right lower lobe. An extensive work-up failed to reveal a definite causative organism. Therefore, the patient underwent fluoroscopically guided percutaneous aspiration of the approximately 1-cm lesion, which revealed *Cryptococcus*.

balance, this appears to be a useful technique, however, and it has become a valuable diagnostic procedure in this patient population.

This technique is also applicable to other immunologically compromised patients, such as those who have received renal transplants and the many patients with neoplasms who are immunologically compromised by virtue of their underlying disease or subsequent treatment. If pulmonary lesions are diffuse throughout the entire lung parenchyma, then this technique can be readily performed at the bedside without the need for fluoroscopic guidance (see Fig. 27–29). Fluoroscopic guidance is employed only for those lesions that are so small that random sampling may miss the area of involvement (Figs. 27–31 and 27–33).

In summary, patients who have received heart transplants are at high risk for infection, and many of the offending organisms are opportunistic in nature. It is important to maintain a high degree of vigilance over such patients and to evaluate aggressively those pulmonary lesions that have a high likelihood of being caused by infection. The radiographic appearance is nonspecific but can often suggest major categories of organisms, thus helping to guide diagnostic approaches or empirical therapy. The technique of fluoroscopically guided percutaneous pulmonary needle aspiration appears to be useful in this clinical setting, determining the etiologic agents in approximately 75 per cent of the patients so studied.

References

1. Bandt, P. D., Blank, N., and Castellino. R. A.: Needle diagnosis of pneumonitis. J.A.M.A. 220:1578–1580, 1972.
2. Blank, N., Castellino, R. A., and Shah, V.: Radiographic aspects of pulmonary infection in patients wth altered immunity. Radiol. Clin. North Am. 11:175–190, 1973.

3. Blank, N., and Castellino, R. A.: The diagnosis of pulmonary infection in patients with altered immunity Semin. Roentgenol. *10*:63–72, 1975.
4. Castellino, R. A., and Blank, N.: Etiologic diagnosis of pulmonary infections in immunocompromised patients by fluoroscopically guided percutaneous needle aspiration, Radiology *132*:563, 1979.
5. Christopherson, L. K., and Lunde, D. T.: Selection of cardiac transplant recipients and their subsequent psychosocial adjustment. Semin. Psychiatr. *3*:1–10, 1971.
6. Goldstein, H. M., Castellino, R. A., Wexler, L., et al.: Roentgenologic aspects of cardiac transplantation: Post-operative pulmonary infections. Am. J. Roentgenol. *111*:476–482, 1971.
7. Griepp, R. B., Stinson, E. B., Dong, E., et al.: Determinants of operative risk in human heart transplantation. Am. J. Surg. *122*:192–197, 1971.
8. Rand, K. H., Pollard, R. B., and Merigan, T. C.: Increased pulmonary superinfections in cardiac transplant patients undergoing primary cytomegalovirus infection. N. Engl. J. Med. *298*:951–953, 1978.
9. Silverman, J. F., Griepp, R. B., and Wexler, L.: Radiographic changes in cardiac contour following cardiac transplantation. Radiology *3*:303–306, 1974.
10. Silverman, J. F., Lipton, M. J., Graham, A., et al.: Coronary arteriography in long-term human cardiac transplantation survivors. Circulation *50*:838–843, 1974.
11. Stinson, E. B., Bieber, C. P., Griepp, R. B., et al.: Infectious complications after cardiac transplantation in man. Ann. Intern. Med. *74*:22–36, 1971.
12. Stinson, E., et al.: Unpublished observations.

INDEX

Page numbers in *italics* denote illustrations; (t) refers to tabular material

i